Review of
Medical
Microbiology

a **LANGE** medical book

1987
Review of
Medical
Microbiology
Seventeenth Edition

Ernest Jawetz, MD, PhD
Professor of Microbiology and Medicine, Emeritus
University of California Medical Center
San Francisco

Joseph L. Melnick, PhD
Distinguished Service Professor and Chairman,
Department of Virology and Epidemiology
Baylor College of Medicine
Houston

Edward A. Adelberg, PhD
Professor of Human Genetics
Yale University School of Medicine
New Haven

In association with

Geo. F. Brooks, MD
Professor of Laboratory Medicine, Medicine,
and Microbiology and Immunology
Chief, Microbiology Section Clinical Laboratories
University of California Medical Center
San Francisco

Janet S. Butel, PhD
Professor of Virology
Baylor College of Medicine
Houston

L. Nicholas Ornston, PhD
Professor of Biology
Yale University
New Haven

**Appleton
&Lange** Norwalk, Connecticut/Los Altos, California

Prentice-Hall of Australia, Pty. Ltd., Sydney
Prentice-Hall Canada, Inc.
Prentice-Hall Hispanoamericana, S.A., Mexico
Prentice-Hall of India Private Limited, New Delhi
Prentice-Hall International (UK) Limited, London
Prentice-Hall of Japan, Inc., Tokyo
Prentice-Hall of Southeast Asia (Pte.) Ltd., Singapore
Whitehall Books Ltd., Wellington, New Zealand
Editora Prentice-Hall do Brasil Ltda., Rio de Janeiro

Spanish Edition: Editorial El Manual Moderno, S.A. de C.V., Av. Sonora 206, Col. Hipodromo, 06100-Mexico, D.F.
German Edition: Springer-Verlag GmbH & Co., Postfach 10 52 80, KG, 6900 Heidelberg 1, West Germany
Italian Edition: Piccin Nuova Libraria, S.p.A., Via Altinate, 107, 35121 Padua, Italy
Portuguese Edition: Editora Guanabara Koogan, S. A., Travessa do Ouvidor, 11, 20,040 Rio de Janeiro - RJ, Brazil
Serbo-Croatian Edition: Skolska Knjiga, Masarykova 28, 41001 Zagreb, Yugoslavia
French Edition: Les Presses de l'Université Laval, Cite Universitaire, C.P. 2447, Quebec G1K 7R4, Canada
Polish Edition: Panstwowy Zaklad Wydawnictw Lekarskich, P.O. Box 379, 00–950 Warsaw, Poland
Japanese Edition: Hirokawa Publishing Company, 27-14, Hongo 3, Bunkyo-ku, Tokyo 113, Japan
Albanian Edition: Department of Microbiology, Faculty of Medicine, University of Pristina, 38000 Pristina, Yugoslavia
Indonesian Edition: CV. E.G.C. Medical Publisher, P. O. Box 4276, 10711 Jakarta, Indonesia
Russian Edition: "Meditsina" Publishing House, Goskomizdat, Petroverigsky per., 6/8, 101838, Moscow, USSR
Greek Edition: Gregory Parisianos, 20, Navarinou Street, GR-106 80 Athens, Greece

Library of Congress Cataloging-in-Publication Data
Main entry under title:
Review of medical microbiology. [1st]–   ed.; 1954–
      Los Altos, Calif., Lange Medical Publications.
          v. ill., diagrs. 26 cm.
      Biennial.
      Vols. for 1954–   by E. Jawetz, J.L. Melnick, and E.A. Adelberg.
      Key title: Review of medical microbiology, ISSN 0486-6118.
          1. Medical microbiology.   I. Jawetz, Ernest, Ed.
      QR46.R47   616.01   60-11336
                                                            MARC-S
      Library of Congress   [r61] rev

ISBN: 0-8385-8432-2

Preface

Review of Medical Microbiology, now in its seventeenth edition, is directed primarily at medical students, house officers, and practicing physicians. The authors' intention in writing it has been to provide comprehensive, accurate, up-to-date coverage of those aspects of medical microbiology that are of significance in the fields of clinical infections and chemotherapy. In general, details of procedure and technique have been omitted. Because of the importance of recent developments in biochemistry, genetics, and other basic sciences, a large part of the book is devoted to relevant topics in these fields. This material will extend the book's usefulness to undergraduate and graduate students in the health sciences.

The book starts with the essential basic science aspects of microbiology: microbial structure, genetics, metabolism, chemotherapy, and immunology. This is followed by a brief survey of those groups of bacteria—including chlamydiae and rickettsiae—that have medical importance; mycology; and diagnostic microbiology. A broad survey of the properties of viruses precedes discussions of groups of viruses of medical significance. The book concludes with a chapter on the protozoal and helminthic parasites important in human disease.

Within each chapter, the description of each organism is followed by an outline of the pathologic features and clinical manifestations of infection, various approaches to prevention, and chemotherapy where applicable. Emphasis has been given to the clinical and public health aspects of infectious diseases.

The seventeenth edition has been substantially revised to incorporate the latest information of relevance to the health sciences. It includes the following new features:

■ The chapters on immunology incorporate the latest advances in the understanding of cell-mediated immunity and its failure in immunocompromised hosts, including patients with organ transplants and those with AIDS.

■ A completely new chapter on AIDS has been added; it includes the latest information on the epidemiology of AIDS and the US Public Health Service's 1986 recommendations on advice to patients with HTLV-III (HIV) infections.

■ Chapters on individual groups of microorganisms have been reorganized and subdivided for easier study and understanding.

■ The roles of cancer chemotherapy, drug treatment, drug addiction, and immunodeficiency have been defined, with emphasis on iatrogenic infection and its management.

■ Integrated presentations of the increasing incidence of sexually transmitted diseases emphasize early diagnosis, treatment, and worldwide prevention, particularly in high-risk groups.

With the seventeenth edition, the authors welcome three associate authors: Dr. G. F. Brooks, Dr. J. S. Butel, and Dr. L. N. Ornston. Besides bringing their own fresh viewpoints and expertise to this edition, these new authors will have an increased responsibility for selecting and updating material in future editions.

The authors and publisher are pleased to report that the sixteen previous editions of *Review of Medical Microbiology* have sold more than 1.2 million copies in English and in translations into Spanish, Portuguese, German, French, Italian, Japanese, Indonesian, Polish, Russian, Serbo-Croatian, Albanian, Turkish, and Greek. A Chinese translation is in progress.

Finally, the authors wish to reaffirm their gratitude to all those whose comments and criticisms have helped to keep each biennial edition of the book accurate and up to date. We would especially like to thank Drs. M. Grossman, C. Halde, F. B. Hollinger, W. Levinson, and L. L. Levintow for their help and support. We must also pay tribute to Dr. Jack D. Lange, who inspired the first edition of this book and who has given unstintingly of his advice and support for a third of a century.

Ernest Jawetz
Joseph L. Melnick
Edward A. Adelberg

San Francisco
October, 1986

SI Units of Measurement in the Biologic Range

Prefix	Abbreviation	Magnitude
kilo-	k	10^3
deci-	d	10^{-1}
centi-	c	10^{-2}
milli-	m	10^{-3}
micro-	μ	10^{-6}
nano-	n	10^{-9}
pico-	p	10^{-12}

These prefixes are applied to metric and other units. For example, a micrometer (μm) is 10^{-6} meter (formerly micron, μ); a nanogram (ng) is 10^{-9} gram (formerly millimicrogram, mμg); and a picogram (pg) is 10^{-12} gram (formerly micromicrogram, $\mu\mu$g). Any of these prefixes may also be applied to seconds, units, mols, equivalents, osmols, etc. The Angstrom (A, 10^{-7}) is now expressed in nanometers (eg, 40 A = 4 nm).

The Microbial World

1

Before the discovery of microorganisms, all known living things were believed to be either plant or animal; no transitional types were thought to exist. During the 19th century, however, it became clear that the microorganisms combine plant and animal properties in all possible combinations. It is now generally accepted that they have evolved, with relatively little change, from the common ancestors of plants and animals.

The compulsion of biologists to categorize all organisms in one of the 2 "kingdoms," plant or animal, resulted in a number of absurdities. The fungi, for example, were classified as plants because they are largely nonmotile, although they have few other plantlike properties and show strong phylogenic affinities with the protozoa.

In order to avoid the arbitrary assignment of transitional groups to one or the other kingdom, Haeckel proposed in 1866 that microorganisms be placed in a separate kingdom, the *Protista*. As defined by Haeckel, the *Protista* included algae, protozoa, fungi, and bacteria. In the middle of the current century, however, the new techniques of electron microscopy revealed that the bacteria differ fundamentally from the other 3 groups in their cell architecture. The latter share with the cells of plants and animals the advanced type of structure called **eukaryotic;** the bacteria possess a more primitive type of structure called **prokaryotic.** (The 2 types of cell structure are described in Chapter 2.) The term protist is currently used to refer only to the eukaryotic microorganisms, the assemblage of bacterial groups being referred to collectively as prokaryotes.

The term algae has long been used to refer to all chlorophyll-containing microorganisms that produce gaseous oxygen as a by-product of photosynthesis. Electron microscopy, however, has revealed that one major group—formerly called blue-green algae—are in fact true prokaryotes, and they have thus been renamed **cyanobacteria.***

Three groups of prokaryotes—methanogens, extreme halophiles, and thermoacidophiles—have been found to share a set of properties that distinguish them clearly from all other prokaryotes. It has been proposed that these organisms represent the most primitive cell types and that they should be classified separately as the **archaebacteria.** All prokaryotes other

Bergey's Manual of Determinative Bacteriology, 8th ed. Williams & Wilkins, 1974.

than archaebacteria and cyanobacteria will be collectively referred to as **eubacteria.** An analysis of the base sequences of ribosomal RNA shows that the archaebacteria are only distantly related to the eubacteria; there are also major differences in the composition of their cell walls and membranes and in their metabolism. Certain features of eukaryotic cells are found in one or another of the archaebacteria, including introns within genes, repetitive DNA sequences, nucleosomes containing histonelike proteins, and modified translation elongation factors. These properties have led to the suggestion that eukaryotic cells evolved from an archaebacterial ancestor.

A current classification of microorganisms might read as follows:

I. Protists (eukaryotic)
    A. Algae
    B. Protozoa
    C. Fungi
    D. Slime molds (sometimes included in the fungi)
II. Prokaryotes
    A. Eubacteria
    B. Archaebacteria
    C. Cyanobacteria

The eubacteria include 2 groups, the **chlamydiae (bedsoniae)** and the **rickettsiae,** which differ from other bacteria in being somewhat smaller ($0.2–0.5\ \mu m$ in diameter) and in being obligate intracellular parasites. The reasons for the obligate nature of their parasitism are not clear; there is some evidence that they depend on their hosts for coenzymes and complex energy-rich metabolites such as ATP, to which their membranes may be permeable.

Viruses are also classed as microorganisms, but they are sharply differentiated from all cellular forms of life. A viral particle consists of a nucleic acid molecule, either DNA or RNA, enclosed in a protein coat, or **capsid.** The capsid serves only to protect the nucleic acid and to facilitate attachment and penetration of the virus into the host cell. Viral nucleic acid is the infectious principle; inside the host cell, it behaves like host genetic material in that it is replicated by the host's enzymatic machinery and also governs the formation of specific (viral) proteins. Maturation consists of assemblage of newly synthesized nucleic acid and protein subunits into mature viral particles; these are liberated into the extracellular environment. Viruses are known to infect a wide variety of specific plant and animal hosts as well as prokaryotes and at least one eukaryotic alga. Viruslike particles (which lack an infectious, extracellular phase) have been found in fungi as well as in a number of genera of algae.

A number of transmissible plant diseases are caused by **viroids,** small, single-stranded, covalently closed circular RNA molecules existing as highly base-paired rodlike structures; they do not possess capsids. Their molecular weights are estimated to fall in the range of 75,000–100,000. It is not known whether they are translated in the host into polypeptides or whether they interfere with host functions directly (as RNA); if the former is true, the largest viroid could only be translated into the equivalent of a single polypeptide containing about 55 amino acids. Viroid RNA is replicated by the DNA-dependent RNA polymerase of the plant host; preemption of this enzyme may contribute to viroid pathogenicity.

The RNAs of viroids have been shown to contain inverted repeated base sequences at their terminuses, a characteristic of transposable elements and retroviruses (see Chapter 4). Thus, it is likely that they have evolved from transposable elements or retroviruses by the deletion of internal sequences.

Scrapie, a degenerative central nervous system disease of sheep, is caused by a filterable agent less than 50 nm in diameter. It is resistant to nucleases and other agents that inactivate nucleic acids but is inactivated by proteases and other agents that react with proteins. The infectious particle has been called a prion; it copurifies with a specific protein, but the presence of nucleic acid within the particle has not been ruled out.

By use of recombinant DNA techniques, the gene encoding the major prion protein has been cloned from hamster brain. The gene—and its corresponding mRNA—are present (and thus expressed) in both normal and scrapie-infected brain tissue. Three competing models exist: (1) Scrapie is a conventional virus with an extremely small nucleic acid genome that has escaped detection; (2) the infectious agent is a small, noncoding RNA molecule that binds to prion protein with high affinity, changing the prion's conformation in a self-propagating manner to a pathologic form; and (3) the prion protein is itself the infectious agent, inducing the synthesis of posttranslational modifying enzymes that convert a normal protein to the pathologic, prion form. These models may also apply to the agents of Creutzfeldt-Jacob disease and kuru, which produce very similar diseases in humans.

The general properties of animal viruses pathogenic for humans are described in Chapter 33. Bacterial viruses are described in Chapter 9.

PROTISTS

The protists share with true plants and animals the type of cell construction called eukaryotic ("possessing a true nucleus"). In such cells, the nucleus contains a set of chromosomes that are separated, following replication, by an elaborate mitotic apparatus. The nuclear membrane is continuous with a ramifying endoplasmic reticulum. The cytoplasm of the cell contains self-replicating organelles (mitochondria and, in photosynthetic cells, chloroplasts) as well as microtubules and microfilaments. Motility organelles (cilia or flagella) are complex multistranded elements.

Algae

The term "algae" refers in general to chlorophyll-containing protists, for descriptions of which the reader is referred to Bold HC, Wynne MJ: *Introduction to the Algae: Structure and Reproduction.* Prentice-Hall, 1978.

Protozoa

The algae include several types of photosynthetic, flagellated, unicellular forms that are sometimes classed with the protozoa. These include members of *Volvocales* in *Chlorophyta,* members of *Euglenophyta,* the dinoflagellates in *Pyrrophyta,* and some of the golden browns in *Chrysophyta.* These are included with the algae because definite phylogenic series are recognized that link them to typical algal forms.

On the other hand, these photosynthetic flagellates probably represent transitional forms between algae and protozoa; according to this view, the protozoa have evolved from various algae by loss of chloroplasts. They thus have a polyphyletic origin (ancestors in many different groups). Indeed, mutations of flagellates from green to colorless have been observed in the laboratory. The resulting forms are indistinguishable from certain protozoa.

The most primitive protozoa are thus the flagellated forms. "Protozoa" are unicellular, nonphotosynthetic protists. From the flagellated forms appear to have evolved the ameboid and the ciliated types; intermediate types are known that have flagella at one stage in the life cycle and pseudopodia (characteristic of the ameba) at another stage. A fourth major group of protozoa consists of the sporozoons, parasites with complex life cycles that include a resting or spore stage. A classification of the protozoa is given in Chapter 48.

Fungi

The fungi are nonphotosynthetic protists growing as a mass of branching, interlacing filaments ("hyphae") known as a mycelium. Although the hyphae exhibit cross-walls, the cross-walls are perforated and allow the free passage of nuclei and cytoplasm. The entire organism is thus a coenocyte (a multinucleate mass of continuous cytoplasm) confined within a series of branching tubes. These tubes, made of polysaccharides such as chitin, are homologous with cell walls. The mycelial forms are called **molds;** a few types, **yeasts,** do not form a mycelium but are easily recognized as fungi by the nature of their sexual reproductive processes and by the presence of transitional forms.

The fungi probably represent an evolutionary offshoot of the protozoa; they are unrelated to the actinomycetes, mycelial bacteria that they superficially resemble. Fungi are subdivided as follows:

Class I: *Zygomycotina* (the phycomycetes). Mycelium usually nonseptate; asexual spores produced in indefinite numbers within a structure called a sporangium. Sexual fusion results in formation of a resting, thick-walled cell termed a zygospore. *Example: Rhizopus nigricans* (no known pathogens).

Class II: *Ascomycotina* (the ascomycetes). Sexual fusion results in formation of a sac, or ascus, containing the meiotic products as 4 or 8 spores (ascospores). Asexual spores (conidia) are borne externally at the tips of hyphae. *Examples: Trichophyton (Arthroderma), Microsporum (Nannizzia), Blastomyces (Ajellomyces).*

Class III: *Basidiomycotina* (the basidiomycetes). Sexual fusion results in formation of a club-shaped organ called a basidium, on the surface of which are borne the 4 meiotic products (basidiospores). Asexual spores (conidia) are borne externally at the tips of hyphae. *Example: Cryptococcus neoformans (Filobasidiella neoformans).*

Class IV: *Deuteromycotina* (the imperfect fungi). This is not a true phylogenic group but rather an artificial class into which are temporarily placed all forms in which the sexual process has not yet been observed. Most of them resemble ascomycetes morphologically. *Examples: Epidermophyton, Sporothrix, Candida.*

The evolution of the ascomycetes from the phycomycetes is seen in a transitional group, members of which form a zygote but then transform this directly into an ascus. The basidiomycetes are believed to have evolved in turn from the ascomycetes.

Although the fungi are classified on the basis of their sexual processes, the sexual stages are difficult to induce and are rarely observed. Descriptions of species thus deal principally with various asexual structures, including the following: (See Figs 31–1 to 31–9 for drawings of some of these structures.)

A. Sporangiospores: Asexual spores borne internally inside a sac known as a sporangium. In terrestrial forms, the sporangium is borne at the tip of a filament called a sporangiophore. These structures are characteristic of the phycomycetes.

B. Conidia: Asexual reproductive units that develop along one of 2 basic pathways. "Blastic" conidia develop from an enlargement of some part of the conidiophore (conidiogenous hypha) prior to delimitation by a septum. "Thallic" conidia differentiate from a whole cell after a septum has formed. The blastic types of conidia show many modifications that may be given specific names. When a sexual stage has not been recognized for a given fungus, the form of conidia it produces is used as a basis for classification within the imperfect fungi.

C. Arthrospores: Thallic conidia formed by segmentation and disarticulation of a filament of a septate mycelium into separate cells. They are properly called **arthroconidia.**

D. Chlamydospores: Thallic conidia formed as enlarged, thick-walled cells within a hypha. They remain a part of the mycelium, surviving after the remainder of the mycelium has died and disintegrated.

E. Blastospores: Simple blastic conidia produced as buds that then separate from the parent cell. They are properly called **blastoconidia.**

Slime Molds

These organisms are characterized by the presence, as a stage in the life cycle, of an ameboid multinucleate mass of cytoplasm called a **plasmodium.** The creeping plasmodium, which reaches macroscopic size, gives rise to walled spores that germinate to produce naked uniflagellate swarm spores or, in some cases, naked nonflagellated amebas ("myxamebae"). These usually undergo sexual fusion before growing into typical plasmodia again.

The plasmodium of a slime mold is analogous to the mycelium of a true fungus. Both are coenocytes; but in the latter, cytoplasmic flow is confined to the branching network of chitinous tubes, whereas in the former the cytoplasm can flow (creep) in all directions.

PROKARYOTES

The prokaryotes form a heterogeneous group of microorganisms distinguished from protists by the following criteria: size range (0.2–2 μm for the smallest diameter), cell construction (see Chapter 2), and unique systems of genetic transfer (see Chapter 4).

Photosynthesis occurs within several subgroups of eubacteria, as well as in all cyanobacteria. The cyanobacteria include a variety of prokaryotic forms that overlap eubacteria and eukaryotic algae in their range of cellular sizes. They possess the same chlorophylls as the eukaryotic algae and oxidize H_2O to gaseous oxygen in their photosynthesis. By these properties they differ from the photosynthetic eubacteria, which have specialized chlorophylls and do not produce gaseous oxygen. The photosynthetic eubacteria use hydrogen donors other than H_2O; for example, one group oxidizes H_2S to free sulfur.

Both the cyanobacteria and the photosynthetic eubacteria contain their photosynthetic pigments in a series of lamellae just under the cell membrane. In some photosynthetic eubacteria, these lamellae differentiate under certain environmental conditions into ovoid or spherical bodies called chromatophores. In contrast, the eukaryotic algae always contain their photosynthetic pigments in autonomous cytoplasmic organelles (chloroplasts). There is strong evidence to support the hypothesis that the chloroplasts of eukaryotic algae and plants evolved from endosymbiotic cyanobacteria.

The cyanobacteria exhibit a type of motility on

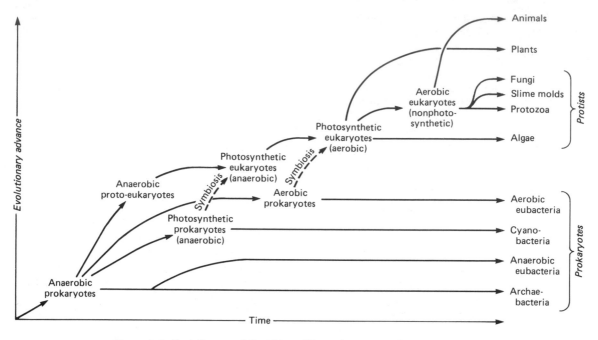

Figure 1–1. Evolutionary relationships of the major groups of microorganisms.

solid surfaces called "gliding"; they cannot swim through liquid medium. Many nonphotosynthetic eubacteria also possess gliding motility; some of these resemble certain cyanobacteria so closely that they are believed to be "colorless blue-greens" that have lost their photosynthetic pigments in the course of evolution.

No further generalizations can be made about the prokaryotes. The reader is referred instead to the descriptions of the various bacterial groups in Chapter 3.

EVOLUTIONARY RELATIONSHIPS

A theory of evolutionary relationships between the above groups is diagrammatically presented in Fig 1–1. Listed at the right are the major groups of present-day microorganisms; the horizontal scale indicates time, and the vertical scale indicates relative evolutionary advance. Thus, the earliest cell type to emerge on earth was presumably anaerobic and prokaryotic. From this ancestral type, 3 parallel lines of evolution diverged, leading to (1) photosynthesis, (2) aerobic respiration, and (3) such eukaryotic structural features as microtubular systems and nuclear complexity ("proto-eukaryotes").

The contemporary eukaryotes are pictured as arising by a sequence of further events: (1) establishment of endosymbiosis between a cyanobacterium and an anaerobic proto-eukaryotic cell, the chloroplast evolving from the endosymbiont; and (2) evolution of the mitochondrion, either from an endosymbiotic aerobic prokaryote or by segregation of part of the eukaryotic nucleus. (Although mitochondria share many properties with bacteria, their DNA more closely resembles that of the eukaryotic nucleus in possessing highly reiterated sequences as well as introns; thus, both theories are at this time equally tenable.)

These 2 events would have produced an aerobic photosynthetic eukaryote comparable to present-day higher algae. Loss of the chloroplast would account for the appearance of protozoa and ultimately of fungi and slime molds.

Anaerobic eubacteria and archaebacteria, according to this line of reasoning, represent forms that have evolved with relatively little change from the earliest prokaryotic groups. The evolutionary origin of present-day viruses, on the other hand, is obscure. A reasonable hypothesis is that they have evolved from their respective host cell genomes, escaping the normal control mechanisms of the cell and acquiring capsids.

REFERENCES

Books

Ainsworth GC, Sparrow FK, Sussman AS (editors): *The Fungi, An Advanced Treatise*. Academic Press, 1973.
Barnett JA, Payne RW, Yarrow D (editors): *Yeasts: Characteristics and Identification*. Cambridge Univ Press, 1984.

Bold HC, Wynne MJ: *Introduction to the Algae: Structure and Reproduction*. Prentice-Hall, 1978.
Carlile MJ, Skehel JJ (editors): *Evolution in the Microbial World: Symposia of the Society for General Microbiology 24*. Cambridge Univ Press, 1974.

Diener TO: *Viroids and Viroid Diseases*. Wiley-Interscience, 1979.

Laskin AT, Lechevalier HA (editors): *CRC Handbook of Microbiology,* 2nd ed. Vol 1: *Bacteria,* 1977; Vol 2: *Fungi, Algae, Protozoa and Viruses,* 1979. CRC Press.

Levandowsky M, Hutner SH (editors): *Biochemistry and Physiology of Protozoa,* 2nd ed. Academic Press, 1980.

Luria SE et al: *General Virology,* 3rd ed. Wiley, 1978.

Margulis L: *Symbiosis in Cell Evolution: Life and Its Environment on the Early Earth.* Freeman, 1981.

Ragan MC, Chapman DJ: *Biochemical Phylogeny of the Protists.* Academic Press, 1978.

Sleigh M: *The Biology of Protozoa.* University Park Press, 1975.

Stanier RY, Adelberg EA, Ingraham J: *The Microbial World,* 4th ed. Prentice-Hall, 1976.

Woese CR, Wolfe RS (editors): *The Bacteria: A Treatise on Structure and Function.* Vol 8. Academic Press, 1985.

Articles & Reviews

Bruenn JA: Virus-like particles of yeast. *Annu Rev Microbiol* 1980;**34:**49.

Cloud P: Evolution of ecosystems. *Am Sci* 1974;**62:**54.

Diener TO: Viroids: Structure and function: *Science* 1979; **205:**859.

Fox GE et al: The phylogeny of prokaryotes. *Science* 1980; **209:**457.

Horowitz NH, Hubbard JS: The origin of life. *Annu Rev Genet* 1974;**8:**393.

Knoll AH, Barghoorn ES: Precambrian eukaryotic organisms: A reassessment of the evidence. *Science* 1975; **190:**52.

Lake JA et al: Eubacteria, halobacteria, and the origin of photosynthesis: The photocytes. *Proc Natl Acad Sci USA* 1985;**82:**3716.

Lemke PA: Viruses of eukaryotic microorganisms. *Annu Rev Microbiol* 1976;**30:**105.

Raff RA, Mahler HR: The nonsymbiotic origin of mitochondria. *Science* 1972;**177:**575.

Robertson HD, Branch AD, Dahlberg JE: Focusing on the nature of the scrapie agent. *Cell* 1985;**40:**725.

Van Valen LM, Maiorana VC: The archaebacteria and eukaryotic origins. *Nature* 1980;**287:**248.

Wallace DC: Structure and evolution of organelle genomes. *Microbiol Rev* 1982;**46:**208.

Woese CR, Magrum LJ, Fox GE: Archaebacteria. *J Mol Evol* 1978;**11:**245.

OPTICAL METHODS

The Light Microscope

The resolving power of the light microscope under ideal conditions is about half the wavelength of the light being used. (Resolving power is the distance that must separate 2 point sources of light if they are to be seen as 2 distinct images.) With yellow light of a wavelength of 0.4 μm, the smallest separable diameters are thus about 0.2 μm. The **useful magnification** of a microscope is the magnification that makes visible the smallest resolvable particles. Microscopes used in bacteriology generally employ a 90-power objective lens with a 10-power ocular lens, thus magnifying the specimen 900 times. Particles 0.2 μm in diameter are therefore magnified to about 0.2 mm and so become clearly visible. Further magnification would give no greater resolution of detail and would reduce the visible area (field).

Further improvement in resolving power can be accomplished only by the use of light of shorter wavelengths of about 0.2 μm, thus allowing resolution of particles with diameters of 0.1 μm. Such microscopes, employing quartz lenses and photographic systems, are too expensive and complicated for general use.

The Electron Microscope

Using a beam of electrons focused by magnets, the electron microscope can resolve particles 0.001 μm apart. Viruses, with diameters of 0.01–0.2 μm, can be easily resolved.

An important technique in electron microscopy is the use of "shadowing." This involves depositing a thin layer of metal (such as platinum) on the object by placing it in the path of a beam of metal ions in a vacuum. The beam is directed obliquely, so that the object acquires a "shadow" in the form of an uncoated area on the other side. When an electron beam is then passed through the coated preparation in the electron microscope and a positive print made from the "negative" image, a 3-dimensional effect is achieved (eg, Figs 2–21, 2–22, and 2–23).

Other important techniques in electron microscopy include the use of ultrathin sections of embedded material; a method of freeze-drying specimens, which prevents the distortion caused by conventional drying procedures; and the use of negative staining with an electron-dense material such as phosphotungstic acid (eg, Fig 33–37).

The **scanning electron microscope** provides 3-dimensional images of the surfaces of microscopic objects (eg, Fig 3–1). The object is first coated with a thin film of a heavy metal and then scanned by a downward-directed electron beam. Electrons scattered by the heavy metal are collected and focused to form the final image.

Darkfield Illumination

If the condenser lens system is arranged so that no light reaches the eye unless reflected from an object on the microscope stage, structures that provide insufficient contrast with the surrounding medium can be made visible. This technique is particularly valuable for observing organisms such as the spirochetes, which are difficult to observe by transmitted light.

Phase Microscopy

The phase microscope takes advantage of the fact that light waves passing through transparent objects, such as cells, emerge in different phases depending on the properties of the materials through which they pass. A special optical system converts difference in phase into difference in intensity, so that some structures appear darker than others. An important feature is that internal structures are thus differentiated in living cells; with ordinary microscopes, killed and stained preparations must be used.

Autoradiography

If cells that have incorporated radioactive atoms are fixed on a slide, covered with a photographic emulsion, and stored in the dark for a suitable period of time, tracks appear in the developed film emanating from the sites of radioactive disintegration. If the cells are labeled with a weak emitter such as tritium, the tracks are sufficiently short to reveal the position of the radioactive label in the cell. This procedure, called autoradiography, has been particularly useful in following the replication of DNA, using tritium-labeled thymidine as a specific tracer (Fig 4–1).

EUKARYOTIC CELL STRUCTURE

The principal features of the eukaryotic cell are shown in the electron micrograph in Fig 2–1. Note the following structures.

The Nucleus

The nucleus is bounded by a membrane (**nm**) that is

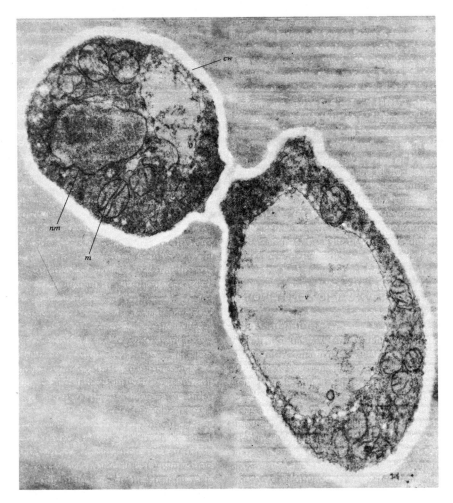

Figure 2–1. Thin section of a eukaryotic cell. A dividing cell of the unicellular yeast *Lipomyces* (17,500 ×). *n* = nucleus; *nm* = nuclear membrane; *v* = vacuole; *m* = mitochondrion; *cw* = cell wall. Electron micrograph taken by Dr CF Robinow. (From Stanier RY, Doudoroff M, Adelberg EA: *The Microbial World,* 2nd ed. Copyright © 1963. By permission of Prentice-Hall, Inc., Englewood Cliffs, NJ.)

continuous with the endoplasmic reticulum. The chromosomes, embedded in the nuclear matrix, are not distinguishable. The mitotic apparatus is not present at this stage in the division cycle.

Cytoplasmic Structures

The cytoplasm of eukaryotic cells is characterized by the presence of an endoplasmic reticulum, vacuoles, self-reproducing plastids, and an elaborate cytoskeleton composed of microtubules, microfilaments, and intermediate filaments about 10 nm in diameter.

The **endoplasmic reticulum** is a network of membrane-bounded channels. In some regions of the endoplasmic reticulum, the membranes are coated with ribosomes; proteins synthesized on these ribosomes pass through the membrane into the channels of the endoplasmic reticulum, through which they can be transported to other parts of the cell. A related structure, the **Golgi apparatus,** pinches off vesicles that can

fuse with the cell membrane, releasing the enclosed proteins into the surrounding medium.

The plastids include **mitochondria,** which contain in their membranes the respiratory electron transport system, and chloroplasts (in photosynthetic organisms). The plastids contain their own DNA, which codes for some (but not all) of their constituent proteins and transfer RNAs.

The cytoskeleton includes arrays of **microtubules,** which play a role in cytoplasmic membrane function and cell shape as well as forming the mitotic spindle and flagellar components; arrays of actin- and myosin-containing **microfilaments,** which provide the mechanism of ameboid motility; and the **intermediate filaments,** whose function is not yet known.

Surface Layers

The cytoplasm is enclosed within a lipoprotein cell membrane, similar to the prokaryotic cell membrane illustrated in Fig 2–11. Most animal cells have no other surface layers; many eukaryotic microorganisms, however, have an outer **cell wall,** which may be composed of a polysaccharide such as cellulose or chitin or may be inorganic, eg, the silica wall of diatoms.

Motility Organelles

Many eukaryotic microorganisms propel themselves through water by means of protein appendages called **cilia** or **flagella** (cilia are short; flagella are long). In almost every case, the organelle consists of a bundle of 9 fibrils surrounding 2 central fibrils (Figs 2–2 and 2–3). The fibrils are assembled from microtubules.

PROKARYOTIC CELL STRUCTURE

The prokaryotic cell is simpler than the eukaryotic cell at every level, with one exception: the cell envelope is more complex.

The Nucleus

The prokaryotic nucleus can be seen with the light microscope in stained material (Fig 2–4). It is Feulgen-positive, indicating the presence of DNA. The negatively charged DNA is at least partially neutral-

ized by small polyamines and magnesium ion, but histonelike proteins exist in bacteria and presumably play a role similar to that of histones in eukaryotic chromatin.

Electron micrographs such as Fig 2–5 reveal the absence of a nuclear membrane and of a mitotic apparatus. The nuclear region is filled with DNA fibrils; the DNA of the bacterial nucleus can be extracted as a single continuous molecule with a molecular weight of $2–3 \times 10^9$ (see Chromosome Structure, p 37). It may thus be considered to be a **single chromosome,** approximately 1 mm long in the unfolded state.

The nucleus can be isolated by gentle lysis of bacteria, followed by centrifugation. The structures thus isolated consist of DNA associated with smaller amounts of RNA, RNA polymerase, and possibly other proteins. The DNA appears to be looped around an RNA core, which serves to hold the DNA in its compact form.

Bacterial DNA, isolated directly on the electron microscope supporting film by gentle lysis of the cells in physiologic salt solution, is seen to have a beaded structure similar to that of eukaryotic chromatin (Fig 2–6).

The electron microscopy of serial thin sections through bacterial cells shows that the DNA is associated at one point with an invagination of the cell mem-

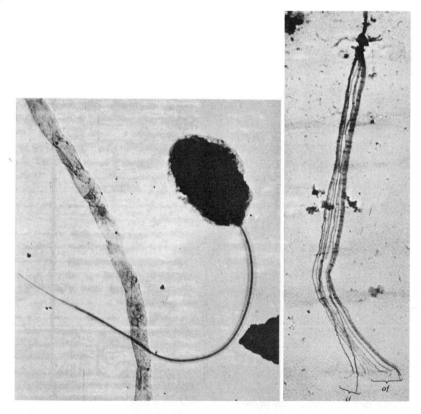

Figure 2–2. Eukaryotic flagella (3000 ×). *Left:* A zoospore of the fungus *Allomyces,* with a single flagellum. *Right:* A partially disintegrated flagellum of *Allomyces,* showing the 2 inner fibrils *(if)* and 9 outer fibrils *(of).* (Courtesy of Manton I et al: *J Exp Bot* 1952;3:204.)

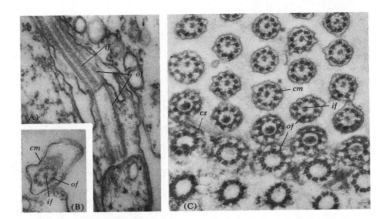

Figure 2–3. Fine structure of eukaryotic flagella and cilia (31,500 ×). *(A)* Longitudinal section of a flagellum of *Bodo,* a protozoon, showing kinetoplast *(k)* from which extend the outer fibrils *(of).* Note the origin of the inner fibrils *(if)* at the cell surface. *(B)* Cross section of same flagellum near the surface of the cell, showing outer fibrils *(of),* inner fibrils *(if),* and extension of cell membrane *(cm).* *(C)* Cross section through surface layer of the ciliate protozoon *Glaucoma,* which cuts across a field of cilia just within the cell membrane (lower half) as well as outside the cell membrane (upper half). *cs* = cell surface. Electron micrographs taken by Dr D Pitelka. (From Stanier RY, Doudoroff M, Adelberg EA: *The Microbial World,* 2nd ed. Copyright © 1963. By permission of Prentice-Hall, Inc., Englewood Cliffs, NJ.)

brane called a mesosome (Fig 2–5). This attachment is thought to play a key role in the segregation of the 2 sister chromosomes following chromosomal replication (see Cell Division, p 28). The genetics and chemistry of the bacterial chromosome are presented in Chapter 4.

Cytoplasmic Structures

Prokaryotic cells lack autonomous plastids, such as mitochondria and chloroplasts. The electron transport enzymes are localized instead in the cell membrane; in photosynthetic organisms, the photosynthetic pigments are localized in **lamellae** underlying the cell membrane (Fig 2–7). In some photosynthetic bacteria, the lamellae may become convoluted and pinch off into discrete particles called **chromatophores.**

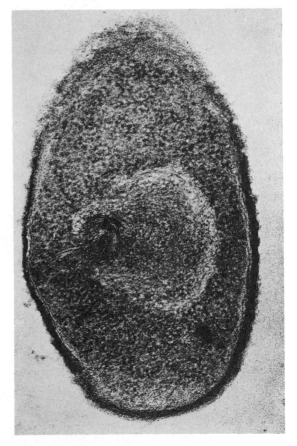

Figure 2–5. Electron micrograph of a thin section of *Bacillus subtilis,* showing the DNA in contact with a mesosome. (From Ryter A, Jacob F: Membrane et ségrégation nucléaire chez les bactéries. Page 267 of: *Proceedings of the 15th Colloquium on Protides of the Biological Fluids.* Vol 15. Peeters H [editor]. 1967.)

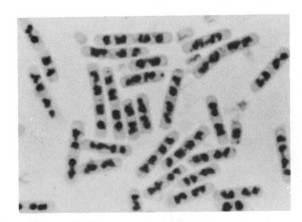

Figure 2–4. Nuclei of *Bacillus cereus* (2500 ×). (Courtesy of Robinow C: *Bacteriol Rev* 1956;20:207.)

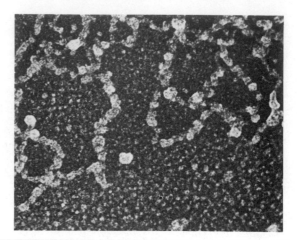

Figure 2–6. Bacteriophage λ DNA prepared by lysing infected cells with lysozyme in NaCl, 150 mmol/L, directly on an electron microscope supporting film. The beaded substructure shows a 13-nm repeating pattern. (From Griffith JD: Visualization of prokaryotic DNA in a regularly condensed chromatinlike fiber. *Proc Natl Acad Sci USA* 1976;**73**:563.)

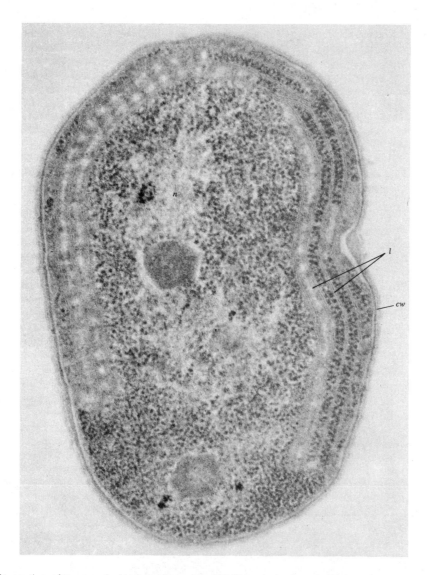

Figure 2–7. Thin section of a cyanobacterium, *Anacystis* (80,500 ×). *l* = lamellae bearing photosynthetic pigments; *cw* = cell wall; *n* = nuclear region. (Reprinted by permission of the Rockefeller Institute Press, from Ris H, Singh RN: *J Biophys Biochem Cytol* 1961;**9**:63.)

Bacteria often store reserve materials in the form of insoluble cytoplasmic **granules,** which are deposited as osmotically inert, neutral polymers. In the absence of a nitrogen source, carbon source material is converted by some bacteria to the polymer **poly-β-hydroxybutyric acid** (Fig 2–8) and by other bacteria to various polymers of glucose such as starch and glycogen. The granules are used as carbon sources when protein and nucleic acid synthesis is resumed. Similarly, certain sulfur-oxidizing bacteria convert excess H_2S from the environment into intracellular granules of elemental **sulfur.** Finally, many bacteria accumulate reserves of inorganic phosphate as granules of polymerized metaphosphate, called **volutin.** Volutin granules are also called **metachromatic granules** because they stain red with a blue dye. They are characteristic features of corynebacteria (see Chapter 15).

Microtubular structures, which are characteristic of eukaryotic cells, are generally absent in prokaryotes. In a few instances, however, the electron microscope has revealed bacterial structures that resemble microtubules.

Certain specialized groups of bacteria contain protein-bounded vesicles in their cytoplasm. These include gas vesicles that control buoyancy in some aquatic bacteria, chlorophyll-containing vesicles in the genus *Chlorobium,* and carboxysomes (containing carboxydismutase) in certain CO_2-fixing forms.

The Cell Envelope

The layers that bound the prokaryotic cell are referred to collectively as the cell envelope. The structure and organization of the cell envelope differ in gram-positive and gram-negative bacteria; in fact, it is this difference that defines these 2 major assemblages of bacterial species. Simplified diagrams of the 2 types of cell envelope are presented in Fig 2–9.

Many bacteria, both gram-positive and gram-negative, possess a 2-dimensional crystalline lattice of protein molecules as their outermost cell layer, underlying the capsule (not shown in Fig 2–9). The function of this **crystalline surface layer (S-layer)** is uncertain; in some cases, however, it has been shown to protect the cell from wall-degrading enzymes, from invasion by *Bdellovibrio bacteriovorus* (a predatory bacterium), and from bacteriophages. It also plays a role in the maintenance of cell shape in some species, and it may be involved in cell adhesion to host epidermal surfaces.

A. The Gram-Positive Cell Envelope: The cell envelope of gram-positive cells is relatively simple, consisting of just 3 layers: the **cytoplasmic membrane,** a thick **peptidoglycan layer,** and a variable outer layer called the **capsule.** The structure and function of these layers are described below.

B. The Gram-Negative Cell Envelope: This is a highly complex, multilayered structure (Fig 2–16). The cytoplasmic membrane (called the **inner membrane** in gram-negative bacteria) is surrounded by a single planar sheet of peptidoglycan to which is anchored a complex layer called the **outer membrane.** An outermost, variable capsule is also present. The space between the inner and outer membrane is called the **periplasmic space.**

The Cytoplasmic Membrane

A. Structure: The bacterial cytoplasmic membrane, also called the cell membrane, is visible in electron micrographs of thin sections (Fig 2–10). It is a typical "unit membrane," composed of phospholipids and proteins; Fig 2–11 illustrates a model of membrane organization. The membranes of prokaryotes are distinguished from those of eukaryotic cells by the absence of sterols, the only exception being mycoplasmas that incorporate sterols into their membranes when growing in sterol-containing media.

Convoluted invaginations of the cytoplasmic membrane form specialized structures called **mesosomes** (Fig 2–12). There are 2 types: septal mesosomes, which function in the formation of cross-walls during cell division; and lateral mesosomes. The bacterial chromosome (DNA) is attached to a septal mesosome (see Cell Division, p 28). More extensive ramifications of the cytoplasmic membrane into the cytoplasm are found in bacteria with exceptionally active electron transport systems (eg, photosynthetic and nitrogen-fixing bacteria).

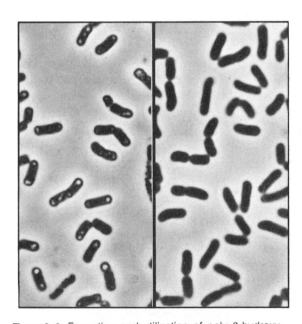

Figure 2–8. Formation and utilization of poly-β-hydroxybutyric acid in *Bacillus megaterium* (1900 ×). *Left:* Cells grown on glucose plus acetate, showing granules (light areas). *Right:* Cells from the same culture after 24 hours' further incubation in the presence of a nitrogen source but without an exogenous carbon source. The polymer has been completely metabolized. Phase contrast photomicrograph taken by Dr JF Wilkinson. (From Stanier RY, Doudoroff M, Adelberg EA: *The Microbial World,* 2nd ed. Copyright © 1963. By permission of Prentice-Hall, Inc., Englewood Cliffs, NJ.)

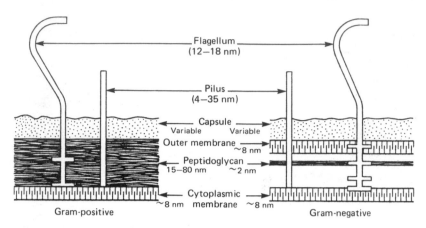

Figure 2–9. Comparison of the structures of gram-positive and gram-negative cell envelopes. The region between the cytoplasmic membrane and the outer membrane of the gram-negative envelope is called the periplasmic space. (From Ingraham JL, Maaløe O, Neidhardt FC: *Growth of the Bacterial Cell.* Sinauer Associates, 1983.)

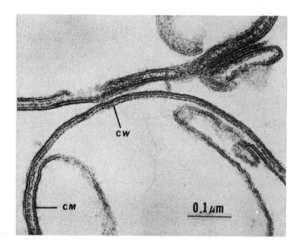

Figure 2–10. The cell membrane. Fragments of the cell membrane (CM) are seen attached to the cell wall (CW) in preparations made from *Escherichia coli.* (From Schnaitman CA: Solubilization of the cytoplasmic membrane of *Escherichia coli* by Triton X-100. *J Bacteriol* 1971; 108:545.)

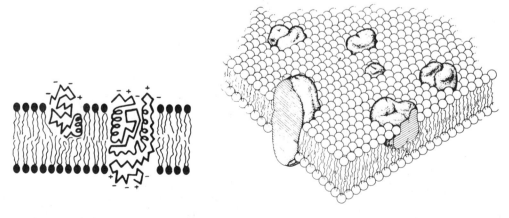

Figure 2–11. A model of membrane structure. Folded polypeptide molecules are visualized as embedded in a phospholipid bilayer, with their hydrophilic regions protruding into the intracellular space, extracellular space, or both. (From Singer SJ, Nicolson AL: The fluid mosaic model of the structure of cell membranes. *Science* 1972;175:720. Copyright © 1972 by the American Association for the Advancement of Science.)

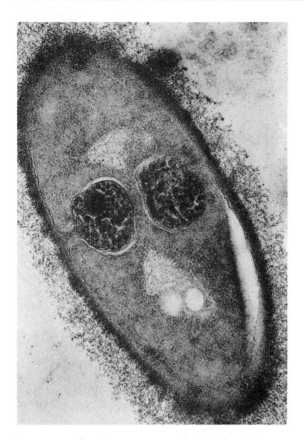

Figure 2–12. Septal mesosomes. A septal mesosome, formed as a concentric fold of the plasma membrane, grows inward. The new transverse septum is seen forming at the base of the concentric mesosome. Cell division will occur by fusion of the membrane layers surrounding the mesosome. (From Ellar DJ, Lundgren D, Slepecky RA: Fine structure of *Bacillus megaterium* during synchronous growth. *J Bacteriol* 1967;**84**:1189.)

B. Function: The major functions of the cytoplasmic membrane are (1) selective permeability and transport of solutes; (2) electron transport and oxidative phosphorylation, in aerobic species; (3) excretion of hydrolytic exoenzymes; (4) bearing the enzymes and carrier molecules that function in the biosynthesis of DNA, cell wall polymers, and membrane lipids; and (5) bearing the receptors and other proteins of the chemotactic and other sensory transduction systems.

At least 50% of the cytoplasmic membrane must be in the semifluid state in order for cell growth to occur. At low temperatures, this is achieved by greatly increased synthesis and incorporation of unsaturated fatty acids.

1. Permeability and transport—The membrane is both a permeability barrier (lipophobic solutes do not penetrate passively) and a permeability link: specific protein systems (permeases) are present that either facilitate the passive diffusion of specific solutes or catalyze energy-dependent active transport against a gradient.

There are 2 types of active transport systems, pri-

mary and secondary. In primary systems ("pumps"), metabolic energy is used to drive solutes through the membrane against their concentration gradients. In aerobic bacteria, the primary pump is the electron transport system, which uses the energy derived from substrate oxidation to export protons (see Chapter 7). As illustrated in Fig 7–32, the exported protons reenter the cell via the membrane ATPase; the energy derived from this ion flow is used by the ATPase to synthesize ATP from ADP plus inorganic phosphate. In anaerobic bacteria, which lack the electron transport system, the system is reversed: proton export takes place through the ATPase, at the expense of energy derived from the breakdown of ATP.

In secondary systems, the energy stored in the cation gradients and membrane potential produced by the pumps is used to actively transport solutes, such as amino acids and sugars, into the cell. This is accomplished by cotransport systems: the carrier binds cation and solute, transporting both simultaneously. Since the cation gradient is directed strongly inward, the combined electrochemical gradient drives the solute into the cell against its own concentration gradient.

The cell also has specific protein carriers in the membrane to facilitate the diffusion of certain solutes either into or out of the cell. Thus, if the cell is placed in a medium containing a high concentration of glycerol, it can equilibrate glycerol by facilitated diffusion in the absence of a coupled energy source.

In gram-negative bacteria, the transport of many nutrients is facilitated by specific **binding proteins** located in the periplasmic space. The nutrient is first bound to its specific binding protein with a dissociation constant in the range of 10^{-6} to 10^{-7} mol/L; it is then passed to a transport carrier protein of the inner membrane. Such systems are called "shock-sensitive," since osmotic shock (sudden dilution of a cell suspension) damages the outer membrane and allows the binding proteins to leak out.

In addition to true transport, in which a solute is moved across the membrane without change in structure, bacteria use a process called **group translocation** (vectorial metabolism) to effect the net uptake of certain sugars (eg, glucose and mannose), the substrate becoming phosphorylated during the transport process. A membrane carrier protein is first phosphorylated in the cytoplasm at the expense of phosphoenolpyruvate; the phosphorylated carrier then binds the free sugar at the exterior membrane face and transports it into the cytoplasm, releasing it as sugar-phosphate. Such systems of sugar transport are called **phosphotransferase systems.**

In *Escherichia coli,* the transport of potassium ion is used to regulate turgor pressure. An increase in external osmolarity at constant K^+ concentration activates the expression of genes coding for a set of K^+ transport proteins and also increases the activity of those proteins.

2. Electron transport and oxidative phosphorylation—The cytochromes and other enzymes of the respiratory chain, including certain dehydrogenases, are located in the cytoplasmic membrane. The bacterial cytoplasmic membrane is thus a functional analog of the mitochondrial inner membrane—a relationship which has been taken by many biologists to support the theory that mitochondria have evolved from symbiotic bacteria. The mechanism by which ATP generation is coupled to electron transport is discussed in Chapter 7.

3. Excretion of hydrolytic exoenzymes–All organisms that rely on macromolecular organic polymers as a source of nutrients (eg, proteins, polysaccharides, lipids) excrete hydrolytic enzymes that degrade the polymers to subunits small enough to penetrate the cytoplasmic membrane. Higher animals excrete such enzymes into the lumen of the digestive tract; bacteria excrete them directly into the external medium (in the case of gram-positive cells) or into the space (the periplasmic space) between the peptidoglycan layer and the outer membrane of the cell wall in the case of gram-negative bacteria (see The Cell Wall, below). Excreted proteins are synthesized on cytoplasmic ribosomes as preproteins carrying a hydrophobic sequence of about 20 amino acids at the N-terminal end. This "leader" or "signal" sequence, acting in concert with specific cytoplasmic and membrane proteins, binds the ribosome to the inner face of the cell membrane early in the process of polypeptide synthesis. Translocation through the membrane, initiated by the leader sequence, then takes place; it is not clear whether this occurs simultaneously with chain elongation or late in the process. Following translocation, the leader sequence is cleaved off by a membrane-bound leader peptidase, and the finished protein is released from the membrane in a final step.

4. Biosynthetic functions–The cytoplasmic membrane is the site of the carrier lipids on which the subunits of the cell wall are assembled (see synthesis of cell wall substances, in Chapter 7), as well as of the enzymes of cell wall biosynthesis. The enzymes of phospholipid synthesis are also localized in the cytoplasmic membrane. Finally, some proteins of the DNA replicating complex are present at discrete sites in the membrane, presumably in the septal mesosomes to which the DNA is attached.

5. Chemotactic systems–Attractants and repellents bind to specific receptors in the bacterial membrane (see Flagella, p 22). There are at least 20 different chemoreceptors in the membrane of *E coli,* some of which also function as a first step in the transport process.

C. Antibacterial Agents Affecting the Cell Membrane: Detergents, which contain lipophilic and hydrophilic groups, disrupt cytoplasmic membranes and kill the cell (see Chapter 5). One class of antibiotics, the polymyxins, consists of detergentlike cyclic peptides that selectively damage membranes containing phosphatidylethanolamine, a major component of bacterial membranes. A number of antibiotics specifically interfere with biosynthetic functions of the cytoplasmic membranes—eg, nalidixic acid, phenylethyl alcohol, and novobiocin inhibit DNA syn-

thesis; and novobiocin also inhibits teichoic acid synthesis.

A third class of membrane-active agents are the ionophores: compounds that permit rapid diffusion of specific cations through the membrane. Valinomycin, for example, specifically mediates the passage of potassium ions. Some ionophores act by forming hydrophilic pores in the membrane; others act as lipid-soluble ion carriers that behave as though they shuttle back and forth within the membrane. Ionophores can kill cells by discharging the membrane potential, which is essential for oxidative phosphorylation as well as for other membrane-mediated processes; they are not selective for bacteria but act on the membranes of all cells.

The Cell Wall

The layers of the cell envelope lying between the cytoplasmic membrane and the capsule are referred to collectively as the "cell wall." In gram-positive bacteria, the cell wall consists mainly of peptidoglycan and teichoic acids (see below); in gram-negative bacteria, the cell wall includes peptidoglycan, lipoprotein, outer membrane, and lipopolysaccharide layers.

The internal osmotic pressure of most bacteria ranges from 5 to 20 atmospheres as a result of solute concentration via active transport. In most environments, this pressure would be sufficient to burst the cell were it not for the presence of a high-tensile-strength cell wall (Fig 2–13). The bacterial cell wall owes its strength to a layer composed of a substance variously referred to as murein, mucopeptide, or **peptidoglycan** (all are synonyms). The structure of peptidoglycan will be discussed below.

Bacteria are classified as gram-positive or gram-negative according to their response to the Gram-staining procedure. This procedure, named for its inventor, was developed in an attempt to selectively stain bacteria in infected tissues. The cells are first stained with crystal violet and iodine and then washed

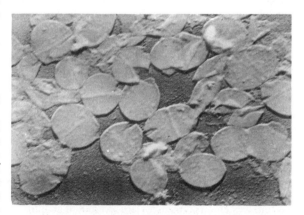

Figure 2–13. Cell walls of *Streptococcus faecalis,* removed from protoplasts by mechanical disintegration and differential centrifugation (11,000 ×). (Courtesy of Salton M, Horne R: *Biochim Biophys Acta* 1951;7:177.)

with acetone or alcohol. The latter step decolorizes gram-negative bacteria but not gram-positive bacteria.

The difference between gram-positive and gram-negative bacteria has been shown to reside in the cell wall: gram-positive cells can be decolorized with acetone or alcohol if the cell wall is removed after the staining step but before the washing step. Although the chemical composition of gram-positive and gram-negative walls is now fairly well known (see below), the reason gram-positive walls block the dye-extraction step is still unclear.

In addition to giving osmotic protection, the cell wall plays an essential role in cell division as well as serving as a primer for its own biosynthesis. Various layers of the wall are the sites of major antigenic determinants of the cell surface, and one layer—the lipopolysaccharide of gram-negative cell walls—is responsible for the nonspecific endotoxin activity of gram-negative bacteria. The cell wall is, in general, nonselectively permeable; one layer of the gram-negative wall, however—the outer membrane—hinders the passage of relatively large molecules (see below).

The biosynthesis of the cell wall and the antibiotics that interfere with this process are discussed in Chapter 7.

A. The Peptidoglycan Layer: Peptidoglycan is a complex polymer consisting, for the purposes of description, of 3 parts: a backbone, composed of alternating N-acetylglucosamine and N-acetylmuramic acid; a set of identical tetrapeptide side chains attached to N-acetylmuramic acid; and a set of identical peptide cross-bridges (Fig 2–14). The backbone is the same in all bacterial species; the tetrapeptide side chains and the peptide cross-bridges vary from species to species, those of *Staphylococcus aureus* being illustrated in Fig 2–14. In many gram-negative cell walls, the cross-bridge consists of a direct peptide linkage between the diaminopimelic acid (DAP) amino group of one side chain and the carboxyl group of the terminal D-alanine of a second side chain.

The tetrapeptide side chains of all species, however, have certain important features in common. Most have L-alanine at position 1 (attached to N-acetylmuramic acid); D-glutamate or substituted D-glutamate at position 2; and D-alanine at position 4. Position 3 is the most variable one: most gram-negative bacteria carry diaminopimelic acid at this position, to which is linked the lipoprotein cell wall component discussed below. Gram-positive bacteria may carry diaminopimelic acid, L-lysine, or any of several other L-amino acids at position 3.

Diaminopimelic acid is a unique element of prokaryotic cell walls and is the immediate precursor of lysine in the bacterial biosynthesis of that amino acid (Fig 7–23). Bacterial mutants that are blocked prior to diaminopimelic acid in the biosynthetic pathway grow normally when provided with diaminopimelic acid in the medium; when given L-lysine alone, however, they lyse, since they continue to grow but are specifically unable to make new cell wall peptidoglycan.

The fact that all peptidoglycan chains are cross-linked means that each peptidoglycan layer is a single giant molecule. In gram-positive bacteria, there are as many as 40 sheets of peptidoglycan, comprising up to 50% of the cell wall material; in gram-negative bacteria, there appear to be only one or 2 sheets, comprising 5–10% of the wall material.

Several prokaryotic groups, collectively called the archaebacteria, lack a peptidoglycan layer. In some species within this group, a similar polymer exists containing N-acetyl sugars and 3 L-amino acids; muramic acid and D-amino acids are absent. In other archaebacteria, a protein layer is present instead. These organisms, which also show major differences in their lipids and RNAs, occupy extreme environments in nature and have been proposed to represent the most primitive forms of cellular life on earth (see Chapter 1).

B. Special Components of Gram-Positive Cell Walls: Most gram-positive cell walls contain considerable amounts of **teichoic** and **teichuronic acids,** which may form up to 50% of the dry weight of the wall and 10% of the dry weight of the total cell. In addition, some gram-positive walls may contain polysaccharide molecules.

1. Teichoic and teichuronic acids–These are water-soluble polymers, containing ribitol or glycerol residues joined through phosphodiester linkages (Fig 2–15A). There are 2 types of teichoic acids: wall teichoic acid, covalently linked to peptidoglycan; and membrane teichoic acid (lipoteichoic acid), covalently linked to membrane glycolipid and concentrated in mesosomes. Some gram-positive species lack wall teichoic acids, but all appear to contain membrane teichoic acids.

The teichoic acids constitute major surface antigens of those gram-positive species that possess them, and their accessibility to antibodies has been taken as evidence that they lie on the outside surface of the peptidoglycan layer. Their activity is often increased, however, by partial digestion of the peptidoglycan; thus, much of the teichoic acid may lie between the cytoplasmic membrane and the peptidoglycan layer, possibly extending upward through pores in the latter (Fig 2–15B). In the pneumococcus *(Streptococcus pneumoniae),* the teichoic acids bear the antigenic determinants called Forssman antigen.

The repeat units of some teichoic acids are shown in Fig 2–15A. The repeat units may be glycerol, joined by 1,3- or 1,2-linkages; ribitol, joined by 1,5-linkages; or more complex units in which glycerol or ribitol is joined to a sugar residue such as glucose, galactose, or N-acetylglucosamine. The chains may be 30 or more repeat units in length, although chain lengths of 10 or less are common.

Most teichoic acids contain large amounts of D-alanine, usually attached to position 2 or 3 of glycerol or position 3 or 4 of ribitol. In some of the more complex teichoic acids, however, D-alanine is attached to one of the sugar residues. In addition to D-alanine, other substituents may be attached to the free hydroxyl groups of glycerol and ribitol: eg, glucose, galactose,

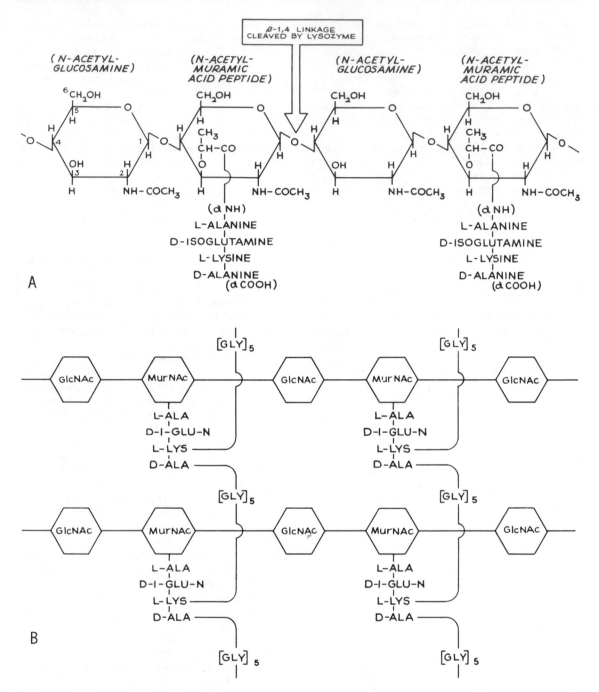

Figure 2–14. *A:* A segment of the peptidoglycan of *Staphylococcus aureus*. The backbone of the polymer consists of alternating subunits of N-acetylglucosamine and N-acetylmuramic acid connected by β-1,4 linkages. The muramic acid residues are linked to short peptides, the composition of which varies from one bacterial species to another. In some species, the L-lysine residues are replaced by diaminopimelic acid, an amino acid that is found in nature only in prokaryotic cell walls. Note the D-amino acids, which are also characteristic constituents of prokaryotic cell walls. The peptide chains of the peptidoglycan are cross-linked between parallel polysaccharide backbones, as shown in Fig 2–14B. *B:* Schematic representation of the peptidoglycan lattice that is formed by cross-linking. Bridges composed of pentaglycine peptide chains connect the α-carboxyl of the terminal D-alanine residue of one chain with the ε-amino group of the L-lysine residue of the next chain. The nature of the cross-linking bridge varies among different species.

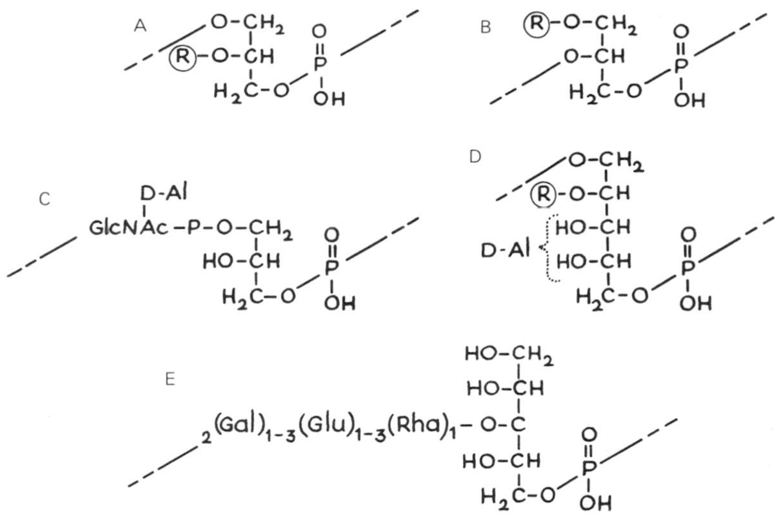

A: $R-O-CH$ with $O-CH_2$, H_2C-O, $P=O$, OH

B: $R-O-CH_2$, $O-CH$, H_2C-O, $P=O$, OH

C: D-Al, $GlcNAc-P-O-CH_2$, $HO-CH$, H_2C-O, $P=O$, OH

D: $O-CH_2$, $R-O-CH$, $HO-CH$, D-Al $HO-CH$, H_2C-O, $P=O$, OH

E: $_2(Gal)_{1-3}(Glu)_{1-3}(Rha)_1-O-C$, $HO-CH_2$, $HO-CH$, $HO-CH$, H_2C-O, $P=O$, OH

Figure 2–15A. Repeat units of some teichoic acids. *A:* Glycerol teichoic acid of *Lactobacillus casei* 7469 (R = D-alanine). *B:* Glycerol teichoic acid of *Actinomyces antibioticus* (R = D-alanine). *C:* Glycerol teichoic acid of *Staphylococcus lactis* 13. D-Alanine occurs on the 6 position of N-acetylglucosamine. *D:* Ribitol teichoic acids of *Bacillus subtilis* (R = glucose) and *Actinomyces streptomycini* (R = succinate). (The D-alanine is attached to position 3 or 4 of ribitol.) *E:* Ribitol teichoic acid of the type 6 pneumococcal capsule.

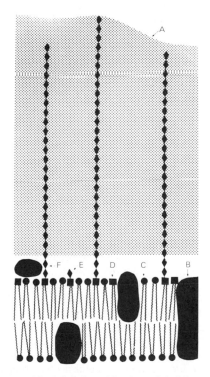

Figure 2–15B. Lipoteichoic acids. A model of the cell wall and membrane of a gram-positive bacterium, showing lipoteichoic acid molecules extending through the cell wall. The wall teichoic acids, covalently linked to muramic acid residues of the peptidoglycan layer, are not shown. A = cell wall; B = protein; C = phospholipid; D = glycolipid; E = phosphatidyl glycolipid; F = lipoteichoic acid. (From Van Driel D et al: Cellular location of the lipoteichoic acids of *Lactobacillus fermenti* NCTC 6991 and *Lactobacillus casei* NCTC 6375. *J Ultrastruct Res* 1971;43:483.)

N-acetylglucosamine, N-acetylgalactosamine, or succinate. A given species may have more than one type of sugar substituent in addition to D-alanine; in such cases, it is not certain whether the different sugars occur on the same or on separate teichoic acid molecules. The composition of the teichoic acid formed by a given bacterial species can vary with the composition of the growth medium.

The teichoic acids bind magnesium ion and play a role in the supply of this ion to the cell. They also play a role in the normal functioning of the cell envelope; thus, replacement of choline by ethanolamine as a component of the teichoic acid of pneumococci causes the cells to resist autolysis and to lose the ability to take up transforming DNA (see Chapter 4).

The teichuronic acids are similar polymers, but the repeat units include sugar acids (such as N-acetylmannosuronic or D-glucosuronic acid) instead of phosphoric acids. They are synthesized in place of teichoic acids when phosphate is limiting.

2. Polysaccharides–The hydrolysis of grampositive walls has yielded, from certain species, neutral sugars such as mannose, arabinose, galactose, rhamnose, and glucosamine and acidic sugars such as glucuronic acid and mannuronic acid. It has been proposed that these sugars exist as subunits of polysaccharides in the cell wall; the discovery, however, that teichoic and teichuronic acids may contain a variety of sugars (Fig 2–15A) leaves the true origin of these sugars uncertain.

C. Special Components of Gram-Negative Cell Walls: Gram-negative cell walls contain 3 components that lie outside of the peptidoglycan layer: lipoprotein, outer membrane, and lipopolysaccharide (Fig 2–16).

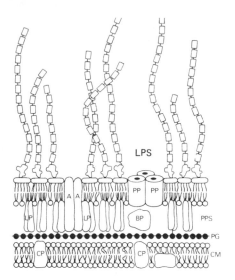

Figure 2–16. Molecular organization of the outer membrane of gram-negative bacteria. LPS, lipopolysaccharide; A, OmpA protein; PP, pore protein (matrix porin); LP, lipoprotein; BP, nutrient-binding protein; PPS, periplasmic space; PG, peptidoglycan; CP, carrier protein; CM, cytoplasmic membrane. (From Lugtenberg B, Van Alphen LV: Molecular architecture and functioning of the outer membrane of *Escherichia coli* and other gram-negative bacteria. *Biochim Biophys Acta* 1983;**737**:51.)

1. Lipoprotein–Molecules of an unusual lipoprotein cross-link the outer membrane and peptidoglycan layers. The protein component contains 57 amino acids, representing repeats of a 15-amino-acid sequence; it is peptide-linked to diaminopimelic acid residues of the peptidoglycan tetrapeptide side chains. The lipid component, consisting of a diglyceride thioether linked to a terminal cysteine, is noncovalently inserted in the outer membrane. Lipoprotein is the most abundant protein of gram-negative cells. Its function (inferred from the behavior of mutants that lack it) is to stabilize the outer membrane and anchor it to the peptidoglycan layer.

2. Outer membrane–The outer membrane is a phospholipid bilayer in which the phospholipids of the outer leaflet are replaced by lipopolysaccharide (LPS) molecules (see below). Like the cytoplasmic membrane, the outer membrane is a fluid mosaic containing a set of specific proteins embedded in a phospholipid matrix.

The outer membrane prevents leakage of the periplasmic proteins and protects the cell (in the case of enteric bacteria) from bile salts and hydrolytic enzymes of the host environment. As described below, the presence of proteinaceous pores in the outer membrane makes it permeable to low-molecular-weight solutes; large antibiotic molecules penetrate it relatively slowly, however, which accounts for the relatively high antibiotic resistance of gram-negative bacteria. The permeability of the outer membrane varies widely from one gram-negative species to another; in *Pseudomonas aeruginosa*, for example, which is extremely resistant to antibacterial agents, the outer membrane is 100 times less permeable than that of *E coli*.

The major proteins of the outer membrane, named according to the genes that code for them, have been placed into several functional categories on the basis of mutants in which they are lacking and on the basis of experiments in which purified proteins have been reconstituted into artificial membranes. The **matrix porins,** exemplified by OmpC, D, and F of *E coli* and *Salmonella typhimurium,* are trimeric proteins that penetrate both faces of the outer membrane. They form relatively nonspecific pores that permit the free diffusion of small hydrophilic solutes across the membrane. The porins of different species have different exclusion limits, ranging from molecular weights of about 600 in *E coli* and *S typhimurium* to more than 3000 in *P aeruginosa*.

Members of a second group of pore-forming proteins, exemplified by LamB and Tsx, show greater specificity: LamB, an inducible porin that is the receptor for lambda bacteriophage, is responsible for most of the transmembrane diffusion of maltodextrins; Tsx, the receptor for T6 bacteriophage, is responsible for the transmembrane diffusion of nucleosides and some amino acids. LamB allows some passage of other solutes, however; its relative specificity may reflect weak interactions of solutes with configuration-specific sites within the channel.

The proteins in a third major group are nonporins: they include OmpA, which participates in the anchoring of the outer membrane to the peptidoglycan layer and is also the sex pilus receptor in F-mediated bacterial conjugation (see Chapter 4).

The outer membrane also contains a set of less abundant, so-called minor proteins, many of which are involved in the transport of specific small molecules such as vitamin B_{12} and the iron siderophores. They show high affinity for their substrates and probably function like the classic carrier transport systems of the inner (cytoplasmic) membrane. The minor proteins include a limited number of enzymes, among them phospholipases and proteases, as well as some penicillin-binding proteins.

The topology of the major proteins of the outer membrane, based on cross-linking studies and analyses of functional relationships, is shown in Fig 2–16. These proteins are synthesized on ribosomes bound to the cytoplasmic surface of the inner membrane; how they are transferred to the outer membrane is still uncertain, but one hypothesis suggests that transfer occurs at regions of adhesion ("Bayer's junctions") between the inner and outer membranes, which regions are visible in the electron microscope.

3. Lipopolysaccharide (LPS)–The lipopolysaccharide of gram-negative cell walls consists of a complex lipid, called lipid A, to which is attached a polysaccharide made up of a core and a terminal series of repeat units (Fig 2–17A).

Lipid A consists of phosphorylated glucosamine disaccharide units to which are attached a number of long-chain fatty acids (Fig 2–17B). β-Hydroxymyris-

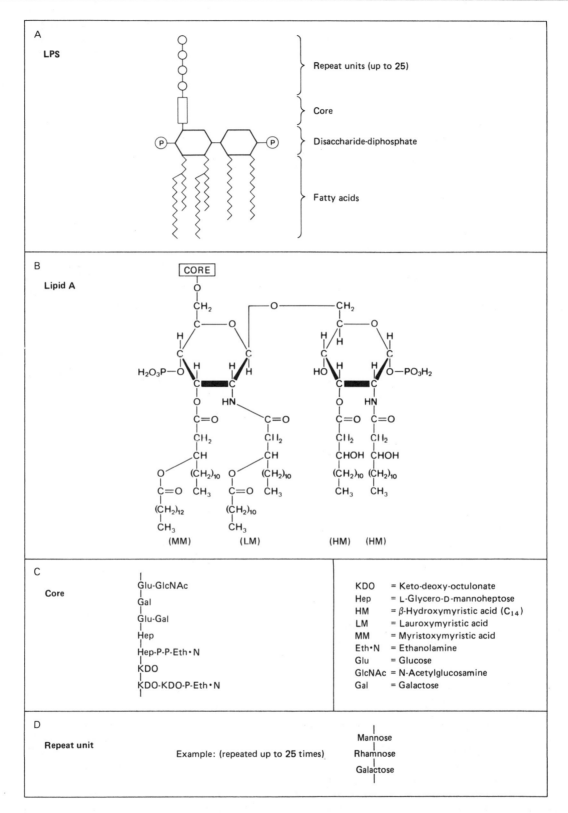

Figure 2–17. The lipopolysaccharide (LPS) of the gram-negative cell envelope. *A:* A segment of the polymer, showing the arrangements of the major constituents. *B:* The structure of lipid A of *Salmonella typhimurium*. *C:* The polysaccharide core. *D:* A typical repeat unit *(Salmonella newington)*.

tic acid, a C_{14} fatty acid, is always present and is unique to this lipid; the other fatty acids, along with substituent groups on the 2 phosphates, vary according to the bacterial species.

The polysaccharide core, shown in Fig 2–17C, is constant in all gram-negative species. Each species, however, contains a unique repeat unit, that of *Salmonella newington* being shown in Fig 2–17D. The repeat units are usually linear trisaccharides or branched tetra- or pentasaccharides.

The negatively charged LPS molecules are noncovalently cross-bridged by divalent cations; this stabilizes the membrane and provides a barrier to hydrophobic molecules. Removal of the divalent cations with chelating agents, or their displacement by polycationic antibiotics such as polymyxins and aminoglycosides, renders the outer membrane permeable to large hydrophobic molecules.

LPS, which is extremely toxic to animals, has been called the **endotoxin** of gram-negative bacteria because it is firmly bound to the cell surface and is released only when the cells are lysed. When LPS is split into lipid A and polysaccharide, all of the toxicity is associated with the former. The polysaccharide, on the other hand, represents a major surface antigen of the bacterial cell—the so-called **O antigen.** Antigenic specificity is conferred by the terminal repeat units, which form a sort of molecular fur on the cell surface. The number of possible antigenic types is very great: over 1000 have been recognized in *Salmonella* alone.

LPS is attached to the outer membrane by hydrophobic bonds. It is synthesized on the cytoplasmic membrane and transported to its final exterior position. The presence of LPS is required for the function of many outer membrane proteins.

4. The periplasmic space—The space between the inner and outer membranes, called the periplasmic space, is filled with a gel consisting of hydrated peptidoglycan. A number of proteins and oligosaccharides are present and are freely diffusible in the gel. The periplasmic proteins include binding proteins for specific substrates, as well as hydrolytic enzymes (eg, alkaline phosphatase and 5′-nucleotidase) that break down nontransportable substrates into transportable ones. The periplasmic oligosaccharides are highly branched polymers of D-glucose, 8–10 residues long. They are variously substituted with glycerol phosphate and phosphatidylethanolamine residues; some contain O-succinyl esters. They appear to play a role in osmoregulation, since cells grown in medium of low osmolarity increase their synthesis of these compounds 16-fold.

D. Enzymes That Attack Cell Walls: The β-1,4 linkage of the peptidoglycan backbone is hydrolyzed by the enzyme **lysozyme,** which is found in animal secretions (tears, saliva, nasal secretions) as well as in egg white. Gram-positive bacteria treated with lysozyme in low-osmotic-strength media lyse; if the osmotic strength of the medium is raised to balance the internal osmotic pressure of the cell, free protoplasts are liberated (Fig 2–l8). The outer membrane of the gram-negative cell wall prevents access of lysozyme unless disrupted by an agent such as EDTA*; in osmotically protected media, cells treated with EDTA-lysozyme form **spheroplasts** that still possess remnants of the complex gram-negative wall, including the outer membrane.

Bacteria themselves possess a number of **autolysins,** hydrolytic enzymes that attack peptidoglycan, including glycosidases, amidases, and peptidases. These enzymes presumably play essential functions in cell growth and division, but their activity is most apparent during the dissolution of dead cells (autolysis).

Enzymes that degrade bacterial cell walls are also found in cells that digest whole bacteria, eg, protozoa and the phagocytic cells of higher animals.

E. Cell Wall Growth: As the protoplast increases in mass, the cell wall is elongated by the intercalation of newly synthesized subunits into the various wall layers. In streptococci, intercalation into the principal antigen-bearing layer is localized to the equatorial region of the cell wall (Fig 2–19); in some gram-negative bacteria, a process of random intercalation has been inferred, although localized intercalation followed by rapid displacement or turnover could produce the same appearance. In *E coli,* growth of the outer membrane framework takes place exclusively at the cell poles, specialized components such as phage receptors and permeases being inserted randomly into this framework. The peptidoglycan layer of *E coli* appears to grow by randomly located intercalations. In *Bacillus subtilis,* pulse-chase experiments have shown that peptidoglycan and teichoic acids exist in blocks, there being fewer than 12 sites per cell for the insertion of newly synthesized material.

F. Protoplasts, Spheroplasts, and L Forms: Removal of the bacterial cell wall may be accomplished by hydrolysis with lysozyme or by blocking peptidoglycan biosynthesis with an antibiotic such as penicillin. In osmotically protective media, such treatments liberate protoplasts from gram-positive cells and spheroplasts (which retain the outer membrane) from gram-negative cells.

If such cells are able to grow and divide, they are called **L forms.** L forms are difficult to cultivate and usually require a medium that is solidified with agar as well as having the right osmotic strength. L forms are produced more readily with penicillin than with lysozyme, suggesting the need for residual peptidoglycan.

Some L forms can revert to the normal bacillary form upon removal of the inducing stimulus. Thus, they are able to resume normal cell wall synthesis. Others, however, are stable and never revert. The factor that determines their capacity to revert may again be the presence of residual peptidoglycan, which normally acts as a primer in its own biosynthesis.

Some bacterial species produce L forms spontaneously. The spontaneous or antibiotic-induced formation of L forms in the host may produce chronic in-

---

*Ethylenediaminetetraacetic acid, a chelating agent.

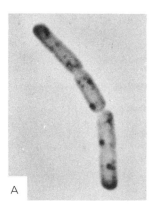
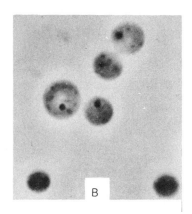
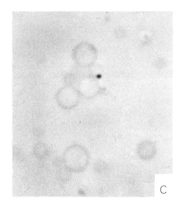

Figure 2–18. *Bacillus megaterium* phase contrast photomicrographs (3000 x). *A:* Before treatment. *B:* Protoplasts liberated following treatment with lysozyme and sucrose. *C:* After treatment with lysozyme alone; the empty structures are cytoplasmic membranes. (Courtesy of Weibull C: *J Bacteriol* 1963;66:688.)

fections, the organisms persisting by becoming sequestered in protective regions of the body. Since L-form infections are relatively resistant to antibiotic treatment, they present special problems in chemotherapy. Their reversion to the bacillary form can produce relapses of the overt infection.

Capsule & Glycocalyx

Many bacteria synthesize large amounts of extracellular polymer when growing in their natural environments. With one known exception (the poly-D-glutamic acid capsule of *Bacillus anthracis*), the extracellular material is polysaccharide (Table 2–1). When the polymer forms a condensed, well-defined layer closely surrounding the cell, it is called the **capsule** (Fig 2–20A); when it forms a loose meshwork of fibrils extending outward from the cell, it is called the **glycocalyx** (Fig 2–20B). In some cases, masses of polymer are formed which appear to be totally detached from the cells but in which cells may be en-

trapped; in these instances, the extracellular polymer may be referred to simply as a "slime layer." Extracellular polymer is synthesized by enzymes located at the surface of the bacterial cell. *Streptococcus mutans*, for example, uses 2 enzymes—glucosyl transferase and fructosyl transferase—to synthesize long-chain dextrans (poly-D-glucose) and levans (poly-D-fructose) from sucrose.

The capsule contributes to the invasiveness of pathogenic bacteria: encapsulated cells are protected from phagocytosis unless they are coated with anticapsular antibody. The glycocalyx plays a major role in the adherence of bacteria to surfaces in their environment, including the cells of their plant and animal hosts. *S mutans*, for example, owes its capacity to adhere tightly to tooth enamel to its glycocalyx. Bacterial cells of the same or different species become entrapped in the glycocalyx, which forms the layer known as plaque on the tooth surface; acidic products excreted by these bacteria cause dental caries (see

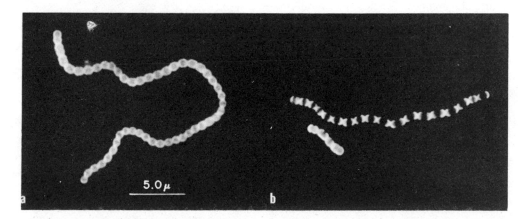

Figure 2–19. Growth of the bacterial cell wall. *(a)* Chains of streptococci, stained with fluorescent antibody directed against cell wall antigens. *(b)* After 15 minutes' growth in the absence of antibody. New cell wall material, unstained by antibody, has been deposited in the equatorial region of each cell. (From Cole RM, Hahn JJ: Cell wall replication in *Streptococcus pyogenes.* Science 1962;**135**:722. Copyright © 1962 by the American Association for the Advancement of Science.)

Table 2–1. Chemical composition of the extracellular polymer in certain bacteria.*

Organism	Polymer	Chemical Subunits
Bacillus anthracis	Polypeptide	D-Glutamic acid
Leuconostoc mesenteroides	Dextran	Glucose
Streptococcus pneumoniae (pneumococcus)	Complex polysaccharides (many types), eg,	
	Type II	Rhamnose, glucose, glucuronic acid
	Type III	Glucose, glucuronic acid
	Type VI	Galactose, glucose, rhamnose
	Type XIV	Galactose, glucose, N-acetylglucosamine
	Type XVIII	Rhamnose, glucose
Streptococcus spp	Hyaluronic acid	N-Acetylglucosamine, glucuronic acid
Streptococcus salivarius	Levan	Fructose
Acetobacter xylinum	Cellulose	Glucose
Enterobacter aerogenes	Complex polysaccharide	Glucose, fucose, glucuronic acid

*From Stanier RY, Doudoroff M, Adelberg EA: *The Microbial World,* 3rd ed. Copyright 1970. By permission of Prentice-Hall, Inc., Englewood Cliffs, NJ.

Chapter 30). The essential role of the glycocalyx in this process—and its formation from sucrose—explains the correlation of dental caries with sucrose consumption by the human population.

Flagella

A. Structure: Bacterial flagella are threadlike appendages composed entirely of protein, 12–30 nm in diameter. They are the organs of locomotion for the forms that possess them. Three types of arrangement are known: **monotrichous** (single polar flagellum), **lophotrichous** (tuft of polar flagella), and **peritrichous** (flagella distributed over the entire cell). The 3 types are illustrated in Figs 2–21, 2–22, and 2–23.

A bacterial flagellum is made up of a single kind of protein subunit called flagellin; the flagellum is formed by the aggregation of subunits to form a hollow cylindric structure. If flagella are removed by mechanically agitating a suspension of bacteria, new flagella are rapidly formed by the synthesis, aggregation, and extrusion of flagellin subunits; motility is restored within 3–6 minutes. The flagellins of different bacterial species presumably differ from one another in primary structure.

The flagellum is attached to the bacterial cell body by a complex structure consisting of a hook and a basal body. The basal body bears a set of rings, one pair in gram-positive bacteria and 2 pairs in gram-negative bacteria. An electron micrograph and interpretative diagrams of the gram-negative structure are shown in Figs 2–24 and 2–25; the rings labeled L and P are absent in gram-positive cells. The complexity of the bacterial flagellum is revealed by genetic studies, which show that over 40 gene products are involved in its assembly and function.

B. Motility: Bacterial flagella are semirigid helical rotors to which the cell imparts a spinning movement. Rotation is driven by the flow of protons into the cell down the gradient produced by the primary proton

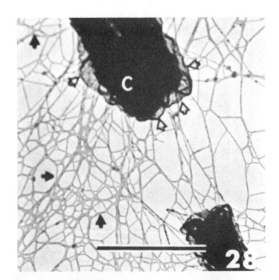

Figure 2–20B. *Klebsiella pneumoniae* cells (C), surrounded by glycocalyx (solid arrows). (From Cagle GD: Fine structure and distribution of extracellular polymer surrounding selected aerobic bacteria. *Can J Microbiol* 1975;21:395.)

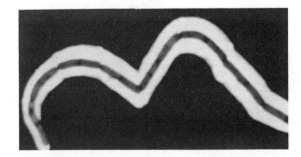

Figure 2–20A. *Bacillus megaterium,* stained by a combination of positive and negative staining (1400 ×). (See section on staining, below.) (Courtesy of Welshimer H: *J Bacteriol* 1953;66:112.)

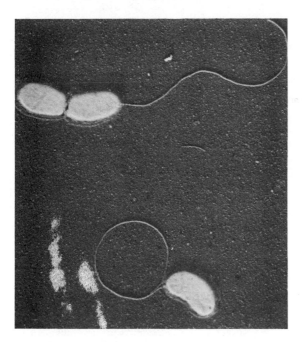

Figure 2–21. *Vibrio metchnikovii*, a monotrichous bacterium (7500 x). (Courtesy of van Iterson W: *Biochim Biophys Acta* 1947;1:527.)

pump (see above); in the absence of a metabolic energy source, it can be driven by a proton motive force generated by ionophores. Bacteria living in alkaline environments (alkalophiles) use the energy of the sodium ion gradient, rather than the proton gradient, to drive the flagellar motor.

All of the components of the flagellar motor are located in the cell envelope. The flagella attached to isolated, sealed cell envelopes rotate normally when the medium contains a suitable substrate for respiration or when a proton gradient is artifically established.

When a peritrichous bacterium swims, its flagella associate to form a posterior bundle that drives the cell forward in a straight line by counterclockwise rotation. At intervals, the flagella reverse their direction of rotation and momentarily dissociate, causing the cell to tumble until swimming resumes in a new, randomly determined direction. This behavior makes possible the property of **chemotaxis:** a cell that is moving away from the source of a chemical attractant tumbles and reorients itself more frequently than one that is moving toward the attractant, the result being the net movement of the cell toward the source. The presence of a chemical attractant (such as a sugar or an amino acid) is sensed by specific receptors located in the cell membrane (in many cases the same receptor also participates in membrane transport of that molecule). The bacterial cell is too small to be able to detect the existence of a spatial chemical gradient (ie, a gradient between its 2 poles); rather, experiments show that it detects temporal gradients, ie, concentrations that decrease with time when the cell is moving away from the attractant source and increase with time when the cell is moving toward it.

Some compounds act as repellents rather than attractants. One mechanism by which cells respond to attractants and repellents involves a cGMP-mediated

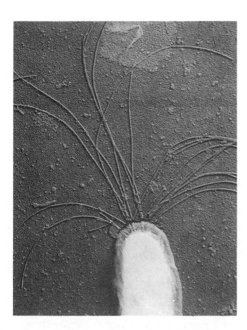

Figure 2–22. Electron micrograph of *Spirillum serpens,* showing lophotrichous flagellation (9000 x). (Courtesy of van Iterson W: *Biochim Biophys Acta* 1947;1:527.)

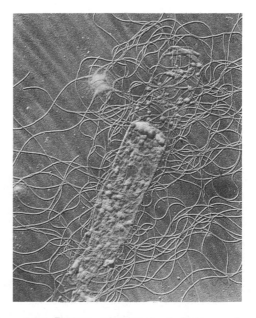

Figure 2–23. Electron micrograph of *Proteus vulgaris,* showing peritrichous flagellation (9000 x). Note basal granules. (Courtesy of Houwink A, van Iterson W: *Biochim Biophys Acta* 1950;5:10.)

methylation and demethylation of specific proteins in the membrane. Attractants cause a transient inhibition of demethylation of these proteins, while repellents stimulate their demethylation.

The mechanism by which a change in cell behavior is brought about in response to a change in the environment is called **sensory transduction.** Sensory transduction is responsible not only for chemotaxis but also for **aerotaxis** (movement toward the optimal oxygen concentration), **phototaxis** (movement of photosynthetic bacteria toward the light), and **electron acceptor taxis** (movement of respiratory bacteria toward alternative electron acceptors, such as nitrate and fumarate). In these 3 responses, as in chemotaxis, net movement is determined by regulation of the tumbling response.

Pili (Fimbriae)

Many gram-negative bacteria possess rigid surface appendages called pili (Latin "hairs") or fimbriae (Latin "fringes"). They are shorter and finer than flagella; like flagella, they are composed of protein subunits. Two classes can be distinguished: ordinary pili, which play a role in the adherence of symbiotic bacteria to host cells; and sex pili, which are responsible for the attachment of donor and recipient cells in bacterial conjugation (see Chapter 4). Pili are illustrated in Fig 2–26, in which the sex pili have been coated with phage particles for which they serve as specific receptors.

The virulence of certain pathogenic bacteria depends on the production not only of toxins but also of "colonization antigens," which are now recognized to be ordinary pili that provide the cells with adherent properties. In enteropathogenic *E coli* strains, both the enterotoxins and the colonization antigens (pili) are genetically determined by transmissible plasmids, as discussed in Chapter 4.

In one group of gram-positive cocci, the streptococci, fimbriae are the site of the major surface antigen, the M protein. Lipoteichoic acid, associated with these fimbriae, is responsible for the adherence of group A streptococci to epithelial cells of their hosts.

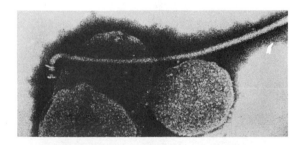

Figure 2–24. Electron micrograph of a negatively stained lysate of *Rhodospirillum molischianum,* showing the basal structure of an isolated flagellum. (From Cohen-Bazire G, London L: Basal organelles of bacterial flagella. *J Bacteriol* 1967;**94**:458.)

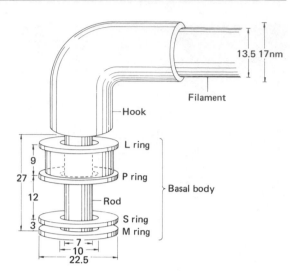

Figure 2–25. Basal structure of the bacterial flagellum. Diagram interpreting the structure seen in Fig 2–24. (From De Pamphilis ML, Adler J: Fine structure and isolation of the hook-basal body complex of flagella from *Escherichia coli* and *Bacillus subtilis. J Bacteriol* 1971;**105**:384.)

Endospores

Members of several bacterial genera are capable of forming endospores (Fig 2–27). The 2 most common are gram-positive rods: the obligately aerobic genus *Bacillus* and the obligately anaerobic genus *Clostridium*. The other bacteria known to form endospores are the gram-positive coccus *Sporosarcina* and the rickettsial agent of Q fever, *Coxiella burnetii*. These organisms undergo a cycle of differentiation in response to environmental conditions: under conditions of nutritional depletion, each cell forms a single internal spore that is liberated when the mother cell undergoes autolysis. The spore is a resting cell, highly resistant to desiccation, heat, and chemical agents; when returned to favorable nutritional conditions and activated (see below), the spore germinates to produce a single vegetative cell.

A. Sporulation: The sporulation process begins when nutritional conditions become unfavorable, depletion of the nitrogen or carbon source (or both) being the most significant factor. Sporulation occurs massively in cultures that have terminated exponential growth as a result of such depletion.

Sporulation involves the production of many new structures, enzymes, and metabolites along with the disappearance of many vegetative cell components. These changes represent a true process of **differentiation:** A series of genes whose products determine the formation and final composition of the spore is activated, while another series of genes involved in vegetative cell function is inactivated. These changes involve alterations in the transcriptional specificity of RNA polymerase, which is determined by the association of the polymerase core protein with one or another

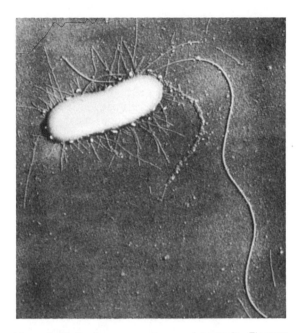

Figure 2–26. Surface appendages of bacteria. Electron micrograph of a cell of *E coli* possessing 3 types of appendages: ordinary pili (short, straight bristles); a sex pilus (longer, flexible, with phage particles attached); and several flagella (longest, thickest). Diameters: Ordinary pili: 7 nm; sex pili: 8.5 nm; flagella: 25 nm. (Courtesy of Dr J Carnahan and Dr C Brinton.)

promoter-specific protein called a sigma factor. Different sigma factors are produced during vegetative growth and sporulation.

The sequence of events in sporulation is highly complex: asporogenous mutants reveal at least 12 morphologically or biochemically distinguishable stages, and at least 30 operons (including an estimated 200 structural genes) are involved. During the process, some bacteria release peptide antibiotics, which may play a role in regulating sporogenesis.

Morphologically, sporulation begins with the isolation of a terminal nucleus by the inward growth of the cell membrane (Fig 2–28). The growth process involves an infolding of the membrane so as to produce a double membrane structure whose facing surfaces correspond to the cell wall-synthesizing surface of the cell envelope. The growing points move progressively toward the pole of the cell so as to engulf the developing spore.

The 2 spore membranes now engage in the active synthesis of special layers that will form the cell envelope: the **spore wall** and **cortex,** lying between the facing membranes; and the **coat** and **exosporium,** lying outside of the facing membranes. In the newly isolated cytoplasm, or **core,** many vegetative cell enzymes are degraded and are replaced by a set of unique spore constituents. A thin section of a sporulating cell is shown in Fig 2–29.

B. Properties of Endospores:

1. Core–The core is the spore protoplast. It contains a complete nucleus (chromosome), all of the components of the protein-synthesizing apparatus, and an energy-generating system based on glycolysis.

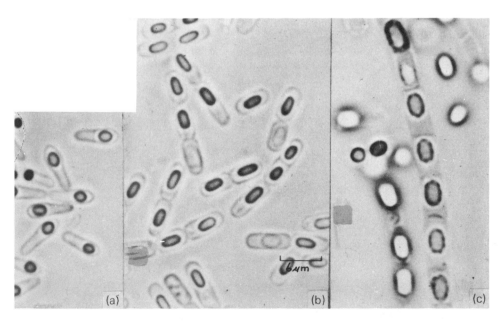

Figure 2–27. Sporulating cells of *Bacillus* species. *A:* Unidentified bacillus from soil. *B: B cereus. C: B megaterium.* (From Robinow CF, in: *Structure.* Vol 1 of: *The Bacteria: A Treatise on Structure and Function.* Gunsalus IC, Stanier RY [editors]. Academic Press, 1960.)

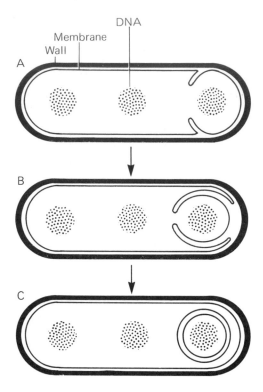

Figure 2–28. The sporulation process. *A:* Inward growth of an invagination of the cell membrane. *B:* Membrane growing points move toward the pole of the cell. *C:* Fusion of membranes completes the isolation of the spore protoplast.

Cytochromes are lacking even in aerobic species, the spores of which rely on a shortened electron transport pathway involving flavoproteins. A number of vegetative cell enzymes are increased in amount (eg, alanine racemase), and a number of unique enzymes are formed (eg, dipicolinic acid synthetase). The energy for germination is stored as 3-phosphoglycerate rather than as ATP.

The heat resistance of spores is due in part to their dehydrated state and in part to the presence in the core of large amounts (5–15% of the spore dry weight) of calcium dipicolinate, which is formed from an intermediate of the lysine biosynthetic pathway (Fig 7–23). In some way not yet understood, these properties result in the stabilization of the spore enzymes, most of which exhibit normal heat lability when isolated in soluble form.

2. Spore wall–The innermost layer surrounding the inner spore membrane is called the spore wall. It contains normal peptidoglycan and becomes the cell wall of the germinating vegetative cell.

3. Cortex–The cortex is the thickest layer of the spore envelope. It contains an unusual type of peptidoglycan, with many fewer cross-links than are found in cell wall peptidoglycan. Cortex peptidoglycan is extremely sensitive to lysozyme, and its autolysis plays a key role in spore germination.

4. Coat–The coat is composed of a keratinlike

protein containing many intramolecular disulfide bonds. The impermeability of this layer confers on spores their relative resistance to antibacterial chemical agents.

5. Exosporium–The exosporium is a lipoprotein membrane containing some carbohydrate.

C. Germination: The germination process occurs in 3 stages: activation, initiation, and outgrowth.

1. Activation–Even when placed in an environment that favors germination (eg, a nutritionally rich medium), bacterial spores will not germinate unless first activated by one or another agent that damages the spore coat. Among the agents that can overcome spore dormancy are heat, abrasion, acidity, and compounds containing free sulfhydryl groups.

2. Initiation–Once activated, a spore will initiate germination if the environmental conditions are favorable. Different species have evolved receptors that recognize different effectors as signaling a rich medium: thus, initiation is triggered by L-alanine in one species and by adenosine in another. Binding of the effector activates an autolysin that rapidly degrades the cortex peptidoglycan. Water is taken up, calcium dipicolinate is released, and a variety of spore constituents are degraded by hydrolytic enzymes.

3. Outgrowth–Degradation of the cortex and outer layers results in the emergence of a new vegetative cell consisting of the spore protoplast with its surrounding wall (Fig 2–30). A period of active biosynthesis follows; this period, which terminates in cell

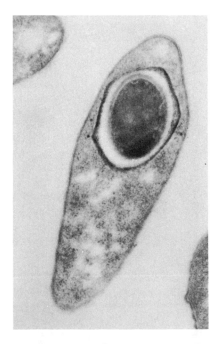

Figure 2–29. Thin section through a sporulating cell of a bacillus (33,000 ×). Electron micrograph taken by Dr CL Hannay. (From Stanier RY, Doudoroff M, Adelberg EA: *The Microbial World*, 2nd ed. Copyright © 1963. By permission of Prentice-Hall, Inc., Englewood Cliffs, NJ.)

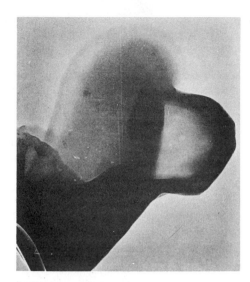

Figure 2–30. Electron micrograph of germinating spore of *Bacillus mycoides.* (Courtesy of Knaysi G, Baker R, Hillier J: *J Bacteriol* 1947;**53**:525.)

division, is called outgrowth. Outgrowth requires a supply of all nutrients essential for cell growth.

STAINING

Stains combine chemically with the bacterial protoplasm; if the cell is not already dead, the staining process itself will kill it. The process is thus a drastic one and may produce artifacts.

The commonly used stains are salts. **Basic** stains consist of a colored cation with a colorless anion (eg, methylene blue$^+$ chloride$^-$); **acidic** stains are the reverse (eg, sodium$^+$ eosinate$^-$). Bacterial cells are rich in nucleic acid, bearing negative charges as phosphate groups. These combine with the positively charged basic dyes. Acidic dyes do not stain bacterial cells and hence can be used to stain background material a contrasting color (see Negative Staining, below).

The basic dyes stain bacterial cells uniformly unless the cytoplasmic RNA is destroyed first. Special staining techniques can be used, however, to differentiate flagella, capsules, cell walls, cell membranes, granules, nuclei, and spores.

The Gram Stain

An important taxonomic characteristic of bacteria is their response to Gram's stain. The Gram-staining property appears to be a fundamental one, since the Gram reaction is correlated with many other morphologic properties in phylogenetically related forms (see Chapter 3). An organism that is potentially gram-positive may appear so only under a particular set of environmental conditions and in a young culture.

The Gram-staining procedure (see Chapter 32 for details) begins with the application of a basic dye, crystal violet. A solution of iodine is then applied; all

bacteria will be stained blue at this point in the procedure. The cells are then treated with alcohol. Gram-positive cells retain the crystal violet-iodine complex, remaining blue; gram-negative cells are completely decolorized by alcohol. As a last step, a counterstain (such as the red dye safranin) is applied so that the decolorized gram-negative cells will take on a contrasting color; the gram-positive cells now appear purple.

The basis of the differential Gram reaction is the structure of the cell wall, as discussed earlier in this chapter.

The Acid-Fast Stain

Acid-fast bacteria are those that retain carbolfuchsin (basic fuchsin dissolved in a phenol-alcohol-water mixture) even when decolorized with hydrochloric acid in alcohol. A smear of cells on a slide is flooded with carbolfuchsin and heated on a steam bath. Following this, the decolorization with acid-alcohol is carried out, and finally a contrasting (blue or green) counterstain is applied. Acid-fast bacteria (mycobacteria and some of the related actinomycetes) appear red; others take on the color of the counterstain.

Negative Staining

This procedure involves staining the background with an acidic dye, leaving the cells contrastingly colorless. The black dye nigrosin is commonly used. This method is used for those cells or structures difficult to stain directly (Fig 2–20A).

The Flagella Stain

Flagella are too fine (12–30 nm in diameter) to be visible in the light microscope. However, their presence and arrangement can be demonstrated by treating the cells with an unstable colloidal suspension of tannic acid salts, causing a heavy precipitate to form on the cell walls and flagella. In this manner, the apparent diameter of the flagella is increased to such an extent that subsequent staining with basic fuchsin makes the flagella visible in the light microscope. Fig 2–31 shows cells stained by this method.

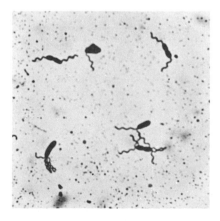

Figure 2–31. Flagella stain of *Pseudomonas* species. (Courtesy of Leifson E: *J Bacteriol* 1951;**62**:377.)

In multitrichous bacteria, the flagella form into bundles during movement, and such bundles may be thick enough to be observed on living cells by dark-field or phase contrast microscopy.

The Capsule Stain

Capsules are usually demonstrated by the negative staining procedure or a modification of it (Fig 2–20A). One such "capsule stain" (Welch method) involves treatment with hot crystal violet solution followed by a rinsing with copper sulfate solution. The latter is used to remove excess stain because the conventional washing with water would dissolve the capsule. The copper salt also gives color to the background, with the result that the cell and background appear dark blue and the capsule a much paler blue.

Staining of Nuclei

Nuclei are stainable with the Feulgen stain, which is specific for DNA.

The Spore Stain

Spores are most simply observed as intracellular refractile bodies in unstained cell suspensions or as colorless areas in cells stained by conventional methods. The spore wall is relatively impermeable, but dyes can be made to penetrate it by heating the preparation. The same impermeability then serves to prevent decolorization of the spore by a period of alcohol treatment sufficient to decolorize vegetative cells. The latter can finally be counterstained. Spores are commonly stained with malachite green or carbolfuchsin.

MORPHOLOGIC CHANGES DURING GROWTH

Cell Division

In general, bacteria reproduce by binary fission. Following elongation of the cell, a transverse cell membrane is formed, and subsequently a new cell wall. In bacteria, the new transverse membrane and wall grow inward from the outer layers, a process in which the septal mesosomes are intimately involved (Fig 2–12). The nuclei, which have doubled in number preceding the division, are distributed equally to the 2 daughter cells.

Although bacteria lack a mitotic spindle, the transverse membrane is formed in such a way as to separate the 2 sister chromosomes formed by chromosomal replication. This is accomplished by the attachment of the chromosome to the cell membrane. According to one model, the completion of a cycle of DNA replication triggers active membrane synthesis between the sites of attachment of the 2 sister chromosomes, which are pushed apart by the inward growth of the transverse membrane (Fig 4–4). The deposition of new cell wall material follows, resulting in the elongation and eventual doubling of the cell envelope.

Cell Groupings

If the cells remain temporarily attached following division, certain characteristic groupings result. Depending on the plane of division and the number of divisions through which the cells remain attached, the following arrangement may occur in the coccal forms: chains (streptococci), pairs (pneumococci), cubical bundles (sarcinae), or flat plates. Rods may form pairs or chains.

Following fission of some bacteria, characteristic postfission movements occur. For example, a "whipping" motion can bring the cells into parallel positions; repeated division and whipping results in the "palisade" arrangement characteristic of diphtheria bacilli.

Life Cycle Changes

As bacteria progress from the dormant to the actively growing state, certain visible changes take place. The cells tend to become larger, granules disappear, and the protoplasm stains more deeply with basic dyes. When growth slows down again, a gradual change in the reverse direction takes place. Finally, in very old cultures there appear morphologically unusual cells called involution forms. These include filaments, buds, and branched cells, many of which are nonviable.

REFERENCES

Books

Aronson S: *Chemical Communication at the Microbial Level.* Vols 1 and 2. CRC Press, 1981.

Beachey EH (editor): *Bacterial Adherence: Receptors and Recognition.* Series B, Vol 6. Chapman & Hall, 1980.

Dring GJ, Ellar DJ, Gould GW (editors): *Fundamental and Applied Aspects of Bacterial Spores.* Academic Press, 1985.

Fuller R, Lovelock DW (editors): *Microbial Ultrastructure: The Use of the Electron Microscope.* Academic Press, 1976.

Goldberger RF: *Molecular Organization and Cell Function.* Plenum, 1980.

Hurst A, Gould GW (editors): *The Bacterial Spore.* Vol 2. Academic Press, 1984.

Inouye M (editor): *Bacterial Outer Membranes: Biogenesis and Functions.* Wiley-Interscience, 1980.

Leive L (editor): *Membranes and Walls of Bacteria.* Dekker, 1973.

Martonosi AS (editor): *The Enzymes of Biological Membranes,* 2nd ed. Vol 1: *Membrane Structure and Dynamics;* Vol 2: *Biosynthesis and Metabolism;* Vol 3: *Membrane Transport;* Vol 4: *Bioenergetics of Electron and Proton Transport.* Plenum, 1984.

Nanninga N (editor): *Molecular Cytology of* Escherichia coli. Academic Press, 1985.

Parish JH: *Developmental Biology of Prokaryotes.* Univ of California Press, 1980.

Rogers H: *Bacterial Cell Structure.* American Society for Microbiology, 1983.

Rosen B: *Bacterial Transport*. Dekker, 1978.

Stanier R et al (editors): *Relations Between Structure and Function in the Prokaryotic Cell. Symposia of the Society for General Microbiology 28.* Cambridge Univ Press, 1978.

Articles & Reviews

Aronson AI, Fitz-James P: Structure and morphogenesis of the bacterial spore coat. *Bacteriol Rev* 1976;**40**:360.

Boyd A, Simon M: Bacterial chemotaxis. *Annu Rev Physiol* 1982;**44**:501.

Burman LG, Park JT: Molecular model for elongation of the murein sacculus of *Escherichia coli. Proc Natl Acad Sci USA* 1984;**81**:1844.

Cagle GD: Fine structure and distribution of extracellular polymer surrounding selected aerobic bacteria. *Can J Microbiol* 1975;**21**:395.

Clasener H: Pathogenicity of the L-phase of bacteria. *Annu Rev Microbiol* 1972;**26**:55.

Costerton JW et al: The bacterial glycocalyx in nature and disease. *Annu Rev Microbiol* 1981;**35**:299.

Doetsch RN, Sjoblad RD: Flagellar structure and function in eubacteria. *Annu Rev Microbiol* 1980;**34**:69.

Doi RH: Genetic contol of sporulation. *Annu Rev Genet* 1977;**11**:29.

Elwell LP, Shipley PL: Plasmid-mediated factors associated with virulence of bacteria to animals. *Annu Rev Microbiol* 1980;**34**:465.

Giesbrecht P, Wecke J, Reinicke B: On the morphogenesis of the cell wall of staphylococci. *Int Rev Cytol* 1976;**44**:225.

Gould GW, Dring GJ: Mechanisms of spore heat resistance. *Adv Microb Physiol* 1974;**11**:137.

Greenawalt JW, Whiteside TL: Mesosomes: Membranous bacterial organelles. *Bacteriol Rev* 1975;**39**:405.

Gunn RB: Co- and counter-transport mechanisms in cell membranes. *Annu Rev Physiol* 1980;**42**:249.

Hancock REW: Alterations in outer membrane permeability. *Annu Rev Microbiol* 1984;**38**:237.

Henning U: Determination of cell shape in bacteria. *Annu Rev Microbiol* 1975;**29**:45.

Hobot JA et al: Periplasmic gel: New concept resulting from the reinvestigation of bacterial cell envelope ultrastructure by new methods. *J Bacteriol* 1984;**160**:143.

Inouye M: Lipoprotein of the outer membrane of *Escherichia coli. Biomembranes* 1979;**10**:141.

Inouye M, Halegoua S: Secretion and membrane localization of proteins in *Escherichia coli. CRC Crit Rev Biochem* 1980;**7**:339.

Kandler O, König H: Chemical composition of the peptidoglycan-free cell walls of methanogenic bacteria. *Arch Microbiol* 1978;**118**:141.

Kennedy EP: Osmotic regulation and the biosynthesis of membrane-derived oligosaccharides in *Escherichia coli. Proc Natl Acad Sci USA* 1982;**79**:1092.

Keynan A: The transformation of bacterial endospores into vegetative cells. *Symp Soc Gen Microbiol* 1973;**23**:85.

Kleppe K, Ovrebö S, Lossius I: The bacterial nucleoid. *J Gen Microbiol* 1979;**112**:1.

Lanyi JK: The role of Na^+ in transport processes of bacterial membranes. *Biochim Biophys Acta* 1979;**559**:377.

Lo TC: The molecular mechanisms of substrate transport in gram-negative bacteria. *Can J Biochem* 1979;**57**:289.

Lugtenberg B et al: Molecular architecture and functionings of the outer membrane of *Escherichia coli* and other gram-negative bacteria. *Biochim Biophys Acta* 1982;**737**:51.

Macnab RM, Aizawa S-I: Bacterial motility and the bacterial flagellar motor. *Annu Rev Biophys Bioeng* 1984;**13**:51.

Neilands JB: Transport functions of the outer membrane of enteric bacteria. *Horiz Biochem Biophys* 1978;**5**:65.

Nikaido H, Vaara M: Molecular basis of bacterial outer membrane permeability. *Microbiol Rev* 1985;**49**:1.

Osborn MJ: Structure and biosynthesis of the bacterial cell wall. *Annu Rev Microbiol* 1969;**38**:501.

Pettijohn DE: Prokaryotic DNA in nucleoid structure. *CRC Crit Rev Biochem* 1976;**4**:175.

Randall LL, Hardy SJS: Export of protein in bacteria. *Microbiol Rev* 1984;**48**:290.

Ryter A: Association of the nucleus and the membrane of bacteria: A morphological study. *Bacteriol Rev 1968;*32:39.

Salton MRJ, Owen P: Bacterial membrane structure. *Annu Rev Microbiol* 1976;**30**:451.

Schleifer KH, Hammes WP, Kandler O: Effect of endogenous and exogenous factors on the primary structure of bacterial peptidoglycan. *Adv Microb Physiol* 1976;**13**:246.

Schleifer KH, Kandler O: Peptidoglycan types of bacterial cell walls and their taxonomic implications. *Bacteriol Rev* 1972;**36**:407.

Shively JM: Inclusion bodies of prokaryotes. *Annu Rev Microbiol* 1974;**2**:167.

Shockman GD, Barrett JF: Structure, function, and assembly of cell walls of gram-positive bacteria. *Annu Rev Microbiol* 1983;**37**:501.

Slater M, Schaechter M: Control of cell division in bacteria. *Bacteriol Rev* 1974;**38**:199.

Sleytr UB, Messner P: Crystalline surface layers on bacteria. *Annu Rev Microbiol* 1983;**37**:311.

Smith H: Microbial surfaces in relation to pathogenicity. *Bacteriol Rev* 1977;**41**:475.

Springer MS, Goy MF, Adler J: Protein methylation in behavioural control mechanisms and in signal transduction. *Nature* 1979;**280**:279.

Takayama K, Qureshi N, Mascagni P: Complete structure of lipid A obtained from the lipopolysaccharides of the heptoseless mutant of *Salmonella typhimurium. J Biol Chem* 1983;**258**:12801.

Taylor BL: Role of proton motive force in sensory transduction. *Annu Rev Microbiol* 1983;**37**:551.

Ward JB: Teichoic and teichuronic acids: Biosynthesis, assembly and location. *Microbiol Rev* 1981;**45**:211.

Warth AD: Molecular structure of the bacterial spore. *Adv Microb Physiol* 1978;**17**:1.

Wilson DB: Cellular transport mechanisms. *Annu Rev Biochem* 1978;**47**:933.

Worcel A, Burgi E: Properties of a membrane-attached form of the folded chromosome of *Escherichia coli. J Mol Biol* 1974;**82**:91.

3   The Major Groups of Bacteria

PRINCIPLES OF CLASSIFICATION

Although it may be said of the higher organisms that no 2 individuals are exactly alike, it is nevertheless true that such individuals tend to form clusters of highly similar types. Furthermore, between any 2 clusters there is generally a sharp discontinuity. It is common practice to speak of each cluster as a **species.** For hundreds of years, biologists have been naming and describing species of plants, animals, and microorganisms. Having at hand a large number of such names and accompanying descriptions, the next step was to compile this information in some orderly and systematic manner, ie, to classify it. In order to understand the problems and limitations of bacterial classification, it is necessary first to discuss 2 fundamental issues: the meaning of the term "species," and the types and purposes of classification.

"Species" Defined

A "species" is a stage in the evolution of a population of organisms. To understand this, it is necessary to consider how species originate in higher plants and animals with obligatory sexual life cycles.

A. Evolution in Higher Organisms: Organisms having obligatory sexual life cycles are characterized by populations that maintain relatively homogeneous gene pools by interbreeding. Divergent evolution occurs when 2 segments of a homogeneous population become geographically isolated from each other: The barrier to interbreeding between the 2 groups allows each to evolve along its own path, eventually becoming sufficiently different in physiology or behavior (or both) to prevent further interbreeding, even if the geographic barrier is overcome. Such populations are said to be "physiologically isolated"; the point in evolution at which physiologic isolation occurs is thus a highly significant one and is therefore chosen as the point at which new species are said to have arisen. A "species" may thus be defined as follows: "A given stage of evolution at which actually or potentially interbreeding arrays of forms become segregated into two or more separate arrays which are physiologically incapable of interbreeding."*

B. Evolution in Bacteria: Unlike higher plants

*Dobzhansky T: *Genetics and the Origin of Species*. Columbia Univ Press, 1957.

and animals, bacteria (and many other microorganisms) multiply almost entirely vegetatively. There is thus no mechanism by which discontinuous "species" can arise; instead, mutations accumulate so as to produce gradients of related types. As bacteria evolve to occupy their niches more and more efficiently, divergent lines of evolution will occur to the extent that the niches differ; groups of related ecologic types can thus often be recognized, but within each group there may be few real discontinuities. The term "species" thus has little meaning when applied to bacteria; it cannot even be defined, as it can for sexually reproducing organisms. Bacterial taxonomists must be purely arbitrary in deciding to what extent 2 types must differ before being classed as different "species."

In recent years, the techniques of molecular genetics have introduced new criteria for determining the degree of evolutionary relatedness between different bacteria. In one such technique, the DNA is extracted from pure cultures of the types in question and their relative base compositions determined. The parameter most often used is the mole percent of guanine (G) plus cytosine (C) in the total DNA; the G + C content may be directly measured or indirectly calculated from buoyant density or melting point determinations. For 2 organisms to be considered closely related, their G + C contents must be closely similar (although such similarity is not proof of relatedness).

Within a well-defined, closely-knit group such as the aerobic spore-forming bacilli, much higher degrees of relatedness can be recognized by the relative abilities of heat-denatured DNAs from different strains to reanneal with each other during slow cooling. Such reannealing reflects the existence in the 2 types of DNA of homologous nucleotide sequences.

A third technique is based on base sequence homologies in ribosomal RNA. The 16S RNA is digested to short oligonucleotides, which are readily sequenced; phylogenetic relatedness is considered to be proportionate to the number of oligonucleotide sequences held in common by 2 species. Since ribosomal RNA sequences have been highly conserved during evolution, such analyses can detect relations between even distantly related species.

Types & Purposes of Classification

While many sorts of systematic compilations are conceivable, only 2 are generally used in taxonomy:

keys, or "artificial classifications"; and phylogenic, or "natural," classifications.

A. Keys: In a "key," descriptive properties are arranged in such a way that an organism on hand may be readily identified. Organisms that are grouped together in a "key" are not necessarily related in the phylogenic sense; they are listed together because they share some easily recognizable property. It would be perfectly reasonable, for example, for a key to bacteria to include a group such as "bacteria forming red pigments," even though this would include such unrelated forms as *Serratia marcescens* and purple sulfur bacteria. The point is that such a grouping would be useful; the investigator having a red-pigmented culture to identify would immediately narrow the search to a relatively few types.

B. Phylogenic Classification: A phylogenic classification groups together types that are **related,** ie, those that share a common ancestor. Species that have arisen through divergent evolution from a common ancestor are grouped together in a single genus; genera with a common origin are grouped in a single family, etc. Recognition of phylogenic relationships in higher organisms is greatly aided by the existence of fossil remnants of common ancestors and by the multitude of morphologic features that can be studied. Bacteria, on the other hand, have not been preserved as recognizable fossils and exhibit relatively few morphologic properties for study. Evolutionary trends are thus difficult to determine or even to guess at, and a valid phylogenic classification of bacteria is a long way from being realized.

Computer Taxonomy of Bacteria

Taxonomy by computer has been developed for groups of bacteria in which a large number of strains exist that can be described in terms of 100 or more clear-cut taxonomic properties (eg, presence or absence of certain enzymes, presence or absence of certain pigments, presence or absence of certain morphologic structures). The computer compares the data and prints out a list of the strains in such an order that each strain is followed in the list by the strain with which it shares the most characteristics. When this is done, the list often reveals several broad subgroups of strains, each subgroup characterized by a large number of shared common characteristics. The median strain within each subgroup can then be arbitrarily considered as a type species.

Bergey's Manual of Systematic Bacteriology

There is no universally accepted natural classification of bacteria, since there is no mechanism for the evolution of discrete bacterial species and we can discern only broad outlines of bacterial evolution. A few groups, such as the photosynthetic bacteria, have been thoroughly classified by studies with enrichment cultures, but we do not know how such major groups are related to each other. The few evolutionary lines that are discernible will be presented later in this chapter.

In spite of these objections, however, an attempt at a phylogenic classification of bacteria has been published in the USA as *Bergey's Manual of Systematic Bacteriology.** First published in 1923, it has now reached its ninth edition. The sixth edition, in 1948, grouped the bacteria in 6 orders containing 36 families. The seventh edition, in 1957, rearranged the genera into 10 orders and 47 families. The eighth edition, in 1974, grouped the bacteria into 19 "parts" (eg, spirochetes, spiral and curved bacteria, gram-negative aerobic rods and cocci), each of which contained numerous genera. In some parts, the genera were grouped into families and orders; in others, they were not. The ninth edition (1984) introduces an entirely new taxonomic scheme.

In view of the divergent views that exist regarding bacterial classification, it is probable that the *Manual* will undergo further major changes with each edition. We will therefore not follow Bergey's classification in this chapter but instead will describe the major groups of bacteria, using common names. We will also refer to the medically important genera, about which there is good agreement among bacteriologists.

Bergey's Manual does serve several useful purposes, however, if we ignore its attempt to represent a phylogeny. First, it represents an exhaustive compilation of names and descriptions; second, the latest edition includes a completely practical although artificial key to the genera, as an aid to identification of newly isolated types. The *Manual* has a companion volume, called *Index Bergeyana,* containing the literature index, the host and habitat index, and descriptions of organisms that the editors consider inadequately described or whose taxonomic positions are uncertain.

In 1980, the International Committee on Systematic Bacteriology published an approved list of bacterial names.[†] This list of about 2500 species replaces a former list that had grown to over 30,000; since January 1, 1980, only the new list of names has been considered valid, and the reinstatement of discarded names, the addition of new ones, or any other changes require publication in *International Journal of Systematic Bacteriology.*

An informal classification of the eubacteria is presented in the following pages and in Table 3–1.

DESCRIPTIONS OF THE PRINCIPAL GROUPS OF BACTERIA

As discussed in Chapter 1, there are 2 major assemblages of prokaryotes: the archaebacteria and the eu-

*Krieg NR (editor): *Bergey's Manual of Systematic Bacteriology,* 9th ed. Williams & Wilkins, 1984. The ninth edition is being published in 4 volumes, starting with Volume 1 in 1984. An abridged version of the eighth edition is available: Holt JG (editor): *The Shorter Bergey's Manual of Determinative Bacteriology.* Williams & Wilkins, 1977.
†Skerman VBD, McGowan V, Sneath PHA (editors): Approved lists of bacterial names. *Int J Systematic Bacteriol* 1980;**30**:225.

Table 3–1. Key to the principal groups of eubacteria (listing the genera that include species pathogenic for humans).

	Genera of Medical Importance
I. Flexible cells, motility conferred by gliding mechanism (gliding bacteria)	
II. Flexible cells, motility conferred by endoflagella (spirochetes)	*Treponema*
	Borrelia
	Leptospira
III. Rigid cells, immotile or motility conferred by flagella	
A. Mycelial (actinomycetes)	*Mycobacterium*
	Actinomyces
	Nocardia
	Streptomyces
B. Simple unicellular	
1. Obligate intracellular parasites	*Rickettsia*
	Coxiella
	Chlamydia
2. Free-living	
a. Gram-positive	
(1) Cocci	*Streptococcus*
	Staphylococcus
(2) Nonsporulating rods	*Corynebacterium*
	Listeria
	Erysipelothrix
(3) Sporulating rods	
Obligate aerobes	*Bacillus*
Obligate anaerobes	*Clostridium*
b. Gram-negative	
(1) Cocci	*Neisseria*
(2) Nonenteric rods	
Spiral forms	*Spirillum*
Straight rods	*Pasteurella*
	Brucella
	Yersinia
	Francisella
	Haemophilus
	Bordetella
	Legionella
(3) Enteric rods	
Facultative anaerobes	*Escherichia* (and related coliform bacteria)
	Salmonella
	Shigella
	Klebsiella
	Proteus
	Vibrio
Obligate aerobes	*Pseudomonas*
Obligate anaerobes	*Bacteroides*
	Fusobacterium
IV. Lacking cells walls (mycoplasmas)	*Mycoplasma*

bacteria. A key to the principal groups of eubacteria is presented in Table 3–1. Four major groups can be recognized on the basis of mechanism of movement and character of cell wall: gliding bacteria, spirochetes, rigid bacteria, and mycoplasmas.

Gliding Bacteria

This heterogeneous group of bacteria, which includes the cyanobacteria as well as nonphotosynthetic forms, have in common a motility mechanism called gliding. Gliding requires contact with a solid substrate; in unicellular forms, it is accompanied by rapid flexing of the cells. The mechanism of gliding differs in the different subgroups. In one group (the genus *Myxococcus*), gliding appears to be caused by localized excretion of a surfactant at the posterior end of the cell, producing asymmetric surface tension forces that propel the cell forward. In other groups, experiments demonstrating rotation and translocation of attached latex beads suggest the existence of subsurface organelles analogous to flagellar motors (see Chapter 2).

There are 3 main assemblages within the nonphotosynthetic gliding bacteria: unicellular forms called **myxobacteria,** characterized by their ability to aggregate into elaborate fruiting structures (Fig 3–1); **cytophagas,** nonfruiting unicellular forms differing markedly from the myxobacteria in the guanine-plus-cytosine content of their DNA; and **filamentous gliding bacteria,** including 2 sulfur-oxidizing genera *(Beggiatoa* and *Thiothrix)* as well as several heterotrophs (eg, *Saprospira, Vitreoscilla,* and *Leucothrix).* None of these groups includes forms that are pathogenic for humans.

Spirochetes

The spirochetes are flexible helical rods. They possess an axial filament, formed from 2 tufts of polar flagella lying between the cell membrane and cell wall (Fig 3–2); it can be freed by enzymatic digestion of the outer envelope (Fig 3–3). Rotation of the endoflagella produces a gyration of the anterior end of the cell, causing a backward-moving spiral wave that propels the cell through the medium. Three genera contain important pathogens for humans: *Treponema, Borrelia,* and *Leptospira* (see Chapter 27).

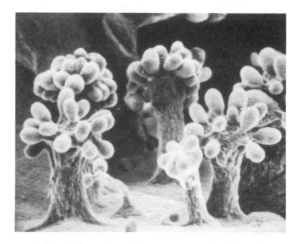

Figure 3–1. Scanning electron micrograph of fruiting bodies of the myxobacterium *Chondromyces crocatus,* prepared by J Pangborn and P Grilione. (From Stanier RY, Adelberg EA, Ingraham JL: *The Microbial World,* 4th ed. Copyright © 1976. By permission of Prentice-Hall, Inc., Englewood Cliffs, NJ.)

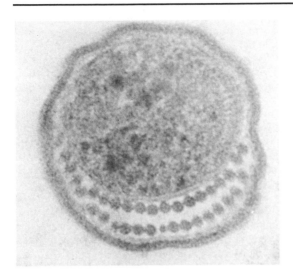

Figure 3–2. Cross section of a large spirochete, showing the location of the flagella between the cell membrane and the cell wall (258,000 ×). (Reproduced, with permission, from Listgarten MA, Socransky SS: Electron microscopy of axial fibrils, outer envelope and cell division of certain oval spirochetes. *J Bacteriol* 1964;**88**:1087.)

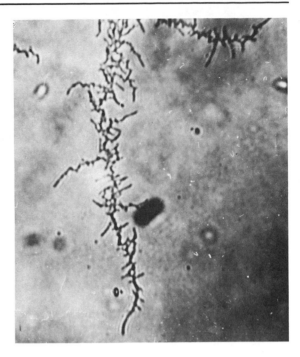

Figure 3–4. The surface growth on agar of *Mycobacterium fortuitum* (600 ×). Photomicrograph by R Gordon and H Lechevalier. (From Stanier RY, Doudoroff M, Adelberg EA: *The Microbial World,* 3rd ed. Copyright © 1970. By permission of Prentice-Hall, Inc., Englewood Cliffs, NJ.)

Rigid Bacteria

This group includes stalked, budding, and mycelial organisms as well as simple unicellular forms. Since there are no pathogens among the stalked and budding forms, they will not be considered further here.

A. Mycelial Forms (Actinomycetes): The mycelial (branching filamentous) growth of these grampositive organisms confers on them a superficial resemblance to the fungi, strengthened by the presence—in higher forms—of external asexual spores, or conidia. The resemblance ends there, however. The actinomycetes are prokaryotic organisms, whereas the fungi are eukaryotic; in the lower actinomycetes (eg, mycobacteria; Fig 3–4), the mycelium breaks up into typical unicellular bacteria. In one group, the *Actino-*

planes, sporangia are formed that rupture to release flagellated bacilli. The bacilli ultimately lose their flagella and initiate new mycelial growth.

1. Mycobacteria—Members of the genus *Mycobacterium,* which includes the agent of tuberculosis, are acid-fast organisms: they are relatively impermeable to dyes, but once stained they resist decolorization with acidified organic solvents. Their acid-fastness, along with their tendency to form a pellicle at the surface of aqueous media, is due to their high content

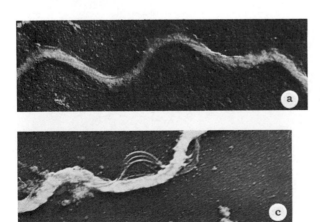

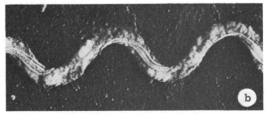

Figure 3–3. *Treponema pallidum.* Electron micrographs showing axial filament. *(a)* Without digestion. *(b)* After 20 minutes of tryptic digestion. *(c)* After 10 minutes of peptic digestion. (Courtesy of Swain RHA: *J Pathol Bacteriol* 1955;**69**:117.)

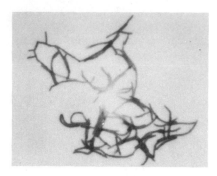

Figure 3–5. Early growth, a species of *Nocardia* (490 ×). (Courtesy of Ordal EJ: *The Biology of Bacteria*, 3rd ed. Heath, 1948.)

of lipids: lipids may account for up to 40% of the dry weight of the cell and up to 60% of the dry weight of the cell wall. They include true waxes along with glycolipids. The only other bacteria containing lipids of these types are corynebacteria and certain nocardiae, which also tend to be acid-fast. The mycobacteria are characterized further in Chapter 26.

2. Nocardia and Actinomyces–These 2 genera form much more advanced mycelia than do the mycobacteria, but they too tend to break up in older cultures to form irregularly shaped cells. A typical young mycelium of *Nocardia* is shown in Fig 3–5.

Actinomyces species are typically anaerobes, but some are facultative anaerobes, tolerating oxygen and capable of growth in air; *Nocardia* species are aerobes, and many are acid-fast. Both groups include pathogens for humans.

3. Higher actinomycetes–Several genera (eg, *Streptomyces, Micromonospora*) remain fully mycelial, reproducing by externally borne asexual spores, or conidia (Fig 3–6). Although their normal habitat is the soil, some *Streptomyces* species may contaminate wounds or scratches and initiate abscesses similar to those caused by nocardiae.

The higher actinomycetes, notably *Streptomyces*, are medically significant principally for their production of a wide array of antibiotics that act against bacteria (see Chapter 10); they possess special mechanisms to protect themselves against the antibiotics they liberate. In *Streptomyces azureus*, for example, which produces the ribosome-binding antibiotic thiostrepton, binding to its own ribosomes is prevented by the methylation of a single adenosine residue in the 23S ribosomal RNA.

B. Unicellular Forms: These bacteria include spheres (cocci), straight rods (bacilli), and helical forms (spirilla), as illustrated in Fig 3–7.

1. Obligate intracellular parasites–Two groups —the rickettsiae (genera *Rickettsia* and *Coxiella*) and the smaller chlamydiae (genus *Chlamydia*)—are obligate intracellular parasites and include pathogens for humans. They are gram-negative. The basis of their obligate parasitism is unknown, although they may depend on the host for energy-rich compounds and coenzymes. Their membranes are the site of a proton ATPase, capable of generating a proton motive force, and an ADP-ATP exchange system that equilibrates the parasite's ADP/ATP ratio with that of its host. These organisms are described more fully in Chapters 28 and 29.

2. Free-living forms–The majority of the bacteria pathogenic for humans fall into this group. The medically important genera are grouped in Table 3–1 according to their Gram-staining properties, their morphology, and (in the case of the gram-negative rods) whether or not they normally inhabit the intestinal tract of humans and other mammals. They are discussed in detail in Chapters 14–24 and Chapter 26.

Mycoplasmas

The mycoplasmas (Fig 3–8) are highly pleomorphic, wall-less bacteria. They resemble the L forms

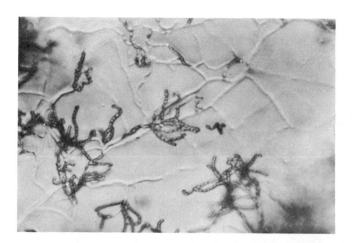
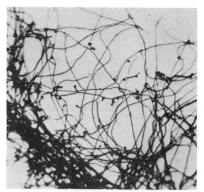

Figure 3–6. *Streptomycetaceae.* **Left:** *Streptomyces,* showing chains of aerial conidia (780 ×). **Right:** *Micromonospora,* showing single conidia on short lateral branches. (From Stanier RY, Doudoroff M, Adelberg EA: *The Microbial World,* 2nd ed. Copyright © 1963. By permission of Prentice-Hall, Inc., Englewood Cliffs, NJ.)

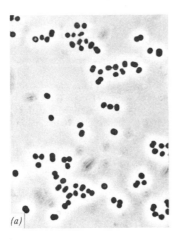
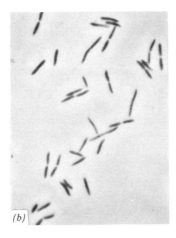
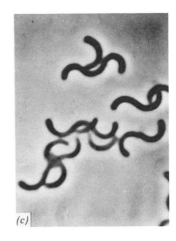

Figure 3–7. The cell shapes that occur among unicellular true bacteria. *(a)* Coccus. *(b)* Rod. *(c)* Spiral. (Phase contrast, 1500 ×.) (From Stanier RY, Doudoroff M, Adelberg EA: *The Microbial World,* 3rd ed. Copyright © 1970. By permission of Prentice-Hall, Inc., Englewood Cliffs, NJ.)

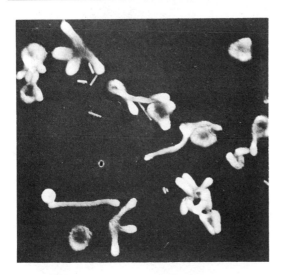

Figure 3–8. Electron micrograph of cells of a member of the *Mycoplasma* group, the agent of bronchopneumonia in the rat (1960 ×). (Reproduced, with permission, from Klieneberger-Nobel E, Cuckow FW: A study of organisms of the pleuropneumonia group by electron microscopy. *J Gen Microbiol* 1955;**12**:99.)

that are produced by the removal of the cell wall of eubacteria; unlike L forms, however, mycoplasmas never revert to the walled state, and there are no antigenic relationships between mycoplasmas and eubacterial L forms.

Six genera have been designated as mycoplasmas, on the basis of their free-living, wall-less state: *Mycoplasma, Ureaplasma, Acholeplasma, Spiroplasma, Thermoplasma,* and *Anaeroplasma. Mycoplasma* and *Ureaplasma* contain animal pathogens; *Spiroplasma* contains plant and insect pathogens. A phylogenetic tree has been constructed based on similarities in ribosomal and transfer RNAs, energy production pathways, and lipid composition. *Mycoplasma, Ureaplasma, Acholeplasma,* and *Spiroplasma* are clustered on a single branch of the tree, which also includes several clostridia; *Thermoplasma,* on the other hand, belongs to the archaebacteria (see Chapter 1). The wall-less state thus arose at least twice during evolution: once within the archaebacteria, and once within the gram-positive eubacteria.

Human pathogens of the genus *Mycoplasma* are described in Chapter 25.

REFERENCES

Books

Alexander M: *Microbial Ecology.* Wiley, 1971.

Barile MF et al (editors): *The Mycoplasmas.* Vol 1: *Cell Biology;* Vol 2: *Human and Animal Mycoplasmas.* Vol 3: *Plant and Insect Mycoplasmas.* Academic Press, 1979.

Goodfellow M, Board RG (editors): *Microbiological Classification and Identification.* Academic Press, l980.

Goodfellow M, Modarski M,Williams ST (editors): *The Biology of the Actinomycetes.* Academic Press, 1984.

Holt JG (editor): *The Shorter Bergey's Manual of Determinative Bacteriology.* Williams & Wilkins, l977.

Krieg NR (editor): *Bergey's Manual of Systematic Bacteriology,* 9th ed. Vol 1. Williams & Wilkins, 1984.

Ratledge C, Stanford J (editors): *The Biology of the Mycobacteria.* Vol l: *Physiology, Identification and Classification.* Academic Press, 1983.

Rosenberg E (editor): *Myxobacteria: Development and Cell Interactions.* Springer-Verlag, 1984.

Sneath PHA, Sokal RR: *Numerical Taxonomy: The Principles and Practice of Numerical Classification.* Freeman, l973.

Stanier RY, Adelberg EA, Ingraham JL: *The Microbial World,* 4th ed. Prentice-Hall, l976.

Starr MP et al (editors): *The Prokaryotes: A Handbook on Habitats, Isolation, and Identification of Bacteria.* Springer-Verlag, l981.

Articles & Reviews

Burchard RP: Gliding motility of prokaryotes: Ultrastructure, physiology and genetics. *Annu Rev Microbiol* 1981; **35:**497.

Harwood CS, Canale-Parola E: The ecology of spirochetes. *Annu Rev Microbiol* 1984;**38:**161.

Holt SC: Anatomy and chemistry of spirochetes. *Microbiol Rev* 1978;**42:**114.

Jones D, Sneath PHA: Genetic transfer and bacterial taxonomy. *Bacteriol Rev* 1970;**34:**40.

Kaiser D et al: Myxobacteria: Cell interactions, genetics, and development. *Annu Rev Microbiol* 1979;**33:**595.

Mandel M: New approaches to bacterial taxonomy: Perspectives and prospects. *Annu Rev Microbiol* 1969;**23:**239.

Maniloff J: Evolution of wall-less prokaryotes. *Annu Rev Microbiol* 1983;**37:**477.

Ormsbee RA: Rickettsiae (as organisms). *Annu Rev Microbiol* 1969;**23:**275.

Razin S: The mycoplasmas. *Microbiol Rev* 1978;**42:**414.

Sanderson KE: Genetic relatedness in the family Enterobacteriaceae. *Annu Rev Microbiol* 1976;**30:**327.

Schachter J, Caldwell HD: Chlamydiae. *Annu Rev Microbiol* 1980;**34:**285.

Schleifer KH, Stackebrandt E: Molecular systematics of prokaryotes. *Annu Rev Microbiol* 1983;**37:**143.

Skerman VBD, McGowan V, Sneath PHA (editors): Approved lists of bacterial names. *Int J Systematic Bacteriol* 1980;**30:**225.

Whitcomb RF: The genus *Spiroplasma*. *Annu Rev Microbiol* 1980;**34:**677.

Woese CR, Magrum LJ, Fox GE: Archaebacteria. *J Mol Evol* 1978;**11:**245.

Woese CR et al: Phylogenetic analysis of the mycoplasmas. *Proc Natl Acad Sci USA* 1980;**77:**494.

Microbial Genetics

4

THE PHYSICAL BASIS OF HEREDITY

In formulating a general concept of mechanisms of inheritance, 2 basic biologic phenomena must be accounted for: **heredity,** or stability of type (eg, the progeny formed by the division of a unicellular organism are generally identical with the parent cell); and the rare occurrence of **heritable variations.** Genetic and cytologic analyses of plant, animal, and microbial cells have established that the physical basis for both of these phenomena is the **gene** (the genetic determinant controlling the properties of organisms). The genes are located along the threadlike **chromosomes** in the cell nucleus. The chromosomes undergo duplication (replication) prior to cell division; when the cell divides, each daughter cell receives an identical set of chromosomes and therefore an identical set of genes. The cell's genes collectively constitute its **genome,** or **genotype;** the structural and physiologic properties of the cell collectively constitute its **phenotype.**

Replication is usually an exact process, which accounts for heredity; any given gene, however, has a low probability of **mutation,** and mutation accounts for variation. Mutated genes are usually stable and are replicated in the new form in subsequent generations. A gene mutation thus causes a heritable change in one or more phenotypic properties of the organism.

In eukaryotic and prokaryotic cells (see Chapter 1), the chemical substance of the chromosome which is responsible for both gene replication and gene function is deoxyribonucleic acid (DNA). In viruses, it can be either DNA or RNA (ribonucleic acid). One of the basic problems of genetics is thus to explain gene replication, mutation, and function in terms of nucleic acid structure. In the following sections this problem will be discussed with particular reference to the prokaryotic chromosome of the bacterium *Escherichia coli*. In general, however, the material to be presented applies equally to the chromosomes of eukaryotes: protozoa, fungi, slime molds, and algae.

The prokaryotic genome may include plasmids, prophages, and transposable elements as well as the chromosome. The eukaryotic genome includes nuclear chromosomes, mitochondrial DNA, and—in photosynthetic cells—chloroplast DNA. It may also include plasmid DNA and transposable elements.

THE PROKARYOTIC CHROMOSOME

Chromosome Structure

The electron micrograph in Fig 2–5 shows the bacterial nucleus to be a packed mass of DNA fibers. When bacterial DNA is extracted and purified by ordinary chemical methods, the preparation obtained has an average molecular weight of about 5×10^6. In the intact cell, however, the bacterial nucleus consists of a single continuous DNA molecule, or chromosome, with a molecular weight of 2 to 3×10^9, which is sheared into several hundred fragments by the extraction procedure. Using gentler methods, Cairns was able to extract the unbroken chromosome of *E coli* (Fig 4–1). Cairns's pictures showed the bacterial chromosome to be a continuous DNA structure approximately 1 mm long. The structure of the DNA molecule is now well known: it consists of a double helix made up of 2 complementary polynucleotide strands in each of which purine and pyrimidine bases are arranged along a backbone made of alternating deoxyribose and phosphate groups (Fig 4–2). The 2 strands are held together by hydrogen bonds between neighboring bases; the stereochemistry is such that hydrogen bonds can be formed only between adenine and thymine (A-T pair) and between guanine and cytosine (G-C pair) (Fig 4–3). Thus, a sequence of bases along one strand such as G-C-C-A-C-T-C-A must be matched on the opposite strand by the complementary sequence of C-G-G-T-G-A-G-T.

The chromosome of *E coli*, with a molecular weight of 2.5×10^9, contains about 4×10^6 base-pairs. It has been shown both by genetic analysis and by autoradiography to be a circular structure. Over 1000 genetic loci (genes) have been mapped on the chromosome of *E coli* strain K12 by means of interrupted conjugation and phage-mediated co-transduction (see below).

Chromosome Replication

In viruses, prokaryotic cells, and eukaryotic cells, DNA has been shown to replicate according to a semiconservative mechanism. The complementary strands separate, each then acting as a **template** on which is assembled a complementary strand by the enzymatic polymerization of nucleotide subunits. The sequence of bases in the new strand is rigidly dictated by the hydrogen bonding possibilities described above; ie, wherever the template carries adenine the new strand

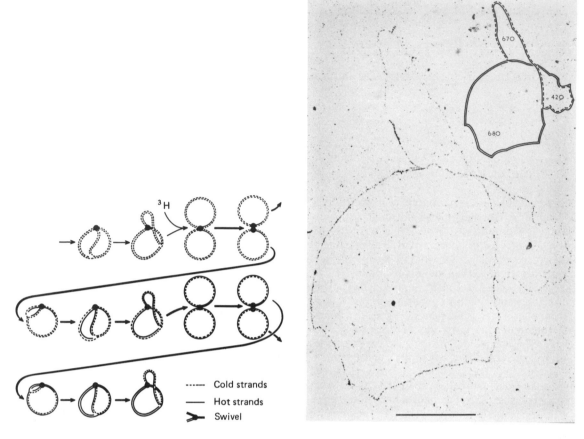

Figure 4–1. Replication of the circular chromosome of *E coli*. *Left:* Diagram showing that introduction of radioactive tritium (³H) toward the end of a replication cycle would lead, 2 cycles later, to a chromosome labeled as found experimentally. Replication begins at the "swivel" and proceeds counterclockwise along the 2 complementary strands of the DNA double helix. *Right:* Autoradiograph of a chromosome extracted from an Hfr cell of *E coli* 2 generations after addition of ³H. Grain counts per unit length in the regions indicated by solid lines are double those in the regions indicated by dashed lines. The numbers in the insert are the lengths (in micrometers) between the 2 forks. (Courtesy of Cairns J: *Cold Spring Harbor Symp Quant Biol* 1963;**28**:43.)

will acquire a thymine, etc. Replication thus leads to the formation of 2 new double helices, each identical with the original double helix. At 37 °C, replication proceeds at a rate of 750 base-pairs per second per replication fork.

Three classes of proteins are required for the correct replication of the bacterial chromosome: **initiation proteins** (including gyrase and RNA polymerase), which direct initiation to the replication origin (*oriC*) and assemble the replication complex; **specificity proteins** (including topoisomerase I and RNase H), which suppress initiation at other sites; and **replication proteins** (including primase and DNA polymerase III holoenzyme), which prime and elongate the polynucleotide chains. Thirteen or more proteins are required altogether.

The bacterial chromosome replicates sequentially along the entire structure, starting at the replication origin, a specific 245-base-pair sequence. According to a model proposed by Jacob and Brenner, the replication origin is attached to a mesosomal site on the cell

membrane; when replication is initiated, the chromosome moves past the membrane attachment site, unwinding and replicating as it goes (Fig 4–4). Separation of the 2 daughter chromosomes is accomplished by localized membrane synthesis; later, a transverse cell wall will form between the DNA attachment sites.

The Jacob-Brenner model is yet to be confirmed experimentally. There is good evidence for the attachment of the replication origin to the cell envelope, including the finding that the *oriC* DNA fragment binds specifically to purified outer membrane preparations; this binding is dependent on the presence of 2 specific outer membrane proteins. Nevertheless, evidence for continuing attachment of the replicating fork (as represented in Fig 4–4) is still inconclusive.

In Figs 4–1 and 4–4, replication is shown to proceed in one direction along the duplex molecule of DNA. Such unidirectional replication has indeed been verified for some circular DNA viruses and is consistent with observations of DNA transfer between conjugating bacteria (Fig 4–14). Vegetative **chromosomal**

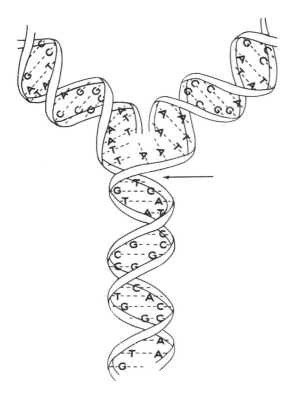

Figure 4–2. Structure and replication of DNA according to the Watson and Crick model. The vertical double strand is unwinding at the point indicated by the arrow, and the 2 arms have acted as templates for the synthesis of complementary strands. Synthesis is proceeding downward along the vertical double strand.

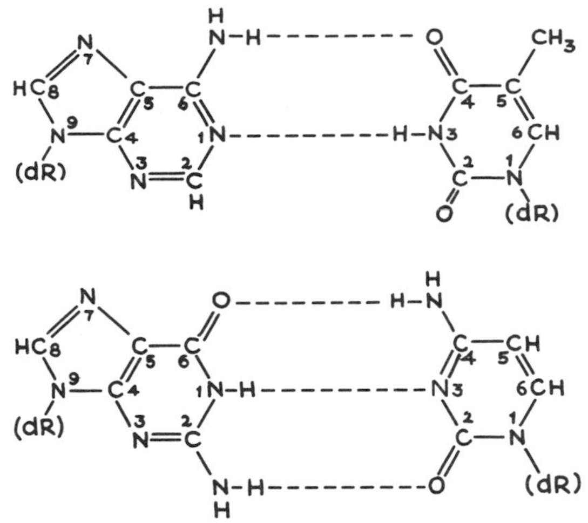

Figure 4–3. Normal base-pairing in DNA. Hydrogen bonds are indicated by dotted lines. (dR = deoxyribose of the sugar-phosphate backbone of DNA.) *Top:* Adenine-thymine pair. *Bottom:* Guanine-cytosine pair.

replication, however, is normally bidirectional: 2 replicating forks may move away simultaneously from the replicator site, meeting approximately halfway around the chromosome at a specific replication terminus. This observation may be reconciled with Fig 4–1 by the finding that the cell is capable of both types of replication (unidirectional and bidirectional), depending on the growth conditions.

In a bacterial cell, several different genetic (DNA) structures may be present and replicating independently at the same time, eg, chromosome, sex factor, and bacteriophage genomes. The term **replicon** has been coined to describe an independent unit of replication.

Chromosome Function

The chromosome, consisting of about 3.8×10^6 nucleotide pairs, is functionally subdivided into segments, each of which determines the amino acid sequence and hence the structure of a discrete protein. These proteins, as enzymes and as components of membranes and other cell structures, determine all the properties of the organism. A segment of chromosomal DNA that determines the structure of a discrete **protein** is called a **gene.** The mechanism by which the sequence of nucleotides in a gene determines the sequence of amino acids in a protein is as follows:

(1) RNA polymerase forms a single polyribonucleotide strand, called "messenger RNA" (mRNA), using DNA as a template; this process is called **transcription.** The mRNA has a nucleotide sequence complementary to one of the strands in the DNA double helix.

(2) Amino acids are enzymatically activated and transferred to specific adapter molecules of RNA, called "transfer RNA" (tRNA). Each adapter molecule has at one end a triplet of bases complementary to a triplet of bases on mRNA, and at the other end its specific amino acid. The triplet of bases on mRNA is called the **codon** for that amino acid.

(3) mRNA and tRNA come together on the surface of the ribosome. As each tRNA finds its complementary nucleotide triplet on mRNA, the amino acid that it carries is put into peptide linkage with the amino acid of the preceding (neighboring) tRNA molecule. The ribosome moves along the mRNA, the polypeptide growing sequentially until the entire mRNA molecule has been translated into a corresponding sequence of amino acids. This process, called **translation,** is diagrammed in Fig 4–5.

Thus, the nucleotide sequence of the DNA gene represents a code that determines, through the mediation of mRNA, the structure of a specific protein. In many cases such proteins act as subunits that polymerize to form active enzymes; many high-molecular-weight enzymes are now known to be made up of subunits having molecular weights in the range of 10^4 to 10^5. The triplet code requires that a gene governing the formation of a protein of molecular weight 40,000 should contain on the order of 1000 nucleotide pairs; the chromosome of *E coli* thus has sufficient DNA for about 4000 such genes.

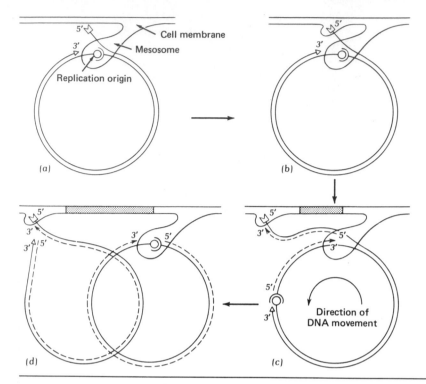

Figure 4–4. Replication of the bacterial chromosome, according to the model of Jacob and Brenner. *(a)* The chromosome is attached to a mesosome at the replication origin site, which serves as a swivel. One of the strands is broken. *(b)* The 5' end of the broken strand attaches to a new site in the membrane. *(c)* The chromosome rotates counterclockwise past the mesosomal attachment site, at which is fixed the replicating enzyme system. Newly synthesized strands are shown as dashed lines. The attachment sites are separated by localized membrane synthesis (shown by shaded area). *(d)* The cycle of replication has been completed. The final step will be the joining of the free ends of one strand of the new chromosome (solid line). (From Stanier RY, Doudoroff M, Adelberg EA: *The Microbial World*, 3rd ed. Copyright © 1970. By permission of Prentice-Hall, Inc., Englewood Cliffs, NJ.)

The prokaryotic genome may also include plasmid and prophage DNA, as described below.

THE EUKARYOTIC GENOME

Chromosome Structure

In contrast to that of the bacterial genome, the DNA of the eukaryotic nucleus is divided among a set of distinct chromosomes. Each chromosome consists of a single continuous, linear DNA molecule, associated tightly with a set of basic proteins called histones and with varying degrees of tightness to a large number of nonhistone proteins. As isolated from the cell, this complex of DNA and proteins is called **chromatin.**

Studies with isolated chromatin show that the DNA molecule is wrapped around histone complexes to form beaded structures called **nucleosomes.** This primary structure is then subject to several further orders of coiling to produce the chromosome as it exists in interphase; at mitosis, a further coiling occurs to bring about the condensation of the chromosomes into their visible, rodlike shapes.

The organization of the DNA in eukaryotic chromosomes differs from that in the prokaryotic chromosome in at least 3 significant ways. First, the genes governing sets of closely related functions appear not to be clustered to form operons, as they are in bacteria; coordinate control of their expression is therefore based on a different mechanism. Second, the genes of eukaryotic organisms are in many cases not continuous base sequences, as they are in prokaryotes; instead, a given gene may be present as a set of DNA segments that are interrupted by intervening sequences, or "introns." The entire sequence is transcribed, but the RNA molecule that is originally formed is processed by enzymes that excise the introns and splice together the coding segments to form the final mRNA molecule. Third, eukaryotic chromosomes contain a high proportion of repetitious DNA: sequences that are repeated in the genome anywhere from 100 times to 100,000 times or more.

Mitosis

Eukaryotic cells undergo a regular cycle of events associated with the division process. Periods of active DNA replication—the S (for "synthesis") phase—alternate with periods of mitosis (M phase), during which the 2 products of chromosomal replication, called chromatids, are segregated into the 2 daughter cells produced by cell division.

At the completion of the S phase, each chromosome is present as a pair of sister chromatids, joined at a specific site called the centromere. At mitosis, a mitotic spindle is formed, and the chromosomes become arranged on the spindle in a flat plane called the metaphase plate. Spindle fibers attach to the chromatids at the centromeres, the chromatids separate, and the 2 chromatids of each chromosome are moved to opposite poles of the cell by the spindle fibers. Cell division segregates the 2 groups of chromatids into the 2 daughter cells; the cycle is completed when they traverse the next S phase. This process ensures that each daughter cell receives a complete set of chromosomes, identical to that of every other mitotic cell.

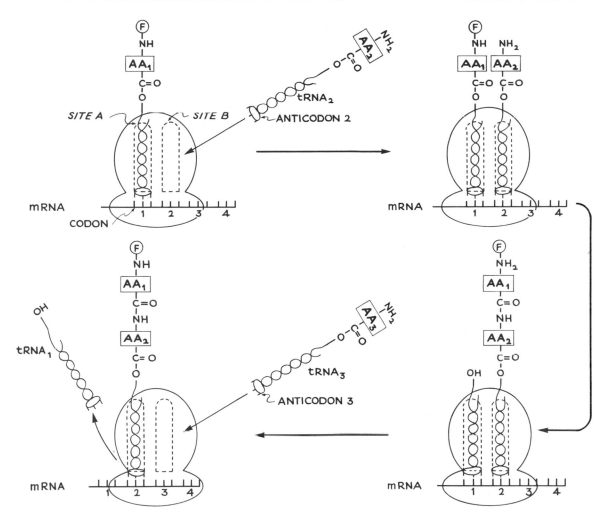

Figure 4–5. Four stages in the lengthening of a polypeptide chain on the surface of a 70S ribosome. *Top left:* A tRNA molecule bearing the anticodon complementary to codon 1 at one end and AA₁ at the other, binds to site A. AA₁ is attached to the tRNA through its carboxyl group; its amino nitrogen bears a formyl group (F). *Top right:* A tRNA molecule bearing AA₂ binds to site B; its anticodon is complementary to codon 2. *Bottom right:* An enzyme complex catalyzes the transfer of AA₁ to the amino group of AA₂, forming a peptide bond. (Note that transfer in the opposite direction is blocked by the prior formylation of the amino group of AA₁.) *Bottom left:* The ribosome moves to the right, so that sites A and B are now opposite codons 2 and 3; in the process, tRNA₁ is displaced and tRNA₂ moves to site A. Site B is again vacant and is ready to accept tRNA₃ bearing AA₃. (When the polypeptide is completed and released, the formyl group is enzymatically removed.) (Redrawn and reproduced by permission of Stanier RY, Doudoroff M, Adelberg EA: *The Microbial World,* 3rd ed. Copyright © 1970. Prentice-Hall, Inc., Englewood Cliffs, NJ.)

Organellar DNA

The early recognized phenomenon of maternal inheritance revealed the existence of genetic determinants in the cytoplasm of eukaryotic cells, and these cytoplasmic determinants were ultimately found to reside in DNA molecules within cytoplasmic organelles: the mitochondria and the chloroplasts of photosynthetic cells.

The mitochondria, for example, contain small circular DNA molecules that code for certain mitochondrial components, including a set of transfer RNAs, ribosomal RNAs, and a number of membrane proteins. Although most mitochondrial proteins are coded by nuclear genes, many mutations that affect mitochondrial function (and thus the phenotype of the cell) can occur in the mitochondrial DNA. In particular, mutations causing resistance of the cell to some of the drugs that inhibit mitochondrial protein synthesis (such as chloramphenicol) have been shown to occur in the mitochondrial DNA.

The mitochondria of eukaryotes share many properties with prokaryotic cells, including membrane-associated electron transport systems, small circular DNA genomes, and ribosomal systems with characteristic structures and patterns of antibiotic sensitivity. These similarities have led to the popular theory of organellar evolution from prokaryotic symbionts of proto-eukaryotic cells. Whether this theory is correct or not, the eukaryotic cell must be viewed as a complex system with at least 2 independent genomes: (1) the set of chromosomes in the nucleus, and (2) the DNA molecules of the cytoplasmic organelles; mutations occurring in either genome can change the phenotype of the cell.

Plasmid DNA

Plasmids are small, circular nucleic acid elements that are replicated autonomously in the host cell; they code for functions that are normally dispensable to the host. Originally described in bacteria (see below), plasmids have since been discovered in yeast and other fungi and may turn out to be widespread in eukaryotic organisms.

The yeast plasmids include the "2 μm plasmid," a DNA plasmid without known gene products; it is widely used as a vector for cloning DNA in yeast (see below). Another yeast element that has been called a plasmid is unusual in that it consists of double-stranded RNA; called the "killer particle," it codes for a protein that kills sensitive cells by forming ion-permeable channels in the cell membrane. The classification of the yeast killer particle as a plasmid has been blurred by the discovery that it is part of a protein-encapsidated viruslike particle (VLP) within the cell. The VLPs contain RNA transcriptase and thus resemble the reoviruses of animal cells; no extracellular, infectious stage has ever been detected, however, in these or other fungal VLPs.

MUTATION

Mutation at the Molecular Level

Any change in the nucleotide sequence of a gene constitutes a mutation. The different forms of a gene produced by mutations are called **alleles.**

A. Types of Sequence Changes: The sequence of nucleotides in DNA can change in either of 2 ways: by the substitution of one base-pair for another as the result of a replication error; or by breakage of the sugar-phosphate backbone, with subsequent deletion or insertion of a DNA segment.

1. Base-pair substitution–The most frequent types are those in which the pyrimidine is replaced by a different pyrimidine and the purine by a different purine, eg, A-T replaced by G-C, or T-A by C-G. These are called **transitions.** In the less frequent type, a pyrimidine is replaced by a purine and vice versa; these are called **transversions.**

2. Insertions and deletions–Occasionally, during replication, a single base-pair or 2 adjacent base-pairs are inserted into or deleted from the DNA structure. This shifts the translation "reading frame" of the coded message from that point on, forming an entirely new set of triplets, or codons. For example, if a portion of the correct message reads —AGG/CTC/CAA/GCC/GAT/TGG—, deletion of the fourth base changes the message to —AGG/TCC/AAG/CCG/ATT/GG—. Such mutations are called **frame shift**

mutations; their effects on translation are discussed below. Much larger insertions and deletions may also occur, involving segments that span one or more entire genes.

B. Spontaneous Mutation:

1. Mechanisms–The most common spontaneous mutations represent replication errors: the template mechanism of replication described earlier may function imperfectly, so that—for example—a G is inserted opposite a T. Such mismatches occur frequently but are usually corrected by a $3' \rightarrow 5'$ exonuclease "proofreading" function of DNA polymerase that recognizes and excises mismatched base-pairs. Base-pair substitutions thus arise as a consequence of failure in template action of the DNA together with failure in the proofreading function of the polymerase.

Base-pair substitutions can also arise as a consequence of a tautomeric shift of electrons in a purine or pyrimidine ring. For example, thymine normally exists in the keto state, in which state it forms 2 hydrogen bonds with adenine. If, however, thymine exists in the rare enol state at the moment that it is acting as a template during replication, it will form 3 hydrogen bonds with guanine instead (Fig 4–6). The new strand will then carry a guanine in place of adenine and will form a G-C pair at the next round of replication, replacing the original A-T pair.

Frame shift mutations (small insertions or deletions) can also arise spontaneously; they are thought to arise as a result of a single-strand nicking of the DNA adjacent to a run of identical base-pairs. The nicked strand may be displaced, looping out a segment carrying one or 2 of the identical bases and leaving a gap which is then filled in by a DNA polymerase; the result is an insertion of one or 2 bases in that strand which is faithfully replicated at future generations. Alternatively, the nick may be widened to a gap by an exonuclease; the gap may then be closed by a displacement and looping out of the opposite strand, leading to a small deletion. Loopouts, with consequent frame shift mutations, can also occur when quasipalindromic DNA sequences re-anneal to form stems with mispaired regions (Fig 4–7).

Large deletions and insertions occur by yet other mechanisms, some of which are mediated by transposons (see below).

2. Mutator genes–A mutator gene is an allele of a normal gene which, by virtue of its altered function, causes a general increase in the spontaneous mutation rate over the entire genome. Three types of mutator genes have been identified: (1) Mutations in DNA polymerase genes, causing either a loss of fidelity of the polymerase or a decrease in $3' \rightarrow 5'$ exonuclease proofreading function. (2) Mutations causing large distortions in the relative pool sizes of the 4 nucleotide triphosphates as a result of alterations in their relative rates of biosynthesis. A large excess of one nucleotide triphosphate leads to an increased rate of substitution of that base for a correct base during replication. (3) Mutations causing a failure in **mismatch repair.** Endonucleases are present in the cell that recognize dis-

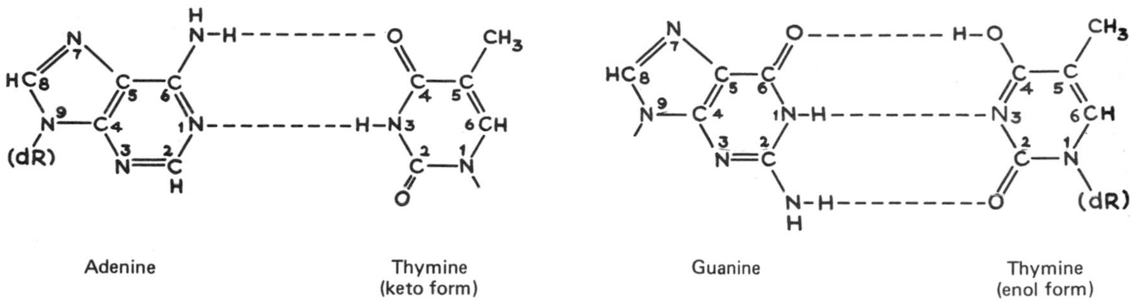

Figure 4–6. Base-pairing in DNA. *Left:* Thymine in its normal (keto) state forms 2 hydrogen bonds with adenine. *Right:* Thymine may exist in the enol state as the result of rare tautomeric shift of electrons. In this state, thymine forms 3 hydrogen bonds with guanine. If the tautomeric shift occurred during replication, guanine would be incorporated into DNA in place of adenine, and a G-C pair would ultimately replace an A-T pair in the nucleotide sequence. (dR = deoxyribose of the sugar-phosphate backbone of DNA.)

tortions in the double helix caused by mismatched base-pairs; they can distinguish between the template strand and the new strand, excising the mismatched base from the latter. The gap thus formed is filled in by a polymerase. Recognition of the new strand is based on the fact that DNA is **methylated:** a methylase adds a methyl group to an occasional purine ring shortly after the new strand has been synthesized. The brief lag in methylation, however, means that the new strand is relatively undermethylated, and it is this state that is recognized by the mismatch repair enzyme system. Mutator alleles include mutants defective in the endonuclease itself as well as mutants defective in methylase: the latter mutants' DNA lacks the methyl groups on which strand recognition depends, so that excision of the correct base (on the template strand) takes place as often as excision of the "wrong" base on the new strand.

C. Mutagenic Agents: Mutations are induced by a variety of physical and chemical agents, which directly or indirectly cause a general increase in the mutation rate.

1. Physical agents–Radiations with wavelengths absorbed by the cell are mutagenic, including visible light, ultraviolet light, and all ionizing radiations. Heat is also mutagenic.

2. Chemical agents–Chemical mutagens can be divided into 2 classes: those that act directly and those that require conversion by cellular enzymes to the active form.

The direct-acting mutagens include nitroso compounds, alkylating agents, base analogs, nitropyrenes, and most anticancer drugs such as methotrexate, bleomycin, and hydroxyurea. The compounds that require activation include polycyclic aromatic hydrocarbons such as benzpyrene and the aflatoxins.

D. Mechanisms of Induced Mutation:

1. Increased frequency of replication errors– A number of mutagens, including base analogs, alkylating agents, and deaminating agents such as nitrous acid, act by increasing the frequency of mismatches during replication.

2. Stabilization of loopouts–A number of muta-

genic compounds, such as acridines, are called stacking agents: They interact with the bases of the double helix so as to stabilize the looped-out single-stranded segments that are intermediates in the frame shift mutation process described above.

3. Error-prone repair–Most agents that damage DNA produce lesions which are recognized by enzymatic repair systems. In some cases, the lesions are removed and the resulting gaps are filled by error-free systems that use the undamaged strand as template. In other cases, however, an undamaged strand is not available. In such cases, the repair system produces a gap that is filled by an **error-prone** system. Ultraviolet light, for example, causes pyrimidine dimer formation on one strand; if the dimer is not removed by an error-free repair system in time, replication past the dimer may produce a duplex carrying a gap opposite a dimer, and gap-filling is accomplished by an error-prone system. Alternatively, the replication polymerase may itself insert a wrong base in the region of a lesion rather than skipping to produce a gap.

The enzymes of the error-prone repair systems are inducible. They are greatly increased in cells that have been treated with DNA-damaging agents.

E. Effects of Mutation on Translation:

1. Nonsense mutations–With 3 exceptions, transfer RNAs are present in the cell for each of the 64 possible nucleotide triplets, or "codons," in messenger RNA. The exceptions are UAG, UAA, and UGA; they are called "nonsense codons." When a ribosome reaches a nonsense codon in the translation process described above, polypeptide chain formation is terminated. One or more of the 3 nonsense codons function as natural chain terminators in the synthesis of proteins; if a nonsense codon is formed within a gene by mutation of a "sense" codon, only a partial polypeptide is produced. Such mutations are called nonsense mutations.

2. Suppressor mutations–A mutation that restores the function of a gene inactivated by a previous mutation is called a suppressor mutation. For example, the frame shift mutation described on p 42, in which a single base was deleted, can be suppressed by

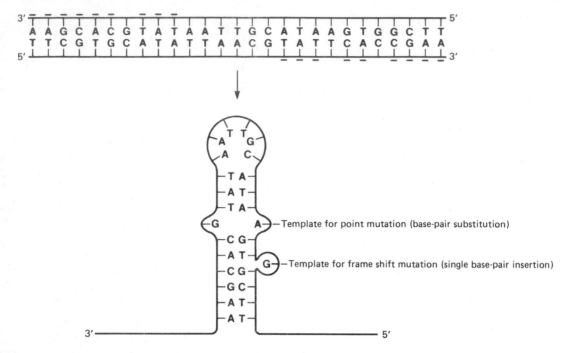

Figure 4–7. *Top:* a quasipalindromic sequence of DNA. (A palindrome reads the same in both directions. The underlined sequences are identical when the top strand is read from left to right and the bottom strand is read from right to left.) *Bottom:* The upper strand has separated and re-annealed to form a stem structure; the mismatches will act as templates for mutations at the next replication cycle. (After de Boer JG, Ripley LS: Demonstration of the production of frameshift and base-substitution mutations by quasipalindromic DNA sequences. *Proc Natl Acad Sci USA* 1984;81:5528.)

a single base insertion at a nearby site. In the above case, imagine that a second frame shift mutation causes insertion of a G between the seventh and eighth bases. The sequence now reads —AGG/TCC/AGA/GCC/GAT/TGG—. Note that the final sequence differs from the normal sequence only in the second and third codons; if these code for amino acids that are not critical to the functioning of the protein produced by this gene, normal activity will have been at least partially restored. In contrast, either frame shift mutation by itself produces an unending string of missense codons within the gene; by random chance, at least one new triplet will be a nonsense codon leading to chain termination.

Suppressor mutations can also occur at other places on the chromosome (**extragenic suppressors**). Some extragenic suppressor loci are genes that code for components of the translation system, such as tRNA; by mutation, they alter the component so as to compensate for the original coding error in the DNA. For example, one suppressor mutation has been shown to act by altering the anticodon in serine tRNA.

Mutation at the Cellular Level

Without DNA sequencing, a gene mutation can only be recognized if it brings about an observable phenotypic change; such changes may be described in terms of gross morphology or physiology, but in most cases it is possible to define the phenotypic change in terms of the loss or gain of a particular protein or its

function (eg, a specific enzyme or its activity). For convenience, we will discuss phenotypic change in terms of enzyme activity only.

A. Phenotypic Expression in Uninucleate Cells:

1. Gain mutations–When a mutation confers on the cell the ability to synthesize an active enzyme, there is no detectable lag between the time of mutation and the beginning of enzyme synthesis.

2. Loss mutations–Most cell proteins are stable. In *E coli,* for example, there is no protein turnover in actively growing cells, and a turnover of only about 5% per hour in resting cells. Thus, when a mutation causes the synthesis of a functional enzyme to stop, the cell remains enzymatically active. If the cell continues to grow, however, the amount of preexisting enzyme per cell is halved at each generation. After 7 generations, the progeny of the original mutant will each have less than 1% of the wildtype enzyme level, usually resulting in the mutant phenotype.

This **phenotypic lag** has certain practical consequences. For example, the sensitivity of bacteria to attack by viruses (bacteriophages, or "phages") depends upon the presence of specific receptor sites in the cell wall. The mutation to phage resistance reflects the loss of synthesis of phage receptor. If such mutations are induced, the phage resistance phenotype will not be detected until a sufficient number of generations has taken place to dilute out the original receptors. In other words, there is a **delay in phenotypic expression.**

B. Phenotypic Expression in Multinucleate Cells:

1. Gain mutations–Many microbial cells are multinucleate. *E coli,* for example, has an average of about 4 nuclei per cell during exponential growth. When a gain mutation occurs in a multinucleate cell, the mutant nucleus synthesizes the new active enzyme and phenotypic expression is immediate. A gain mutation is thus **dominant;** the active form ("allele") of the gene is expressed, and the inactive allele is not.

2. Loss mutations–When a loss mutation occurs in a multinucleate cell, only the mutant nucleus ceases to make active enzyme, whereas the other nuclei continue. The loss mutation is thus **recessive** and is not expressed in the original cell. After several generations, however, the mutant nucleus will have segregated into a separate cell (Fig 4–8). Phenotypic expression of a loss mutation must thus await both phenotypic lag and nuclear segregation.

Mutation at the Population Level
A. Mutant Frequency and Mutation Rate:
1. Relation between frequency and rate–The proportion of mutants in a cell population is the **mutant frequency.** Frequencies ranging from 1×10^{-5} to 1×10^{-10} are commonly observed when individual phenotypes are considered. The frequency of mutants in a given culture reflects 3 independent parameters: (1) The probability that a cell will mutate during a given interval, such as a generation. This is the **mutation rate.** (2) The distribution in time of mutational events over the growth period of the culture. For example, exceptionally early mutations will produce extremely large **clones** of mutant progeny. (A clone constitutes the total progeny of a single cell.) (3) The growth rates of the mutant cells relative to the parental type.

2. Measurement of mutation rate–The mutation rate can be related to average mutant frequencies by a complex equation that takes into account all of the above parameters. However, there are methods (such as the one described below) that permit a direct determination of the number of mutations which have occurred in a culture (as opposed to the number of mutant cells in the culture) and thus permit a simple estimation of the mutation rate.

The mutation rate is commonly expressed in units of "mutations per cell per generation"; ie, the probability that a mutation will occur during the event of a single cell doubling in size and dividing to become 2 cells. When one cell goes through 2 successive generations to become 4 cells, for example, 3 such "cell-doubling events" occur (Fig 4–8). In general terms, when N_0 cells increase to form N_1 cells, the number of doubling events is equal to $N_1 - N_0$. The mutation rate **(a)** is thus expressed by the simple formula

$$a = \frac{M}{N_1 - N_0}$$

where **M** $=$ the number of mutations occurring during the growth of N_0 cells to form N_1 cells.

The number of mutations (M) that have occurred in a culture during a measured interval of growth can be determined by depositing an inoculum on a membrane filter and placing the filter on top of an agar medium that permits every cell to initiate colony formation. After a limited period of incubation, during which the colonies develop to only microscopic size, the membrane is moved to a different agar medium that permits only the desired mutant type to continue growth. Each large colony that ultimately develops represents a **single mutational event** that occurred when N_0 cells (the inoculum) increased to N_1 cells (the number of cells present at the time that the medium was changed).

B. Selection:
1. Relative selection–Although any given type of mutant may be present in a culture at very low frequency (eg, 10^{-6}), small differences between the mutant and parent in either growth rate or death rate can lead to tremendous population shifts. For example, consider a culture containing 10^7 penicillin-sensitive (pen-s) cells and 10^1 penicillin-resistant (pen-r) cells. If the pen-s cells have a generation (doubling) time of 60 minutes and the pen-r cells a generation time of 50 minutes, then after 3 transfers of the culture, permitting 30 generations of the pen-s cells, the frequency of pen-r cells will have changed from 1×10^{-6} to 1×10^{-4}—a 100-fold increase. After 3 more transfers, 1% of the culture will be penicillin-resistant.

2. Absolute selection–In medical or microbiologic practice, microbial populations are commonly subjected to absolute selection, either consciously or unconsciously. For example, growth of the above-described culture in the presence of penicillin will lead to the death of all pen-s cells, so that the final culture will be 100% pen-r after one transfer. Since most mutants occur in cultures at very low frequencies, absolute selection is generally employed for their detec-

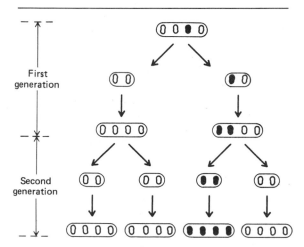

Figure 4–8. Segregation of a mutant nucleus. The nucleus containing the mutation is shown in black. If the mutation occurs in a cell with 4 nuclei, 2 generations are required before a pure mutant cell is produced.

First generation

Second generation

tion. The usual practice is to plate the culture on an agar medium that will permit only the sought-for mutant type to form colonies.

INTERCELLULAR DNA TRANSFER & GENETIC RECOMBINATION IN BACTERIA

The Formation of Bacterial Zygotes

In eukaryotic organisms, the diploid cell formed by the fusion of 2 haploid sexual cells (gametes) is called the **zygote.** Zygotes may also be formed in bacteria, but true cell fusion does not normally take place; instead, part of the genetic material of a donor cell is transferred to a recipient cell, and the recipient thus becomes diploid for only a part of its genetic complement. In the partial zygote, the genetic fragment from the donor is called the **exogenote** and the genetic complement of the recipient is called the **endogenote.** Exogenote and endogenote usually pair and recombine immediately after transfer. This recombinational step occurs by breakage and reunion of the paired genotes (Figs 4–9 and 4–10).

During succeeding nuclear and cell divisions, the **recombinant chromosome** is segregated into a single haploid cell. This cell can be experimentally detected by plating the partial zygotes on a selective medium on which only recombinants can grow.

The 3 processes by which recombination normally occurs in bacteria differ from each other primarily in the mechanism of the transfer process. These processes—transformation, transduction, and plasmid-mediated conjugation—are summarized in the following sections.

Protoplast Fusion

Although DNA transfer and partial zygosis are the normal processes by which bacteria recombine, complete zygosis can be artificially induced by removing the bacterial cell wall and fusing the resulting protoplasts with an agent such as polyethylene glycol. In *Bacillus subtilis,* for example, up to 10% of the treated protoplasts yield cells that, after reversion to walled bacilli, contain both parental genomes. These biparental types segregate true recombinants as well as parental segregants during further cell divisions.

Mechanism of Recombination

A model for the mechanism of recombination between 2 DNA molecules is shown in Fig 4–10. Evidence for this model comes from electron micrographs of DNA molecules extracted from cells (or from in vitro preparations) in which plasmid recombination was taking place: structures are seen that correspond to the intermediates labeled F and G in the figure.

The formation of the recombinational intermediates shown in Fig 4–10 requires the participation of several proteins, including DNA synaptase (a catalytic, ATP-independent enzyme acting on double-stranded substrates), the recA protein (the product of the *recA* gene), and topoisomerase I, which relaxes supercoiled DNA. The recA protein binds stoichiometrically to a single-stranded region of duplex DNA in an ATP-requiring reaction; the recA protein-coated single-stranded region then invades a homologous region of another, double-stranded DNA molecule, following which recombination takes place. The recA protein promotes both the initial pairing step and a second step of strand transfer, which is represented by stages C, D, and E of Fig 4–10.

Restriction & Modification

Bacterial cells of many species contain 2 enzymes with complementary functions. One enzyme **modifies** all the DNA in the cell by methylating bases at a few specific sites on the DNA. The other enzyme degrades all DNA that is not so modified; this process is called **restriction.** Restriction and modification may have

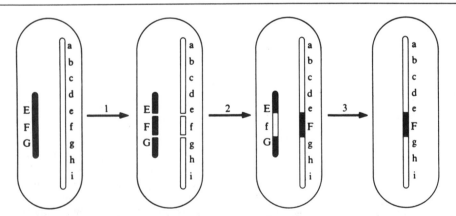

Figure 4–9. Genetic recombination in partial zygotes. The open bar represents the recipient cell chromosome, with genes lettered a–i. The solid bar represents an exogenote that has been transferred from a donor cell. An exchange of segments bearing the alleles of gene f, followed by cell division and segregation, leads to a recombinant cell. See Fig 4–10 for the detailed mechanism by which broken ends are reciprocally rejoined. (From Stanier RY, Doudoroff M, Adelberg EA: *The Microbial World,* 2nd ed. Copyright © 1963. By permission of Prentice-Hall, Inc., Englewood Cliffs, NJ.)

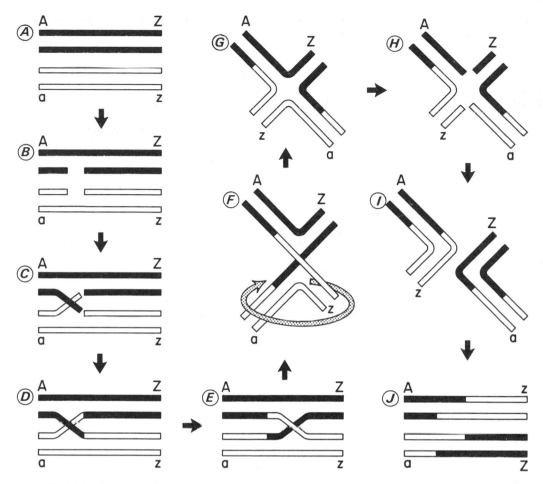

Figure 4–10. Model for the mechanism of recombination. Two parental DNA duplexes are represented by the pairs of shaded and unshaded bars, with one duplex carrying the markers A and Z; the other, a and z. *(A)* Duplexes pair. *(B)* Breakage of 2 strands occurs. *(C)*, *(D)* The broken segments are reciprocally rejoined. *(E)* The crossover point is laterally displaced. *(F)*, *(G)* Rearrangement of the diagram. *(H)* The other strands are broken and partially digested. *(I)* Localized repair and reciprocal rejoining. *(J)* Rearrangement of the diagram to show the heterozygosity within each duplex at the site of crossing over, a phenomenon that can be demonstrated readily in certain phage crosses. (After Potter H, Dressler D: In vitro system from *Escherichia coli* that catalyzes generalized genetic recombination. *Proc Natl Acad Sci USA* 1978; 75:3698.)

evolved to protect the cell from the lytic attack of DNA viruses (bacteriophages; see Chapter 9).

The degrading enzymes are called **restriction endonucleases;** the DNA site recognized by a particular restriction endonuclease is a specific sequence of 6–8 base-pairs that constitute a palindrome, ie, the sequence reads the same in both directions, starting from the 3' end of each strand. For example, the restriction endonuclease of *E coli* called EcoR1 recognizes the sequence

$$
\begin{array}{c}
\downarrow \quad * \\
- - \text{G A A T T C} - - \\
- - \text{C T T A A G} - - \\
* \quad \uparrow
\end{array}
$$

cutting it at the symmetric sites indicated by the arrows. The asterisks represent the sites that are methyl-

ated by the modifying enzyme of *E coli*, thus protecting the sequence from endonuclease attack.

When a zygote is formed by the transfer of DNA between bacterial strains with different specificities of restriction and modification, the DNA that penetrates the recipient is rapidly degraded in most of the cells. In a few cells, however, the exogenote may escape restriction and recombination can take place.

For example, conjugation between *E coli* strain B and *E coli* strain K12 yields recombinants at an extremely low frequency. From such crosses, however, a few recombinants can be isolated that are K12 strains carrying strain B's genes for modification and restriction. Such recombinants show high frequencies of recombination with *E coli* strain B. Restriction and modification similarly affect the transfer of phages from one strain of bacterium to another (see p 128).

Almost every bacterial species produces a unique

restriction endonuclease in terms of its DNA recognition site. The availability of this large series of specific enzymes has made possible the technologies of genetic engineering based on recombinant DNA, as discussed on pp 61–63.

TRANSFORMATION

In transformation, the recipient cell takes up soluble DNA released from the donor cell. In some cases, transforming DNA is released spontaneously; eg, it is found in the extracellular slime of certain *Neisseria* species. Usually, however, it is necessary to extract the DNA from donor cells by chemical procedures and to protect it from degradation by DNases.

Transformation occurs only in bacteria that are capable of taking up high-molecular-weight DNA from the medium. Originally discovered in the pneumococcus, it was subsequently discovered to occur in a number of other bacterial species, both gram-positive and gram-negative. Gram-positive species include the pneumococcus *(Streptococcus pneumoniae)* and *B subtilis;* gram-negative species include the gonococcus *(Neisseria gonorrhoeae)* and *Haemophilus influenzae.* Transformation also occurs in *E coli* in the presence of high concentrations of calcium ion. In some species, transformable cells are capable of taking up DNA from any source, although they form genetic recombinants only if the donor is a closely related organism. This specificity reflects the requirement of endogenote and exogenote to pair before exchanges can take place: pairing of DNA molecules demands close homology of nucleotide sequences.

Transformation may be considered to occur in 3 steps: binding of high-molecular-weight DNA to the cell surface; uptake of the bound DNA through the cell membrane; and integration of the donor DNA fragment into the recipient cell's chromosome. Only the first 2 stages occur in transformation with plasmid DNA, which becomes reestablished in the recipient cell as an autonomous replicon.

In *Neisseria,* cells are competent to bind DNA at all times; in the other transformable species, competence develops only at certain stages in the cell cycle or under a particular growth regimen and requires formation of competence factors by the cell. These factors include specific DNA-binding proteins of the cell envelope as well as poly-β-hydroxybutyrate in the cell membrane.

Transformation in Gram-Positive Bacteria

During the late exponential phase of growth, streptococcal cells excrete a low-molecular-weight protein called competence factor, which induces other cells in the culture to synthesize 8–10 new competence proteins, one of which is an autolysin that exposes a membrane-bound DNA-binding protein. Competence factor has not yet been demonstrated in other species.

Gram-positive cells bind both homologous and heterologous DNA. Once bound to the membrane, double-stranded DNA is nicked by a membrane-associated endonuclease at intervals of 6–8 kilobases. Entry is then initiated, at which time the nicks become double-stranded breaks. Driven by the cell's proton motive force, entry proceeds with digestion of one of the 2 strands, each cell taking up 5 or 6 bound molecules. The intact strand (if homologous) displaces one strand of the recipient cell's double-stranded DNA, forming a heteroduplex that, if not repaired, segregates a recombinant daughter duplex at the next round of DNA replication.

When circular plasmid DNA is bound, it is first linearized and then taken up by the process described above. The plasmid molecules taken up are often less than full length; restoration of complete circular plasmids in the recipient involves recombination between overlapping donor molecules or between a plasmid molecule and a region of homology in the recipient's chromosome (if such a region is present).

Transformation in Gram-Negative Bacteria

Transformation in gram-negative bacteria differs from that in gram-positive bacteria in the following respects: (1) Homologous DNA is taken up at a much higher rate than is heterologous DNA, reflecting different numbers of recognition sequences. (2) The double-stranded DNA fragments are sequestered in membranous surface structures called **transformasomes;** transfer from transformasomes into the cell interior is accompanied by the degradation of one strand. Again, only a single strand takes part in the final recombination step.

The uptake specificity is determined by a series of specific sites in the donor DNA. In *Haemophilus,* these sites are repeats of an 11-base-pair sequence that occurs at about 600 randomly distributed locations in the donor chromosome: roughly one per 4 kilobases.

In *Pseudomonas stutzeri,* a transformation process has been observed that is 1000 times more effective in the presence of donor cells than in the presence of an equivalent concentration of free DNA. This indicates that the donor cells play an active role, which may be DNA extrusion during replication.

TRANSDUCTION BY BACTERIOPHAGE

In transduction, a fragment of donor chromosome is carried to the recipient by a bacteriophage that has been produced in the donor cell. Transduction is generally observed with temperate bacteriophages, ie, those capable of forming prophages (see Chapter 9); certain mutants of virulent phages, however, may also effect transduction.

Transduction occurs in many bacterial genera, both gram-negative and gram-positive. Transduction may be generalized or restricted: in **generalized transduction,** the phage has a roughly equal chance of carrying any segment of the donor's chromosome; in **restricted transduction,** the transducing particles carry only those segments that are immediately adjacent to the site of prophage attachment.

Restricted Transduction

The mechanism of prophage attachment is shown in Fig 9–4, for phage λ (lambda). When λ is induced, λ DNA is detached from the chromosome by the reversal of the steps shown in Fig 9–4; detachment is followed by phage replication, maturation, and host cell lysis. As a rare event (about 10^{-6} to 10^{-5} of the cells), the crossover event occurs at a different position, generating a circle of DNA in which part of the λ genome has been replaced by a segment of host chromosome (Fig 4–11). The recombinant circles, lacking certain essential phage genes, are usually defective; they cannot replicate or mature unless the cell is simultaneously infected with a normal phage that supplies the missing phage gene products. When this occurs, the cell lyses and liberates both normal phage particles and "transducing particles."

When a transducing particle is adsorbed by a recipient cell, it injects its DNA in the normal fashion. The recipient thus receives a segment of the donor's chromosome as part of a phage genome; the latter integrates with the recipient's chromosome to become a prophage. The transduced donor genes are expressed in the recipient cell, even though they are inserted within a prophage.

Generalized Transduction

Although generalized transducing phages may oc-

casionally incorporate host DNA by the mechanism described above, the great majority of their transducing particles contain only host DNA; it thus appears that phage heads can be assembled around condensed segments of host DNA as well as around condensed phage genomes. The products of certain phage genes are essential for normal head assembly; presumably these "morphopoietic factors" complex with phage DNA and provide a matrix for assembly of the head subunits. Transducing phage particles may thus arise when morphopoietic factors complex with fragments of host DNA of the right size. As in restricted transduction, only about one particle in 10^5 or 10^6 is a transducing particle.

It has been found that phage P1, a typical generalized transducing phage, does not form a prophage that is integrated into the host chromosome. Instead, the prophage occupies an independent site in the cell. This difference is compatible with the different mechanisms of formation of transducing particles.

In generalized transduction, part of the donor cell DNA is degraded within the recipient cell; the rest is integrated into the recipient cell's chromosome as a double-stranded fragment. The frequency with which 2 or more genetic markers are co-transduced within the same phage particle defines the relative positions on the donor chromosome of closely linked genes; co-transduction is the principal method used for fine-structure mapping of the bacterial chromosome.

In the pneumococcus, a phage-associated gene transfer process has been discovered that exhibits

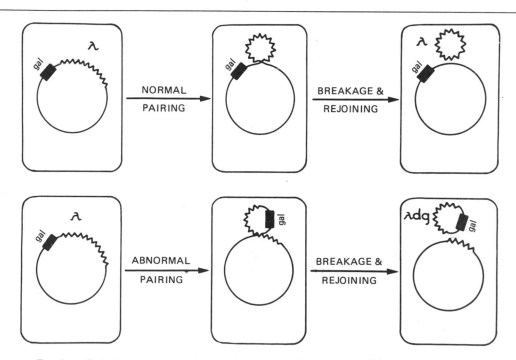

Figure 4–11. *Top Row:* Detachment of λ prophage to form a normal λ vegetative DNA. *Bottom Row:* Detachment of λ prophage to form λ dg DNA, which will mature as a transducing particle. ("λ dg" is an abbreviation for "lambda defective carrying gal genes.")

transformationlike as well as transductionlike properties. In this system, host genes are packaged in DNase-resistant particles that adsorb to recipient cells in a phagelike manner. Unlike transduction, however, entry of the DNA requires recipient competence and endonuclease action and becomes DNase-sensitive. It is not known whether this mixed mode of transfer occurs in other host-phage systems.

High-Frequency Transduction

In restricted transduction, the transducing particle contains part of a phage genome linked to a segment of host DNA. When this is injected into the recipient, the entire DNA structure becomes integrated into the bacterial chromosome. The transduced recipient then produces a clone of cells, every one of which carries the defective prophage plus the extra segment of donor DNA. If these cells also carry a normal prophage (as a result of simultaneous infection of the original recipient by a normal particle and a transducing particle), then, on induction, a lysate is produced in which half of the particles are transducing particles. This is the phenomenon of "high-frequency transduction."

Abortive Transduction

In many generalized transductions, failure of the exogenote to be integrated may lead to persistence without replication. Thus, when the zygote divides, only one of the daughter cells receives the exogenote. In further cell generations, the exogenote is again transmitted without replicating, so that only one cell in the clone at any given time is a partial diploid. This situation is called "abortive transduction"; the exogenote appears to be maintained in circular form by a host cell protein, accounting for its resistance to nuclease attack.

In abortive transduction, the genes of the exogenote function normally. Thus, if a gal$^+$/gal$^-$ cell is produced by an abortive transduction, the cell in which the nonreplicating gal$^+$ gene resides will produce the galactose-fermenting enzyme. During further generations, the clone of cells arising from each gal$^-$ segregant will produce no more enzyme, and the enzyme will be diluted out by the cell division process. If a gal$^+$/gal$^-$ abortive transductant is plated on a medium in which galactose is the sole source of carbon and energy, it will produce a minute colony (containing about 10^6 cells) after 4 days of growth as a result of the limited production of the galactose-fermenting enzyme. (A normal gal$^+$ cell would produce a very large colony, containing over 10^9 cells, in 2 days of growth.) The production of a minute colony as the result of abortive transduction is shown in Fig 4–12.

PLASMID-MEDIATED CONJUGATION

Plasmids

Bacteria are hosts to small, extrachromosomal genetic elements called plasmids, which are dispensable to the cell under ordinary conditions of growth.

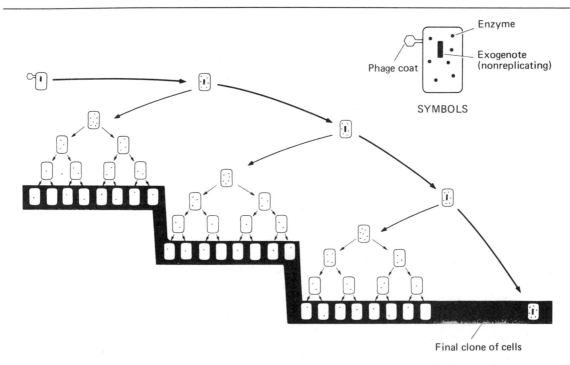

Figure 4–12. Abortive transduction. At each division, only one of the daughter cells receives the active gene. The other cell goes through a few cell divisions, until the active gene product (eg, enzyme) is diluted out. Plating an abortive transductant produces a minute colony in which only one cell is capable of further growth and division. (From Stanier RY, Doudoroff M, Adelberg EA: *The Microbial World*, 3rd ed. Copyright © 1970. By permission of Prentice-Hall, Inc., Englewood Cliffs, NJ.)

Plasmids share many properties with bacterial viruses (phages), from which they differ chiefly in their lack of an encapsidated, extracellular phase. They are of major clinical significance, not only because they may carry genes for resistance to therapeutic drugs and for virulence factors, as discussed below, but also because many of them mediate gene transfer—a process that leads to the emergence of bacterial strains with new combinations of drug resistance, antigens, and virulence mechanisms.

A. Physical Properties: Most plasmids discovered to date are circular, double-stranded DNA molecules. Their molecular weights range from 3×10^6 to 1×10^8, which is sufficient to code for 5–160 average polypeptides.

B. Replication: Plasmid DNA replicates while maintaining a supercoiled, circular state. Replicating plasmid DNA can be isolated in the form of "relaxation complexes," in which the DNA is bound to proteins that appear to provide the following functions: (1) binding of the DNA to the membrane replicator site; (2) nicking and unwinding of the strands to permit replication; and (3) resealing of the nicks. Replication is bidirectional in some plasmids and unidirectional in others; its mechanism is generally similar to that of chromosomal replication.

Plasmids regulate their own replication in such a way that each plasmid exhibits a typical copy-number ratio (ratio of plasmid copies to chromosome copies in the cell). In general, the small nonconjugative plasmids have high copy-number ratios whereas the large conjugative plasmids have copy-number ratios close to 1. Plasmid replication is unusually sensitive to inhibition by such agents as acridine dyes and ultraviolet light; by using these agents at threshold doses, cells can be "cured" of their plasmids.

Even in plasmids having a copy-number ratio of 1, partition between daughter cells following replication is highly efficient. This is effected by a plasmid DNA site called *par*, which is the functional equivalent of the eukaryotic chromosomal centromere. It may act by binding to a cell membrane site or, alternatively, by associating with the host chromosome. The plasmid of *E coli* strain K12, called F, has an additional mechanism for ensuring its partition: a set of plasmid gene products interact to inhibit host cell division when only one plasmid copy is present; the inhibition is reversed when the plasmid copy-number rises to 2 or more.

C. Incompatibility: Plasmids can be classified into a number of incompatibility groups; 2 members of the same group cannot coexist in the same cell. In several cases, the genes which determine incompatibility have been shown to produce inhibitors of replication specific for that incompatibility group. In one case, the incompatibility gene contains 3 repeats of a 19-base-pair sequence that bind to, and thus titrate out, an essential replication protein. In other cases, the incompatibility gene produces an untranslated mRNA that anneals with the mRNA for a replication protein and thus inhibits its translation. Members of the same incompatibility group are closely related, as indicated by the extensive hybridization of their DNAs.

D. Self-Transfer:

1. Gram-negative bacteria—Many—but not all—plasmids of gram-negative bacteria are conjugative: they carry the genes (called the *tra* genes) mediating their own transfer by the process of cell conjugation. There are 12 or more *tra* genes arranged in an operon (see below); some of these code for the production of the **sex pilus.** One *tra* gene codes for a DNA helicase, an enzyme that, prior to transfer of DNA, unwinds the DNA duplex by an ATP-dependent mechanism.

Plasmid transfer in gram-negative bacteria begins with the extrusion of a sex pilus, a protein thread several times the length of the cell. The tip of the sex pilus adheres to the outer membrane of gram-negative cell walls. Any gram-negative cell that it touches becomes tethered to the plasmid-containing cell; shortly thereafter, the 2 cells become bound together at a point of direct wall-to-wall contact, possibly by retraction of the pilus into the donor cell (Fig 4–13).

Binding of the recipient cell to the donor pilus requires the presence of specific receptor sites on the recipient cell's surface. In certain conjugation-deficient mutants, one of the major proteins of the outer membrane is missing and the lipopolysaccharide is altered, indicating a role for both of these components in pair formation.

Following specific pair formation, the plasmid undergoes a special type of replication called "transfer replication," one parental strand passing into the recipient and the other remaining in the donor cell (Fig 4–14). Complementary strands are synthesized in the donor and recipient simultaneously with transfer. The daughter molecules are circularized by ligase action immediately after transfer replication is complete.

No cytoplasm, nor any cell material other than DNA, passes from donor to recipient. The mating couples eventually break apart, resulting in 2 plasmid-containing cells where there had been one before.

2. Gram-positive bacteria—Several antibiotics produced by members of the genus *Streptomyces* have been found to be determined by plasmid genes, and some of these plasmids are transferable from one streptomycete to another. The process resembles conjugation in that direct hyphal contact is necessary. The best known such plasmid is SCP1, which carries the genes for the biosynthetic pathway producing the antibiotic methylenomycin. SCP1 also carries the genes responsible for transfer by a mechanism which has some similarities to that of plasmid-mediated chromosome transfer in gram-negative bacteria.

Plasmid-mediated conjugation also occurs in members of the gram-positive genera *Bacillus* and *Streptococcus*. In *Streptococcus lactis*, the ability to ferment lactose is conjugally transmitted as a plasmid-borne β-galactosidase (*lac*) gene. A series of conjugative plasmids have been analyzed in *Streptococcus faecalis*, carrying genes for hemolysin, bacteriocin, and single or multiple drug resistance. These plasmids can

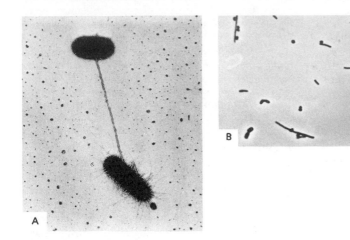
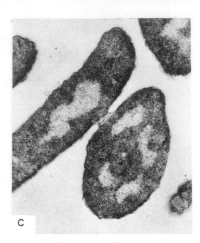

Figure 4–13. *(A)* A male and a female cell joined by an F pilus. The F pilus has been "stained" with male-specific RNA phage particles. The male cell also possesses ordinary pili, which do not adsorb male-specific phages and are not involved in mating. *(B)* Mating pairs of *E coli* cells. Hfr cells are elongated. *(C)* Electron micrograph of a thin section of a mating pair. The cell walls of the mating partners are in intimate contact in the "bridge" area. (Electron micrograph [A] by Carnahan J and Brinton C. From Stanier RY, Doudoroff M, Adelberg EA: *The Microbial World,* 3rd ed. Copyright © 1970. By permission of Prentice-Hall, Inc., Englewood Cliffs, NJ. Photographs [B] and [C] from Gross JD and Caro LG: DNA transfer in bacterial conjugation. *J Mol Biol* 1966;**16**:269.)

mobilize other (nonconjugative) plasmids as well as chromosomal markers.

An unusual feature of the *S faecalis* mating system is the production by recipient cells of specific **sex pheromones**—diffusible proteins that stimulate donor cell aggregation (with each other and with recipient cells) and, if the donor cells are preinduced by the pheromone, increase the frequency of donor plasmid transfer as much as a million-fold. When a recipient cell acquires a given plasmid, it ceases to produce the pheromone specific for that plasmid but continues to excrete pheromones that act on donor cells harboring other conjugative plasmids.

E. Recombination: Plasmids undergo crossing over with each other and with the host chromosome, depending on the extent of their base sequence homologies or on the presence of transposable elements (see below). Since both plasmids and chromosome are circular, an odd number of crossovers serves to integrate the 2 DNA structures, which then replicate as a single unit. An even number of crossovers, on the other hand, brings about an exchange of segments.

A plasmid capable of integrating with the bacterial chromosome is called an **episome.** When integration occurs, a double replicon is formed bearing both a chromosomal and a plasmid replicator site. In some cases, replication continues to start at the chromosomal replicator; in others (eg, at nonpermissive temperatures in mutants temperature-sensitive for DNA synthesis), replication of the entire structure is taken over by the plasmid replicator, a phenomenon known as "integrative suppression."

F. Mobilization: If a gram-negative cell harbors 2 plasmids, one self-transferable and the other not, the former may bring about the simultaneous transfer of the latter—ie, the latter is "mobilized." Mobilization is brought about when the 2 plasmids are either permanently or transiently integrated by a crossover; mobilization can also occur without integration if the nontransferable plasmid simply lacks one or more gene functions (eg, pilus formation) that the self-transferable plasmid can provide.

The bacterial chromosome may also be mobilized by integration with a self-transferable plasmid. If the integration is relatively stable, the cell in which it has occurred may give rise to a clone, every cell in which is capable of chromosome transfer. The strain obtained by isolation of such a clone is called **Hfr,** for "high-frequency recombination"; chromosome transfer by Hfr strains is described below.

G. Population Dynamics: Plasmids are occasionally irreversibly lost by their host cells and hence would ultimately disappear from bacterial populations in nature if their loss were not compensated by cell-to-cell transfer and replication. As discussed above, such transfer may occur either by conjugation or by phage transduction. The rates of loss and transfer are such as to maintain each type of plasmid in a small percentage of the natural host population at any given time. When selection is applied, however, as in the case of R factor selection by antibiotics, a majority of host cells may harbor a given type of plasmid (see below).

The transmission frequency of plasmids is limited mainly by the efficiency of pilus formation, which in most host strains is repressed to a level of 10^{-5} per cell, and by species specificity. For example, F (the conjugative plasmid of *E coli* K12), which is totally nonrepressed, is transferred from one *E coli* strain to another with a frequency of 1.0, but from *E coli* to *Proteus mirabilis* at a frequency of 1×10^{-5} or less.

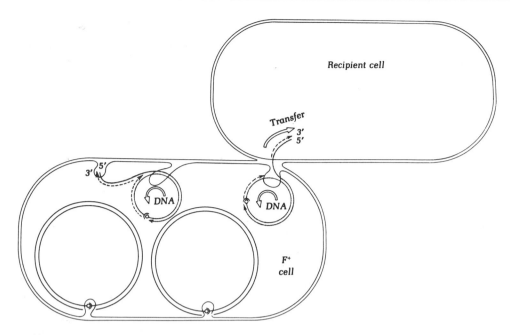

Figure 4–14. An F⁺ cell, containing 2 autonomous F replicons and 2 chromosomes, is shown conjugating with a recipient cell. Replication of F is proceeding according to the mechanism outlined in Fig 4–4. The F at the left is replicating within the host cell; the F at the right is being driven into the recipient by replication. (From Stanier RY, Doudoroff M, Adelberg EA: *The Microbial World,* 3rd ed. Copyright © 1970. By permission of Prentice-Hall, Inc., Englewood Cliffs, NJ.)

H. Cell Properties Determined by Plasmid Genes:

1. Drug resistance–In gram-negative bacteria, genes governing resistance to such agents as neomycin, kanamycin, streptomycin, chloramphenicol, tetracyclines, penicillins, and sulfonamides are found on one or another plasmid in various combinations. In the gram-positive staphylococci, genes governing resistance to such agents as penicillin, erythromycin, and heavy metals (eg, Hg^{2+} and Co^{2+}) are found on plasmids. Genes conferring resistance to the same agents may also be found on the chromosome, but in such cases they do so by different mechanisms. Most plasmid-governed resistance is mediated by enzymatic inactivation of the drug (eg, by acetylation or phosphorylation), whereas chromosome-mediated resistance usually reflects a lowered affinity of its target molecule for the drug. These findings are compatible with the fact that plasmids are (by definition) dispensable to the cell: Only chromosomal genes can confer resistance by structurally altering the binding site for the drug, since the genes determining the structures of indispensable cell components must themselves be indispensable. Table 4–1 compares the mechanisms of resistance determined by a number of plasmid and chromosomal genes.

The conjugative drug-resistance plasmids of gram-negative bacteria are called **R factors.** In many cases, the R factor reversibly dissociates into 2 or more smaller units: an element called **resistance transfer factor (RTF),** carrying the genes that govern the process of intercellular transfer; and one or more separate elements called **R determinants,** carrying the resistance genes. Many—perhaps all—R determinants are transposons (see below).

As mentioned earlier, not all plasmids are conjugative. The penicillinase-determining plasmids of the staphylococci, which can be transferred from cell to cell only by transformation or phage-mediated transduction, are notable examples of nonconjugative plasmids.

2. Virulence–A number of plasmids carry genes whose products contribute to, or may be essential for, the virulence of the pathogenic host cell. Some plasmids carry genes that code for toxins, eg, the enterotoxins of enteropathogenic strains of *E coli,* the exfoliative toxin of staphylococci, the toxin of *Bacillus anthracis,* the neurotoxin of *Clostridium tetani,* and the insect-killing endotoxin of *Bacillus thuringiensis.* Others carry genes whose products contribute to invasiveness. These include plasmids of *Yersinia enterocolitica, Shigella flexneri,* and "*Shigella*-like" *E coli* strains that produce dysentery; plasmids of *Yersinia pestis*; and plasmids of enteropathogenic *E coli* strains, in which plasmid genes determine the adhesive colonization antigens (pili).

Plasmid-borne genes can contribute to host cell virulence in other ways. The colicinogenic plasmid Col V, for example, determines enzymes that synthesize cell-associated, hydroxamate-containing iron-sequestering compounds which are induced in media containing low concentrations of iron. It is believed that invasiveness of symbiotic bacteria depends heavily on the ability of the bacteria to compete with their mammalian host cells for iron; most *E coli* strains isolated from bacteremias carry Col V, suggesting a role for

Table 4–1. Some mechanisms of bacterial resistance to drugs.

Target	Drug	Chromosomal Mutation	Plasmid Product	Plasmid Action
Ribosome	Chloramphenicol.	Altered 23S ribosomal RNA.	Acetyltransferase.	Detoxification (acetylation of −OH groups).
	Tetracyclines.	Increased drug efflux due to amplified (repeated) gene.	Membrane protein.	Active drug efflux.
	Erythromycin.	Lowered affinity of ribosomal protein; altered 23S ribosomal RNA.	Methylase.	Methylation of 23S ribosomal RNA.
	Aminoglycosides (eg, streptomycin).	Lowered affinity of ribosomal protein; 16S RNA methylation (kasugamycin).	O-phosphotransferase. O-adenyltransferase. N-acetyltransferase.	Interference with drug binding to target.
Cell wall synthesis	β-Lactams (penicillin, cephalosporins).	Lowered affinity of penicillin-binding proteins; increase in β-lactamase.	β-Lactamase.	Drug degradation.
	D-Cycloserine.	Decreased transport.	—	—
Membrane	Polymyxins.	? (rare).	—	—
Folate synthesis	Sulfonamides.	Lowered affinity of dihydropteroate synthase.	Sulfa-resistant synthase.	Substitute resistant enzyme.
	Trimethoprim.	Thymine auxotrophy (spares folate).	Drug-resistant dihydrofolate reductase.	Substitute resistant enzyme.
−SH groups in proteins	Mercury, organomercurials.	—	Reductases, hydrolases.	Detoxification.
DNA gyrase	Nalidixic acid, novobiocin.	Lowered affinity of gyrase.	?	?
RNA polymerase	Rifampin.	Lowered affinity of β subunit.	—	—

the Col V-determined iron-sequestering system in host cell virulence.

Plasmids determine an intricate relationship between certain tumorigenic plant pathogens and their hosts. The best studied of these is the Ti plasmid of *Agrobacterium tumefaciens*. When *A tumefaciens* transfers this plasmid to plant host cells, one genetic region of the plasmid converts the host cell to malignancy, so that a tumor forms; and other genetic regions of the plasmid cause the tumor cells to excrete opines, unusual amino acids that the bacteria then utilize as energy sources by means of still other enzymes determined by Ti plasmid genes. The Ti plasmid is an important vector in plant genetic engineering (see below).

3. Production of antimicrobial agents–Antimicrobial agents include antibiotics, which are the products of metabolic pathways, and polypeptide toxins. A number of these agents are encoded by plasmid genes, including many antibiotics of *Streptomyces* and microcins—oligopeptides produced by certain strains of *E coli*.

Plasmids determine a special class of antimicrobial agents called **bacteriocins,** proteins that are active only against other strains of the same bacterial species (see p 235). **Colicins,** for example, are produced by *E coli* cells harboring small, nonconjugative plasmids called **Col factors;** a given Col factor determines not only the colicin but also a protein that protects the

donor cell from the colicin it produces. Some colicins act by forming ion-permeable channels in the membrane of sensitive cells, collapsing the essential membrane potential.

4. Metabolic activities–Some plasmids carry sets of genes determining metabolic pathways; some examples are listed in Table 4–2. The enzyme for nylon degradation is particularly interesting: it attacks the amide bond of this synthetic compound but not those of any naturally occurring compound tested. The gene for this enzyme appears to have evolved recently by duplication and extensive mutation.

5. Chromosome transfer–As mentioned above, some conjugative plasmids are able to integrate with the host cell's chromosome; in the conjugation process, both plasmid and chromosomal DNA are transferred from the donor to the recipient cell. Plasmids capable of mobilizing the chromosome in this way are often called **sex factors;** the best known sex factor is **F,** the plasmid first isolated from *E coli* strain K12; chromosome transfer by F-bearing cells of *E coli* is described below.

I. Relation to Viruses: Bacterial viruses possess all of the properties described above for plasmids; a *Pseudomonas* phage has even been found to promote conjugation. The major difference thus appears to be the ability of phages to form mature, protein-coated virions that can be liberated and passed to other cells through the medium. Their many similarities suggest a

Table 4-2. Examples of metabolic activities determined by plasmids.

Organism	Activity
Pseudomonas spp	Degradation of camphor, toluene, octane, salicylic acid.
Bacillus stearothermophilus	α-Amylase.
Alcaligenes eutrophus	Utilization of H_2 as oxidizable energy source.
Escherichia coli	Sucrose uptake and metabolism, citrate uptake.
Klebsiella spp	Nitrogen fixation.
Streptococcus (group N)	Lactose utilization, galactose phosphotransferase system, citrate metabolism.
Rhodospirillum rubrum	Synthesis of photosynthetic pigment.
Flavobacterium spp	Nylon degradation.

close evolutionary relationship between phages and plasmids.

J. Clinical Significance: The ease with which plasmids can transfer from cell to cell and the strong selection that chemotherapy has exerted for drug resistance have combined to produce striking effects. Some examples of this impact are given on p 135.

RTFs (plasmids carrying the genes for self-transfer but not for drug resistance) have also been discovered to be extremely common in the bacterial flora of humans and animals. For example, 20 out of 60 *E coli* strains isolated from healthy humans and animals were found in one study to carry RTFs, as did 15 out of 21 enteropathogenic strains isolated from patients. (RTFs are detected in the following way: strain A, which is being screened for the presence of an RTF, is mated with strain B, which carries only a nontransferable R determinant. Strain B is then mated with a third strain—strain C—which is plasmid-free. The transfer of the R determinant from strain B to strain C reveals the presence of an RTF acquired from strain A.)

Roughly 20% of *Enterobacteriaceae* strains collected between 1917 and 1954 (the "pre-antibiotic era") have been found to carry conjugative plasmids; all but a few of these plasmids are free of R determinants. Thus, conjugative plasmids were as common in *Enterobacteriaceae* then as now, but they only rarely carried genes for drug resistance.

Chromosome Transfer

A. The F⁻, F⁺, and Hfr States: Cells of *E coli* K12 which carry F are called F⁺; those which have lost it are called F⁻. F⁺ cells will transfer replicas of their sex factors to F⁻ cells by the process described above.

In a population of F⁺ cells, the integration of F and chromosome occurs about once per 10^5 cells at each generation; integration occurs by crossing over, in a manner analogous to the integration of λ prophage (Fig 9–4). The cells in which this occurs, and the clones that arise from them, are called Hfr (see above).

Integration does not always occur at the same site on the bacterial chromosome. There are 8 or 10 preferred sites, containing insertion sequences (see below) or base-pair regions homologous with regions on F.

The integration process is reversible; in a population of Hfr cells, detachment by a second crossover occurs about once per 10^5 cells at each generation. Thus, every F⁺ population contains a few Hfr cells, and every Hfr population contains a few F⁺ cells.

B. DNA Transfer by Hfr Donors: When a suspension of Hfr cells is mixed with an excess of F⁻ cells, every Hfr cell will attach to an F⁻ cell and initiate replicative transfer. Since F and the chromosome have merged to form a single replicon, chromosomal DNA as well as F DNA passes into the recipient (Fig 4–15).

The order in which chromosome markers move into the recipient depends on the chromosomal site at which F has become integrated, as illustrated in Fig 4–16.

DNA transfer proceeds at a constant rate in each mating pair: approximately 4×10^4 base-pairs per minute at 37 °C. Transfer is interrupted by spontaneous breakage of the DNA molecule at random times; thus, the chance of a given marker's being transferred decreases exponentially with its distance from the transfer origin. A marker close to the origin will be transferred with a probability of 1.0, while the terminal marker will be transferred with a probability of less than 0.01.

Conjugal DNA transfer can also be interrupted artificially, using violent agitation of a suspension of conjugating cells to shear apart mating couples. When the mating of a given Hfr × F⁻ pair is interrupted at a series of precise times, the earliest time at which a given marker appears within a recombinant defines its distance from the "transfer origin" (the Hfr breakage point shown in Fig 4–16). Such "time-of-entry" data constitute one of the principal bases for constructing the **genetic maps** of bacterial species capable of conjugation. In *E coli* strain K12, the entire chromosome requires about 100 minutes to be transferred at 37 °C; the time-of-entry method can resolve markers about 0.5 minute apart. For mapping within regions so short that they take less than 0.5 minute to be transferred, co-transduction frequencies are used (see above).

C. Formation and Transfer of F Genotes: As a very rare event (10^{-8}–10^{-6} per cell per generation), an Hfr cell will undergo F detachment by a crossover in an abnormal region, in a manner analogous to the detachment of λ dg shown in Fig 4–11. The F that is formed includes within its circular structure a segment of chromosomal DNA; it is called an **F genote,** and the cell that carries it is called F′ (F prime), rather than F⁺.

The cell in which the F genote arose is called a primary F′ cell; its chromosome has a deletion corresponding to the segment on the F genote. Transfer of the F genote to a normal F⁻ cell gives rise to a secondary F′ strain, in which part of the chromosome is present in the diploid state. Crossing over occurs at a high rate in such cells, so that the F genote undergoes

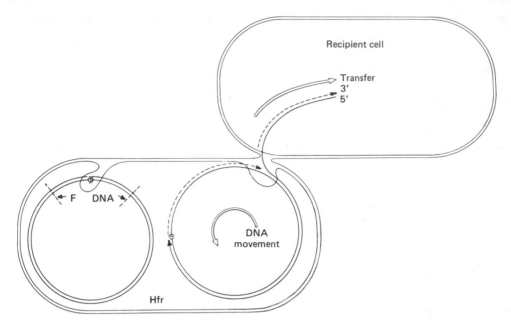

Figure 4–15. DNA transfer by an Hfr cell. Since F and chromosome are integrated, F replicative transfer causes the sequential transfer of chromosomal DNA. (From Stanier RY, Doudoroff M, Adelberg EA: *The Microbial World,* 3rd ed. Copyright © 1970. By permission of Prentice-Hall, Inc., Englewood Cliffs, NJ.)

alternate integration and detachment from the chromosome.

When a culture of a secondary F′ strain is mated with an F⁻, 2 types of transfer take place: some cells (those in which F is at that moment detached) transfer only the F genote; others (those in which F is integrated) transfer both F genote DNA and contiguous chromosomal DNA.

RECOMBINATION IN EUKARYOTIC MICROORGANISMS

Meiotic Recombination

The cells of protists (algae, protozoa, fungi, and slime molds) have typical eukaryotic nuclei, each nucleus containing several chromosomes. Following chromosomal replication, which converts each chromosome into a pair of identical chromatids, nuclear division takes place by mitosis. The mitotic processes segregate one chromatid of each pair into each daughter cell.

Some eukaryotic protists multiply in the diploid state, a clone of diploid cells arising from a zygote formed by the fusion of 2 haploid gametes. Each diploid nucleus thus contains 2 haploid sets of chromosomes, one from each parent. The 2 homologs of a particular chromosome will often differ by mutation at several genetic loci, ie, the cell will be heterozygous for those genes.

Just after replication, then, each chromosome of a diploid cell is represented by 4 chromatids, one pair from each parent. At meiosis, 2 sequential divisions segregate the 4 chromatids into 4 separate nuclei. The cells containing these nuclei may act immediately as gametes, fusing to restore the diploid condition, or—in some species—may give rise to clones of haploid cells, delaying the fusion event to a later stage in the life cycle.

New combinations of genes are produced during meiosis in 2 ways: (1) the random segregation of the chromatids during the division events scrambles the original parental sets of chromosomes, so that a given meiotic product receives some chromatids from one set and some from the other; and (2) during the first meiotic division, the 2 homologs of each chromosome pair and a chromatid from one homolog may exchange segments with a chromatid from the other homolog by a recombinational (crossing over) event. The molecular mechanism of such recombination is presumably identical to that described above for prokaryotic organisms.

Gene Conversion

Consider a heterozygous marker on one of the chromosomes in the diploid cell. Call the dominant allele **A** and the recessive allele **a**; the 4 chromatids must carry the set **A, A, a, a** both at the start and at the end of meiosis. In exceptional cases, however, the 4 products of meiosis are found to carry the alleles **A, A, A, a**: ie, one of the **a** alleles has been converted to the **A** form during the meiotic process. This phenomenon, called gene conversion, may be explained by the following sequence of events: (1) Single-strand breaks occur in 2 neighboring chromatids, one carrying allele **A** and the other allele **a**; (2) the nick in the latter chromatid is widened by exonuclease action, destroying allele **a** on one strand; (3) a single-stranded segment

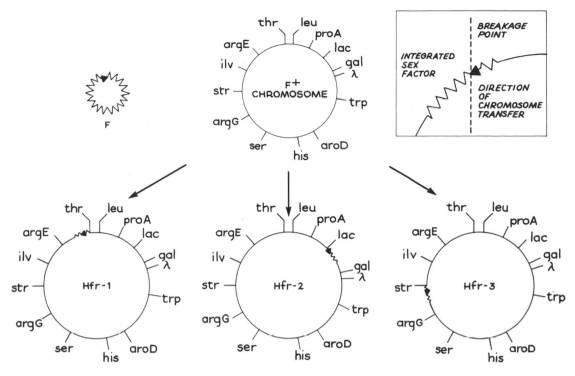

Figure 4–16. Integration of the sex factor and F⁺ chromosome to produce 3 different Hfr males. The upper circle represents the F⁺ chromosome; only a few of the known genetic loci, or "markers," are shown. The lower circles represent cases in which the sex factor (F) has integrated with the chromosome between argE and thr, between lac and gal, and between str and argG, respectively. (The 3- and 4-letter symbols represent genes governing biochemical activities of the cell, eg, "lac," the set of loci governing the utilization of β-galactosides; "his," the set of loci governing the biosynthesis of histidine, etc.)

from the other parental chromatid is transferred into the gap, thus replacing allele **a** with allele **A;** (4) the transferred strand is replaced in the donor **A** chromatid by DNA polymerase action. The net result of this sequence of events is the conversion of an **a** chromatid into an **A/a** heteroduplex, which can segregate an **A** allele in a future replication cycle. Such gene conversions occur frequently in the region of a crossover but may also occur elsewhere on the chromosome. Gene conversion can occur during mitosis as well as during meiosis.

Mitotic Recombination

During the multiplication of heterozygous diploid cells by mitosis, homologous chromosomes do not normally pair. As a rare event, however, they may do so, and in the process chromatids may exchange segments just as in meiosis. As shown in Fig 4–17, the ensuing random segregation of chromatids will result—in 50% of cases—in daughter cells that are homozygous for all loci distal to the crossover. The cell receiving the homozygous recessive alleles will then show a change from the dominant phenotype of the heterozygous parent to the recessive phenotype.

Heterokaryosis & Parasexuality in Fungi

Many fungi multiply in the haploid condition. When 2 mutationally different strains of the same spe-

cies come into contact, hyphal fusion may occur to produce a mycelium in which the 2 parental types of nuclei commingle. Such a mycelium is called a **heterokaryon.**

On rare occasions, nuclear fusion may occur, producing a truly diploid heterozygous nucleus. When this nucleus is segregated into a uninucleate spore, germination will give rise to a diploid heterozygous mycelium. During mitotic growth, successive losses of one homolog of each chromosome pair may restore the haploid condition. The resulting haploids are genetic recombinants, since homolog loss is random with respect to parental origin; furthermore, genetic exchanges may have occurred by mitotic crossing over.

This cycle of events—the fusion of haploid nuclei to form a diploid nucleus and the return to haploidy by homolog loss—is called **parasexuality.** It provides a mechanism for genetic recombination in imperfect fungi but may be of less importance in fungi with a sexual stage in their life cycle.

Recombination in Cytoplasmic Organelles

The mitochondrial ribosomes of yeast are sensitive to certain inhibitors of protein synthesis such as chloramphenicol, erythromycin, and spiramycin that have no effect on cytoplasmic ribosomes. Mutants resistant to these inhibitors have been isolated and the muta-

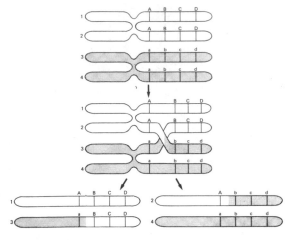

Figure 4–17. Mitotic recombination. *(Top)* Two homologs of a heterozygous cell, carrying dominant (A, B, C, D) and recessive (a, b, c, d) alleles at 4 loci, pair at mitosis. *(Center)* Crossing over between heterologous chromatids occurs. *(Bottom)* Chromatids separate at mitosis. If chromatids 2 and 4 segregate together (a random event occurring in 50% of such mitoses), a daughter is produced that is **homozygous recessive** at all loci distal to the crossover site.

tions shown to reside in mitochondrial DNA. When different mitochondrial mutants of the yeast *Saccharomyces cerevisiae* are crossed and the resulting diploid cells allowed to undergo meiosis, the haploid progeny are found to contain recombinant mitochondria, with new combinations of mitochondrial genes.

The chloroplasts of algae and higher plants also contain their own DNA. In the unicellular green alga *Chlamydomonas,* mutants resistant to inhibitors of chloroplast ribosomal synthesis of protein have been isolated; the mutations reside in the chloroplast DNA. In experiments analogous to those done with yeast, sexual crosses between haploid algal cells carrying different chloroplast mutations yield progeny containing genetically recombinant chloroplasts.

GENES OF STRUCTURE & GENES OF REGULATION

A gene that determines the structure of a particular protein (eg, an enzyme) is called a **structural gene.** The activity of a structural gene, in terms of production of messenger RNA for enzyme synthesis, is strictly regulated in the cell. It has been shown that many structural genes lie adjacent to specific sites concerned with the regulation of structural gene activity. Such a site is called an **operator.** Under certain conditions the cell produces cytoplasmic proteins called **repressors;** when an operator binds its specific repressor, the structural gene adjacent to it is prevented from producing mRNA and is thus inactivated. In many cases, a series of structural genes determining a series of coordinated enzymes (eg, the enzymes of a particular metabolic pathway) form a continuous segment of

DNA under the control of a single adjacent operator. A gene sequence under the coordinated control of a single operator is called an **operon.**

Each specific type of repressor molecule of the cell must, of course, be formed by its own structural gene. A gene concerned with the production of a repressor is called a **regulator gene.** Both operators and regulator genes can be detected when they occur in mutant form. For example, the operator can mutate to a state in which it is unable to bind repressor. The operon now functions under all conditions and is said to be "derepressed."

Mutations of the regulator gene produce phenotypes similar to those produced by mutations of the corresponding operator. For example, a mutated regulator gene may fail to make repressor, giving rise to the derepressed phenotype (Fig 4–18). Regulator genes can be distinguished from operator, however, by the behavior of diploid cells carrying one normal gene and one mutated gene. In such diploids, the derepressed state is dominant if the mutation has altered the operator but recessive if the mutation has inactivated the regulator gene.

Regulation may be positive rather than negative. For example, the operon containing the genes for arabinose utilization in *E coli* is transcribed only when its operator binds an "activator" protein (the product of the regulatory *araC* gene) which in turn has bound an arabinose molecule.

Note that the set of structural genes which make up an operon is transcribed as a unit, forming a polygenic mRNA molecule. Transcription begins at the operator end of the operon; a nonsense mutation in one of the genes proximal to the operator may stop translation not only of that gene but also of all genes in the operon distal to it. Such mutations are called **polar mutations;** the polarity of nonsense mutations reflects the inability of a ribosome, once discharged from the mRNA, to reinitiate translation further downstream.

Operons are characteristic of prokaryotic cells; they are rare or absent in eukaryotic organisms.

TRANSPOSABLE ELEMENTS

Transposable elements are specific DNA sequences, copies of which move to new positions in the genome; their replication and movement are catalyzed by enzymes they themselves encode. These events have profound effects on both genome evolution and gene expression.

The existence of such elements was first recognized in the 1930s by McClintock, who observed the movement of genetic controlling elements in maize. The discovery of transposable elements in bacteria in the 1960s made possible an analysis of their molecular structure and function; similar elements have been found in yeast, in the worm *Caenorhabditis elegans,* and in *Drosophila;* and close structural relationships between such elements and the mammalian tumor viruses have been recognized.

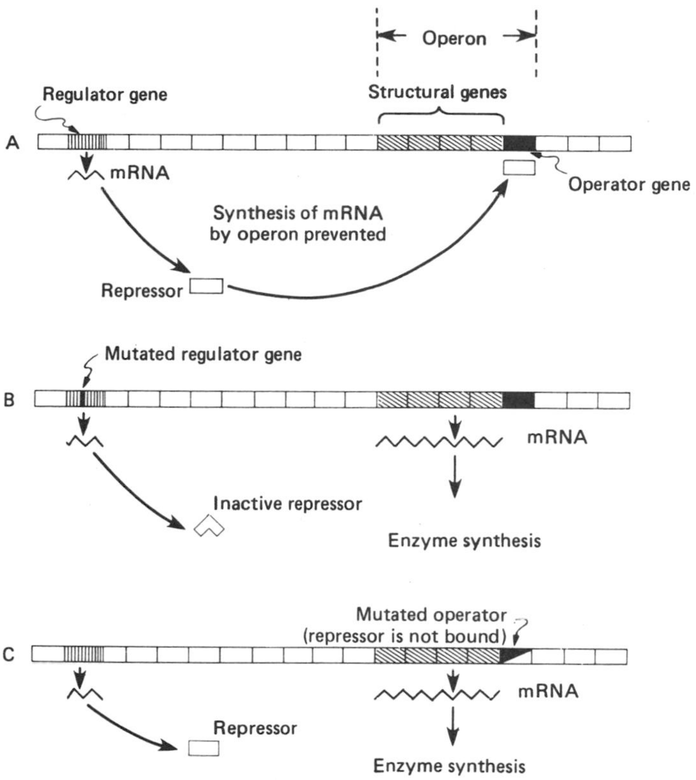

Figure 4–18. Genetic regulation of enzyme synthesis. The product of the regulator gene, the repressor, prevents the functioning of the operon, which it controls by binding to the operator site. Mutations at either the regulator gene or the operator can interfere with repression, thus permitting enzyme synthesis. (*Note:* Enzyme inducers generally act by inactivating repressors. In feedback repression of biosynthetic enzymes, however, the repressor is normally inactive and must be activated by the biosynthetic end product. See p 105.)

Transposable Elements in Prokaryotes

A. Structure: Transposable elements in prokaryotes were discovered when a series of polar mutations in an *E coli* operon were found to represent the insertions of specific DNA sequences 800–1400 base-pairs in length. By heteroduplex analysis and DNA-DNA hybridizations, it was found that copies of a small number of these specific sequences (called **insertion sequences** or **ISs**) are present at numerous sites on the *E coli* chromosome as well as on many plasmids and phage genomes. ISs are transposed as discrete elements and are integrated at new sites by mechanisms that are independent of DNA sequence homology.

Soon after the discovery of ISs, it was found that many of the R determinants of R factors are similarly transposable; in every such case, the R determinant is flanked by repeated sequences. In some cases, these repeated sequences are known ISs; the R determinant for kanamycin resistance, for example, is flanked by 2 copies of IS1 (Fig 4–19). Such elements, consisting of repeated sequences flanking a gene coding for an unrelated function, are called **transposons.**

All ISs and transposons terminate in **inverted repeats** 20–40 base-pairs long. These repeats serve as recognition sites for enzymes that mediate a variety of reactions, including not only replication and transposition but also the deletion of DNA segments adjacent to the transposable element. When such an element is transposed from one replicon to another within the same cell, replicon fusion may occur as an intermediate step. Replicon fusion can also occur by normal recombination between replicons carrying the identical element, the 2 copies of the element providing sequence homology.

Transposons code for one or more proteins, including an enzyme ("transposase") that catalyzes their own transposition. The transposon Tn3, for example, encodes for β-lactamase (conferring penicillin resistance), transposase, and a repressor of the transposase. Probably all transposable elements, including ISs, code for their own transposases. If that is the case, the distinction between ISs and transposons becomes a minor one, a transposon being an insertion sequence that carries one or more additional genes coding for functions unrelated to the transposition process itself.

Transposons may range in complexity from types such as Tn3, which carries only one transposition-unrelated function, to Mu, a transposon carrying an entire phage genome. A transposon found in *S faecalis* carries all the genetic information needed for conjugation, catalyzing its own transfer from cell to cell at low frequency.

B. Transposition: Transposition takes place by a process that combines recombination and replication: At the completion of the process, the original transposable element remains in position, and a new copy has been inserted within a "target site" elsewhere in the genome. The new copy may appear within the same replicon or in a different replicon; in the latter case, a cointegrate structure—representing the fusion of the 2 replicons—may occur as an intermediate stage in the transposition process. In all cases, the process

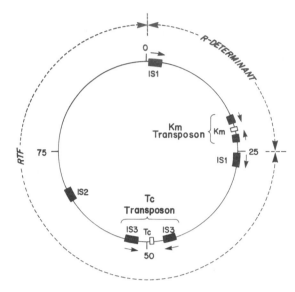

Figure 4–19. Map of the R factor R6-5. The coordinates (0, 25, 50, 75) are distances in kilobases. The R determinant carrying the kanamycin resistance (Km) gene is bounded by 2 direct repeats of IS1; a copy of IS2 is present in the RTF region. A tetracycline resistance (Tc) transposon, bounded by reverse repeats of IS3, is also inserted in the RTF region. Km is itself part of a transposon; the inverted repeats that bound it have not been identified with any of the known IS elements. (After Cohen SN, Kopecko DJ: *Fed Proc* 1976;**35**:2031.)

results in the generation of short (5–11 base-pairs long) direct repeats of target DNA on each side of the transposed sequence.

Transposable elements show a wide range of specificity for target sites, ranging from elements having no detectable specificity to those having only a single integration site.

Despite the existence of mechanisms for the movement of transposable elements between replicons and for the transfer of DNA from one bacterial species to another, a given transposable element may have a very limited distribution in nature. IS2, for example, several copies of which are present in the chromosome of *E coli* strain K12, was not detected when 15 other species of gram-negative bacteria were screened for its presence by DNA hybridization.

C. Deletion: Deletions of DNA segments immediately adjacent to a transposable element occur at rates 100- to 1000-fold higher than the spontaneous background for the remainder of the genome. Two types of IS-mediated deletions have been observed: In type I, which involves small duplications and is dependent on the recA gene product, the IS element itself is deleted along with adjacent DNA. In type II, which is independent of duplications and of recA, only adjacent DNA is deleted.

D. Excision: When a transposable element inserts within a functional gene, that gene is inactivated for normal expression. Such events appear as loss mutations such as auxotrophy. The mutant genes are fre-

quently found to revert back to normal expression; when they do, the transposed element is found to have been precisely eliminated. This elimination is not associated with further transposition but rather appears to be a specific deletion event that is independent of transposase action.

Transposable Elements in Protists

A transposable element called Ty1 has been discovered in *S cerevisiae*. Ty1 is a 5.6-kilobase sequence that is present in the yeast genome in about 35 copies. It carries a repeated sequence 338 base-pairs long at each end; this sequence, in turn, is present in the genome in about 100 copies. Ty1 generates 5-base-pair repeats of target DNA and can inactivate functional genes by insertion.

S cerevisiae has a locus controlling mating type, depending on which allele—a or α—is present. A given strain may switch between the a and α phenotypes, but this change does not reflect mutation. Rather, the a and α genes are separately and silently stored at other specific loci; a copy of the a or α gene is occasionally transposed into the mating-type locus, displacing the preexisting allele and becoming expressed. The a and α genes thus belong to a special class of transposable elements.

Genetic Roles of Transposable Elements

A. Gene Expression: Transposable elements contain transcriptional promoters, transcriptional termination signals, and nonsense codons. Their insertion adjacent to (or within) a functional gene can thus lead to the switching on or switching off of that gene's expression.

The long-known phenomenon of flagellar phase variation in *Salmonella* is explained by the presence of an 800-base-pair sequence that seems closely related to the transposable elements. This sequence, called PD, lies immediately adjacent to an operon containing the gene for the H2 type of flagellin and a repressor of the unlinked gene for the H1 type of flagellin. PD contains a transcriptional promoter; when present in the correct orientation, PD's promoter switches on the H2 gene and the H1 repressor, so that the flagella are made exclusively of the H2 flagellin. Occasionally, however, the PD sequence inverts; now, neither the H2 gene nor the H1 repressor is expressed, and the flagella are made exclusively of H1 flagellin. The inversion event is controlled by a *trans*-acting, closely-linked gene called *rh2*; *rh2* presumably codes for the enzyme catalyzing the inversion.

It has been proposed that sequences closely related to—and perhaps evolved from—transposable elements govern the orderly sequence of gene expression changes that take place during differentiation and that aberrant transposition events may be responsible for the abnormal gene expression associated with some malignant transformations. These are areas of intensive current investigation.

B. Genome Evolution: Evolution depends on the forces of selection acting upon new genes arising by mutation and upon new combinations of genes arising by recombination. In mitotic and meiotic crossing over, recombination takes place by breakage and reunion events within regions of DNA homology. Transposable elements are now seen to provide another mechanism of evolution: blocks of genes become rearranged through transpositions, replicon fusions, deletions, and inversions, independent of sequence homologies. Such rearrangements have apparently played a major role in the evolution of viruses, plasmids, and prokaryotic genomes. The emergence of new, multiple drug resistance R factors is a modern manifestation of this phenomenon.

MOLECULAR CLONING OF DNA

Only part of the DNA of any genome is directly involved in coding for amino acid sequences in proteins. Other, noncoding regions function in such processes as DNA replication, recombination, the control of gene expression, and the structural organization of the chromosome. In many cases, this is accomplished by short base-pair sequences in the DNA that serve as binding sites for specific proteins or RNA molecules; in other cases, it seems likely that recognition sites are provided by secondary structures in the DNA, formed by internal base-pairing in regions of repeated base sequences.

To obtain definitive information concerning such processes, it is necessary to perform a **functional analysis of DNA structure:** Specific segments of DNA of known base-pair sequence must be altered and rearranged in known ways, then reintroduced into host cells or put into in vitro systems to determine the effects of the changes on specific functions. Such functional analysis has been made possible by 3 major technical advances: (1) the ability to determine the complete base-pair sequence of DNA molecules ("DNA sequencing"); (2) the ability to synthesize DNA sequences 20 or more base sequences in length (performed by automatic machines); and (3) the ability to carry out the **molecular cloning of DNA.** These techniques not only permit the functional analysis of DNA structure but also make possible the production in large quantities of almost any desired gene product, eg, otherwise scarce hormones, enzymes, and antigens.

Principles of Molecular Cloning

Molecular cloning involves the following steps, the details of which are discussed below: (1) DNA from any desired source is cleaved into fragments of appropriate size. (2) The fragments are spliced into a **vector,** ie, a circular replicon such as a plasmid or a viral genome. (3) By the process of transformation, the vector is introduced into a host cell in which it can replicate. (4) After replication of the cell and vector, which provides an enormous amplification of the original DNA fragment, the vector is isolated and the inserted

fragment cleaved back out and purified. Alternatively, the host-vector system may be designed so as to permit the efficient expression of genes carried by the foreign DNA segment, with the aim of isolating the gene product rather than the gene itself.

The techniques of molecular cloning are commonly referred to as "recombinant DNA technology."

DNA Splicing

The fragments of DNA to be spliced are provided with **cohesive ends**—short, single-stranded extensions complementary to each other. This can be done by adding complementary homopolymers such as poly-dA to the $3'$ ends of one molecule and poly-dT to the $3'$ ends of another; usually, however, it is done by cleaving the DNA with a **restriction endonuclease.**

The production of cohesive ends by restriction endonucleases is based on their property of making staggered cuts in short palindromic sequences, as illustrated in Fig 4–20. Bacteria produce a wide variety of species-specific endonucleases, each recognizing a different palindromic sequence; by screening through a battery of such enzymes, one can usually find an enzyme that cleaves the vector at a single site and cuts the donor DNA into fragments without cleaving within the base sequence of interest. The fragments and the linearized vector, cleaved with the same restriction endonuclease, are mixed under conditions that promote the annealing (hydrogen bonding) of their complementary ends, following which the gaps are sealed by polynucleotide ligase (Fig 4–20).

Vectors

Molecular cloning of DNA can be done in any propagatable host cells, provided that a suitable vector is available. Animal virus genomes, for example, can be used to clone DNA in animal tissue culture cells, and plasmids are available for cloning in yeast. In bacteria, the vector may be either a plasmid or a bacteriophage genome (bacteriophages are described in Chapter 9).

A. Plasmid Vectors: When a plasmid vector is reintroduced into a host bacterium, it establishes itself as an independent replicon. The "infected" cell then gives rise to a clone, every cell of which contains one or more copies of the vector with its foreign DNA insert. The clone can be expanded by large-scale mass culture, the plasmid DNA reextracted, and the foreign DNA reisolated.

Plasmid vectors have been specially engineered for this purpose. Those in general use now have some or all of the following properties: (1) The plasmid may be amplified to reach 40–50% of the total cellular DNA (up to 2000 copies per cell) by providing a final period of incubation in the presence of chloramphenicol. (2) The plasmid contains one each of several different restriction sites, so that a restriction enzyme suitable for the donor DNA may be chosen. (3) Markers are present that permit the selection of vectors with inserted DNA sequences as well as the selection of host cells that have been infected with the vector. (4) If ex-

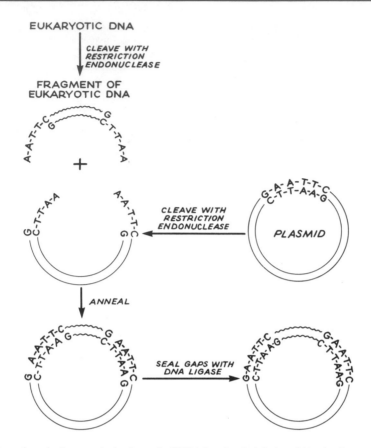

Figure 4–20. The insertion of a fragment of eukaryotic DNA into a bacterial plasmid by in vitro procedures. See text.

pression of an inserted gene is desired, the insertion site is adjacent to a high-efficiency promotor of transcription. (5) The vector contains a minimum of essential plasmid DNA, making room for larger inserts. (An upper size limit is imposed by increasing instability as the size of the overall vector is increased.)

B. Bacteriophage Vectors: The sequence of a bacteriophage such as lambda (see Chapter 9) can be isolated, cleaved with a restriction endonuclease, and spliced to a foreign DNA insert. The phage DNA can then be reintroduced into bacterial host cells, where it undergoes a lytic cycle of infection; the host cells eventually burst, each liberating several hundred infectious virions (protein-coated phage genomes). After repeated cycles of infection have destroyed all host cells, the virions are harvested and their DNA extracted. Alternatively, a phage vector may be used which has been engineered so that it may be propagated either lytically, as described above, or as a nonlytic plasmid.

For virion production, the process by which phage DNA is packaged with the capsid (phage coat) limits to about 10% the amount of DNA that can be added. However, lambda contains a dispensable region amounting to about 25% of its total DNA; replacing this region with foreign DNA allows a total of about 35%, or about 17,000 base-pairs, to be cloned. This method has the added advantage that infectious parti-

cles are formed only from phage genomes carrying DNA inserts, since the correct amount of DNA must be present for packaging to proceed.

Selection of Cloned DNA Segments

In some cases, the segment of DNA to be cloned may be available as a relatively pure material—eg, as cDNA (reverse transcripts of highly purified messenger RNAs), as synthetic DNA molecules, or as DNA fragments that can be purified on the basis of their high copy-number in vivo. In many cases, however, a "shotgun" approach is used: Total DNA is cleaved, all possible fragments are spliced into a population of vector molecules, and this mixture is used to transform host cells. The problem, then, is to detect those clones of bacteria (or phage plaques) that carry the particular sequence of interest.

If a cloned gene is expressed in the host cell, it is often possible to devise a technique that will permit only those cells carrying the desired gene to form colonies. In most cases, however, the gene is not expressed and can only be detected by the use of a "probe," consisting of radioactive RNA or DNA complementary to the sequence of interest. Colonies of cells or phage plaques are produced on nitrocellulose filters, denatured in situ, and their DNA allowed to anneal with the probe. The filters are washed to remove excess, nonannealed probe; autoradiography then reveals those clones containing DNA complementary to the probe, and live cells or viruses are recovered from replica plates made beforehand.

Radioactive probes depend on the availability of a small amount of a radioactive RNA or DNA complementary to part or all of the sequence of interest. In many cases, such probes are obtained as mRNA (or DNA made by reverse transcription of mRNA), isolated from specialized cells in which that mRNA is a major species. The availability of techniques for synthesizing DNA molecules of any desired sequence up to 20 or more bases in length, however, adds another approach: If one knows the amino acid sequence of the polypeptide coded for by the gene in question, the DNA sequence of that gene can be deduced and a portion of it synthesized for use as a probe.

Expression of Cloned DNA

Transcription of the cloned DNA will occur if the inserted fragment carries its own promoter (RNA polymerase binding site) or if the vector carries a properly spaced promoter adjacent to the insertion site. The correct translation of eukaryotic sequences, however, requires that the host system possess the enzyme for processing RNA transcripts; thus, prokaryotic host cells cannot be used to express cloned eukaryotic genes that contain introns. For such genes, translation

in bacterial host cells is made possible by the cloning of cDNA made from mRNA that has already been processed in the eukaryotic donor cell.

Genes & DNA Segments Cloned

The rapid development of improvements in cloning techniques has made the list of cloned segments much too long to tabulate here, and the list is increasing rapidly. The techniques lend themselves to commercial applications, since microorganisms expressing genes that code for useful products can be grown on a scale of tens of thousands of gallons. The commercial production of a variety of medically useful hormones and antigens, as well as many industrially useful enzymes, is being developed using microorganisms carrying cloned segments of DNA.

Recombinant DNA technology is also being used to produce improved strains of microorganisms for use in industrial processes such as fermentations and biochemical conversions. It will almost certainly be used to produce improved strains of plants, thanks to the Ti plasmid of *A tumefaciens,* and holds promise for animal husbandry as well. Finally, recombinant DNA technology opens the way to future applications in the treatment of human genetic disease as a source of normal genes for gene replacement therapy.

REFERENCES

Books

Adelberg E (editor): *Papers on Bacterial Genetics,* 2nd ed. Little, Brown, 1966.

Alberts B et al: *Molecular Biology of the Cell.* Garland, 1983.

Bennett PM, Grinsted J (editors): *Methods in Microbiology.* Vol 17: *Plasmid Technology.* Academic Press, 1984.

Bryan LE (editor): *Antimicrobial Drug Resistance.* Academic Press, 1984.

Caskey CT, White RL (editors): *Recombinant DNA Applications to Human Disease.* Cold Spring Harbor Laboratory, 1983.

Cold Spring Harbor Symposia on Quantitative Biology: Vol 45: *Moveable Genetic Elements,* 1981; Vol 47: *Structures of DNA,* 1983. Cold Spring Harbor Laboratory.

Dubnau DA (editor): *The Molecular Biology of the Bacilli.* Vol 1, 1982; Vol 2, 1985. Academic Press.

Emery A: *An Introduction to Recombinant DNA.* Wiley, 1985.

Freifelder D: *Molecular Biology: A Comprehensive Introduction to Prokaryotes and Eukaryotes.* Science Books International, 1983.

Ganesan AT, Chang S, Hoch JA: *Molecular Cloning and Gene Regulation in Bacilli.* Academic Press, 1982.

Goldberger RF (editor): *Biological Regulation and Development.* Vol 1: *Gene Expression,* 1978; Vol 2: *Molecular Organization and Cell Function,* 1980. Plenum.

Hardy K: *Bacterial Plasmids.* American Society for Microbiology, 1981.

Hofschneider PH, Goebel W (editors): *Gene Cloning in Organisms Other Than* Escherichia coli. Springer-Verlag, 1982.

Hubscher U (editor): *Proteins Involved in DNA Replication.* Plenum, 1984.

Inouye M (editor): *Experimental Manipulation of Gene Expression.* Academic Press, 1983.

King RC, Stansfield WD: *A Dictionary of Genetics,* 3rd ed. Oxford Univ Press, 1985.

Kornberg A: *DNA Replication.* Freeman, 1980.

Kornberg A: *1982 Supplement to DNA Replication.* Freeman, 1982.

Kosuge T, Nester E (editors): *Plant-Microbe Interactions: Molecular and Genetic Perspectives.* Vol 1. Macmillan, 1984.

Levy SB, Clowes RC, Koenig EL (editors): *Molecular Biology, Pathogenicity and Ecology of Bacterial Plasmids.* Plenum, 1981.

Lewin B: *Gene Expression.* Vol 1: *Bacterial Genomes,* 1974; Vol 2: *Eukaryotic Chromosomes,* 2nd ed. 1980; Vol 3: *Plasmids and Phages,* 1977. Wiley-Interscience.

Maniatis T: *Molecular Cloning: A Laboratory Manual.* Cold Spring Harbor Laboratory, 1982.

Miller JH, Reznikoff WS: *The Operon,* 2nd ed. Cold Spring Harbor Laboratory, 1980.

Mitsuhashi S, Hashimoto H (editors): *Microbial Drug Resistance.* Vol 1, 1976; Vol 2, 1979. University Park Press.

Morrow J: *Eukaryotic Cell Genetics.* Academic Press, 1983.

Oliver SG, Brown TA: *Microbial Extrachromosomal Genetics.* American Society for Microbiology, 1985.

Ray D (editor): *The Initiation of DNA Replication.* Academic Press, 1981.

Razin AM, Cedar H, Riggs AD (editors): *DNA Methylation: Biochemistry and Biological Significance.* Springer-Verlag, 1984.

Scaife J, Leach D (editors): *Genetics of Bacteria.* Academic Press, 1985.

Setlow JK, Hollander A (editors): *Genetic Engineering, Prin-*

ciples and Methods. Vol 1, 1979; Vol 2, 1980; Vol 3, 1981; Vol 4, 1982; Vol 5, 1983; Vol 6, 1984. Plenum.

Shapiro JA (editor): *Mobile Genetic Elements.* Academic Press, 1983.

Simon M, Herskowitz I (editors): *Genome Rearrangement.* Alan R. Liss, 1985.

Spencer JFT, Spencer DM, Smith ARW (editors): *Yeast Genetics: Fundamental and Applied Aspects.* Springer-Verlag, 1983.

Stein G, Stein J (editors): *Recombinant DNA and Cell Proliferation.* Academic Press, 1984.

Stent GS, Calendar R: *Molecular Genetics, An Introductory Narrative,* 2nd ed. Freeman, 1978.

Strathern JN et al (editors): *The Molecular Biology of the Yeast* Saccharomyces. Cold Spring Harbor Laboratory, 1981.

Trautner TA (editor): *Methylation of DNA.* Springer-Verlag, 1984.

Watson JD: *The Molecular Biology of the Gene,* 3rd ed. Benjamin, 1976.

Watson JD, Tooze J, Kurtz DT: *Recombinant DNA: A Short Course.* Freeman, 1983.

Whitehouse HLK: *Genetic Recombination: Understanding the Mechanism.* Wiley, 1982.

Williamson R: *Genetic Engineering.* Vols 1 and 2, 1981; Vol 3, 1982; Vol 4, 1983. Academic Press.

Wu R, Grossman L, Moldave K (editors): *Recombinant DNA,* Parts B and C. Vols 100 and 101 of: *Methods in Enzymology.* Academic Press, 1983.

Articles & Reviews

Bachmann BJ: Linkage map of *Escherichia coli* K-12, edition 7. *Microbiol Rev* 1983;**47:**180.

Bevan MW, Chilton MD: T-DNA of the *Agrobacterium* Ti and Ri plasmids. *Annu Rev Genet* 1982;**16:**357.

Birky CW: Transmission genetics of mitochondria and chloroplasts. *Annu Rev Genet* 1978;**12:**471.

Botstein D, Maurer R: Genetic approaches to the analysis of microbial development. *Annu Rev Genet* 1982;**16:**61.

Brill WJ: Biochemical genetics of nitrogen fixation. *Microbiol Rev* 1980;**44:**499.

Calos MP, Miller JH: Transposable elements. *Cell* 1980;**20:**579.

Campbell A: Evolutionary significance of accessory DNA elements in bacteria. *Annu Rev Microbiol* 1981;**35:**55.

Chernin LS et al: Effects of plasmids on chromosome metabolism in bacteria. *Plasmid* 1981;**6:**119.

Clark AJ, Warren GJ: Conjugal transmission of plasmids. *Annu Rev Genet* 1979;**13:**99.

Clewell DB: Plasmids, drug resistance, and gene transfer in the genus *Streptococcus. Microbiol Rev* 1981;**45:**409.

Cohen SN, Shapiro JA: Transposable genetic elements. *Sci Am* (Feb) 1980;**242:**40.

Crosa JH: The relationship of plasmid-mediated iron transport and bacterial virulence. *Annu Rev Microbiol* 1984;**38:**69.

Dawid IB et al: Application of recombinant DNA technology to questions of developmental biology: A review. *Dev Biol* 1979;**69:**305.

Dressler D, Potter H: Molecular mechanisms in genetic recombination. *Annu Rev Biochem* 1982;**51:**727.

Elander RP: New genetic approaches to industrially important fungi. *Biotechnol Bioeng* 1980;**22(Suppl 1):**49.

Elwell LP, Shipley PL: Plasmid-mediated factors associated with virulence of bacteria to animals. *Annu Rev Microbiol* 1980;**34:**465.

Foster TJ: Plasmid-determined resistance to antimicrobial

drugs and toxic metal ions in bacteria. *Microbial Rev* 1983;**47:**361.

Goodgal SH: DNA uptake in *Haemophilus* transformation. *Annu Rev Genet* 1982;**16:**169.

Gunge N: Yeast DNA plasmids. *Annu Rev Microbiol* 1983;**37:**253.

Hardy KG: Colicinogeny and related phenomena. *Bacteriol Rev* 1975;**39:**464.

Helinski DR: Bacterial plasmids: Autonomous replication and vehicles for gene cloning. *CRC Crit Rev Biochem* 1979;**7:**83.

Henner BJ et al: *The Bacillus subtilis* chromosome. *Microbiol Rev* 1980;**44:**57.

Herskowitz I: Cellular differentiation, cell lineages and transposable genetic cassettes in yeast. *Curr Top Dev Biol* 1983;**18:**1.

Hopwood DA: Extrachromosomally determined antibiotic production. *Annu Rev Microbiol* 1978;**32:**373.

Hopwood DA: Genetic studies with bacterial protoplasts. *Annu Rev Microbiol* 1981;**35:**237.

Kimball RF: The relation of repair phenomena to mutation induction in bacteria. *Mutat Res* 1978;**55:**85.

Kleckner N: Transposable elements in prokaryotes. *Annu Rev Genet* 1981;**15:**341.

Loeb LA, Kunkel TA: Fidelity of DNA synthesis. *Annu Rev Biochem* 1982;**52:**429.

Miller JH: Mutational specificity in bacteria. *Annu Rev Genet* 1983;**17:**215.

Nester EW, Kosuge T: Plasmids specifying plant hyperplasias. *Annu Rev Microbiol* 1981;**35:**531.

Nossal NG: Prokaryotic DNA replication systems. *Annu Rev Biochem* 1983;**52:**581.

Pemberton JM: Degradative plasmids. *Int Rev Cytol* 1983;**84:**155.

Petes TD: Molecular genetics of yeast. *Annu Rev Biochem* 1980;**49:**845.

Piggot PJ, Hoch JA: Revised genetic linkage map of *Bacillus subtilis. Microbiol Rev* 1985;**49:**158.

Potter H et al: Mechanisms in generalized genetic recombination. *Prog Clin Biol Res* 1982;**102:**109.

Radding CM: Homologous pairing and strand exchange in genetic recombination. *Annu Rev Genet* 1982;**16:**405.

Radding CM: Recombination activities of *Escherichia coli* recA protein. *Cell* 1981;**25:**3.

Radman M, Wagner R: Effects of DNA methylation on mismatch repair, mutagenesis and recombination in *Escherichia coli. Curr Top Microbiol Immunol* 1984;**108:**23.

Radman M et al: Replication fidelity: Mechanisms of mutation avoidance and mutation fixation. *Cold Spring Harbor Symp Quant Biol* 1979;**43:**937.

Riggs AD et al: Synthesis, cloning and expression of hormone genes in *Escherichia coli. Recent Prog Horm Res* 1980;**36:**261.

Ripley LS: The specificity of DNA polymerase. *Basic Life Sci* 1983;**23:**83.

Roberts RJ: Restriction and modification enzymes and their recognition sequences. *Gene* 1980;**8:**329.

Sanderson KE, Roth JR: Linkage map of *Salmonella typhimurium. Microbiol Rev* 1983;**47:**410.

Schwesinger MD: Additive recombination in bacteria. *Bacteriol Rev* 1977;**41:**872.

Scott JR: Regulation of plasmid replication. *Microbiol Rev* 1984;**48:**1.

Shapiro JA: Changes in gene order and gene expression. *Natl Cancer Inst Monogr* 1982;**60:**87.

Singer B: Mutagenic effects of nucleic acid modification repair assessed by in vitro transcription. *Basic Life Sci* 1983;**23**:1.

Singer B, Kusmierek JT: Chemical mutagenesis. *Annu Rev Biochem* 1982;**52**:655.

Smith GR: Chi hotspots of generalized recombination. *Cell* 1983;**34**:709.

Smith HO, Danner DB, Deich RA: Genetic transformation. *Annu Rev Biochem* 1981;**50**:41.

Walker GC: Mutagenesis and inducible responses to DNA damage in *Escherichia coli*. *Microbiol Rev* 1984;**48**:60.

Walker GC et al: Regulation and function of cellular gene products involved in UV and chemical mutagenesis in *Escherichia coli*. *Basic Life Sci* 1983;**23**:181.

Willetts N, Skurray R: The conjugation system of F-like plasmids. *Annu Rev Genet* 1980;**14**:41.

Willetts N et al: Processing of plasmid DNA during bacterial conjugation. *Microbiol Rev* 1984;**48**:24.

Williamson VM: Transposable elements in yeast. *Int Rev Cytol* 1983;**83**:1.

5

The Growth, Survival, & Death of Microorganisms

SURVIVAL OF MICROORGANISMS IN THE NATURAL ENVIRONMENT

The population of microorganisms in the biosphere is roughly constant: growth is counterbalanced by death. The survival of any microbial group within its niche is determined in large part by successful competition for nutrients and by maintenance of a pool of living cells during nutritional deprivation. It is increasingly evident that many microorganisms exist in consortia formed by representatives of different genera. Other microorganisms, often characterized as single cells in the laboratory, form cohesive colonies in the natural environment.

Most of our understanding of microbial physiology has come from the study of isolated cell lines growing under optimal conditions, and this knowledge forms the basis for this section. Nevertheless, it should be remembered that many microorganisms compete in the natural environment while under nutritional stress, a circumstance that may lead to a physiologic state quite unlike that observed in the laboratory. Furthermore, it should be recognized that a vacant microbial niche in the environment will soon be filled. Public health procedures that eliminate pathogenic microorganisms by clearing their niche are likely to be less successful than methods that leave the niche occupied by successful nonpathogenic competitors.

THE MEANING OF GROWTH

Growth is the orderly increase in the sum of all of the components of an organism. Thus, the increase in size that results when a cell takes up water or deposits lipid or polysaccharide is not true growth. Cell multiplication is a consequence of growth; in unicellular organisms, growth leads to an increase in the number of individuals making up a population or culture.

The Measurement of Microbial Concentrations

Microbial concentrations can be measured in terms of cell concentration (the number of viable cells per unit volume of culture) or of biomass concentration (dry weight of cells per unit volume of culture). These 2 parameters are not always equivalent, because the average dry weight of the cell varies at different stages in the history of a culture. Nor are they of equal

significance: in studies of microbial genetics or the inactivation of cells, cell concentration is the significant quantity; in studies on microbial biochemistry or nutrition, biomass concentration is the significant quantity.

A. Cell Concentration: The viable cell count (Table 5–1) is usually considered the measure of cell concentration. However, for many purposes the turbidity of a culture, measured by photoelectric means, may be related to the viable count in the form of a **standard curve.** A rough visual estimate is sometimes possible: a barely turbid suspension of *Escherichia coli* contains about 10^7 cells per milliliter, and a fairly turbid suspension contains about 10^8 cells per milliliter. In using turbidimetric measurements, it must be remembered that the correlation between turbidity and viable count can vary during the growth and death of a culture; cells may lose viability without producing a loss in turbidity of the culture.

B. Biomass Density: In principle, biomass can be measured directly by determining the dry weight of a microbial culture after it has been washed with distilled water. In practice, this procedure is cumbersome, and the investigator customarily prepares a standard curve that correlates dry weight with turbidity. Alternatively, the concentration of biomass can be estimated indirectly by measuring an important cellular component such as protein or by determining the volume occupied by cells that have settled out of suspension.

EXPONENTIAL GROWTH

The Growth Rate Constant

The growth rate of cells unlimited by nutrient is first-order: the rate of growth (measured in grams of biomass produced per hour) is the product of the

Table 5–1. Example of a viable count.

Dilution	Plate Count*
Undiluted	Too crowded
10^{-1}	to count
10^{-2}	510
10^{-3}	72
10^{-4}	6
10^{-5}	1

*Each count is the average of 3 replicate plates.

growth rate constant, k, and the biomass concentration, B:

$$\frac{dB}{dt} = kB \qquad \ldots (1)$$

Rearrangement of equation (1) demonstrates that the growth rate constant is the rate at which cells are producing more cells:

$$k = \frac{Bdt}{dB} \qquad \ldots (2)$$

A growth rate constant of 4.3 h^{-1}, one of the highest recorded, means that each gram of cells produces 4.3 g of cells per hour during this period of growth. Slowly growing organisms may have growth rate constants as low as 0.02 h^{-1}. With this growth rate constant, each gram of cells in the culture produces 0.02 g of cells per hour.

Integration of equation (1) yields

$$\ln \frac{B_1}{B_0} = 2.3 \log_{10} \frac{B_1}{B_0} = k(t_1 - t_0) \qquad \ldots (3)$$

The logarithm of the ratio of B_1 (the biomass at time 1 [t_1]) to B_0 (the biomass at time zero [t_0]) is equal to the product of the growth rate constant (k) and the difference in time ($t_1 - t_0$). Growth obeying equation (3) is termed exponential because biomass increases exponentially with respect to time. Linear plots of exponential growth can be produced by plotting the logarithm of biomass concentration (B) as a function of time (t).

Calculation of the Growth Rate Constant & Prediction of the Amount of Growth

Many bacteria reproduce by binary fission, and the average time required for the population, or the biomass, to double is known as the **generation time** or **doubling time** (t_D). Usually the t_D is determined by plotting the amount of growth on a semilogarithmic scale as a function of time; the time required for doubling the biomass is t_D (Fig 5–1). The growth rate constant can be calculated from the doubling time by substituting the value 2 for B_1/B_0 and t_D for ($t_1 - t_0$) in equation (3), which yields

$$\ln 2 = kt_D$$

$$k = \frac{\ln 2}{t_D} \qquad \ldots (4)$$

A rapid doubling time corresponds to a high growth rate constant. For example, a doubling time of 0.16 h corresponds to a growth rate constant of 4.3 h^{-1}. The relatively long doubling time of 35 hours corresponds to a growth rate constant of 0.02 h^{-1}.

The calculated growth rate constant can be used either to determine the amount of growth that will occur

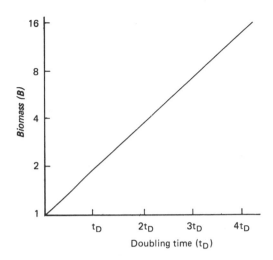

Figure 5–1. Exponential growth. The biomass (B) doubles with each doubling time (t_D).

in a specified period of time or to calculate the amount of time required for a specified amount of growth.

The amount of growth within a specified period of time can be predicted on the basis of the following rearrangement of equation (3):

$$\log_{10} \frac{B_1}{B_0} = \frac{k(t_1 - t_0)}{2.3} \qquad \ldots (5)$$

For example, it is possible to determine the amount of growth that would occur if a culture with a growth rate constant of 4.3 h^{-1} grew exponentially for 5 hours:

$$\log_{10} \frac{B_1}{B_0} = \frac{4.3 \text{ h}^{-1} \times 5 \text{ h}}{2.3} \qquad \ldots (6)$$

In this example, the increase in biomass is 2×10^9; a single bacterial cell with a dry weight of 2×10^{-13} g would give rise to 0.4 mg of biomass, a quantity that would densely populate a 5-mL culture. Clearly, this rate of growth cannot be sustained for a long period of time. Another 5 hours of growth at this rate would produce 8×10^5 g dry weight of biomass, roughly a ton of cells.

Another rearrangement of equation (3) allows calculation of the amount of time required for a specified amount of growth to take place. In equation (7), shown below, N, cell concentration, is substituted for B, biomass concentration, to permit calculation of the time required for a specified increase in cell number.

$$t_1 - t_0 = \frac{2.3 \log_{10} (N_1/N_0)}{k} \qquad \ldots (7)$$

Using equation (7), it is possible, for example, to determine the time required for a slowly growing organism with a growth rate constant of 0.02 h^{-1} to grow from a single cell into a barely turbid cell suspension with a concentration of 10^7 cells/mL.

$$t_1 - t_0 = \frac{2.3 \times 7}{0.02h^{-1}} \qquad \ldots (8)$$

Solution of equation (8) reveals that about 800 hours—slightly more than a month—would be required for this amount of growth to occur. The survival of slowly growing organisms implies that the race for biologic survival is not always to the swift—those species flourish that compete successfully for nutrients and avoid annihilation by predators and other environmental hazards.

THE GROWTH CURVE

If a liquid medium is inoculated with microbial cells taken from a culture that has previously been grown to saturation and the number of viable cells per milliliter determined periodically and plotted, a curve of the type shown in Fig 5–2 is usually obtained. The curve may be discussed in terms of 6 phases, represented by the letters A–F (Table 5–2).

The Lag Phase (A)

The lag phase represents a period during which the cells, depleted of metabolites and enzymes as the result of the unfavorable conditions that obtained at the end of their previous culture history, adapt to their new environment. Enzymes and intermediates are formed and accumulate until they are present in concentrations that permit growth to resume.

If the cells are taken from an entirely different medium, it often happens that they are genetically incapable of growth in the new medium. In such cases a long lag may occur, representing the period necessary for a few mutants in the inoculum to multiply sufficiently for a net increase in cell number to be apparent.

The Exponential Phase (C)

During the exponential phase, the mathematics of which has already been discussed, the cells are in a

Table 5–2. Phases of microbial death curve.

Section of Curve	Phase	Growth Rate
A	Lag	Zero
B	Acceleration	Increasing
C	Exponential	Constant
D	Retardation	Decreasing
E	Maximum stationary	Zero
F	Decline	Negative (death)

steady state. New cell material is being synthesized at a constant rate, but the new material is itself catalytic, and the mass increases in an exponential manner. This continues until one of 2 things happens: Either one or more nutrients in the medium become exhausted, or toxic metabolic products accumulate and inhibit growth. For aerobic organisms, the nutrient that becomes limiting is usually oxygen: When the cell concentration exceeds about 1×10^7/mL (in the case of bacteria), the growth rate will decrease unless oxygen is forced into the medium by agitation or by bubbling in air. When the bacterial concentration reaches $4-5 \times 10^9$/mL, the rate of oxygen diffusion cannot meet the demand even in an aerated medium, and growth is progressively slowed.

The Maximum Stationary Phase (E)

Eventually, the exhaustion of nutrients or the accumulation of toxic products causes growth to cease completely. In most cases, however, cell turnover takes place in the stationary phase: there is a slow loss of cells through death, which is just balanced by the formation of new cells through growth and division. When this occurs, the total cell count slowly increases although the viable count stays constant.

The Phase of Decline (The Death Phase, F)

After a period of time in the stationary phase, which varies with the organism and with the culture conditions, the death rate increases until it reaches a steady level. The mathematics of steady-state death are discussed below. Frequently, after the majority of cells have died, the death rate decreases drastically, so that a small number of survivors may persist for months or even years. This persistence may in some cases reflect cell turnover, a few cells growing at the expense of nutrients released from cells that die and lyse.

THE MAINTENANCE OF CELLS IN EXPONENTIAL PHASE

Cells can be maintained in exponential phase by transferring them repeatedly into fresh medium of identical composition while they are still growing exponentially. Two devices have been invented for carrying out this process automatically: the chemostat and the turbidostat.

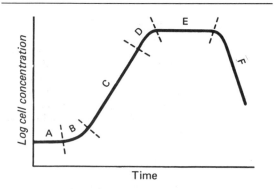

Figure 5–2. Cell concentration curve.

The Chemostat

This device consists of a culture vessel equipped with an overflow siphon and a mechanism for dripping in fresh medium from a reservoir at a regulated rate. The medium in the culture vessel is stirred by a stream of sterile air; each drop of fresh medium that enters causes a drop of culture to siphon out.

The medium is prepared so that one nutrient limits growth yield. The vessel is inoculated, and the cells grow until the limiting nutrient is exhausted; fresh medium from the reservoir is then allowed to flow in at such a rate that the cells use up the limiting nutrient as fast as it is supplied. Under these conditions, the cell concentration remains constant and the growth rate is directly proportionate to the flow rate of the medium.

The chemostat thus provides a steady-state culture of exponentially growing cells and permits regulation of the growth rate. However, its disadvantage is that growing cells are always in a state of semistarvation for one nutrient and must be grown at less than maximum rate to achieve good regulation. These disadvantages are not present in the turbidostat.

The Turbidostat

This device resembles the chemostat except that the flow of medium is controlled by a photoelectric mechanism that measures the turbidity of the culture. When the turbidity exceeds the chosen level, fresh medium is allowed to flow in. Thus, the cells can grow at maximum rate at a constant cell concentration. The growth rate can be controlled in the turbidostat only by varying the nature of the medium or the culture conditions (eg, temperature).

SYNCHRONOUS GROWTH

In ordinary cultures, the cells are growing nonsynchronously: at any moment, cells are present in every possible stage of the division cycle. The culture must be synchronized if one is to study the sequence of events occurring in a single cell during the division cycle.

Synchrony has been achieved for a variety of microorganisms by several techniques. Some microorganisms, for example, go through one or 2 synchronous divisions when diluted from a stationary phase culture into fresh medium. In many cases, however, it is necessary to bring the cells into synchrony by a more involved process. Pneumococci, for example, will divide synchronously after several alternating periods of incubation at high and low temperature. E coli has been synchronized by 2 different methods: in one, a thymine-requiring mutant is starved for thymine until viability begins to drop. Replacing thymine in the culture then causes the surviving cells to undergo several synchronous divisions. In the other method, a heavy cell suspension is deposited in a filter paper pile. As the adsorbed cells divide, the newly formed daughter cells are released from the filter paper; they can be recovered as a synchronously dividing population by washing the paper briefly with warm medium.

Synchrony only persists for 1–4 cycles. After that time, the cells become more and more out of phase until their division times become completely random.

GROWTH PARAMETERS

Physiologic studies may be carried out by introducing controlled variations in individual environmental factors and then quantitatively determining the effect of such variations on bacterial growth. To be most useful, experiments of this type should involve determination of meaningful growth parameters. Growth parameters that may be determined include total growth and exponential growth rate.

Total Growth

A culture eventually stops growing when one of 3 things occurs: (1) one or more nutrients are exhausted; (2) toxic products accumulate; or (3) an unfavorable ion equilibrium develops (eg, unfavorable pH).

If total growth (G) is limited by exhaustion of a nutrient, then

$$G = KC \qquad \ldots (9)$$

where K is a constant and C is the initial concentration of the limiting nutrient. Such an equation implies a straight-line relationship between C and G.

Exponential Growth Rates

If some nutrient is initially present at a sufficiently low concentration, metabolic intermediates will be formed at a limited rate and the overall growth rate will be a function of the concentration of the limiting nutrient. Experiments show that a hyperbolic curve results, in accordance with the following general equation:

$$R = R_K \frac{C}{C_1 + C} \qquad \ldots (10)$$

where R = Growth rate
R_K = Maximum rate reached with increasing concentration of nutrient
C = Concentration of the limiting nutrient
C_1 = Value of C at which $R = \frac{1}{2} R_K$

Total growth is a useful parameter in many microbial assays, for example, in the assay of a vitamin or a carbon source in some natural material. For most physiologic studies, however, growth rate is the most meaningful parameter. One method, for example, is to compare concentrations of nutrients or inhibitors that give half-maximal growth rates.

DEFINITION & MEASUREMENT OF DEATH

The Meaning of Death

For a microbial cell, death means the irreversible loss of the ability to reproduce (grow and divide). The empiric test of death is the culture of cells on solid media: a cell is considered dead if it fails to give rise to a colony on any medium. Obviously, then, the reliability of the test depends upon choice of medium and conditions: A culture in which 99% of the cells appear "dead" in terms of ability to form colonies on one medium may prove to be 100% viable if tested on another medium. Furthermore, the detection of a few viable cells in a large clinical specimen may not be possible by directly plating a sample, as the sample fluid itself may be inhibitory to microbial growth. In such cases, the sample may have to be diluted first into liquid medium, permitting the outgrowth of viable cells before plating.

The conditions of incubation in the first hour following treatment are also critical in the determination of "killing." For example, if bacterial cells are irradiated with ultraviolet light and plated immediately on any medium, it may appear that 99.99% of the cells have been killed. If such irradiated cells are first incubated in a suitable buffer for 20 minutes, however, plating will indicate only 10% killing. In other words, irradiation determines that a cell will "die" if plated immediately but will live if allowed to repair radiation damage before plating.

A microbial cell that is not physically disrupted is thus "dead" only in terms of the conditions used to test viability.

The Measurement of Death

When dealing with microorganisms, one does not customarily measure the death of an individual cell but the death of a population. This is a statistical problem: Under any condition that may lead to cell death, the probability of a given cell's dying is constant per unit time. For example, if a condition is employed that causes 90% of the cells to die in the first 10 minutes, the probability of any one cell dying in a 10-minute interval is 0.9. Thus, it may be expected that 90% of the surviving cells will die in each succeeding 10-minute interval, and a death curve similar to those shown in Fig 5–3 will be obtained.

The number of cells dying in each time interval is thus a function of the number of survivors present, so that death of a population proceeds as an exponential process according to the general formula

$$S = S_0e^{-kt} \qquad \ldots (11)$$

where S_0 is the number of survivors at time zero, and S is the number of survivors at any later time t. As in the case of exponential growth, $-k$ represents the rate of exponential death when the fraction $ln\ (S/S_0)$ is plotted against time.

The one-hit curve shown in Fig 5–3A is typical of the kinetics of inactivation observed with many an-

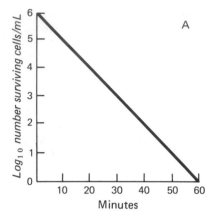

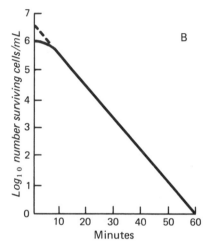

Figure 5–3. Death curve of microorganisms. *A:* Single-hit curve. *B:* Multi-hit curve. The straight-line portion extrapolates to 6.5, corresponding to 4×10^6 cells. The number of targets is thus 4×10^6, or 4 per cell.

timicrobial agents. The fact that it is a straight line from time zero (dose zero)—rather than exhibiting an initial shoulder—means that a single "hit" by the inactivating agent is sufficient to kill the cell, ie, only a single target must be damaged in order for the entire cell to be inactivated. Such a target might be the chromosome of a uninucleate bacterium or the cell membrane; conversely, it could not be an enzyme or other cell constituent that is present in multiple copies.

A cell that contains several copies of the target to be inactivated exhibits a multi-hit curve of the type shown in Fig 5–3B. Extrapolation of the straight-line portion of the curve to the ordinate permits an estimate of the number of targets (eg, 4 in Fig 5–3B).

Sterilization

In practice, we speak of "sterilization" as the process of killing all of the organisms in a preparation. From the above considerations, however, we see that no set of conditions is guaranteed to sterilize a preparation. Consider Fig 5–3, for example. At 60 minutes, there is one organism (10^0) left per milliliter. At 70 minutes there would be 10^{-1}, at 80 minutes 10^{-2}, etc. By 10^{-2} organisms per milliliter we mean that in a total volume of 100 mL, one organism would survive. How long, then, does it take to "sterilize" the culture? All we can say is that after any given time of treatment, the probability of having any surviving organisms in 1 mL is that given by the curve. After 2 hours, in the above example, the probability is 1×10^{-6}. This would usually be considered a safe sterilization time, but a thousand-liter lot might still contain one viable organism.

Note that such calculations depend upon the curve's remaining unchanged in slope over the entire time range. Unfortunately, it is very common for the curve to bend upward after a certain period, as a result of the population being heterogeneous with respect to sensitivity to the inactivation agent. Extrapolations are dangerous and can lead to errors such as those encountered in early preparations of sterile poliovaccine.

The Effect of Drug Concentration

When antimicrobial substances (drugs) are used to inactivate microbial cells, it is commonly observed that the concentration of drug employed is related to the time required to kill a given fraction of the population by the following expression:

$$C^n t = K \qquad \ldots (12)$$

In this equation, C is the drug concentration, t is the time required to kill a given fraction of the cells, and n and K are constants.

This expression says that, for example, if $n = 5$ (as it is for phenol), then doubling the concentration of the drug will reduce the time required to achieve the same extent of inactivation 32-fold. That the effectiveness of a drug varies with the fifth power of the concentration suggests that 5 molecules of the drug are required to inactivate a cell, although there is no direct chemical evidence for this conclusion.

In order to determine the value of n for any drug, inactivation curves are obtained for each of several concentrations, and the time required at each concentration to inactivate a fixed fraction of the population is determined. For example, let the first concentration used be C_1 and the time required to inactivate 99% of the cells be t_1. Similarly, let C_2 and t_2 be the second concentration and time required to inactivate 99% of the cells. From equation (12), we see that

$$C_1{}^n t_1 = C_2{}^n t_2 \qquad \ldots (13)$$

Solving for n gives

$$n = \frac{\log t_2 - \log t_1}{\log C_1 - \log C_2}$$

Thus, n can be determined by measuring the slope of the line that results when $\log t$ is plotted against $\log C$ (Fig 5–4). If n is experimentally determined in this manner, K can be determined by substituting observed values for C, t, and n in equation (12).

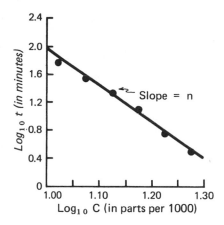

Figure 5–4. Relationship between drug concentration and time required to kill a given fraction of a cell population.

ANTIMICROBIAL AGENTS

Definitions

The following terms are commonly employed in connection with antimicrobial agents and their uses.

A. Bacteriostatic: Having the property of inhibiting bacterial multiplication; multiplication resumes upon removal of the agent.

B. Bactericidal: Having the property of killing bacteria. Bactericidal action differs from bacteriostasis only in being irreversible; ie, the "killed" organism can no longer reproduce, even after being removed from contact with the agent. In some cases the agent causes lysis (dissolving) of the cells; in other cases the cells remain intact and may even continue to be metabolically active.

C. Sterile: Free of life of every kind. Sterilization may be accomplished by filtration (in the case of liquids or air) or by treatment with microbicidal agents. Since the criterion of death for microorganisms is the inability to reproduce, sterile material may contain intact, metabolizing microbial cells.

D. Disinfectant: A chemical substance used to kill microorganisms on surfaces but too toxic to be applied directly to tissues.

E. Septic: Characterized by the presence of pathogenic microbes in living tissue.

F. Aseptic: Characterized by absence of pathogenic microbes.

Modes of Action

A. Damage to DNA: A number of antimicrobial agents act by damaging DNA; these include ionizing radiations, ultraviolet light, and DNA-reactive chemicals. Among the last category are alkylating agents and other compounds that react covalently with purine and pyrimidine bases to form DNA adducts or interstrand cross-links. Radiations damage DNA in several ways: ultraviolet light, for example, induces cross-linking between adjacent pyrimidines on one or the other of the 2 polynucleotide strands, forming pyrimidine dimers; ionizing radiations produce breaks in single and double strands. Radiation- and chemically-induced DNA lesions kill the cell mainly by interfering with DNA replication.

All living cells possess both constitutive and inducible **DNA repair enzyme systems.** For example, bacteria possess several systems for the repair of DNA that contains pyrimidine dimers. One system, called **photoreactivation,** consists of an enzyme that cleaves the pyrimidine dimers. This enzyme is activated by visible light; hence, cells that have been "killed" by ultraviolet light can be reactivated by exposure to intense light of wavelength 400 nm. A second system is called the **excision repair system.** It requires the action of 4 enzymes operating in succession: (1) a specific endonuclease, which makes single-strand cuts on either side of the dimer, excising it from the DNA; (2) a 3′ exonuclease, which widens the gap in the DNA strand by sequential digestion; (3) DNA polymerase, which fills in the gap by lengthening the 3′ end, using the opposite strand as template; and (4) polynucleotide ligase, which rejoins the free ends.

Both photoreactivation and excision repair function in nonreplicated DNA duplexes. Replication of DNA past an unrepaired lesion (pyrimidine dimer) will usually be lethal, since it will produce a new duplex with a gap opposite a dimer; nevertheless, one or more repair systems exist for **postreplicative repair.** One of these systems is recombinational: it catalyzes the exchange of undamaged segments between daughter duplexes. Another system, called "SOS repair," is part of a complex, induced set of reactions to DNA damage collectively called the **SOS response.** The SOS response begins with enzymatic cleavage and partial digestion of one DNA strand, leaving a single-stranded region on the other. The recA protein (product of the *recA* gene) binds to the single-stranded DNA and is converted to an active form with 2 unrelated functions: It initiates recombinational events, and it acts as a protease, cleaving certain repressors. Some of these are repressors of prophages, such as λ; others are repressors of genes whose products are involved in DNA repair. The end result of the SOS response is thus 3-fold: (1) the rate of recombination is greatly increased; (2) prophages are induced to enter the vegetative phase (see Chapter 9); and (3) DNA repair systems are induced.

One or more of the inducible repair systems is **error-prone,** resulting in the appearance of induced mutations (see Chapter 4). The induced error-prone system appears to involve a modified DNA polymerase system that is capable of replicating past a pyrimidine dimer to form an intact daughter strand but does so with less fidelity than the normal polymerase system.

Bacteria also possess inducible systems for the removal of alkyl groups that have been added to DNA by alkylating agents. One of these consists of an enzyme (methyltransferase) that stoichiometrically transfers methyl groups to itself; another is a DNA glycosylase that removes N-methylated purines. In the latter case, an endonuclease cuts the strand bearing the depuri-

nated site; the gap is then widened and ultimately repaired by the excision repair system described above.

Enzyme systems also exist for the repair of single- and double-strand breaks and cross-links, but less is known about their mechanisms. The relative resistance of different bacterial strains to radiation and other agents that directly damage DNA is due to the relative effectiveness of their repair enzyme systems.

B. Protein Denaturation: Proteins exist in a folded, 3-dimensional state determined by intramolecular covalent disulfide linkages and a number of noncovalent linkages such as ionic, hydrophobic, and hydrogen bonds. This state is called the **tertiary structure** of the protein; it is readily disrupted by a number of physical or chemical agents, causing the protein to become nonfunctional. The disruption of the tertiary structure of a protein is called protein denaturation.

C. Disruption of Cell Membrane or Wall: The cell membrane acts as a selective barrier, allowing some solutes to pass through and excluding others. Many compounds are actively transported through the membrane, becoming concentrated within the cell. The membrane is also the site of enzymes involved in the biosynthesis of components of the cell envelope. Substances that concentrate at the cell surface may alter the physical and chemical properties of the membrane, preventing its normal functions and therefore killing or inhibiting the cell.

The cell wall acts as a corseting structure, protecting the cell against osmotic lysis. Thus, agents that destroy the wall (eg, lysozyme) or prevent its normal synthesis (eg, penicillin) may bring about lysis of the cell.

D. Removal of Free Sulfhydryl Groups: Enzyme proteins containing cysteine have side chains terminating in sulfhydryl groups. In addition to these, at least one key coenzyme (coenzyme A, required for acyl group transfer) contains a free sulfhydryl group. Such enzymes and coenzymes cannot function unless the sulfhydryl groups remain free and reduced. Oxidizing agents thus interfere with metabolism by tying neighboring sulfhydryls in disulfide linkages:

$$R-SH + HS-R \xrightarrow{-2H} R-S-S-R$$

Many metals such as mercuric ion likewise interfere by combining with sulfhydryls:

$$\begin{matrix} R-SH \\ + \\ R-SH \end{matrix} \quad \begin{matrix} Cl \\ | \\ Hg \\ | \\ Cl \end{matrix} \longrightarrow \begin{matrix} R-S \\ \\ R-S \end{matrix}\!\!>\!\!Hg + 2HCl$$

There are many sulfhydryl enzymes in the cell; therefore, oxidizing agents and heavy metals do widespread damage. The exact reason for the requirement of free sulfhydryl groups is not certain, although in many cases (eg, coenzyme A) they probably represent the normal site of substrate attachment.

E. Chemical Antagonism: The interference by a chemical agent with the normal reaction between a specific enzyme and its substrate is known as "chemical antagonism." The antagonist acts by combining with some part of the holoenzyme (either the protein apoenzyme, the mineral activator, or the coenzyme), thereby preventing attachment of the normal substrate. ("Substrate" is here used in the broad sense to include cases in which the inhibitor combines with the apoenzyme, thereby preventing attachment to it of coenzyme.)

An antagonist combines with an enzyme because of its chemical affinity for an essential site on that enzyme. Enzymes perform their catalytic function by virtue of their affinity for their natural substrates; hence any compound structurally resembling a substrate in essential aspects may also have an affinity for the enzyme. If this affinity is great enough, the "analog" will displace the normal substrate and prevent the proper reaction from taking place.

Many holoenzymes include a mineral ion as a bridge either between enzyme and coenzyme or between enzyme and substrate. Chemicals that combine readily with these minerals will again prevent attachment of coenzyme or substrate; for example, carbon monoxide and cyanide ($-C\equiv N$) combine with the iron atom in the porphyrin enzymes and prevent their function in respiration.

Chemical antagonists can be conveniently discussed under 2 headings: antagonists of energy-yielding processes, and antagonists of biosynthetic processes. The former include poisons of respiratory enzymes (carbon monoxide, cyanide) and of oxidative phosphorylation (dinitrophenol); the latter include analogs of the building blocks of proteins (amino acids) and of nucleic acids (nucleotides). In some cases the analog simply prevents incorporation of the normal metabolite (eg, 5-methyltryptophan prevents incorporation of tryptophan into protein), and in other cases the analog replaces the normal metabolite in the macromolecule, causing it to be nonfunctional. The incorporation of p-fluorophenylalanine in place of phenylalanine in proteins is an example of the latter type of antagonism.

Reversal of Antibacterial Action

In the section on definitions, the point was made that bacteriostatic action is, by definition, reversible. Reversal can be brought about in several ways:

A. Removal of Agent: When cells that are inhibited by the presence of a bacteriostatic agent are removed by centrifugation, washed thoroughly in the centrifuge, and resuspended in fresh growth medium, they will resume normal multiplication.

B. Reversal by Substrate: When a chemical antagonist of the analog type forms a dissociating complex with the enzyme, it is possible to displace it by adding a high concentration of the normal substrate. Such cases are termed "competitive inhibition." The ratio of inhibitor concentration to concentration of substrate reversing the inhibition is called the **antimicrobial index;** it is usually very high (100–10,000), indicating a much greater affinity of enzyme for its normal substrate.

C. Inactivation of Agent: An agent can often be inactivated by adding to the medium a substance that combines with it, preventing its combination with cellular constituents. For example, mercuric ion can be inactivated by addition to the medium of sulfhydryl compounds such as thioglycolic acid.

D. Protection Against Lysis: Osmotic lysis can be prevented by making the medium isotonic for naked bacterial protoplasts. Concentrations of 10–20% sucrose are required. Under such conditions penicillin-induced protoplasts remain viable and continue to grow as L forms.

Resistance to Antibacterial Agents

The ability of bacteria to become resistant to antibacterial agents is an important factor in their control. The mechanisms by which resistance is acquired are discussed in Chapters 4 and 10.

Physical Agents

A. Heat: Application of heat is the simplest means of sterilizing materials, provided the material is itself resistant to heat damage. A temperature of 100 °C will kill all but spore forms of bacteria within 2–3 minutes in laboratory-scale cultures; a temperature of 121 °C for 15 minutes is utilized to kill spores. Steam is generally used, both because bacteria are more quickly killed when moist and because steam provides a means for distributing heat to all parts of the sterilizing vessel. Steam must be kept at a pressure of 15 lb/sq in above atmospheric pressure to obtain a temperature of 121 °C; autoclaves or pressure cookers are used for this purpose. For sterilizing materials that must remain dry, circulating hot air electric ovens are available; since heat is less effective on dry material, it is customary to apply a temperature of 160–170 °C for 1 hour or more.

Under the conditions described above (ie, excessive temperatures applied for long periods of time), heat acts by denaturing cell proteins and nucleic acids and by disrupting cell membranes.

B. Radiation: Ultraviolet light and ionizing radiations have various applications as sterilizing agents. Their modes of action are discussed on p 71.

Chemical Agents

Because antibacterial agents must be safe for the host organism under the conditions employed (selective toxicity), the number of commonly used antibacterial agents is much lower than the number of cell poisons and inhibitors available. Thus cyanide, arsenic, and other poisons are not included below because of the limitations on their practical usefulness.

A. Alcohols: Compounds with the structure $R-CH_2OH$ (where R means "alkyl group") are toxic to cells at relatively high concentrations. Ethyl alcohol (CH_3CH_2OH) and isopropyl alcohol ($[CH_3]_2CHOH$) are commonly used. At the concentrations generally employed (70% aqueous solutions), they act as protein denaturants.

B. Phenol: Phenol and many phenolic compounds are strong antibacterial agents. At the high concentrations generally employed (1–2% aqueous solutions), they denature proteins.

C. Heavy Metal Ions: Mercury, copper, and silver salts are all protein denaturants at high concentrations but are too injurious to human tissues to be used in this manner. They are commonly used at very low concentrations, under which conditions they act by combining with sulfhydryl groups. Mercury can be made safer for external use by combining it with organic compounds (eg, Mercurochrome, Merthiolate). Except when used on clean skin surfaces, these organic mercurials are of doubtful practical value, since they are readily inactivated by extraneous organic matter.

D. Oxidizing Agents: Strong oxidizing agents inactivate cells by oxidizing free sulfhydryl groups. Useful agents include hydrogen peroxide, iodine, hypochlorite, chlorine, and compounds slowly liberating chlorine (chloride of lime).

E. Alkylating Agents: A number of agents react with compounds in the cell to substitute alkyl groups for labile hydrogen atoms. The 2 agents of this type that are commonly used for disinfection purposes are formaldehyde (sold as the 37% aqueous solution **formalin**) and **ethylene oxide.** Ethylene oxide gas, rendered inexplosive by mixture with 90% CO_2 or a fluorocarbon, is the most reliable disinfectant available for dry surfaces. It is extensively used for the disinfection of surgical instruments and materials, which must be placed in special vacuum chambers for the purpose.

F. Detergents: Compounds that have the property of concentrating at interfaces are called "surface-active agents," or "detergents." The interface between the lipid-containing membrane of a bacterial cell and the surrounding aqueous medium attracts a particular class of surface-active compounds, namely, those possessing both a fat-soluble group and a water-soluble group. Long-chain hydrocarbons are very fat-soluble, while charged ions are very water-soluble; a compound possessing both structures will thus concentrate at the surface of the bacterial cell.

Two general types of such surface-active agents, or detergents, are known: anionic and cationic.

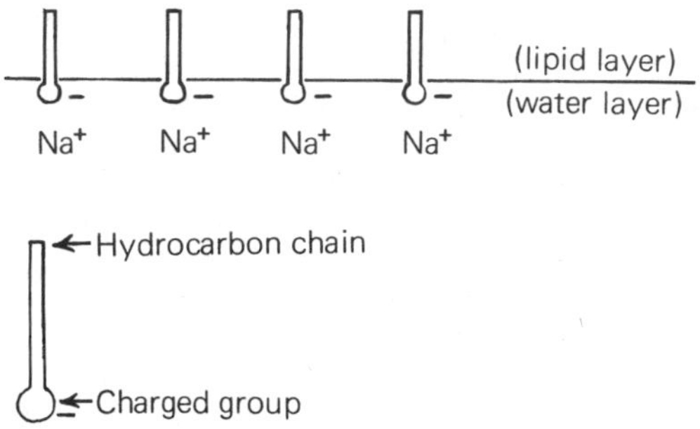

1. Anionic detergents–Detergents in which the long-chain hydrocarbon has a negative charge are called "anionic." These include soaps (sodium salts of long-chain carboxylic acids); synthetic products resembling soaps except that the carboxyl group is replaced by a sulfonic acid group; and bile salts, in which the fat-soluble portion has a steroid structure. Some examples are shown in Figs 5–6, 5–7, and 5–8.

The synthetic detergents have advantages in solubility and cost over the natural soaps (obtained by saponification of animal fat). Bile salts are notable in that they completely dissolve pneumococcal cells, thus providing an aid in identification.

2. Cationic detergents–The fat-soluble moiety can be made to have a positive charge by combining it with a quaternary (valence = +5) nitrogen atom (Fig 5–5).

Since the detergents concentrate at the cell membrane, and since the latter is a delicate, essential cell component, the inference is drawn that detergents act by disrupting the normal function of the cell membrane. Support for this view comes from experiments

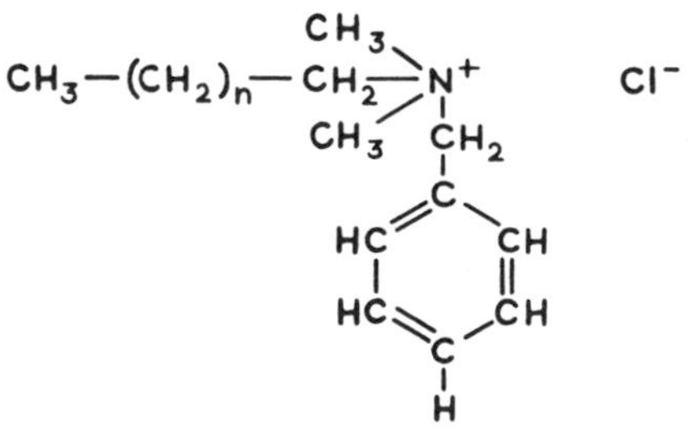

Figure 5–5. Alkyldimethylbenzylammonium chloride.

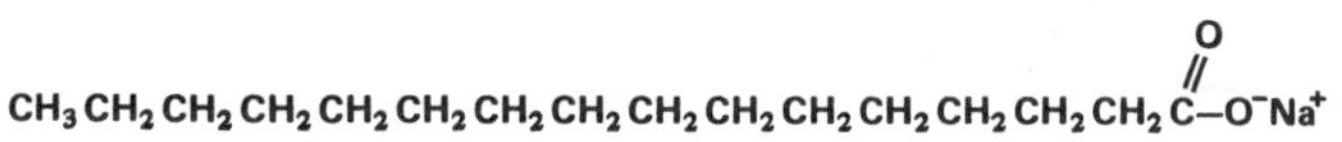

Figure 5–6. Sodium salt of palmitic acid (a soap).

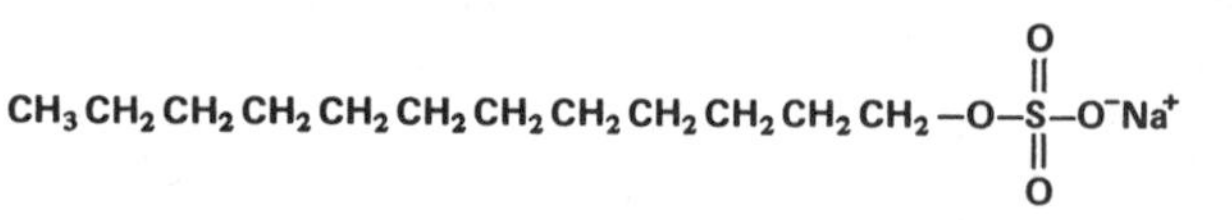

Figure 5–7. Sodium lauryl sulfate (a synthetic anionic detergent, Duponol WA).

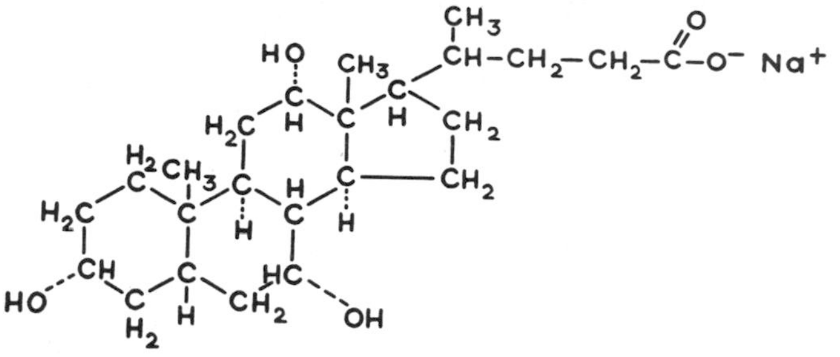

Figure 5–8. Sodium salt of cholic acid (a bile salt).

showing that cells exposed to detergents leak soluble nitrogen and phosphorus compounds into the medium.

Chemotherapeutic Agents

To be a useful chemotherapeutic agent, a compound must be either bacteriostatic or bactericidal in vivo (action not reversed by substances in host tissues or fluids) and at the same time remain noninjurious to the host. These requirements for in vivo effectiveness and selective toxicity narrow the list of important chemotherapeutic agents to a very few compounds, including the sulfonamides, the antibiotics, and the antituberculosis agents.

The natures and modes of action of these drugs are discussed in Chapter 10.

REFERENCES

Books

Block SS (editor): *Disinfection, Sterilization, and Preservation,* 2nd ed. Lea & Febiger, 1977.

Gerhardt P (editor): *Manual of Methods for General Bacteriology.* American Society for Microbiology, 1981.

Gunsalus IC, Stanier RY (editors): *The Bacteria.* Vol 4: *Physiology of Growth.* Academic Press, 1962.

Hanawalt PC et al (editors): *DNA Repair Mechanisms.* Academic Press, 1978.

Hugo WB (editor): *Inhibition and Destruction of the Microbial Cell.* Academic Press, 1971.

Ingraham JL, Maaløe O, Neidhardt FC: *Growth of the Bacterial Cell.* Sinauer Associates, 1983.

Mandelstam J, McQuillen K (editors): *The Biochemistry of Bacterial Growth,* 3rd ed. Wiley, 1981.

Rehm H-J, Reed G (editors): *Biotechnology.* Vol 1: *Microbial Fundamentals.* Verlag Chemie, 1982.

Russell AD: *The Destruction of Bacterial Spores.* Academic Press, 1982.

Articles & Reviews

Franklin WA, Haseltine WA: Removal of UV light-induced pyrimidine-pyrimidone(6-4) products from *Escherichia coli* DNA requires the *uvrA, uvrB,* and *uvrC* gene products. *Proc Natl Acad Sci USA* 1984;**81:**3821.

Howard-Flanders P: Inducible repair of DNA. *Sci Am* (Nov) 1981;**245:**72.

Huisman O, D'Ari R, Gotterman S: Cell-division control in *Escherichia coli:* Specific induction of the SOS function SfiA protein is sufficient to block septation. *Proc Natl Acad Sci USA* 1984;**81:**4490.

Lambert PA: Membrane-active antimicrobial agents. *Progr Med Chem* 1978;**15:**87.

Lehmann AR, Bridges BA: DNA repair. *Essays Biochem* 1977;**13:**71.

Lindahl T: DNA repair enzymes. *Annu Rev Biochem* 1982; **51:**61.

Novick A: Growth of bacteria. *Annu Rev Microbiol* 1955; **9:**97.

Scherbaum OH: Synchronous division of microorganisms. *Annu Rev Microbiol* 1960;**14:**283.

Tempest DW, Niejssel OM: The status of YATP and maintenance energy as biologically interpretable phenomena. *Annu Rev Microbiol* 1984;**38:**459.

Witkin EM: Ultraviolet mutagenesis and DNA repair in *Escherichia coli. Bacteriol Rev* 1976;**40:**869.

Cultivation of Microorganisms

Cultivation is the process of propagating organisms by providing the proper environmental conditions. Growing microorganisms are making replicas of themselves, and they require the elements present in their chemical composition. Nutrients must provide these elements in metabolically accessible form. In addition, the organisms require metabolic energy in order to synthesize macromolecules and maintain essential chemical gradients across their membranes. Factors that must be controlled during growth include the nutrients, pH, temperature, aeration, salt concentration, and ionic strength of the medium.

REQUIREMENTS FOR GROWTH

Most of the dry weight of microorganisms is organic matter containing the elements carbon, hydrogen, nitrogen, oxygen, phosphorus, and sulfur. In addition, inorganic ions such as potassium, sodium, iron, magnesium, calcium, and chloride are required to facilitate enzymatic catalysis and to maintain chemical gradients across the cell membrane.

For the most part, the organic matter is in macromolecules formed by **anhydride bonds** between building blocks. Synthesis of the anhydride bonds requires chemical energy, which is provided by the 2 phosphodiester bonds in ATP (adenosine triphosphate; see Chapter 7). Additional energy required to maintain a relatively constant cytoplasmic composition during growth in a range of extracellular chemical environments is derived from the **proton motive force.** The proton motive force is the potential energy that can be derived by passage of a proton across a membrane. In eukaryotes, the membrane may be part of the mitochondrion or the chloroplast. In prokaryotes, the membrane is the cytoplasmic membrane of the cell.

The proton motive force is an electrochemical gradient with 2 components: a difference in pH (hydrogen ion concentration) and a difference in ionic charge. The charge on the outside of the bacterial membrane is more positive than the charge on the inside, and the difference in charge contributes to the free energy released when a proton enters the cytoplasm from outside the membrane. Metabolic processes that generate the proton motive force are discussed in Chapter 7. The free energy may be used to move the cell, to maintain ionic or molecular gradients across the membrane, to synthesize anhydride bonds in ATP, or for a combination of these purposes. Alternatively, cells given a source of ATP may use its anhydride bond energy to create a proton motive force that in turn may be used to move the cell and to maintain chemical gradients.

In order to grow, an organism requires all of the elements in its organic matter and the full complement of ions required for energetics and catalysis. In addition, there must be a source of energy to establish the proton motive force and to allow macromolecular synthesis. Microorganisms vary widely in their nutritional demands and their sources of metabolic energy.

SOURCES OF METABOLIC ENERGY

The 3 major mechanisms for generating metabolic energy are fermentation, respiration, and photosynthesis. At least one of these mechanisms must be employed if an organism is to grow.

Fermentation

The formation of ATP in fermentation is not coupled to the transfer of electrons. Fermentation is characterized by **substrate phosphorylation,** an enzymatic process in which a pyrophosphate bond is donated directly to ADP (adenosine diphosphate) by a phosphorylated metabolic intermediate. The phosphorylated intermediates are formed by metabolic rearrangement of a fermentable substrate such as glucose, lactose, or arginine. Because fermentations are not accompanied by a change in the overall oxidation-reduction state of the fermentable substrate, the elemental composition of the products of fermentation must be identical to those of the substrates. For example, fermentation of a molecule of glucose ($C_6H_{12}O_6$) by the Embden-Meyerhof pathway (see Chapter 7) yields a net gain of 2 pyrophosphate bonds in ATP and produces 2 molecules of lactic acid ($C_3H_6O_3$).

Respiration

Respiration is analogous to the coupling of an energy-dependent process to the discharge of a battery. Chemical reduction of an oxidant (electron acceptor) through a specific series of electron carriers in the membrane establishes the proton motive force across the bacterial membrane. The reductant (electron donor) may be organic or inorganic: for example, lactic acid serves as a reductant for some organisms, and hydrogen gas is a reductant for other organisms. Gaseous oxygen (O_2) often is employed as an oxidant, but alternative oxidants that are employed by some organisms include carbon dioxide (CO_2), sulfate (SO_4^{2-}), and nitrate (NO_3^-).

Photosynthesis

Photosynthesis is similar to respiration in that the reduction of an oxidant via a specific series of electron carriers establishes the proton motive force. The difference in the 2 processes is that in photosynthesis the reductant and oxidant are created photochemically by light energy absorbed by pigments in the membrane; thus, photosynthesis can continue only as long as there is a source of light energy. Plants and some bacteria are able to invest a substantial amount of light energy in making water a reductant for carbon dioxide. Oxygen is evolved in this process, and organic matter is produced. Respiration, the energetically favorable oxidation of organic matter by an electronic acceptor such as oxygen, can provide photosynthetic organisms with energy in the absence of light.

NUTRITION

Nutrients in growth media must contain all the elements necessary for the biologic synthesis of new organisms. In the following discussion, nutrients are classified according to the elements that they supply.

Carbon Source

As mentioned above, plants and some bacteria are able to use photosynthetic energy to reduce carbon dioxide at the expense of water. These organisms belong to the group of **autotrophs,** creatures that do not require organic nutrients for growth. Other autotrophs are the **chemolithotrophs,** organisms that use an inorganic substrate such as hydrogen or thiosulfate as a reductant and carbon dioxide as a carbon source.

Heterotrophs require organic carbon for growth, and the organic carbon must be in a form that can be assimilated. Naphthalene, for example, can provide all the carbon and energy required for respiratory heterotrophic growth, but very few organisms possess the metabolic pathway necessary for naphthalene assimilation. Glucose, on the other hand, can support the fermentative or respiratory growth of many organisms. It is important that growth substrates be supplied at levels appropriate for the microbial strain that is being grown: levels that will support the growth of one organism may inhibit the growth of another organism.

Carbon dioxide is required for a number of biosynthetic reactions. Many respiratory organisms produce more than enough carbon dioxide to meet this requirement, but others require a source of carbon dioxide in their growth medium.

Nitrogen Source

Nitrogen is a major component of proteins and nu-

Table 6–1. Sources of nitrogen in microbial nutrition.

Compound	Valence of N
NO_3^-	+5
NO_2^-	+3
N_2	0
NH_4^+	−3
$R-NH_2$*	−3

*R = Organic radical.

cleic acids, accounting for about 10% of the dry weight of a typical bacterial cell. Nitrogen may be supplied in a number of different forms (Table 6–1), and microorganisms vary in their abilities to assimilate nitrogen. The end product of all pathways for nitrogen assimilation is the most reduced form of the element, ammonium ion (NH_4^+).

Many microorganisms possess the ability to assimilate nitrate (NO_3^-) and nitrite (NO_2^-) reductively by conversion of these ions to ammonia (NH_3). These pathways for **assimilation** differ from pathways used for **dissimilation** of nitrate and nitrite. The dissimilatory pathways are used by organisms that employ the ions as terminal electron acceptors in respiration; this process is known as **denitrification,** and its product is nitrogen gas (N_2), which is evolved into the atmosphere.

The ability to assimilate N_2 reductively via NH_3, which is called **nitrogen fixation,** is a property unique to prokaryotes, and relatively few bacteria possess this metabolic capacity. The process requires a large amount of metabolic energy and is readily inactivated by oxygen. The capacity for nitrogen fixation is found in widely divergent bacteria that have evolved quite different biochemical strategies to protect their nitrogen-fixing enzymes from oxygen.

Most microorganisms can use NH_4^+ as a sole nitrogen source, and many organisms possess the ability to produce NH_4^+ from amines ($R-NH_2$). Ammonia is introduced into organic matter by biochemical pathways involving glutamate and glutamine. These pathways are discussed in Chapter 7.

Sulfur Source

Like nitrogen, sulfur is a component of many organic cell substances. It forms part of the structure of several coenzymes and is found in the cysteinyl and methionyl side chains of proteins. Most microorganisms can use sulfate (SO_4^{2-}) as a sulfur source, reducing the sulfate to the level of hydrogen sulfide (H_2S). Some microorganisms can assimilate H_2S directly from the growth medium, but this compound can be toxic to many organisms. Direct assimilation of H_2S occurs by the O-acetylserine sulfhydrolase reaction:

O-Acetylserine + H_2S → L-Cysteine + Acetate

Metabolically formed reduced sulfur (H_2S) is transferred directly from a metabolic carrier to O-acetylserine.

Phosphorus Source

Phosphate (PO_4^{3-}) is required as a component of ATP, nucleic acids, and such coenzymes as NAD, NADP, and flavins. In addition, many metabolites and some proteins are phosphorylated. Phosphate is always assimilated as free inorganic phosphate (P_i).

Mineral Sources

Numerous minerals are required for enzyme function. Magnesium ion (Mg^{2+}) and ferrous ion (Fe^{2+}) are also found in porphyrin derivatives: magnesium in the chlorophyll molecule, and iron as part of the coenzymes of the cytochromes and peroxidases. Mg^{2+} and K^+ are both essential for the function and integrity of ribosomes. Ca^{2+} is required as a constituent of gram-positive cell walls, although it is dispensable for gram-negative bacteria. Many marine organisms require Na^+ for growth. In formulating a medium for the cultivation of most microorganisms, it is necessary to provide sources of potassium, magnesium, calcium, and iron, usually as their ions (K^+, Mg^{2+}, Ca^{2+}, and Fe^{2+}). Many other minerals (eg, Mn^{2+}, Mo^{2+}, Co^{2+}, Cu^{2+}, and Zn^{2+}) are required; these frequently can be provided in tap water or as contaminants of other medium ingredients.

The uptake of iron, which forms insoluble hydroxides at neutral pH, is facilitated in many bacteria and fungi by their production of **siderochromes**—compounds that chelate iron and promote its transport as a soluble complex. These include hydroxamates ($-CONH_2OH$) called sideramines, and derivatives of catechol (eg, 2,3-dihydroxybenzoylserine). Plasmid-determined siderochromes play a major role in the invasiveness of some bacterial pathogens (see Chapter 4).

Growth Factors

A growth factor is an organic compound which a cell must contain in order to grow but which it is unable to synthesize. Many microorganisms, when provided with the nutrients listed above, are able to synthesize all of the building blocks for macromolecules (Fig 6–1): amino acids; purines, pyrimidines, and pentoses (the metabolic precursors of nucleic acids); additional carbohydrates (precursors of polysaccharides); and fatty acids and isoprenoid compounds. In addition, free-living organisms must be able to synthesize the complex vitamins that serve as precursors of coenzymes.

Each of these essential compounds is synthesized by a discrete sequence of enzymatic reactions; each enzyme is produced under the control of a specific gene. When an organism undergoes a gene mutation resulting in failure of one of these enzymes to function, the chain is broken and the end product is no longer produced. The organism must then obtain that compound from the environment: the compound has become a **growth factor** for the organism. This type of mutation can be readily induced in the laboratory.

Different microbial species vary widely in their growth factor requirements. The compounds involved are found in and are essential to all organisms; the differences in requirements reflect differences in synthetic abilities. Some species require no growth factors, while others—like some of the lactobacilli—have lost, during evolution, the ability to synthesize as many as 30–40 essential compounds and hence require them in the medium.

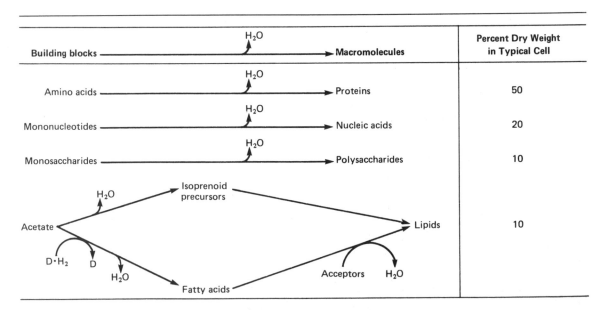

Figure 6–1. Macromolecular synthesis. Polymerization of building blocks into macromolecules is achieved largely by the introduction of anhydride bonds. Formation of fatty acids from acetate requires several steps of biochemical reduction using organic hydrogen donors. (D • H_2).

ENVIRONMENTAL FACTORS AFFECTING GROWTH

A suitable growth medium must contain all the nutrients required by the organism to be cultivated, and such factors as pH, temperature, and aeration must be carefully controlled. A liquid medium is used; the medium can be gelled for special purposes by adding agar or silica gel. Agar, a polysaccharide extract of a marine alga, is uniquely suitable for microbial cultivation because it is resistant to microbial action and because it dissolves at 100 °C but does not gel until cooled below 45 °C; cells can be suspended in the medium at 45 °C and the medium quickly cooled to a gel without harming them.

Nutrients

On the previous pages, the function of each type of nutrient is described and a list of suitable substances presented. In general, the following must be provided: (1) Hydrogen donors and acceptors: about 2 g/L. (2) Carbon source: about 1 g/L. (3) Nitrogen source: about 1 g/L. (4) Minerals: sulfur and phosphorus, about 50 mg/L of each; trace elements, 0.1–1 mg/L of each. (5) Growth factors: amino acids, purines, pyrimidines, about 50 mg/L of each; vitamins, 0.1–1 mg/L of each.

For studies of microbial metabolism, it is usually necessary to prepare a completely synthetic medium in which the characteristics and concentration of every ingredient are exactly known. Otherwise, it is much cheaper and simpler to use natural materials such as yeast extract, protein digest, or similar substances. Most free-living microbes will grow well on yeast extract; parasitic forms may require special substances found only in blood or in extracts of animal tissues.

For many organisms, a single compound (such as an amino acid) may serve as energy source, carbon source, and nitrogen source; others require a separate compound for each. If natural materials for nonsynthetic media are deficient in any particular nutrient, they must be supplemented.

Hydrogen Ion Concentration (pH)

Most organisms have a fairly narrow optimal pH range. The optimal pH must be empirically determined for each species. Most organisms (neutrophiles) grow best at a pH of 6.0–8.0, although some forms (acidophiles) have optima as low as pH 3.0 and others (alkalophiles) have optima as high as pH 10.5.

Microorganisms regulate their internal pH over a wide range of external pH values. Acidophiles maintain an internal pH of about 6.5 over an external range of 1.0–5.0; neutrophiles maintain an internal pH of about 7.5 over an external range of 5.5–8.5; and alkalophiles maintain an internal pH of about 9.5 over an external range of 9.0–11.0. Internal pH is regulated by a set of proton transport systems in the cytoplasmic membrane, including a primary, ATP-driven proton pump and a Na^+/H^+ exchanger. A K^+/H^+ exchange system has also been proposed to contribute to internal pH regulation in neutrophiles.

Temperature

Different microbial species vary widely in their optimal temperature ranges for growth: psychrophilic forms grow best at low temperatures (15–20 °C); mesophilic forms grow best at 30–37 °C; and most thermophilic forms grow best at 50–60 °C. Most organisms are mesophilic; 30 °C is optimal for many free-living forms, and the body temperature of the host is optimal for symbionts of warm-blooded animals.

The upper end of the temperature range tolerated by any given species correlates well with the general thermal stability of that species' proteins as measured in cell extracts. Microorganisms share with plants and animals the **heat-shock response:** transient synthesis of a set of "heat-shock proteins" when exposed to a sudden rise in temperature above the growth optimum. These proteins appear to be unusually heat-resistant and to stabilize the heat-sensitive proteins of the cell.

The relationship of growth rate to temperature for any given microorganism is seen in a typical Arrhenius plot (Fig 6–2). Arrhenius showed that the logarithm of the velocity of any chemical reaction (log k) is a linear function of the reciprocal of the temperature (1/T); since cell growth is the result of a set of chemical reactions, it might be expected to show this relationship. Fig 6–2 shows this to be the case over the normal range of temperatures for a given species: log k decreases linearly with 1/T. Above and below the normal range, however, log k drops rapidly, so that maximum and minimum temperature values are defined.

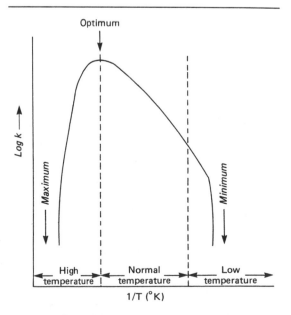

Figure 6–2. General form of an Arrhenius plot of bacterial growth. (After Ingraham JL, Maaløe O, Neidhardt FC: *Growth of the Bacterial Cell.* Sinauer Associates, 1983.)

Beyond their effects on growth rate, extremes of temperature kill microorganisms. Extreme heat is used to sterilize preparations (see Chapter 5); extreme cold also kills microbial cells, although it cannot be used safely for sterilization. Bacteria also exhibit a phenomenon called **cold shock:** the killing of cells by rapid—as opposed to slow—cooling. For example, the rapid cooling of *Escherichia coli* from 37 °C to 5 °C can kill 90% of the cells. A number of compounds protect cells from either freezing or cold shock; glycerol and dimethylsulfoxide are most commonly used.

Aeration

The role of oxygen as hydrogen acceptor is discussed in Chapter 7. Many organisms are obligate aerobes, specifically requiring oxygen as hydrogen acceptor; some are facultative, able to live aerobically or anaerobically; and others are obligate anaerobes, requiring a substance other than oxygen as hydrogen acceptor and being sensitive to oxygen inhibition.

The toxicity of O_2 results from its reduction by enzymes in the cell (such as flavoproteins) to hydrogen peroxide (H_2O_2) and by ferrous ion to the even more toxic free radical, superoxide (O_2^-). Aerobes and aerotolerant anaerobes are protected from these products by the presence of superoxide dismutase, an enzyme that catalyzes the reaction

$$2O_2^- + 2H^+ \rightarrow O_2 + H_2O_2$$

and by the presence of catalase, an enzyme that catalyzes the reaction

$$2H_2O_2 \rightarrow 2H_2O + O_2$$

One exception to this rule is the lactic acid bacteria, aerotolerant anaerobes that do not contain catalase. This group relies instead on peroxidases, which reduce H_2O_2 to $2H_2O$ at the expense of oxidizable organic substrates. All strict anaerobes lack both superoxide dismutase and catalase; the former enzyme is indispensable for survival in the presence of O_2.

Hydrogen peroxide owes much of its toxicity to the damage it causes to DNA. DNA repair-deficient mutants are exceptionally sensitive to hydrogen peroxide; the *recA* gene product, which functions in both genetic recombination and repair, has been shown to be more important than either catalase or superoxide dismutase in protecting *E coli* cells against hydrogen peroxide toxicity.

The supply of air to cultures of aerobes is a major technical problem. Vessels are usually shaken mechanically to introduce oxygen into the medium, or air is forced through the medium by pressure. The diffusion of oxygen often becomes the limiting factor in growing aerobic bacteria; when a cell concentration of $4-5 \times 10^9$/mL is reached, the rate of diffusion of oxygen to the cells sharply limits the rate of further growth.

Obligate anaerobes, on the other hand, present the problem of oxygen exclusion. Many methods are available for this: reducing agents such as sodium thioglycolate can be added to liquid cultures; tubes of agar can be sealed with a layer of petrolatum and paraffin; the culture vessel can be placed in a container from which the oxygen is removed by evacuation or by chemical means; or the organism can be handled within an anaerobic glove-box.

Ionic Strength & Osmotic Pressure

To a lesser extent, such factors as osmotic pressure and salt concentration may have to be controlled. For most organisms, the properties of ordinary media are satisfactory; but for marine forms and organisms adapted to growth in strong sugar solutions, for example, these factors must be considered. Organisms requiring high salt concentrations are called **halophilic;** those requiring high osmotic pressures are called **osmophilic.**

Most bacteria are able to tolerate a wide range of external osmotic pressures and ionic strengths because of their ability to regulate internal osmolality and ion concentration. Osmolality is regulated by the active transport of K^+ ions into the cell; internal ionic strength is kept constant by a compensating excretion of the positively charged organic polyamine putrescine. Since putrescine carries several positive charges per molecule, a large drop in ionic strength is effected at only a small cost in osmotic strength.

CULTIVATION METHODS

Two problems will be considered: the choice of a suitable medium and the isolation of a bacterial organism in pure culture.

The Medium

The technique used and the type of medium selected depend upon the nature of the investigation. In general, 3 situations may be encountered: (1) one may need to raise a crop of cells of a particular species that is on hand; (2) one may need to determine the numbers and types of organisms present in a given material; or (3) one may wish to isolate a particular type of microorganism from a natural source.

A. Growing Cells of a Given Species: Microorganisms observed microscopically to be growing in a natural environment may prove exceedingly difficult to grow in pure culture in an artificial medium. Certain parasitic forms, for example, have never been cultivated outside the host. In general, however, a suitable medium can be devised by carefully reproducing the conditions found in the organism's natural environment. The pH, temperature, and aeration are simple to duplicate; the nutrients present the major problem. The contribution made by the living environment is important and difficult to analyze; a parasite may require an extract of the host tissue, and a free-living form may require a substance excreted by a microorganism with which it is associated in nature. Considerable experimentation may be necessary in order to determine the requirements of the organism, and success depends upon providing a suitable source of each category of nutrient listed at the beginning of this chapter. The cultivation of obligate parasites such as rickettsiae is discussed in Chapter 34.

B. Microbiologic Examination of Natural Materials: A given natural material may contain many different microenvironments, each providing a niche for a different species. Plating a sample of the material under one set of conditions will allow a selected group of forms to produce colonies but will cause many other types to be overlooked. For this reason, it is customary to plate out samples of the material using as many different media and conditions of incubation as is practicable. Six to 8 different culture conditions are not an unreasonable number if most of the forms present are to be discovered.

Since every type of organism present must have a chance to grow, solid media are used and crowding of colonies is avoided. Otherwise, competition will prevent some types from forming colonies.

C. Isolation of a Particular Type of Microorganism: A small sample of soil, if handled properly, will yield a different type of organism for every microenvironment present. For fertile soil (moist, aerated, rich in minerals and organic matter) this means that hundreds or even thousands of types can be isolated. This is done by selecting for the desired type. One gram of soil, for example, is inoculated into a flask of liquid medium that has been made up for the purpose of favoring one type of organism, eg, aerobic nitrogen fixers (*Azotobacter*). In this case, the medium contains no combined nitrogen and is incubated aerobically. If cells of *Azotobacter* are present in the soil, they will grow well in this medium; forms unable to fix nitrogen will grow only to the extent that the soil has introduced contaminating fixed nitrogen into the medium. When the culture is fully grown, therefore, the percentage of *Azotobacter* in the total population will have increased greatly; the method is thus called "enrichment culture." Transfer of a sample of this culture to fresh medium will result in further enrichment of *Azotobacter;* after several serial transfers, the culture can be plated out on a solidified enrichment medium and colonies of *Azotobacter* isolated.

Liquid medium is used to permit competition and hence optimal selection, even when the desired type is represented in the soil as only a few cells in a population of millions. Advantage can be taken of "natural enrichment." For example, in looking for kerosene oxidizers, oil-laden soil is chosen, since it is already an enrichment environment for such forms.

Enrichment culture, then, is a procedure whereby the medium is prepared so as to duplicate the natural environment ("niche") of the desired microorganism, thereby selecting for it. An important principle involved in such selection is the following: The organism selected for will be the type whose nutritional requirements are barely satisfied. *Azotobacter*, for example, grows best in a medium containing organic nitrogen, but its minimum requirement is the presence of N_2; hence it is selected for in a medium containing N_2 as the sole nitrogen source. If organic nitrogen is added to the medium, the conditions no longer select for *Azotobacter* but rather for a form for which organic nitrogen is the minimum requirement.

When searching for a particular type of organism in a natural material, it is advantageous to plate the organisms obtained on a differential medium if available. A differential medium is one that will cause the colonies of a particular type of organism to have a distinctive appearance. For example, colonies of *E coli* have a characteristic iridescent sheen on agar containing the dyes eosin and methylene blue (EMB agar). EMB agar containing a high concentration of one sugar will also cause organisms which ferment that sugar to form reddish colonies. Differential media are used for such purposes as recognizing the presence of enteric bacteria in water or milk and the presence of certain pathogens in clinical specimens.

Table 6–2 presents examples of enrichment culture conditions and the types of bacteria they will select.

Isolation of Microorganisms in Pure Culture

In order to study the properties of a given organism, it is necessary to handle it in pure culture free of all other types of organisms. To do this, a single cell must be isolated from all other cells and cultivated in such a manner that its collective progeny also remain isolated. Several methods are available.

A. Plating: Unlike cells in a liquid medium, cells in or on a gelled medium are immobilized. Therefore, if few enough cells are placed in or on a gelled medium, each cell will grow into an isolated colony. The ideal gelling agent for most microbiologic media is **agar,** an acidic polysaccharide extracted from certain red algae. A 1.5–2% suspension in water dissolves at 100 °C, forming a clear solution that gels at 45 °C. Thus, a sterile agar solution can be cooled to 50 °C, bacteria or other microbial cells added, and then the solution quickly cooled below 45 °C to form a gel. (Although most microbial cells are killed at 50 °C, the time-course of the killing process is sufficiently slow at this temperature to permit this procedure. See Fig 5–3.) Once gelled, agar will not again liquefy until it is heated above 80 °C, so that any temperature suitable for the incubation of a microbial culture can subsequently be used. In the pour-plate method, a suspension of cells is mixed with melted agar at 50 °C and poured into a Petri dish. When the agar solidifies, the cells are immobilized in the agar and grow into colonies. If the cell suspension was sufficiently dilute, the colonies will be well separated, so that each has a high probability of being derived from a single cell. To make certain of this, however, it is necessary to pick a colony of the desired type, suspend it in water, and replate. Repeating this procedure several times ensures that a pure culture will be obtained.

Alternatively, the original suspension can be streaked on an agar plate with a wire loop. As the streaking continues, fewer and fewer cells are left on

Table 6–2. Some enrichment cultures.

Constituents of all media: $MgSO_4$, K_2HPO_4, $FeCl_3$, $CaCl_2$, $CaCO_3$, trace elements.

Nitrogen Source	Carbon Source	Atmosphere	Illumination	Predominant Organism Initially Enriched
N₂	CO₂	Aerobic or anaerobic	Dark	None
			Light	Cyanobacteria
	Alcohol, fatty acids, etc	Anaerobic	Dark	None
		Air	Dark	*Azotobacter*
	Glucose	Anaerobic	Dark	*Clostridium pasteurianum*
		Air	Dark	*Azotobacter*
NaNO₃	CO₂	Aerobic or anaerobic	Dark	None
			Light	Green algae and cyanobacteria
	Alcohol, fatty acids, etc	Anaerobic	Dark	Denitrifiers
		Air	Dark	Aerobes
	Glucose	Anaerobic	Dark	Fermenters
		Air	Dark	Aerobes
NH₄Cl	CO₂	Anaerobic	Dark	None
		Aerobic	Dark	*Nitrosomonas*
		Aerobic or anaerobic	Light	Green algae and cyanobacteria
	Alcohol, fatty acids, etc	Anaerobic	Dark	Sulfate or carbonate reducers
		Aerobic	Dark	Aerobes
	Glucose	Anaerobic	Dark	Fermenters
		Aerobic	Dark	Aerobes

the loop, and finally the loop may deposit single cells on the agar. The plate is incubated and any well-isolated colony is then removed, resuspended in water, and again streaked on agar. If a suspension (and not just a bit of growth from a colony or slant) is streaked, this method is just as reliable as and much faster than the pour-plate method.

B. Dilution: A much less reliable method is that of extinction dilution. The suspension is serially diluted and samples of each dilution are plated. If only a few samples of a particular dilution exhibit growth, it is presumed that some of these cultures started from single cells. This method is not used unless plating is for some reason impossible. An undesirable feature of this method is that it can only be used to isolate the predominant type of organism in a mixed population.

REFERENCES

Books

Alexander M: *Microbial Ecology.* Wiley, 1971.

Cohen G, Greenwald RA (editors): *Oxy Radicals and Their Scavenger Systems.* Vol 1: *Molecular Aspects.* Vol 2: *Cellular and Medical Aspects.* Elsevier, 1983.

Gerhardt P (editor): *Manual of Methods for General Bacteriology:* American Society for Microbiology, 1981.

Lichstein H (editor): *Bacterial Nutrition.* Benchmark Papers in Microbiology, No. 19. Hutchinson Ross, 1983.

Oberley LW: *Superoxide Dismutase.* CRC Press, 1982.

Pirt SJ: *Principles of Microbe and Cell Cultivation.* Wiley, 1975.

Precht H et al (editors): *Temperature and Life.* Springer, 1974.

Schlegel HG (editor): *Enrichment Culture and Mutant Selection.* Fischer (Stuttgart), 1965.

Stanier RY, Adelberg EA, Ingraham JL: *The Microbial World,* 4th ed. Prentice-Hall, 1976.

Articles & Reviews

Alexander M: Why microbial predators and parasites do not eliminate their prey and hosts. *Annu Rev Microbiol* 1981; **35**:113.

Baross JA, Deming JW: Growth of "black smoker" bacteria at temperatures of at least 250 °C. *Nature* 1983;**303**:423.

Brown AD: Aspects of bacterial response to the ionic environment. *Bacteriol Rev* 1964;**28**:296.

Carlsson J, Carpenter VS: The *recA*+ gene product is more important than catalase and superoxide dismutase in protecting *Escherichia coli* against hydrogen peroxide toxicity. *J Bacteriol* 1980;**142**:319.

Fridovich I: Oxygen, boon and bane. *Am Sci* 1975;**63**:54.

Harder W, Dijkhuizen L: Physiological responses to nutrient limitation. *Annu Rev Microbiol* 1983;**37**:1.

Hutner SH: Inorganic nutrition. *Annu Rev Microbiol* 1972; **26**:313.

Minton KE et al: Non-specific stabilization of stress susceptible proteins by stress-resistant proteins: A model for the biological role of heat-shock proteins. *Proc Natl Acad Sci USA* 1982;**79**:7107.

Morris JG: The physiology of obligate anaerobiosis. *Adv Microb Physiol* 1975;**12**:169.

Nielands JB: Hydroxamic acids in nature. *Science* 1967; **156**:1443.

Padan E, Zilberstein D, Schuldiner S: pH homeostasis in bacteria. *Biochim Biophys Acta* 1981;**650**:151.

Wang CC, Newton A: Iron transport in *Escherichia coli:* Roles of energy-dependent uptake and 2,3-dihydroxybenzoylserine. *J Bacteriol* 1969;**98**:1142.

7

Microbial Metabolism

THE ROLE OF METABOLISM IN BIOSYNTHESIS & GROWTH

Microbial growth requires the polymerization of biochemical building blocks into proteins, nucleic acids, polysaccharides, and lipids. The building blocks must come preformed in the growth medium or must be synthesized by the growing cells. Additional biosynthetic demands are placed by the requirement for coenzymes that participate in enzymatic catalysis. Biosynthetic polymerization reactions demand the transfer of anhydride bonds from ATP. Growth demands a source of metabolic energy for the synthesis of anhydride bonds and for the maintenance of transmembrane gradients of ions and metabolites.

The biosynthetic origins of building blocks and coenzymes can be traced to relatively few precursors, called **focal metabolites.** Figs 7–1, 7–2, 7–3, and 7–4 illustrate how the respective focal metabolites glucose 6-phosphate, phosphoenolpyruvate, oxaloacetate, and α-ketoglutarate give rise to most biosynthetic end products. Microbial metabolism can be divided into 4 general categories: (1) pathways for the interconversion of focal metabolites, (2) assimilatory pathways for the formation of focal metabolites, (3) biosynthetic sequences for the conversion of focal metabolites to end products, and (4) pathways that yield metabolic energy for growth and maintenance.

When provided with building blocks and a source of metabolic energy, a cell synthesizes macromolecules. The sequence of building blocks within a macromolecule is determined in one of 2 ways. In nucleic acids and proteins, it is **template-directed:** DNA serves as the template for its own synthesis and for the synthesis of the various types of RNA; messenger RNA serves as the template for the synthesis of proteins. In carbohydrates and lipids, on the other hand, the arrangement of building blocks is determined entirely by enzyme specificities. Once the macromolecules have been synthesized, they self-assemble to form the supramolecular structures of the cell, eg, ribosomes, membranes, cell wall, flagella, pili.

FOCAL METABOLITE	INTERMEDIATES	END PRODUCTS

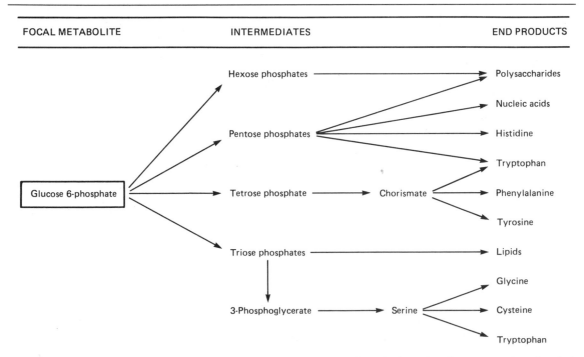

Figure 7–1. Biosynthetic end products formed from glucose 6-phosphate. Carbohydrate phosphate esters of varying chain length serve as intermediates in the biosynthetic pathways.

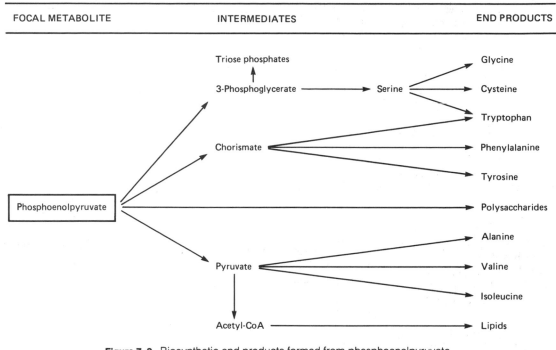

Figure 7–2. Biosynthetic end products formed from phosphoenolpyruvate.

The rate of macromolecular synthesis and the activity of metabolic pathways must be regulated so that biosynthesis is balanced. All of the components required for macromolecular synthesis must be present for orderly growth, and control must be exerted so that the resources of the cell are not expended on products that do not contribute to growth or survival.

This chapter contains a review of microbial metabolism and its regulation. Microorganisms represent extremes of evolutionary divergence, and a vast array of metabolic pathways are found within the group. For example, any of more than half a dozen different metabolic pathways may be used for assimilation of a relatively simple compound, benzoate, and a single pathway for benzoate assimilation may be regulated by any of more than half a dozen control mechanisms. Our goal will be to illustrate the principles that underlie metabolic pathways and their regulation. The primary principle that determines metabolic pathways is that they are achieved by organizing relatively few biochemical type reactions in a specific order. Many biosynthetic pathways can be deduced by examining the chemical structures of the starting material, the end product, and, perhaps, one or 2 metabolic intermediates. The primary principle underlying metabolic regulation is that enzymes tend to be called into play only when their catalytic activity is demanded. The activity of an enzyme may be changed by varying either the amount of enzyme or the amount of substrate. In some cases, the activity of enzymes may be altered by the binding of specific **effectors,** metabolites that modulate enzyme activity.

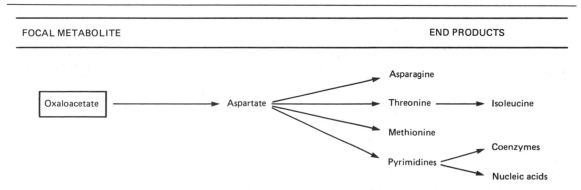

Figure 7–3. Biosynthetic end products formed from oxaloacetate. The end products threonine and pyrimidines serve as intermediates in the synthesis of additional compounds.

| FOCAL METABOLITE | INTERMEDIATES | END PRODUCTS |

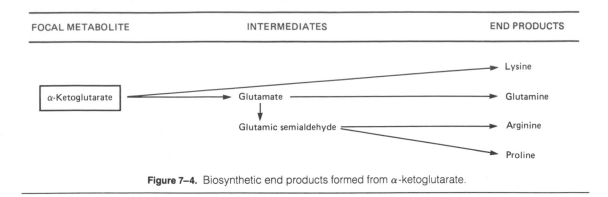

Figure 7–4. Biosynthetic end products formed from α-ketoglutarate.

FOCAL METABOLITES & THEIR INTERCONVERSION

Glucose 6-Phosphate & Carbohydrate Interconversions

Fig 7–1 illustrates that glucose 6-phosphate is converted to a range of biosynthetic end products via phosphate esters of carbohydrates with different chain lengths. Carbohydrates possess the empirical formula $(CH_2O)_n$, and the primary objective of carbohydrate metabolism is to change n, the length of the carbon chain. Mechanisms by which the chain lengths of carbohydrate phosphates are interconverted are summarized in Fig 7–5. In one case, oxidative reactions are used to remove a single carbon from glucose 6-phosphate, producing the pentose derivative ribulose 5-phosphate. Isomerase and epimerase reactions interconvert the most common biochemical forms of the pentoses: ribulose 5-phosphate, ribose 5-phosphate, and xylulose 5-phosphate. Transketolases transfer a 2-carbon fragment from a donor to an acceptor molecule. These reactions allow pentoses to form or to be formed from carbohydrates of varying chain lengths. As shown in Fig 7–5, two pentose 5-phosphates (n=5) are interconvertible with triose 3-phosphate (n=3) and heptose 7-phosphate (n=7); pentose 5-phosphate (n=5) and tetrose 4-phosphate (n=4) are interconvertible with triose 3-phosphate (n=3) and hexose 6-phosphate (n=6).

The 6-carbon hexose chain of fructose 6-phosphate can be converted to two 3-carbon triose derivatives by the consecutive action of a kinase and an aldolase on fructose 6-phosphate. Alternatively, aldolases, acting in conjunction with phosphatases, can be used to lengthen carbohydrate molecules: triose phosphates give rise to fructose 6-phosphate; a triose phosphate and tetrose 4-phosphate form heptose 7-phosphate. The final form of carbohydrate chain length interconversion is the transaldolase reaction, which interconverts heptose 7-phosphate and triose 3-phosphate with tetrose 4-phosphate and hexose 6-phosphate.

The coordination of different carbohydrate rearrangement reactions to achieve an overall metabolic goal is illustrated by the hexose monophosphate shunt (Fig 7–6). This metabolic cycle is used by blue-green bacteria for the reduction of NAD^+ to NADH, which serves as a reductant for respiration in the dark. Many organisms use the hexose monophosphate shunt to reduce $NADP^+$ to NADPH, which is used for biosynthetic reduction reactions. The first steps in the hexose monophosphate shunt are the oxidative reactions that shorten six hexose 6-phosphates (abbreviated as 6 C_6 in Fig 7–6) to six pentose 5-phosphates (abbreviated 6 C_5). Carbohydrate rearrangement reactions convert the 6 C_5 molecules to 5 C_6 molecules so that the oxidative cycle may continue.

Clearly, all reactions for interconversion of carbohydrate chain lengths are not called into play at the same time. Selection of specific sets of enzymes, essentially the determination of the metabolic pathway taken, is dictated by the source of carbon and the biosynthetic demands of the cell. For example, a cell given triose phosphate as a source of carbohydrate will use the aldolase-phosphatase combination to form fructose 6-phosphate; the kinase that acts on fructose 6-phosphate in its conversion to triose phosphate would not be expected to be active under these circumstances. If demands for pentose 5-phosphate are high, as is the case in photosynthetic carbon dioxide assimilation, transketolases that can give rise to pentose 5-phosphates are very active.

In sum, glucose 6-phosphate can be regarded as a focal metabolite because it serves both as a direct precursor for metabolic building blocks and as a source of carbohydrates of varying length that are used for biosynthetic purposes. Glucose 6-phosphate itself may be generated from other phosphorylated carbohydrates by selection of pathways from a set of reactions for chain length interconversion. The reactions chosen are determined by the genetic potential of the cell, the primary carbon source, and the biosynthetic demands of the organism. Metabolic regulation is required to ensure that reactions which meet the requirements of the organism are selected.

Formation & Utilization of Phosphoenolpyruvate

Triose phosphates, formed by the interconversion of carbohydrate phosphoesters, are converted to phosphoenolpyruvate by the series of reactions shown in

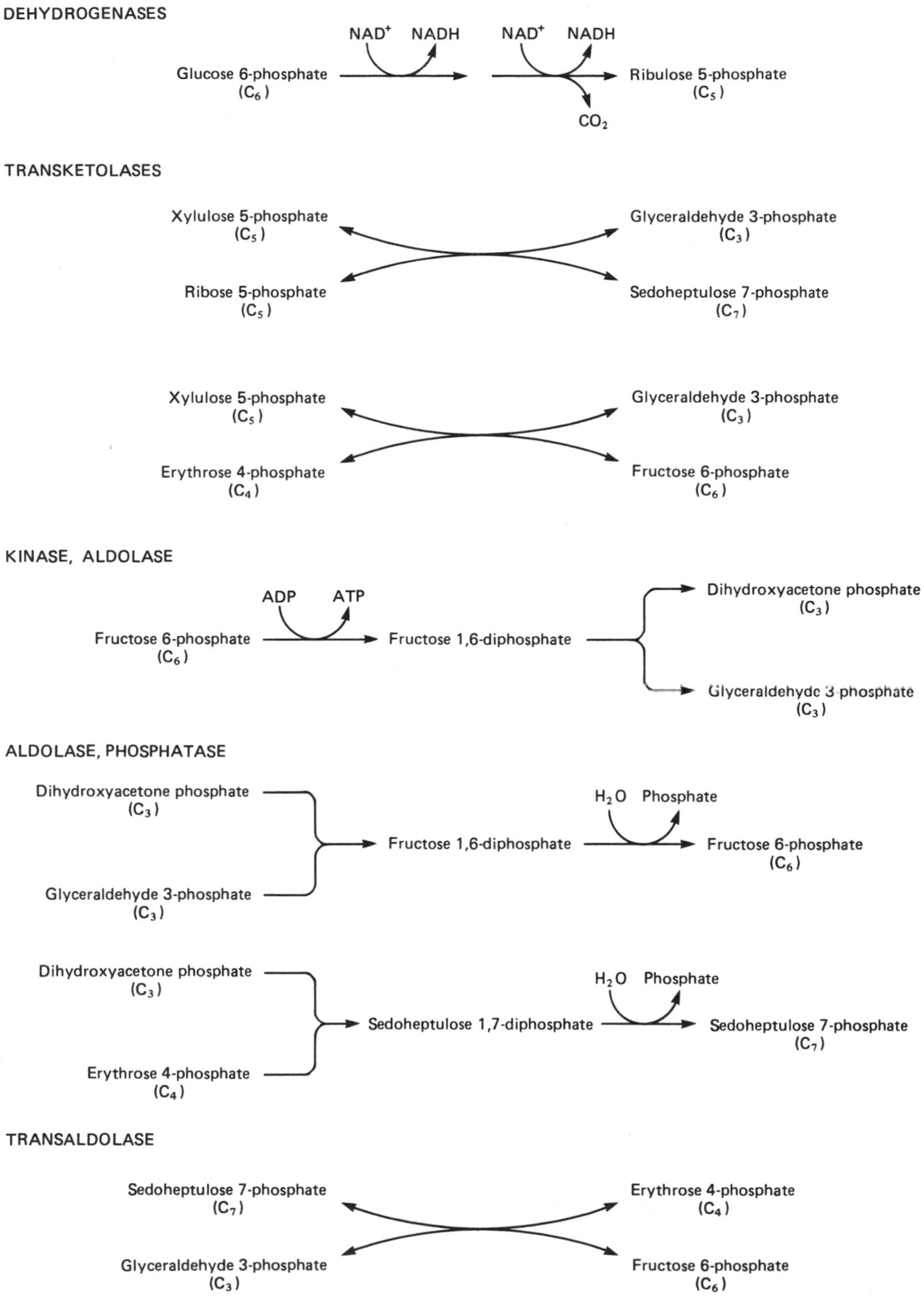

DEHYDROGENASES

$$
\text{Glucose 6-phosphate} \atop (C_6) \quad \xrightarrow{\text{NAD}^+ \quad \text{NADH}} \quad \xrightarrow{\text{NAD}^+ \quad \text{NADH} \atop CO_2} \quad \text{Ribulose 5-phosphate} \atop (C_5)
$$

TRANSKETOLASES

Xylulose 5-phosphate
(C_5)

Ribose 5-phosphate
(C_5)

Glyceraldehyde 3-phosphate
(C_3)

Sedoheptulose 7-phosphate
(C_7)

Xylulose 5-phosphate
(C_5)

Erythrose 4-phosphate
(C_4)

Glyceraldehyde 3-phosphate
(C_3)

Fructose 6-phosphate
(C_6)

KINASE, ALDOLASE

$$
\text{Fructose 6-phosphate} \atop (C_6) \quad \xrightarrow{\text{ADP} \quad \text{ATP}} \quad \text{Fructose 1,6-diphosphate}
$$

Dihydroxyacetone phosphate
(C_3)

Glyceraldehyde 3-phosphate
(C_3)

ALDOLASE, PHOSPHATASE

Dihydroxyacetone phosphate
(C_3)

Glyceraldehyde 3-phosphate
(C_3)

$$
\longrightarrow \text{Fructose 1,6-diphosphate} \xrightarrow{H_2O \quad \text{Phosphate}} \text{Fructose 6-phosphate} \atop (C_6)
$$

Dihydroxyacetone phosphate
(C_3)

Erythrose 4-phosphate
(C_4)

$$
\longrightarrow \text{Sedoheptulose 1,7-diphosphate} \xrightarrow{H_2O \quad \text{Phosphate}} \text{Sedoheptulose 7-phosphate} \atop (C_7)
$$

TRANSALDOLASE

Sedoheptulose 7-phosphate
(C_7)

Glyceraldehyde 3-phosphate
(C_3)

Erythrose 4-phosphate
(C_4)

Fructose 6-phosphate
(C_6)

Figure 7–5. Biochemical mechanisms for changing the length of carbohydrate molecules. The general empirical formula for carbohydrate phosphate esters, $(C_nH_{2n}O_n)$-N-phosphate, is abbreviated (C_n) in order to emphasize changes in chain length.

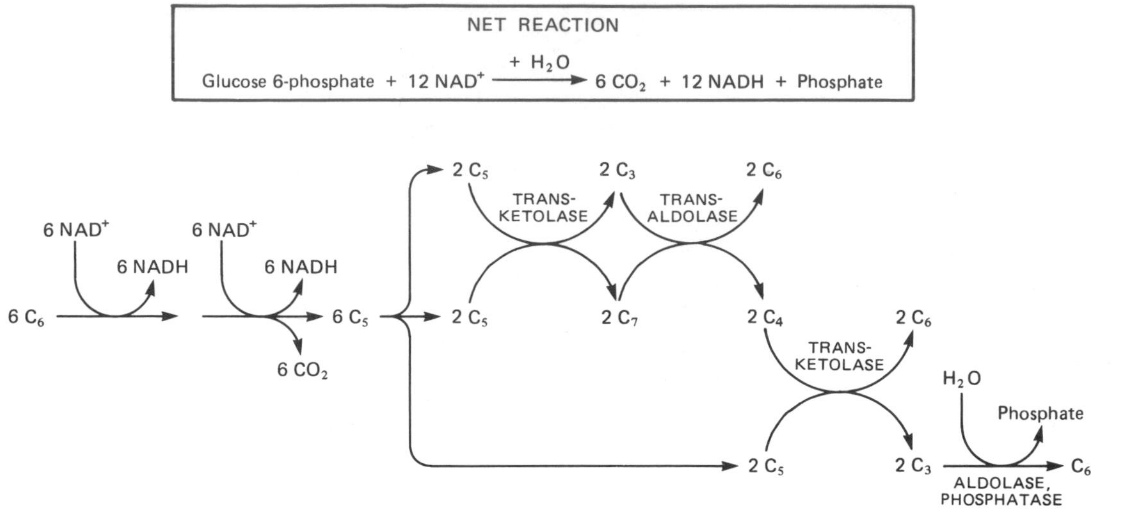

NET REACTION

$$\text{Glucose 6-phosphate } + 12 \text{ NAD}^+ \xrightarrow{\ + \text{ H}_2\text{O}\ } 6 \text{ CO}_2 + 12 \text{ NADH } + \text{ Phosphate}$$

Figure 7–6. The hexose monophosphate shunt. Oxidative reactions (Fig 7–5) reduce NAD^+ and produce CO_2, resulting in the shortening of the six hexose phosphates (abbreviated C_6) to six pentose phosphates (abbreviated C_5). Carbohydrate rearrangements (Fig 7–5) convert the pentose phosphates to hexose phosphates so that the oxidative cycle may continue.

Fig 7–7. Oxidation of glyceraldehyde 3-phosphate by NAD^+ is accompanied by the formation of the acid anhydride bond on the 1-carbon of 1,3-diphosphoglycerate. This phosphate anhydride is transferred in a **substrate phosphorylation** to ADP, yielding an energy-rich bond in ATP. Another energy-rich phosphate bond is formed by dehydration of 2-phosphoglycerate to phosphoenolpyruvate; and via another substrate phosphorylation, phosphoenolpyruvate can donate the energy-rich bond to ADP, yielding ATP and pyruvate. Thus, 2 energy-rich bonds in ATP can be obtained by the metabolic conversion of triose phosphate to pyruvate. This is an oxidative process,

and in the absence of an exogenous electron acceptor, the NADH generated by oxidation of glyceraldehyde 3-phosphate must be oxidized to NAD^+ by pyruvate or by metabolites derived from pyruvate. The products formed as a result of this process vary and, as described later in this chapter, can be used in the identification of clinically significant bacteria.

Formation of phosphoenolpyruvate from pyruvate (Fig 7–8) requires a substantial amount of metabolic energy, and 2 anhydride ATP bonds invariably are invested in the process. Some organisms—*Escherichia coli*, for example—directly phosphorylate pyruvate with ATP, yielding AMP and inorganic phosphate

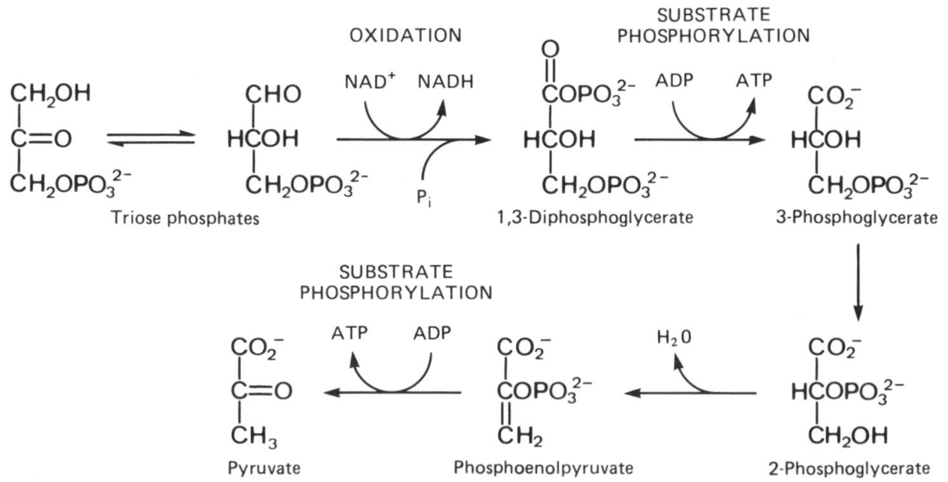

Figure 7–7. Formation of phosphoenolpyruvate and pyruvate from triose phosphate. The figure draws attention to 2 sites of substrate phosphorylation and to the oxidative step that results in the reduction of NAD^+ to NADH. Repetition of this energy-yielding pathway demands a mechanism for oxidizing NADH to NAD^+. Fermentative organisms achieve this goal by using pyruvate or metabolites derived from pyruvate as oxidants.

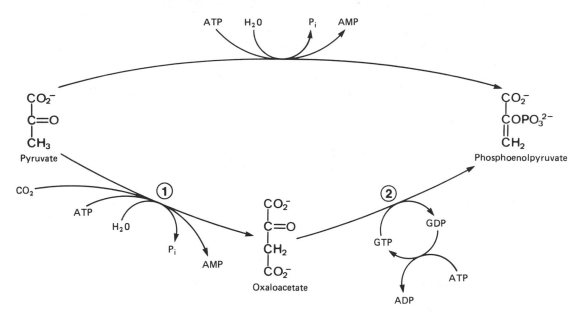

Figure 7–8. Two mechanisms for the conversion of pyruvate to phosphoenolpyruvate. This reaction requires the thermodynamic investment of 2 pyrophosphate bonds. Some organisms carry out the reaction in a single step in which the phosphorylation of pyruvate is enzymatically coupled to the hydrolysis of a pyrophosphate bond. Other organisms invest pyrophosphate bonds in each of 2 consecutive metabolic steps: (1) the ATP-dependent carboxylation of pyruvate to oxaloacetate, and (2) the GTP-dependent decarboxylation of oxaloacetate to phosphoenolpyruvate.

(P_i). Other organisms use 2 metabolic steps: one ATP pyrophosphate bond is invested in the carboxylation of pyruvate to oxaloacetate, and a second pyrophosphate bond (often carried in GTP rather than ATP) is used to generate phosphoenolpyruvate from oxaloacetate.

Formation & Utilization of Oxaloacetate (Fig 7–9)

As described above, many organisms form oxaloacetate by the ATP-dependent carboxylation of pyruvate (Fig 7–8). Other organisms, such as *E coli,* which

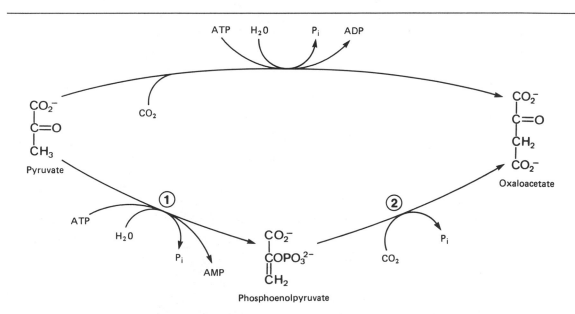

Figure 7–9. Formation of oxaloacetate from pyruvate. As described in Fig 7–8, some organisms carboxylate pyruvate directly to oxalacetate in an ATP-dependent reaction. The organisms that convert pyruvate directly to phosphoenolpyruvate (Fig 7–8) carboxylate phosphoenolpyruvate to oxaloacetate.

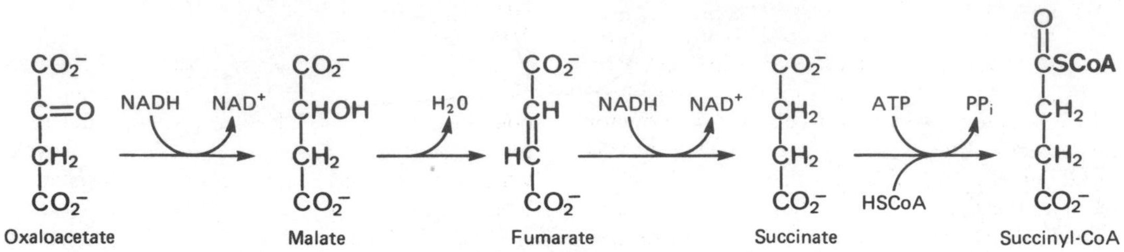

Figure 7–10. Reductive conversion of oxaloacetate to succinyl-CoA. This reductive series of reactions is used as a biosynthetic route in organisms that do not employ a conventional tricarboxylic acid cycle (Fig 7–13), and the direction of metabolic flow is the reverse of that found in the tricarboxylic acid cycle. The reactions that result in the oxidation of NADH are used by some fermentative organisms to generate NAD$^+$ so that the energy-yielding metabolism of triose phosphates (Fig 7–7) can continue.

form phosphoenolpyruvate directly from pyruvate, synthesize oxaloacetate by carboxylation of phosphoenolpyruvate (Fig 7–9).

Succinyl-CoA is a required biosynthetic precursor for the synthesis of porphyrins and other essential compounds. Some organisms form succinyl-CoA by reduction of oxaloacetate via malate and fumarate (Fig 7–10). These reactions represent a reversal of the metabolic flow observed in the conventional tricarboxylic acid cycle (Fig 7–13).

Formation of α-Ketoglutarate From Pyruvate (Fig 7–11)

Conversion of pyruvate to α-ketoglutarate requires a metabolic pathway that diverges and then converges (Fig 7–11). In one branch, oxaloacetate is formed by

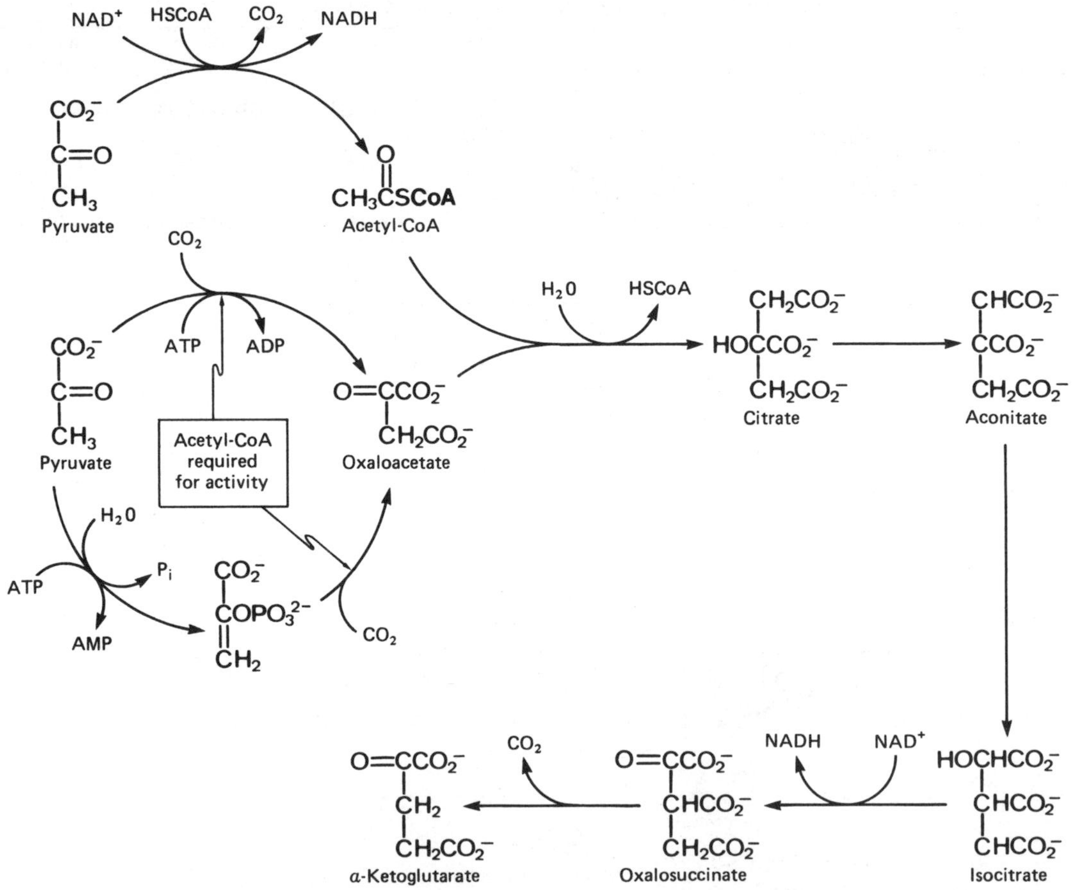

Figure 7–11. Conversion of pyruvate to α-ketoglutarate. Pyruvate is converted to α-ketoglutarate by a branched biosynthetic pathway. In one branch, pyruvate is oxidized to acetyl-CoA; in the other, pyruvate is carboxylated to oxaloacetate. As noted in Fig 7–9, the latter conversion can proceed through either of 2 mechanisms.

carboxylation of pyruvate or phosphoenolpyruvate. In the other branch, pyruvate is oxidized to acetyl-CoA. It is noteworthy that, regardless of the enzymatic mechanism used for the formation of oxaloacetate, acetyl-CoA is required as a positive metabolic effector for this process. Thus, the synthesis of oxaloacetate is balanced with the production of acetyl-CoA. Condensation of oxaloacetate with acetyl-CoA yields citrate. Isomerization of the citrate molecule produces isocitrate, which is oxidatively decarboxylated to α-ketoglutarate.

ASSIMILATORY PATHWAYS

Growth With Acetate

Acetate is metabolized via acetyl-CoA, and many organisms possess the ability to form acetyl-CoA (Fig 7–12). Acetyl-CoA is used in the biosynthesis of α-ketoglutarate, and in most respiratory organisms, the acetyl fragment in acetyl-CoA is oxidized completely to carbon dioxide via the tricarboxylic acid cycle (Fig 7–13). The ability to utilize acetate as a net source of carbon, however, is limited to relatively few microorganisms and plants. Net synthesis of biosynthetic precursors from acetate is achieved by coupling reactions of the tricarboxylic acid cycle with 2 additional reactions catalyzed by isocitrate lyase and malate synthase. As shown in Fig 7–14, these reactions allow the *net* oxidative conversion of 2 acetyl moieties from acetyl-CoA to one molecule of succinate. Succinate may be used for biosynthetic purposes after its conversion to oxaloacetate, α-ketoglutarate, phosphoenolpyruvate, or glucose 6-phosphate.

Growth With Carbon Dioxide: The Calvin Cycle

Like plants and algae, a number of microbial species can use carbon dioxide as a sole source of carbon. In almost all of these organisms, the primary route of carbon assimilation is via the Calvin cycle, in which carbon dioxide and ribulose diphosphate combine to form 2 molecules of 3-phosphoglycerate (Fig 7–15A). 3-Phosphoglycerate is phosphorylated to 1,3-diphosphoglycerate, and this compound is reduced to the triose derivative, glyceraldehyde 3-phosphate. Carbohydrate rearrangement reactions (Fig 7–5) allow triose phosphate to be converted to the pentose derivative ribulose 5-phosphate, which is phosphorylated to regenerate the acceptor molecule, ribulose 1,5-diphosphate (Fig 7–15B). Additional reduced carbon, formed by the reductive assimilation of carbon dioxide, is converted to focal metabolites for biosynthetic pathways.

Cells that can use carbon dioxide as a sole source of carbon are termed **autotrophic,** and the demands for this pattern of carbon assimilation can be summarized briefly as follows: In addition to the primary assimilatory reaction giving rise to 3-phosphoglycerate, there must be a mechanism for regenerating the acceptor molecule, ribulose 1,5-diphosphate. This process demands the energy-dependent reduction of 3-phosphoglycerate to the level of carbohydrate. Thus, autotrophy requires carbon dioxide, ATP, NADPH, and a specific set of enzymes.

Depolymerases

Many potential growth substrates occur as building blocks within the structure of biologic polymers. These large molecules are not readily transported

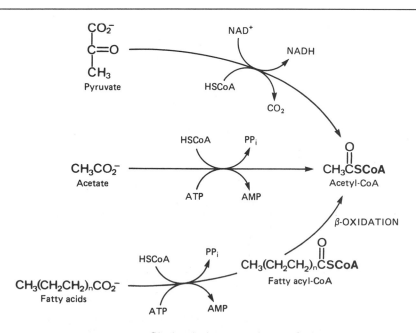

Figure 7–12. Biochemical sources of acetyl-CoA.

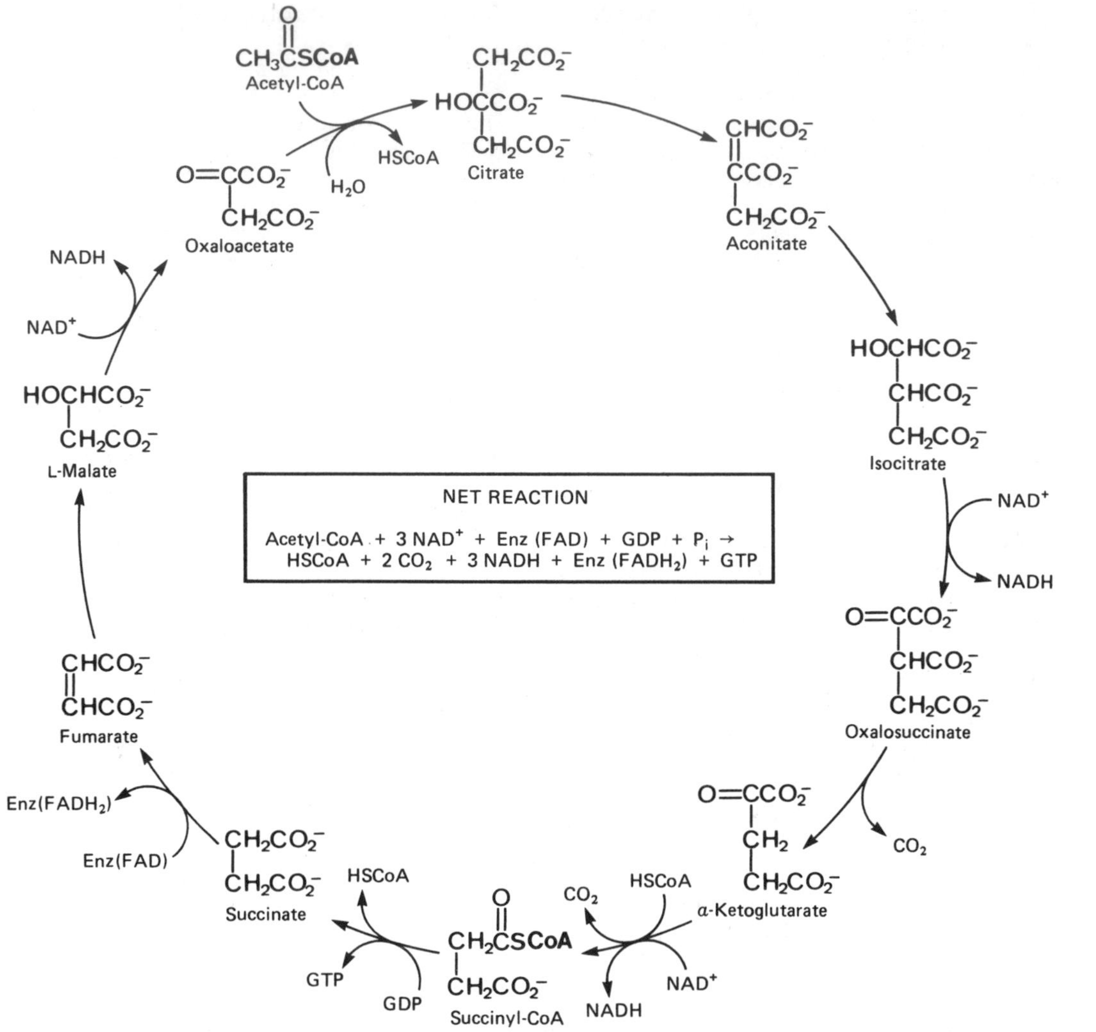

Figure 7–13. The tricarboxylic acid cycle. There are 4 oxidative steps, 3 giving rise to NADH and one giving rise to a reduced flavoprotein, Enz(FADH$_2$). The cycle can continue only if electron acceptors are available to oxidize the NADH and reduced flavoprotein.

across the cell membrane and often are affixed to even larger cellular structures. Many microorganisms elaborate extracellular depolymerases that hydrolyze proteins, nucleic acids, polysaccharides, and lipids. The pattern of depolymerase production can be useful in the identification of microorganisms.

Oxygenases

Many compounds in the environment are relatively resistant to enzymatic modification, and utilization of these compounds as growth substrates demands a special class of enzymes, oxygenases. These enzymes directly employ the potent oxidant molecular oxygen as a substrate in reactions that convert a relatively intractable compound to a form in which it can be assimilated by thermodynamically favored reactions. The action of oxygenases is illustrated in Fig 7–16, which shows the role of 2 different oxygenases in the utilization of benzoate.

Reductive Pathways

Some microorganisms live in extremely reducing environments that favor chemical reactions which would not occur in organisms using oxygen as an electron acceptor. In these organisms, powerful reductants can be used to drive reactions that allow the assimilation of relatively intractable compounds. An example is the reductive assimilation of benzoate (Fig 7–17), a process in which the aromatic ring is reduced and opened to form the dicarboxylic acid pimelate. Further metabolic reactions convert pimelate to focal metabolites.

Nitrogen Assimilation

The reductive assimilation of molecular nitrogen (Fig 7–18) is required for continuation of life on our planet. Nitrogenase, the enzyme catalyzing the reaction, is found only in bacteria and demands a substantial amount of metabolic energy: 12–15 molecules of

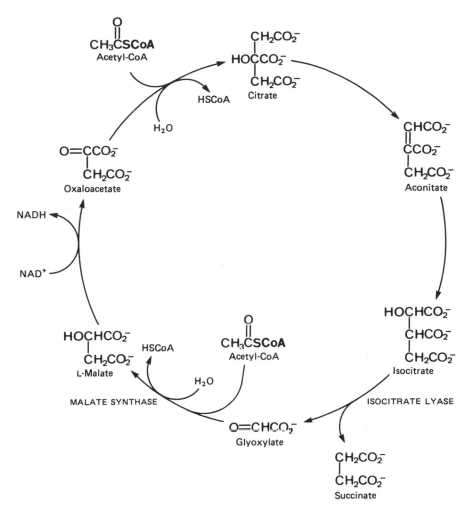

Figure 7–14. The glyoxylate cycle. Note that the reactions which convert malate to isocitrate are shared with the tricarboxylic acid cycle (Fig 7–13). Metabolic divergence at the level of isocitrate and the action of 2 enzymes, isocitrate lyase and malate synthase, modify the tricarboxylic acid cycle so that it reductively converts 2 molecules of acetyl-CoA to succinate.

ATP are hydrolyzed as a single N_2 molecule is reduced to 2 molecules of NH_3 by 3 molecules of NADPH.

Additional physiologic demands are placed by the fact that nitrogenase is readily inactivated by oxygen. Aerobic organisms that employ nitrogenase have developed elaborate mechanisms to protect the enzyme against inactivation. Some form specialized cells in which nitrogen fixation takes place, and others have developed elaborate electron transport chains to protect nitrogenase against inactivation by oxygen. The most significant of these bacteria in agriculture are the *Rhizobiaceae,* organisms that fix nitrogen symbiotically in the root nodules of leguminous plants.

The capacity to use ammonia as a nitrogen source is widely distributed among organisms. The primary portal of entry of nitrogen into carbon metabolism is glutamate, which is formed by reductive amination of α-ketoglutarate. As shown in Fig 7–19, there are 2 biochemical mechanisms by which this can be achieved. One, the single-step reduction catalyzed by glutamate dehydrogenase (Fig 7–19A), is effective in environments in which there is an ample supply of ammonia. The other, a 2-step process in which glutamine is an intermediate (Fig 7–19B), is employed in environments in which ammonia is in short supply. The latter mechanism allows cells to invest the free energy formed by hydrolysis of a pyrophosphate bond in ATP into the assimilation of ammonia from the environment.

The amide nitrogen of glutamine, an intermediate in the 2-step assimilation of ammonia into glutamate (Fig 7–19B), is also transferred directly into organic nitrogen appearing in the structures of purines, pyrimidines, arginine, tryptophan, and glucosamine. The activity and synthesis of glutamine synthase are regulated by the ammonia supply and by the availability of metabolites containing nitrogen derived directly from the amide nitrogen of glutamine.

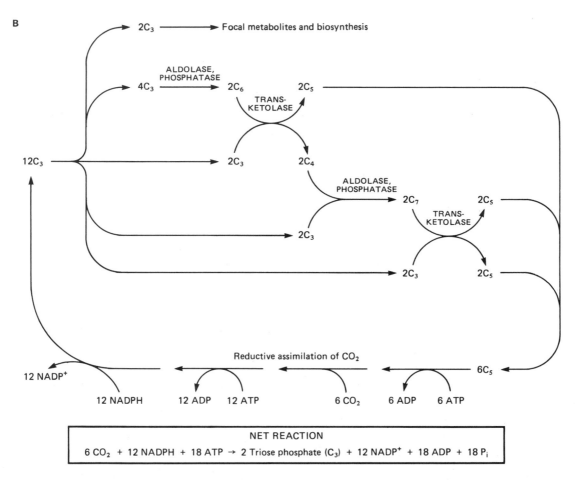

Figure 7–15. The Calvin cycle. **A:** Reductive assimilation of CO_2. ATP and NADPH are used to reductively convert pentose 5-phosphate (C_5) to 2 molecules of triose phosphate (C_3). **B:** The Calvin cycle is completed by carbohydrate rearrangement reactions (Fig 7–5) that allow the net synthesis of carbohydrate and the regeneration of pentose phosphate so that the cycle may continue.

Most of the organic nitrogen in cells is derived from the α-amino group of glutamate, and the primary mechanism by which the nitrogen is transferred is **transamination,** illustrated in Fig 7–20. The usual acceptor in these reactions is an α-keto acid, which is transformed to the corresponding α-amino acid. α-Ketoglutarate, the other product of the transamination reaction, may be converted to glutamate by reductive amination (Fig 7–19).

BIOSYNTHETIC PATHWAYS

Tracing the Structures of Biosynthetic Precursors: Glutamate & Aspartate

In many cases, the carbon skeleton of a metabolic end product may be traced to its biosynthetic origins. Glutamine, an obvious example, clearly is derived from glutamate (Fig 7–21). The glutamate skeleton in the structures of arginine and proline (Fig 7–21) is less

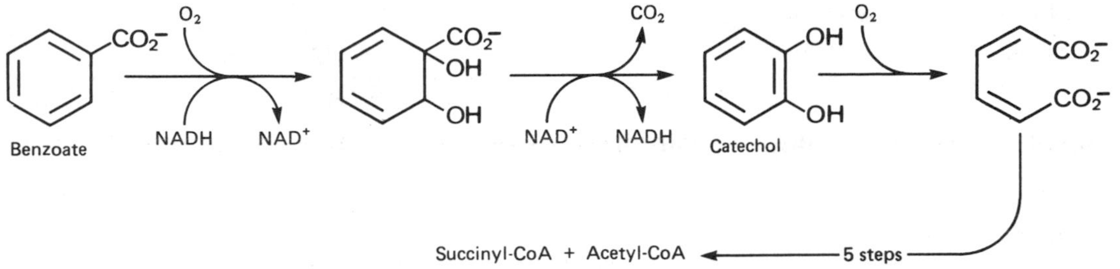

Figure 7–16. The role of oxygenases in aerobic utilization of benzoate as a carbon source. Molecular oxygen participates directly in the reactions that disrupt the aromaticity of benzoate and catechol.

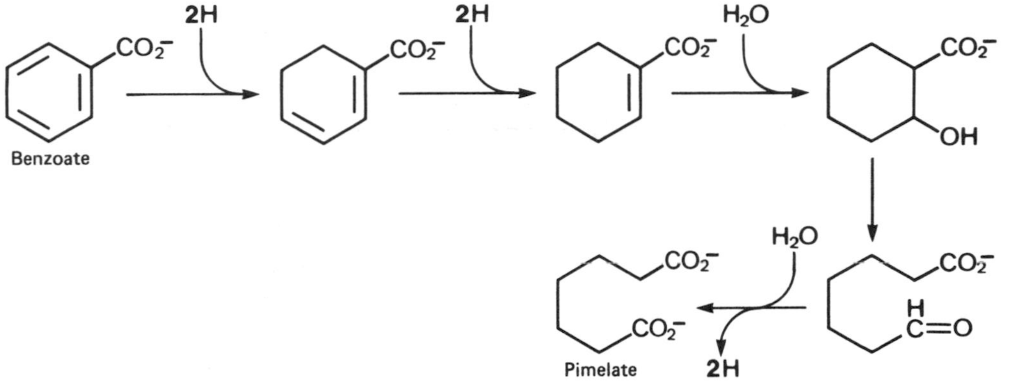

Figure 7–17. Reductive reactions in anaerobic utilization of benzoate as a carbon source. Individual steps in the pathway are somewhat speculative; for example, benzoate may be metabolized as its CoA thioester. The metabolic sequence illustrates that, in a strongly reducing environment, the aromatic ring of benzoate can be reduced, with the result that the dicarboxylate pimelate is produced as a source of carbon.

obvious but readily discernible. Similarly, the carbon skeleton of aspartate, directly derived from the focal metabolite oxaloacetate, is evident in the structures of asparagine, threonine, methionine, and pyrimidines (Fig 7–22). In some cases, different carbon skeletons combine in a biosynthetic pathway. For example, aspartate semialdehyde and pyruvate combine to form the metabolic precursor of lysine, diaminopimelic acid, and dipicolinic acid (Fig 7–23). The latter 2 compounds are found only in prokaryotes. Diami-

nopimelic acid is a component of peptidoglycan in the cell wall, and dipicolinic acid represents a major portion of endospores.

Synthesis of Cell Wall Peptidoglycan

The structure of peptidoglycan is shown in Fig 2–14; the pathway by which it is synthesized is shown in simplified form in Fig 7–24. The synthesis of peptidoglycan begins with the stepwise synthesis in the cytoplasm of UDP–N-acetylmuramic acid–pentapeptide. N-Acetylglucosamine is first attached to UDP and then converted to UDP–N-acetylmuramic acid by condensation with phosphoenolpyruvate and reduction. The amino acids of the pentapeptide are sequentially added, each addition catalyzed by a different enzyme and each involving the split of ATP to ADP + P_i.

The UDP–N-acetylmuramic acid–pentapeptide is attached to bactoprenol (a lipid of the cell membrane) and receives a molecule of N-acetylglucosamine from UDP. The pentaglycine derivative is next formed in a series of reactions using glycyl-tRNA as the donor; the completed disaccharide is polymerized to an oligomeric intermediate before being transferred to the growing end of a glycopeptide polymer in the cell wall.

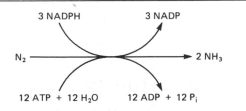

Figure 7–18. Reduction of N_2 to 2 molecules of NH_3. In addition to reductant, the nitrogenase reaction requires a substantial amount of metabolic energy. The number of ATP molecules required for reduction of a single nitrogen molecule to ammonia is uncertain; the value appears to lie between 12 and 15.

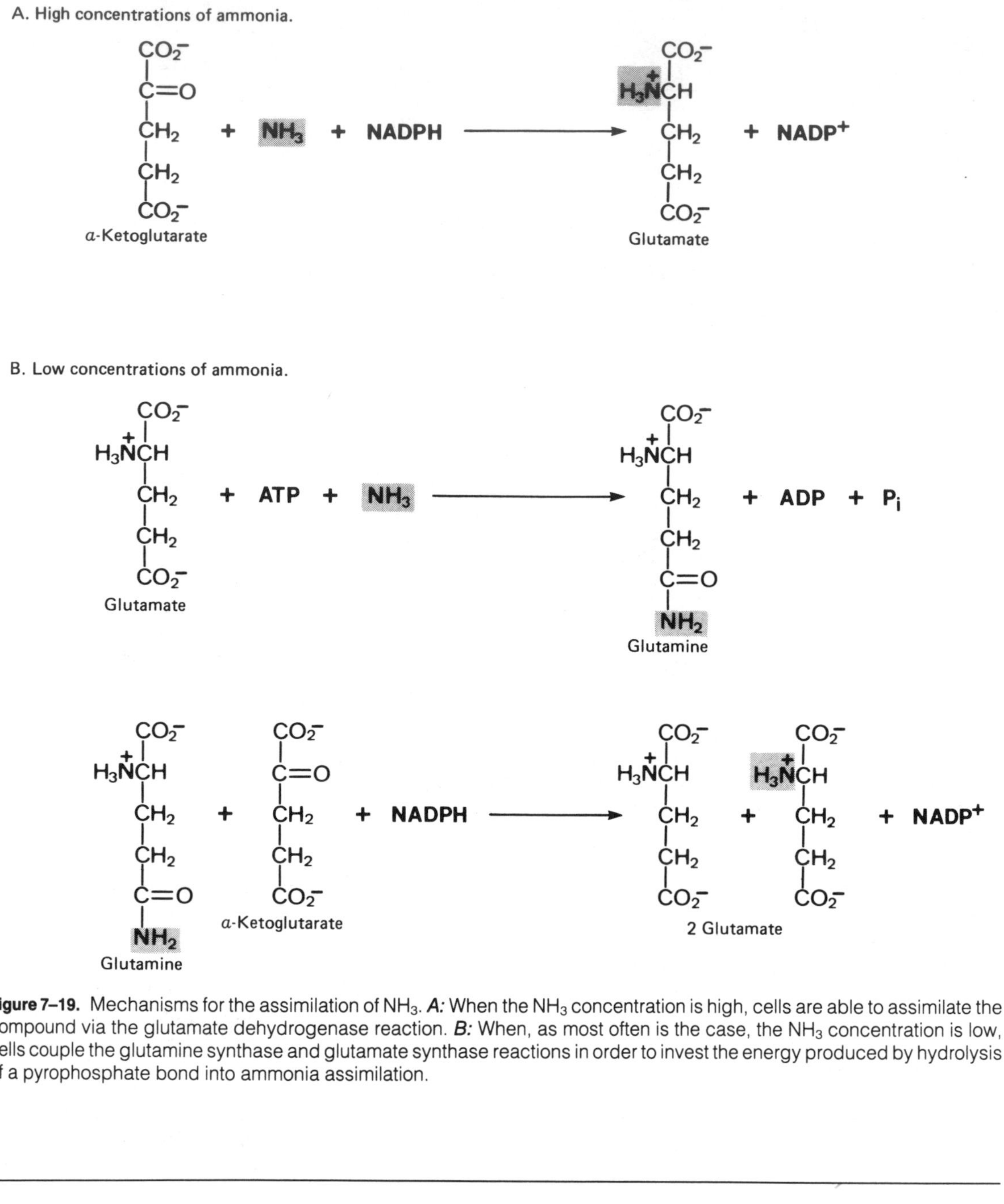

A. High concentrations of ammonia.

B. Low concentrations of ammonia.

Figure 7–19. Mechanisms for the assimilation of NH_3. *A:* When the NH_3 concentration is high, cells are able to assimilate the compound via the glutamate dehydrogenase reaction. *B:* When, as most often is the case, the NH_3 concentration is low, cells couple the glutamine synthase and glutamate synthase reactions in order to invest the energy produced by hydrolysis of a pyrophosphate bond into ammonia assimilation.

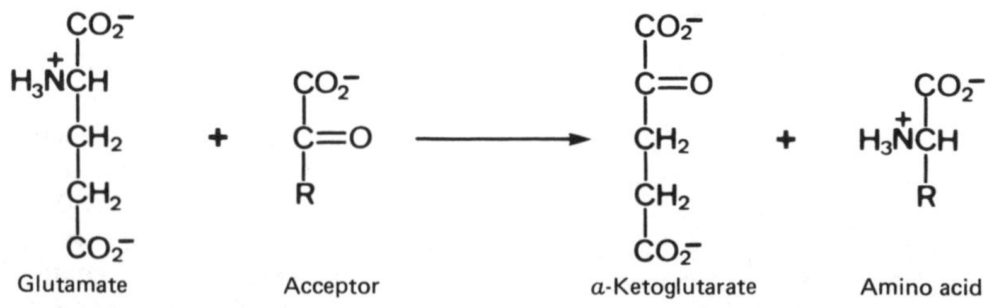

Figure 7–20. Transamination, the major mechanism for forming the α-amino group of amino acids. R, organic radical.

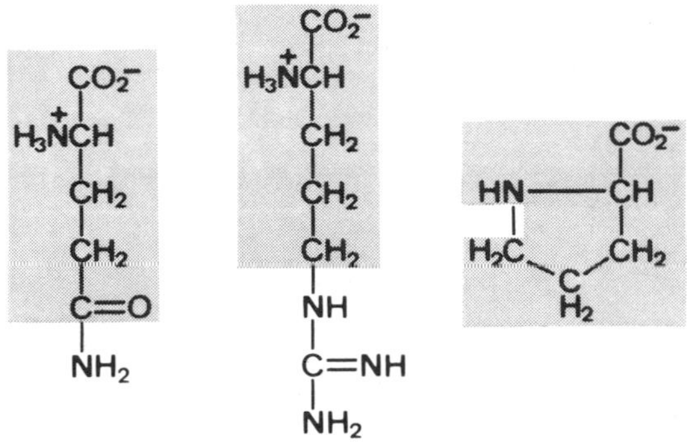

Figure 7–21. Amino acids formed from glutamate.

Final cross-linking is accomplished by a transpeptidation reaction in which the free amino group of a pentaglycine residue displaces the terminal D-alanine residue of a neighboring pentapeptide. Transpeptidation is catalyzed by one of a set of enzymes called penicillin-binding proteins (PBPs). PBPs bind penicillin and other β-lactam antibiotics covalently; they have both transpeptidase and carboxypeptidase activities, their relative rates perhaps controlling the degree of cross-linking in peptidoglycan (a factor important in cell septation).

The biosynthetic pathway is of particular importance in medicine, as it provides a basis for the selective antibacterial action of several chemotherapeutic agents. Unlike their host cells, bacteria are not isotonic with the body fluids. Their contents are under high osmotic pressure, and their viability depends on the integrity of the peptidoglycan lattice in the cell wall being maintained throughout the growth cycle. Any compound that inhibits any step in the biosynthesis of peptidoglycan causes the wall of the growing bacterial cell to be weakened and the cell to lyse. The sites of action of several antibiotics are shown in Fig 7–24.

Synthesis of Cell Wall Lipopolysaccharide

The general structure of the antigenic lipopolysaccharide of gram-negative cell walls is shown in Fig 2–17.The biosynthesis of the repeating end-group, which gives the cell wall its antigenic specificity, is shown in Fig 7–25. Note the resemblance to peptidoglycan synthesis: in both cases, a series of subunits is assembled on a lipid carrier in the membrane and then transferred to open ends of the growing polymer fabric of the cell wall.

Synthesis of Extracellular Capsular Polymers

The capsular polymers, a few examples of which are listed in Table 2–1, are enzymatically synthesized from activated subunits. No membrane-bound lipid carriers have been implicated in this process. The presence of a capsule is often environmentally determined: dextrans and levans, for example, can only be synthesized using the disaccharide sucrose (fructose-glucose) as the source of the appropriate subunit, and their synthesis thus depends on the presence of sucrose in the medium.

Synthesis of Reserve Food Granules

When nutrients are present in excess of the requirements for growth, bacteria convert certain of them to intracellular reserve food granules. The principal ones are starch, glycogen, poly-β-hydroxybutyrate (PBHB), and volutin, which consists mainly of inorganic polyphosphate. The type of granule formed is species-specific. The granules are degraded when exogenous nutrients are depleted.

PATTERNS OF MICROBIAL ENERGY-YIELDING METABOLISM

As described in Chapter 6, there are 2 major metabolic mechanisms for generating the energy-rich acid pyrophosphate bonds in ATP: **substrate phosphorylation** (the direct transfer of a phosphate anhydride bond from an organic donor to ADP) and phosphorylation of ADP by inorganic phosphate. The latter reaction is energetically unfavorable and must be driven by a transmembrane electrochemical gradient: the **proton motive force.** In respiration, the electrochemical gradient is created from externally supplied reductant and oxidant. Energy released by transfer of electrons from the reductant to the oxidant through membrane-bound carriers is coupled to the formation

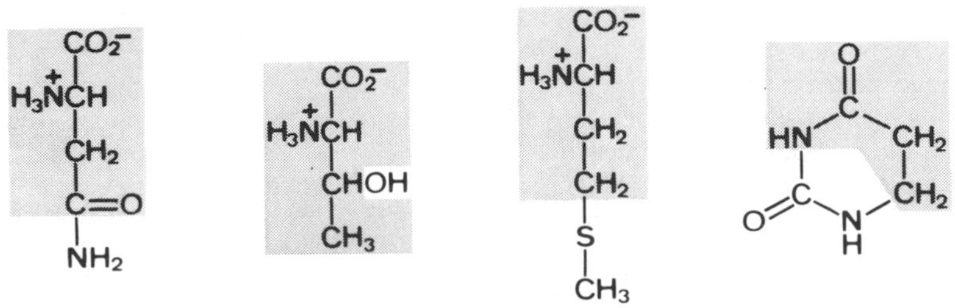

Figure 7–22. Biosynthetic end products formed from aspartate.

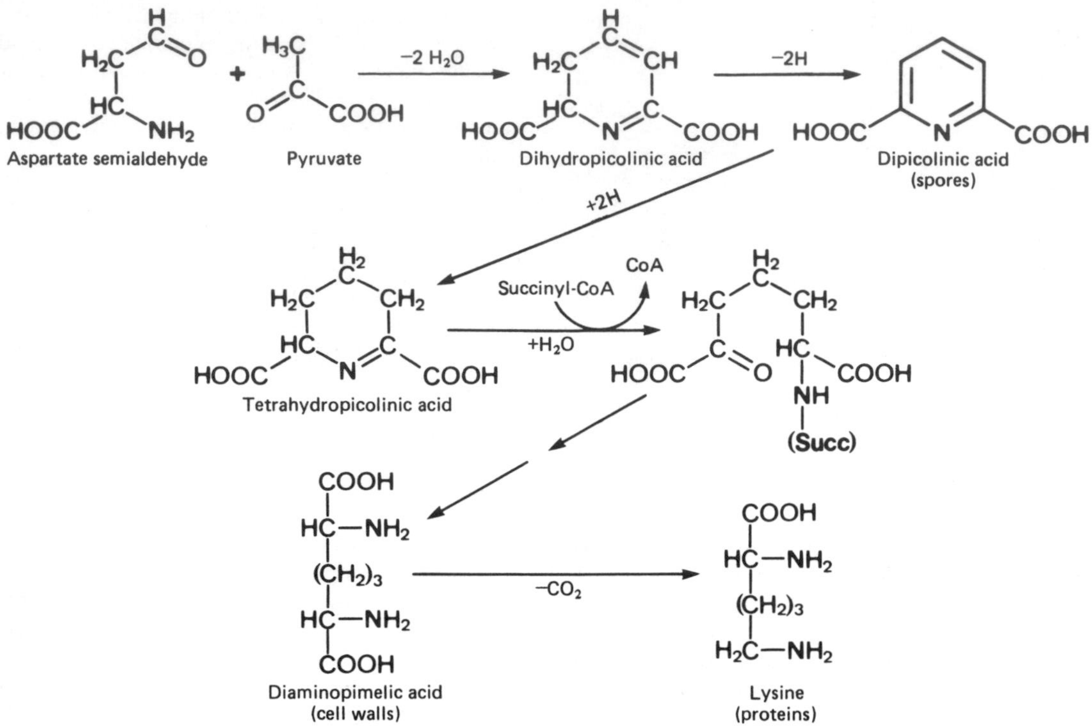

Figure 7–23. Biosynthetic end products formed from aspartate semialdehyde and pyruvate.

of the transmembrane electrochemical gradient. In photosynthesis, light energy generates membrane-associated reductants and oxidants; the proton motive force is generated as these electron carriers return to the ground state. These processes are discussed below.

Pathways of Fermentation

A. Strategies for Substrate Phosphorylation: In the absence of respiration or photosynthesis, cells are entirely dependent upon substrate phosphorylation for their energy: generation of ATP must be coupled to chemical rearrangement of organic compounds. Many compounds can serve as fermentable growth substrates, and many pathways for their fermentation have evolved. These pathways have the following 3 general stages: (1) Conversion of the fermentable compound to the phosphate donor for substrate phosphorylation. This stage often contains metabolic reactions in which NAD$^+$ is reduced to NADH. (2) Phosphorylation of ADP by the energy-rich phosphate donor. (3) Metabolic steps that bring the products of the fermentation into chemical balance with the starting materials. The most frequent requirement in the last stage is a mechanism for oxidation of NADH, generated in the first stage of fermentation, to NAD$^+$ so that the fermentation may proceed. In the following sections, examples of each of the 3 stages of fermentation are considered.

B. Fermentation of Glucose: The diversity of fermentative pathways is illustrated by consideration

of some of the mechanisms used by microorganisms to achieve substrate phosphorylation at the expense of glucose. In principle, the phosphorylation of ADP to ATP can be coupled to either of 2 chemically balanced transformations:

$$\text{Glucose} \longrightarrow \text{2 Lactic acid}$$
$$(C_6H_{12}O_6) \qquad\qquad (C_3H_6O_3)$$

or

$$\text{Glucose} \longrightarrow \text{2 Ethanol} + \text{2 Carbon dioxide}$$
$$(C_6H_{12}O_6) \qquad\qquad (C_2H_6O) \qquad\qquad (CO_2)$$

The biochemical mechanisms by which these transformations are achieved vary considerably.

In general, the fermentation of glucose is initiated by its phosphorylation to glucose 6-phosphate. There are 2 mechanisms by which this can be achieved: (1) Extracellular glucose may be transported across the cytoplasmic membrane into the cell and then phosphorylated by ATP to yield glucose 6-phosphate and ADP (Fig 7–26A). (2) In many microorganisms, extracellular glucose is phosphorylated as it is being transported across the cytoplasmic membrane by an enzyme system in the cytoplasmic membrane that phosphorylates extracellular glucose at the expense of phosphoenolpyruvate, producing intracellular glucose 6-phosphate and pyruvate (Fig 7–26B). The latter process is an example of **vectorial metabolism,** a set of biochemical reactions in which both the structure and the

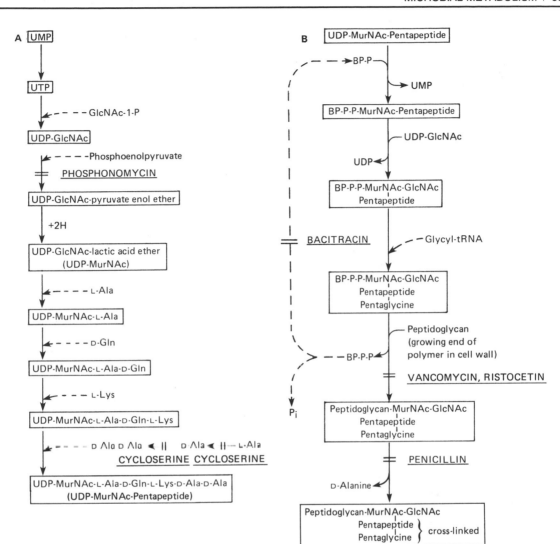

Figure 7–24. The biosynthesis of cell wall peptidoglycan, showing the sites of action of 6 antibiotics. BP = bactoprenol; MurNAc = N-acetylmuramic acid; GlcNAc = N-acetylglucosamine. *(A)* Synthesis of UDP–acetylmuramic acid–pentapeptide. *(B)* Synthesis of peptidoglycan from UDP–acetylmuramic acid–pentapeptide, UDP–N-acetylglucosamine, and glycyl residues. (See Fig 2–14 for structure of peptidoglycan.)

location of a substrate are altered. It should be noted that the choice of ATP or phosphoenolpyruvate as a phosphorylating agent does not alter the ATP yield of fermentation, because phosphoenolpyruvate is used as a source of ATP in the later stages of fermentation (Fig 7–7).

C. The Embden-Meyerhof Pathway: This pathway (Fig 7–27), a commonly encountered mechanism for the fermentation of glucose, uses a kinase and an aldolase (Fig 7–5) to transform the hexose (C_6) phosphate to 2 molecules of triose (C_3) phosphate. Four substrate phosphorylation reactions accompany the conversion of the triose phosphate to 2 molecules of pyruvate. Thus, taking into account the 2 ATP pyrophosphate bonds required to form triose phosphate from glucose, the Embden-Meyerhof pathway produces a net yield of 2 ATP pyrophosphate bonds. For-

mation of pyruvate from triose phosphate is an oxidative process, and the NADH formed in the first metabolic step (Fig 7–27) must be converted to NAD^+ for the fermentation to proceed; 2 of the simpler mechanisms for achieving this goal are illustrated in Fig 7–28. Direct reduction of pyruvate by NADH produces lactate as the end product of fermentation and thus results in acidification of the medium. Alternatively, pyruvate may be decarboxylated to acetaldehyde, which is then used to oxidize NADH, resulting in production of the neutral product ethanol. The pathway taken is determined by the evolutionary history of the organism and, in some microorganisms, by the growth conditions.

D. The Entner-Doudoroff and Heterolactate Fermentations: Alternative pathways for glucose fermentation include some specialized enzyme reac-

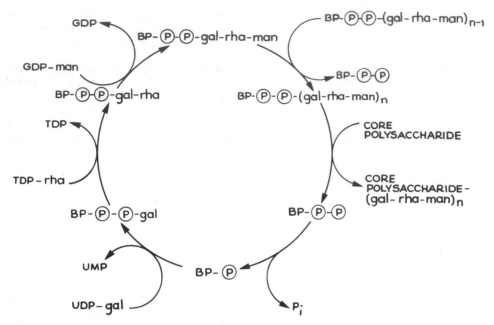

Figure 7–25. Synthesis of the repeating unit of the polysaccharide side chain of *Salmonella newington* and its transfer to the lipopolysaccharide core. BP = bactoprenol.

tions, and these are shown in Fig 7–29. The Entner-Doudoroff pathway diverges from other pathways of carbohydrate metabolism by a dehydration of 6-phosphogluconate followed by an aldolase reaction that produces pyruvate and triose phosphate (Fig 7–29A). The heterolactate fermentation and some other fermentative pathways depend upon a phosphoketolase reaction (Fig 7–29B) that phosphorolytically cleaves a ketose-phosphate to produce acetyl phosphate and triose phosphate. The acid anhydride acetyl phosphate may be used to synthesize ATP or may allow the oxidation of 2 NADH molecules to NAD^+ as it is reduced to ethanol.

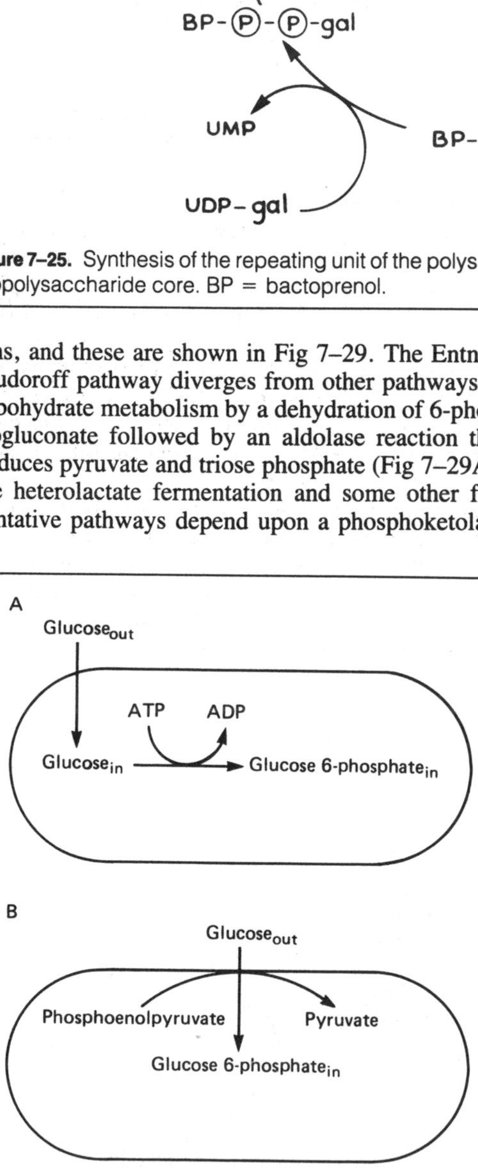

The overall outlines of the respective Entner-Doudoroff and heterolactate pathways are shown in Figs 7–30 and 7–31. The pathways yield only a single molecule of triose phosphate from glucose, and the energy yield is correspondingly low: unlike the Embden-Meyerhof pathway, the Entner-Doudoroff and heterolactate pathways yield only a single net substrate phosphorylation of ADP per molecule of glucose fermented. Why have the alternative pathways for glucose fermentation been selected in the natural environment? In answering this question, 2 facts should be kept in mind. First, in direct growth competition between 2 microbial species, the rate of substrate utilization can be more important than the amount of growth. Second, glucose is but one of many carbohydrates encountered by microorganisms in their natural environment. Pentoses, for example, can be fermented quite efficiently by the heterolactate pathway.

E. Additional Variations in Carbohydrate Fermentations: Pathways for carbohydrate fermentation can accommodate many more substrates than described here, and the end products may be far more diverse than suggested thus far. For example, there are numerous mechanisms for oxidation of NADH at the expense of pyruvate. One such pathway is the reductive formation of succinate (Fig 7–10). Many clinically significant bacteria form pyruvate from glucose via the Embden-Meyerhof pathway, and they may be distinguished on the basis of reduction products

Figure 7–26. Phosphorylation of glucose to form glucose 6-phosphate. *A:* After transport across the cell membrane, glucose is phosphorylated by a kinase. *B:* Glucose is phosphorylated by phosphoenolpyruvate as it crosses the cell membrane.

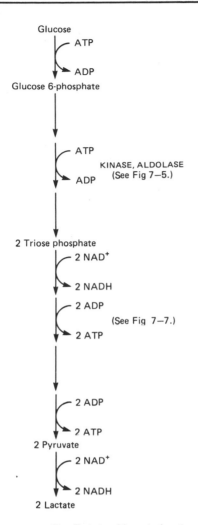

Figure 7–27. The Embden-Meyerhof pathway.

formed from pyruvate, reflecting the enzymatic constitution of different species. The major products of fermentation, listed in Table 7–1, form the basis for many diagnostic tests.

F. Fermentation of Other Substrates: Carbohydrates are by no means the only fermentable substrates. Metabolism of amino acids, purines, and pyrimidines may allow substrate phosphorylations to occur. For example, arginine may serve as an energy source by giving rise to carbamoyl phosphate, which can be used to phosphorylate ADP to ATP. Some organisms ferment pairs of amino acids, using one as an electron donor and the other as an electron acceptor:

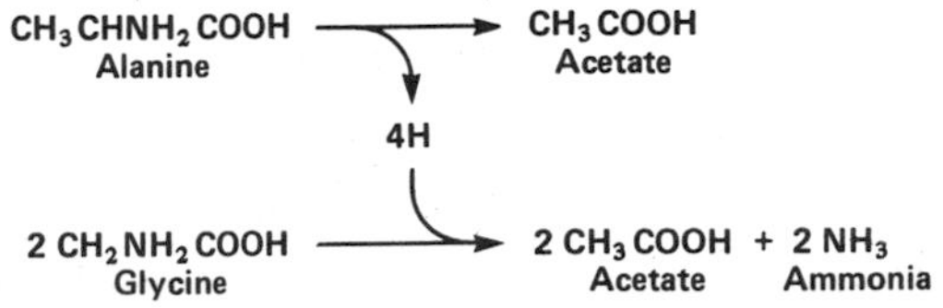

$$CH_3CHNH_2COOH \longrightarrow CH_3COOH$$
Alanine   Acetate

4H

$$2\,CH_2NH_2COOH \longrightarrow 2\,CH_3COOH + 2\,NH_3$$
Glycine   Acetate   Ammonia

Patterns of Respiration

Respiration requires a closed membrane. In bacteria, the membrane is the cell membrane. Electrons are passed from a chemical reductant to a chemical oxidant through a specific set of electron carriers within the membrane, and as a result, the proton motive force is established (Fig 7–32); return of protons across the membrane is coupled to the synthesis of ATP. As suggested in Fig 7–32, the biologic reductant for respiration frequently is NADH, and the oxidant often is oxygen.

Tremendous microbial diversity is exhibited in the sources of reductant used to generate NADH, and many microorganisms can use electron acceptors other than oxygen. Organic growth substrates are converted

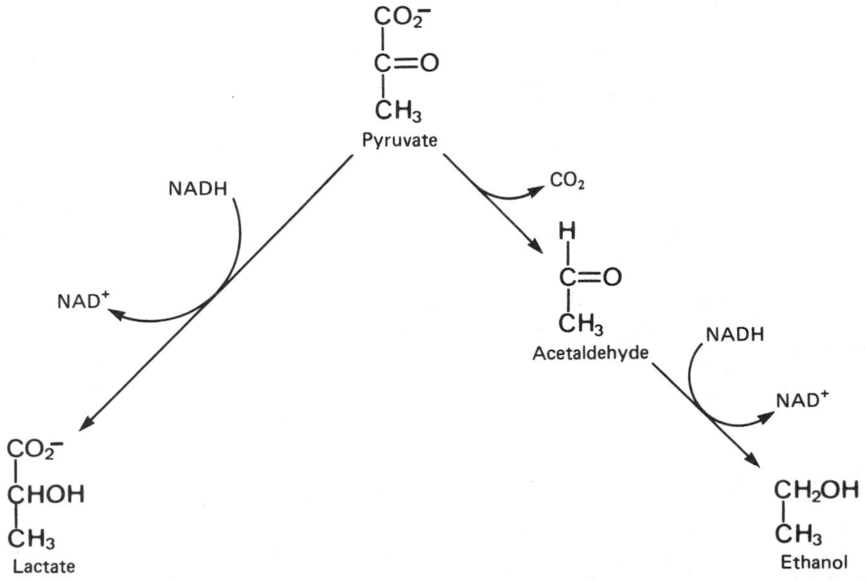

Figure 7–28. Two biochemical mechanisms by which pyruvate can oxidize NADH. *Left:* Direct formation of lactate, which results in net production of lactic acid from glucose. *Right:* Formation of the neutral products carbon dioxide and ethanol.

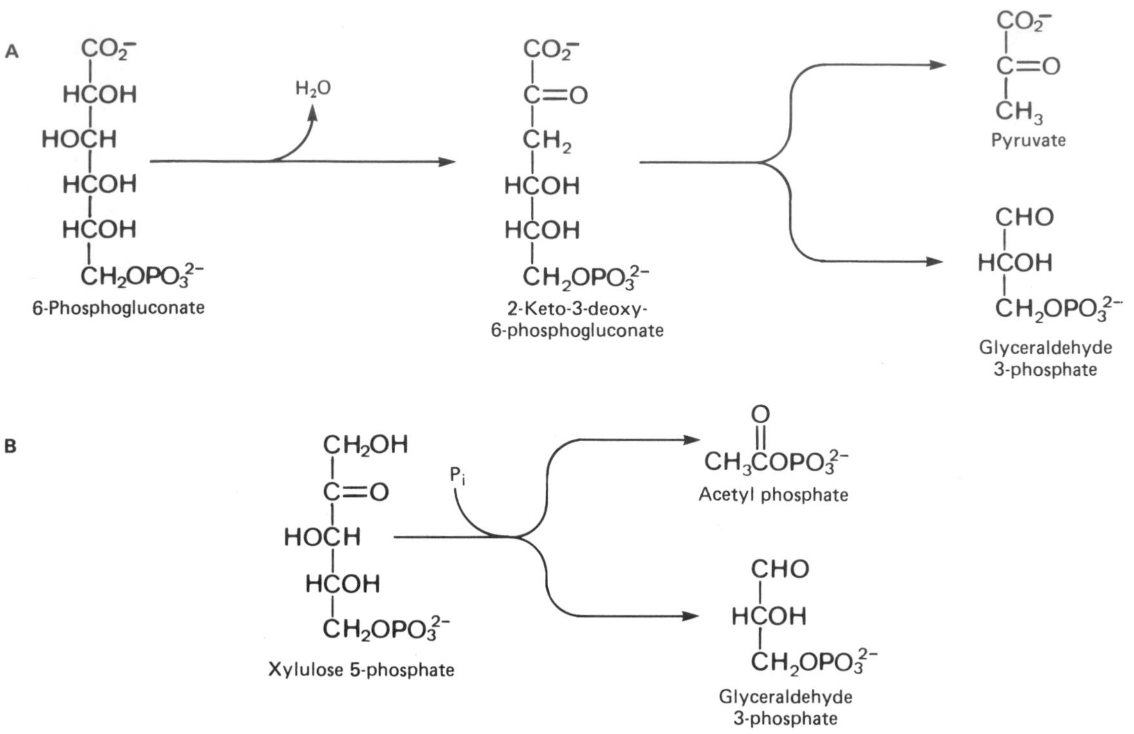

A

6-Phosphogluconate → (H₂O) → 2-Keto-3-deoxy-6-phosphogluconate → Pyruvate + Glyceraldehyde 3-phosphate

B

Xylulose 5-phosphate → (Pᵢ) → Acetyl phosphate + Glyceraldehyde 3-phosphate

Figure 7–29. Reactions associated with specific pathways of carbohydrate fermentation. *A:* Dehydratase and aldolase reactions used in the Entner-Doudoroff pathway. *B:* The phosphoketolase reaction. This reaction, found in several pathways for fermentation of carbohydrates, generates the mixed acid anhydride acetyl phosphate, which can be used for substrate phosphorylation of ADP.

Table 7–1. Microbial fermentations based on the Embden-Meyerhof pathway.

Fermentation	Organisms	Products
Ethanol	Some fungi (notably some yeasts)	Ethanol, CO_2.
Lactate (homofermentation)	*Streptococcus* Some species of *Lactobacillus*	Lactate (accounting for at least 90% of the energy source carbon).
Butylene glycol	*Enterobacter* *Aeromonas* *Bacillus polymyxa*	Ethanol, acetoin, 2,3-butylene glycol, CO_2, lactate, acetate, formate. (Total acids = 21 mol.*)

Propionate	*Clostridium propionicum*
	 Propionibacterium
	 Corynebacterium diphtheriae
	 Some species of:
	   Neisseria
	   Veillonella
	   Micromonospora
		Propionate, acetate, succinate, CO_2.

Mixed acid	*Escherichia* *Salmonella* *Shigella* *Proteus*	Lactate, acetate, formate, succinate, H_2, CO_2, ethanol. (Total acids = 159 mol.*)

Butanol-butyrate	*Butyribacterium*
	 Zymosarcina maxima
	 Some species of:
	   Clostridium
	   Neisseria
		Butanol, butyrate, acetone, isopropanol, acetate, ethanol, H_2, CO_2.

*Per 100 mol of glucose fermented.

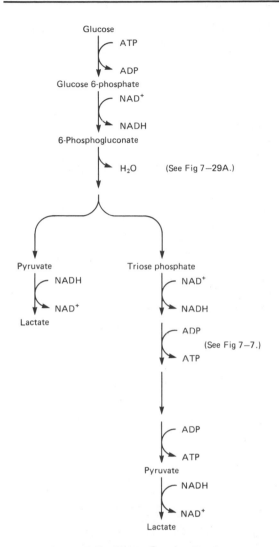

Figure 7–30. The Entner-Duodoroff pathway.

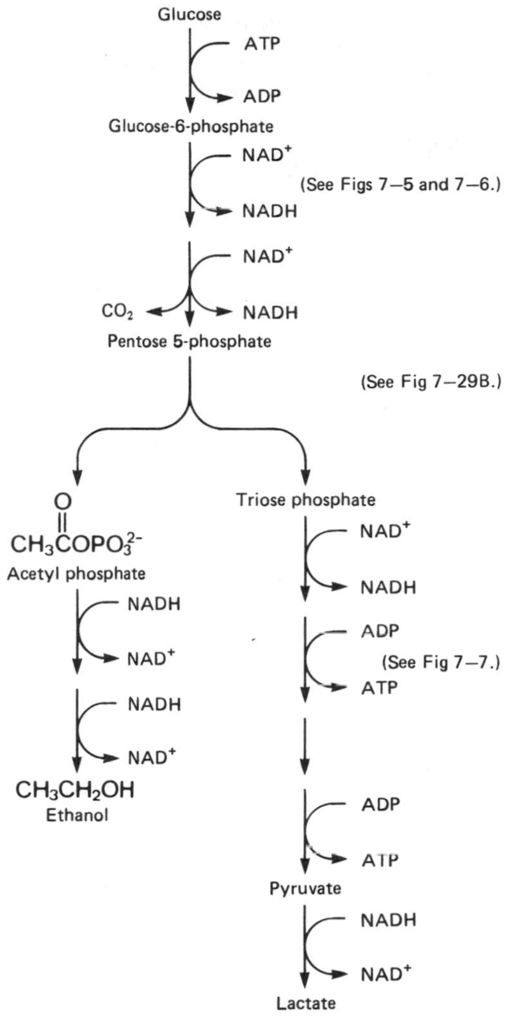

Figure 7–31. The heterolactic fermentation of glucose.

to focal metabolites that may reduce NAD$^+$ to NADH either by the hexose monophosphate shunt (Fig 7–6) or by the tricarboxylic acid cycle (Fig 7–13). Additional reductant may be generated during the breakdown of some growth substrates, eg, fatty acids (Fig 7–12).

Some bacteria, called **chemolithotrophs,** are able to use inorganic reductants for respiration. These energy sources include hydrogen, ferrous iron, and several reduced forms of sulfur and nitrogen. ATP derived from respiration and NADPH generated from the reductants can be used to drive the Calvin cycle (Fig 7–15).

Compounds and ions other than O_2 may be used as terminal oxidants in respiration. This ability, the capacity for **anaerobic respiration,** is a widespread microbial trait. Suitable electron acceptors include nitrate, sulfate, and carbon dioxide. Respiratory metabolism dependent upon carbon dioxide as an electron **acceptor is a** property found among representatives of

a large and recently defined microbial group, the **archaebacteria.** Representatives of this group possess, for example, the ability to reduce carbon dioxide to acetate as a mechanism for generating metabolic energy.

Bacterial Photosynthesis

Photosynthetic organisms use light energy to separate electronic charge, to create membrane-associated reductants and oxidants as a result of a photochemical event. Transfer of electrons from the reductant to the oxidant creates a proton motive force. Many bacteria carry out a photosynthetic metabolism that is entirely independent of oxygen. Light is used as a source of metabolic energy, and carbon for growth is derived either from organic compounds or from a combination of an inorganic reductant (eg, thiosulfate) and carbon dioxide. These bacteria possess a single photosystem that, although sufficient to provide energy for the synthesis of ATP and for the generation of essential transmembrane ionic gradients, does not allow the

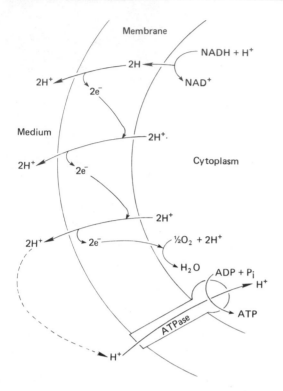

Figure 7–32. The coupling of electron transport in respiration to the generation of ATP. The indicated movements of protons and electrons are mediated by carriers (flavoprotein, quinone, cytochromes) associated with the membrane. The flow of protons down their electrochemical gradient, via the membrane ATPase, furnishes the energy for the generation of ATP from ADP and P_i. See text for explanation. (After Harold FM: Chemiosmotic interpretation of active transport in bacteria. *Ann NY Acad Sci* 1974; **227**:297.)

highly exergonic reduction of $NADP^+$ at the expense of water. This process, essential for oxygen-evolving photosynthesis, rests upon additive energy derived from the coupling of 2 different photochemical events, driven by 2 independent photochemical systems. Among prokaryotes, this trait is found solely in the cyanobacteria (blue-green bacteria). Among eukaryotic organisms, the trait is shared by algae and plants in which the essential energy-providing organelle is the chloroplast.

THE REGULATION OF METABOLIC PATHWAYS

In their normal environment, microbial cells generally regulate their metabolic pathways so that no intermediate is made in excess. Each metabolic reaction is regulated not only with respect to all others in the cell but also with respect to the concentrations of nutrients in the environment. Thus, when a sporadically available carbon source suddenly becomes abundant, the enzymes required for its catabolism increase in both

amount and activity; conversely, when a building block (such as an amino acid) suddenly becomes abundant, the enzymes required for its biosynthesis decrease in both amount and activity.

The regulation of enzyme activity as well as enzyme synthesis provides both fine control and coarse control of metabolic pathways. For example, the inhibition of enzyme activity by the end product of a pathway constitutes a mechanism of fine control, since the flow of carbon through that pathway is instantly and precisely regulated. The inhibition of enzyme synthesis by the same end product, on the other hand, constitutes a mechanism of coarse control. The preexisting enzyme molecules continue to function until they are diluted out by further cell growth, although unnecessary protein synthesis ceases immediately.

The mechanisms by which the cell regulates enzyme activity and enzyme synthesis are discussed in the following sections.

The Regulation of Enzyme Activity

A. Enzymes as Allosteric Proteins: In many cases, the activity of an enzyme catalyzing an early step in a metabolic pathway is inhibited by the end product of that pathway. Such inhibition cannot depend on competition for the enzyme's substrate binding site, however, because the structures of the end product and the early intermediate (substrate) are usually quite different. Instead, inhibition depends on the fact that regulated enzymes are **allosteric:** each enzyme possesses not only a catalytic site, which binds substrate, but also one or more other sites that bind small regulatory molecules, or **effectors.** The binding of an effector to its site causes a conformational change in the enzyme such that the affinity of the catalytic site for the substrate is reduced (allosteric inhibition) or increased (allosteric activation).

Allosteric proteins are usually oligomeric. In some cases, the subunits are identical, each subunit possessing both a catalytic site and an effector site; in other cases, the subunits are different, one type possessing only a catalytic site and the other only an effector site.

B. Feedback Inhibition: The general mechanism which has evolved in microorganisms for regulating the flow of carbon through biosynthetic pathways is the most efficient that one can imagine. The end product in each case allosterically inhibits the activity of the first—and only the first—enzyme in the pathway. For example, the first step in the biosynthesis of isoleucine not involving any other pathway is the conversion of L-threonine to α-ketobutyric acid, catalyzed by threonine deaminase. Threonine deaminase is allosterically and specifically inhibited by L-isoleucine and by no other compound (Fig 7–33); the other 4 enzymes of the pathway are not affected (although their synthesis is repressed, as discussed below).

C. Allosteric Activation: In some cases, it is advantageous to the cell for an end product or an intermediate to activate rather than inhibit a particular enzyme. In the breakdown of glucose by *E coli*, for ex-

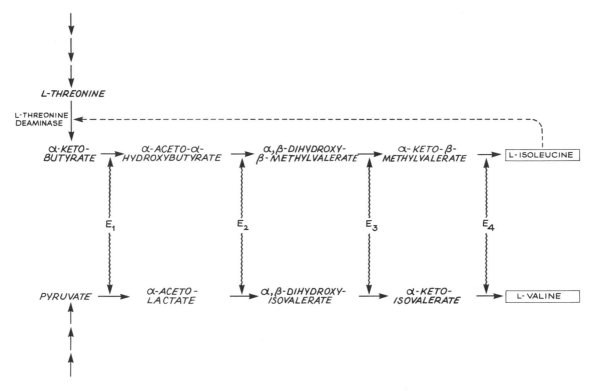

Figure 7–33. Feedback inhibition of L-threonine deaminase by L-isoleucine (dashed line). The pathways for the biosynthesis of isoleucine and valine are mediated by a common set of 4 enzymes, as shown.

ample, overproduction of the intermediates glucose 6-phosphate and phosphoenolpyruvate signals the diversion of some glucose to the pathway of glycogen synthesis; this is accomplished by the allosteric activation of the enzyme converting glucose 1-phosphate to ADP-glucose (Fig 7–34).

D. Cooperativity: Many oligomeric enzymes, possessing more than one substrate binding site, show cooperative interactions of substrate molecules. The binding of substrate by one catalytic site increases the affinity of the other sites for additional substrate molecules. The net effect of this interaction is to produce an exponential increase in catalytic activity in response to an arithmetic increase in substrate concentration.

The Regulation of Enzyme Synthesis

A. Regulatory Proteins: As discussed in Chapter 4, enzyme synthesis is controlled by regulatory proteins, each produced by a specific regulator gene (Fig 4–18). The regulatory proteins are allosteric: one site binds to an operator region of DNA, either potentiating transcription of an adjacent region or blocking it; the other site binds an effector molecule, which alters the affinity of the DNA binding site. Regulatory proteins that potentiate gene transcription—and thus enzyme synthesis—are called **activators;** those that block enzyme synthesis by interfering with transcription are called **repressors.**

B. Enzyme Induction: In microorganisms,

many of which have evolved the ability to use a variety of sporadically occurring carbon sources, the enzymes for the catabolism of these carbon sources are **inducible:** they are synthesized only when the carbon source is present in the medium. Most such enzymes are under "negative control," ie, their synthesis is normally blocked by specific repressors. Induction of enzyme synthesis occurs when an inducer molecule (usually an intermediate in the catabolic pathway) binds to the effector site of the repressor; such binding alters the repressor so that it can no longer bind to its cognate site on DNA, and enzyme synthesis begins.

In a few cases, inducible enzymes have been found to be under "positive control," ie, transcription requires the binding to DNA of an activator protein, which is in turn activated by the binding (at an effector site) of the inducer molecule.

C. End Product Repression: The regulation of biosynthetic pathways demands a response opposite to that found in catabolic pathways: instead of enzyme synthesis being induced when the substrate of the pathway becomes available, enzyme synthesis is repressed when the end product of the pathway is made in excess or becomes available as a nutrient. Thus, the repressor of a biosynthetic enzyme is normally unable to bind to the operator site on DNA and gains this ability only when it has bound its specific effector, ie, the end product of the pathway.

Feedback repression, as we may call this phenomenon, differs from feedback inhibition of enzyme

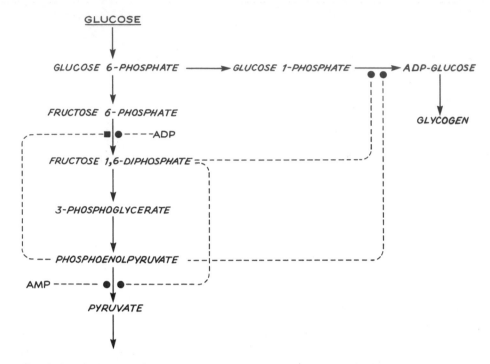

Figure 7–34. Regulation of glucose utilization by a combination of allosteric activation (...●) and allosteric inhibition (...■). (After Stanier RY, Adelberg EA, Ingraham JL: *The Microbial World,* 4th ed. Prentice-Hall, 1976.)

activity in that the synthesis of every enzyme in the pathway is repressed. In some cases (notably in bacteria), this is accomplished by the action of a repressor on an **operon** (see Chapter 4), blocking transcription of a polygenic messenger RNA (mRNA).

D. Attenuation: Base sequence analysis of several polygenic mRNAs for amino acid biosynthesis operons has revealed the presence of a leader sequence rich in codons for the amino acid in question—eg, the mRNA for the tryptophan operon has a leader sequence containing 2 adjacent tryptophan codons (UGG). The mRNA also contains sequences that give it 2 mutually exclusive, alternate base-pairing configurations. This situation has led to a proposed model of feedback repression called "translational control of transcription termination," or **attenuation.** According to the model, when the tryptophan concentration is high, for example, all tryptophan tRNA molecules are charged, and translation of the leader sequence proceeds normally until the ribosome reaches a terminator codon. The presence of a ribosome at this site blocks one of the alternative base-pairing configurations; the other configuration is thus permitted and acts as a transcription termination signal. Alternatively, when the tryptophan concentration is low, uncharged tryptophan tRNA molecules cause stalling of the ribosomes in the leader region. Base-pairing then occurs in the other configuration, and transcription proceeds to completion.

In *E coli,* the regulation of 5 amino acid operons (phenylalanine, histidine, leucine, threonine, and isoleucine) is accomplished solely by attenuation. One operon (tryptophan) is regulated by both attenuation and repression.

E. Catabolite Repression: Many of the enzymes of catabolic pathways are subject to a regulation process called **catabolite repression.** If the cell is provided with a rapidly metabolizable energy source, such as glucose, the enzymes that degrade alternative sources of energy cease to be synthesized. For example, β-galactosidase, which hydrolyzes lactose, is not synthesized by cells when glucose is present.

The synthesis of all enzymes subject to catabolite repression is under the positive control of a protein called CAP (catabolite activator protein). CAP binds to DNA at sites adjacent to each gene governing a catabolite-repressible enzyme and activates the gene's transcription; CAP, in turn, is activated by 3′, 5′-cAMP. When a rapidly metabolizable substrate such as glucose binds to the cell membrane, the internal concentration of cAMP falls and synthesis of the catabolite-repressible enzymes ceases.

Patterns of Regulation in Branched Biosynthetic Pathways

Many biosynthetic pathways are branched, each branch leading to a different, indispensable end product. Aspartic acid, for example, is the starting point for a pathway that branches out to form lysine, methionine, threonine, and isoleucine (Fig 7–35). It would clearly be fatal if the presence in excess of any one of these end products were to shut off the entire pathway starting at aspartate, yet to be efficient the cell

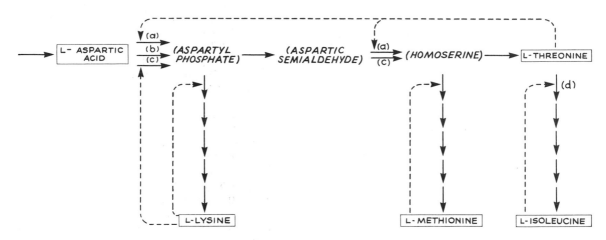

Figure 7–35. Regulation of a branched pathway by feedback inhibition (dashed lines). (a), (b), and (c) are isofunctional aspartokinases; (a) and (c) also catalyze the third step in the pathway. (d) is L-threonine deaminase. Feedback repression of enzyme synthesis is not shown. (After Stanier RY, Adelberg EA, Ingraham JL: *The Microbial World,* 4th ed. Prentice-Hall, 1976.)

must regulate the early steps in the pathway as well as the late ones.

A number of different solutions to this problem have evolved:

A. Isofunctional Enzymes: The first step in the pathway is catalyzed by 2 or more different enzymes with the same catalytic activity. For example, there are 3 aspartokinases in *E coli,* labeled (a), (b), and (c) in Fig 7–35. Enzymes (a) and (c) also catalyze the third step in the pathway, reducing aspartic semialdehyde to homoserine. Enzyme (a) is both inhibited and repressed by threonine; enzyme (b) is repressed by methionine; and enzyme (c) is both inhibited and repressed by lysine. Thus, if one of the 3 end products of the branched pathway is present in excess, the flow of carbon through the common pathway is proportionately reduced. (Note in Fig 7–35 that the final branches of the pathway are separately controlled by their respective end products.)

B. Sequential Feedback Inhibition: Fig 7–36 illustrates a second solution to the problem of regulating the early steps of a branched pathway. The 2 end products inhibit the first steps in their own branches, causing the accumulation of a common intermediate. The latter compound then serves as the feedback inhibitor of the first step in the common pathway.

C. Concerted and Cumulative Feedback Inhibition: In still other cases, the enzyme catalyzing the first step of a branched pathway possesses 2 or more effector sites, each binding a different end product. In **concerted feedback inhibition,** all effector sites must be occupied for the enzyme to be inhibited. In **cumulative feedback inhibition,** each end product causes partial inhibition; the effects of binding more than one end product are additive. The latter is the more efficient of the 2 mechanisms.

D. The Diversity of Microbial Regulatory Systems: Different groups of microorganisms have evolved different mechanisms for regulating the same

pathway. In the aspartate pathway shown in Fig 7–35, for example, aspartokinase is regulated by the use of separately inhibited isofunctional enzymes in the enteric bacteria but by concerted feedback inhibition in *Pseudomonas.* Thus, regulatory systems appear to have developed late in the evolution of the different microbial groups.

THE REGULATION OF RNA SYNTHESIS

The mechanisms described above for the regulation of enzyme (protein) synthesis all act at the level of transcription and hence regulate messenger RNA (mRNA) synthesis. The 2 classes of stable RNA—ribosomal (rRNA) and transfer (tRNA)—are regulated together by a different set of mechanisms that are as yet poorly understood. However, the following gener-

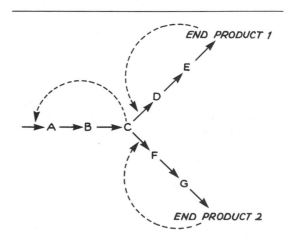

Figure 7–36. Regulation of a branched biosynthetic pathway by sequential feedback inhibition (dashed lines).

alizations can be made: (1) The synthesis of stable RNA is closely geared to the growth rate of the cell as determined by nutrient supply. In rich media, allowing high rates of protein synthesis and short doubling times, the rate of synthesis of stable RNA increases; in poor media, allowing only low rates of protein synthesis and long doubling times, the rate of synthesis of stable RNA decreases. At all growth rates, the amount of stable RNA made by the cell is precisely that which is sufficient to support the permitted level of protein synthesis. (2) Regulation of stable RNA synthesis is not effected by varying the concentration of RNA precursors (nucleotide triphosphates) but by varying the number of RNA polymerase molecules actively engaged in transcribing the *rRNA* and *tRNA* genes.

One mechanism by which stable RNA synthesis is coupled to protein synthesis has been partially elucidated. When protein synthesis is arrested—eg, by depriving the cell of an essential amino acid—2 regulatory molecules are rapidly synthesized on the ribosomes: ppGpp and ppGppp.* These molecules, in turn, effect the repression of stable RNA synthesis. In *E coli,* a mutation in the gene called **rel** (for "relaxed synthesis of RNA") abolishes the production of the 2 guanosine polyphosphates, and stable RNA synthesis continues in the absence of protein synthesis.

Additional mechanisms must exist for the regulation of stable RNA synthesis, however, since the modulation of such synthesis as a function of growth rate is normal in the **rel** mutants.

THE REGULATION OF DNA SYNTHESIS & CELL DIVISION

In bacteria, the rate of DNA polymerization is constant at a given temperature. In *E coli* cells growing at 37 °C, for example, chromosome replication takes 40 minutes. In rich media, however, cells may double in as few as 20 minutes; this increase, which requires a corresponding increase in the rate of DNA synthesis, does not reflect a change in the rate of polymerization but rather an increase in the number of replication forks. In other words, a new round of replication begins before the previous round has been completed.

There is a precise relationship between the timing of DNA replication and cell division. For example, in *E coli* at 37 °C, cell division occurs 20 minutes after completion of chromosomal replication. Since both (R), the replication period, and (D), the period between replication and division, are constant, totaling 60 minutes, the following situations may occur: (1) At doubling times of less than 60 minutes, a second round of replication begins during D and each daughter cell receives a chromosome containing a replication fork. (2) At a doubling time of 60 minutes or longer, each daughter cell receives a chromosome without a replication fork.

Thus, the *E coli* cell is so regulated that (1) rounds of DNA replication are initiated at intervals equal to the doubling time of the culture, and (2) a cell division event occurs at a precise interval (eg, 60 minutes at 37 °C) after each initiation event. If DNA synthesis is selectively inhibited, cell elongation continues but cell division is prevented.

The regulation of DNA replication and cell division appears to be achieved through the synthesis of specific proteins; if protein synthesis is blocked, ongoing rounds of DNA replication are completed, but the initiation of new rounds of replication is blocked, as is cell division.

*ppGpp: guanosine-3′, 5′-di(diphosphate); ppGppp: guanosine-3′-diphosphate-5′-triphosphate.

REFERENCES

Books

Chakrabarty AM (editor): *Biodegradation and Detoxification of Environmental Pollutants.* CRC Press, 1982.

Cohen GN: *Biosynthesis of Small Molecules.* Harper, 1967.

Gottschalk A: *Bacterial Metabolism.* Springer-Verlag, 1978.

Gunsalus IC, Stanier RY (editors): *The Bacteria: A Treatise on Structure and Function.* Vol 2: *Metabolism,* 1961; Vol 3: *Biosynthesis,* 1962. Academic Press.

Ingraham JL, Maaløe O, Neidhardt FC: *Growth of the Bacterial Cell.* Sinauer Associates, 1983.

Kornberg A: *DNA Replication.* Freeman, 1980.

Kulaev IS, Tempest DW, Dawes EA (editors): *Environmental Regulation of Microbial Metabolism.* Academic Press, 1985.

Laskin AI, Lechevalier HA (editors): *CRC Handbook of Microbiology,* 2nd ed. Vol 3: *Microbial Composition: Amino Acids, Proteins and Nucleic Acids;* Vol 4: *Microbial Composition: Carbohydrates, Lipids and Minerals.* CRC Press, 1981.

Mandelstam J, McQuillen K, Dawes I: *Biochemistry of Bacterial Growth.* Blackwell, 1982.

Nicholls DG: *Bioenergetics: An Introduction to the Chemiosmotic Theory.* Academic Press, 1983.

Ornston LN, Sokatch JR (editors): *Bacterial Diversity.* Vol 6 of: *The Bacteria: A Treatise on Structure and Function.* Gunsalus IC, Stanier RY (editors). Academic Press, 1978.

Postgate JR: *Fundamentals of Nitrogen Fixation.* Cambridge Univ Press, 1983.

Rosen BP: *Bacterial Transport.* Dekker, 1978.

Sokatch JR, Ornston LN (editors): *Mechanisms of Adaptation.* Vol 7 of: *The Bacteria: A Treatise on Structure and Function.* Gunsalus IC, Stanier RY (editors). Academic Press, 1979.

Stryer L: *Biochemistry,* 2nd ed. Freeman, 1981.

Watson JD: *Molecular Biology of the Gene,* 3rd ed. Benjamin, 1976.

Woese CR, Wolfe RS (editors): *Archaebacteria.* Vol 8 of: *The Bacteria: A Treatise on Structure and Function.* Gunsalus IC, Stanier RY (editors). Academic Press, 1985.

Articles & Reviews

Bourgeois S et al: Repressors. *Adv Protein Chem* 1976;**30**:1.

Dagley S: A biochemical approach to some problems of environmental pollution. Pages 81–138 in: *Essays in Biochemistry*. Vol 11. Campbell PN, Aldridge WN (editors). Academic Press, 1975.

Dawes EA, Senior PJ: The role and regulation of energy reserve polymers in microorganisms. *Adv Microb Physiol* 1973;**10**:136.

Downie JA et al: Membrane adenosine triphosphatases of prokaryotic cells. *Annu Rev Biochem* 1979;**48**:103.

Evans WC: Biochemistry of the bacterial catabolism of aromatic compounds in anaerobic environments. *Nature* 1977;**270**:17.

Finnerty WR: Physiology and biochemistry of bacterial phospholipid metabolism. *Adv Microb Physiol* 1978;**18**:177.

Giesbrecht P et al: On the morphogenesis of the cell wall of staphylococci. *Int Rev Cytol* 1976;**44**:225.

Harold FM: Membranes and energy transduction in bacteria. *Curr Top Bioenerg* 1977;**6**:83.

Iaccarino M et al: Regulation of isoleucine and valine biosynthesis. *Curr Top Cell Regul* 1978;**14**:29.

Ingledew WJ, Poole RK: The respiratory chains of *Escherichia coli*. *Microbiol Rev* 1984;**48**:222.

Kinoshita N, Unemoto T, Kobayashi H: Sodium stimulated ATPase in *Streptococcus faecalis*. *J Bacteriol* 1984;**158**:844.

Lamond AI: The control of stable RNA synthesis in bacteria. *Trends Biochem Sci* 1985;**10**:271.

Mitchell P: Vectorial chemiosmotic processes. *Annu Rev Biochem* 1977;**46**:996.

Mizino T, Chou M-Y, Inouye M: A unique mechanism regulating gene expression: Translational inhibition by a complementary DNA transcript (micRNA). *Proc Natl Acad Sci USA* 1984;**81**:1966.

Morris JG: The physiology of obligate anaerobiosis. *Adv Microb Physiol* 1975;**12**:169.

Nierlich DP: Regulation of bacterial growth, RNA and protein synthesis. *Annu Rev Microbiol* 1978;**32**:393.

Priest FG: Extracellular enzyme synthesis in the genus *Bacillus*. *Bacteriol Rev* 1977;**41**:711.

Tabor CW, Tabor H: Polyamines in microorganisms. *Microbiol Rev* 1985;**49**:81.

Tang M-S, Helmstetter CE: Coordination between chromosome replication and cell division in *Escherichia coli*. *J Bacteriol* 1980;**144**:1148.

Troy FA: The chemistry and biosynthesis of selected bacterial capsular polymers. *Annu Rev Microbiol* 1979;**33**:519.

Umbarger HE: Amino acid biosynthesis and its regulation. *Annu Rev Biochem* 1978;**47**:532.

Waxman DJ, Strominger JL: Penicillin-binding proteins and the mechanism of action of β-lactam-antibiotics. *Annu Rev Biochem* 1983;**52**:825.

Yanofsky C, Killey RL, Horn V: Repression is relieved before attenuation in the *trp* operon of *Escherichia coli* as tryptophan starvation becomes increasingly severe. *J Bacteriol* 1984;**158**:1018.

8

The Microbiology of Special Environments

WATER

Methods of Study

A. Quantitative Analysis: Bacteria cannot be accurately counted by microscopic examination unless there are at least 100 million (10^8) cells per milliliter. Natural bodies of water, however, rarely contain more than 10^5 cells per milliliter. The method employed is therefore the plate count: A measured volume of water is serially diluted (see below), following which 1 mL from each dilution tube is plated in nutrient agar and the resulting colonies counted. Since only cells able to form colonies are counted, the method is also known as the "viable count."

A typical example of serial dilution would be the following: One milliliter of the water sample is aseptically transferred by pipette to 9 mL of sterile water. The mixture is thoroughly shaken, yielding a 1:10 dilution. (For obvious reasons, this is also known as the "10^{-1}" dilution.) The process is repeated serially until a dilution is reached that contains between 30 and 300 colony-forming cells per milliliter, at which point several 1-mL samples are plated in a nutrient medium. Since the original sample may have contained up to 1 million (10^6) viable bacteria, it is necessary to dilute all the way to 10^{-5}, plate 1-mL samples from each dilution tube, and then count the colonies only on those plates containing 30–300 colonies. The reasons for these numerical limits are that with over 300 colonies the plate becomes too crowded to permit each cell to form a visible colony, whereas with below 30 colonies the percent counting error becomes too great. (The statistical error of sampling can be calculated as follows: The standard deviation of the count equals the square root of N, where N equals the average of many samples. Ninety-five percent of all samples will give counts within 2 standard deviations of the average. For example, if the average count is 36, then 95% of all samples will lie between 24 and 48 [36 ± 12]. In other words, within 95% confidence limits, a sample count of 36 has an error of plus or minus 33%.)

B. Qualitative Analysis: The methods of plating and enrichment culture (see Chapter 6) are used to obtain a picture of the aquatic bacterial population. Although such methods are satisfactory for general biologic studies, they are inadequate for the purpose of sanitary water analysis; this involves the detection of intestinal bacteria in water, since their presence indicates sewage pollution and the consequent danger of the spread of enteric diseases (see Chapter 18). Since any enteric bacteria would be greatly outnumbered by other types present in the water samples, a selective technique is necessary in order to detect them. Two widely used procedures for sanitary water analysis are as follows:

1. Tube method–Dilutions of a water sample are inoculated into tubes of a medium which is selective for coliform bacteria and in which all coliform bacteria but few noncoliform bacteria will form acid and gas. Such media include MacConkey's medium, which contains bile salts as inhibitors of noncoliform bacteria; lactose-containing media; and glutamate-containing media. Cultures showing both acid and gas may then be subjected to further tests to confirm the presence of *Escherichia coli* or closely related enteric gram-negative rods. Such tests include streaking cultures on a lactose-peptone agar containing eosin and methylene blue (EMB agar), on which *E coli* forms characteristic blue-black colonies with a metallic sheen; subculturing at 44 °C; and a series of diagnostic biochemical tests (see p 234).

2. Membrane filtration method–A large measured volume of water is filtered through a sterilized membrane of a type that retains bacteria on its surface while permitting the rapid passage of smaller particles and water. The membrane is then transferred to the surface of an agar plate containing a selective differential medium for coliform bacteria. Upon incubation, coliform bacteria give rise to typical colonies on the surface of the membrane. The advantages of this method are speed (the complete test takes less than 24 hours) and quantitation, the number of coliform cells being determined for a given volume of water.

Nature of the Environment & of the Microbial Population

A. The Environment: Natural bodies of water contain nutrients in sufficient quantities to support populations of specialized groups of microorganisms. Few if any of these cause diseases in humans; the presence of human pathogens in water indicates contamination either from the soil or from the deliberate discharge of sewage.

B. The Microbial Population: Pathogens that reach the water from soil represent organisms liberated from animal or human excrement or from the bodies of animals or humans who have died of infectious disease. Of the latter group, only the spores of the anthrax bacillus *(Bacillus anthracis)* are able to survive in the soil for a significant length of time. The major pathogens in water, then, are those originating in excreta: *Salmonella typhi* and other salmonellae, *Vibrio cholerae, Shigella dysenteriae, Escherichia,* and *Leptospira* among the bacteria; a number of enteric viruses, including infectious hepatitis and poliovirus; and the protozoon *Entamoeba histolytica. Francisella tularensis,* the agent of tularemia, may also be transmitted in drinking water contaminated by infected animals. Waterborne diseases may be acquired by drinking or washing food utensils in contaminated water or by eating shellfish that concentrate pathogenic microorganisms when filter-feeding in contaminated water.

When sufficiently diluted in a large body of water, coliform bacteria survive for only short periods of time; a positive test for such bacteria may usually be taken as evidence of recent contamination. Some rivers and harbors are now so polluted with sewage-derived organic nutrients, however, that coliform bacteria may not only survive but may maintain significant populations by slow multiplication.

Bacteria that enter the soil from septic tanks or other sources of human excrement are rapidly filtered out in fine soils or sandstone, but in coarse soils or in limestone formations, enteric bacteria may pollute water supplies several miles from the source of contamination. In general, contamination is limited to the upper layers of the soil; deep waters contain very low numbers of bacteria, usually of the harmless types that survive well in soil.

Control of Microorganisms in Water

Microorganisms are controlled in water only in connection with sanitation measures. Three problems are encountered: the sanitation of drinking water, the sanitation of swimming pools, and the purification of sewage.

A. Sanitation of Drinking Water: Since drinking water supplies may at any time become contaminated with sewage and cause an epidemic of enteric disease, water supplies for large cities are usually filtered and chlorinated. The presence of only 0.5 parts per million of free chlorine will rid the water of enteric pathogens. Before chlorination, however, the majority of the bacteria are usually removed by filtration through beds of sand. In "slow sand filters," removal of bacteria is actually accomplished by their adsorption on the gelatinous film of slime-forming microbes that builds up in the sand layers. In "rapid sand filters," chemicals are first added to coagulate organic matter and bacteria; after the precipitate is settled out or is removed mechanically, rapid filtration through clean sand completes the purification.

B. Sanitation of Swimming Pools: The rapidity with which bathers may exchange pathogenic organisms makes the sanitation of swimming pools a major problem. The problem is effectively handled by maintaining free chlorine concentrations of 0.5 parts per million. Coliform bacteria are used as indicators of pollution, as in the case of drinking water, but staphylococci of human origin persist longer than coliforms in chlorine-treated water, and their presence is thus a more sensitive indicator of pollution.

C. Sewage Purification: In modern cities, domestic sewage is pumped through a disposal plant that accomplishes the following general objectives:

1. Screening—Bulky, nondecomposable material is screened and removed (bottles, paper, boxes, gravel, etc).

2. Sludge formation—The screened sewage is allowed to settle in large tanks. The sediment, containing much of the organic matter and microorganisms, is called **sludge.** It is drained off at the bottom of the tank and separated from the supernatant, which still contains large amounts of putrescible organic matter. The sludge and supernatant are then treated separately as described below.

The amount of organic matter in the supernatant can be greatly reduced if, instead of simply allowing sludge to form by settling, an activated sludge is caused to form by aeration of the sewage. As air is forced through the sewage, a floc, or precipitate, is formed, the particles of which teem with actively oxidizing microbes. After a period of time, during which the organic matter is oxidized to a very great extent, the sludge is allowed to settle. The supernatant and part of the sludge are removed for treatment as described below, and part of the sludge is returned to the tank to activate fresh sewage.

3. Sludge digestion—The sludge obtained by either process described above consists of organic matter rich in bacteria and other microbes. It is then pumped to anaerobic tanks where fermentation is allowed to go on for weeks or months. Much of the organic matter is converted to gases (CO_2, CH_4, NH_3, H_2, and H_2S). The methane content of the gas may be as high as 75%, and the collected gas may consequently be burned, with the production of useful heat. When fermentation is complete, the sludge is removed and disposed of in one of several ways: it may be dried and discarded or dried and sold as fertilizer (nitrogen may have to be added), or it may be pumped into a large body of water.

4. Disposal of supernatant—The supernatant, after chlorination, may be pumped into a large body of water. When none is nearby, however, the supernatant must be treated to remove remaining putrescible material as well as enteric bacteria. This is accomplished by aerating and filtering the fluid: it is sprayed over a bed of sand or broken stone, which then filters it as in the process described earlier for drinking water purification. The aeration is necessary to ensure formation of an oxidizing microbial film on the filter-bed particles.

MILK

Methods of Study

A. Quantitative Analysis: Bacteria in milk are counted either directly under the microscope or by plate count. The direct procedure has been rigidly standardized and is known as the "Breed count." The plate count method employs a medium containing skimmed milk in addition to other ingredients, ensuring maximal development of colonies of milk-inhabiting organisms.

Most procedures connected with the bacteriologic analysis of milk have been devised as tests of the safety of the product for human consumption. In addition to the counting procedures, a rough index of bacterial activity in milk is provided by the reductase test. Bacteria contain many enzymes that reduce various substrates. Various dyes are available that are susceptible to bacterial reduction ("reductase activity") and change color when reduced. These dyes thus serve as indicators; in a typical test, a standard amount of a dye such as methylene blue is added to a measured volume of milk, and the time necessary for it to change from blue to colorless is determined. Grade A raw milk that is to be pasteurized, for example, should show a reduction time under standard conditions of 6 hours or more.

B. Qualitative Analysis: The types of organisms present in milk are determined by the procedures described above for water bacteriology. Although coliform bacteria are frequently present in milk, they are derived from the cow and are not usually pathogenic for humans. They are thus not useful indicators of contamination with human pathogens.

Nature of the Environment & of the Microbial Population

A. The Environment: Milk constitutes an ideal microbial habitat, consisting of emulsified fat droplets and physiologic concentrations of salts, sugars, and proteins dissolved in water. Milk also contains enzymes originating in the animal. Sugar is present in the form of lactose, a disaccharide in which glucose is linked to one of its stereoisomers, galactose. The pH of fresh milk is about 6.8, which is within the optimal range for most bacteria. As normally handled (in filled containers), milk tends to be anaerobic.

B. The Microbial Population: Because microorganisms invade milk as dust-borne contaminants, almost any type may be present. Milk constitutes a typical enrichment culture medium, however, and so only the most suited types will predominate. The first organism to flourish in milk is usually *Streptococcus lactis,* which ferments the lactose principally to lactic acid. As the pH drops, other species, such as *Lactobacillus casei* and *Lactobacillus acidophilus,* may replace *S lactis* as the predominant type. If the milk is kept at body temperature, *Enterobacter (Aerobacter) aerogenes* and *Escherichia coli* may be favored.

Other organisms that may develop in milk under special conditions include anaerobic sporeformers (clostridia), *Streptococcus faecalis* and related enterococci, *Pseudomonas aeruginosa* (producing blue pigment), and lactose-fermenting yeasts. The presence of pathogens in milk is discussed below.

Ecology

A. Effect of the Environment on Microorganisms: The environmental factors that most affect the microbial population are the degree of anaerobiosis, the temperature, the presence of lactose as the principal sugar, and the pH (which drops as fermentation ensues). The selective effect of these factors has been described above.

B. Effect of Microorganisms on Milk:

1. Souring–Milk, whether raw or pasteurized (see below), will sour on standing, mainly as a result of the production of lactic acid by *S lactis* or by the lactobacilli. Many dairy products are purposely allowed to sour in this way, as in the manufacture of buttermilk, butter, sour cream, yogurt, and cheese. When *E coli* or *E aerogenes* propagates, mixed acid or butylene glycol fermentations take place; these organisms produce less acidity than lactic acid bacteria but cause the production of gas and unpleasant flavors.

2. "Abnormal fermentations"–All changes due to microbial activity other than souring are referred to as "abnormal fermentations," although many of the processes involved are not fermentative. Included are gas formation by yeasts or bacteria; "ropiness," due to gum secretion by bacteria; "sweet curdling," due to secretion by bacteria of the protein-coagulating enzyme rennin; various color productions due to pigment-forming bacteria; and digestion of milk proteins and fats by bacterial enzymes (proteolytic and lipolytic).

Control of Microorganisms in Milk

It has not yet proved economically feasible to sterilize milk completely except by drastic heating, and this destroys the flavor of fresh milk. (Heat sterilization is used in the production of canned evaporated milk.) However, because contaminated milk is a means of transmission of many diseases, rigid control is necessary.

A. Diseases Transmitted by Milk: Two general classes of disease may be transmitted by milk: those transmitted from the animal, the causative microbe being able to infect both animals and humans; and those transmitted from other contaminating sources, which are ultimately derived from infected persons.

1. Transmission from the animal–Tuberculosis and brucellosis (undulant fever) are the most important of these diseases. Both are transmissible from animal to animal or from animal to human. The route from the animal's tissues to the milk is not definitely known, but it is possible that brucellae may be secreted directly from the bloodstream into the udder.

Cows are also subject to infections with group A streptococci, salmonellae, *Staphylococcus aureus,* and *Coxiella burnetii,* the agent of Q fever; any of these may be shed from the udder directly into the milk, reaching densities of 10^3/mL or higher, and may cause outbreaks of disease in human populations. *S aureus* is liberated in milk by cows suffering from mastitis and produces an enterotoxin that causes a well-known type of food poisoning (see p 161).

2. Transmission from infected persons–Milk that is not handled under scrupulously clean conditions may at any time become contaminated by dust or droplets bearing pathogenic microorganisms. Still more likely is direct infection from diseased milk handlers and dairy workers. The diseases most commonly transmitted by contaminated milk are typhoid fever and other salmonelloses, dysentery, tuberculosis, streptococcal infections, and infectious hepatitis.

B. Control of Pathogenic Microorganisms in Milk: Since many diseases transmitted by milk are the result of milk contamination, an obvious control measure is to insist on sanitary procedures in milk production and bottling. Communities that enforce the provisions of their own Medical Milk Commission with regard to "Certified Raw Milk" or of the USPHS with regard to "Grade A Raw Milk" supervise the production of milk under sanitary conditions. However, even the most sanitary handling procedures cannot prevent the transmission of tuberculosis or brucellosis from infected animals, and the only safe milk is therefore that which has been pasteurized. In the USA, it is the general practice to check all dairy cattle by the tuberculin test; an agglutinin test is used to detect infection with *Brucella*.

Pasteurization may be carried out by maintaining the milk at 62 °C for 30 minutes and then rapidly cooling it; this will kill all pathogenic bacteria that may be present, although many harmless forms (eg, *S lactis*) survive. Alternatively, pasteurization can be accomplished by heating an extremely thin layer of milk for a very short time at a much higher temperature, eg, 71.7 °C for 15 seconds, or 90 °C for 0.5 second. Pasteurization is the only procedure that renders milk absolutely safe without destroying its flavor and palatability. Even the heating processes used in producing dried milk products are insufficient to guarantee freedom from pathogens; salmonellae have been detected in such products, and staphylococcal food poisoning outbreaks have been traced to batches of dried milk. The refrigeration "shelf life" of some dairy products is extended by exposing them to ultrahigh temperatures (UHT) for short times, eg, 138 °C for at least 2 seconds.

C. Safety Standards: A very sensitive, practical method used to determine whether milk has been properly pasteurized is known as the **phosphatase test,** which consists of quantitatively determining the activity of the enzyme phosphatase in a sample of the milk. Because this enzyme is more resistant than any pathogenic bacterium to pasteurization, its destruction indicates that the milk is safe. Phosphatase activity indicates improper pasteurization or adulteration with raw milk.

A satisfactory phosphatase test, however, does not guarantee that the milk has not become contaminated by handlers after pasteurization. To determine this, milk is analyzed for the presence of coliform organisms by the procedures described in the section on water microbiology, above. Even a negative coliform test does not eliminate the possibility that diphtheria or streptococcal organisms may have been introduced. The best protection against this danger is the insistence on sanitary procedures of dairies and medical examination of milk handlers.

FOODS

Methods of Study

The plate count and enrichment culture methods are also used for the examination of foods. Solid food samples must be ground and suspended in liquid for dilution and plating; care must be taken to avoid introducing microorganisms from other sources during preparation of the sample. Coliform analysis is carried out on food samples as well as on water and milk to determine whether fecal contamination has occurred. A rough method for assaying the extent of microbial contamination of foods involves the addition of ^{14}C-glucose to a sample and measuring the amount of radioactive CO_2 produced by microbial metabolism.

Nature of the Environment & of the Microbial Population

A. Meat: The interior of intact meat is usually sterile or nearly so unless the meat was taken from an infected animal. The surface, however, becomes contaminated from dust or from handling immediately upon dismemberment of the animal. Any organotrophic bacterium may be found, including those from soil, dung, or human handlers.

B. Ground Meat: The grinding process introduces the surface contaminants into the interior of the meat and may also warm the meat enough to encourage considerable bacterial multiplication. The interior of the meat is somewhat anaerobic, and fermentative organisms are enriched for. The number of bacteria in ground meat is so high that a count of 10 million per gram is considered a safe maximum. (Since such counts are made on aerobic plates, the many obligate anaerobes present are not included in this figure.)

C. Fish: The general picture is similar to that for unground meat, but the bacterial population will include many marine halophilic and psychrophilic forms. The "phosphorescence" of spoiling fish is due to the growth of luminescent marine bacteria (such as *Achromobacter*) on the surface.

D. Shellfish: These become contaminated during handling, but they also bear organisms acquired from their marine environment. Shellfish gathered near a sewage outlet will contain numbers of sewage organisms, including both pathogenic enterobacteria and viruses. Outbreaks of typhoid fever have frequently arisen from the consumption of contaminated shellfish, and outbreaks of infectious hepatitis have been traced to oysters contaminated with the viral agent of this disease. Oysters are often "planted" near sewage outlets because they fatten rapidly on sewage. In recent years it has become mandatory that such oysters be transported to clean water and left there long enough to have cleansed themselves of sewage organisms before they are marketed.

E. Fruits and Vegetables: Most vegetables have a considerable surface contamination of soil organisms. Fruits acquire a surface flora through dust contamination and handling. Fruits and vegetables with tough skins are fairly proof to penetration by bacteria unless bruised; soft fruits and vegetables will spoil much more readily. Acid fruits offer a selective environment for yeasts and molds; otherwise, a typical array of soil microorganisms is found.

The number of microbial cells contaminating the surfaces of fruits and vegetables varies over a wide range. For example, on the unwashed surfaces of leafy vegetables, the count may be as high as $2 \times 10^6/g$. On the unwashed surfaces of tomatoes, counts as high as $5 \times 10^3/cm^2$ have been recorded; on washed tomatoes, the counts vary between 4 and $7 \times 10^2/cm^2$.

F. Eggs: Bacteria may be incorporated into eggs from infected ovaries or oviducts; otherwise, the interiors of eggs are usually sterile. The surface becomes contaminated immediately after laying, but penetration of the egg by bacteria is normally prevented by a dry, mucilaginous coating on the surface. This coating is easily removed, however, by washing or overhandling, in which case the interior of the egg becomes contaminated. Bacteria on eggs come from soil and from the feces of the birds. A mixed flora is common, but fermenters predominate inside the egg. Egg products, like ground meat, show the result of mixing surface contaminants throughout the material; counts are similar to those of ground meat.

G. Bread: The flour from which bread is made contains polysaccharide carbohydrates and protein; fats are added in the form of "shortening." Hydrolysis of the polysaccharides by the yeast added to make the bread rise, and partial hydrolysis of the protein by enzymes in the flour, yield a mixture that is ideal for bacterial growth. Baking kills most microorganisms, but spores of bacilli, clostridia, and fungi persist and will germinate to produce a new flora unless preservatives are added.

Ecology

A. Effect of the Environment on the Microbial Population: When organisms begin to grow in food products, selection will determine the predominant type (eg, fermentative organisms are selected for in the anaerobic interior of ground meat). Variables that most affect microbial growth are moisture, pH, redox potential, temperature, factors permitting penetration (bruising of fruits, washing of eggs, etc), and autolysis ("self-dissolving"). As cells die, enzymes are released that dissolve cell walls and protoplasts to a variable extent depending upon the tissue and the environmental conditions; the "ripening" or "tenderizing" of meat, for example, is a result of autolysis. Autolysis results in digestion of polysaccharides, proteins, and fats,

rendering the product much more susceptible to microbial growth.

The moisture content of food preparations is a major limitation to microbial growth. The parameter used to describe moisture content is "water activity" (a_w), defined as the vapor pressure of pure water. Few microorganisms can grow at a_w values below 0.90; the exceptions are *S aureus*, which has a lower limit of 0.84; some molds, which can grow at a_w values down to 0.80; and halophiles, which can grow at a_w values down to 0.75.

B. Effect of Microorganisms on Food: The interest in food microbiology is focused on spoilage and disease transmission. Since pathogens affect the consumer rather than the food, only spoilage need be considered here. Disease transmission is discussed below.

Spoilage is the result of microbial growth in or on food. The metabolic activity associated with growth causes both a breakdown of the food substance and the release of the products of fermentation, digestion, and other processes. Spoilage may be defined as the process by which food is rendered aesthetically unfit for human consumption. Only rarely is spoilage accompanied by actual poisoning of the food. (The term food poisoning is restricted to infection by enteric pathogens contaminating food, or ingestion of food containing exotoxins produced by staphylococci or *Clostridium botulinum*.)

Unpleasant odors and tastes are produced by "putrefactive" organisms, ie, those that digest proteins and produce H_2S, sulfhydryl compounds, or amines. These compounds, while not poisonous in the concentrations involved, have vile smells. Molds produce a musty odor and taste, and some bacteria produce great quantities of slime (as in "ropy bread"). Eggs have a high sulfur content, and their spoilage results in H_2S production, rendering them completely unpalatable.

Control of Microorganisms in Food

A. Prevention of Spoilage: For some foods, such as meats, much can be accomplished to prevent contamination through the use of sanitary procedures. Fruits and vegetables, however, already have a rich surface flora from their natural environment, and contamination during handling plays a relatively minor role. In the case of meat, fruit, eggs, and vegetables, it is important to prevent penetration of the food by bacteria (see above). Most effort, however, is directed toward preservative measures; the following measures are used either singly or in combination.

1. Irradiation—Ultraviolet light is used to reduce surface contamination of food materials and equipment in many types of food processing but is relatively ineffective. Irradiation with high-penetration gamma rays has proved to be much more effective and is used to extend the "shelf life" of packaged nonsterilized food products, including those preserved by chilling, freezing, drying, heating, or the addition of chemical preservatives.

2. Low temperature—Bacterial activity is markedly slowed at refrigeration temperatures and virtually negligible at temperatures below freezing. Refrigeration and freezing are well-known methods of food preservation and need no further discussion here.

3. Drying—Foods kept completely dry will stay preserved indefinitely, since moisture is essential to microbial activity. Examples of dried foods are hay, raisins, "cured" meat, powdered eggs, and powdered milk. All of these contain dormant microorganisms and will spoil if exposed to humidity.

4. Heat—A temperature of 121 °C for 15 minutes is utilized to kill heat-resistant bacterial spores. Such conditions are obtainable with steam at a pressure of 7 kg/2.5 cm² (15 lb/sq in) above atmospheric pressure. Industrial autoclaves and home pressure cookers are used for heat sterilization of canned foods.

The USDA requires that egg products be pasteurized in order to destroy salmonellae.

5. Salt—Most bacteria are unable to grow at high salt concentrations. Meat and fish are often "salt-cured" by immersion in brine or by rubbing salt into the surface.

6. Sugar—High sugar concentrations produce osmotic pressures that are too high for most bacteria, although permitting the growth of molds. Many fruits are packed in syrup, and meat is sometimes rubbed with or mixed with sugar instead of salt ("sugar-cured" ham).

7. Smoking—Smoke contains volatile bactericidal substances that are gradually absorbed by the meat or fish being smoked. The smoking process is slow, however, and the food is often salt-treated first to prevent spoilage early in the process.

8. Chemical preservatives—Only a few chemicals are useful preservatives at concentrations harmless to humans. Calcium propionate, for example, is used to prevent growth of molds in bread; sodium benzoate is used in cider and some vegetable products; and sulfur dioxide is used to preserve sausages, pickles, and soft fruits used in the manufacture of jams, jellies, and alcoholic beverages. Nitrites, used in the curing of meats, are bacteriostatic. Sorbic acid, a 6-carbon unsaturated fatty acid, and sorbates are used as fungistatic agents in various foods, particularly cheeses. Esters of p-hydroxybenzoate are used as preservatives in beer and wine.

A number of agents, including butylated hydroxyanisole (BHA) and diphenyl, are used to treat packaging materials in order to retard microbial growth; the growth of microorganisms in packaged foods may also be controlled by the use of a vacuum or a CO_2 atmosphere. The sterilization of certain foods by ethylene oxide, propylene oxide, or methylbromide has been approved by the FDA.

9. Acids—Many foods that are soured for the purpose of flavor are thereby preserved, since few bacteria can tolerate the pH values produced by the lactic acid or acetic acid bacteria. Examples are buttermilk, pickles, sauerkraut, and vinegar.

B. Prevention of Disease Transmission: Since few of the preservative measures listed above are bactericidal, it is essential that pathogenic organisms be prevented from contaminating food. The principal infectious diseases transmissible by food are *Shigella* and *Salmonella* infections, dysentery, streptococcal infections, and infectious hepatitis. Salmonellae other than *S typhi* are widespread contaminants of poultry and eggs in the USA.

The principal bacterial toxins that may be produced in food and cause poisoning are those of staphylococci, *Clostridium perfringens, C botulinum, E coli, Vibrio parahaemolyticus,* and *Bacillus cereus. C botulinum* is an obligate anaerobe; it is usually found in improperly sterilized canned foods. Since the canning industry now observes rigid standards of sterilization, most cases of botulism arise from home-canned foods, although outbreaks of botulism from ingestion of commercially canned foods have occurred recently. Proper methods of autoclaving (pressure-cooking) foods can prevent botulism. Although foods suspected of containing botulinus toxin can probably be made safe by boiling for more than 20 minutes at 100 °C, the extreme potency of the toxin suggests that no reliance should be placed on this procedure and that suspect foods should be discarded.

Staphylococci grow well in meats and dairy products, where they produce a potent exotoxin. This can usually be prevented by careful refrigeration and sanitary measures to prevent their introduction into foods.

Many fungi that may grow in food produce poisonous substances called **mycotoxins,** which cause serious—sometimes fatal—diseases if ingested. They also produce a variety of **hallucinogens,** such as lysergic acid. The mycotoxins of importance to humans include the toxins of the poisonous mushrooms, the toxins of *Claviceps purpurea* (ergot, a parasite of rye), and the **aflatoxins.**

The aflatoxins are produced by the fungus *Aspergillus flavus;* they are highly toxic (as well as carcinogenic) for animals. Aflatoxins have caused serious damage to livestock when their feed has become contaminated with *A flavus.* The risk to humans is unknown; there is strong circumstantial evidence, however, based on epidemiologic data, that aflatoxins may cause cirrhosis and cancer of the liver in parts of the world where human foodstuffs are subject to aflatoxin contamination (eg, India and Africa). Aflatoxins have been found in the food and in the urine of children in India who exhibited cirrhosis of the liver.

AIR

The air does not constitute a microbial habitat; microbial cells exist in the air as accidental contaminants or as air-dispersed fungal spores. Many pathogens are transmitted through the air on dust particles or on the dry residues of saliva droplets, and control measures are attempted for this reason.

Types of Infectious Particles

In addition to naturally dispersed fungal spores, pathogenic microorganisms occur in the air associated with 2 types of particles: the residues of evaporated exhalation droplets (**droplet nuclei**), and the much larger **dust particles**. These 2 types of particles are very different with respect to their source, their settling behavior, their significance in disease, and the methods needed to assess them and to control them. Some of these differences are summarized in Table 8–1.

Viability of Airborne Organisms

Both dust-borne and droplet nuclei-borne organisms lose viability in air, and the kinetics of survival are similar to those shown in Fig 5–3. Usually the curve changes slope sharply, revealing the presence of a more resistant fraction, even in experiments dealing with a single type of organism. The presence of 2 populations with different death rates probably reflects differences in the microenvironments of the particles rather than genetic differences in the organisms. The death rates are markedly affected by the humidity and temperature of the air, and there are great differences in death rates among different species of organisms. In general, organisms that are normally airborne (eg, *Mycobacterium tuberculosis*) are more resistant to inactivation than organisms that are normally waterborne (eg, *E coli*).

Epidemiology of Droplet Nuclei-Borne Infections

In propagated epidemics, succeeding crops of cases, or "generations," occur as a result of the incubation period that intervenes between successive cases. At each generation, the relationship between the number of new cases (C), the number of infectors (I), and the number of susceptibles (S) is given by the equation*

$$C = KIS \qquad \ldots (1)$$

*The equations in this section are from Riley R, O'Grady F: *Airborne Infection*. Macmillan, 1961.

where K is a constant representing the effective contact rate.

For droplet nuclei-borne infections, K is related to the volume of air (s) breathed by a susceptible, the number of infectious doses (i) liberated by an infector, and the volume of air (V) that passes through the space in which contact occurs, all measured over the same interval of time, by the equation

$$K = si/V \qquad \ldots (2)$$

For an epidemic to occur, C/I must exceed 1; the greater the ratio C/I, the more severe the epidemic. Since equation (1) can be rearranged as

$$C/I = KS \qquad \ldots (3)$$

it is seen that the severity of an epidemic is directly proportionate to K, the effective contact rate, and to S, the number of susceptibles.

These simple equations have been used to make some illuminating calculations. For example, in a measles epidemic occurring in a school where contact took place only in a well-defined classroom area, K was estimated by equation (1) to be 0.1. Since both s and V were known, i could be calculated from equation (2); it was found to be 270. Thus, each infector liberated enough measles virus to infect 270 persons. This represented about one infectious dose per 3000 cubic feet of air, which was the volume breathed by 10 children during the time interval used for the calculation. Thus, under such conditions, one child in 10 could be expected to be infected. (Since, however, the distribution of particles in air is random, there is about one chance in 3 under such conditions that no child would be infected. Chance thus may play a significant part in deciding whether an epidemic will occur.)

Table 8–1. Characteristics of and control measures for airborne infections.

	Droplet Nuclei	Dust Particles
Source of particles in air	Evaporation of droplets expelled from the respiratory tract by sneezing, coughing, and talking (in decreasing order of effectiveness).	Movements that cause the shedding of particles from skin and clothing; air turbulence sufficient to redistribute previously settled dust.
Settling behavior	Remain suspended indefinitely as a result of minor air turbulence (average settling velocity in still air, 1.2 cm/min).	Settle rapidly to the ground (average settling velocity, 46 cm/min). Redistributed by major air turbulence.
Organisms per particle	Rarely more than one.	Usually many.
Access to susceptible tissues and significance in disease	Deposited in lungs; probably responsible for most pulmonary infections.	Deposited on external surfaces and in upper respiratory tract.
Epidemiologic characteristics	Propagated epidemics (disease transmitted serially from person to person).	Epidemics associated with specific places as reservoirs of infection.
Control measures	Ventilation; ultraviolet irradiation of the air; evaporation of glycols.	Prevention of accumulation of infectious material (eg, by sterilization of clothing and bedding); prevention of dispersal (eg, by oiling of floors and bedding, and by proper design of ventilation system).

Epidemiology of Infections Associated With Air-Dispersed Fungal Spores

A number of serious respiratory diseases (mycoses) result from the inhalation of fungal cells that have been dispersed as airborne spores or as contaminants of airborne dust particles. These diseases include infections with *Coccidioides immitis, Histoplasma capsulatum,* and *Blastomyces dermatitidis* (see Chapter 31). Fungal cells are also the agents of a number of occupational allergic diseases: Farmer's lung, for example, is a form of allergic alveolitis caused by thermophilic actinomycetes growing in moldy hay, and a significant percentage of farmers working with harvested grain develop allergies to a variety of fungal spores.

Control of Indoor Airborne Infections

Some control measures for dust-borne infections are indicated in Table 8-1. The accumulation of infectious organisms on fabrics can be minimized by a bactericidal rinse at the end of the laundering process or by heat sterilization when feasible. The dispersal of dust can be minimized by the oiling or other wetting of blankets and floors; however, the design of the ventilation system often limits what can be accomplished by such measures.

The control measures for droplet nuclei-borne infections include the following:

A. Sanitary Ventilation: If equations (2) and (3) above are combined, it is found that

$$C/I = si/V_s \qquad \ldots (4)$$

where V_s is the volume of air per susceptible. Thus, the severity of an epidemic as well as its probability of being initiated (which is proportionate to C/I) is inversely proportionate to V_s. In order to achieve a value of C/I less than 1, the corresponding V_s may require one **air change per minute** under ordinary circumstances of room size and occupancy. This is more than 5 times that supplied by ordinary ventilation systems. A very large improvement can be achieved by the use of laminar flow ventilation systems.

B. Ultraviolet Irradiation: The use of ultraviolet light can accomplish the equivalent of one air change per minute by the killing of airborne organisms. This can be done either by installing high-intensity ultraviolet lamps in the air supply ducts or by irradiating the air in the upper levels of the room by indirect lamps. The latter method requires good mixing of upper and lower air, but this condition does obtain in many situations. Ultraviolet barriers, or "curtains," can also be set up at room entrances so that personnel can pass through quickly and avoid radiation injury.

C. Chemical Disinfection: Propylene glycol and some related compounds are effective germicides in the vapor phase. They presumably act by condensing on droplet nuclei and dehydrating the nuclei-borne organisms. This method is only successful within a narrow range of relative humidities and is therefore not always reliable.

D. Evaluation: Control measures against dust-borne and droplet nuclei-borne infections must be separately evaluated by methods that assay only the appropriate particles. The best criterion of success is the lowering of the incidence of disease; in practice, however, it is almost impossible to design valid controls for comparison. For this reason, there are very few data that permit a valid evaluation of the efficacies of the methods listed above, and in some trials neither ultraviolet irradiation systems nor chemical vapor disinfection was found to reduce the incidence of airborne infections.

When the data indicate that a control measure has failed, it can mean either that the transmission route being controlled is not significant in the spread of the disease being studied or that the exposure to the disease is taking place outside of the controlled area.

SOIL

The earth is covered with green plants that rapidly convert nitrate, sulfate, and CO_2 into organic matter. The plants die—or are eaten by animals that in turn die—and so return the elements to the soil in organic form. The nitrogen and sulfur are then present principally as the amino ($-NH_2$) and sulfhydryl ($-SH$) groups of proteins; the carbon is present principally in the form of the reduced "carbon skeletons" of carbohydrates, proteins, fats, and nucleic acids.

Without a mechanism for the "mineralization" of these elements, the surface of the earth would long ago have been depleted of the nitrate, sulfate, and CO_2 needed for plant growth, and life on the earth would have ceased. But, as we have seen in the previous sections on metabolism, such a mechanism does exist in the form of microbial metabolic activities. Thus, nitrogen, sulfur, and carbon are constantly undergoing cycles of transformation from the oxidized, inorganic state to the reduced, organic state and back again.

One other major element, phosphorus (as phosphate), is converted to organic form during plant growth, being incorporated chiefly into nucleic acids. On return to the soil, nucleic acids are hydrolyzed by microbial enzymes, again liberating free phosphate. No oxidation or reduction is involved.

These cycles, and hence all life on earth, are completely dependent on the metabolic activities of soil microorganisms. A gram of typical fertile soil contains on the order of several million bacteria, a million fungal spores, 50,000 algae, and 25,000 protozoa. The top 6 inches of such soil may contain more than 2 tons of microorganisms per acre.

The Nitrogen Cycle (Fig 8-1.)

A. Decomposition: The proteins of organic matter are digested by many microorganisms to free amino acids, from which ammonia (NH_3) is then liberated by deamination. Urea, the principal form in which higher animals excrete nitrogen, is hydrolyzed to NH_3 and CO_2 by various urea-decomposing bacteria.

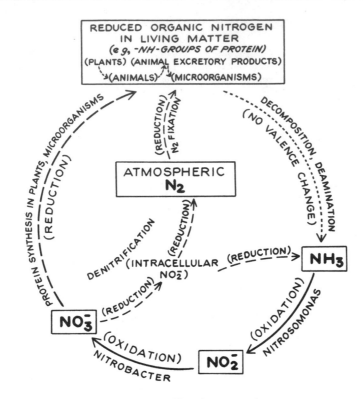

Figure 8–1. The nitrogen cycle.

B. Oxidation of Ammonia: Soil rich in ammonia from decomposing organic matter is abundantly occupied by cells of *Nitrosomonas,* which obtain their energy for growth by oxidizing NH_3 to nitrite (NO_2^-). As nitrite is formed, the *Nitrobacter* cells that are present multiply and convert the nitrite to nitrate (NO_3^-).

C. Nitrate Reduction and Denitrification: Nitrate serves as the final hydrogen acceptor for various anaerobic bacteria, being reduced by some to NH_3 and by others to gaseous N_2. In the former case, no nitrogen is lost from the soil, since the ammonia usually stays in solution as ammonium ion (NH_4^+); N_2 escapes, however, and the latter process is hence termed "denitrification."

D. Conversion of Nitrate to Organic Nitrogen: Green plants, as well as many microorganisms, convert nitrate to organic nitrogen and reduce it once again to amino groups, thus completing the cycle.

E. Nitrogen Fixation: One other important source of nitrogen is the atmosphere. Atmospheric nitrogen is reduced to organic nitrogen by nitrogen-fixing bacteria, balancing the losses due to denitrification. This process, although a reduction, is not a mechanism for anaerobic respiration but rather a means of obtaining nitrogen. Many nitrogen fixers, in fact, are aerobes.

The Sulfur Cycle (Fig 8–2.)

A. Decomposition: Following digestion, the sulfur-containing amino acids are broken down by many microorganisms, and in the process H_2S is released.

B. Oxidation of H₂S to Free Sulfur: H_2S spontaneously oxidizes to S in the presence of oxygen; in addition, it is oxidized as an energy source by certain chemolithotrophs and as a hydrogen donor by some photosynthetic bacteria.

C. Oxidation of S to SO₄²⁻: Certain chemolithotrophs and photosynthetic bacteria oxidize sulfur to sulfate.

D. Conversion of Sulfate to Organic Sulfur: This process is analogous to the conversion of nitrate to organic nitrogen in the nitrogen cycle.

E. Sulfate Reduction: *Desulfovibrio* uses SO_4^{2-} as the final hydrogen acceptor in anaerobic respiration.

The Carbon Cycle (Fig 8–3.)

The valence changes of carbon are frequently associated with valence changes of oxygen, hence the inclusion of an "oxygen cycle." Since anaerobic respiration of organic matter may involve electron transfer from carbon to sulfate or nitrate, the sulfur and nitrogen cycles are also "geared" to the carbon cycle. By "gearing" we mean that the organic carbon oxidation is coupled with a reduction of nitrate or sulfate by electron transfer.

A. Green Plant Photosynthesis and Aerobic Oxidation: For each molecule of CO_2 reduced in photosynthesis, one molecule of O_2 is produced from H_2O. This process just balances the reduction of O_2 to

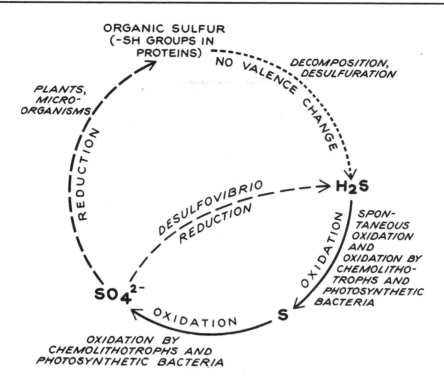

Figure 8–2. The sulfur cycle.

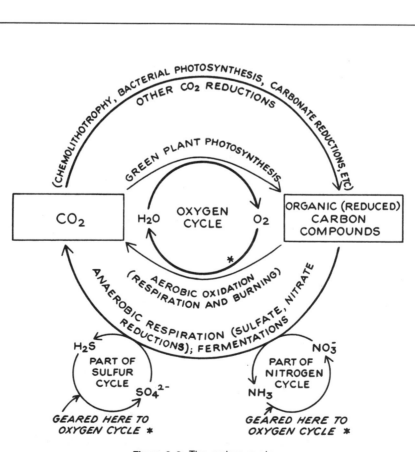

Figure 8–3. The carbon cycle.

H_2O in aerobic oxidations, so that the oxygen content of the atmosphere remains remarkably constant at about 20%.

B. Other CO_2 Reductions: A relatively small amount of CO_2 is reduced to organic carbon by processes that do not result in the formation of oxygen. These processes include chemolithotrophic reduction, bacterial photosynthesis, carbonate reduction in anaerobic respiration, and CO_2 fixations in chemoorganotrophic nutrition.

C. Anaerobic Respiration: Anaerobic organotrophs oxidize carbon compounds to CO_2 with nitrate, sulfate, or organic molecules as electron acceptors. When nitrate or sulfate is reduced, their respective cycles are affected; reoxidation of the nitrogen and sulfur is usually accomplished aerobically, causing a half-turn of the oxygen cycle.

REFERENCES

Books

Atlas RM, Bartha R: *Microbial Ecology: Fundamentals and Applications.* Addison-Wesley, 1981.

Banwart GJ: *Basic Food Microbiology.* Avi, 1981.

Block SS (editor): *Disinfection, Sterilization, and Preservation,* 2nd ed. Lea & Febiger, 1977.

Corry J, Roberts D, Skinner FA (editors): *Isolation and Identification Methods for Food Poisoning Organisms.* Academic Press, 1983.

Graham HD (editor): *The Safety of Foods,* 2nd ed. Avi, 1980.

Gregory PH: *The Microbiology of the Atmosphere,* 2nd ed. Wiley, 1973.

Gregory PH, Monteith JL (editors): *Airborne Microbes.* Cambridge Univ Press, 1967.

Harrigan WF, McCance ME: *Laboratory Methods in Food and Dairy Microbiology.* Academic Press, 1976.

Hawker LE, Linton AH (editors): *Micro-organisms: Function, Form and Environment,* 2nd ed. University Park Press, 1979.

Hers JFP, Winkler KC (editors): *Airborne Transmission and Airborne Infection: 6th International Symposium on Aerobiology.* Wiley, 1973.

Hugo WB (editor): *Inhibition and Destruction of the Microbial Cell.* Academic Press, 1971.

Klug MJ, Reddy CA (editors): *Current Perspectives in Microbial Ecology.* American Society for Microbiology, 1984.

Lynch JM, Poole NJ: *Microbial Ecology: A Conceptual Approach.* Wiley, 1979.

Reimann H, Bryan FL (editors): *Food-borne Infections and Intoxications,* 2nd ed. Academic Press, 1979.

Riley R, O'Grady F: *Airborne Infection.* Macmillan, 1961.

Roberts TA, Skinner FA: *Food Microbiology: Advances and Prospects.* Academic Press, 1983.

Slater JH, Whittenbury R, Wimpenny JWT (editors): *Microbes in Their Natural Environments.* Cambridge Univ Press, 1983.

Stanier RY, Adelberg EA, Ingraham JL: *The Microbial World,* 4th ed. Prentice-Hall, 1976.

Tyrell DAJ: *Airborne Microbes.* Cambridge Univ Press, 1967.

Articles & Reviews

Cundell AM: Rapid counting methods for coliform bacteria. *Adv Appl Microbiol* 1981;**27**:169.

Diet and aflatoxin toxicity. *Nutr Rev* 1971;**29**:181.

Focht DD, Verstraete W: Biochemical ecology of nitrification and denitrification. *Adv Microb Ecology* 1977;**1**:135.

Harrison AP Jr: The acidophilic thiobacilli and other acidophilic bacteria that share their habitat. *Annu Rev Microbiol* 1984;**38**:265.

Jannasch HW, Taylor CD: Deep-sea microbiology. *Annu Rev Microbiol* 1984;**38**:487.

Nakamura M, Schulze JA: *Clostridium perfringens* food poisoning. *Annu Rev Microbiol* 1970;**24**:359.

Salyers AA: Bacteroides of the human lower intestinal tract. *Annu Rev Microbiol* 1984;**38**:293.

Stark AA: Mutagenicity and carcinogenicity of mycotoxins: DNA binding as a possible mode of action. *Annu Rev Microbiol* 1980;**34**:235.

Taber WA: Wastewater microbiology. *Annu Rev Microbiol* 1976;**30**:263.

Bacteriophage

9

Bacteria are host to a special group of viruses called bacteriophage, or "phage." Although any given phage is highly host-specific, it is probable that every known type of bacterium serves as host to one or more phages. Phages have not been successfully used in therapy. They are important, however, because they furnish ideal materials for studying host-parasite relationships, virus multiplication, and molecular genetics.

LIFE CYCLES OF PHAGE & HOST

Fig 9–1 summarizes the potential life cycles of bacterial cells infected with double-stranded DNA phages. Single-stranded DNA phages and RNA phages are discussed in later sections.

Fig 9–1 shows the following:

(1) Life cycle of uninfected bacterium: An uninfected bacterium may reproduce by binary fission, showing no involvement with phage.

(2) Adsorption of free phage: When an uninfected bacterium is exposed to free phage, infection will take place if the cell is sensitive. Bacteria may also be genetically resistant to phage infection; such cells lack the necessary receptors on their surfaces. (Contrast this with "immunity" due to the presence of prophage. See p 126.)

When infection takes place, the phage is adsorbed onto the cell surface, and the nucleic acid of the phage penetrates the cell. In this state, the phage nucleic acid is called "vegetative phage."

(3) Lytic infection: The injected vegetative phage material may be reproduced, forming many

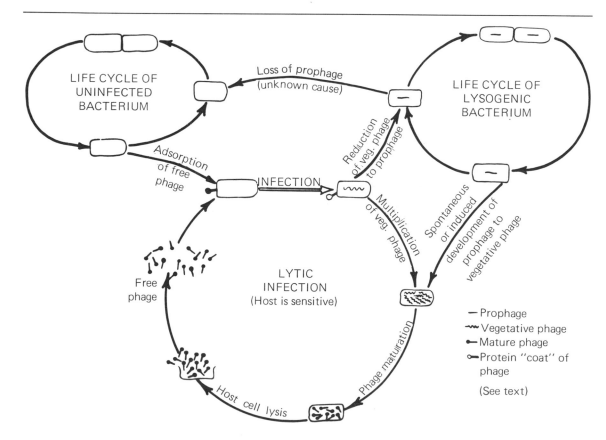

Figure 9–1. Phage-host life cycles.

replicas. These mature by acquisition of protein coats, following which the host cell lyses and free phage is liberated.

(4) Reduction of vegetative phage to prophage: Many phages, termed "temperate," are capable of reduction to prophage as an alternative to producing a lytic infection. The bacterium is now lysogenic (see pp 125–128); after an indeterminate number of cell divisions, one of its progeny may lyse and liberate infective phage.

(5) Loss of prophage: Occasionally a lysogenic bacterium may lose its prophage, remaining viable as an uninfected cell.

METHODS OF STUDY

Assay

Since phages (like all viruses) multiply only within living cells, and since their size precludes direct observation except with the electron microscope, it is necessary to follow their activities by indirect means. For this purpose, advantage is taken of the fact that one phage particle introduced into a crowded layer of dividing bacteria on a nutrient agar plate will produce a more or less clear zone of lysis in the opaque film of bacterial growth. This zone of lysis is called a "plaque"; it results from the fact that the initially infected host cell bursts (lyses) and liberates dozens of new phage particles, which then infect neighboring cells. This process is repeated cyclically until bacterial growth on the plate ceases as a result of exhaustion of nutrients and accumulation of toxic products. When handled properly, each phage particle produces one plaque; any material containing phage can thus be titrated by making suitable dilutions and plating measured samples with an excess of sensitive bacteria. The plaque count is analogous to the colony count for bacterial titration.

Isolation & Purification

In order to study the physical and chemical properties of phage, it is necessary to prepare a large batch of purified virus as free as possible of host cell material. For this purpose, a culture of the host bacterium is inoculated with phage and incubated until the culture is completely lysed. The now clear culture fluid, or lysate, contains in suspension only viral particles and bacterial debris. These materials are easily separated from each other by differential centrifugation. The centrifuged pellet of phage material can be resuspended and washed in the centrifuge as often as needed and may then be used for chemical and physical analysis in the laboratory or for electron microscopy.

PROPERTIES OF PHAGE

One group of phages has been studied more extensively than any other: certain phages that attack *Es-*

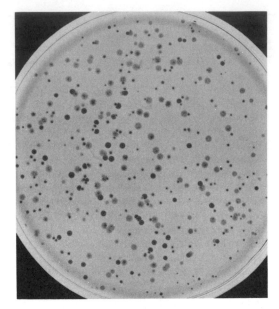

Figure 9–2. Different phage plaque types.(Courtesy of Stent GS.)

cherichia coli strain B (coliphages). Of the numerous coliphages, 7 have been selected for intensive study. Unless otherwise noted, the information given below applies to this group, which has been numbered T1 through T7.

Morphology

A typical phage particle consists of a "head" and a "tail." The head represents a tightly packed core of nucleic acid surrounded by a protein coat, or **capsid.** The protein capsid of the head is made up of identical subunits, packed to form a prismatic structure, usually hexagonal in cross section. The smallest known phage has a head diameter of 25 nm; others range from 55×40 nm up to 100×70 nm.

The phage tail varies tremendously in its complexity from one phage to another. The most complex tail is found in phage T2 and in a number of other coli and typhoid phages. In these phages, the tail consists of at least 3 parts: a hollow core, ranging from 6 to 10 nm in width; a contractile sheath, ranging from 15 to 25 nm in width; and a terminal base-plate, hexagonal in shape, to which may be attached prongs, tail fibers, or both. Electron micrographs of phage preparations embedded in electron-dense material such as phosphotungstate show the phages to exist in 2 states: in one, the head contrasts highly with the medium, the sheath is expanded, and the base-plate appears to have a series of prongs. In the second state, the head is of low contrast, the sheath is contracted, and the base-plate is now revealed to have 6 fibers attached to it. The former state represents active phage, containing nucleic acid; the latter state represents phage that has ejected its nucleic acid (eg, into a host cell). These 2 states are diagrammed in Fig 9–3.

PHAGE T2

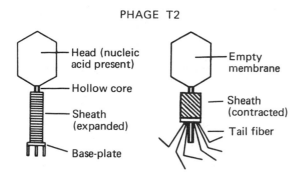

Figure 9–3. Diagrams of phage T2 based on electron micrographic observation.

A number of other tail morphologies have been reported. In some of these, sheaths are visible but the contracted state has not been observed; and in one case, no sheath can be seen. The phages also vary with respect to the terminal structure of the tail: some have base-plates, some have "knobs," and some appear to lack specific terminal structures.

The phage tail is the adsorption organ for those phages that possess them. Some phages lack tails altogether; in the RNA phages, for example, the capsid is a simple icosahedron.

Chemistry

Phage particles contain only protein and one kind of nucleic acid. Most phages contain only DNA; however, phages that contain only RNA are also known. In the T-even phages, the nucleic acid makes up about 50% of the dry weight and consists of a single molecule (called the phage chromosome) with a molecular weight of 1.3×10^8, sufficient to code for about 200 different proteins of molecular weight 30,000. In phages T2, T4, and T6, a unique base (hydroxymethylcytosine) is present to which are attached short chains of glucose units. This pyrimidine has never been found in the nucleic acid of the uninfected bacterial host.

The proteins that make up the head, the core, the sheath, and the tail fibers are distinct from each other; in each case, the structure appears to be made of repeating subunits.

An unusual phage called PM2 has been isolated from a culture of a marine pseudomonad. PM2 is a double-stranded DNA phage in which the virion is surrounded by a lipoprotein membrane and contains 2 enzymes: an endonuclease that converts the phage DNA to the linear form within the host, and a DNA-dependent RNA polymerase.

PHAGE REPRODUCTION

Adsorption

The kinetics of phage adsorption have been thoroughly analyzed, and the process has been shown to be a first-order reaction; the rate of adsorption is proportional to the concentration of both the phage and the bacterium. Under optimal conditions, the observed rates are compatible with the assumption that almost every collision between phage and host cell results in adsorption. If the bacteria are mixed with an excess of phage, adsorption will continue until as many as 300 particles are adsorbed per cell.

Before the phage can be adsorbed onto the host cell, the phage surface must be modified by attachment of positively charged cations (the nature and number of cations varying from one phage to another) and, in some cases, the amino acid tryptophan. Each phage is quite specific with regard to the cofactors required for adsorption.

The bacterial surface, ie, the cell wall, is complex and heterogeneous. In gram-negative bacteria, there are 3 distinct layers: an inner layer composed of peptidoglycan, the outer membrane, and lipopolysaccharide (see Chapter 2). Different bacterial strains are highly specific with regard to the phages that they will adsorb. The factors in the cell wall responsible for adsorption constitute discrete, localized "receptors"; the receptors for phages T3, T4, and T7 reside in the lipopolysaccharide layer, whereas the receptors for phages T2 and T6 reside in the outer membrane. Ability to adsorb phage is obviously a factor in the determination of bacterial sensitivity to infection.

In certain phages (eg, phages T2, T4, T6), the attachment of phage particles (or of empty phage capsids) causes a profound change in the cell membrane: at low phage multiplicities, the membrane becomes permeable to small molecules; and at high multiplicities, the cell lyses ("lysis from without"). Even a single phage or ghost particle will affect the membrane, causing not only a permeability change but also inhibition of host DNA and protein synthesis.

Penetration

Phages with contractile tails, such as the T-even phages (Fig 9–3), behave as hypodermic syringes, injecting the phage DNA into the cell. In phage T4, it has been found that the triggering of DNA injection requires the maintenance of a membrane potential by the host cell. It is not known whether host metabolic energy is required for the penetration process.

Intracellular Development of DNA Phages

Some phages always lyse their host cells shortly after infection, generally in a matter of minutes and usually before the host cell can divide again . (See "lytic infection" cycle in Fig 9–1.) The process of intracellular development is as follows:

(1) For several minutes following infection (eclipse period), active phage is not detectable by artifically induced premature lysis (eg, by sonic oscillation). During this period, a number of new proteins ("early proteins") are synthesized. These include certain enzymes necessary for the synthesis of phage DNA: a new DNA polymerase, a new kinases for the formation of nucleoside triphosphates, and a new

thymidylate synthetase. The T-even phages (T2, T4, T6), which incorporate hydroxymethylcytosine instead of cytosine into their DNA, also cause the appearance of a series of enzymes needed for the synthesis of hydroxymethylcytosine, as well as an enzyme that destroys the deoxycytidine triphosphate of the host. Later on in the eclipse period, "late proteins" appear, which include the subunits of the phage head and tail as well as lysozyme that degrades the peptidoglycan layer of the host cell wall. All of these enzymes and phage proteins are synthesized by the host cell using the genetic information provided by the phage DNA. The switch from synthesis of cell proteins to synthesis of phage proteins involves a phage-induced modification of the RNA polymerase core.

(2) During the eclipse period, up to several hundred new phage chromosomes are produced; as fast as they are formed, they undergo random exchanges of genetic material (see below).

In many phages, the linear DNA molecule that enters the cell has cohesive ends consisting of short complementary base sequences. Base-pairing of these cohesive ends converts the DNA from the linear to the circular form; circularization is completed by a ligase-catalyzed sealing of the single-stranded gaps. Replication then occurs in the circular state, by either a simple-circle or a rolling-circle mechanism.

(3) The protein subunits of the phage head and tail aggregate spontaneously (self-assemble) to form the complete capsid. In the case of a complex capsid such as that of phageT4, capsid formation results from the coming together of 3 independent subassembly lines: one each for the head, the tail, and the tail fibers. Each subassembly proceeds in a defined sequence of protein additions.

(4) Maturation consists of irreversible combination of phage nucleic acid with a protein coat. The mature particle is a morphologically typical infectious virus and no longer reproduces in the cell in which it was formed. If the cells are artificially lysed late in the eclipse period, immature phage particles are found in which the DNA and protein are not yet irreversibly attached, so that the DNA is easily removed.

Lysis & Liberation of New Phage

Phage synthesis continues until the cell disintegrates, liberating infectious phage. The cell bursts as a result of osmotic pressure after the cell wall has been weakened by the phage lysozyme.

FILAMENTOUS PHAGES

Although most phages have the head-and-tail structure described above, some filamentous phages have been discovered that have a very different morphology. Three of these (M13, fd, and f1) have been studied in detail; they are rod-shaped structures measuring about 6 nm in diameter and 800 nm in length. Each consists of a circular, single-stranded DNA molecule complexed with protein.

The phage adsorbs to the tip of the bacterial sex pilus, moves to the base of the pilus by an unknown mechanism, and penetrates the cell wall in intact form. The major protein of the phage coat is deposited on the cell membrane, which is penetrated by the phage DNA.

The DNA is replicated by a "rolling-circle" mechanism; during this period, the major coat protein is synthesized in large quantities and inserted into the cell membrane, where it temporarily becomes an integral membrane protein. Replication involves first the production of a double-stranded replicative form, from which new single-stranded elements are copied. As they are synthesized, the single-stranded copies are covered by a phage-encoded DNA-binding protein, forming a structure resembling a virion. At the cell membrane, binding protein is exchanged for the major coat protein plus 4 phage-encoded minor proteins; this process forms a virion that is extruded into the medium without cell death.

The product of a bacterial gene called *fip* is required for phage assembly. Computer comparison of the base sequence of the cloned gene with known sequences in a central data bank showed the *fip* gene product to be thioredoxin, a hydrogen-transferring coenzyme: apparently a cycle of oxidation and reduction is involved in the phage assembly process.

REPLICATION OF RNA PHAGES

When a molecule of viral RNA enters the cytoplasm of the host cell, it is immediately recognized as messenger RNA by the ribosomes, which bind to it and initiate its translation into viral proteins. One such viral protein is a complex enzyme, RNA polymerase. This enzyme brings about the replication of the viral RNA: it polymerizes the ribonucleoside triphosphates of adenine, guanine, cytosine, and uracil, using viral RNA as template.

The first step in the process of RNA replication is the formation of double-stranded intermediates, in which the entering viral RNA strand (called the "plus" strand) is hydrogen-bonded to the complementary "minus" strand synthesized by the polymerase. The polymerase now uses the double-stranded molecule as a template for the repeated synthesis of new plus strands, each new plus strand displacing the previous one from the double-stranded intermediate.

As the newly synthesized plus strands are released from the replicative intermediate, they are either used by the polymerase to form a new double-stranded intermediate or are assembled into mature virions by the attachment of coat protein subunits.

The complete nucleotide sequence of one RNA phage, MS2, has been determined. It is a single molecule, 3566 nucleotides in length, and contains 3 functional genes coding respectively for the RNA polymerase, the coat protein, and a third protein called the "A protein." The single-stranded RNA molecule is capable of folding back on itself and forming double-stranded regions by base-pairing; the secondary structure that results appears to play a role in the regulation of viral RNA replication and translation.

PHAGE GENETICS

Phage particles exhibit the same 2 fundamental genetic properties that are characteristic of organized cells: general stability of type and a low rate of heritable variation (see Chapter 4).

Phage Mutation

All phage properties are controlled by phage genes and are subject to change through gene mutation. The mechanisms of gene mutation described in Chapter 4 apply equally well to phages; indeed, most of our knowledge concerning the chemical basis of mutation comes from studies on phage genetics.

Phage Recombination

If a bacterium simultaneously adsorbs 2 related but slightly different DNA phage particles, both can infect and reproduce; on lysis, the cell releases both types. When this occurs, many of the progeny are observed to be recombinants. Recombination takes place between pairs of phage DNA molecules and is repeated many times between different, random pairs of replicating phage DNA before maturation. Three-way recombinants are therefore possible in a cell simultaneously infected with 3 parental phage types.

Genetic Maps

The relative positions on the phage chromosome of mutant loci involved in phage structure or phage reproduction can be determined by a combination of genetic and physical mapping procedures. In genetic mapping, 2 different mutants are propagated simultaneously in the same host cell, and the frequency of their recombination is measured: the lower the frequency, the shorter the distance between the 2 loci. In physical mapping, heteroduplexes are made between single strands of DNA from normal phage and deletion mutants; examination in the electron microscope reveals the location of the deletion in the form of a non-base-paired region.

An example of a phage genetic map is given in Fig 9–5 for the phage λ. The genes lettered A–W on the map were originally identified as conditional lethal mutations that were suppressed in a host strain carrying a particular suppressor gene; their functions were later identified by electron microscopy and biochemical analyses.

Phage genomes vary widely in size. The smallest known phage genome, that of the RNA phage MS2, has only 3 genes, as described above. In contrast, the largest phages contain sufficient DNA to code for about 200 proteins of average size; genes are present for coat proteins, morphogenesis, enzymes and regulators of phage replication, glycosylation of phage DNA, inhibitors of host restriction enzymes, enzymes that degrade host DNA, DNA repair enzymes, recombination enzymes, and proteins involved in integration and excision of prophage DNA.

LYSOGENY

Prophage

Earlier in this chapter, it was mentioned that some phages ("temperate phages") fail to lyse the cells they infect and then appear to reproduce synchronously with the host for many generations. Their presence can be demonstrated, however, because every so often one of the progeny of the infected bacterium will lyse and liberate infectious phage. To detect this event, it is necessary to use a sensitive indicator strain of bacterium, ie, one that is lysed by the phage. The bacteria that liberate the phage are called "lysogenic"; when a few lysogenic bacteria are plated with an excess of sensitive bacteria, each lysogenic bacterium grows into a colony in which are liberated a few phage particles. These particles immediately infect neighboring sensitive cells, with the result that plaques appear in the film of bacterial growth; in the center of each plaque is a colony of the lysogenic bacterium.

A culture of lysogenic bacteria can also be centrifuged, removing the cells and leaving the temperate phage particles in the supernatant. Their number can be measured by plating suitable dilutions of the supernatant on a sensitive bacterial indicator strain and counting typical plaques.

The release of infectious phage in a culture of lysogenic bacteria is restricted to a very few cells of any given generation. For example, in one bacterial type, about 1 in 200 lyse and liberate phage during each generation; in another type, it may be 1 in 50,000. The remainder of the cells, however, retain the potentiality to produce active phage and transmit this potentiality to their offspring for an indefinite number of generations.

With the rare exceptions mentioned, lysogenic bacteria contain no detectable phage, either as morphologic, serologic, or infectious entities. However, the fact that they carry the potentiality to produce, generations later, phage with a predetermined set of characteristics means that each cell must contain one or more specific noninfectious structures endowed with genetic continuity. This structure is termed "prophage."

The Nature of Prophage

Two entirely different prophage states are found in different phages. In one state, discovered in phage λ, the prophage consists of a molecule of DNA integrated with the host chromosome. The chromosomes of *E coli* and of phage λ are circular; the length of the phage chromosome is about one-fiftieth that of the bacterial chromosome. Both the phage and bacterial chromosomes carry a specific **attachment site.** The bacterial attachment site is immediately adjacent to the *gal* locus (Fig 4–16); the phage attachment site is similarly located at a specific point on the phage genetic map. When λ infects a cell of *E coli*, recombination between the 2 attachment sites occurs, with the result that the 2 circles are integrated (Fig 9–4). This integration process requires the action of a phage gene product: phage mutants defective in this gene (the *int* locus) are unable to lysogenize the cell.

A number of coliphages are of the λ type: their prophages integrate with the host chromosome at specific attachment sites. One phage, called Mu, is unusual in that it is capable of integrating at totally random sites on the chromosome, including sites within bacterial genes. Such integrations result in the inactivation of the gene in question and produce the appearance of mutations. Phage Mu owes its unusual behavior to the fact that it is also a transposon (see Chapter 4).

In the other state, discovered in phage P1, the phage chromosome circularizes and enters a state of "quiescent" replication synchronous with that of the host; no phage proteins are formed. The prophage in the "P1 type" of system is not integrated with the chromosome; its replication is analogous to that of plasmids.

Further Properties of the Lysogenic System

A. Immunity: Lysogenic bacteria are immune to infection by phage of the type already carried in the cell as prophage. When nonlysogenic cells are exposed to temperate phage, many permit phage multiplication and are lysed, while other cells are lysogenized. Once a cell carries prophage, however, neither it nor its progeny can be lysed by homologous phage. Adsorption takes place, but the adsorbed phage simply persists without reproducing and is quickly "diluted out" by continued cell division.

It has been shown that temperate phages cause the appearance in the cytoplasm of a repressor substance that inhibits multiplication of vegetative phage. Repressor also blocks the detachment of prophage (which otherwise would occur by the reversal of the integration process described above) as well as the expression of other phage genes (eg, formation of phage proteins). The establishment of the lysogenic state is thus dependent on the production and action of repressor. The λ repressor has been isolated and characterized as a protein that specifically binds to λ DNA (see below).

The immunity of a lysogenic cell to homologous phage, mediated by a repressor, is clearly different from the phenomenon of "resistance" to virulent phage exhibited by certain bacteria. In the latter case, resistance is caused by failure to adsorb the phage.

B. Induction: "Vegetative phage" is defined as rapidly reproducing phage on its way to mature infective phage, whereas "prophage" reproduces synchronously with the host cell. On rare occasions, prophage "spontaneously" develops into vegetative (and later into mature) phage. This accounts for the sporadic cell lysis and liberation of infectious particles in a lysogenic culture. However, the prophage of practically every cell of certain lysogenic cultures can be induced by various treatments to form and liberate infectious phage. For example, ultraviolet light will induce phage formation and liberation by most of the cells in a lysogenic culture at a dose that would kill very few nonlysogenic bacteria.

Induction requires the inactivation or destruction of repressor molecules present in the cell. Phage mutants have been obtained that produce thermolabile repressors: these phages can be induced simply by raising the temperature to 44 °C. Agents such as ultraviolet light that damage host DNA induce prophage development by the following series of reactions, the end result of which is the inactivation of phage repressor: (1) The DNA lesions are recognized by specific endonucleases that digest a short segment of one strand. (2) The single-stranded regions thus formed bind and activate a protein called the recA protein (product of the *recA* gene), which acts as a protease. (3) The recA protein cleaves the phage repressor molecules, which have also bound to the single-stranded regions of DNA. Oligonucleotides, produced in the first step, are required to activate repressor cleavage.

C. Mutation to Virulence: When virulent phage is mixed with bacterial cells, all of the infected cells

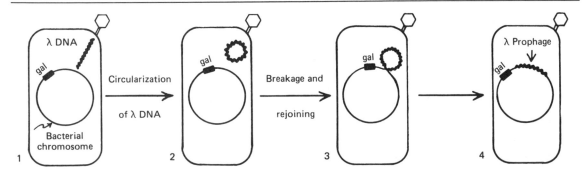

Figure 9–4. The integration of prophage and host chromosome. *(1)* The phage DNA is injected into the host. *(2)* The ends of the phage DNA are covalently joined to form a circular element. *(3)* Pairing occurs between a sequence of bases adjacent to the *gal* locus and a homologous sequence on the phage DNA. *(4)* Breakage and reciprocal rejoining ("crossing over") within the region of pairing integrates the 2 circular DNA structures. The integrated phage DNA is called prophage. The length of λ DNA has been exaggerated for diagrammatic purposes. It is actually 1–2% of the chromosomal length.

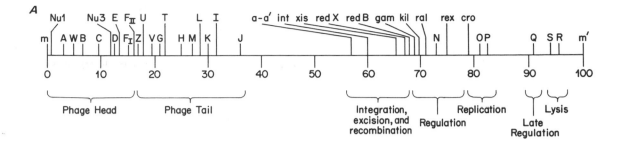

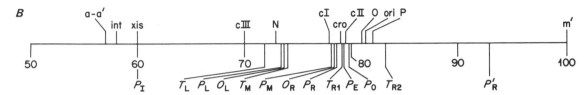

Figure 9–5. *A.* Genetic map of λ phage. During the replication phase, the 2 ends of the DNA (m–m') are joined to form a circular molecule. The regulatory genes controlling transcription are omitted, being shown in *B*, below. For the functions of the different loci, see the reference given at the end of this caption. Note the clustering of genes for related structures and activities. *B.* Map of λ genes regulating gene activity. See text for explanation. (After Echols H, Murialdo H: Genetic map of bacteriophage lambda. *Microbiol Rev* 1978;**42**:577.)

lyse. When temperate phage is mixed with nonlysogenic bacteria, some of the cells reproduce the phage and are lysed, while others are lysogenized.

Temperate phage can mutate to the virulent state. Two types of virulent mutants have been found. In one type, the mutation has made the phage resistant to the repressor, so that it can multiply even in lysogenic cells that are otherwise immune; in the other type, the phage has lost the ability to produce repressor. Virulent mutants of temperate phages are quite different from the naturally virulent phages such as T2. The latter cause the appearance of enzymes that degrade host DNA and stop the synthesis of ribosomal RNA, whereas the former do not interfere with the normal metabolism of the host in this manner.

D. Effect on Genotype of Host: When a lysogenic phage, grown on host "A," infects and lysogenizes host "B" of a different genotype, some of the cells of host "B" may acquire one or more closely linked genes from host "A." For example, if phage grown in a lactose-fermenting host is used to infect a lactose-nonfermenting host, about 1 in every million cells infected becomes lactose-fermenting. The transferred property is heritable. This phenomenon, called "transduction," is described in more detail in Chapter 4.

In other instances, phage genes may themselves determine new host properties. For example, the toxin of *Corynebacterium diphtheriae* and the toxins of many clostridia are determined by genes carried in prophage DNA. In *Salmonella*, phage infection confers a new antigenic surface structure on the host cell. The acquisition of new cell properties as the result of phage infection is called "phage conversion." Phage conversion differs from transduction in that the genes

controlling the new properties are found only in the phage genome and never in the chromosome of the host bacterium.

Genetic Regulation of Phage Reproduction

The vegetative and prophage modes of temperate phage reproduction are regulated by a complex series of genes that govern the transcription of different segments of the phage DNA. One such system of regulation, for the phage λ, is shown in Fig 9–5.

It should be recalled that λ DNA is circularized immediately after penetration of the cell membrane and that the circular DNA may be replicated and ultimately combined with coat proteins to form mature virions, or alternatively may be integrated into the host chromosome by a recombinational event.

In Fig 9–5B, transcriptional promoters (sites of initiation of mRNA synthesis) are indicated by the letter *P*; termination sites for transcription are indicated by the letter *T*; and operator sites are indicated by the letter *O*. These symbols are shown on the map in italics to distinguish them from the genes A–W, which code for various phage proteins not directly involved in transcription regulation.

A. Regulation of Vegetative Replication and Maturation: Gene activity involved in productive phage growth occurs in 3 phases: (1) In the "immediate-early" phase, transcription initiates at promoters P_L and P_R, proceeds left and right respectively, and terminates at the ends of the N and cro genes. These termination sites are designated T_L and T_{R1}; some rightward transcripts extend further, to termination site T_{R2}. (2) In the "delayed-early" phase, the N gene product (protein) acts as an antitermination factor, allowing the above transcriptions to extend further through the genes for replication, recombination, and regulation. (3) In the "late" phase, the cro protein acts at operators O_L and O_R to reduce the initiation of early mRNA transcription from promoters P_L and P_R respectively. Also, Q protein activates rightward transcription from the promoter P'_R, which continues through the lysis, head, and tail genes. (Remember that the genome is circular, the m and m' ends being joined during this phase.)

B. Regulation of Lysogenic Development: Different genes are involved in the establishment and maintenance of lysogeny: (1) In the "establishment" phase, the cII and cIII proteins activate leftward transcription from the promoters P_E and P_I, thus transcribing the cI and int genes; the cII and cIII proteins also inhibit rightward transcription of the lysis genes. (2) In the "maintenance" phase, the cI protein acts at operators O_L and O_R to repress nearly all transcription from promoters P_L and P_R. The cI protein also regulates its own synthesis by controlling leftward transcription from the promoter P_M. Transcription from this site is stimulated by low cI protein concentrations and inhibited by high cI protein concentrations.

The choice between the lytic and lysogenic modes of phage development depends on the mutually antagonistic effects of the cI protein ("repressor") and the cro protein. Both bind to the same 3 sites within the O_R operator, but with different patterns of affinity. The binding of repressor shuts off transcription of all other genes, including cro, and the cell is stably lysogenized. When the repressor is inactivated during prophage induction, however, the cro gene is transcribed; the cro protein that is formed binds to the operator's 3 sites in such a pattern as to block further repressor synthesis (which occurs by leftward transcription) while allowing rightward transcription through the cro gene to continue. The cell is now irreversibly switched to the lytic state.

C. DNA Replication: Replication starts at the site marked ori and requires the activities of the proteins coded by phage genes O and P.

D. Integration and Excision of Prophage: The a–a' attachment site is recognized by the int protein, catalyzing integration by crossing over at a specific attachment site on the host chromosome. Excision, brought about by a second crossover event, requires the activities of both the int and xis proteins.

E. Cleavage of the Circular DNA: Prior to its packaging in virions, the circular DNA must be cleaved at a specific site (m–m') to form linear molecules. This requires the activity of the A protein as well as the presence of phage head precursors.

Restriction & Modification

The phenomena of restriction and modification, as described in Chapter 4, were discovered as a result of their effects on phage multiplication. It was observed that if phage λ is grown in *E coli* strain K12, only about 1 in 10^4 particles can multiply in strain B. The few that succeed, however, liberate progeny that infect B with an efficiency of 1.0 but infect strain K12 with an efficiency of 10^{-4}.

It was shown that DNA of particles formed in K12 is modified by a K12 enzyme so as to be immune to degradation in K12. In strain B, however, the DNA of such particles is rapidly degraded by the restricting enzyme of the host. The few particles that escape restriction are modified by the specific modification enzyme of strain B; the progeny formed are now susceptible to degradation in K12 but not in B. The modifying enzymes have been shown to act by methylating bases within the target sites of the specific restriction endonucleases.

Certain temperate phages carry genes that govern the formation of new modification and restriction enzymes in the host. Thus, *E coli* cells carrying P1 prophage will degrade all DNA not modified in a P1-containing cell.

As discussed in Chapter 4, a given restricting enzyme recognizes a particular site on DNA and causes cleavage at that site unless the site has already been protected by the homologous modifying enzyme. Restriction appears to be a mechanism by which a cell protects itself against invasion by foreign DNA. Some phages have been found to have mechanisms for resisting restriction: Phages T3 and T7, for example, produce an early protein that inhibits the host restriction endonuclease; in other cases, the phage codes for enzymes that modify its DNA (eg, by glycosylation) so as to block the action of the restriction enzymes.

REFERENCES

Books

Freifelder D: *Molecular Biology: A Comprehensive Introduction to Prokaryotes and Eukaryotes.* Science Books International, 1983.

Hayes W: *The Genetics of Bacteria and Their Viruses,* 2nd ed. Blackwell, 1976.

Hendrix RW et al (editors): *Lambda II.* Cold Spring Harbor Laboratory, 1982.

Mathews CK et al (editors): *Bacteriophage T4.* American Society for Microbiology, 1983.

Stent G (editor): *Papers on Bacterial Viruses,* 2nd ed. Little, Brown, 1965.

Stent G, Calendar R: *Molecular Genetics,* 2nd ed. Freeman, 1978.

Zinder N (editor): *RNA Phages.* Cold Spring Harbor Laboratory, 1975.

Articles & Reviews

Barksdale L, Arden SB: Persisting bacteriophage infection, lysogeny, and phage conversion. *Annu Rev Microbiol* 1976;**28**:265.

Bernstein C: DNA repair in bacteriophage. *Microbiol Rev* 1981;**45**:72.

Broker TR, Doermann AH: Molecular and genetic recombination of bacteriophage T4. *Annu Rev Genet* 1975;**9**:213.

Echols H, Murialdo H: Genetic map of bacteriophage lambda. *Microbiol Rev* 1978;**42**:577.

Friedman DI et al: Interactions of bacteriophage and host macromolecules in the growth of bacteriophage lambda. *Microbiol Rev* 1984;**48**:299.

Gottesman S: Lambda site-specific recombination: The att site. *Cell* 1982;**25**:585.

Hayes W: Portraits of viruses: Bacteriophage lambda. *Intervirology* 1980;**13**:133.

Hemphill HE, Whiteley HR: Bacteriophages of *Bacillus subtilis*. *Bacteriol Rev* 1975;**39**:257.

Herskowitz I, Hagen D: The lysis-lysogeny decision of phage λ: Explicit programming and responsiveness. *Annu Rev Genet* 1980;**14**:399.

Horne RW, Wildy P: Symmetry in virus structure. *Virology* 1961;**15**:348.

Johnson AD et al: λ Repressor and Cro: Components of an efficient molecular switch. *Nature* 1981;**294**:217.

Koerner JF et al: Shutoff of host macromolecular synthesis after T-even bacteriophage infection. *Microbiol Rev* 1979;**43**:199.

Lemke PA: Viruses of eukaryotic microorganisms. *Annu Rev Microbiol* 1976;**30**:105.

Lindberg AA: Bacteriophage receptors. *Annu Rev Microbiol* 1973;**27**:205.

Lwoff A: The concept of virus. *J Gen Microbiol* 1957;**17**:239.

Marvin DA, Wachtel E: Structure and assembly of filamentous bacterial viruses. *Nature* 1975;**253**:19.

Miller RC: Replication and molecular recombination of T-phage. *Annu Rev Microbiol* 1975;**29**:355.

Ptashne M, Johnson AD, Pabo CO: A genetic switch in a bacterial virus. *Sci Am* (Nov) 1982;**247**:128.

Ptashne M et al: How the lambda repressor and cro work. (Review.) *Cell* 1980;**19**:1.

Sternberg N, Hoess R: The molecular genetics of bacteriophage P1. *Annu Rev Genet* 1983;**17**:123.

Szybalski EH et al: A comprehensive molecular map of bacteriophage lambda. *Gene* 1979;**7**:217.

Valentine R, Ward R, Strand M: The replication cycle of RNA bacteriophages. *Adv Virus Res* 1969;**15**:1.

Witmer HJ: Regulation of bacteriophage T4 gene expression. *Prog Mol Subcell Biol* 1976;**4**:53.

Zinder ND, Horiuchi K: Multiregulatory element of filamentous bacteriophages. *Microbiol Rev* 1985;**49**:101.

Antimicrobial Chemotherapy

Although various chemicals have been used for the treatment of infectious diseases since the 17th century (eg, quinine for malaria and emetine for amebiasis), chemotherapy as a science began with Paul Ehrlich. He was the first to formulate the principles of selective toxicity and to recognize the specific chemical relationships between parasites and drugs, the development of drug-fastness in parasites, and the role of combined therapy in combating this development. Ehrlich's experiments in the first decade of the 20th century led to the arsphenamines, the first major triumph of planned chemotherapy.

The current era of rapid development in antimicrobial chemotherapy began in 1935, with the discovery of the sulfonamides by Domagk. In 1940, Chain and Florey demonstrated that penicillin, which had been observed in 1929 by Fleming, could be made into an effective chemotherapeutic substance. During the next 25 years, chemotherapeutic research largely centered around antimicrobial substances of microbial origin called antibiotics. The isolation, concentration, purification, and mass production of penicillin were followed by the development of streptomycin, tetracyclines, chloramphenicol, and many other agents. Although these substances were all originally isolated from filtrates of media in which their respective molds (*Streptomyces*) had grown, several have subsequently been synthesized. In recent years, chemical modification of molecules by biosynthesis has been a prominent method of new drug development. Brief summaries of antimicrobial agents commonly employed in medical treatment are presented at the end of this section.

MECHANISMS OF ACTION OF CLINICALLY USED ANTIMICROBIAL DRUGS

Selective Toxicity

An ideal antimicrobial agent exhibits *selective toxicity*. This term implies that a drug is harmful to a parasite without being harmful to the host. Often, selective toxicity is relative rather than absolute; this implies that a drug in a concentration tolerated by the host may damage a parasite.

Selective toxicity may be a function of a specific receptor required for drug attachment, or it may depend on the inhibition of biochemical events essential to the parasite but not to the host. The mechanism of action of most antimicrobial drugs is not completely under-stood. However, it is convenient to present these mechanisms of action under 4 headings:

(1) Inhibition of cell wall synthesis.

(2) Alteration of cell membrane permeability or inhibition of active transport across cell membrane.

(3) Inhibition of protein synthesis (ie, inhibition of translation and transcription of genetic material).

(4) Inhibition of nucleic acid synthesis.

Antimicrobial Action Through Inhibition of Cell Wall Synthesis
(*Examples:* Bacitracin, Cephalosporins, Cycloserine, Penicillins, Ristocetin, Vancomycin.)

In contrast to animal cells, bacteria possess a rigid outer layer, the cell wall. It maintains the shape of the microorganism and "corsets" the bacterial cell, which has a high internal osmotic pressure. The internal pressure is 3–5 times greater in gram-positive than in gram-negative bacteria. Injury to the cell wall (eg, by lysozyme) or inhibition of its formation may lead to lysis of the cell. In a hypertonic environment (eg, 20% sucrose), damaged cell wall formation leads to formation of spherical bacterial "protoplasts" from gram-positive organisms or "spheroplasts" from gram-negative organisms; these forms are limited by the fragile cytoplasmic membrane. If such "protoplasts" or "spheroplasts" are placed in an environment of ordinary tonicity, they may explode.

The cell wall contains a chemically distinct complex polymer "mucopeptide" ("murein," "peptidoglycan") consisting of polysaccharides and a highly cross-linked polypeptide. The polysaccharides regularly contain the amino sugars N-acetylglucosamine and acetylmuramic acid. The latter is found only in bacteria. To the amino sugars are attached pentapeptide chains. The final rigidity of the cell wall is imparted by cross-linking of the peptide chains (eg, through pentaglycine bonds) as a result of transpeptidation reactions carried out by several enzymes. The peptidoglycan layer is much thicker in the cell wall of gram-positive bacteria than in the cell wall of gram-negative bacteria.

All penicillins and all cephalosporins (β-lactam drugs) are selective inhibitors of bacterial cell wall synthesis. This is only one of several different activities of these drugs, but it is the best understood. The initial step in drug action consists of binding of the drug to cell receptors ("penicillin-binding proteins," PBPs). There are 3–6 PBPs (MW 4–12×10^5), some of which are transpeptidation enzymes. Different receptors have different affinities for a drug, and each may mediate a different effect. For example, attachment of penicillin to one PBP may result chiefly in abnormal elongation of the cell, whereas attachment to another PBP may lead to a defect in the periphery of the cell wall, with resulting cell lysis. PBPs are under chromosomal control, and mutations may alter their number or their affinity for β-lactam drugs.

After a β-lactam drug has attached to its receptor or receptors, the transpeptidation reaction is inhibited and peptidoglycan synthesis is blocked. The next step probably involves the removal or inactivation of an inhibitor or autolytic enzymes in the cell wall. This activates the lytic enzyme and results in lysis if the environment is isotonic. In a markedly hypertonic environment (eg, 20% sucrose), the cells change to protoplasts or spheroplasts, covered only by the fragile cell membrane. In such protoplasts or spheroplasts, synthesis of proteins and nucleic acids may continue for some time.

The inhibition of the transpeptidation enzymes by penicillins and cephalosporins may be due to a structural similarity of these drugs to acyl-D-alanyl-D-alanine. The transpeptidation reaction involves loss of a D-alanine from the pentapeptide.

The remarkable lack of toxicity of penicillins to mammalian cells must be attributed to the absence of a bacterial type cell wall, with its peptidoglycan, in animal cells. The difference in susceptibility of gram-positive and gram-negative bacteria to various penicillins or cephalosporins probably depends on structural differences in their cell walls (eg, amount of peptidoglycan, presence of receptors and lipids, nature of cross-linking, activity of autolytic enzymes) that determine penetration, binding, and activity of the drugs.

Amdinocillin (mecillinam) is an amidinopenicillanic acid derivative that differs from other penicillins in that it binds *only* to penicillin-binding protein 2 (PBP-2) and is more active against gram-negative than against gram-positive bacteria. Amdinocillin can act synergistically with other β-lactam drugs (penicillins, cephalosporins) that attach to other PBPs, and such synergism may be clinically applicable.

Insusceptibility to penicillins is in part determined by the organism's production of penicillin-destroying enzymes (β-lactamases). Beta-lactamases open the β-lactam ring of penicillins and cephalosporins and abolish their antimicrobial activity. Certain penicillins (eg, cloxacillin) and other compounds (eg, clavulanic acid) have a high affinity for the β-lactamase produced by some gram-negative bacteria, eg, *Haemophilus*. They bind the enzyme but are not hydrolyzed by it and thus protect simultaneously present hydrolyzable penicillins (eg, ampicillin) from destruction. This is a form of "synergism" of known mechanism (see p 140). A fixed combination of clavulanic acid, 250 mg, with amoxicillin, 500 mg, given orally 3 times daily, is used to treat β-lactamase-producing *Haemophilus influenzae* infections.

Two other types of resistance mechanisms may exist. One is due to the absence of some penicillin receptors (PBPs) and occurs as a result of chromosomal mutation; the other results from failure of the β-lactam drug to activate the autolytic enzymes in the cell wall. As a result, the organism is inhibited but not killed. Such "tolerance" has been observed especially with staphylococci and certain streptococci.

Several other drugs, including bacitracin, vancomycin, ristocetin, and novobiocin, inhibit early steps in the biosynthesis of the peptidoglycan. Since the early stages of synthesis take place inside the cytoplasmic membrane, these drugs must penetrate the membrane to be effective. For these drugs, inhibition of peptidoglycan synthesis is not a main basis of antibacterial action.

Cycloserine, an analog of D-alanine, also interferes with peptidoglycan synthesis. This drug blocks the action of alanine racemase, an essential enzyme in the incorporation of D-alanine in the pentapeptide of peptidoglycan. Phosphonopeptides also inhibit enzymes needed for early synthesis of peptidoglycans.

Antimicrobial Action Through Inhibition of Cell Membrane Function
(*Examples:* Amphotericin B, Colistin, Imidazoles, Nystatin, Polymyxins.)

The cytoplasm of all living cells is bounded by the cytoplasmic membrane, which serves as a selective permeability barrier, carries out active transport functions, and thus controls the internal composition of the cell. If the functional integrity of the cytoplasmic membrane is disrupted, macromolecules and ions escape from the cell, and cell damage or death ensues. The cytoplasmic membrane of bacteria and fungi has a structure different from that of animal cells and can be more readily disrupted by certain agents. Consequently, selective chemotherapeutic activity is possible.

The outstanding examples of this mechanism are the polymyxins acting on gram-negative bacteria (polymyxins selectively act on membranes rich in phosphatidylethanolamine and act like cationic detergent) and the polyene antibiotics acting on fungi. However, polymyxins are inactive against fungi, and polyenes are inactive against bacteria. This is because sterols are present in the fungal cell membrane and absent in the bacterial cell membrane. Polyenes must interact with a sterol in the fungal cell membrane prior to exerting their effect. Bacterial cell membranes do not contain that sterol and (presumably for this reason) are resistant to polyene action—a good example of cell individuality and of selective toxicity. Conversely, polymyxins will not act on the sterol-containing cell membranes of fungi. The antifungal imidazoles impair the integrity of fungal cell membranes by inhibiting the biosynthesis of membrane lipids.

Antimicrobial Action Through Inhibition of Protein Synthesis
(*Examples:* Chloramphenicol, Erythromycins, Lincomycins, Tetracyclines; Aminoglycosides: Amikacin, Gentamicin, Kanamycin, Neomycin, Netilmicin, Streptomycin, Tobramycin, Etc.)

It is established that chloramphenicol, tetracyclines, aminoglycosides, erythromycins, and lincomycins can inhibit protein synthesis in bacteria. Puromycin is an effective inhibitor of protein synthesis in animal and other cells. The concepts of protein synthesis are undergoing rapid change, and the precise mechanism of action is not fully established for these drugs.

Bacteria have 70S ribosomes, whereas mammalian cells have 80S ribosomes. The subunits of each type of ribosome, their chemical composition, and their functional specificities are sufficiently different to explain why antimicrobial drugs can inhibit protein synthesis in bacterial ribosomes without having a major effect on mammalian ribosomes.

In normal microbial protein synthesis, the mRNA message is simultaneously "read" by several ribosomes, which are strung out along the mRNA strand. These are called polysomes.

A. Aminoglycosides: The mode of action of streptomycin has been studied far more than that of other aminoglycosides (kanamycin, neomycin, gentamicin, tobramycin, amikacin, etc), but probably all act similarly. The first step is the attachment of the aminoglycoside to a specific receptor protein (P 12 in the case of streptomycin) on the 30S subunit of the microbial ribosome. Second, the aminoglycoside blocks the normal activity of the "initiation complex" of peptide formation (mRNA + formyl methionine + tRNA). Third, the mRNA message is misread on the "recognition region" of the ribosome, and as a result, the wrong amino acid is inserted into the peptide, resulting in a nonfunctional protein. Fourth, aminoglycoside attachment results in the breakup of polysomes and their separation into "monosomes" incapable of protein synthesis. These activities occur more or less simultaneously, and the overall effect is usually an irreversible event—killing of the cell.

Chromosomal resistance of microbes to aminoglycosides principally depends on the lack of a specific protein receptor on the 30S subunit of the ribosome. Plasmid-dependent resistance to aminoglycosides depends on the production by the microorganism of adenylylating, phosphorylating, or acetylating enzymes that destroy the drugs. A third type of resistance consists of a "permeability defect," an outer membrane change that reduces active transport of the aminoglycoside into the cell so that the drug cannot reach the ribosome. Sometimes at least, this is plasmid-mediated.

B. Tetracyclines: Tetracyclines bind to the 30S subunit of microbial ribosomes. They inhibit protein synthesis by blocking the attachment of charged aminoacyl-tRNA. Thus, they prevent introduction of new amino acids to the nascent peptide chain. The action is usually inhibitory and reversible upon withdrawal of the drug. Resistance to tetracyclines results from changes in permeability of the microbial cell envelope. In susceptible cells, the drug is concentrated from the environment and does not readily leave the cell. In resistant cells, the drug is not actively transported into the cell or leaves it so rapidly that inhibitory concentrations are not maintained. This is often plasmid-controlled. Mammalian cells do not actively concentrate tetracyclines.

C. Chloramphenicol: Chloramphenicol binds to the 50S subunit of the ribosome. It interferes with the binding of new amino acids to the nascent peptide chain, largely because chloramphenicol inhibits peptidyl transferase. Chloramphenicol is mainly bacteriostatic, and growth of microorganisms resumes (ie, drug action is reversible) when the drug is withdrawn. Microorganisms resistant to chloramphenicol produce the enzyme chloramphenicol acetyltransferase, which destroys drug activity. The production of this enzyme is usually under control of a plasmid.

D. Macrolides (Erythromycins, Oleandomycins): These drugs bind to the 50S subunit of the ribosome, and the binding site is a 23S rRNA. They may interfere with formation of initiation complexes for peptide chain synthesis or may interfere with aminoacyl translocation reactions. Some macrolide-resistant bacteria lack the proper receptor on the ribosome (through methylation of the rRNA). This may be under plasmid or chromosomal control.

E. Lincomycins (Lincomycin, Clindamycin): Lincomycins bind to the 50S subunit of the microbial ribosome and resemble macrolides in binding site, antibacterial activity, and mode of action. There may be mutual interference between these drugs. Chromosomal mutants are resistant because they lack the proper binding site on the 50S subunit.

Antimicrobial Action Through Inhibition of Nucleic Acid Synthesis
(*Examples:* Nalidixic Acid, Novobiocin, Pyrimethamine, Rifampin, Sulfonamides, Trimethoprim.)

Drugs such as the actinomycins are effective inhibitors of DNA synthesis. Actually, they form complexes with DNA by binding to the deoxyguanosine residues. The DNA-actinomycin complex inhibits the DNA-dependent RNA polymerase and blocks mRNA formation. Actinomycin also inhibits DNA virus replication. Mitomycins result in the firm cross-linking of complementary strands of DNA and subsequently block DNA replication. Both actinomycins and mitomycins inhibit bacterial as well as animal cells and are not sufficiently selective to be employed in antibacterial chemotherapy.

Rifampin inhibits bacterial growth by binding strongly to the DNA-dependent RNA polymerase of bacteria. Thus, it inhibits bacterial RNA synthesis. Rifampin resistance results from a change in RNA polymerase due to a chromosomal mutation that occurs with high frequency. The mechanism of rifampin action on viruses is different. It blocks a late stage in the assembly of poxviruses.

The halogenated pyrimidines, eg, IUDR (5-iodo-2'-deoxyuridine, idoxuridine, IDU) can block the synthesis of functionally intact DNA and thus interfere with the replication of infective DNA viruses. IUDR can interfere with the incorporation of thymidine into viral DNA, and IUDR itself may be incorporated to form nonfunctional DNA. The systemic administration of IUDR is not feasible because of severe toxicity. Local application of IUDR to DNA virus-producing cells (in herpes simplex keratitis) can result in significant suppression of viral replication in vivo. Other inhibitors of DNA replication, eg, vidarabine or acyclovir, are used in systemic antiviral chemotherapy (see p 158).

Nalidixic and oxolinic acid, used principally as urinary antiseptics, are potent inhibitors of DNA synthesis. They block DNA gyrase. Whether the effect in vivo depends solely on this action is not known.

For many microorganisms, p-aminobenzoic acid (PABA) is an essential metabolite. It is used by them as a precursor in the synthesis of folic acid, which serves as an important step in the synthesis of nucleic acids. The specific mode of action of PABA involves an adenosine triphosphate (ATP)-dependent condensation of a pteridine with PABA to yield dihydropteroic acid, which is subsequently converted to folic acid. Sulfonamides are structural analogs of PABA and inhibit dihydropteroate synthetase.

| p-Aminobenzoic acid (PABA) | Basic ring structure of sulfonamides |

Sulfonamides can enter into the reaction in place of PABA and compete for the active center of the enzyme. As a result, nonfunctional analogs of folic acid are formed, preventing further growth of the bacterial cell. The inhibiting action of sulfonamides on bacterial growth can be counteracted by an excess of PABA in the environment (competitive inhibition). Animal cells cannot synthesize folic acid and must depend upon exogenous sources. Some bacteria, like animal cells, are not inhibited by sulfonamides. Many other bacteria, however, synthesize folic acid as mentioned above and consequently are susceptible to action by sulfonamides.

Tubercle bacilli are not markedly inhibited by sulfonamides, but their growth is inhibited by PAS (p-aminosalicylic acid). Conversely, most sulfonamide-

susceptible bacteria are resistant to PAS. This suggests that the receptor site for PABA differs in different types of organisms.

Trimethoprim (3,4,5-trimethoxybenzyl pyrimidine) inhibits dihydrofolic acid reductase 50,000 times more efficiently in bacteria than in mammalian cells. This enzyme reduces dihydrofolic to tetrahydrofolic acid, a stage in the sequence leading to the synthesis of purines and ultimately of DNA. Sulfonamides and trimethoprim each can be used alone to inhibit bacterial growth. If used together, they produce sequential blocking, resulting in a marked enhancement (synergism) of activity. Such sulfonamide (5 parts) + trimethoprim (1 part) mixtures have been used in the treatment of *Pneumocystis* pneumonia, malaria, *Shigella* enteritis, systemic *Salmonella* infections, urinary tract infections, and many others.

Pyrimethamine (Daraprim) also inhibits dihydrofolate reductase, but it is more active against the enzyme in mammalian cells and therefore is more toxic than trimethoprim. Pyrimethamine plus sulfonamide is the current treatment of choice in toxoplasmosis and some other protozoal infections.

RESISTANCE TO ANTIMICROBIAL DRUGS

There are many different mechanisms by which microorganisms might exhibit resistance to drugs. The following are fairly well supported.

(1) Microorganisms produce enzymes that destroy the active drug. *Examples:* Staphylococci resistant to penicillin G produce a β-lactamase that destroys the drug. Other β-lactamases are produced by gram-negative rods. Gram-negative bacteria resistant to aminoglycosides (by virtue of a plasmid) produce adenylylating, phosphorylating, or acetylating enzymes that destroy the drug. Gram-negative bacteria may be resistant to chloramphenicol if they produce a chloramphenicol acetyltransferase.

(2) Microorganisms change their permeability to the drug. *Examples:* Tetracyclines accumulate in susceptible bacteria but not in resistant bacteria. Resistance to polymyxins is also associated with a change in permeability to the drugs. Streptococci have a natural permeability barrier to aminoglycosides. This can be partly overcome by the simultaneous presence of a cell-wall-active drug, eg, a penicillin. Resistance to amikacin and to some other aminoglycosides may depend on a lack of permeability to the drugs, apparently due to an outer membrane change that impairs active transport into the cell.

(3) Microorganisms develop an altered structural target for the drug (see also ¶5, below). *Examples:* Chromosomal resistance to aminoglycosides is associated with the loss or alteration of a specific protein in the 30S subunit of the bacterial ribosome that serves as a binding site in susceptible organisms. Erythromycin-resistant organisms have an altered receptor on the 50S subunit of the ribosome, resulting from methylation of

a 23S ribosomal RNA. Resistance to some penicillins may be a function of the loss or alteration of PBPs.

(4) Microorganisms develop an altered metabolic pathway that bypasses the reaction inhibited by the drug. *Example:* Some sulfonamide-resistant bacteria do not require extracellular PABA but, like mammalian cells, can utilize preformed folic acid.

(5) Microorganisms develop an altered enzyme that can still perform its metabolic function but is much less affected by the drug than the enzyme in the susceptible organism. *Example:* In some sulfonamide-susceptible bacteria, the tetrahydropteroic acid synthetase has a much higher affinity for sulfonamide than for PABA. In sulfonamide-resistant mutants, the opposite is the case.

ORIGIN OF DRUG RESISTANCE

The origin of drug resistance may be genetic or nongenetic.

Nongenetic Origin

Active replication of bacteria is usually required for most antibacterial drug actions. Consequently, microorganisms that are metabolically inactive (nonmultiplying) may be phenotypically resistant to drugs. However, their offspring are fully susceptible. *Example:* Mycobacteria often survive in tissues for many years after infection yet are restrained by the host's defenses and do not multiply. Such "persisting" organisms are resistant to treatment and cannot be eradicated by drugs. Yet if they start to multiply (eg, following corticosteroid treatment of the patient), they are fully susceptible to the same drugs.

Microorganisms may lose the specific target structure for a drug for several generations and thus be resistant. *Example:* Penicillin-susceptible organisms may change to L forms during penicillin administration. Lacking most cell wall, they are then resistant to cell wall inhibitor drugs (penicillins, cephalosporins) and may remain so for several generations as "persisters." When these organisms revert to their bacterial parent forms by resuming cell wall production, they are again fully susceptible to penicillin.

Genetic Origin

Most drug-resistant microbes emerge as a result of genetic change and subsequent selection processes by antimicrobial drugs. The mechanisms by which genetic changes occur are discussed in Chapter 4.

A. Chromosomal Resistance: This develops as a result of spontaneous mutation in a locus that controls susceptibility to a given antimicrobial drug. The presence of the antimicrobial drug serves as a selecting mechanism to suppress susceptible organisms and favor the growth of drug-resistant mutants. Spontaneous mutation occurs with a frequency of 10^{-7} to 10^{-12} and thus is an infrequent cause of the emergence of clinical drug resistance in a given patient. However, chromosomal mutants resistant to rifampin occur with high frequency (about 10^{-5}), and consequently, treatment of bacterial infections with rifampin alone usually fails. Chromosomal mutants are most commonly resistant by virtue of a change in a structural receptor for a drug. Thus, the P 12 protein on the 30S subunit of the bacterial ribosome serves as a receptor for streptomycin attachment. Mutation in the gene controlling that structural protein results in streptomycin resistance. A narrow region of the bacterial chromosome contains structural genes that code for a number of drug receptors, including those for erythromycin, lincomycin, aminoglycosides, and others.

B. Extrachromosomal Resistance: Bacteria often contain extrachromosomal genetic elements called plasmids. Their features are described in Chapter 4.

R factors are a class of plasmids that carry genes for resistance to one—and often several—antimicrobial drugs and heavy metals. Plasmid genes for antimicrobial resistance often control the formation of enzymes capable of destroying the antimicrobial drugs. Thus, plasmids determine resistance to penicillins and cephalosporins by carrying genes for the formation of β-lactamases. Plasmids code for enzymes that destroy chloramphenicol (acetyltransferase); for enzymes that acetylate, adenylylate, or phosphorylate various aminoglycosides; for enzymes that determine the active transport of tetracyclines across the cell membrane; and for others (Table 4–1).

Genetic material and plasmids can be transferred by the following mechanisms (see Chapter 4 for detailed descriptions):

1. Transduction–Plasmid DNA is enclosed in a bacterial virus and transferred by the virus to another bacterium of the same species. *Example:* The plasmid carrying the gene for β-lactamase production can be transferred from a penicillin-resistant to a susceptible *Staphylococcus* if carried by a suitable bacteriophage. Similar transduction occurs in salmonellae.

2. Transformation–Naked DNA passes from one cell of a species to another cell, thus altering its genotype. This can occur through laboratory manipulation (eg, in recombinant DNA technology; see pp 61–63) and perhaps spontaneously.

3. Conjugation–A unilateral transfer of genetic material between bacteria of the same or different genera occurs during a mating (conjugation) process. This is mediated by a fertility (F) factor that results in the extension of sex pili from the donor (F^+) cell to the recipient. Plasmid or other DNA is transferred through these protein tubules from the donor to the recipient cell. A series of closely linked genes, each determining resistance to one drug, may thus be transferred from a resistant to a susceptible bacterium. This is the commonest method by which multidrug resistance spreads among different genera of gram-negative bacteria. Transfer of resistance plasmids also occurs among some gram-positive cocci.

4. Transposition–A transfer of short DNA sequences (transposons, transposable elements) occurs between one plasmid and another or between a plasmid and a portion of the bacterial chromosome within a bacterial cell.

Cross-Resistance

Microorganisms resistant to a certain drug may also be resistant to other drugs that share a mechanism of action. Such relationships exist mainly between agents that are closely related chemically (eg, polymyxin B–colistin; erythromycin-oleandomycin; neomycin-kanamycin), but they may also exist between unrelated chemicals (erythromycin-lincomycin). In certain classes of drugs, the active nucleus of the chemical is so similar among many congeners (eg, tetracyclines, cephalosporins) that extensive cross-resistance is to be expected.

Limitation of Drug Resistance

Emergence of drug resistance in infections may be minimized in the following ways: (1) maintain sufficiently high levels of the drug in the tissues to inhibit both the original population and first step mutants; (2) simultaneously administer 2 drugs that do not give cross-resistance, each of which delays the emergence of mutants resistant to the other drug (eg, rifampin and isoniazid in the treatment of tuberculosis); and (3) avoid exposure of microorganisms to a particularly valuable drug by restricting its use, especially in hospitals and in animal feeds (see below).

Clinical Implications of Drug Resistance

A few examples will illustrate the impact of the emergence of drug-resistant organisms and their selection by the widespread use of antimicrobial drugs.

(1) Gonococci: When sulfonamides were first employed in the late 1930s for the treatment of gonorrhea, virtually all isolates of gonococci were susceptible and most infections were cured. A few years later, most strains had become resistant to sulfonamides, and gonorrhea was rarely curable by these drugs. Most gonococci were still highly susceptible to penicillin. Over the next decades, there was a gradual increase in resistance to penicillin, but large doses of that drug were still curative. In the 1970s, β-lactamase-producing gonococci appeared, first in the Philippines and in West Africa, and then spread to form endemic foci in the USA, Britain, and elsewhere. Such infections could not be treated effectively by penicillin but were somewhat contained by public health measures and the use of spectinomycin. Resistance to spectinomycin is now appearing.

(2) Meningococci: Until 1962, meningococci were uniformly susceptible to sulfonamides, and these drugs were effective for both prophylaxis and therapy. Subsequently, sulfonamide-resistant meningococci spread widely, and the sulfonamides have now lost most of their usefulness against meningococcal infections. Penicillins remain effective for therapy, and rifampin is employed for prophylaxis. However, rifampin-resistant meningococci persist in about 1% of individuals who have received rifampin for prophylaxis.

(3) Staphylococci: In 1944, most staphylococci were susceptible to penicillin, although a few resistant strains had been observed. After massive use of penicillin, 65–85% of staphylococci isolated from hospitals in 1948 were β-lactamase producers and thus resistant to penicillin G. The advent of β-lactamase-resistant penicillins (eg, methicillin) provided a temporary respite, but outbreaks of infections due to methicillin-resistant staphylococci now occur intermittently. In 1986, penicillin-resistant staphylococci include not only those acquired in hospital but also 80% of those isolated in the community. These organisms also tend to be resistant to other drugs, eg, tetracyclines.

(4) Pneumococci: Until 1963, pneumococci were uniformly susceptible to penicillin G; in that year, some relatively penicillin-resistant pneumococci were found in New Guinea. Such organisms have been encountered since 1977 in hospital outbreaks, first in South Africa and then elsewhere. While they do not produce β-lactamase, they are insusceptible to penicillin G, probably because of altered PBPs; this makes treatment of meningitic infections difficult.

(5) Gram-negative enteric bacteria: Most drug resistance in enteric bacteria is attributable to the widespread transmission of resistance plasmids among different genera. In Japan, the frequency of multi-resistant *Shigella* strains rose from 10–20% in 1955 to 80% in 1968. A similar rise in *Shigella* resistance caused epidemics in Central America at the same time.

Salmonellae carried by animals have developed resistance also, particularly to drugs (especially tetracyclines) incorporated in animal feeds. The practice of incorporating drugs into animal feeds caused farm animals to grow more rapidly but was associated with an increase in drug-resistant enteric organisms in the fecal flora of farm workers. A concomitant rise in drug-resistant *Salmonella* infections in Britain led to a restriction on antibiotic supplements in animal feeds. Continued use of tetracycline supplements in animal feeds in the USA may contribute to the spread of resistance plasmids and of drug-resistant salmonellae.

Plasmids carrying drug resistance genes occur in many gram-negative bacteria of the normal gut flora. The abundant use of antimicrobial drugs—particularly in hospitalized patients—leads to the suppression of drug-susceptible organisms in the gut flora and favors the persistence and growth of drug-resistant bacteria, including *Enterobacter, Klebsiella, Proteus, Pseudomonas, Serratia,* and fungi. Such organisms present particularly difficult problems in granulopenic and immunocompromised patients. The closed environment of hospitals favors transmission of such resistant organisms through personnel and fomites as well as by direct contact.

(6) Tubercle bacilli: To a limited extent, drug-resistant mutants have arisen in tuberculosis. They may complicate the treatment of individual patients in whom they arise and may be transmitted to contacts, giving rise to primary drug-resistant infections. This problem has been important among migrants from Southeast Asia, where indiscriminate distribution of antituberculosis drugs is rampant.

DRUG DEPENDENCE

Certain organisms are not only resistant to a drug but require it for growth. This has been best demonstrated for streptomycin. When streptomycin-dependent meningococci are injected into mice, progressive fatal disease results only if the animals are treated simultaneously with streptomycin. In the absence of streptomycin, the microorganisms cannot proliferate, and the animals remain well. This phenomenon probably plays no role in human infection. Drug-dependent bacteria have been used in live vaccines for animals.

ANTIMICROBIAL ACTIVITY IN VITRO

Antimicrobial activity is measured in vitro in order to determine (1) the potency of an antibacterial agent in solution, (2) its concentration in body fluids or tissues, and (3) the sensitivity of a given microorganism to known concentrations of the drug.

Measurement of Antimicrobial Activity

Determination of these quantities may be undertaken by one of 2 principal methods: dilution or diffusion.

Using an appropriate standard test organism and a known sample of drug for comparison, these methods can be employed to estimate either the potency of antibiotic in the sample or the "sensitivity" of the microorganism.

A. Dilution Tests: Graded amounts of antimicrobial substances are incorporated into liquid or solid bacteriologic media. The media are subsequently inoculated with test bacteria and incubated. The end point is taken as that amount of antimicrobial substance required to inhibit the growth of, or to kill, the test bacteria. Agar-dilution susceptibility tests are time-consuming, and their use is limited to special circumstances. Broth-dilution tests were cumbersome and little used when dilutions had to be made in test tubes; however, the advent of prepared broth-dilution series for many different drugs in microtiter plates has greatly enhanced and simplified the method. The advantage of microtiter broth-dilution tests is that they permit a quantitative result to be reported, indicating the amount of a given drug necessary to inhibit (or kill) the microorganisms tested.

B. Diffusion Method: A filter paper disk, a porous cup, or a bottomless cylinder containing measured quantities of drug is placed on a solid medium that has been heavily seeded with the test organisms. After incubation, the diameter of the clear zone of inhibition surrounding the deposit of drug is taken as a measure of the inhibitory power of the drug against the particular test organism. Obviously, this method is subject to many physical and chemical factors in addition to the simple interaction of drug and organisms (eg, nature of medium and diffusibility, molecular size, and stability of drug). Nevertheless, standardization of conditions permits quantitative assay of drug potency or sensitivity of the organism.

When determining bacterial sensitivity by the diffusion method, most laboratories use disks of antibiotic-impregnated filter paper. A concentration gradient of antibiotic is produced in the medium by diffusion from the disk. As the diffusion is a continuous process, the concentration gradient is never stable for long; but some stabilization can be achieved by allowing diffusion to start before bacterial growth begins. The greatest difficulties arise from the varying growth rates of different microorganisms and must be corrected by varying the density of the inoculum.

Interpretation of the results of diffusion tests must be based on comparisons between dilution and diffusion methods. Such comparisons have led to the establishment of international reference standards. Linear regression lines can express the relationship between log of minimum inhibitory concentration in dilution tests and diameter of inhibition zones in diffusion tests.

Use of a single disk for each antibiotic with careful standardization of the test conditions permits the report of S (susceptible) or R (resistant) for a microorganism by comparing the size of the inhibition zone against a standard of the same drug (Kirby-Bauer method).

It is fundamentally wrong to regard inhibition around a disk containing a certain amount of antibiotic as implying sensitivity to the same concentration of the antibiotic per millimeter of medium, blood, or urine.

Factors Affecting Antimicrobial Activity

Among the many factors that affect antimicrobial activity in vitro, the following must be considered, because they significantly influence the results of tests.

A. pH of Environment: Some drugs are more active at acid pH (eg, nitrofurantoin); others, at alkaline pH (eg, aminoglycosides, sulfonamides).

B. Components of Medium: Sodium polyanethol sulfonate and other anionic detergents inhibit aminoglycosides. PABA in tissue extracts antagonizes sulfonamides. Serum proteins bind penicillins in varying degrees, ranging from 40% for methicillin to 98% for dicloxacillin.

C. Stability of Drug: At incubator temperature, several antimicrobial agents lose their activity. Chlortetracycline is inactivated rapidly and penicillins more slowly, whereas aminoglycosides, chloramphenicol, and polymyxin B are quite stable for long periods.

D. Size of Inoculum: In general, the larger the bacterial inoculum, the lower the apparent "sensitivity" of the organism. Large bacterial populations are less promptly and completely inhibited than small ones. In addition, the likelihood of the emergence of a resistant mutant is much greater in large populations.

E. Length of Incubation: In many instances, microorganisms are not killed but only inhibited upon short exposure to antimicrobial agents. The longer incubation continues, the greater the chance for resistant mutants to emerge or for the least susceptible members of the antimicrobial population to begin multiplying as the drug deteriorates.

F. Metabolic Activity of Microorganisms: In general, actively and rapidly growing organisms are more susceptible to drug action than those in the resting phase. "Persisters" are metabolically inactive organisms that survive long exposure to a drug but whose offspring are fully susceptible to the same drug. A specialized form of "persisters" might be L forms of bacteria. Under treatment with drugs that inhibit cell wall formation, cell-wall-deficient forms may develop in certain tissues possessing suitable osmotic properties (eg, medulla of kidney). These protoplasts could persist in tissues while the drug (eg, penicillin) was administered and might later revert to intact bacterial forms, causing relapse of disease.

ANTIMICROBIAL ACTIVITY IN VIVO

The problem of the activity of antimicrobial agents is much more complex in vivo than in vitro. It involves not only drug and parasite but also a third factor, the host. The interrelationships of host, drug, and parasite are diagrammed in Figure 10–1. Drug-parasite and host-parasite relationships are discussed in the following paragraphs. Host-drug relationships (absorption, excretion, distribution, metabolism, and toxicity) are dealt with mainly in pharmacology texts.

DRUG-PARASITE RELATIONSHIPS

Several important interactions between drug and parasite have been discussed in the preceding pages. The following are additional important in vivo factors.

Environment

The environment in the test tube is constant for all members of a microbial population. In the host, how-ever, varying environmental influences are brought to bear on microorganisms located in different tissues and in different parts of the body. Therefore, the response of the microbial population is much less uniform within the host than in the test tube.

A. State of Metabolic Activity: In the test tube, the state of metabolic activity is relatively uniform for the majority of microorganisms. In the body, it is diverse; undoubtedly, many organisms are at a low level of biosynthetic activity and are thus relatively insusceptible to drug action. These "dormant" microorganisms often survive exposure to high concentrations of drugs and subsequently may produce a clinical relapse of the infection. Alternatively, cell-wall-deficient forms may be insusceptible to drugs that inhibit cell wall formation.

B. Distribution of Drug: In the test tube, all microorganisms are equally exposed to the drug. In the body, the antimicrobial agent is unequally distributed in tissues and fluids. Many drugs do not reach the central nervous system effectively. The concentration in urine is often much greater than the concentration in blood or tissue. The tissue response induced by the microorganism may protect it from the drug. Necrotic tissue or pus may adsorb the drug and thus prevent its contact with bacteria.

C. Location of Organisms: In the test tube, the microorganisms come into direct contact with the drug. In the body, they may often be located within tissue cells. Drugs enter tissue cells at different rates. Some (eg, tetracyclines) reach about the same concentration inside monocytes as in the extracellular fluid. With others (eg, streptomycin), the intracellular concentration is only a small fraction (perhaps 5–10%) of the extracellular concentration.

D. Interfering Substances: In the test tube, drug activity may be impaired by binding of the drug to protein or to lipids or by interaction with salts. The biochemical environment of microorganisms in the body is very complex and results in significant interference with drug action. The drug may be bound by blood and tissue proteins or phospholipids; it may also react with nucleic acids in pus and may be physically adsorbed onto exudates, cells, and necrotic debris. In necrotic tissue, the pH may be highly acid and thus unfavorable for drug action (eg, aminoglycosides).

Concentration

In the test tube, microorganisms are exposed to an essentially constant concentration of drug. In the body, this is not so.

A. Absorption: The absorption of drugs from the intestinal tract (if taken by mouth) or from tissues (if injected) is irregular. There is also a continuous excretion as well as inactivation of the drug. Consequently, the available levels of drug in body compartments fluctuate continuously, and the microorganisms are exposed to varying concentrations of the antimicrobial agent.

B. Distribution: The distribution of drugs varies greatly with different tissues. Some drugs penetrate

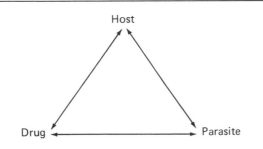

Figure 10–1. Interrelationships of host, drug, and parasite.

certain tissues poorly (eg, central nervous system, prostate). Drug concentrations following systemic administration may therefore be inadequate for effective treatment. In such situations, the drug may be administered locally (eg, injection of drugs into the central nervous system). On surface wounds or mucous membranes, local (topical) application of poorly absorbed drugs permits highly effective local concentrations without toxic side effects. Drug concentrations in urine are often much higher than in blood.

C. Variability of Concentration: The critical consideration in antimicrobial therapy is the necessity of maintaining an effective concentration of the drug in contact with microorganisms at their site of proliferation or establishment in the tissues for a sufficient length of time to cause eradication of infecting organisms. Because the drug is administered intermittently and is absorbed and excreted irregularly, the levels constantly fluctuate at the site of infection. In order to maintain sufficient drug concentrations for a sufficient time, the time-dose relationship has to be considered. The larger each individual drug dose, the longer the permissible interval between doses. The smaller the individual dose, the shorter the interval that will ensure adequate drug levels. A good general rule in antimicrobial therapy is as follows: Give a sufficiently large amount of an effective drug as early as possible and continue treatment long enough to ensure eradication of infection; but give an antimicrobial drug only when it is indicated by rational choice.

HOST-PARASITE RELATIONSHIPS

Host-parasite relationships may be altered by antimicrobial drugs in several ways.

Alteration of Tissue Response

The inflammatory response of the tissue to infections may be altered if the drug suppresses the multiplication of microorganisms but does not eliminate them from the body, and an acute process may in this way be transformed into a chronic one. Conversely, the suppression of inflammatory reactions in tissues by corticosteroids may reduce the effectiveness of bacteriostatic drugs. Anticancer drugs depress inflammatory reactions and immune responses and consequently cause enhanced susceptibility to infection and diminished response to antimicrobial drugs.

Alteration of Immune Response

If an infection is modified by an antimicrobial drug, the immune response of the host may also be altered. An example will suffice to illustrate this phenomenon:

Infection with β-hemolytic group A streptococci is followed frequently by the development of antistreptococcal antibodies and occasionally by rheumatic fever. If the infective process can be interrupted early and completely with antimicrobial drugs, the development of an immune response and of rheumatic fever can be prevented (presumably by rapid elimination of the antigen). Drugs and doses that rapidly eradicate the infecting streptococci (eg, penicillin) are more effective in preventing rheumatic fever than those that merely suppress the microorganisms temporarily (eg, tetracycline).

Alteration of Microbial Flora

Antimicrobial drugs affect not only the infecting microorganisms but also susceptible members of the normal microbial flora of the body. An imbalance is thus created that in itself may lead to disease. A few examples will serve:

(1) In hospitalized patients who receive antimicrobials, the normal microbial flora is suppressed. This creates a partial void that is filled by the organisms most prevalent in the environment, particularly drug-resistant gram-negative aerobic bacteria (eg, *Pseudomonas*), staphylococci, fungi, etc. Such superinfecting organisms subsequently may produce serious drug-resistant infections.

(2) In women taking tetracycline antibiotics by mouth, the normal vaginal flora may be suppressed, permitting marked overgrowth of *Candida*. This leads to unpleasant local inflammation (vaginitis) and itching that is difficult to control.

(3) In the presence of urinary tract obstruction, the tendency to bladder infection is great. When such urinary tract infection due to a sensitive microorganism (eg, *Escherichia coli*) is treated with an appropriate chemotherapeutic drug, the organism may be eradicated. However, very often a reinfection due to drug-resistant *Proteus, Pseudomonas,* or *Enterobacter* occurs after the drug-sensitive microorganisms are eliminated. A similar process accounts for respiratory tract superinfections in patients given antimicrobials for chronic bronchitis or bronchiectasis.

(4) In persons receiving antimicrobial drugs by mouth for several days, parts of the normal intestinal flora may be suppressed. Drug-resistant organisms may establish themselves in the bowel in great numbers and may precipitate serious enterocolitis (*Clostridium difficile,* staphylococci, etc).

CLINICAL USE OF ANTIBIOTICS

Selection of Antibiotics

The rational selection of antimicrobial drugs depends upon the following:

A. Diagnosis: A specific etiologic diagnosis must be formulated. This can often be done on the basis of a clinical impression. Thus, in typical lobar pneumonia or acute urinary tract infection, the relationship between clinical picture and causative agent is sufficiently constant to permit selection of the antibiotic of choice on the basis of clinical impression alone. Even in these cases, however, as a safeguard against diagnostic error, it is preferable to obtain a representative specimen for bacteriologic study before giving antimicrobial drugs.

In most infections, the relationship between causative agent and clinical picture is not constant. It is therefore important to obtain proper specimens for bacteriologic identification of the causative agent. As soon as such specimens have been secured, chemotherapy can be started on the basis of the "best guess." Once the causative agent has been identified by laboratory procedures, empiric chemotherapy can be modified as necessary.

The "best guess" of a causative organism is based on the following considerations, among others: (1) the site of infection (eg, pneumonia, urinary tract infection); (2) the age of the patient (eg, meningitis; neonatal, young child, adult); (3) the place where the infection was acquired (hospital, community); (4) mechanical predisposing factors (intravenous drip, urinary catheter, respirator, exposure to vector); and (5) predisposing host factors (immunodeficiency, corticosteroids, transplant, cancer chemotherapy, etc).

When the causative agent of a clinical infection is known, the drug of choice can often be selected on the basis of current clinical experience (Table 10–2). At other times, laboratory tests for antibiotic sensitivity (see below) are necessary to determine the drug of choice.

B. Sensitivity Tests: Laboratory tests for antibiotic sensitivity are indicated in the following circumstances: (1) when the microorganism recovered is of a type that is often resistant to antimicrobial drugs (eg, gram-negative enteric bacteria); (2) when an infectious process is likely to be fatal unless treated specifically (eg, meningitis, septicemia); (3) in certain infections where eradication of the infectious organisms requires the use of drugs that are rapidly bactericidal, not merely bacteriostatic (eg, infective endocarditis). The laboratory aspects of antibiotic sensitivity testing are discussed in Chapter 32.

C. Serum Assay of Bactericidal Activity: This test determines directly whether adequate amounts of the correct drugs are being administered to the patient from whom a causative organism has been isolated. Serum is obtained during therapy, diluted, inoculated with the organism previously isolated from the patient, and incubated. Subcultures at intervals must indicate bactericidal activity in significant serum dilutions (depending upon inoculum size and time after drug administration, usually at least 1:5) to suggest adequate therapy (see Chapter 32).

Dangers of Indiscriminate Use

(1) Widespread sensitization of the population, with resulting hypersensitivity, anaphylaxis, rashes, fever, blood disorders, cholestatic hepatitis, and perhaps connective tissue diseases.

(2) Changes in the normal flora of the body, with disease resulting from "superinfection" due to overgrowth of drug-resistant organisms.

(3) Masking serious infection without eradicating it. For example, the clinical manifestations of an abscess may be suppressed while the infectious process continues.

(4) Direct drug toxicity, particularly with prolonged use of certain agents. Important examples are aplastic anemia due to inappropriate use of chloramphenicol; renal damage or auditory nerve damage due to aminoglycoside antibiotics.

(5) Development of drug resistance in microbial populations, chiefly through the elimination of drug-sensitive microorganisms from antibiotic-saturated environments (eg, hospitals) and their replacement by drug-resistant microorganisms.

ANTIMICROBIAL DRUGS USED IN COMBINATION

Indications

Possible reasons for employing 2 or more antimicrobials simultaneously instead of a single drug are as follows:

(1) To give prompt treatment in desperately ill patients suspected of having a serious microbial infection. A good guess about the most probable 2 or 3 pathogens is made, and drugs are aimed at those organisms. Before such treatment is started, it is essential that adequate specimens be obtained for identifying the etiologic agent in the laboratory. Suspected gram-negative or staphylococcal sepsis in immunocompromised patients and bacterial meningitis in children are foremost indications in this category.

(2) To delay the emergence of microbial mutants resistant to one drug in chronic infections by the use of a second or third non-cross-reacting drug. The most prominent example is active tuberculosis of an organ, with large microbial populations.

(3) To treat mixed infections, particularly those following massive trauma or those involving vascular structures. Each drug is aimed at an important pathogenic microorganism.

(4) To achieve bactericidal synergism (see below). In a few infections, eg, enterococcal sepsis, a combination of drugs is more likely to eradicate the infection than either drug used alone. Unfortunately, such synergism is unpredictable, and a given drug pair may be synergistic for only a single microbial strain. Occasionally, simultaneous use of 2 drugs permits significant reduction in dose and thus avoids toxicity but still provides satisfactory antimicrobial action.

Disadvantages

The following disadvantages of using antimicrobial drugs in combinations must always be considered:

(1) The physician may feel that since several drugs are already being given, everything possible has been done for the patient. This attitude leads to relaxation of the effort to establish a specific diagnosis. It may also give a false sense of security.

(2) The more drugs that are administered, the greater the chance for drug reactions to occur or for the patient to become sensitized to drugs.

(3) The cost is unnecessarily high.

(4) Antimicrobial combinations usually accomplish no more than an effective single drug.

(5) Very rarely, one drug may antagonize a second drug given simultaneously (see below).

Mechanisms

When 2 antimicrobial agents act simultaneously on a homogeneous microbial population, the effect may be one of the following: (1) indifference, ie, the combined action is no greater than that of the more effective agent when used alone; (2) addition, ie, the combined action is equivalent to the sum of the actions of each drug when used alone; (3) synergism, ie, the combined action is significantly greater than the sum of both effects; (4) antagonism, ie, the combined action is less than that of the more effective agent when used alone. All these effects may be observed in vitro (particularly in terms of bactericidal rate) and in vivo.

Antagonism is sharply limited by time-dose relationships and is therefore a rare event in clinical antimicrobial therapy. Antagonism resulting in higher morbidity and mortality rates has been most clearly demonstrated in bacterial meningitis. It occurred when a bacteriostatic drug (which inhibited protein synthesis in bacteria) such as chloramphenicol or tetracycline was given with a bactericidal drug such as a penicillin or an aminoglycoside. Antagonism occurred mainly if the bacteriostatic drug reached the site of infection before the bactericidal drug, if the killing of bacteria was essential for cure, and if only minimal effective doses of either drug in the pair were present. Antagonism can be overcome by large excess amounts of one or both drugs in the pair—a common event clinically—and it very rarely affects the outcome of clinical therapy.

Synergism

Antimicrobial synergism can occur in several types of situations. Synergistic drug combinations must be selected by complex laboratory procedures.

(1) Two drugs may sequentially block a microbial metabolic pathway. Sulfonamides inhibit the use of extracellular p-aminobenzoic acid by some microbes for the synthesis of folic acid. Trimethoprim or pyrimethamine inhibits the next metabolic step, the reduction of dihydro- to tetrahydrofolic acid. The simultaneous use of a sulfonamide plus trimethoprim is effective in some bacterial infections (*Shigella, Salmonella, Serratia*) and in some other parasitic infections (*Pneumocystis carinii,* malaria). Pyrimethamine plus a sulfonamide is used in toxoplasmosis.

(2) One drug may greatly enhance the uptake of a second drug and thereby greatly increase the overall bactericidal effect. Penicillins enhance the uptake of aminoglycosides by enterococci. Thus, a penicillin plus an aminoglycoside may be essential for the eradication of *Streptococcus faecalis* or *Streptococcus* group B infections, particularly sepsis or endocarditis. Similarly, ticarcillin plus gentamicin may be synergistic against some strains of *Pseudomonas*. Cell wall inhibitors (penicillins and cephalosporins) may enhance

the entry of aminoglycosides into other gram-negative bacteria and thus produce synergistic effects.

(3) One drug may affect the cell membrane and facilitate the entry of the second drug. The combined effect may then be greater than the sum of its parts. Polymyxins have been synergistic with trimethoprim-sulfamethoxazole or rifampin against *Serratia,* and amphotericin has been synergistic with flucytosine against certain fungi, eg, *Cryptococcus, Candida*.

(4) One drug may prevent the inactivation of a second drug by microbial enzymes. Thus, inhibitors of β-lactamase (eg, clavulanic acid) can protect amoxicillin from inactivation by β-lactamase-producing *H influenzae* and other β-lactamase-producing organisms. In such circumstances, a form of synergism takes place.

The effects that can be achieved with combinations of antimicrobial drugs vary with different combinations and are specific for each strain of microorganism. Thus, no combination is uniformly synergistic. Combined effects cannot be predicted from the behavior of the microorganism toward single drugs.

Combined therapy should not be used indiscriminately; every effort should be made to employ the single antibiotic of choice. In resistant infections, detailed laboratory study can at times define synergistic drug combinations that may be essential to eradicate the microorganisms.

ANTIMICROBIAL CHEMOPROPHYLAXIS

Anti-infective chemoprophylaxis implies the administration of antimicrobial drugs to prevent infection. In a broader sense, it also includes the use of antimicrobial drugs soon after the acquisition of pathogenic microorganisms (eg, after compound fracture) but before the development of signs of infection.

Useful chemoprophylaxis is limited to the action of a specific drug on a specific organism. An effort to prevent all types of microorganisms in the environment from establishing themselves only selects the most drug-resistant organisms as the cause of a subsequent infection. In all proposed uses of prophylactic antimicrobials, the risk of the patient's acquiring an infection must be weighed against the toxicity, cost, inconvenience, and enhanced risk of superinfection resulting from the "prophylactic" drug.

Prophylaxis in Persons of Normal Susceptibility Exposed to a Specific Pathogen

In this category, a specific drug is administered to prevent one specific infection. Outstanding examples are the injection of benzathine penicillin G, 1.2 million units intramuscularly once every 3–4 weeks, to prevent reinfection with group A hemolytic streptococci in rheumatic patients; prevention of meningitis by eradicating the meningococcal carrier state with rifampin, 600 mg orally twice daily for 2 days, or minocycline, 100 mg every 12 hours for 5 days; prevention of syphilis by the injection of benzathine penicillin G, 2.4 million units intramuscularly, within 24 hours of exposure; prevention of plague pneumonia in those exposed to infectious droplets by administration of tetracycline, 0.5 g twice daily for 5 days; and prevention of clinical rickettsial disease (but not of infection) by the daily ingestion of 1 g of tetracycline during exposure.

Early treatment of an asymptomatic infection is sometimes called "prophylaxis." Thus, administration of isoniazid, 6–10 mg/kg/d (maximum, 300 mg daily) orally for 6–12 months, to an asymptomatic person who converts from a negative to a positive tuberculin skin test may prevent later clinically active tuberculosis.

Prophylaxis in Persons of Increased Susceptibility

Certain anatomic or functional abnormalities predispose to serious infections. It may be feasible to prevent or abort such infections by giving a specific drug for short periods. Some important examples are listed below:

A. Heart Disease: Persons with heart valve abnormalities or with prosthetic heart valves are unusually susceptible to implantation of microorganisms circulating in the bloodstream. This bacterial endocarditis can sometimes be prevented if the proper drug can be used during periods of bacteremia. Large numbers of viridans streptococci are pushed into the circulation during dental procedures and operations on the mouth or throat. At such times, the increased risk warrants the use of a prophylactic antimicrobial drug aimed at viridans streptococci, eg, procaine penicillin G, 600,000 units injected intramuscularly 1–2 hours before the procedure and once daily for 2 days thereafter. In addition, 600,000 units of aqueous penicillin G is injected intramuscularly just prior to the procedure. It may be that an aminoglycoside should be given together with penicillin for optimal bactericidal effect. Alternatively, penicillin V, 2 g orally, can be given before the procedure, followed by 500 mg every 6 hours for 8 doses afterward. In persons hypersensitive to penicillin or those receiving daily doses of penicillin for prolonged periods (for rheumatic fever prophylaxis), erythromycin, 2 g daily orally, can be substituted to cover penicillin-resistant viridans streptococci in the throat.

Enterococci cause 5–15% of cases of bacterial endocarditis. They reach the bloodstream from the urinary or gastrointestinal tract or from the female genital tract. During surgical procedures in these areas, persons with heart valve abnormalities can be given prophylaxis directed against enterococci, eg, penicillin G, 5 million units, plus gentamicin, 3 mg/kg intramuscularly daily, beginning on the day of surgery and continuing for 2 days.

During and after cardiac catheterization, blood cultures may be positive in 10–20% of patients. Many of these persons also have fever, but very few acquire en-

docarditis. Prophylactic antimicrobials do not appear to influence these events.

B. Respiratory Tract Disease: Persons with functional and anatomic abnormalities of the respiratory tract—eg, emphysema or bronchiectasis—are subject to attacks of "recurrent chronic bronchitis." This is a recurrent bacterial infection, often precipitated by acute viral infections and resulting in respiratory decompensation. The most common organisms are pneumococci and *H influenzae*. Chemoprophylaxis consists of giving tetracycline or ampicillin, 1 g daily orally, during the "respiratory disease season." This is successful only in patients who are not hospitalized; otherwise, superinfection with *Pseudomonas, Proteus,* or yeasts is common. Simple prophylaxis of bacterial infection has been applied to children with mucoviscidosis who are not hospitalized. In spite of this, such children contract complicating infections caused by *Pseudomonas* and staphylococci. Trimethoprim-sulfamethoxazole is effective as a prophylactic against *P carinii* pneumonia in immunocompromised persons.

C. Recurrent Urinary Tract Infection: In certain women who are subject to frequently recurring urinary tract infections, the daily oral intake of nitrofurantoin, 200 mg, or trimethoprim (40 mg)-sulfamethoxazole (200 mg) can markedly reduce the frequency of symptomatic recurrences over periods of many months—perhaps years—until resistant microorganisms appear.

Certain women frequently develop symptoms of cystitis after sexual intercourse. The ingestion of a single dose of antimicrobial drug (nitrofurantoin, 200 mg; cephalexin, 250 mg; etc) can prevent this postcoital cystitis by early inhibition of growth of bacteria moved into the proximal urethra or bladder from the introitus during intercourse.

D. Opportunistic Infections in Severe Granulocytopenia: Patients with leukemia or neoplasm develop profound leukopenia while being given anticancer chemotherapy. When the neutrophil count falls below 1000/μL, they become unusually susceptible to opportunistic infections, most often gram-negative sepsis. In some cancer centers, such individuals are given a drug combination (eg, vancomycin, gentamicin, cephalosporin) directed at the most prevalent opportunists at the earliest sign—or even without clinical evidence—of infection. This is continued for several days until the granulocyte count rises again. Retrospective studies suggest that there is some benefit to this procedure.

In other centers, such patients are given oral insoluble antimicrobials (neomycin + polymyxin + nystatin) during the period of granulopenia to reduce the incidence of gram-negative sepsis. Some benefit has been reported from this approach.

Prophylaxis in Surgery

A major portion of all antimicrobial drugs used in hospitals is employed on surgical services with the stated intent of "prophylaxis." The administration of antimicrobials before and after surgical procedures is sometimes viewed as "banning the microbial world" both from the site of the operation and from other organ systems that suffer postoperative complications. Regrettably, the provable benefit of antimicrobial prophylaxis in surgery is much more limited.

Several general features of "surgical prophylaxis" merit consideration:

(1) In clean elective surgical procedures (ie, procedures during which no tissue bearing normal flora is traversed, other than the prepared skin), the disadvantages of "routine" antibiotic prophylaxis (allergy, toxicity, superinfection) generally outweigh the possible benefits.

(2) Prophylactic administration of antibiotics should generally be considered only if the expected rate of infectious complications approaches or exceeds 5%. An exception to this rule is the elective insertion of prostheses (cardiovascular, orthopedic), where a possible infection would have a catastrophic effect.

(3) If prophylactic antimicrobials are to be effective, a sufficient concentration of a drug must be present at the operative site to inhibit or kill bacteria that might settle there. Thus, it is essential that drug administration begin 1–3 hours before operation.

(4) Prolonged administration of antimicrobial drugs tends to alter the normal flora of organ systems, suppressing the susceptible microorganisms and favoring the implantation of drug-resistant ones. Thus, antimicrobial prophylaxis should last only 1–3 days after the procedure to prevent superinfection.

(5) Systemic levels of antimicrobial drugs usually do not prevent wound infection, pneumonia, or urinary tract infection if physiologic abnormalities or foreign bodies are present.

In major surgical procedures, the administration of a "broad-spectrum" bactericidal drug from just before until 1 day after the procedure has been found effective. Thus, cefazolin, 1 g given intramuscularly or intravenously 2 hours before gastrointestinal, pelvic, or orthopedic procedures and again at 2, 10, and 18 hours after the end of the operation, results in a demonstrable lowering of the risk of deep infection at the operative site. Similarly, in cardiovascular surgery, antimicrobials directed at the commonest organisms producing infection are begun just prior to the procedure and continued for 2 or 3 days thereafter. While this prevents drug-susceptible organisms from producing endocarditis, pericarditis, or similar complications, it may favor the implantation of drug-resistant bacteria or fungi.

Other forms of surgical prophylaxis attempt to reduce normal flora or existing bacterial contamination at the site. Thus, the colon is routinely prepared not only by mechanical cleansing through cathartics and enemas but also by the oral administration of insoluble drugs (eg, neomycin, 1 g, plus erythromycin, 1 g, every 6 hours) for 1 day before operation. In the case of a perforated viscus resulting in peritoneal contamination, there is little doubt that immediate treatment with an aminoglycoside, a penicillin, or clindamycin re-

duces the impact of seeded infection. Similarly, grossly infected compound fractures or war wounds benefit from a penicillin or cephalosporin plus an aminoglycoside. In all these instances, the antimicrobials tend to reduce the likelihood of rapid and early invasion of the bloodstream and tend to help localize the infectious process—although they generally are incapable of preventing it altogether. The surgeon must be watchful for the selection of the most resistant members of the flora, which tend to manifest themselves 2 or 3 days after the beginning of such "prophylaxis"—which is really an attempt at very early treatment.

In all situations where antimicrobials are administered with the hope that they may have a "prophylactic" effect, the risk from these same drugs (allergy, toxicity, selection of superinfecting microorganisms) must be evaluated daily, and the course of prophylaxis must be kept as brief as possible.

Topical antimicrobials (intravenous tube site, catheter, closed urinary drainage, within a surgical wound, acrylic bone cement, etc) may have limited usefulness but must always be scrutinized with suspicion.

DISINFECTANTS

Disinfectants and antiseptics differ from systemically active antimicrobials in that they possess little selective toxicity: they are toxic not only for microbial parasites but for host cells as well. Therefore, they can be used only to inactivate microorganisms in the inanimate environment or, to a limited extent, on skin surfaces; but they cannot be administered systemically and are not active in tissues.

The antimicrobial action of disinfectants is determined by concentration, time, and temperature; and the evaluation of their effect may be complex. The known modes of action of several classes of chemical disinfectants are described in chapter 5. A few examples of disinfectants that are used in medicine or public health are listed in Table 10–1.

ANTIMICROBIAL DRUGS FOR SYSTEMIC ADMINISTRATION

PENICILLINS

The penicillins are derived from molds of the genus *Penicillium* (eg, *Penicillium notatum*) and obtained by extraction of submerged cultures grown in special media. The most widely used natural penicillin at present is penicillin G. From fermentation brews of *Penicillium,* 6-aminopenicillanic acid has been isolated on a large scale. This makes it possible to synthesize an almost unlimited variety of penicillinlike compounds by

Table 10–1. Practical chemical disinfectants.

Disinfection of inanimate environment

Table tops, instruments	5% Lysol or other phenolic compound 1–10% formaldehyde 2% aqueous glutaraldehyde 0.1% mercury bichloride Quaternary ammonium compounds (0.1%)
Excreta, bandages, bedpans	1% sodium hypochlorite 5% Lysol or other phenolic compound
Air	Propylene glycol mist or aerosol Formaldehyde vapor
Heat-sensitive instruments	Ethylene oxide gas (Alkylates nucleic acids. Residual gas must be removed by aeration.)

Disinfection of skin or wounds

	Washing with soap and water Soaps or detergents containing 2% hexachlorophene or 1.5% trichlorocarbanilide or chlorhexidine 2% tincture of iodine 70% ethyl alcohol; 70–90% isopropyl alcohol Povidone-iodine (water-soluble) Nitrofurazone, 0.2% jelly or solution

Topical application of drugs to skin or mucous membranes

In candidiasis	Gentian violet, 1:2000 Nystatin cream, 100,000 units/g Candicidin ointment, 0.6 mg/g Miconazole, 2% cream
In burns	Silver nitrate, 0.5% Mafenide acetate cream Silver sulfadiazine
In dermatophytosis	Undecylenic acid powder or 5–10% cream Tolnaftate cream, 1%
In pyoderma	Ammoniated mercury, 2–5% ointment Bacitracin-neomycin-polymyxin ointment Potassium permanganate, 0.01%

Topical application of drugs to eyes

For gonorrhea prophylaxis	1% silver nitrate
For bacterial conjunctivitis	Sulfacetamide ointment Chloramphenicol ointment

coupling the free amino group of the penicillanic acid to free carboxyl groups of different radicals.

All penicillins share the same basic structure (see 6-aminopenicillanic acid in Fig 10–2). A thiazolidine ring (a) is attached to a β-lactam ring (b) that carries a free amino group (c). The acidic radicals attached to the amino group can be split off by bacterial and other amidases. The structural integrity of the 6-aminopenicillanic acid nucleus is essential to the biologic activity of the compounds. If the β-lactam ring is enzymatically cleaved by β-lactamases (penicillinases), the resulting product, penicilloic acid, is devoid of antibacterial activity. However, it carries an antigenic determinant of the penicillins and acts as a sensitizing hapten when attached to carrier proteins.

The different radicals (R) attached to the aminopenicillanic acid determine the essential pharmacologic properties of the resulting drugs. The clinically important penicillins in 1986 fall into 4 principal

groups: (1) Highest activity against gram-positive organisms, spirochetes, and some others but susceptible to hydrolysis by β-lactamases and acid-labile (eg, penicillin G). (2) Relatively resistant to β-lactamases but lower activity against gram-positive organisms and inactive against gram-negatives (eg, nafcillin). (3) Relatively high activity against both gram-positive and gram-negative organisms but destroyed by β-lactamases (eg, ampicillin, carbenicillin, ticarcillin). (4) Relatively stable to gastric acid and suitable for oral administration (eg, penicillin V, cloxacillin, amoxicillin). Some representatives are shown in Fig 10–2. Most penicillins are dispensed as sodium or potassium salts of the free acid. Potassium penicillin G contains about 1.7 meq of K^+ per million units (2.8 meq/g). Procaine salts and benzathine salts of penicillin provide repository forms for intramuscular injection. In dry form, penicillins are stable, but solutions rapidly lose their activity and must be prepared fresh for administration.

Antimicrobial Activity

The initial step in penicillin action is binding of the drug to cell receptors. These receptors are penicillin-binding proteins (PBPs), and at least some of them are enzymes involved in transpeptidation reactions. From 3 to 6 (or more) PBPs per cell can be present. After penicillin molecules have attached to the receptors, peptidoglycan synthesis is inhibited as final transpeptidation is blocked. A final bactericidal event is the removal or inactivation of an inhibitor of autolytic enzymes in the cell wall. This activates the autolytic enzymes and results in cell lysis. Organisms with defective autolysin function are inhibited but not killed by β-lactam drugs, and they are said to be "tolerant."

Since active cell wall synthesis is required for penicillin action, metabolically inactive microorganisms, L forms, or mycoplasmas are insusceptible to such drugs.

Penicillin G and penicillin V are often measured in units (1 million = 0.6 g), but the semisynthetic penicillins are measured in grams. Whereas 0.002–1 μg/mL of penicillin G is lethal for a majority of susceptible gram-positive organisms, 10–100 times more is required to kill gram-negative bacteria (except neisseriae). The activity of penicillins also varies with the degree to which they are bound to serum proteins, which ranges from 40% to more than 95% for different drugs.

Resistance

Resistance to penicillins falls into several categories: (1) Production of β-lactamases by staphylococci, gram-negative bacteria, *Haemophilus,* gonococci, and others. More than 50 different β-lactamases are known, most of them produced under the control of bacterial plasmids. Some β-lactamases are inducible by the newer cephalosporins. (2) Lack of penicillin receptors (PBPs) or inaccessibility of receptors because of permeability barriers of bacterial outer membranes. These are often under chromosomal con-

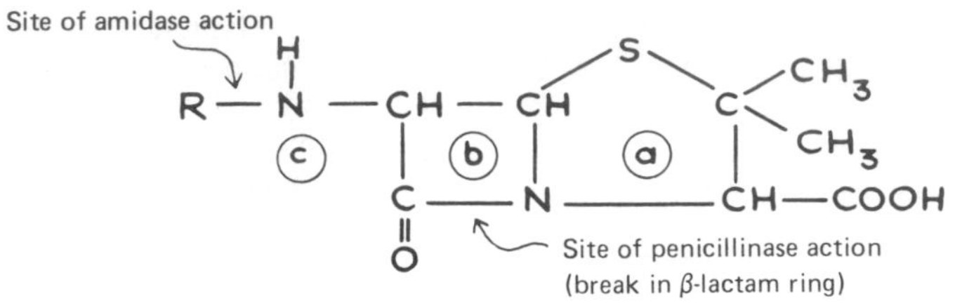

6-Aminopenicillanic acid

The following structures can each be substituted at the R to produce a new penicillin.

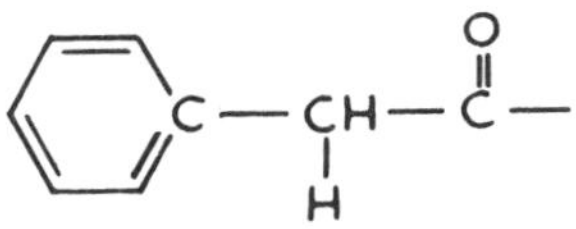

Penicillin G (benzylpenicillin):
High activity against gram-positive bacteria. Low activity against gram-negative bacteria. Acid-labile. Destroyed by β-lactamase; 60% protein-bound.

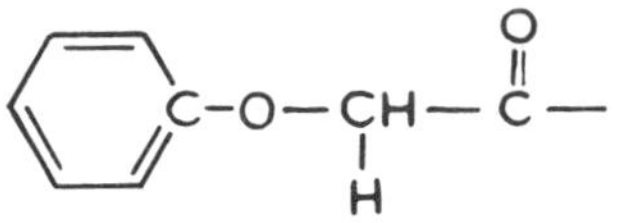

Penicillin V (phenoxymethyl penicillin):
Similar to penicillin G, but relatively acid-resistant.

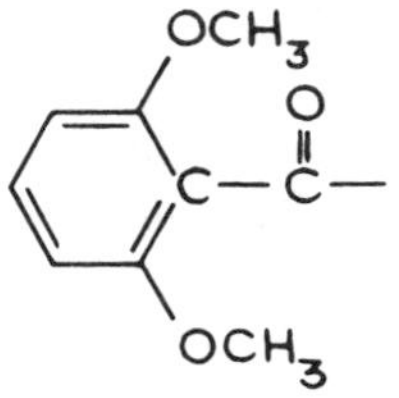

Methicillin (dimethoxyphenylpenicillin):
Lower activity than penicillin G but resistant to penicillinase. Acid-labile. 40% protein-bound.

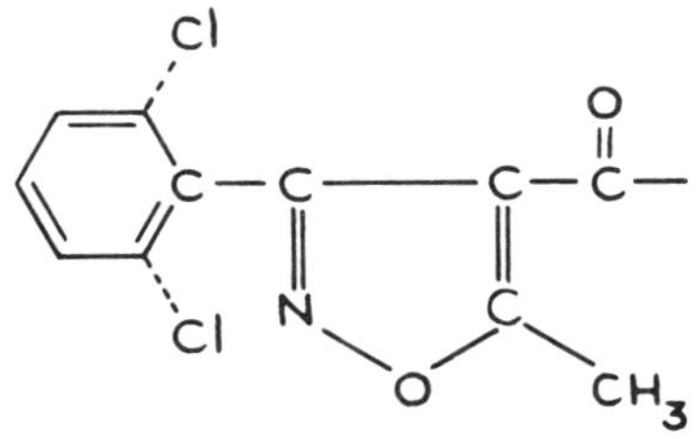

Oxacillin; cloxacillin (one Cl in structure); dicloxacillin (2 Cls in structure); flucloxacillin (one Cl and one F in structure) (isoxazolyl penicillins): Similar to methicillin in penicillinase resistance, but acid-stable. Highly protein-bound (95–98%).

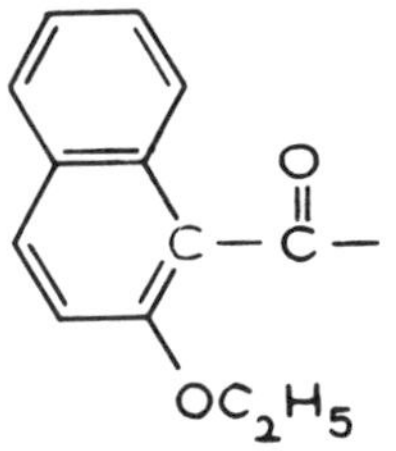

Nafcillin (ethoxynaphthamidopenicillin):
Similar to isoxazolyl penicillins; less strongly protein-bound (90%); less nephrotoxic than methicillin.

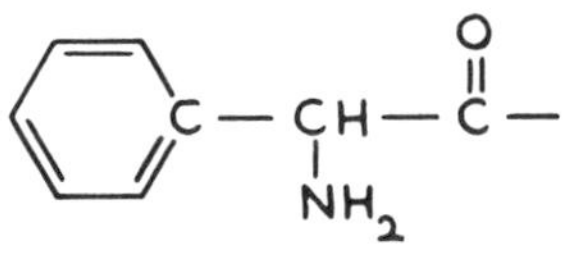

Ampicillin (alpha-aminobenzylpenicillin):
Similar to penicillin G (destroyed by β-lactamase), but acid-stable and more active against gram-negative bacteria. Carbenicillin has —COONa instead of the —NH₂ group.

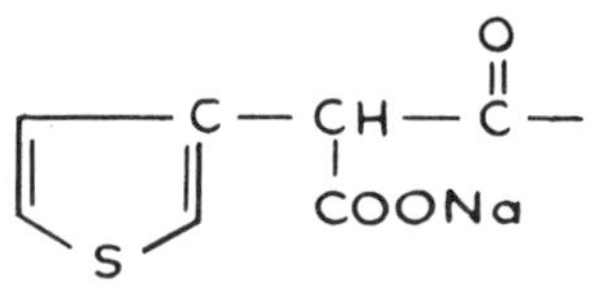

Ticarcillin:
Similar to carbenicillin but gives higher blood levels. Piperacillin, azlocillin, and mezlocillin resemble ticarcillin in action against gram-negative aerobic rods.

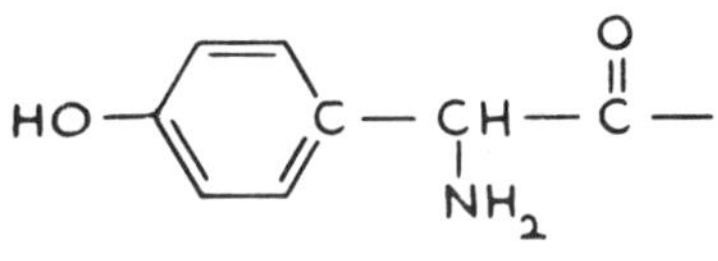

Amoxicillin:
Similar to ampicillin but better absorbed; gives higher blood levels.

Figure 10–2. Structures of some penicillins.

trol. (3) Failure of activation of autolytic enzymes in cell wall can result in inhibition without killing bacteria, eg, "tolerance" of some staphylococci. (4) Failure to synthesize peptidoglycans, eg, in mycoplasmas, L forms, or metabolically inactive bacteria.

Absorption, Distribution, & Excretion

After intramuscular or intravenous administration, absorption of most penicillins is rapid and complete. After oral administration, only 5–30% of the dose is absorbed, depending on acid stability, binding to foods, presence of buffers, etc. After absorption, penicillins are widely distributed in tissues and body fluids. Protein binding is 40–60% for penicillin G, ampicillin, and methicillin; 90% for nafcillin; and 95–98% for oxacillin and dicloxacillin. For most rapidly absorbed penicillins, a parenteral dose of 3–6 g/24 h yields serum levels of approximately 1–6 μg/mL.

Special dosage forms have been designed for delayed absorption to yield drug levels for long periods. After a single intramuscular dose of benzathine penicillin, 1.5 g (2.4 million units), serum levels of 0.03 unit/mL are maintained for 10 days and levels of 0.005 unit/mL for 3 weeks. Procaine penicillin given intramuscularly yields therapeutic levels for 24 hours.

In many tissues, penicillin concentrations are similar to those in serum. Lower levels occur in eyes, the prostate, and the central nervous system. However, in meningitis, penetration is enhanced, and levels of 0.2 μg/mL occur in the cerebrospinal fluid with a daily parenteral dose of 12 g. Thus, meningococcal and pneumococcal meningitis are treated with systemic penicillin, and intrathecal injection has been abandoned.

Most of the absorbed penicillin is rapidly excreted by the kidneys. About 10% of renal excretion is by glomerular filtration and 90% by tubular secretion. The latter can be partially blocked by probenecid to achieve higher systemic and cerebrospinal fluid levels. In the newborn and in persons with renal failure, penicillin excretion is reduced and systemic levels remain elevated longer.

Clinical Uses

Penicillins are the most widely used antibiotics, particularly in the following areas.

Penicillin G is the drug of choice in infections caused by streptococci, pneumococci, meningococci, spirochetes, clostridia, aerobic gram-positive rods, nonpenicillinase-producing staphylococci and gonococci, *Actinomyces,* and *Bacteroides* (except *Bacteroides fragilis*). Most of these infections respond to daily doses of penicillin G, 0.4–4 g, often given by intermittent intramuscular injection. Much larger amounts (6–50 g/d) are given by intermittent addition (every 2–6 hours) to an intravenous infusion in serious or complicated infections due to susceptible organisms. Sites for such intravenous infusions are subject to thrombophlebitis and superinfection; they must be kept scrupulously clean and changed every 2–3 days.

Oral administration of penicillin V in daily doses of 1–4 g is indicated in minor infections. Oral administration is subject to so many variables that it should not be relied upon in seriously ill patients unless serum levels are monitored.

Penicillin G is inhibitory for enterococci *(S faecalis)*, but for bactericidal effects (eg, in enterococcal endocarditis), an aminoglycoside must be added. Penicillin G in ordinary doses is excreted into the urine in sufficiently high concentrations to inhibit some gram-negative organisms in urinary tract infections, particularly *Proteus mirabilis*. However, this treatment fails in the presence of large numbers of β-lactamase-producing bacteria in urine.

Benzathine penicillin G is a salt of very low solubility given intramuscularly for low but prolonged drug levels. A single injection of 1.2 million units (0.7 g) is satisfactory treatment for group A streptococcal pharyngitis. The same injection once every 3–4 weeks is satisfactory prophylaxis against group A streptococcal reinfection in rheumatic patients. A dose of 2.4 million units 1–3 times at weekly intervals is effective in early syphilis.

Infection with β-lactamase-producing staphylococci is the only indication for the use of lactamase-resistant penicillins, eg, nafcillin or oxacillin (6–12 g intravenously for adults, 50–100 mg/kg/d intravenously for children); cloxacillin or nafcillin, 2–6 g/d by mouth, can be given for milder staphylococcal infections. Staphylococci resistant to methicillin and nafcillin probably lack drug receptors.

Ampicillin, 2–3 g/d, can be given orally for treatment of some urinary tract infections with coliforms. In larger doses, ampicillin suppresses *Salmonella* enteric fevers. For bacterial meningitis in small children, ampicillin, 300 mg/kg/d intravenously, is a present choice, but the increase in lactamase-producing *H influenzae* necessitates the concomitant initial administration of chloramphenicol. Moxalactam (see p 148) is an alternative drug. Oral amoxicillin is better absorbed than ampicillin and yields higher levels. Amoxicillin given together with clavulanic acid may control lactamase-producing *H influenzae* (see p 131). Carbenicillin resembles ampicillin but is more active against *Pseudomonas* and *Proteus*. Up to 30 g intravenously is given daily, usually in conjunction with gentamicin, 5 mg/kg/d. Ticarcillin is more active than carbenicillin, and the daily dose is therefore 12–16 g/d. Piperacillin, mezlocillin, and azlocillin are somewhat more effective against aerobic gram-negative rods, especially *Pseudomonas*.

Side Effects

Penicillins possess less direct toxicity than any of the other antimicrobial drugs. Most serious side effects are due to hypersensitivity.

A. Toxicity: Very high doses (more than 30 g/d intravenously) may produce central nervous system concentrations that are irritating. In patients with renal failure, smaller doses may produce encephalopathy, delirium, and convulsions. With such doses, direct

Table 10–2. Drug selection, 1985–1986.

Suspected or Proved Etiologic Agent	Drug(s) of First Choice	Alternative Drug(s)
Gram-negative cocci		
Gonococcus	Penicillin,[1] ampicillin, tetracycline[2]	Spectinomycin, cefoxitin
Meningococcus	Penicillin[1]	Chloramphenicol, sulfonamide[7]
Gram-positive cocci		
Pneumococcus (Streptococcus pneumoniae)	Penicillin[1]	Erythromycin,[3] cephalosporin[4]
Streptococcus, hemolytic groups A, B, C, G	Penicillin[1]	Erythromycin,[3] cephalosporin[4]
Streptococcus viridans	Penicillin[1] + aminoglycoside(?)[5]	Cephalosporin,[4] vancomycin
Staphylococcus, nonpenicillinase-producing	Penicillin[1]	Cephalosporin,[4] vancomycin
Staphylococcus, penicillinase-producing	Penicillinase-resistant penicillin[6]	Vancomycin, cephalosporin[4]
Streptococcus faecalis (enterococcus)	Ampicillin + aminoglycoside[5]	Vancomycin
Gram-negative rods		
Acinetobacter (Mima-Herellea)	Aminoglycoside[5]	Minocycline
Bacteroides (except B fragilis)	Penicillin,[1] chloramphenicol	Clindamycin, cephalosporin[4]
Bacteroides fragilis	Metronidazole, clindamycin	Cefoxitin, chloramphenicol
Brucella	Tetracycline[2] + streptomycin	Streptomycin + sulfonamide[7]
Enterobacter	Aminoglycoside,[5] new cephalosporin[8]	Chloramphenicol
Escherichia		
Escherichia coli sepsis	Aminoglycoside[5]	New cephalosporin,[8] ampicillin
Escherichia coli urinary infection (first attack)	Sulfonamide,[9] TMP-SMX[10]	Ampicillin, cephalosporin[4]
Haemophilus (meningitis, respiratory infections)	Chloramphenicol + ampicillin	New cephalosporin[8]
Klebsiella	New cephalosporin,[8] aminoglycoside[5]	Chloramphenicol
Legionella pneumophila (pneumonia)	Erythromycin[3]	Tetracycline,[2] rifampin
Pasteurella (Yersinia) (plague, tularemia)	Streptomycin, tetracycline[2]	Sulfonamide,[7] chloramphenicol
Proteus		
Proteus mirabilis	Ampicillin	New cephalosporin,[8] aminoglycoside[5]
Proteus vulgaris and other species	Aminoglycoside[5]	Chloramphenicol
Pseudomonas		
Pseudomonas aeruginosa	Aminoglycoside[5] + ticarcillin, piperacillin, or azlocillin	New cephalosporin,[8] polymyxin
Pseudomonas pseudomallei (melioidosis)	Tetracycline,[2] TMP-SMX[10]	Chloramphenicol
Pseudomonas mallei (glanders)	Streptomycin + tetracycline[2]	Chloramphenicol
Salmonella	Chloramphenicol, ampicillin	TMP-SMX[10]
Serratia, Providencia	Aminoglycoside[5]	TMP-SMX[10] + polymyxin
Shigella	TMP-SMX,[10] chloramphenicol	Ampicillin, tetracycline[2]
Vibrio (cholera, others)	Tetracycline[2]	TMP-SMX[10]
Gram-positive rods		
Actinomyces	Penicillin[1]	Tetracycline[2]
Bacillus (eg, anthrax)	Penicillin[1]	Erythromycin[3]
Clostridium (eg, gas gangrene, tetanus)	Penicillin[1]	Metronidazole, cephalosporin[4]
Corynebacterium	Erythromycin[3]	Penicillin,[1] cephalosporin[4]
Listeria	Ampicillin + aminoglycoside[5]	Tetracycline[2]

[1]Penicillin G is preferred for parenteral injection; penicillin V for oral administration. Only highly sensitive microorganisms should be treated with oral penicillin.

[2]All tetracyclines have similar activity against microorganisms and comparable therapeutic activity and toxicity. Dosage is determined by the rates of absorption and excretion of different preparations.

[3]Erythromycin estolate is the best-absorbed oral form but carries greatest risk of hepatitis. Also erythromycin stearate, erythromycin ethylsuccinate.

[4]Cefazolin, cephapirin, cephalothin, cefamandole, and cefoxitin are older parenteral cephalosporins; cephalexin and cephradine the best oral forms.

[5]Aminoglycoside: Gentamicin, tobramycin, amikacin, netilmicin, selected by local pattern of susceptibility.

[6]Parenteral nafcillin or oxacillin. Oral dicloxacillin, cloxacillin, or oxacillin.

[7]Trisulfapyrimidines and sulfisoxazole have the advantage of greater solubility in urine over sulfadiazine for oral administration; sodium sulfadiazine is suitable for intravenous injection in severely ill persons.

[8]New cephalosporins (1985–1986): Cefotaxime, moxalactam, cefoperazone, cefuroxime, ceftizoxime, etc.

[9]For previously untreated urinary tract infection, a highly soluble sulfonamide such as sulfisoxazole or trisulfapyrimidines is the first choice. TMP-SMX[10] is acceptable.

[10]TMP-SMX is a mixture of 1 part trimethoprim + 5 parts sulfamethoxazole.

[11]Either or both.

Table 10–2. (cont'd). Drug selection, 1985–1986.

Suspected or Proved Etiologic Agent	Drug(s) of First Choice	Alternative Drug(s)
Acid-fast rods		
Mycobacterium tuberculosis	INH + rifampin, INH + ethambutol[11]	Other antituberculosis drugs
Mycobacterium leprae	Dapsone + rifampin, clofazimine	Amithiozone
Mycobacteria, atypical	Rifampin + ethambutol + INH	Combinations
Nocardia	Sulfonamide[7]	Minocycline
Spirochetes		
Borrelia (relapsing fever)	Tetracycline[2]	Penicillin[1]
Leptospira	Penicillin[1]	Tetracycline[2]
Treponema (syphilis, yaws)	Penicillin[1]	Erythromycin,[3] tetracycline[2]
Mycoplasma	Tetracycline[2]	Erythromycin[3]
Chlamydia trachomatis, Chlamydia psittaci	Tetracycline[2]	Erythromycin[3]
Rickettsiae	Tetracycline[2]	Chloramphenicol

[1]Penicillin G is preferred for parenteral injection; penicillin V for oral administration. Only highly sensitive microorganisms should be treated with oral penicillin.

[2]All tetracyclines have similar activity against microorganisms and comparable therapeutic activity and toxicity. Dosage is determined by the rates of absorption and excretion of different preparations.

[3]Erythromycin estolate is the best-absorbed oral form but carries greatest risk of hepatitis. Also erythromycin stearate, erythromycin ethylsuccinate.

[4]Cefazolin, cephapirin, cephalothin, cefamandole, and cefoxitin are older parenteral cephalosporins; cephalexin and cephradine the best oral forms.

[5]Aminoglycoside: Gentamicin, tobramycin, amikacin, netilmicin, selected by local pattern of susceptibility.

[6]Parenteral nafcillin or oxacillin. Oral dicloxacillin, cloxacillin, or oxacillin.

[7]Trisulfapyrimidines and sulfisoxazole have the advantage of greater solubility in urine over sulfadiazine for oral administration; sodium sulfadiazine is suitable for intravenous injection in severely ill persons.

[8]New cephalosporins (1985–1986): Cefotaxime, moxalactam, cefoperazone, cefuroxime, ceftizoxime, etc.

[9]For previously untreated urinary tract infection, a highly soluble sulfonamide such as sulfisoxazole or trisulfapyrimidines is the first choice. TMP-SMX[10] is acceptable.

[10]TMP-SMX is a mixture of 1 part trimethoprim + 5 parts sulfamethoxazole.

[11]Either or both.

cation toxicity (K^+) may also occur. Lactamase-resistant penicillins occasionally cause granulocytopenia. Oral penicillins can cause diarrhea. Carbenicillin may cause a bleeding tendency.

B. Allergy: All penicillins are cross-sensitizing and cross-reacting. Any material (including milk, cosmetics) containing penicillin may induce sensitization. The responsible antigens are degradation products, eg, penicilloic acid, bound to host protein. Skin tests with penicilloyl-polylysine, with alkaline hydrolysis products, and with undegraded penicillin identify many hypersensitive persons. Among positive reactors to skin tests, the incidence of major immediate allergic reactions is high. Such reactions are associated with cell-bound IgE antibodies. IgG antibodies to penicillin are common and are not associated with allergic reactions except rare hemolytic anemia. A history of a penicillin reaction in the past is not reliable, but the drug must be administered with caution to such persons, or a substitute drug should be chosen.

Allergic reactions may occur as typical anaphylactic shock, typical serum sickness type reactions (urticaria, joint swelling, angioneurotic edema, pruritus, respiratory embarrassment within 7–12 days of penicillin dosage), and a variety of skin rashes, fever, nephritis, eosinophilia, vasculitis, etc. The incidence of hypersensitivity to penicillin is negligible in children but may be 1–5% among adults in the USA.

Acute anaphylactic life-threatening reactions are very rare (0.05%). Corticosteroids can sometimes suppress allergic manifestations to penicillins.

CEPHALOSPORINS

Fungi of *Cephalosporium* species yield several antibiotics called cephalosporins. They resemble penicillins, are resistant to β-lactamases, and are active against both gram-positive and gram-negative bacteria. The nucleus of the cephalosporins, 7-aminocephalosporanic acid, closely resembles the nucleus of penicillin, 6-aminopenicillanic acid. The cephamycin drugs are similar but are made by actinomycetes.

The intrinsic activity of the natural cephalosporins is low, but attachment of various R groups to the cephalosporanic acid nucleus has yielded several compounds of high therapeutic activity and low toxicity. The cephalosporins have molecular weights of about 420; they are freely soluble in water and relatively stable. Cephalexin, cephradine, and cefadroxil are relatively well absorbed from the gut. Urinary and respiratory tract infections can be treated, but these oral drugs are rarely suitable for treatment of major systemic infections. Most other cephalosporins are not well absorbed from the gut and must be administered parenterally, most often as a bolus of 1–2 g added to an intravenous infusion every 2–4 hours. They are then widely distributed in tissues. The earlier cephalosporins (eg, cephalothin, cefazolin, cephapirin, cefamandole, cefoxitin) did not penetrate the central nervous system and were ineffective in meningitis. The newer cephalosporins (eg, cefotaxime, cefoperazone, cefuroxime, moxalactam) do diffuse into the central nervous system and cerebrospinal fluid and can be considered for the treatment of meningitis due to gram-negative aerobic bacteria; the dosage is 150–200 mg/kg/d intravenously.

Activity

Cephalosporins are β-lactam drugs with mechanisms of action comparable to those of the penicillins, including attachment to receptors and inhibition of the final transpeptidation of bacterial cell wall peptidoglycan. Cephalosporins resist inactivation by β-lactamases in varying degrees. They tend to be bactericidal in vitro in concentrations of 1–20 μg/mL for many gram-positive bacteria except enterococci, and in concentrations of 5–30 μg/mL for many gram-negative bacteria.

Proteus, Pseudomonas, Serratia and other organisms tend to be resistant to the earlier cephalosporins but susceptible to the newer ("third-generation") cephalosporins. The latter, especially cefotaxime, cefoperazone, moxalactam, and ceftizoxime, are being intensively promoted in 1986 for their wide spectrum of activity, including effectiveness against many gram-negative bacteria that cause hospital-acquired infections. Some cephalosporins, eg, cefoxitin and cefuroxime, are active against anaerobes—including *Bacteroides*—and also against lactamase-producing *Neisseria gonorrhoeae*. Cefazolin and other cephalosporins with high tissue levels and a long half-life are drugs of choice for short-term surgical prophylaxis. The newer cephalosporins are also often considered (alone or in combination with an aminoglycoside) for use in suspected sepsis in immunodeficient or immunosuppressed individuals. However, the primary indications for the newer cephalosporins are not well defined in 1986, and their very high cost must be considered.

Side Effects

A. Allergy: Cephalosporins can be sensitizing, and specific hypersensitivity reactions, including anaphylaxis, can occur. Because of the chemical difference in drug nucleus structure, the antigenicity of cephalosporins differs from that of penicillins. Consequently, many individuals who are hypersensitive to penicillins can tolerate cephalosporins. The degree of cross-allergenicity between penicillins and cephalosporins remains controversial (6–16%). Some cross-antigenicity can be demonstrated in vitro.

B. Toxicity: Pain on injection, thrombophlebitis, rashes, granulocytopenia, and hypoprothrombinemia occur intermittently. Diarrhea and nausea and vomiting may occur with the oral cephalosporins.

C. Superinfection: Several of the newer cephalosporins have diminished activity against gram-positive organisms, especially enterococci and staphylococci. Consequently, superinfection with such organisms may occur during treatment of gram-negative bacterial infections with such drugs.

TETRACYCLINES

The tetracyclines have virtually identical antimicrobial properties and give complete cross-resistance. However, they differ in physical and pharmacologic characteristics. All tetracyclines are readily absorbed from the intestinal tract and distributed widely in tissues but penetrate poorly into the cerebrospinal fluid.

Cephalosporanic acid

Cefotaxime

Moxalactam

Some can also be administered intramuscularly or intravenously. They are excreted in stool and into bile and urine at varying rates. With doses of tetracycline hydrochloride, 2 g daily orally, blood levels reach 8 μg/mL. Demeclocycline, methacycline, minocycline, and doxycycline are excreted more slowly; similar blood levels are achieved by daily doses of 0.6, 0.3, 0.2, and 0.1 g, respectively.

The tetracyclines have the basic structure shown below. The following radicals occur in the different chemical forms:

	R	R_1	R_2	Renal Clearance (mL/min)
Tetracycline	—H	—CH_3	—H	65
Chlortetracycline	—Cl	—CH_3	—H	35
Oxytetracycline	—H	—CH_3	—OH	90
Demeclocycline	—Cl	—H	—H	35
Methacycline	—H	=CH_2 *	—OH	31
Doxycycline	—H	—CH_3	—OH	16
Minocycline	—N(CH_3)$_2$	—H	—H	< 10

*No hydroxyl at C6.

Tetracyclines

Activity

Tetracyclines are concentrated by susceptible bacteria and inhibit protein synthesis by inhibiting the binding of aminoacyl-tRNA to the 30S unit of bacterial ribosomes. Resistant bacteria fail to concentrate the drug. This resistance is under the control of transmissible plasmids.

The tetracyclines are principally bacteriostatic agents. They inhibit the growth of susceptible gram-positive and gram-negative bacteria (inhibited by 0.1–10 μg/mL) and are drugs of choice in infections caused by rickettsiae, chlamydiae, and *Mycoplasma pneumoniae*. Tetracyclines are used in cholera to shorten excretion of vibrios, and in shigellosis. They are effective in gonococcal infections provided dosage is continued for 5 days, but such therapy does not attack coexisting syphilis. Tetracyclines are sometimes employed in combination with streptomycin to treat *Brucella, Yersinia,* and *Francisella* infections. Minocycline is often active against *Nocardia* and can eradicate the meningococcal carrier state, but it induces vestibular damage. Low doses of tetracycline for many months are given for acne to suppress both skin bacteria and their lipases, which promote inflammatory changes.

Tetracyclines do not inhibit fungi and may even stimulate the growth of yeasts. They temporarily suppress parts of the normal bowel flora. Their therapeutic usefulness is limited by the occurrence of "superinfections": while one microorganism is suppressed, another is permitted to multiply freely and produce pathogenic effects. This has occurred particularly with tetracycline-resistant *Psuedomonas, Proteus,* staphylococci, and yeasts.

Side Effects

The tetracyclines produce varying degrees of gastrointestinal upset (nausea, vomiting, diarrhea), skin rashes, mucous membrane lesions, and fever in many patients, particularly when administration is prolonged and dosage high. It is not definitely known what part is played by allergy and what part by direct toxicity. Replacement of bacterial flora (see above) occurs commonly. Overgrowth of yeasts on anal and vaginal mucous membranes during tetracycline administration leads to inflammation and pruritus. Overgrowth of organisms in the intestine may lead to enterocolitis.

Tetracyclines are deposited in bony structures and teeth, particularly in the fetus and during the first 6 years of life. Discoloration and fluorescence of the teeth occur in newborns if tetracyclines are taken for prolonged periods by pregnant women. In pregnancy, hepatic damage may occur. Outdated tetracycline can produce renal damage. Demeclocycline causes photosensitization. Minocycline can cause marked vestibular disturbances.

Bacteriologic Examination

Because of its instability in vitro, chlortetracycline often appears less active than the other members of the group. Antimicrobial efficacy of the tetracyclines is virtually identical, so that only one stable tetracycline need be included in antibiotic sensitivity tests. Cross-resistance of microorganisms to tetracyclines is extensive; an organism resistant to one of the drugs may be assumed to be resistant to the others also.

CHLORAMPHENICOL

Chloramphenicol is a substance produced originally from cultures of *Streptomyces venezuelae* but now manufactured synthetically.

Chloramphenicol

Crystalline chloramphenicol is a stable compound that is rapidly absorbed from the gastrointestinal tract and widely distributed into tissues and body fluids, including the central nervous system and cerebrospinal fluid; it penetrates cells well. Most of the drug is inactivated in the liver by conjugation with glucuronic acid or by reduction to inactive arylamines. Excretion is mainly in the urine, 90% in inactive form. Although chloramphenicol is usually administered orally (2 g daily gives blood levels up to 10 μg/mL), the succinate can be injected intravenously in similar dosage.

Activity

Chloramphenicol is a potent inhibitor of protein synthesis in microorganisms. It blocks the attachment of amino acids to the nascent peptide chain on the 50S unit of ribosomes by interfering with the action of peptidyl transferase. Chloramphenicol is principally bacteriostatic, and its spectrum is similar to that of the tetracyclines. Dosage and blood levels are similar to those of the tetracyclines. Chloramphenicol is a drug of possible first choice in (1) symptomatic *Salmonella* infections, eg, typhoid fever (although resistant strains are increasing); (2) *H influenzae* infections due to β-lactamase-producing strains; (3) meningococcal infections in patients hypersensitive to penicillin; (4) anaerobic or mixed infections in the central nervous system, eg, brain abscess; (5) severe rickettsial infections, and (6) eye infections except chlamydial infections (the drug is applied topically to the eye).

Chloramphenicol resistance is due to destruction of the drug by an enzyme (chloramphenicol acetyltransferase) that is under plasmid control.

Side Effects

Chloramphenicol infrequently causes gastrointestinal upsets. However, prolonged administration of more than 3 g daily to adults regularly results in abnormalities of early forms of red blood cells, elevation of serum iron, and anemia. These changes are reversible upon discontinuance of the drug. Very rare individuals exhibit an apparent idiosyncrasy to chloramphenicol and develop severe or fatal depression of bone marrow function. The mechanism of this aplastic anemia is not understood, but it is distinct from the dose-related reversible effect described above. For these reasons, the use of chloramphenicol is generally restricted to those infections where it is clearly the most effective drug by laboratory test or experience.

In premature and newborn infants, chloramphenicol can induce collapse ("gray syndrome") because the normal mechanism of detoxification (glucuronide conjugation in the liver) is not yet developed.

Bacteriologic Examination

Chloramphenicol is very stable and diffuses well in agar media. For these reasons, it tends to give larger zones of growth inhibition by the "disk test" than the tetracyclines, even when tube dilution tests show identical effectiveness. An enzymatic assay (using acetyltransferase) permits estimation of chloramphenicol concentration in body fluids.

ERYTHROMYCINS (Macrolides)

Erythromycin is obtained from *Streptomyces erythreus* and has the chemical formula $C_{37}H_{67}NO_{13}$. Drugs related to erythromycin are spiramycin, oleandomycin, and others. These drugs give complete cross-resistance but are less effective than erythromycin.

Erythromycins attach to a receptor (a 23S rRNA) on the 50S subunit of the bacterial ribosome. They inhibit protein synthesis by interfering with translocation reactions and the elongation of the peptide chain. Resistance to erythromycins results from an alteration (methylation) of the rRNA receptor. This is under control of a transmissible plasmid. The activity of erythromycins is greatly enhanced at alkaline pH.

Erythromycins in concentrations of 0.1–2 μg/mL are active against gram-positive bacteria, including pneumococci, streptococci, and corynebacteria. *Mycoplasma, Chlamydia trachomatis, Legionella pneumophila,* and *Campylobacter jejuni* are also susceptible. Resistant variants occur in susceptible microbial populations and tend to emerge during treatment, especially in staphylococcal infections.

Erythromycins may be drugs of choice in infections caused by the organisms listed above and are substitutes for penicillins in persons hypersensitive to the latter. Erythromycin stearate, succinate, or estolate, 0.5 g every 6 hours orally, yields serum levels of 0.5–2 μg/mL. Special forms (erythromycin glucep-

Table 10–3. Blood levels of some commonly used antibiotics at therapeutic dosage in adults.

	Route	Daily Dose	Expected Mean Concentration per mL Blood or per gram Tissue
Penicillin	IM	0.6–1 million units	1 unit (0.6 μg)
	Oral	0.6 million units	0.2 unit
Nafcillin	IV	6–12 g	5–30 μg
Cloxacillin, dicloxacillin	Oral	2–4 g	3–12 μg
Ampicillin	Oral	2–3 g	3–4 μg
	IV	4–6 g	10–40 μg
Carbenicillin	IV	30 g	100–200 μg
Ticarcillin	IV	18 g	100–200 μg
Cephalothin	IV	8–12 g	10–20 μg
Cefazolin	IM	2–4 g	20–50 μg
Cefoxitin, cefamandole	IV	4–12 g	40–80 μg
Tetracyclines	Oral	2 g	6–8 μg
Chloramphenicol	Oral	2 g	8–10 μg
Erythromycin	Oral	2 g	0.5–2 μg
Amikacin	IM	1 g	20–30 μg
Gentamicin, tobramycin	IM	0.3 g	3–6 μg
Vancomycin	IV	2 g	10–20 μg
Clindamycin	IV	2.4 g	3–6 μg
Polymyxin B	IV	0.15 g	1–3 μg

tate or lactobionate) are given intravenously in a dose of 0.5 g every 8–12 hours (40 mg/kg/d).

Undesirable side effects are drug fever, mild gastrointestinal upsets, and cholestatic hepatitis as a hypersensitivity reaction, especially to the estolate. Hepatotoxicity may be increased during pregnancy.

CLINDAMYCIN & LINCOMYCIN

Lincomycin (derived from *Streptomyces lincolnensis*) and clindamycin (a chlorine-substituted derivative) resemble erythromycins in mode of action, antibacterial spectrum, and ribosomal receptors but are chemically distinct. Clindamycin is very active against *Bacteroides* and other anaerobes.

The drugs are acid-stable and can be given by mouth or by injection of 600 mg intravenously 3–4 times daily (20–30 mg/kg/d). Serum levels reach 3–6 μg/mL, and the drugs are widely distributed in tissues, except the central nervous system. Excretion is mainly through liver, bile, and urine.

Probably the most important indication for intravenous clindamycin is the treatment of severe anaerobic infections, including those caused by *B fragilis*. Lincomycins have also been suggested for treatment of gram-positive coccal infections in persons hypersensitive to penicillins, but erythromycins may be preferable. Successful treatment of staphylococcal infections of bone with lincomycins has been recorded. Lincomycins should not be used in meningitis. Clindamycin has been prominent in antibiotic-associated colitis caused by *C difficile*. This organism is generally clindamycin-resistant and gains prominence in bowel flora during treatment with this—or occasionally other—drugs. It produces a necrotizing toxin and results in pseudomembranous colitis, which may be fatal. Early diagnosis and treatment with oral vancomycin are necessary.

VANCOMYCIN

Vancomycin is an amphoteric material produced by *Streptomyces orientalis,* dispensed as the hydrochloride. It has a high molecular weight (1450) and is poorly absorbed from the intestine.

Vancomycin is markedly bactericidal for staphylococci, enterococci, and some clostridia. The drug inhibits early stages in cell wall mucopeptide synthesis. Drug-resistant strains do not emerge rapidly. The dosage is 0.5 g every 6–12 hours intravenously (injected in a 30-minute period) for serious systemic staphylococcal or enterococcal infections, including endocarditis, especially if resistant to nafcillin. Oral vancomycin, 0.25–0.5 g, is indicated in antibiotic-associated pseudomembranous colitis (see Clindamycin and p 212).

Undesirable side effects are thrombophlebitis, skin rashes, nerve deafness, and occasionally kidney damage.

BACITRACIN

Bacitracin is a polypeptide obtained from a strain of *Bacillus subtilis* (Tracy strain). It is stable and poorly absorbed from the intestinal tract or from wounds. Its best use is for topical application to skin, wounds, or mucous membranes.

Bacitracin is mainly bactericidal for gram-positive bacteria, including penicillin-resistant staphylococci. For topical use, concentrations of 500–2000 units per milliliter of solution or gram of ointment are used. In combination with polymyxin B or neomycin, bacitracin is useful for the suppression of mixed bacterial flora in surface lesions.

Bacitracin is toxic for the kidney, causing proteinuria, hematuria, and nitrogen retention. For this reason, it has no place in systemic therapy. Bacitracin is said not to induce hypersensitivity readily.

POLYMYXINS

Polymyxin B and polymyxin E (colistin) are basic polypeptides, poorly absorbed from the intestinal tract but readily absorbed after injection. They are not widely distributed in tissues and body fluids. Unless locally introduced, they do not reach the spinal fluid or pleural or joint space. Colistin is dispensed as a methanesulfonate complex and produces fewer side effects than polymyxin B sulfate.

Activity

The polymyxins are strongly bactericidal against gram-negative bacilli, including *Pseudomonas,* that are resistant to other antibiotics. Polymyxins coat the bacterial cell membrane and destroy its active transport, functioning as a selective permeability barrier. They act like cationic detergents.

In tissues, polymyxins are strongly bound to membranes rich in phosphatidylethanolamine and are inhibited by pus. This limits their availability for antibacterial action. They have been largely supplanted by more effective and less toxic drugs.

Side Effects

The polymyxins produce reversible central nervous system side effects, including drowsiness, abnormal sensations, and ataxia. With doses exceeding 2.5 mg/kg/d, damage to the kidney may occur, particularly if renal function is impaired.

Bacteriologic Examination

The polymyxins are large molecules and diffuse poorly through agar. Consequently, inhibition zones in "disk tests" are always very small, even when the organism is shown to be highly sensitive by the tube dilution test. Organisms highly sensitive in vitro (inhibited by 0.1–1 μg/mL) may not respond in vivo if parenchymatous organs are involved in the infection. In susceptible strains of bacteria, resistance to polymyxins rarely develops.

AMINOGLYCOSIDES

Aminoglycosides are a group of drugs sharing chemical, antimicrobial, pharmacologic, and toxic characteristics. At present, the group includes streptomycin, neomycin, kanamycin, amikacin, gentamicin, tobramycin, sisomicin, netilmicin, and others. All inhibit protein synthesis of bacteria by attaching to and inhibiting the function of the 30S subunit of the bacterial ribosome. Resistance is based on (1) a deficiency of the ribosomal receptor (chromosomal mutant), (2) enzymatic destruction of the drug (plasmid-mediated transmissible resistance of clinical importance), or (3) lack of permeability to the drug molecule and lack of active transport into the cell. The last factor can be chromosomal in nature (eg, streptococci are relatively impermeable to aminoglycosides), or it can be plasmid-mediated (clinically significant resistance among gram-negative enteric bacteria). Anaerobic bacteria are often resistant to aminoglycosides because transport through the cell membrane is an energy-requiring process that is oxygen-dependent.

All aminoglycosides are more active at alkaline pH than at acid pH. All are potentially ototoxic and nephrotoxic, though to different degrees. All can accumulate in renal failure; therefore, marked dosage adjustments must be made when nitrogen retention occurs. Aminoglycosides are used most widely against gram-negative enteric bacteria or when there is suspicion of sepsis. In the treatment of bacteremia or endocarditis caused by fecal streptococci or some gram-negative bacteria, the aminoglycoside is given together with a penicillin that enhances permeability and facilitates the entry of the aminoglycoside. Aminoglycosides are selected according to recent susceptibility patterns in a given area or hospital until susceptibility tests become available on a specific isolate. All positively charged aminoglycosides and polymyxins are inhibited in blood cultures by sodium polyanethol sulfonate and other polyanionic detergents. Some aminoglycosides (especially streptomycin) are useful as antimycobacterial drugs.

1. NEOMYCIN & KANAMYCIN

Kanamycin is a close relative of neomycin, with similar activity and complete cross-resistance. Paromomycin is also closely related and is used in amebiasis. These drugs are stable, poorly absorbed from the intestinal tract, readily absorbed and distributed after intramuscular injection, and slowly excreted in the urine. Kanamycin is less toxic than neomycin, and only kanamycin is used systemically in children.

Kanamycin is bactericidal for many gram-negative bacilli, including some strains of *Proteus*, but ineffective against *Pseudomonas* and *Serratia*. Kanamycin, 15 mg/kg/d, is administered in serious infections due to gram-negative organisms that are resistant to other drugs. Oral doses of 4–6 g daily are used for reduction of intestinal flora preoperatively but are ineffective in most bacterial diarrheas except those caused by enteropathogenic *E coli*. Neomycin is limited to topical application to skin wounds or gut.

Neomycin and kanamycin may cause renal damage and nerve deafness without warning signs. Intraperitoneal administration of 3–5 g can induce respiratory paralysis that may be reversed by calcium gluconate or neostigmine.

2. AMIKACIN

Amikacin is a semisynthetic derivative of kanamycin. It is relatively resistant to several of the enzymes that inactivate gentamicin and tobramycin and therefore can be employed against some microorganisms resistant to the latter drugs. However, bacterial resistance due to impermeability to amikacin is increasing. Many gram-negative enteric bacteria, including many strains of *Proteus, Pseudomonas, Enterobacter,* and *Serratia,* are inhibited in vitro by amikacin, 1–20 μg/mL. After the injection of amikacin, 500 mg intramuscularly every 12 hours (15 mg/kg/d), peak levels in serum are 10–30 μg/mL. Some infections caused by gram-negative bacteria resistant to gentamicin respond to amikacin. Central nervous system infections require intrathecal or intraventricular injection of 1–10 mg daily.

Like all aminoglycosides, amikacin is nephrotoxic and ototoxic (particularly for the auditory portion of the eighth nerve). Its level should be monitored in patients with renal failure.

3. GENTAMICIN

In concentrations of 0.5–5 μg/mL, gentamicin is bactericidal for many gram-positive and gram-negative bacteria, including many strains of *Proteus, Serratia,* and *Pseudomonas*. Gentamicin is ineffective against streptococci and *Bacteroides*.

After intramuscular injection of 3–5 mg/kg/d, serum levels reach 3–6 μg/mL and the drug is widely distributed. Gentamicin is indicated in serious infections caused by gram-negative bacteria insusceptible to other drugs, when up to 7 mg/kg/d has been used. Gentamicin may precipitate with carbenicillin in vitro, but enhancement of bactericidal action against *Pseudomonas* occurs sometimes in vivo.

Gentamicin is nephrotoxic and ototoxic, particularly in the presence of impaired renal function, which predisposes to cumulation and toxic effects. Gentamicin sulfate, 0.1%, has been used topically in creams or solutions for infected burns or skin lesions. Such creams tend to select gentamicin-resistant bacteria, and patients receiving them must remain in strict isolation.

4. TOBRAMYCIN

This aminoglycoside closely resembles gentamicin but is more active than the latter against *Pseudomonas* species. Although there is some cross-resistance between gentamicin and tobramycin, it is unpredictable in individual strains. Separate laboratory susceptibility tests are therefore necessary.

The pharmacologic properties of tobramycin are virtually identical to those of gentamicin. The daily dose of tobramycin is 3–5 mg/kg/d intramuscularly, divided in 3 equal amounts and given every 8 hours. Such dosage produces blood levels of 2–5 μg/mL in the presence of normal renal function. About 80% of the drug is excreted by glomerular filtration into the urine within 24 hours of administration. In uremia, the drug dosage must be reduced. A formula for such dosage is 1 mg/kg every (6 × serum creatinine level) hours. However, monitoring of blood levels is desirable in uremia.

Like other aminoglycosides, tobramycin is ototoxic but perhaps less nephrotoxic than gentamicin. It should not be used concurrently with other drugs having similar adverse effects or with diuretics, which tend to enhance aminoglycoside tissue concentrations.

5. NETILMICIN

This aminoglycoside shares many characteristics with gentamicin and tobramycin. However, the addition of an ethyl group to the 1-amino position of the 2-deoxystreptamine ring (see below) sterically protects the netilmicin molecule from enzymatic degradation at the 2-hydroxyl and 3-amino positions. Consequently netilmicin is not inactivated by many bacteria that are resistant to gentamicin and tobramycin.

The dosage (5–7 mg/kg/d) and routes of administration are the same as for gentamicin. The principal indication for netilmicin may be iatrogenic infections in immunocompromised and severely ill patients at very high risk for gram-negative bacterial sepsis in the hospital setting.

Netilmicin may prove to be less ototoxic and possibly less nephrotoxic than the other aminoglycosides.

6. STREPTOMYCIN

Streptomycin was the first aminoglycoside—it was discovered in the 1940s as a product of *Streptomyces griseus*. It was studied in great detail and became the prototype of this class of drugs. For this reason, its properties are listed here, although widespread resistance among microorganisms has greatly reduced its clinical usefulness. Dihydrostreptomycin has been abandoned altogether because of excessive ototoxicity.

After intramuscular injection, streptomycin is rapidly absorbed and widely distributed in tissues except the central nervous system. Only 5% of the extracellular concentration of streptomycin reaches the interior of the cell. Absorbed streptomycin is excreted by glomerular filtration into the urine. After oral administration, it is poorly absorbed from the gut; most of it is excreted in feces.

Activity

Like other aminoglycosides, streptomycin inhibits protein synthesis in bacteria.

Streptomycin is bactericidal against susceptible microorganisms (inhibited in vitro by 0.1–20 μg/mL). The therapeutic effectiveness of streptomycin is limited by the rapid emergence of resistant mutants.

Streptomycin may be given in a dosage of 1 g/d intramuscularly with a penicillin in enterococcal endocarditis to enhance bactericidal action. In tularemia and plague, it is given with tetracyclines. In tuberculosis, 1 g is injected intramuscularly twice weekly (or daily), together with one or 2 other antituberculosis drugs (isoniazid, rifampin).

Resistance

All microbial strains produce streptomycin-resistant chromosomal mutants with relatively high frequency. Chromosomal mutants have an alteration in the P 12 receptor on the 30S ribosomal subunit. Plasmid-mediated resistance results in enzymatic destruction of the drug. In tuberculosis, combination of streptomycin with other antituberculosis drugs results in a marked delay in the emergence of resistance.

Side Effects

A. Allergy: Fever, skin rashes, and other allergic manifestations may result from hypersensitivity to streptomycin. This occurs most frequently upon prolonged contact with the drug, in patients receiving a protracted course of treatment (eg, for tuberculosis), or in personnel preparing and handling the drug. (Nurses preparing solutions should wear gloves.)

B. Toxicity: Streptomycin is markedly toxic for the vestibular portion of the eighth cranial nerve, causing tinnitus, vertigo, and ataxia, which are often irreversible. It is moderately nephrotoxic.

Streptomycin

Bacteriologic Examination

When sensitivity determinations with streptomycin are carried out in liquid media, a single resistant organism in the inoculum may grow out rapidly, although the bulk of the population is streptomycin-sensitive. Conversely, testing on solid media may fail to reveal the presence of resistant mutants in the population unless a very large inoculum is employed.

SPECTINOMYCIN

This is an aminocyclitol antibiotic (related to aminoglycosides) for intramuscular administration. Its sole application is in the treatment of gonorrhea caused by β-lactamase-producing gonococci or occurring in individuals hypersensitive to penicillin. One injection of 2 g (40 mg/kg) produces blood levels of 60–90 μg/mL. About 5–10% of gonococci are probably resistant. There is usually pain at the injection site, and there may be nausea and fever.

ISONIAZID
(Isonicotinic Acid Hydrazide, INH)

Isoniazid has little effect on most bacteria but is strikingly active against mycobacteria, especially *Mycobacterium tuberculosis*. Most tubercle bacilli are inhibited and killed in vitro by isoniazid, 0.1–1 μg/mL, but large populations of tubercle bacilli usually contain some isoniazid-resistant organisms. For this reason, the drug is employed in combination with other antimycobacterial agents (especially ethambutol or rifampin) to reduce the emergence of resistant tubercle bacilli. Isoniazid acts on mycobacteria by inhibiting the synthesis of mycolic acids. Isoniazid and pyridoxine are structural analogs. Patients receiving isoniazid excrete pyridoxine in excessive amounts, which results in peripheral neuritis. This can be prevented by the administration of pyridoxine, 0.3–0.5 g daily, which does not interfere with the antituberculosis action of isoniazid.

Isoniazid is rapidly and completely absorbed from the gastrointestinal tract and is in part acetylated and in part excreted in the urine. In the ordinary systemic dose of 4–6 mg/kg/d, toxic manifestations (eg, hepatitis) are infrequent, and blood levels reach an average of 0.5 μg/mL. Isoniazid freely diffuses into tissue fluids, including the cerebrospinal fluid. In tuberculous meningitis, 8–10 mg/kg/d is given for many weeks.

In converters from negative to positive tuberculin skin tests who have no evidence of disease, isoniazid, 300 mg daily for 1 year, may be used "prophylactically."

ETHAMBUTOL

Ethambutol is a synthetic, water-soluble, heat-stable D-isomer of the structure shown below.

$$H-\overset{\overset{\displaystyle CH_2OH}{|}}{\underset{\underset{\displaystyle C_2H_5}{|}}{C}}-NH-(CH_2)_2-HN-\overset{\overset{\displaystyle C_2H_5}{|}}{\underset{\underset{\displaystyle CH_2OH}{|}}{C}}-H$$

Ethambutol

Many strains of *M tuberculosis* and of "atypical" mycobacteria are inhibited in vitro by ethambutol, 1–5 μg/mL. The mechanism of action is not known.

Ethambutol is well absorbed from the gut. Following ingestion of 15 mg/kg, a blood level peak of 1–4 μg/mL is reached in 2–4 hours. About 20% of the drug is excreted in feces and 50% in urine, in unchanged form. Excretion is delayed in renal failure. About 15% of absorbed drug is metabolized by oxidation and conversion to a dicarboxylic acid. In meningitis, ethambutol appears in the cerebrospinal fluid.

Resistance to ethambutol emerges fairly rapidly among mycobacteria when the drug is used alone. Therefore, ethambutol is always given in combination with other antituberculosis drugs.

Ethambutol, 15 mg/kg, is usually given as a single daily dose. Hypersensitivity to ethambutol occurs infrequently. The commonest side effects are visual disturbances: reduction in visual acuity, optic neuritis, and perhaps retinal damage occur in some patients given 25 mg/kg/d for several months. Most of these changes apparently regress when ethambutol is discontinued. However, periodic visual acuity testing is mandatory during treatment. With 15 mg/kg/d, visual disturbances are very rare.

Isoniazid

Pyridoxine

RIFAMPIN

Rifampin is a semisynthetic derivative of rifamycin, an antibiotic produced by *Streptomyces mediterranei*. It is active in vitro against some gram-positive and gram-negative cocci, some enteric bacteria, mycobacteria, chlamydiae, and poxviruses. Although many meningococci and mycobacteria are inhibited by less than 1 $\mu g/mL$, highly resistant mutants occur in all microbial populations in a frequency of 10^{-5} to 10^{-6}. The prolonged administration of rifampin as a single drug permits the emergence of these highly resistant mutants. There is no cross-resistance to other antimicrobial drugs.

Rifampin binds strongly to DNA-dependent RNA polymerase and thus inhibits RNA synthesis in bacteria and chlamydiae. It blocks a late stage in the assembly of poxviruses, perhaps interfering with envelope formation. Rifampin penetrates phagocytic cells well and can kill intracellular organisms. Rifampin-resistant mutants exhibit an altered RNA polymerase.

Rifampin is well absorbed after oral administration, widely distributed in tissues, and excreted mainly through the liver and to a lesser extent into the urine. With oral doses of 600 mg, serum levels exceed 5 $\mu g/mL$ for 4–6 hours and urine levels may be 10–100 times higher.

In tuberculosis, a single oral dose of 600 mg daily (10–20 mg/kg/d) is administered together with ethambutol, isoniazid, or another antituberculosis drug in order to delay the emergence of rifampin-resistant mycobacteria. A similar regimen may apply to atypical mycobacteria. In short-term treatment schedules for tuberculosis, rifampin, 600 mg orally, is given first daily (together with isoniazid) and then 2 or 3 times weekly for 6–9 months. However, no less than 2 doses weekly should be given to avoid a "flu syndrome" and anemia. Rifampin used in conjunction with a sulfone (see p 156) is effective in leprosy.

An oral dose of rifampin, 600 mg twice daily for 2 days, can eliminate a majority of meningococci from carriers. Unfortunately, some highly resistant meningococcal strains are selected out by this procedure. Close contacts of children with *H influenzae* infections (eg, in the family or in day-care centers) can receive rifampin, 20 mg/kg/d for 4 days, as prophylaxis. In urinary tract infections and in chronic bronchitis, rifampin is not useful because resistance emerges promptly.

Rifampin imparts an orange color to urine, sweat, and contact lenses, which is harmless. Occasional adverse effects include rashes, thrombocytopenia, light chain proteinuria, and impairment of liver function.

AMINOSALICYLIC ACID (PAS)

p-Aminosalicylic acid closely resembles *p*-aminobenzoic acid and sulfonamides. Most bacteria are not inhibited by PAS, but tubercle bacilli are usually inhibited by PAS, 1–5 $\mu g/mL$, whereas atypical mycobacteria are resistant. In susceptible mycobacterial populations, PAS-resistant mutants tend to emerge. The simultaneous use of a second antituberculosis drug inhibits this development.

Aminosalicylic acid

PAS, 8–12 g daily orally, was commonly given in combination with streptomycin or isoniazid as antituberculosis therapy. However, full oral doses of PAS were commonly associated with severe gastrointestinal side effects. Therefore, the use of PAS has been largely abandoned.

AMPHOTERICIN B

Amphotericin B is a complex antibiotic polyene produced by a *Streptomyces* species and has negligible antibacterial properties. It strongly inhibits the growth of several pathogenic fungi in vitro and in vivo. Amphotericin binds to sterols on the fungal cell membranes and disturbs their function. The microcrystals of the drug are dispensed with sodium deoxycholate and a buffer to be dissolved in dextrose solution. It is injected intravenously in daily doses of 0.4–0.7 mg/kg/d (with an initial dose of 5 mg/d) and can be given intrathecally in doses up to 0.5 mg every other day in meningitis. Amphotericin B appears to be the most effective agent available for the treatment of disseminated coccidioidomycosis, blastomycosis, histoplasmosis, cryptococcosis, and candidiasis. It frequently produces marked toxic effects, including fever, chills, nausea and vomiting, renal failure, hypokalemia, and anemia. When it is used together with flucytosine, synergism may occur, particularly against *Cryptococcus* and *Candida* infections.

FLUCYTOSINE

5-Fluorocytosine is an oral antifungal compound of relatively low toxicity. Flucytosine, 5 $\mu g/mL$, inhibits many strains of *Candida, Cryptococcus,* and *Torulopsis* and some other yeasts. Oral doses of 150 mg/kg/d are well absorbed and widely distributed in tissues, including cerebrospinal fluid. Although the drug is relatively well tolerated, prolonged high serum levels often cause depression of bone marrow, loss of hair, skin rashes, and abnormal liver function. With 3–8 g administered daily in divided doses, there has been prolonged remission of fungemia and meningitis caused by susceptible organisms. Resistant mutants occur frequently, and, for this reason, simultaneous use of amphotericin B has been proposed. This delays resistance and may result in synergistic antifungal action, especially in cryptococcal meningitis and disseminated candidiasis.

GRISEOFULVIN

Griseofulvin is an antibiotic obtained from certain *Penicillium* species. It has no effect on bacteria or fungi producing systemic mycoses but suppresses dermatophytes, particularly *Microsporum audouini* and *Trichophyton rubrum*. Daily oral doses of 1 g are given for weeks or months. The absorbed drug is deposited in diseased skin, bound to keratin. Toxic effects include headache, drowsiness, skin rashes, and gastrointestinal disturbances. Ultramicrosized griseofulvin (Gris-Peg) is absorbed nearly twice as effectively as microsized griseofulvin.

ANTIFUNGAL IMIDAZOLES

These are drugs that increase membrane permeability and inhibit synthesis of sterols (ergosterol) in fungal cell membranes, among other actions. Clotrimazole, 10-mg troches orally 5 times daily, can suppress oral candidiasis. Miconazole, 2% cream, is used in dermatophytosis and vaginal candidiasis. Miconazole has been given intravenously in systemic micosis but is quite toxic. **Ketoconazole,** 200–600 mg orally once daily for many weeks, dramatically improves chronic mucocutaneous candidiasis, vaginal candidiasis, and paracoccidioidomycosis. It has therapeutic benefits in pulmonary coccidioidomycosis and histoplasmosis or blastomycosis but not in meningitis due to these fungi or to *Cryptococcus*.

Adverse effects include nausea, vomiting, headache, skin rashes, elevations in transaminase levels, inhibition of adrenal steroid synthesis, and gynecomastia.

CYCLOSERINE

Cycloserine is an antibiotic active against many types of microorganisms, including coliform bacteria, *Proteus,* and tubercle bacilli. It acts by inhibiting the incorporation of D-alanine into peptidoglycan of bacterial cell walls by blocking alanine racemase. It is occasionally used in urinary tract infections (15–20 mg/kg/d orally) but often causes neurotoxic side effects or shock and is therefore rarely used.

THE NITROFURANS

The nitrofurans are synthetic nitrofuraldehyde compounds that are strongly bactericidal in vitro for many gram-positive and gram-negative bacteria. Most nitrofurans are very insoluble in water. Some compounds (eg, nitrofuraldehyde semicarbazone, Furacin) are effective topical antibacterial agents used in surgical dressings and virtually unabsorbed.

Nitrofurantoin (Furadantin) is absorbed after oral administration and excreted in the urine. With daily doses of 400 mg, urine concentrations reach 100–200 μg/mL, sufficient to inhibit most organisms commonly encountered in urinary tract infections. Activity is limited to the urine. There is no antibacterial activity in blood or tissues. Thus, nitrofurantoin has no effect on systemic infections but is a good urinary antiseptic (see below).

Gastrointestinal intolerance is the commonest side effect of orally administered nitrofurantoin, but occasionally hemolytic anemia, skin rashes, hepatitis, pneumonitis, and other effects have been observed.

SULFONAMIDES

The sulfonamides are a large group of compounds with the basic formula shown on p 133. By substituting various R-radicals, a series of compounds is obtained with somewhat varying physical, pharmacologic, and antibacterial properties. The basic mechanism of action of all of these compounds is the competitive inhibition of *p*-aminobenzoic acid (PABA) utilization. The simultaneous use of sulfonamides with trimethoprim results in the inhibition of sequential metabolic steps and possible antibacterial synergism (see p 133).

The sulfonamides are bacteriostatic for some gram-negative and gram-positive bacteria, chlamydiae, nocardiae, and some protozoa. Several special sulfones (eg, dapsone) are employed in the treatment of leprosy.

The "soluble" sulfonamides (eg, trisulfapyrimidines, sulfisoxazole) are readily absorbed from the intestinal tract after oral administration of 4–8 g daily and are distributed in all tissues and body fluids (required blood levels: 8–12 mg/dL). The sodium salts of sulfonamides may be injected intravenously. Most sulfonamides are excreted rapidly in the urine. Some (eg, sulfamethoxypyridazine) are excreted very slowly and thus tend to be toxic. At present, sulfonamides are particularly useful in the treatment of nocardiosis and first attacks of urinary tract infections due to coliform bacteria. By contrast, many meningococci, shigellae, group A streptococci, and organisms causing recurrent urinary tract infections are now resistant. A mixture of 5 parts sulfamethoxazole plus 1 part trimethoprim is widely used in urinary tract infections, shigellosis, and salmonellosis and may be effective in treating other gram-negative bacterial infections and *P carinii* pneumonia.

Trimethoprim alone, 100 mg orally every 12 hours, can be effective treatment for uncomplicated urinary tract infections. Its widespread use in Finland has led to widespread bacterial resistance there.

The "insoluble" sulfonamides (eg, phthalylsulfathiazole, succinylsulfathiazole) are poorly absorbed from the intestinal tract and exert their action largely by inhibiting the microbial population within the lumen of the tract. They are given in a dosage of 8–15 g orally daily for 4–7 days to prepare the large bowel for surgery.

Resistance

Microorganisms that do not use extracellular PABA but, like mammalian cells, can use preformed folic acid are resistant to sulfonamides. In some sulfonamide-resistant mutants, the tetrahydropteroic acid synthetase has a much higher affinity for PABA than for sulfonamides. The opposite is true for sulfonamide-susceptible organisms.

Side Effects

The soluble sulfonamides may produce side effects that fall into 2 categories:

A. Allergic Reactions: Many individuals develop hypersensitivity to sulfonamides after initial contact with these drugs and, on reexposure, may develop fever, hives, skin rashes, and chronic vascular diseases such as polyarteritis nodosa.

B. Direct Toxic Effects: There may be fever, skin rashes, gastrointestinal disturbances, depression of the bone marrow leading to anemia or agranulocytosis, hemolytic anemia, and toxic effects on the liver and kidney. Some of the toxic action on the kidney can be prevented by keeping the urine alkaline and the water intake adequate; by using mixtures of sulfonamides such as trisulfapyrimidines (which are relatively more soluble than a single drug); or by employing sulfisoxazole, which is highly soluble in urine.

Bacteriologic Examination

When culturing specimens from patients receiving sulfonamides, the incorporation of PABA (5 mg/dL) into the medium overcomes sulfonamide inhibition.

METRONIDAZOLE

Metronidazole is an antiprotozoal drug used in treating *Trichomonas, Giardia,* and amebic infections. The usual dosage is 250–500 mg 3 times daily orally for 7–10 days. It also has striking effects against anaerobic bacteria, especially *Bacteroides* species, and against *Gardnerella vaginalis*. It may be effective in preoperative preparation of the colon. Adverse effects include stomatitis, diarrhea, and nausea. There is a question about possible teratogenic activity.

URINARY ANTISEPTICS

These are drugs with antibacterial effects limited to the urine. They fail to produce significant levels in tissues and thus have no effect on systemic infections. However, they effectively lower bacterial counts in the urine and thus greatly diminish the symptoms of lower urinary tract infection. They are used only in the management of urinary tract infections.

The most prominent urinary antiseptics are methenamine mandelate (Mandelamine) or hippurate, nitrofurantoin, and nalidixic acid. The active compounds are liberated in the urine only and have no systemic effect. Therefore, it is meaningless to perform and report sensitivity tests with these substances in any systemic infection. Nalidixic acid is effective in the urine, but microbial resistance tends to emerge rapidly. Oxolinic acid is similar. Other materials, such as amino acids (methionine) or hippuric acid (cranberry juice), may be ingested in large doses to provide an acid, bacteriostatic urine.

ANTIVIRAL DRUGS

Viruses, because of their structure and method of replication, are not affected by the common antibacterial drugs. However, viral multiplication may be interrupted by a variety of chemicals at various stages. In addition to specific antibody globulins that block penetration of extracellular virus into the cell, several chemicals have found limited application in the treatment of viral infections. The following substances are currently used in the management of clinical viral disease.

Amantadine Hydrochloride

This tricyclic symmetric amine (and its congener rimantadine) inhibits the penetration into susceptible cells, or uncoating, of certain myxoviruses, especially influenza A, but not influenza B. A daily oral dose of 200 mg of amantadine hydrochloride for 3 days before and 7 days after influenza A virus infection reduces the incidence and severity of symptoms. The most marked side effects noted with this drug are insomnia, dizziness, and ataxia, especially in elderly persons. Rimantadine is equally effective and perhaps less toxic.

Idoxuridine (5-Iodo-2'-deoxyuridine)

This halogenated pyrimidine can inhibit the replication of DNA viruses by becoming incorporated into viral DNA in place of thymidine. Topical application to herpetic keratitis can result in marked improvement. The topically applied drug remains localized in the avascular cornea and inhibits herpesvirus replication. For the treatment of herpetic keratitis, 1 drop of 0.1% solution is instilled into the conjunctival sac every 2 hours around the clock. Ointments containing 0.5% idoxuridine can be applied less frequently. Some toxic effects on corneal epithelium occur after prolonged use.

Idoxuridine is too severely cytotoxic for use in generalized virus infections.

Cytarabine (cytosine arabinoside, arabinofuranosylcytosine) also inhibits replication of DNA viruses. It has been used topically in herpetic keratitis and systemically in varicella-zoster, but it is more toxic than idoxuridine. It appears to be ineffective in disseminated herpes zoster.

Vidarabine (Adenine Arabinoside, Ara-A)

Vidarabine is the least toxic and most effective of the available purine and pyrimidine analogs. Vidarabine is phosphorylated in the cell to the triphosphate derivative, which inhibits viral DNA polymerase much more effectively than it inhibits mammalian DNA polymerase. In vivo, vidarabine is rapidly metabolized to hypoxanthine arabinoside, which has only slight antiviral action. In experimental models, the simultaneous use of vidarabine and an adenosine deaminase inhibitor enhances the antiviral action of vidarabine.

As a 3% ointment, vidarabine is more effective than idoxuridine in herpetic keratitis. Vidarabine, 10–15 mg/kg/d intravenously, can suppress progression of disseminated herpes zoster or herpes simplex. It can arrest herpetic encephalitis if administered early, before onset of coma. If started later, it may reduce the mortality rate, but the neurologic sequelae may be devastating. Among the older antiviral drugs tried systemically, vidarabine is relatively well tolerated. However, if vidarabine is given for prolonged periods (eg, for suppression of the viremia of hepatitis B), significant untoward effects are encountered.

Acyclovir (Acycloguanosine)

Acyclovir is a guanine derivative that is phosphorylated in herpesvirus-infected cells 30–100 times faster than in uninfected cells. This is due to the action of a virus-specific thymidine kinase. The resulting acycloguanosine triphosphate inhibits herpesvirus DNA polymerase 10–30 times more effectively than it inhibits normal cellular DNA polymerase and thus inhibits herpesvirus replication.

In intravenous doses of 15 mg/kg/d, acyclovir can prevent or limit mucocutaneous lesions of herpes simplex in transplant patients and other immunocompromised patients. Acyclovir can also reduce the pain and accelerate the healing of herpes zoster lesions and of primary herpes simplex genital infection. However, it does not affect the establishment of viral latency or the frequency of recurrence. Acyclovir, 200 mg 5 times daily orally, has therapeutic effects similar to those achieved when the drug is administered intravenously. Oral acyclovir is equally effective in primary herpes simplex genital infections. When taken prophylactically for 4–6 months, it can reduce the frequency and severity of recurrent lesions during this period. Acyclovir is somewhat more effective than vidarabine in herpetic encephalitis and disseminated neonatal herpes but is not beneficial in cytomegalovirus or Epstein-Barr herpesvirus infections. Topical application of 5% acyclovir ointment can limit mucocutaneous lesions of herpes simplex in immunosuppressed individuals but not in patients with normal immunity. It can also shorten healing time and reduce pain in primary genital herpes but not in recurrent lesions. It has no effect on frequency of recurrence.

Acyclovir-resistant herpesviruses that are thymidine-kinase-deficient may emerge during treatment, but this need not greatly alter the clinical response.

Ribavirin

Ribavirin is a synthetic nucleoside that inhibits DNA and RNA viruses. When administered as an aerosol to infants suffering from respiratory syncytial virus infection, it reduces the length and severity of illness. The aerosolized ribavirin also benefits patients with symptomatic influenza B virus infections.

Methisazone (N-Methylisatin-β-thiosemicarbazone)

This drug can block replication of poxviruses, probably by inhibiting the formation of a structural protein. Administered to contacts of smallpox cases within 1–2 days after exposure, 2–4 g/d orally for 3–4 days (100 mg/kg/d for children) gave striking protection against smallpox.

Generalized or progressive vaccinia in immunodeficient individuals can also be treated with methisazone.

The principal side effect is vomiting.

Interferons

Interferons are a group of antiviral substances generated by human cells. The human interferons employed in clinical studies until 1982 were prepared from pooled blood leukocytes or from human lymphoid cell lines. Since 1982, recombinant DNA technology has been applied to greatly increase the yields of several interferons for clinical trials. Interferons inhibit virus replication by inducing at least 3 enzymes: (1) a protein kinase that leads to phosphorylation of elongation factor EF-2, resulting in inhibition of peptide chain growth; (2) oligoisonadenylate, which ultimately results in activation of an RNase that degrades viral mRNA; and (3) a phosphodiesterase that leads to inhibition of peptide elongation. In addition, some interferons act as immunomodulators, and it is this feature that is being tested in cancer therapy trials.

In immunosuppressed patients, human interferons can prevent dissemination of herpes zoster and herpes simplex. They can also suppress the viremia of chronic active hepatitis B. If given before trigeminal ganglion surgery for neuralgia, interferons can temporarily suppress the appearance of recurrent lesions of herpes simplex. Other possible antiviral applications of interferons will be explored.

REFERENCES

Balfour HH: Intravenous acyclovir therapy for varicella in immunocompromised children. *J Pediatr* 1984;**104**:134.

Bauer AW et al: Antibiotic susceptibility testing by a standardized single disc method. *Am J Clin Pathol* 1966;**45**:493.

Beeuwkes H, Rutgers VH: A combination of amoxicillin and clavulanic acid in the treatment of respiratory tract infections caused by amoxicillin-resistant *Haemophilus influenzae*. *Infection* 1981;**9**:244.

Bennett JE et al: A comparison of amphotericin B alone and combined with flucytosine in the treatment of cryptococcal meningitis. *N Engl J Med* 1979;**301**:126.

Bennett WM et al: Drug therapy in renal failure. *Ann Intern Med* 1980;**93**:62.

Blumberg PM, Strominger JL: Interaction of penicillin with the bacterial cell: Penicillin-binding proteins and penicillin-sensitive enzymes. *Bacteriol Rev* 1974;**38**:291.

Datta N (editor): Antibiotic resistance in bacteria. *Br Med Bull* 1984;**40**:1. [Entire issue.]

Davis SD: Polymyxins, colistin, vancomycin and bacitracin. In: *Antimicrobial Therapy,* 3rd ed. Kagan BM (editor). Saunders, 1980.

Dolin R et al: A controlled trial of amantadine and rimantadine in the prophylaxis of influenza A infection. *N Engl J Med* 1982;**307**:580.

Douglas JM et al: A double-blind study of oral acyclovir for suppression of recurrences of genital herpes simplex virus infection. *N Engl J Med* 1984;**310**:1551.

Elion GB: Mechanism of action and selectivity of acyclovir. *Am J Med* 1982;**73**:7.

Falkow S: *Infectious Multiple Drug Resistance.* Pion Ltd, 1975.

Finland M: Emergence of antibiotic resistance in hospitals, 1935–75. *Rev Infect Dis* 1979;**1**:4.

Gale EF et al: *The Molecular Basis of Antibiotic Action,* 2nd ed. Wiley, 1981.

Goldman P: Metronidazole. *N Engl J Med* 1980;**303**:1212.

Hall CB et al: Aerosolized ribavirin treatment of infants with respiratory syncytial viral infection. *N Engl J Med* 1983;**308**:1443.

Hirsch MS, Swartz MN: Antiviral drugs. (2 parts.) *N Engl J Med* 1980;**302**:903, 949.

Holmberg SD et al: Drug-resistant *Salmonella* from animals fed antimicrobials. *N Engl J Med* 1984;**311**:617.

Jackson GG: Considerations of antibiotic prophylaxis in nonsurgical high risk patients. *Am J Med* 1981;**70**:467.

Jacobs MR et al: Emergence of multiply resistant pneumococci. *N Engl J Med* 1978;**299**:735.

Jawetz E: The doctor's dilemma. In: *Current Clinical Topics in Infectious Diseases.* Remington JS, Swartz MN (editors). McGraw-Hill, 1981.

Katzung BG (editor): *Basic & Clinical Pharmacology,* 2nd ed. Lange, 1984.

Kaufman RH et al: Treatment of genital herpes simplex infection with photodynamic inactivation. *Am J Obstet Gynecol* 1979;**132**:861.

McCormack WM, Finland M: Spectinomycin. *Ann Intern Med* 1976;**84**:712.

McDonnell RW et al: Conjugational transfer of gentamicin resistance plasmids intra- and interspecifically in staphylococci. *Antimicrob Agents Chemother* 1983;**23**:151.

Merigan TC: Interferon: The first quarter century. *JAMA* 1982;**248**:2513.

Merigan TC et al: Human leukocyte interferon for the treatment of herpes zoster in patients with cancer. *N Engl J Med* 1978;**298**:981.

Meyers JD et al: Multicenter collaborative trial of intravenous acyclovir for treatment of mucocutaneous herpes simplex in the immunocompromised host. *Am J Med* 1982;**73**:229.

Moellering RC Jr, Nelson JD, Neu HC (editors): An international review of amdinocillin: A new beta-lactam antibiotic. (Symposium.) *Am J Med* 1983;**75(No. 2A)**:1. [Entire issue.]

Neu HC: The new beta-lactamase-stable cephalosporins. *Ann Intern Med* 1982;**97**:408.

O'Brien TF et al: International comparison of prevalence of resistance to antibiotics. *JAMA* 1978;**239**:1518.

Parker CW: Drug allergy. (3 parts.) *N Engl J Med* 1975;**292**:511, 732, 957.

Petz LD: Immunologic cross-reactivity between penicillins and cephalosporins: A review. *J Infect Dis* 1978;**137(Suppl)**:S74.

Rahal JJ: Antibiotic combinations: The clinical relevance of synergy and antagonism. *Medicine* 1978;**57**:179.

Restrepo A, Stevens DA, Utz JP (editors): Symposium on ketoconazole. *Rev Infect Dis* 1980;**2**:519.

Ronald AR, Harding KM: Urinary infection prophylaxis in women. *Ann Intern Med* 1981;**94**:268.

Rubin RH, Swartz MN: Trimethoprim-sulfamethoxazole. *N Engl J Med* 1980;**303**:426.

Russell AD, Hugo WB, Ayliffe GAJ (editors): *Principles and Practice of Disinfection, Preservation and Sterilization.* Blackwell, 1982.

Sabath LD et al: A new type of penicillin resistance of *Staphylococcus aureus. Lancet* 1977;**1**:443.

Sanders CC, Sanders WE: Microbial resistance to newer generation β lactam antibiotics. *J Infect Dis* 1985;**151**:399.

Siegel D: Tetracyclines: New look at an old antibiotic. *NY State J Med* 1978;**78**:950.

Sivonen A et al: The effect of chemoprophylactic use of rifampin and minocycline on rates of carriage of *Neisseria meningitidis* in army recruits in Finland. *J Infect Dis* 1978;**137**:238.

Snavely SR, Hodges GR: The neurotoxicity of antibacterial agents. *Ann Intern Med* 1984;**101**:92.

Spruance SL, Crumpacker CS: Topical 5 percent acyclovir in polyethylene glycol for herpes simplex labialis: Antiviral effect without clinical benefit. *Am J Med* 1982;**73**:315.

Tipper DJ: Mode of action of beta-lactam antibiotics. *Rev Infect Dis* 1979;**1**:39.

Weinstein L, Dalton AC: Host determinants of response to antimicrobial agents. *N Engl J Med* 1968;**279**:467.

Wendel GD et al: Penicillin allergy and desensitization in serious infections during pregnancy. *N Engl J Med* 1985;**312**:1229.

Whitley RJ et al: Herpes simplex encephalitis: Vidarabine therapy and diagnostic problems. *N Engl J Med* 1981;**304**:313.

Whitley RJ et al: Infections caused by herpes simplex virus in the immunocompromised host: Natural history and topical acyclovir therapy. *J Infect Dis* 1984;**150**:323.

Whitley RJ et al: Vidarabine therapy of neonatal herpes simplex infection. *Pediatrics* 1980;**66**:495.

Winston DJ et al: Infectious complications of human bone marrow transplantation. *Medicine* 1979;**58**:1.

Host-Parasite Relationships

A parasite is an organism that resides on or within another living organism in order to find the environment and nutrients it requires for growth and reproduction. This does not imply that a parasite must harm its host. On the contrary, the most successful parasites achieve a balance with the host that ensures the survival, growth, and propagation of both parasite and host. Thus a majority of host-parasite interactions do not result in disease: the infection remains latent or subclinical.

The relationship between parasite and host is determined both by those characteristics of the parasite that favor establishment of the parasite and damage to the host and by the various host mechanisms that oppose these processes. Among the parasite's attributes are infectivity, invasiveness, pathogenicity, and toxigenicity. These are described below. If the parasite injures the host to a sufficient degree, disturbances will result in the host that manifest themselves as disease.

INFECTION

Infection is the process whereby the parasite enters into a relationship with the host. Its essential component steps in humans and animals are the following:

(1) Entrance of the parasite into the host– The most frequent portals of entry are the respiratory tract (mouth and nose), the gastrointestinal tract, the genitourinary tract, and breaks in the superficial mucous membranes and skin. Surface components of the microbe determine its ability to adhere to epithelial cells. Such adhesins may be surface proteins (eg, K88 in enteropathic *Escherichia coli*), lipoteichoic acids (in group A streptococci), or others. Surface receptors on epithelial cells bind adhesins; for example, fibronectin, a glycoprotein on buccal cells, attaches streptococci. Some parasites can penetrate intact mucous membrane and skin; still others are passively introduced by arthropods through these layers directly into the lymphatic channels or the bloodstream.

(2) Establishment and multiplication of the parasite within the host–From the portal of entry, the parasite may spread directly through the tissues or may proceed via the lymphatic channels to the bloodstream, which distributes it widely and permits it to reach tissues particularly suitable for its multiplication. The biochemical environment of the tissues ultimately determines the susceptibility or resistance of a certain host to a given parasite.

Although the process of infection is of paramount interest to medicine, there are 2 other requirements for the perpetuation of a parasitic species: a satisfactory portal of exit of the parasite from the host and an effective mechanism for transmission to new hosts.

ATTRIBUTES OF MICROORGANISMS THAT ENABLE THEM TO CAUSE DISEASE

There is no sharp semantic distinction between the terms "pathogenicity" and "virulence." **Pathogenicity** denotes the ability of microorganisms to cause disease or to result in the production of progressive lesions. **Virulence** introduces the concept of degree, ie, virulent organisms exhibit pathogenicity when introduced into the host in very small numbers. These properties may be subdivided into **toxigenicity** (ability to produce toxic substances) and **invasiveness** (ability to enter host tissues, multiply there, and spread). Different pathogenic microorganisms possess these attributes in varying degrees. Toxigenicity and invasiveness may be under separate genetic control. The production of most exotoxins is controlled by genes in plasmids or in bacterial viruses rather than by the chromosomal genes of bacteria.

Virulence is measured in terms of the number of microorganisms or micrograms of toxin necessary to kill a given host when administered by a certain route. It is usually expressed as the LD_{50}, ie, the number of organisms or micrograms of toxin that must be administered to kill 50% of the animals.

A few representative substances known to play a role in the production of disease by microorganisms are mentioned below.

Toxins

Microbial toxins are usually grouped as exotoxins or endotoxins. The essential features of each group are listed in Table 11–1. Several exotoxins consist of 2 moieties: one aids entrance of the exotoxin into host cells, and the other exerts the toxin effect per se.

Pathogenetic Mechanisms in Some Disorders Caused by Microbial Exotoxins

A. Diphtheria: The microorganism *Corynebacterium diphtheriae* grows in the upper respiratory tract or wounds, and lysogenic strains produce toxin. The

Table 11–1. Differentiation of exotoxins and endotoxins.

Exotoxins	Endotoxins
Excreted by living cells; found in high concentrations in fluid medium.	Integral part of microbial cell walls of gram-negative organisms liberated upon their disintegration.
Polypeptides, molecular weight 10,000–900,000.	Lipopolysaccharide complexes. Lipid A portion probably responsible for toxicity.
Relatively unstable; toxicity often destroyed rapidly by heat over 60° C.	Relatively stable; withstand heat over 60° C for hours without loss of toxicity.
Highly antigenic; stimulate the formation of high-titer antitoxin. Antitoxin neutralizes toxin.	Do not stimulate formation of antitoxin; stimulate formation of antibodies to polysaccharide moiety.
Converted into antigenic, nontoxic toxoids by formalin, acid, heat, etc.	Not converted into toxoids.
Highly toxic; fatal for laboratory animals in micrograms or less.	Weakly toxic; fatal for laboratory animals in hundreds of micrograms.
Do not produce fever in host.	Often produce fever in host.

toxin is absorbed, inhibits protein synthesis, and results in necrosis of epithelium, heart muscle, kidney, and nerve tissue.

Diphtheria toxin is a polypeptide (MW 62,000) that can be lethal in a dose of 40 ng. The essential action is inhibition of peptide chain elongation by inactivating the elongation factor EF-2 (formerly called transferase II). The toxin inactivates EF-2 by catalyzing a reaction that yields free nicotinamide plus an inactive adenosine diphosphate-ribose-EF-2 complex. The arrest of protein synthesis may bring about disruption of normal physiologic functions. Some strains of *Pseudomonas aeruginosa* produce a toxin that has the same mode of action as diphtheria toxin.

B. Tetanus: *Clostridium tetani* contaminates wounds, and the spores germinate in an anaerobic environment (devitalized tissue). Vegetative forms produce toxin (MW 150,000) that reaches the central nervous system by retrograde axon transport and is bound to gangliosides. Toxin increases reflex excitability in neurons of the spinal cord by blocking release of an inhibitory mediator in motor neuron synapses. The toxin may also affect synaptic transmission at the myoneural junction, perhaps because of accumulation of acetylcholine. Muscle spasms result.

C. Gas Gangrene: Spores of *Clostridium perfringens* and other clostridia (especially *Clostridium ramosum, Clostridium bifermentans, Clostridium histolyticum, Clostridium sporogenes, Clostridium novyi*) are introduced into wounds by soil or feces. In the presence of necrotic tissue (anaerobic environment), spores germinate and vegetative cells produce toxins. Many of these are necrotizing and hemolytic and, together with distention of tissue by gas formed from carbohydrates and interference with blood supply, favor the spread of gangrene. *Clostridium difficile*, and perhaps other clostridia, can produce a necrotizing toxin in the gut that leads to antibiotic-associated colitis.

The alpha toxin of *C perfringens* is a lecithinase that damages cell membranes by splitting lecithin to phosphocholine and diglyceride. Theta toxin also has a necrotizing effect. Collagenases and DNases are produced by various clostridia. Some strains of *C perfringens* also produce an enterotoxin (see below).

D. Botulism: *Clostridium botulinum* grows in anaerobic foods (canned, vacuum-packed, etc) and produces a neurotoxin (MW 150,000) of 6 antigenic types. The toxin is absorbed from the gut and carried by the blood to motor nerves. Toxin blocks the release of acetylcholine at synapses and neuromuscular junctions, producing diplopia, dysphagia, respiratory paralysis, and other motor paralyses.

E. Staphylococcal Food Poisoning: Certain strains of *Staphylococcus aureus* produce an enterotoxin while growing in meat, dairy, or bakery products. This enterotoxin (MW 40,000) is resistant to heating at 100 °C for 20 minutes. After ingestion, enterotoxin is absorbed in the gut, where it stimulates neural receptors. From there, impulses are transmitted to medullary centers of gut motility. Vomiting, often projectile, results within hours. Diarrhea is less frequent.

F. Cholera: *Vibrio cholerae* from feces of infected persons contaminates food or drink. Vibrios grow in the small intestine, producing a heat-labile enterotoxin (MW 80,000) that binds to ganglioside receptors on villi of the small intestine. The enterotoxin causes a large increase in adenylate cyclase activity and in the concentration of cAMP in the gut. This results in massive hypersecretion of chloride and water and impaired absorption of sodium in the jejunum and ileum. The effect is massive diarrhea and acidosis.

G. Other Food Poisons: Some strains of *C perfringens, E coli, Vibrio parahaemolyticus, Bacillus cereus,* and others can produce enterotoxins that result in massive diarrhea. Enterotoxin production is often controlled by plasmid genes.

H. Streptococcal Erythrogenic Toxin: Some strains of hemolytic lysogenic streptococci produce a toxin that results in a punctate maculopapular erythematous rash, as in scarlet fever. The precise mode of action is uncertain. Production of erythrogenic toxin is under genetic control of a temperate bacteriophage. If phage is lost, the streptococci cannot produce toxin.

Toxin stimulates antitoxin formation, which neutralizes the toxin effect. Thus, a person possessing antitoxin may have pharyngitis when infected with streptococci producing erythrogenic toxin but not get scarlet fever.

I. Toxic Shock Syndrome (TSST-1): Some staphylococci growing in wounds or on mucous membranes elaborate TSST-1, which appears to be identical to exotoxin C and enterotoxin F (see pp 219 and 220). The resulting illness is characterized by high fever, vomiting, watery diarrhea, a diffuse red rash that later desquamates, and hypotensive shock with renal and cardiac failure. The staphylococci typically do not reach the bloodstream.

J. Other Exotoxins: Other exotoxins are described in Chapters 14, 16, 17, 18, 19, and 21.

Extracellular Enzymes

Certain bacteria produce substances that are not directly toxic but do play an important role in the infectious process.

A. Collagenase: *C perfringens* produces, in addition to a lecithinase, proteolytic enzymes (collagenases) capable of disintegrating collagen. This promotes the spread of bacilli in tissues.

B. Coagulase: Many pathogenic staphylococci produce a substance (coagulase) that, in conjunction with certain serum factors, coagulates plasma. Coagulase contributes to the formation of fibrin walls around staphylococcal lesions, which help them to persist. Coagulase also causes a deposit of fibrin on the surface of individual staphylococci, which may protect them from phagocytosis or from destruction within phagocytic cells.

C. Hyaluronidases: Hyaluronidases (enzymes that hydrolyze hyaluronic acid, a constituent of the ground substance of connective tissue) are produced by many bacteria (eg, staphylococci, clostridia, streptococci, pneumococci) and aid in their spread through tissues.

D. Streptokinase (Fibrinolysin): Many hemolytic streptococci produce a substance (streptokinase) that activates a proteolytic enzyme of the plasma (plasminogen → plasmin). This enzyme (also called fibrinolysin) is then able to dissolve coagulated plasma and probably aids in the spread of streptococci through tissues.

E. Hemolysins and Leukocidins: Many microorganisms produce substances that dissolve red blood cells (hemolysins) or kill tissue cells or leukocytes (leukocidins). Streptolysin O, for example, is produced by group A hemolytic streptococci and is lethal for mice in addition to being hemolytic for a variety of red cells. This substance is readily oxidized and thereby inactivated, but it is reactivated by reducing agents. It is antigenic. The same streptococci also produce oxygen-stable streptolysin S, which is nonantigenic. Clostridia produce a variety of hemolysins, among them the lecithinase described above. Hemolysins are also produced by staphylococci and many gram-negative rods.

F. Proteases: Many organisms produce proteases that can hydrolyze immunoglobulins. Thus, *Neisseria* species or *Streptococcus* species can cleave local secretory IgA antibodies, preventing adherence, opsonization, and phagocytosis.

Factors in the Invasiveness of Microorganisms

A continuous scale of invasiveness could be drawn up for microorganisms. One end of this scale would be occupied by noninvasive toxin producers like those that cause tetanus or diphtheria; the other, by highly invasive organisms like anthrax or plague bacilli, with staphylococci and streptococci in between. The toxin producers are pathogenic principally because of elaboration of poisonous chemical substances without much tissue invasion. Plague or anthrax bacilli produce disease and death because they are able to invade tissues rapidly and multiply extensively, with the production of several toxic materials. Pneumococci or meningococci also spread widely throughout the body. The invasiveness of such organisms may be aided by enzymes favoring spread, such as hyaluronidase or streptokinase, but invasiveness is not clearly related to toxic properties. A part of the invasiveness of microorganisms may be attributed to certain surface components that protect the bacteria from phagocytosis and destruction. Such surface substances may be polysaccharide capsules (eg, pneumococci, meningococci, *Klebsiella pneumoniae, Haemophilus influenzae*), hyaluronic acid capsules and surface "M" proteins (β-hemolytic streptococci), or a surface polypeptide (anthrax bacilli). Certain microorganisms may be invasive and "virulent" because they survive within phagocytic cells and are resistant to enzymatic attack. Although these various factors contribute to the observed invasiveness of microorganisms, it must be concluded that this behavior is an expression of inherent biochemical properties not yet understood. On the other hand, invasiveness as such is by no means synonymous with disease production. Some infectious agents, eg, viruses, may be widely distributed in the body without causing illness.

How can one prove that a given microorganism really causes a disease? Traditionally, the causative relationship between a microorganism and a disease is established by fulfilling "Koch's postulates": (1) The microorganism must regularly be isolated from cases of the illness. (2) It must be grown in pure culture in vitro. (3) When such a pure culture is inoculated into susceptible animal species, the typical disease must result. (4) From such experimentally induced disease, the microorganism must again be isolated.

Although these postulates were adequate to prove the causes of some bacterial and fungal diseases, they had to be modified for other infections, particularly for diseases caused by viruses that replicate only in humans and not in other animals.

ATTRIBUTES OF THE HOST THAT DETERMINE RESISTANCE TO MICROORGANISMS

The various factors that operate to prevent infection of a host can be arranged in 2 groups: nonspecific factors operating against a variety of parasites and specific factors based on immunologic responses toward specific agents.

SOME MECHANISMS OF NONSPECIFIC HOST RESISTANCE

Physiologic Barriers at the Portal of Entry

A. The Skin: Few microorganisms are capable of penetrating the intact skin, but many can enter sweat or sebaceous glands and hair follicles and establish themselves there. Sweat and sebaceous secretions, by virtue of their acid pH and possibly chemical substances (especially fatty acids), have antimicrobial properties that tend to eliminate pathogenic organisms. Lysozyme, an enzyme that dissolves some bacterial cell walls, and perhaps other enzymes are also present on the skin. Lysozyme is also present in tears and respiratory and cervical secretions.

Skin resistance may vary with age. For example, children are highly susceptible to ringworm infection. After puberty, resistance to such fungi increases markedly with the increased content of saturated fatty acids in sebaceous secretions.

B. Mucous Membranes: In the respiratory tract, a film of mucus covers the surface and is constantly being driven upward by ciliated cells toward the natural orifices. Bacteria tend to stick to this film. Mucus and tears also contain lysozyme and other substances with antimicrobial properties. For some microorganisms, the first step in infection is their attachment to surface epithelial cells by means of adhesins and cell receptors (see above). If such cells have IgA antibody on their surfaces, attachment may be prevented—a host resistance mechanism. In turn, if the organism breaks down the antibody with a protease, this constitutes a "virulence factor." When organisms enter the mucous membrane, they tend to be taken up by phagocytes and transported into regional lymphatic channels that carry them to lymph nodes. These act as barriers toward further spread and can dispose of large numbers of bacteria. The mucociliary apparatus for removal of bacteria in the respiratory tract is aided by pulmonary macrophages. This entire defense system can be suppressed by alcohol, narcotics, cigarette smoke, hypoxia, acidosis, and other harmful influences. Special protective mechanisms in the respiratory tract include the hairs at the nares and the cough reflex, which prevents aspiration.

In the gastrointestinal tract, saliva contains numerous hydrolytic enzymes; the acidity of the stomach inactivates many ingested bacteria (eg, *V cholerae*); and the small intestine contains many proteolytic enzymes and active macrophages.

It must be remembered that most mucous membranes of the body carry a constant normal microbial flora that itself opposes the establishment of pathogenic microorganisms ("bacterial interference") and has important physiologic functions. For example, in the adult vagina, an acid pH is maintained by normal lactobacilli that interfere with the establishment of yeasts, anaerobes, and gram-negative organisms.

Phagocytosis

The main functions of phagocytic cells include migration, chemotaxis, ingestion, and microbial killing. Microorganisms (and other particles) that enter the lymphatics, lung, bone marrow, or bloodstream are engulfed by any of a variety of phagocytic cells. Among them are polymorphonuclear leukocytes, phagocytic monocytes (macrophages), and fixed macrophages of the reticuloendothelial system (see below). Many microorganisms elaborate chemotactic factors that attract phagocytic cells. Defects in chemotaxis may account for hypersusceptibility to certain infections (eg, Job's syndrome), or they may be familial in nature. Phagocytosis can occur in the absence of serum antibodies, particularly if aided by the architecture of tissue. Thus, phagocytic cells are inefficient in large, smooth, open spaces like pleura, pericardium, or joint but may be more effective in ingesting microorganisms that are trapped in small tissue spaces (eg, alveoli) or on rough surfaces. Such "surface phagocytosis" occurs early in the infectious process before antibodies are available.

Phagocytosis is made more efficient by the presence of antibodies (opsonins) that coat the bacterial surface and facilitate the ingestion of bacteria by the phagocyte. Opsonization can occur by 3 mechanisms: (1) Antibody alone can act as opsonin. (2) Antibody plus antigen can activate complement via the classic pathway to yield opsonins. (3) Opsonin may be produced by a heat-labile system where immunoglobulin or other factors activate C3 via the alternative pathway. Macrophages have receptors on their membrane for the Fc portion of antibody and for the C3 component of complement. This aids the phagocytosis of antibody-coated particles.

Hyperosmolality (eg, in the renal medulla) inhibits phagocytosis. Hypophosphatemia depletes ATP in granulocytes and reduces the efficiency of phagocytosis. Neutrophils from patients with diabetes (and perhaps other metabolic disorders) ingest bacteria normally but then are deficient in the ability to kill them. By contrast, during acute infections, the killing power of neutrophils may be increased.

The ingestion of foreign particles, eg, microorganisms, has the following effects on phagocytic granulocytes: (1) Oxygen consumption increases and there is an increased generation of superoxide anion (O_2^-) and an increased release of H_2O_2. (2) Glycolysis increases via the hexose monophosphate shunt. (3) Lysosomes rupture, and their hydrolytic enzymes are discharged into the phagocytic vacuole to form a digestive vacuole, or "phagolysosome." Morphologically, this process appears as **"degranulation"** of granulocytes.

Granulocytes (polymorphonuclear leukocytes) contain at least 2 types of granules: lysosomes that appear to be "bags" of hydrolytic enzymes, and granules consisting of basic proteins that have antibacterial effects but no known enzymatic function, eg, phagocytin or lactoferrin.

The functional mechanisms of intracellular killing of microorganisms in phagocytic granulocytes are not fully known. They include nonoxidative mechanisms (eg, activation of hydrolytic enzymes in contact with microorganisms, action of basic proteins) and oxidative mechanisms. Among the latter, the following have been implicated:

(1) The increased oxidative activity results in accumulation of H_2O_2. In the presence of oxidizable cofactors (halides such as iodine, bromine, chlorine), an acid pH, and the enzyme myeloperoxidase, intensive oxidation results in microbial death.

Children suffering from "granulomatous disease" have granulocytes that ingest microbes normally but lack the subsequent respiratory burst and normal intracellular killing (see below). In Chédiak-Higashi syndrome, most microorganisms are phagocytosed normally, but intracellular killing is impaired, perhaps because myeloperoxidase is not released from (abnormal) lysosomes. Ascorbate can correct this defect.

(2) In normal granulocytes, superoxide anion (O_2^-) is generated upon phagocytosis of particles and destroyed by superoxide dismutase. The superoxide radical may be directly lethal for many microorganisms. "Granulomatous disease" granulocytes have a greatly reduced capacity for generation of superoxide radicals after ingestion of microorganisms. Perhaps this defect is responsible for the impaired killing ability of granulocytes from such patients, which promotes their susceptibility to infections, especially those due to staphylococci.

When the bone marrow of patients is suppressed by disease, drugs, or radiation, the number of functional granulocytes falls. If the level drops below 500 polymorphonuclear neutrophils per microliter, the patient is highly susceptible to "opportunistic" infections by bacteria. Such patients may have their antibacterial defenses boosted temporarily by granulocyte transfusions.

Corticosteroids probably increase the stability of lysosomal membranes. This may contribute to the diminished ability of phagocytes to eradicate bacterial and fungal infection in persons receiving high doses of corticosteroids.

In bacterial infections, the number of circulating neutrophilic leukocytes often increases. In addition, these neutrophils reduce colorless nitroblue tetrazolium (NBT) to intracellular blue-black formazan granules. The presence of more than 10% NBT-positive neutrophils suggests the presence of bacterial infection. Depressed NBT responses occur in patients with defective phagocytic immune mechanisms, eg, chronic granulomatous disease. However, the correlation is not good between defective bactericidal activity and increased NBT-positive neutrophils.

Macrophages (circulating phagocytic monocytes) are derived from monocyte stem cells in bone marrow, have a longer life span than circulating granulocytic phagocytes, and continue their activity at lower pH.

Macrophages (mononuclear phagocytes) in blood can be activated by a variety of "activators," or stimulants (Fig 11–1), including microbes and their products, antigen-antibody complexes, inflammation, sensitized T lymphocytes, lymphokines (see below), injury, and others. Activated macrophages have an increased number of lysosomes and produce and release interleukin-1, a substance or mixture of substances with a wide range of activity in inflammation. Interleukin-1 participates in the production of fever and in the activation of other phagocytic cells and T cells and B cells to produce their resulting effects (Fig 11–1).

Intracellular killing in macrophages probably includes mechanisms similar to those described above for granulocytes. However, the role of superoxide anion is less well defined.

All types of phagocytic cells (granulocytes, macrophages in blood, and fixed macrophages of the reticuloendothelial system) may kill ingested microorganisms or may permit their prolonged survival or even their intracellular multiplication. It is evident that the outcome of phagocytosis is determined by a complex set of factors, including the specific nature of the microorganism and the genetic and functional makeup and the preconditioning of phagocytic cells.

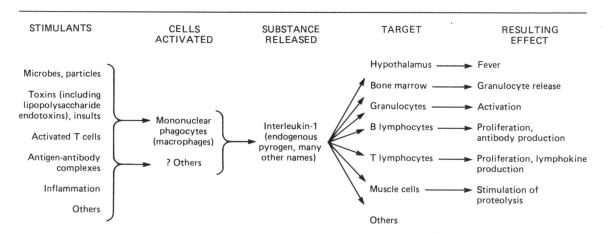

Figure 11–1. Scheme of interleukin-1 production and some of its effects, including fever.

Reticuloendothelial System

This refers to a functional concept of mononuclear phagocytic cells in blood, lymphoid tissue, liver, spleen, bone marrow, lung, and other tissues that are efficient in uptake and removal of particulate matter from lymph and bloodstream. It includes cells lining blood and lymph sinuses (Kupffer cells in the liver) and histiocytes of tissues (macrophages). An important function of the spleen, bone marrow, and other reticuloendothelial organs is the filtering of microorganisms from the bloodstream. Patients whose spleens were removed or are nonfunctional (eg, in sickle cell disease) often suffer from bacterial sepsis, particularly with pneumococci. Phagocytosis by reticuloendothelial cells is greatly enhanced by opsonins.

Biochemical Tissue Constituents

Certain animal tissues are resistant to specific bacteria (eg, *Bacillus anthracis*) because of their content of basic polypeptides, which have antibacterial properties. Such biochemical constituents may determine tissue resistance to infection. Beta lysin of serum can kill some gram-positive bacteria. The nutritional status of the host plays an important role in susceptibility or resistance to a given infection.

The role of interferon in resistance to virus infections is discussed in Chapter 33.

Many normal tissues have a high inherent ability to inhibit proliferation of microorganisms. This resistance is severely impaired by trauma, foreign bodies, disturbances in fluid and electrolyte balance, and depressed inflammatory response (x ray radiation, corticosteroids, anticancer drugs, lymphomas).

Inflammatory Response

Any injury to tissue, such as that following the establishment and multiplication of microorganisms, calls forth an inflammatory response. This begins with dilation of local arterioles and capillaries, from which plasma escapes. Edema fluid accumulates in the area of injury, and fibrin forms a network and occludes the lymphatic channels, tending to limit the spread of organisms. Polymorphonuclear leukocytes in the capillaries stick to the walls, then migrate out of the capillaries toward the irritant. This migration is stimulated by substances in the inflammatory exudate (chemotaxis). The phagocytes engulf the microorganisms, and intracellular digestion begins. Soon the pH of the inflamed area becomes more acid, and the cellular proteases tend to induce lysis of the leukocytes. Large mononuclear macrophages arrive on the site and, in turn, engulf leukocytic debris as well as microorganisms and pave the way for resolution of the local inflammatory process.

Among probable mediators of the inflammatory response are lymphokines (see below) and derivatives of arachidonic acid, including prostaglandins, leukotrienes, and thromboxanes. Drugs that inhibit the synthesis of prostaglandins (by blocking the enzyme cyclooxygenase) act as anti-inflammatory agents.

Different stages in the inflammatory sequence may predominate with different microorganisms as the inciting cause of the inflammation. The early edema fluid may actually promote bacterial growth. The degree of local fixation depends on the nature of the organism: staphylococci tend to limit their spread through extensive lymphatic thrombi, fibrin walls, etc, precipitated by coagulase, whereas hemolytic streptococci, through the activity of streptokinase (fibrinolysin) and hyaluronidase, tend to spread rapidly through the tissue. Phagocytosis and intracellular residence are destructive to some bacteria (some pyogenic cocci), whereas for others (eg, tubercle bacilli) they serve as a means of transport and protection and even of multiplication.

Fever

Fever is certainly the most common systemic manifestation of the inflammatory response and a cardinal symptom of infectious diseases. Possible mechanisms of fever production must therefore be discussed.

A. Possible Mechanisms of Fever Production: The ultimate regulators of body temperature are the thermoregulatory centers in the hypothalamus. They are subject to physical and chemical stimuli. Direct mechanical injury or the application of chemical substances to these centers results in fever. Neither of these obvious forms of stimulation is present in the many types of fever that are associated with infection, neoplasms, hypersensitivity, and other processes that cause inflammation.

Among the substances capable of inducing fever are the endotoxins of gram-negative bacteria and extracts of cells—especially monocytes and macrophages—called interleukin-1. These 2 substances differ as follows:

1. Endotoxins—Endotoxins are heat-stable lipopolysaccharides. After intravenous injection, there is a 60- to 90-minute latent period until the onset of fever. Repeated intravenous injection of endotoxin makes the recipient **tolerant:** no response occurs to further injections of endotoxin.

2. Interleukin-1—Interleukin-1 (endogenous pyrogen, lymphocyte activating factor, many other terms depending on its effect) is heat-labile (destroyed by 90 °C for 30 minutes). After intravenous injection, fever begins in a few minutes, even in endotoxin-tolerant recipients. Repeated injection of interleukin-1 does not induce unresponsiveness.

It appears that a variety of activators can act upon mononuclear phagocytes and perhaps other cells and induce them to release interleukin-1. Among the activators (Fig 11–1) are microbes and their products; toxins, including microbial endotoxins; antigen-antibody complexes; inflammatory processes; and many others. The released interleukin-1 is carried in the bloodstream to the thermoregulatory center in the hypothalamus, where physiologic responses are initiated that result in fever, eg, increased heat production, reduced heat loss. Associated effects of interleukin-1 are mentioned below.

Lymphokines are regulatory mediators that are

produced by certain lymphoid cells and influence other lymphoid cells. Interleukin-1 promotes lymphocyte proliferation in addition to inducing fever (see above and Fig 11–1). Interleukin-2 (formerly called T cell growth factor) is produced by T cells. Gamma interferon, also produced by T cells, is another lymphokine with numerous immunomodulating functions. Several other lymphokines exist (see p 196).

Interleukin-1 appears to be a protein with a molecular weight of 15,000 and an isoelectric point near 6.9. It is inactivated rapidly by pH above 8.0 or heat and is stabilized by sulfhydryl-reducing agents. It induces no tolerance (see above) when administered repeatedly, and its activity is greatly augmented when it is injected directly into the hypothalamus. Interleukin-1 can stimulate muscle proteolysis (muscle wasting during fever) by increasing the production of prostaglandin E_2 (PGE_2). Cyclooxygenase inhibitors can prevent this.

It is possible to demonstrate some beneficial effects of fever on the control of infection in isolated instances. For example, antibody production and T cell proliferation are more efficient at elevated than at normal body temperatures. Poikilothermic lizards can resist bacterial infection at elevated environmental temperatures but will die of the same infection in a cool environment. In humans, no consistent benefits can be attributed to fever for the control of infection. Suppression of fever by drugs (eg, aspirin) is not harmful during infections and often makes febrile patients more comfortable.

B. Some Causes of Persistent Fever of Unknown Origin (FUO) Lasting More Than 3 Weeks: If the usual diagnostic procedures (including thorough bacteriologic and serologic studies) fail to reveal the diagnosis, consider early biopsy. Some causes of persistent fever of unknown origin are listed in Table 11–2.

Table 11–2. Some causes of persistent fever of unknown origin lasting more than 3 weeks.

Infections (bacterial, fungal, parasitic, viral)—Especially mycobacterial infection, liver and biliary tract disease, infective endocarditis, abscesses, urinary tract disease.

Neoplasms—Especially those involving the kidneys, lungs, thyroid, liver, pancreas; lymphomas, leukemias, myeloma.

Hypersensitivity diseases—Visceral angiitis, disseminated lupus erythematosus, polyarteritis nodosa, scleroderma, dermatomyositis, rheumatic fever, drug fever, rheumatoid arthritis.

Granulomatous diseases—Regional enteritis, granulomatous hepatitis.

Neurogenic or endocrine disorders—Lesions of brain stem and thalamus; encephalitis, hyperthyroidism; exaggerated circadian temperature variation.

Factitious fever—Malingering.

Miscellaneous—Sarcoidosis, thrombophlebitis, infarction, poisons, drugs, etc.

RESISTANCE & IMMUNITY

In the preceding section were described various properties of the host that give nonspecific resistance to infection. The term "immunity" signifies all those properties of the host that confer resistance to a specific infectious agent. This resistance may be of all degrees, from almost complete susceptibility to complete insusceptibility. Therefore, "resistance" and "immunity" are relative terms implying only that one host is more or less susceptible to a given infection than another host. No inference can be drawn regarding the possible mechanisms of this resistance.

Immunity may be natural or acquired. Acquired immunity may be passive or active.

NATURAL IMMUNITY

Natural immunity is that type of immunity which is not acquired through previous contact with the infectious agent (or with a related species) but is largely genetically determined. Little is known about the mechanism responsible for this form of resistance.

Species Immunity

A given pathogenic microorganism is often capable of producing disease in one animal species but not in another. *Mycobacterium leprae* can produce disease in humans but not in monkeys or apes; *B anthracis* infects humans but not chickens (perhaps because of the higher body temperatures of fowl); *Neisseria gonorrhoeae* infects humans and chimpanzees but no other animal species.

Racial Basis of Immunity

Within one animal species, there may be marked racial and genetic differences in susceptibility. Some dark-skinned human races have a 10 times greater chance of developing disseminated coccidioidomycosis following primary infection than light-skinned races. Certain strains of mice are highly susceptible to viral and resistant to bacterial infections; with other strains, the opposite is true.

In a few instances, the biochemical basis of racial (genetic) immunity is known. For example, a hereditary deficiency of glucose 6-phosphate dehydrogenase (G6PD) occurs in the red blood cells of certain individuals. Such persons are markedly less susceptible to *Plasmodium falciparum* malaria but more susceptible to red cell hemolysis after certain drugs (sulfonamides, primaquine, nitrofurans) than persons with normal G6PD content. Persons with sickle cell anemia are highly resistant to *P falciparum* infection. Blacks may be resistant to *Plasmodium vivax* infection if their red blood cells lack the Duffy surface antigen, which may act as a receptor for the parasite. The genetic basis of several specific defects of immune responses is under study. (See the discussion of HLA immune response genes on p 168.)

Individual Resistance

As with any biologic phenomenon, resistance to infection varies with different individuals of the same species and race, following a distribution curve for the host population. Thus, certain individuals may be discovered within a "highly susceptible population" who unaccountably cannot be infected with a certain microorganism even though they have had no previous contact with it. Other individuals have genetic defects (see above) in immunologic responsiveness, antibody production, or phagocyte function that make them unusually susceptible to infections. Nutritional status (eg, protein deficiency may enhance susceptibility; microorganisms may be pathogenic by competing for iron with the host), exposure to ionizing radiation or immunosuppressive drugs, and hormonal balance all greatly influence individual susceptibility.

Differences Due to Age

In general, the very young and the elderly are more susceptible to bacterial disease than persons in other age groups. Many age differences in specific infections can be related to physiologic factors. Thus, bacterial meningitis during the first month of life is often caused by coliform bacteria because bactericidal antibodies to these bacteria are IgM and thus fail to cross the placenta. Gonococcal vaginitis occurs mainly in small girls: near puberty, estrogen production results in epithelial cell cornification and a more acid pH, which induce relative resistance.

Some virus infections (eg, rubella) damage the fetus severely but otherwise produce only mild disease. Rickettsial infections are, by contrast, more severe with advancing age. There are many other examples.

Hormonal & Metabolic Influences

Many known hormones influence susceptibility to infection. Only 2 examples are listed here.

In diabetes mellitus, there is increased susceptibility to infections of the vagina and pyogenic infections of tissue. The latter may be due in part to altered metabolism, elevated glucose, lowered pH, reduced influx of phagocytic cells, and diminished bactericidal activity of phagocytic cells.

Both in hypoadrenal (Addison's disease) and in hyperadrenal (Cushing's disease) states, susceptibility to infection is increased. Administration of corticosteroids in high doses has similar effects. Bacterial infections are enhanced because of the suppression of the inflammatory response by glucocorticoids. Viral infections (herpes keratitis, varicella) are aggravated by corticosteroids, perhaps because of suppression of interferon production. Huge doses of corticosteroids can directly suppress antibody formation.

Certain clinical associations between an underlying constitutional disorder and a supervening infection are so frequent as to deserve listing:

Sickle cell anemia: *Salmonella* osteomyelitis, pneumococcal bacteremia, meningitis.

Splenectomy: pneumococcal bacteremia.

Diabetes **mellitus** (especially ketosis): mucormycosis (zygomycosis), probably also increased susceptibility to urinary tract infection; papillary necrosis with pyelonephritis; malignant external otitis caused by *P aeruginosa*.

Cirrhosis, nephrosis: pneumococcal peritonitis.

Hypoparathyroidism: candidiasis.

Pulmonary alveolar proteinosis: nocardiosis.

Lymphocytic leukemia: disseminated herpes zoster, cytomegalovirus.

Immunosuppression by drugs: many "opportunistic" infections—viral, bacterial, fungal, protozoal.

ACQUIRED IMMUNITY

Passive Immunity

"Passive immunity" means a state of relative temporary insusceptibility to an infectious agent that has been induced by the administration of antibodies preformed against that agent in another host rather than formed actively by the individual. Because the antibody molecules are decaying steadily while no new ones are being formed, passive protection lasts only a short time—usually a few weeks at most. On the other hand, the protective mechanism is in force immediately upon administration of antibody: there is no lag period such as is required for the formation of active immunity. Antibodies play only a limited role in invasive bacterial infections, and passive immunization (eg, the administration of convalescent serum or globulin) is rarely useful in that type of disease. On the other hand, when an illness is largely attributable to a toxin (eg, diphtheria, tetanus, botulism), the passive administration of antitoxin is of the greatest use because large amounts of antitoxin can be made immediately available for neutralization of the toxin. In certain virus infections (eg, measles, hepatitis A), specific antibodies that are found in normal human plasma or pooled gamma globulin (immune globulin USP) can be injected during the incubation period to limit viral replication and to prevent or modify the clinical disease.

Passive immunity resulting from the in utero transfer to the fetus of antibodies formed earlier in the mother protects the newborn child during the first months of life against some common infections. Passive immunity (acquired from the mother's blood) may be reinforced by antibodies taken up by the child in mother's milk (mainly colostrum), but that immunity wanes at age 4–6 months.

Active Immunity

Active immunity is a state of resistance built up in an individual following effective contact with foreign antigens, eg, microorganisms or their products. "Effective contact" may consist of clinical or subclinical infection, injection with live or killed microorganisms or their antigens, or absorption of bacterial products (eg, toxins, toxoids). In all these instances, the host actively produces antibodies, and the host's cells learn to respond to the foreign material. Active immunity develops slowly over a period of days or weeks but tends to persist, usually for years. A few of the mechanisms that make up the resistance of acquired immunity can be defined.

A. Humoral Immunity: Active production of **antibodies** against antigens of microorganisms or their products. These antibodies may induce resistance because they (1) neutralize toxins or cellular products; (2) have direct bactericidal or lytic effect with complement; (3) block the infective ability of microorganisms or viruses; (4) agglutinate microorganisms, making them more subject to phagocytosis; or (5) opsonize microorganisms, ie, combine with surface antigens that normally interfere with phagocytosis and thus contribute to the ingestion of parasites.

Antibody formation is disturbed in certain individuals with agammaglobulinemia, B cell deficiency, or T cell dysfunction (see Chapter 12).

B. Cellular Immunity: Although antibodies arise in response to foreign antigens, they often play only a minor role in the defense of the organism against invading microbes. The central position in such defenses is occupied by cell-mediated immune responses of great complexity, combining immunologically specific and nonspecific features. Circulating thymus-dependent lymphoid cells (see T and B cells, Chapter 12) recognize materials as foreign and initiate a chain of responses that include mononuclear inflammatory reactions, cytotoxic destruction of invading cells (microbial, graft, or neoplastic), "activation" of phagocytic macrophages (see p 164), and delayed type hypersensitivity reactions in tissues. In the course of these events, foreign microorganisms or cells are fixed at their point of entry, thus limiting invasiveness (see tuberculosis, p 286); the phagocytic capacity of cells (polymorphonuclears, macrophages, reticuloendo-thelial) is enhanced; ingested microbes or cells are more effectively killed, especially in "activated" macrophages (see p 164); and the biochemical environment in tissues is made less favorable for spread and multiplication of the parasite.

GENETIC INFLUENCES

Natural and acquired immunity and predisposition toward specific disease states have a genetic component. Disease susceptibility is related to genes closely associated with the major histocompatibility complex (see Chapter 13), particularly the HLA-D region located on chromosome 6 in humans. Genes in this region are particularly involved in disorders suspected of having an immunologic component; therefore, this region is believed to carry immune response (Ir) genes. An example of a specific correlation is the association of HLA-B27 with ankylosing spondylitis and juvenile arthritis in humans; the association of multiple sclerosis with HLA-Dw2 and of juvenile-onset diabetes with HLA-DR3 and -DR4 is less regular. The basis for this association of specific genes with specific disease susceptibility is not clear. Possible explanations are that (1) HLA antigens may serve as cell-surface receptors for viruses or toxins; (2) HLA antigen may be incorporated into a viral coat protein; (3) HLA antigens may not themselves be responsible but may be linked to immune response genes that do determine actual susceptibility; and (4) HLA antigens may cross-react with the antigens of bacteria, viruses, or other inciting agents to trigger "autoimmune responses." It is evident that increasing attention will focus on genetic features linking disease susceptibility to major histocompatibility antigens.

REFERENCES

Atkins E: Fever: New perspectives on an old phenomenon. *N Engl J Med* 1983;**308:**958.

Bach FH, van Rood JJ: The major histocompatibility complex: Genetics and biology. (3 parts.) *N Engl J Med* 1976;**295:**806, 872, 927.

Bartlett JG, Onderdonk AB: Virulence factors of anaerobic bacteria. *Rev Infect Dis* 1979;**1:**398.

Beisel WR et al: Single-nutrient effects on immunologic functions. *JAMA* 1981;**245:**53.

Boxer LA et al: Correction of leukocyte function in Chédiak-Higashi syndrome by ascorbate. *N Engl J Med* 1976;**295:**1041.

Chandra RK: Nutritional deficiency and susceptibility to infection. *Bull WHO* 1979;**57:**167.

Densen P, Mandell GL: Phagocyte strategy vs microbial tactics. *Rev Infect Dis* 1980;**2:**817.

Dinarello CA: Interleukin-1 and the pathogenesis of the acute-phase reaction. *N Engl J Med* 1984;**311:**1413.

Dinarello CA, Wolff SM: Molecular basis of fever in humans. *Am J Med* 1982;**72:**799.

Elsbach P: Degradation of microorganisms by phagocytic cells. *Rev Infect Dis* 1980;**2:**106.

Evans AS: Causation and disease: The Henle-Koch postulates revisited. *Yale J Biol Med* 1976;**49:**175.

Gardner ID: The effect of aging on susceptibility to infection. *Rev Infect Dis* 1980;**2:**801.

Gross RL, Newborne PM: Role of nutrition in immunologic functions. *Physiol Rev* 1980;**60:**188.

Herzig RH et al: Successful granulocyte transfusion therapy for gram-negative septicemia. *N Engl J Med* 1977;**296:**701.

Hocking WG, Golde DW: The pulmonary-alveolar macrophage. (2 parts.) *N Engl J Med* 1979;**301:**580, 639.

Klebanoff SJ: Oxygen metabolism and the toxic properties of phagocytes. *Ann Intern Med* 1980;**93:**480.

Matula G, Paterson PY: Reduction of nitroblue-tetrazolium by neutrophils in infection. *N Engl J Med* 1971;**285:**311.

McDevitt H: Regulation of the immune response by the major histocompatibility system. *N Engl J Med* 1980;**303:**1514.

Mills EL, Quie PG: Congenital disorders of the functions of polymorphonuclear neutrophils. *Rev Infect Dis* 1980;**2:**505.

Nathan CF et al: The macrophage as an effector cell. *N Engl J Med* 1980;**303:**622.

Newhouse M et al: Lung defense mechanisms. (2 parts.) *N Engl J Med* 1976;**295:**990, 1045.

Olley PM: The prostaglandins. *Am J Dis Child* 1980;**134:**688.

Orskov F: Virulence factors of the bacterial cell surface. *J Infect Dis* 1978;**137:**630.

Peterson PK, Quie PG: Bacterial surface components and the pathogenesis of infectious diseases. *Annu Rev Med* 1981; **32:**29.

Plaut AG: Microbial IgA proteases. *N Engl J Med* 1978; **298:**1459.

Pollack MS, Rich RR: The HLA complex and the pathogenesis of infectious diseases. *J Infect Dis* 1985;**151:**1.

Repine JE et al: Bactericidal function of neutrophils from patients with acute bacterial infections and from diabetics. *J Infect Dis* 1980;**142:**869.

Ritzmann SE: HLA patterns and disease associations. *JAMA* 1976;**236:**2305.

Ryan GB: Inflammation and localization of infection. *Surg Clin North Am* 1976;**56:**831.

Stossel TP: Phagocytosis. (3 parts.) *N Engl J Med* 1974;**290:** 717, 774, 833.

Immunology: I. Antigens & Antibodies

DEFINITIONS & CELLULAR BASIS OF IMMUNE RESPONSES

DEFINITIONS

An **antigen (Ag)** is a substance that stimulates the formation of an **antibody (Ab)** by cells which specifically react with that antigen in a particular animal. Most complete antigens are proteins, but some are polysaccharides or polypeptides. Most antigens are macromolecules with a molecular weight over 10,000. To act as antigens, substances must be recognized as "foreign" or "nonself" by an animal, since, in general, animals do not produce antibodies to their own ("self") proteins.

Antigenic determinants are those portions of antigen molecules that determine the specificity of antigen-antibody reactions. The term **epitope** denotes the simplest form of an antigenic determinant. The size of the antigenic determinant group may be quite small in relation to the size of the whole antigen molecule, eg, 4–7 amino acid residues or glucose residues.

Haptens are chemicals of low molecular weight that do not by themselves elicit the formation of antibodies but can combine with antibodies elicited by a large molecule that possesses a structural unit similar to or identical with the hapten. Many simple chemicals and drugs can function as haptens. They bind to host proteins or other carriers to form complete antigens.

Antibodies are proteins that are formed in response to an antigen and react specifically with that antigen or one very closely related to it. Only vertebrates make antibodies. Antibodies are specialized proteins, the immunoglobulins. The behavior of these antibodies depends to some extent on the class of immunoglobulins to which they belong.

An **idiotype** is a unique antigenic determinant that is present in the variable domain of a homogeneous antibody. It represents the antigenicity of the antigen-binding site. Anti-idiotype antibodies can be prepared by the use of elaborate absorption procedures.

THE CELLULAR BASIS OF IMMUNE RESPONSES

The capacity to respond to immunologic stimuli rests principally in cells of the lymphoid system. In order to make clear normal immune responses as well as clinically occurring immune deficiency syndromes and their possible management, a brief outline of current concepts of the development of the lymphoid system must be presented.

During embryonic life, a stem cell develops in fetal liver and other organs. This stem cell probably resides in bone marrow in postnatal life. Under the differentiating influence of various environments, it can be induced to differentiate along several different lines. Within fetal liver and later in bone marrow, the stem cell may differentiate into cells of the red cell series or of the granulocyte series. Alternatively, the stem cell may turn into a lymphoid stem cell that may differentiate to form at least 2 distinct lymphocyte populations. One population (called T lymphocytes) is dependent on the presence of a functioning thymus; the other (B lymphocytes, analogous to lymphocytes derived in birds from the bursa of Fabricius) is independent of the thymus. Some characteristics of B and T lymphocytes are described below, and some major differences between these 2 types of cells are listed in Table 12–1. Some cells lack the identifying features of B or T cells and are called null cells. Among null cells are killer cells (K cells), which exhibit antibody-dependent cytotoxicity in vitro, and natural killer cells (NK cells), which function without antibody and participate in lysis of tumor cells or virus-infected cells.

B Lymphocytes

These constitute about 20–25% of the recirculating pool of small lymphocytes, being mostly restricted to lymphoid tissue. Their life span is short (days or weeks). The mammalian equivalent of the avian bursa is not known, but it is believed that gut-associated lymphoid tissue (eg, tonsils, Peyer's patches, appendix) may be an important source of B lymphocytes. B cells are produced abundantly in the absence of a thymus. B cells have abundant membrane-bound immunoglobulin molecules (about 10^5 per cell). Most B cells have only one class of immunoglobulin (Ig) (see p 174) present on the surface, with IgM **predominat-**

Table 12–1. Some differences between T and B cells.

	T Cells	B Cells
Frequency in blood, average	70%	20%*
Frequency in spleen	50%	50%
Immunoglobulins on surface	±	+++
Method of counting	Rosette formation with sheep red cells.	Immunofluorescence with anti-Ig.
Secretion of antibody	–	+
Effector in cell-mediated reactions	+	–
Inactivated by x-ray radiation	–	+
Inactivated by anti-lymphocytic serum	+	–
Recognition of determinants on	Carrier	Hapten

*When T cells and B cells are counted by the methods shown in this table, the sum usually adds up to less than 100% of the total lymphocyte count. The remaining few percent of lymphocytelike cells are null cells.

ing, but some B cells carry both IgM and IgD. In addition, most B cells have a receptor for the Fc portion of immunoglobulin molecules (Fc receptor) and diverse complement receptors. B cells are counted by using fluorescent-labeled anti-immunoglobulin antibody.

When antigen attaches to the surface immunoglobulin or when antigen-antibody complexes attach to the Fc receptors of B cells, the B cells are stimulated to proliferate, differentiate, and mature into plasma cells, large lymphocytes that synthesize the same immunoglobulin that was carried by their B cell precursors. B cell activation and differentiation sometimes require helper T cell activity (see below). Mature B

cells can revert to small lymphocytes that have a long life and serve as B memory cells.

B cell populations are the source of specific immunoglobulins and of antibody production in the host. B cell deficiencies (absence, insufficient numbers, defective function) result in defects in immunoglobulin synthesis (Table 12–2). With certain antigens, especially large polymers (eg, pneumococcal polysaccharide), B cells are stimulated to produce antibodies without the assistance of helper T cells. However, with most antigens that have a smaller number of determinants and require a carrier, T cell cooperation with B cells is needed for antibody production.

B cell overactivity may result from a failure of suppressor T cell control and may lead to autoimmune disorders.

T Lymphocytes

T cells constitute 65–80% of the recirculating pool of small lymphocytes. Their life span is long (months or years). Although they are derived from stem cells in the bone marrow, they require an intact thymus for functional maturation. In early life, the thymus may be a main intermediate source of T lymphocytes that originated in the bone marrow. In later life, the thymus presumably controls T cells through peptide hormones.

T cells do not have surface immunoglobulin receptors and do not differentiate into immunoglobulin-synthesizing cells. However, many human T lymphocytes have membrane receptors for the Fc portion of IgG and monomeric IgM. Virtually all T cells have the ability to form rosettes with sheep erythrocytes, and this feature is used to count T cells.

In mice and humans, T cells have surface antigens (cell membrane markers) that permit definition of T

Table 12–2. Examples of clinical immunodeficiencies.*

Disorder	Postulated Cell Defect		Observed Immunologic Defect
	B	T	
Congenital X-linked agammaglobulinemia (Bruton's)	+	–	Absent plasma cells, all classes of immunoglobulins extremely deficient. Cellular immunity normal.
Transient hypogammaglobulinemia of infancy	+	–	Usually self-limited.
Selective immunoglobulin deficiency (IgA, IgM, or IgG subclass)	+	(–)	IgA-, IgM-, or IgG-producing plasma cells absent, respective immunoglobulin absent. Cellular immunity normal.
Thymic hypoplasia (DiGeorge's syndrome)	–	+	Immunoglobulins normal but some antibody responses deficient. Cellular immunity defective.
(?) Chronic mucocutaneous candidiasis	–	+	
Immunodeficiency with ataxia-telangiectasia	+	+	Variable deficiency in immunoglobulins and antibodies. Cellular immunity defective for some antigens.
Immunodeficiency with thrombocytopenia and eczema (Wiskott-Aldrich syndrome)	(+)	+	Variable deficiency in immunoglobulins and antibodies. Cellular immunity defective for some antigens.
Immunodeficiency (eg, with thymoma; with short-limbed dwarfism; autosomal recessive, combined, X-linked).	+	+	Extremely deficient antibodies. Cellular immunity defective for all antigens.

*Modified from Cooper MD et al: Classification of primary immunodeficiencies. N Engl J Med 1973;**288**:966.
(–) means that there is occasionally a coexisting T cell defect. (+) means that the defect is predominantly T cell but that B cell defects occur also.

cell subsets by the use of monoclonal antibodies specific for these antigens. In mice, one such group of antigens is the Lyt (lymphocyte alloantigen) series; in humans, a similar series is known as either Leu (leukocyte alloantigens) or OKT. The OKT series of monoclonal antibodies is frequently used to identify human T cell subsets, with OKT4 (Leu-3) identifying helper/inducer T cells and OKT8 (Leu-2) identifying suppressor/cytotoxic T cells (see below).

T lymphocytes recognize specific antigens and become able to respond to them; ie, they become "immunologically committed." T cells develop cell-mediated responses that are of particular importance in controlling intracellular parasites (eg, mycobacteria, fungi, viruses, certain protozoa and bacteria) and neoplastic cells. A deficiency of the T cell system manifests itself as an impairment in cell-mediated immunity, particularly against the types of intracellular parasites mentioned above. Because helper T cells are essential in B cell function, a T cell defect may also result in impaired antibody production in spite of an intact B cell system.

A few of the main functions of the T cell system and some important subsets of T lymphocytes are described briefly below:

A. Cell-Mediated Immune Responses: T cells are responsible for delayed type hypersensitivity reactions to many different antigens, in particular those of intracellular parasites (see above) and contact allergens. In delayed type hypersensitivity, some stimulated T cells release soluble substances ("lymphokines") that modulate the behavior of other cells.

B. Cytotoxicity, Tumor Rejection, & Graft Rejection: Some T cells (identified in mice by the Lyt-2,3$^+$ marker and in humans by OKT5) are cytotoxic or lethal for cells that carry specific antigens, Such "killer" (K) cells may damage virus-infected cells, tumor cells, or grafted cells and may also mediate the graft-versus-host reaction.

C. Immunologic Memory: Some T cells divide to form a population of antigen-sensitive cells that have a long life span and contribute importantly to immunologic memory. When such T cells encounter the same antigen later, they are promptly stimulated to proliferate and provide T cell responses.

D. Helper T Cells: (Fig 12–1.) Certain subsets of T cells exert essential "helper" functions for B cells and other T cells. At least some of these helper T cells in humans carry surface molecules that are identified by monoclonal antibody OKT4 (Leu-3). Helper T cell cooperation with B cells is essential in order for the latter to produce antibody responses to many nonpolymer antigens; B cells can interact with haptens but are unable to produce antibodies to them until the hapten carrier has interacted with helper T cells. Helper T cells also cooperate with other T cell populations and modulate their behavior.

E. Suppressor T Cells: Certain subsets of T cells exert important "suppressor" functions on B cells and other T cells. At least some of these suppressor T cells in humans carry surface molecules that are identified

by monoclonal antibody OKT8 (Leu-2). Such cells play a role in immune tolerance; the failure of "suppressor" cell activity on B cells may give rise to autoimmune phenomena. Suppressor T cells also modulate the responses of other T cell populations. Overactivity of suppressor T cells (shown by an inverted OKT4/OKT8 ratio) can result in immunodeficiency states with prominent opportunistic intracellular infections (eg, *Pneumocystis* pneumonia) or with neoplasms (eg, Kaposi's sarcoma), as seen in acquired immune deficiency syndrome (AIDS), and carries a high mortality rate (see Chapter 13).

F. Mitogen Activity: Many T cells undergo blastogenic transformation in vitro when they are exposed to concanavalin A or phytohemagglutinin. These mitogens do not affect B cells.

G. Anatomic Location: Different subpopulations of T lymphocytes occur with different frequency in defined anatomic locations. Thus, OKT8-reactive suppressor T cells predominate in human bone marrow and gut epithelium, and OKT4-reactive helper T cells predominate in thymic medulla, tonsils, and blood.

Cellular Interactions in the Immune Response

The activation of immunocompetent cells and the modulation of their expression is regulated by complex interactions between different cell types. The principal events may be summarized as follows: (1) Macrophages carry antigen on their surface and present it to T lymphocytes. (2) Helper T cells permit activation of B cells, which become antibody-producing plasma cells. (3) Helper T cells enable other T cell subsets to become specifically activated to initiate cell-mediated immune reactions that result in delayed type hypersensitivity, liberation of lymphokines, cell-to-cell interactions, cytotoxicity, etc. (4) Suppressor T cells modulate the response of both B cells and T cell subsets to regulate the magnitude of effect.

Genetic Control of Immune Responses

The responses of lymphoid cells appear to be controlled by "immune response" (Ir) genes. These genes are in the region of the major histocompatibility complex (in humans, HLA-D, which is located on human chromosome 6).

Genes that control the constant (C) and the variable (V) regions of immunoglobulins (Fig 12–4) are both expressed by B cells as they synthesize antibody. T cells also express V genes that code for antigen-binding regions, but they may have different C genes. It is likely that cellular interactions—including helper T cell and suppressor T cell functions—are also controlled by Ir genes. Several disease states that result from defects in lymphocyte cell interactions are associated with specific HLA-D subtypes. These subtypes, in turn, are probably associated with definite Ir genes.

Examples of Clinical Immunodeficiency

In a majority of individuals with **clinical im-**

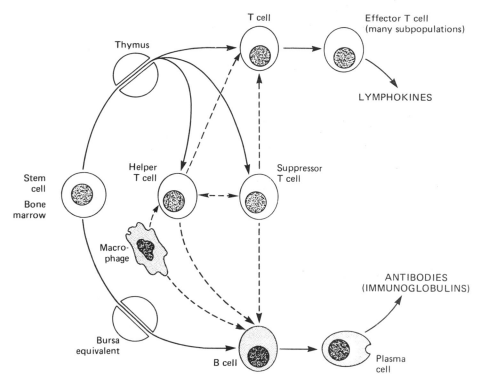

Figure 12–1. Schematic diagram of interactions of the immune system.

munodeficiency, there are complex functional impairments, often involving both B cell and T cell functions. In a few clinical syndromes, the defect is relatively well defined, as illustrated by the examples given in Table 12–2.

Hypersensitivity Reactions

Hypersensitivity or allergic reactions occur in individuals whose reactivity to an antigen has been altered. Reexposure to the same (or a closely related) antigen results in a variety of abnormal reactions. Hypersensitivity reactions are of 2 types: (1) antibody-mediated, or immediate type, reactions and (2) cell-mediated, or delayed type, reactions. Some important

differences between the 2 groups are listed in Table 12–3.

From the standpoint of pathogenesis, hypersensitivity reactions have been classified by Gell and Coombs into 4 major types:

I. Anaphylactic Type Hypersensitivity: A special class of antibody (cytotropic antibody, mainly IgE) binds to mast cells and basophils through the Fc fragment. When antigen reacts with these antibodies, vasoactive amines and other mediators are liberated and elicit the reaction (see Chapter 13).

II. Cytotoxic Type Hypersensitivity: Antigens on the cell surface combine with antibody. This may lead to opsonization and phagocytosis without com-

Table 12–3. Differences between immediate and delayed hypersensitivity reactions.

	Ab-Mediated or Immediate Type	Cell-Mediated or Delayed Type
Clinical examples	Anaphylactic shock; allergy to pollen, with asthma; serum sickness; some allergies to antibiotics; asthma reaction.	Tuberculin hypersensitivity; allergy to fungi (Histoplasma), parasites (trichina), Rhus plants (poison ivy or oak), chemicals (nickel); skin graft rejection.
Timing	The reaction begins immediately, ie, within minutes after contact with the allergen, and disappears within 1 hour.	The reaction is delayed. It begins within several hours after contact with the allergen and may last for days.
Histology	The main pathologic reaction consists of dilatation of capillaries and arterioles, with prominent erythema and edema and only limited polymorphonuclear leukocyte infiltration.	The main pathologic reaction consists of inflammatory change with predominant mononuclear cell infiltration and tissue induration.
Passive transfer	The reaction is associated with circulating antibodies and can be transferred passively by means of serum.	The reaction is not associated with circulating Abs and cannot be transferred passively by means of serum. It can often be transferred passively by means of lymphoid cells or their extracts.

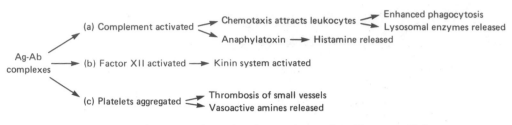

Figure 12–2. Sequence of reactions in complex-mediated hypersensitivity.

plement, may facilitate attack by killer cells, or may lead to binding of complement, which promotes immune adherence to phagocytes; or the lytic effect may result in membrane damage by complement (see Chapter 13).

III. Complex-Mediated Hypersensitivity: Antigens combine with antibody to form complexes that in turn activate complement and factor XII (Hageman factor) and aggregate platelets, with the consequences shown in Fig 12–2.

IV. Cell-Mediated Hypersensitivity: T lymphocytes carrying specific antigen receptors become activated by contact with that antigen, proliferate, transform, and release a variety of mediators (lymphokines) which in turn act on macrophages, lymphocytes, and other cells to yield the reactions of delayed type hypersensitivity (see Chapter 13).

A preliminary fifth type of hypersensitivity reaction has been proposed:

V. Stimulatory Hypersensitivity: Non-complement-binding antibody against cell surface components may actually stimulate the cell. For example, autoantibody to thyrotropin (thyroid-stimulating hormone, TSH) receptor on thyroid cells stimulates cell activity, producing Graves' disease. The antibody action resembles that of TSH.

ANTIBODIES: STRUCTURE & FORMATION

Antibodies are immunoglobulins that can react specifically with the antigen that stimulated their production. Immunoglobulins comprise about 20% of total serum proteins, and a variable proportion of immunoglobulins have antibody activity. Antibodies may be characterized by their chemical, physical, and immunologic properties. Among the prominent physicochemical properties used for classifying antibodies are solubility in salts and solvents, electrophoretic mobility, molecular size, and sedimentation in the ultracentrifuge. Electrophoretically, most antibodies move with the γ and β_2 fractions and a few with α globulins.

In terms of molecular weight (by ultracentrifugal analysis), antibodies fall into 3 main groups: (1) molecular weight 150,000, 7S; (2) 900,000, 19S; and (3) 170,000–400,000, 7S to 11S.

Electrophoresis permits the separation of proteins by migration in an electrical field in paper, starch, gel, etc. From anode toward cathode, albumins migrate slowly the shortest distance, α and β globulins somewhat farther, and γ globulins faster and farther than the others. **Immunoelectrophoresis** is an important tool in immunoglobulin and antibody identification. The techniques described in this chapter (and others) have indicated that antibodies exhibit considerable heterogeneity. Some of this heterogeneity is based on the facts that antibodies to the same antigens are made by different clones of B cells (see below) and that they belong to different immunoglobulin classes. Immunoglobulins are arranged into 5 main classes (Table 12–4).

STRUCTURE OF IMMUNOGLOBULINS

In response to a single pure antigen, a large, heterogeneous population of antibody molecules arises from different clones of cells, ie, they are **polyclonal**. This made study of the chemical structure of immunoglobulins (Igs) virtually impossible until myeloma proteins were isolated. Myelomas are tumors originating as a clone from a single cell. The immunoglobulins produced by myelomas are homogeneous and thus permit chemical analysis of IgG, IgA, IgD, and IgE. In Waldenström's macroglobulinemia (clinically distinct from typical myelomas), a monoclonal IgM is produced. Now, unlimited quantities of pure **monoclonal antibodies** can be made artificially by the "hybridoma" technique. This involves the fusion of plasmacytoma (tumor) cells with isolated spleen cells stimulated by a given antigen. The fused "hybridoma" continues to produce the selected monoclonal antibodies in cell culture for long periods. From the study of myeloma proteins and other monoclonal antibodies, the following generalizations about immunoglobulin structure were derived.

All immunoglobulins have similar structural patterns but great diversity of antigenic properties and amino acid sequences. Immunoglobulin molecules are made up of light (small) and heavy (large) polypeptide chains. Each chain consists of a constant (C) carboxy terminal portion and a variable (V) amino terminal

Table 12–4. Some characteristics of immunoglobulins.

	IgG	IgM	IgA	IgD	IgE
Sedimentation coefficient	7S	19S	7S or 11S*	7S	8S
Molecular weight	150,000	900,000	170,000 or 400,000*	180,000	190,000
Heavy chain symbol	γ	μ	α	δ	ϵ
Average concentration in normal serum (mg/dL)	1000–1500	60–180	100–400	3–5	0.03
Half-life in serum (days)	23	5	6	3	2.5
Prominent in external secretions	–	–	++	–	+
Percent carbohydrate	4	15	10	18	18
Crosses placenta	+	–	–	?	–
Fixes complement	+	+	–	–	–
Examples of antibodies	Many Abs to toxins, bacteria, viruses; especially late in Ab response.	Many Abs to infectious agents, especially early in Ab response; antipolysaccharide Ab; cold agglutinins.	Important as secretory antibody on mucous membranes.	No proved Ab activity; main immunoglobulin on surface of β lymphocytes in newborn.	Binds to mast and basophil cells; raised in allergic and parasitic infections.

*11S, molecular weight 400,000 IgA in external secretions; 7S, molecular weight 170,000 IgA in serum.

portion, each of which, in turn, is genetically determined. Thus, each immunoglobulin chain is coded by separate gene clusters, one for the constant region and 2 or more for the variable region (see p 178). Heavy and light chains are held together by disulfide bonds (Fig 12–3) and can be isolated by reduction followed by chromatography at acid pH. The chains are folded 3-dimensionally with disulfide bonds to form **domains**. There are **variable** and **constant** domains.

Light (L) Chains

These always belong to one of 2 types: κ (kappa) and λ (lambda), with molecular weights of 25,000. Both types occur in all classes of immunoglobulin, but any one molecule contains only one type of L chain. Some myeloma tumors secrete homogeneous L chains, either κ or λ type, called Bence Jones proteins, which are excreted in urine. The hereditary human globulin marker Km is located on κ L chains. In primary amyloidosis, the amyloid fibrils contain L chains, possibly fragments of autoantibodies.

Heavy (H) Chains

Each of the 5 immunoglobulin classes has an antigenically distinct set of H chains (isotypes) with molecular weights of 50,000–70,000. The 5 heavy chain types are called γ in IgG, μ in IgM, α in IgA, δ in IgD, and ϵ in IgE. The portion of H chains that is not involved in the antibody combining site (Fc fragment) carries the sites for various effector reactions (biologic activity), eg, complement fixation, placental transfer, attachment to phagocytic cells, degranulation of mast cells, and skin fixation. It also is the site of the human genetic Gm markers on IgG (with which rheumatoid factors react) and of most of the carbohydrate moiety of immunoglobulins. In "heavy chain disease," H chains linked by disulfide bonds are excreted in urine.

Immunoglobulin fragments resulting from enzymatic treatment of immunoglobulin molecules are shown schematically in Fig 12–3.

Treatment of a 7S IgG molecule with papain results in the production of 3 fragments. Two of these are identical antigen-binding Fab fragments (each of which is univalent, containing a single antigen-binding site). The third is the Fc fragment, which carries no antibody activity but a variety of effector reactions (see above).

Treatment of the IgG molecule with pepsin results

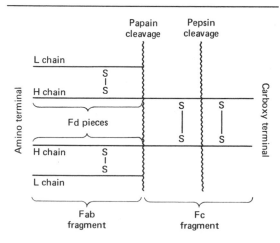

Figure 12–3. Schematic representation of a 7S immunoglobulin (IgG) molecule.

in similar fragments (Fig 12–3). Thus, Fab fragments are joined to the Fc fragments by peptide bonds that are readily cleaved by proteases. These act mainly in the "hinge" region.

The piece of heavy chain within the Fab fragment is called the Fd piece.

Combining Site

The biologic activity of an antibody molecule centers on its ability to specifically bind antigens. The combining site is located on the amino terminal end of the antibody molecule (Fig 12–4) and is composed of certain **hypervariable** folded segments within the variable regions of both L and H chains. The active sites of certain antibodies are estimated to be just large enough to accommodate 4–6 glucose residues. It has been estimated that of the approximately 650 amino acid residues of an L chain–H chain pair, between 15 and 30 amino acid residues may be involved in each antibody combining site. Antibody specificity is a function of both the amino acid sequence and its 3-dimensional configuration.

Immunoglobulin G (IgG)

IgG comprises about 75% of immunoglobulins in normal human sera. Each molecule of IgG consists of 2 L chains and 2 H chains (Fig 12–4) linked by 20 to 25 –S–S– bonds. There are 4 subclasses of IgG (IgG-1 to IgG-4), based on antigenic differences in H chains. Each IgG molecule has only one type of L chain and one type of H chain. IgG is the *only* immunoglobulin to cross the placenta and to produce passive cutaneous anaphylaxis. IgG synthesis in humans is about 35 mg/kg/d, and its half-life is about 23 days. Normal adult serum levels (1000–1500 mg/dL) are reached at 2 years of age and decrease from the fourth decade onward.

IgG molecules are probably Y-shaped, with a "hinge region" near the middle of the heavy chain connecting the 2 Fab segments to the Fc segment. The IgG molecule can probably assume various angles at the "hinge." Since each Fab segment has one antigen-binding site, an IgG molecule has a valence of 2. Carbohydrate is less abundant in IgG (4%) than in other immunoglobulin classes. Carbohydrate (located on the Fc and occasionally also on Fab segments) may provide binding sites for receptors and may play a role in immunoglobulin secretion by plasma cells.

The heterogeneity between IgG subclasses (in antigenicity or amino acid sequence) is less than that between different immunoglobulin classes. There are small differences in effector functions among subclasses because of different H chains.

IgG antibodies can probably attach to various cells through the Fc fragment and participate in anaphylactic (immediate) type reactions.

Immunoglobulin M (IgM)

IgM comprises about 10% of the immunoglobulin in normal human sera. The greater size of IgM molecules (19S, MW 900,000) is due to 5 units (each similar to one IgG unit) linked through –S–S– bonds near their "hinge regions." Reducing agents (eg, mercaptoethanol) tend to break these linking disulfide bonds

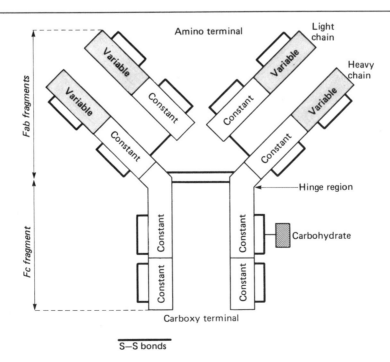

Figure 12–4. Schematic representation of an IgG molecule indicating the location of the constant and the variable regions on the light and the heavy chains.

and dissociate IgM molecules into 5 subunits of 7–8S. IgM can usually be distinguished from IgG and other immunoglobulin classes because treatment with mercaptoethanol results in a loss of agglutinating activity.

Each subunit of IgM consists of 2 L chains and 2 H chains. In addition, there is one J chain (MW 15,000) per 10 L chains of IgM molecules. The J chain is acidic and differs in antigenicity and amino acid composition from the other chains. It probably aids in polymerization and stabilization of IgM (and IgA) molecules. IgM molecules may also contain a secretory component (see below).

Since each IgM molecule has 10 Fab segments, it can combine with up to 10 antigenic sites. It has a valence of from 5 (due to steric hindrance) to 10 (Fig 12–5).

IgM molecules are the earliest antibodies synthesized in response to antigenic stimulation. They fix complement well in the presence of antigen. The rate of IgM synthesis is about 8 mg/kg/d, and the half-life in serum is about 5 days. The fetus synthesizes IgM in utero. Since IgM does not cross the placenta, IgM antibodies in the newborn are thus considered a sign of intrauterine infection. Adult serum levels (60–180 mg/dL) are reached at 6–9 months after birth.

Immunoglobulin A (IgA)

The basic structural unit of IgA corresponds to that of IgG, with 2 H and 2 L chains. While IgG is uniformly a monomer, IgA can occur as a 7S monomer or a 9S dimer. IgA comprises about 15% of the immunoglobulin in human serum. It occurs mainly as a monomer, and its average concentration is 100–400 mg/dL. Serum IgA is synthesized at the rate of approximately 35 mg/kg/d, and it is rapidly catabolized. In humans and other mammals, IgA is the principal immunoglobulin in external secretions of the respiratory, intestinal, and genitourinary tracts and in tears, saliva, and milk. This secretory IgA is produced by plasma cells within mucous membranes at the various locations. It exists mainly as a dimer that contains a J chain (see above) and also a polypeptide chain (MW 60,000) called **secretory component.** The secretory component appears to be synthesized in specialized cells in the epithelium and linked to the IgA dimer as it is transported through the mucous membrane epithelium. The production of secretory IgA is stimulated more effectively by local than by systemic infection or antigen administration. IgA (serum or secretory) does *not* fix complement in the presence of antigen but may activate C3 by the alternative pathway. Secretory IgA can neutralize viruses and can inhibit attachment of bacteria to epithelial cells unless cleaved by microbial proteases.

Immunoglobulin D (IgD)

This immunoglobulin was first encountered as a myeloma protein and then found in trace amounts (3–5 mg/dL) in normal sera. IgD is rapidly catabolized and has a half-life of only 3 days. IgD has not been proved to have antibody activity. IgD (with IgM) has been demonstrated on the surface of B lymphocytes in cord blood and also on cells in certain lymphatic leukemias.

Immunoglobulin E (IgE)

In normal sera, IgE is found only in minute concentration (0.03 mg/dL). Intact IgE molecules are 8S, with a molecular weight of 190,000. The H chains of IgE are longer than those of IgG by about 100 amino acid residues, perhaps indicating a special function. IgE mediates allergic reactions in skin and other tissues and, with the Fc fragment, binds to mast cells and basophils. The latter degranulate upon exposure to the specific antigen, with the liberation of mediators (see pp 191–192). Whereas most immunoglobulins are quite heat-stable, IgE loses the ability to sensitize skin after being heated for 4 hours at 56 °C.

In persons with allergic reactivity of the antibody-mediated (immediate) type, the serum concentrations of IgE are greatly increased. In such individuals, IgE also appears in external secretions and mediates local allergic reactions. The serum level of IgE is increased in parasitic infections (helminthiases).

One or more immunoglobulins may be present in abnormally high concentration in neoplasms of plasma cells (myelomas), in liver disease, in chronic protozoal or microbial infections, and in autoimmune diseases. Deficiencies of specific immunoglobulins often have a hereditary basis and can be due to absence of specific cells, impaired synthesis, or increased catabolism (see previous section).

Antibody Formation

The mechanism by which antibodies are formed has been debated for years. The **instructive theory** proposed that the specificity of an antibody molecule was determined not by its amino acid sequence but by

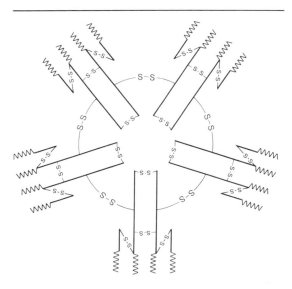

Figure 12–5. Schematic diagram of the pentameric structure of human IgM.

the molding of the peptide chain around the antigenic determinant; the presence of antigen was required to serve as a template. This theory was abandoned when it became apparent that antibody-forming cells were devoid of antigen and that antibody specificity was a function of amino acid sequence.

At present, the **clonal selection theory** is accepted. It holds that an immunologically responsive cell can respond to only one antigen or a closely related group of antigens and that this property is inherent in the cell before the antigen is encountered. According to the clonal selection theory, each individual is endowed with a large pool of lymphocytes (about 10^7), each of which is capable of responding to a different antigen; when the antigen enters the body, it selects the lymphocyte that has the best "fit" by virtue of a surface receptor. The antigen binds to this antibodylike receptor, and the cell is stimulated to proliferate and form a clone of cells (clonal amplification). Thus, selected B cells quickly differentiate into plasma cells and secrete antibody that is specific for the antigen which served as the original selecting agent (or a closely related group of antigens).

Synthesis of Antibodies

The initial step in antibody formation is the phagocytosis of antigen by macrophages. These macrophages present the antigen to B cells and helper T cells. B cells that carry on their surface the immunoglobulin which matches the antigen become stimulated to proliferate, form clones, and differentiate into plasma cells. The latter synthesize antibody proteins.

Immunoglobulin genes occur on widely separated fragments of DNA. There is one gene for the constant (C) region and 2 or more gene segments—V, D, J (see below)—for the variable (V) region of chains. During cell differentiation, the DNA is rearranged to form functional genes for antibody production. In a given mature B cell producing immunoglobulin, one gene is assembled for the production of a single type of L chain (either κ or λ) and one gene for the production of a single type of H chain. After mRNA has been transcribed from each gene, H and L chains are synthesized on polyribosomes. The chains are then linked by disulfide bonds in the form of H_2L_2 units, and the sugar moiety is added before the immunoglobulin molecule is released from the cell.

The remarkable diversity of antibodies, ie, the enormous number of antibody specificities, arises from several factors, including (1) multiple gene regions; (2) rearrangement of DNA to bring together V, J (junction), and D (diversity) segments in H chain sequences; and (3) independence of L and H chain structures.

Although a given cell produces only one immunoglobulin type at one time, the so-called **IgM-IgG switch** may occur: initially, IgM is synthesized; later, the genes controlling the variable regions of the H chain of IgM may recombine with genes controlling the constant regions of IgG so that the IgG later produced is of the same specificity as the earlier IgM.

With certain antigens, the induction of an antibody response requires the cooperation of B cells with T cells as well as with macrophages. Helper T cells that recognize the T-dependent antigen by means of surface receptor molecules interact with antigen-specific B cells. Conversely, "suppressor" T cells may inhibit responses by B cells. HLA-linked immune response genes control this B cell–T cell interaction.

The Primary Response

When an animal or human is injected with an antigen—and if this represents the individual's first contact with that antigen—there is a rise in detectable antibody in serum within several days, depending on the route of injection and the dose and nature of the antigen. The antibody concentration then rises to a peak within 1–10 weeks, then drops, and may fall below detectable levels (Fig 12–6). In general, IgM antibodies appear earlier than IgG antibodies in the primary response. IgM antibody concentrations decline more rapidly than IgG antibody concentrations because IgM and IgA are normally catabolized more rapidly than IgG. Antibodies made some time after immunization tend to bind antigen more firmly than antibody made soon after immunization—ie, the affinity and avidity of antibody increase with time. However, cross-reactivity may also increase with time.

The Secondary Response

When an animal is reinjected with the same antigen weeks, months, or even years after the primary antibody levels have subsided, there is a more rapid antibody response to a higher level—and for a longer period—than in the primary response. This is presumably based on persistence of a substantial number of antigen-sensitive "memory" cells after initial contact with the antigen. The memory for secondary antibody response resides in B cells and, for certain antigens, in both B and T cells. During the secondary response, IgM antibody production may be similar to that in the primary response, whereas IgG antibody

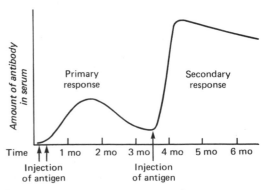

Figure 12–6. Rate of antibody production following initial antigen administration and "booster" injection.

production is usually far greater. A secondary response may be elicited with an antigen that is identical with or related to the antigen eliciting the primary response in that individual. This phenomenon ("original antigenic sin") can be employed in serologic epidemiology of infectious diseases caused by antigenically related but not identical agents (eg, influenza viruses).

Interference With Antibody Formation

When 2 or more antigens are injected simultaneously, the host reacts by producing antibodies to each. Competition of antigens for antibody-producing mechanisms has been observed experimentally, but it plays no practical role. Combined immunization with several antigens is widely used (eg, diphtheria and tetanus toxoids with pertussis vaccine, and live measles-mumps-rubella virus vaccines). The passive administration of a specific antibody may interfere with the active production of that same specific antibody by the host. A practical application is the injection of human antibody to Rh antigen into Rh-negative women with Rh-positive partners and children. If the Rh-negative woman is permitted to form antibodies to the fetus's Rh-positive red cells, these antibodies are likely to produce Rh disease in the offspring; but if the Rh-negative woman receives concentrated Rh antibodies before she begins to synthesize Rh antibodies, the antigen is bound, her antibody production is inhibited, and Rh disease of the newborn is prevented (see below).

Human Gamma Globulin

Immune globulin USP is a preparation of gamma globulin derived from large pools of human plasma by low-temperature ethanol fractionation. The preparation contains about 165 mg of gamma globulin per milliliter of solution, representing a 25-fold concentration of antibody-containing globulins of plasma, glycine as stabilizer, and an antibacterial agent. This concentrated gamma globulin is administered intramuscularly or subcutaneously. For intravenous administration, immune gamma globulin can be treated at acid pH with pepsin, or a 5% solution of gamma globulin can be mixed with 10% maltose. The recommended intravenous dose is 0.2 g/kg. Immune globulin may be employed clinically in the following conditions:

A. Hypo- or Dysgammaglobulinemia With Recurrent Bacterial Infections: Inject 0.6–1 mL/kg body weight (100–165 mg immune globulin per kilogram) once each month, but twice initially. Antimicrobial drugs must also be used.

B. Measles: To prevent clinical disease in nonimmunized children, give 0.25 mL/kg as soon as possible after exposure. To attenuate the disease (and permit development of active immunity), give 0.04 mL/kg within 8 days of exposure. Immune globulin has no effect after the rash has appeared. Attenuation markedly reduces the incidence of complications, but (ideally) all susceptible individuals (except severely

immunosuppressed persons) should be vaccinated with live attenuated vaccine (see p 189).

C. Hepatitis A: Use of 0.02 mL/kg once or twice during the incubation period may prevent or modify the disease without interfering with the development of immunity. For prolonged exposure, give 0.1 mL/kg every 6 months.

Specific Human Gamma Globulins

These are obtained from the blood of individuals who have been immunized with a given antigen and have acquired high concentrations of specific antibody. A few specific indications are listed below.

A. Tetanus: For prevention of tetanus after injury in nonimmunized individuals, 250–500 units of tetanus immune globulin USP injected intramuscularly will yield serum levels of more than 0.01 unit/mL for several weeks. For treatment of tetanus, up to 10,000 units has been administered.

B. Vaccinia: Vaccinia immune globulin USP (VIG), 0.6–1 mL/kg, can be used in the rare individual who develops progressive vaccinia gangrenosum following smallpox vaccination. Such a person is usually immunodeficient.

C. Rabies: Rabies immune globulin USP (RIG) is prepared from plasma pools with high rabies antibody titer obtained from immunized volunteers. The recommended dose is 20 units/kg. Up to half should be infiltrated around the wound and the rest injected intramuscularly. Usually given in conjunction with injections of diploid-cell-grown inactivated rabies vaccine, as indicated by the manufacturer, for postexposure immunization against rabies.

D. Mumps: Limited evidence suggests that 20 mL of mumps immune globulin (not available in the USA) may prevent orchitis in adult males.

E. Chickenpox: Varicella-zoster immune globulin (VZIG), 0.15 mL/kg intramuscularly, can prevent the disease when injected into high-risk children within 72–96 hours of exposure.

F. Rh Disease: $Rh_0(D)$ immune globulin USP can be injected into an Rh-negative mother following delivery of an Rh-positive infant. This prevents Rh isoimmunization of the mother and reduces the risk of hemolytic Rh disease in her next Rh-positive infant.

G. Pertussis: Pertussis immune globulin (2–3 mL) may reduce the mortality rate in debilitated infants or unimmunized children under 3 years of age. It is not available in the USA.

H. Hepatitis: Hepatitis B immune globulin USP (HBIG) may be given within 7 days of parenteral or mucous membrane exposure to HBsAg-positive material. This is repeated (0.06 mL/kg) 3–4 weeks later. Newborn infants of mothers who became HBsAg-positive late in pregnancy or who are HBeAg-positive at delivery should receive HBIG soon after birth and hepatitis B vaccine thereafter.

ANTIGEN-ANTIBODY REACTIONS

Antigens have been defined as substances that can elicit the formation of antibodies in a living animal. An animal does not generally produce antibodies against its own antigens, ie, it differentiates between "self" and "nonself." Exceptions are discussed in Chapter 13.

Antigenic Specificity

Reactions of antigens with antibodies are highly specific. This means that an antigen will react only with antibodies elicited by its own kind or by a closely related kind of antigen. The majority of antigenic substances are species-specific, and some are even organ-specific within an animal species. Human proteins can easily be distinguished from the proteins of other animals by antigen-antibody reactions and will cross-react only with the proteins of closely related species (eg, anthropoid apes). Within a single species, kidney protein may be distinguished from lung protein, etc. Exceptions to this species-specificity are certain antigens that are widely distributed among animals, particularly protein of the lens of the eye and the so-called **heterophil antigen**, which is present in the organs of mice, dogs, cats, horses, fish, and chickens as well as in the red cells of sheep and in some bacteria.

Antigenic specificity is a function of the antigenic determinants, small defined chemical areas on a large antigen molecule. The antigenic determinant may be a small group that is an essential part of the molecule and may repeat itself (eg, egg albumin has about 5 determinants). Alternatively, the antigenic determinant may be a hapten, a small molecule linked to a larger carrier. Coupling simple chemical groups like $-COOH$, $-SO_3H$, or $-AsO_3H_2$ on a benzene ring with serum protein (by diazo reactions) showed that each of these groups conferred specificity upon the antigen, depending particularly on the position of the radical (ortho-, meta-, or para-) in the aromatic compound.

Antigen-antibody reactions are highly specific. Antibodies usually can distinguish between the homologous antigen (which stimulated their formation) and heterologous, related antigen. The **specificity** of an antibody population depends on its ability to discriminate between antigens of related structure by combining with them to a different extent.

The binding of antigen to antibody does *not* involve covalent bonds but only relatively weak, short-range forces (electrostatic, coulombic, hydrogen bonding, van der Waals forces, etc). The strength of antigen-antibody bonds depends to a large extent on the closeness of fit between the configuration of the antigenic determinant site and the combining site of the antibody. The combining sites on antibody formed against a given antigenic determinant are not all perfect fits. Any antiserum thus contains some antibodies with very close fit and relatively strong binding forces and some with poor fit and weaker binding forces. Antibodies with the best fit and the strongest binding are said to have high **affinity** for the antigen. They have little tendency to dissociate from antigen after binding it (ie, they have high **avidity**). Antibodies of low avidity tend to dissociate more readily from the antigen. Early in the process of immunization, antibody may have relatively low affinity; as immunization proceeds, antibody of increasingly higher affinity is made.

In spite of the very great antigenic specificity, cross-reactions occur between antigenic determinants of closely related structure and their antibodies. The sharing of similar antigenic determinants by molecules of different origin leads to unexpected and unpredictable cross-reactions, eg, between human group A red blood cells and type 14 pneumococci. Many microorganisms share antigens (eg, *Haemophilus* and *Escherichia coli* O75:K100).

When antigenic proteins are denatured by heating or by chemical treatment, the molecular configuration is somewhat changed. This usually results in the loss of the original antigenic determinants and often leads to the uncovering of new antigenic determinants. Formaldehyde-treated proteins acquire an added antigenicity, and their antisera tend to cross-react with other formaldehyde-treated proteins. However, with gentle formaldehyde treatment of toxins, the original antigenicity may also be preserved, whereas the toxicity of the molecule (eg, exotoxins) may be abolished and the molecule thus converted to a **"toxoid"** that is immunogenic but nontoxic.

Most microorganisms contain not just one but many antigens to each of which antibodies may develop in the course of infection. Among these antigens may be capsular polysaccharides, somatic proteins or lipoprotein-carbohydrate complexes, protein exotoxins, and enzymes produced by the organism. All enzymes appear to be antigenic, and in some but not all cases that portion of the molecule which combines with specific antibody appears to be distinct from the portion of the molecule responsible for enzymatic activity. Many hormones are also antigenic.

Alloantigens (Blood Group Substances)

In general, antibodies are elicited only by antigens foreign to the injected animal species (heteroantibodies). However, animals may produce "alloantibodies" against "alloantigens," ie, antigens derived from other individuals of the same species. Outstanding among alloantigens are the blood group substances present in the red cells. There are 4 combinations of the 2 antigens present in erythrocytes. Their presence is under genetic control. The serum contains antibody against the absent antigens. As shown in Table 12–5, antigen and corresponding antibody do not coexist in the same blood. To avoid antigen-antibody reactions that would result in serious transfusion accidents, all bloods must be carefully matched for transfusion.

In addition to these major alloantigens, certain red blood cells contain other blood group substances capa-

Table 12–5. Determination of blood group by cross-match.

Group	Ags in Red Cell	Abs in Plasma	Determinant Group of Blood Group Ag
O	. . .	a, b	L-Fucose
A	A	b	α-N-Acetyl-galactos-aminoyl-galactose
B	B	a	α-D-Galactosyl-galactose
AB	AB	. . .	. . .

ble of stimulating antibodies. Among them is the Rh substance. Antibodies to Rh are developed when an Rh-negative person is transfused with Rh-positive blood or when an Rh-negative pregnant woman absorbs Rh substance from her Rh-positive fetus who inherited the *D* gene from the father. The development of high-titer anti-Rh_0D antibodies in the mother can lead to transplacental passage of IgG to the fetus, with resulting erythroblastosis of the newborn.

Apart from certain "sequestered" antigens—eg, thyroid or lens protein—that can definitely serve as autoantigens, it is not clear what may bring about the autoantigenicity of other organ antigens. Perhaps mobilization from the fixed site or slight alteration of structure, eg, by infection, may predispose to autoimmunization, with consequent disease (see Autoimmune Diseases in Chapter 13).

Rate of Absorption & Elimination of Antigen

One of the features that determines the effectiveness of an antigen as a stimulus for antibody production is its rate of absorption and elimination from the site of administration. Antigens differ greatly in their rate of excretion, but the major portion of injected antigen is often eliminated from the host within hours or days. In general, the antibody response will be higher and more sustained if the antigen is absorbed slowly from its "depot" at the site of injection. For this reason, many immunizing preparations employ physical methods to delay absorption. Toxoids are often adsorbed onto aluminum hydroxide. Bacterial or viral suspensions are sometimes prepared with adjuvants that delay absorption and promote tissue reaction to "fix" the antigen at its site of injection. (Adjuvants are discussed in Chapter 13.)

Following intravenous injection of a soluble antigen, the following phases in elimination are observed: (1) equilibration between intra- and extravascular compartments; (2) slow degradation of the antigen; (3) rapid immune elimination, as newly formed antibody combines with persisting antigen to form complexes that are phagocytosed by macrophages and digested.

Kinds of Antibodies

Antibodies are generally described in terms of their reactions with antigen:

A. Antitoxins: Antibodies to toxins or toxoids that neutralize or flocculate with the antigen.

B. Agglutinins: Antibodies that aggregate cells, forming clumps. Agglutinins can only be demonstrated if the antigen is particulate or if it is adsorbed onto the surface of a visible particle of uniform size (red blood cell, latex, bentonite, etc).

C. Precipitins: Antibodies that form complexes with antigen molecules in solution, forming precipitates. Precipitins can only be demonstrated if the antigen is soluble.

D. Lysins: Antibodies that, usually together with complement, dissolve the antigenic cells.

E. Opsonins: Antibodies that combine with surface components of microbial and other particles so that they are more readily taken up by phagocytes.

F. Neutralizing (Nt, Protective) Antibodies: Antibodies that render the antigenic infective agent (commonly viruses) noninfective.

G. Complement-Fixing (CF) Antibodies: Detected by the consumption of complement by the antigen-antibody complex. These reactions are discussed in detail below.

H. "Blocking," Inhibitory, and Other Nonprecipitating Antibodies: These combine with antigen but are not grossly detectable unless they are shown to inhibit or "block" a reaction or unless the protein species of antibody can be identified.

Different types of reactions may sometimes be demonstrated with the same antigen and antibody. Often one reaction may be more efficient than another. In general, antigens are multivalent with respect to antibody. Antibody valence is 2 (for IgG, IgA, IgE) or 5–10 (for IgM). In many reactions, antigen and antibody may combine in multiple proportions (see Danysz Phenomenon, p 184).

SEROLOGIC REACTIONS

Serology attempts to quantitate reactions between an antigen and its antibody by keeping one reagent constant and diluting the other.

Serologic reactions can be used to identify antigens or antibodies, if either of these reagents is known. They are also used to estimate the relative quantity of these reactants. Because of the specificity and sensitivity of antigen-antibody reactions, they find wide application in medicine. Examples are the diagnosis of an infection by detection of antibody titer rise against an etiologic agent (eg, *Salmonella*); the detection of circulating antigen in infection (eg, hepatitis B surface antigen [HBsAg]) by serum of known antibody; the "matching" of red blood cells against the serum antibodies of a potential recipient; and many others.

The type of antigen-antibody reaction applicable to a given situation depends largely on the physical state of the available antigen (see above). Each of the common types of antigen-antibody reactions is taken up in some detail on the following pages. Because the precipitin reaction permits the most accurate chemical quantitative work, it has been studied in the greatest detail. Some of the characteristics observed in precipitin reactions apply generally to all antigen-antibody reactions.

PRECIPITATION REACTIONS

A simple way to demonstrate the presence of antibody against an antigen in solution is to layer a small volume of one over the other in a tube. At the interface, precipitation will occur, forming a ring. This gives qualitative evidence of an antigen-antibody reaction but does not indicate whether one or several antigen-antibody systems are present. If, however, the reaction takes place not in solution but in a semisolid gel, then different antigens and antibodies are likely to diffuse at different rates. As a result, optimal proportions for precipitation occur at different sites in the agar, and distinct multiple bands of precipitate form. Double diffusion gel precipitation methods based on this principle are described below. They are used for many different immunologic tests.

Precipitation reactions involving single antigen-antibody systems can be performed quantitatively. A measured quantity of a given antibody is placed in a series of test tubes; varying amounts of the corresponding pure antigen are added, mixed, and allowed to react. A precipitate forms in some tubes, and the quantity of this precipitate, after sedimentation and washing, can be measured accurately in several ways. For example, a total nitrogen determination can be made on the precipitate and the (known) amount of antigen nitrogen subtracted from the total to yield the amount of antibody nitrogen. Or the antigen can be labeled with a radioactive isotope and the amount of radioactivity in the precipitate measured. Other methods can be used as well. When the precipitate is removed and the supernatant examined, 3 zones of antigen-antibody interaction, shown schematically in Fig 12–7, can be discerned:

(1) A zone of antibody excess, in which uncombined antibody is present.

(2) A zone of equivalence, in which both antigen and antibody are completely precipitated and no uncombined antigen or antibody is present. In this zone there is also maximal complement fixation.

(3) A zone of antigen excess, in which all antibody has combined with antigen and additional uncombined antigen is present. In this zone, precipitation is partly or completely inhibited because soluble antigen-antibody complexes form in the presence of excess antigen.

The field of immunochemistry provides methods for absolute quantitative measurement of antibody that can be applied to a large variety of theoretical and practical problems.

The initial combination of antigen and antibody takes place almost immediately upon mixing of the reactants. The subsequent formation of larger, visible aggregates requires an hour or more and depends

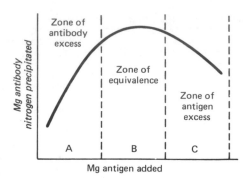

Figure 12–7. The main zones of antigen-antibody interactions.

somewhat on the temperature and the total volume of the mixture. The reaction is fastest in the zone of equivalence, where optimal proportions between antigen and antibody exist. The speed of gross precipitation is an index of the zone of equivalence, where complete precipitation of both antigen and antibody takes place and neither is present in excess.

GEL DIFFUSION TESTS

These tests are based on the diffusion of antigen and antibody through a semisolid medium to form stable complexes that can be analyzed visually. The Ouchterlony plate (an agar-coated plate in which wells have been cut to hold antigen and antibody) may be used to identify immunologically active substances and detect their components and relationships. Antigens and antibodies diffusing in all directions will form lines of precipitate when equivalent concentrations of each meet. Typical reaction patterns in angular **double diffusion** are shown in Fig 12–8. These reaction patterns permit the identification of identical antigens, nonidentical antigens, and antigens of partial identity that cross-react.

Single radial diffusion can be used to quantitate an antigen, eg, an immunoglobulin in a mixture. Radial diffusion is based on the quantitative relationship between the amount of antigen placed in a well cut into agar and the diameter of the ring of precipitate that forms with antibody incorporated in the agar. These are then compared to a standard curve obtained with known amounts of antigen and the same antibody-containing plate.

AGGLUTINATION REACTIONS

Whereas the antigen is in solution in precipitation tests, it is particulate in agglutination reactions. It may consist of suspensions of microorganisms, cells (eg, red blood cells), or uniform particles like latex or bentonite onto which antigens have been adsorbed. When mixed with specific antiserum, these cells or particles

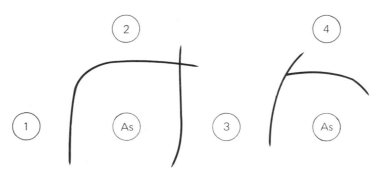

As = Antiserum in wells
1, 2, 3, 4 = Antigens in wells

1 and 2 = Reaction of identity
2 and 3 = Reaction of nonidentity
3 and 4 = Reaction of partial identity (cross-reaction; the "spur"
is caused by the fraction of antibody that was not precipitated by antigen 4)

Figure 12–8. Double diffusion precipitin reactions in gel.

become clumped; the clumps aggregate and finally settle as large, visible clumps, leaving the supernatant clear. If one of the reagents is known, the reaction may be employed for the identification of either antigen or antibody. Thus, the reaction is commonly used to identify, by means of known antisera, microorganisms cultured from clinical specimens. The agglutination reaction is also used to estimate the titer of antibacterial agglutinins in the serum of patients with unknown disease. A rise in antibody titer directed against a specific microorganism occurring during an illness strongly suggests a causal relationship.

Microorganisms possess a variety of antigens, and antibodies to one or more of these may be present in antiserum. A simple example is provided by the antibody response to infection by flagellated bacteria. Antibodies may be directed against the flagellar surface antigen, the somatic antigens, or both. The type of macroscopic agglutination may also be distinctive; the flagellar antigen-antibody complex appears coarse and floccular, whereas the somatic complex is fine and granular.

Agglutination is aided by elevated temperature (37–56 °C) and by movement (eg, shaking, stirring, centrifuging), which increases the contact between antigen and antibody. The aggregation of clumps requires the presence of salts. In the zone of antibody excess (ie, concentrated serum), agglutination may be inhibited owing to the presence of blocking antibody (see Brucellae, p 266). Such a prozone may give the impression that antibodies are absent; this error can be avoided only by using serial dilutions of serum.

The agglutination test may be performed microscopically by mixing a loopful of serum with a suspension of microorganisms on a slide and inspecting the result through the low-power objective. This is commonly done for the identification of unknown cultures. For the estimation of the "titer" of agglutinating antibody in an unknown serum, a macroscopic tube dilution test or a microtiter dilution test may be done: a suitable fixed amount of antigen is added to each tube

of a series of serum dilutions, and after thorough shaking, the tubes are incubated at 37 °C for 1–2 hours. The result is determined by looking for sedimented clumps and clear supernatant fluid. The "titer" of the serum is the highest dilution with clearly visible agglutination.

In **co-agglutination,** the Fc fragment of almost any antibody fixes to protein A of staphylococci. Thus, staphylococci with a given attached antibody are agglutinated when mixed with the specific antigen.

THE ANTIGLOBULIN (COOMBS) TEST

This is an indirect agglutination test for the detection of cell-bound or incomplete antibodies. Such antibodies are by themselves incapable of agglutinating particles but can bind to them firmly. By adding an antibody against the globulin species (eg, antihuman globulin prepared in rabbits), agglutination of the coated particles results. This test has found greatest application in the detection of various anti-red-blood-cell antibodies in hemolytic anemias.

TOXIN-ANTITOXIN REACTIONS

The toxin-antitoxin reactions described below apply only to exotoxins, as exemplified by the toxins of diphtheria, tetanus, or botulism. The following examples of definitions of units apply to diphtheria toxin:

International Unit of antitoxin (IU): The amount of antitoxin in 0.0628 mg of a standard dried antitoxin maintained at the Serum Institute, Copenhagen.

L+ dose: The smallest amount of toxin that, when mixed with 1 unit of antitoxin and injected subcutaneously into a guinea pig weighing 250 g, will cause death within 4 days.

Lf dose (flocculating unit): That amount of toxin which flocculates most rapidly with 1 unit of antitoxin in a series of mixtures containing constant amounts of antitoxin and varying amounts of toxin. (This value is calculated from experimental results.)

Antitoxic potency can be measured by the ability to neutralize the toxin when the mixture is injected into animals or to precipitate toxin in vitro.

Any preparation of toxin contains some molecules of full toxicity and others of low or no toxicity but persistent antigenicity (toxoid). Dried antitoxin, however, is constant in its ability to combine with toxin or toxoid molecules. For this reason, antitoxin is taken as the constant standard for biologic estimation of toxic or antitoxic potency. The L+ dose is usually relied upon. The Lf unit is independent of the toxic activity of a given preparation and is only a function of its antigenic combining power. Thus, it remains constant when a toxin is converted to toxoid by formalin or heat. It is of great importance in the standardization of antigenic quantities of toxoid.

Toxin-antitoxin flocculations are similar to precipitin reactions but show a very sharp zone of equivalence. The reaction is inhibited by both antigen excess and antibody excess; soluble complexes result from either.

Danysz Phenomenon

If toxin is added to antitoxin in several fractions with time intervals between them, then more antitoxin (or less toxin) is necessary to give a neutral end point in injected animals than if all the toxin had been added at once. This is explained by the ability of toxin to combine with antitoxin in multiple proportions. The first fraction of toxin combines with a relatively large amount of the antitoxin present, so that little antitoxin is left to combine with the second fraction. After some time, however, an equilibrium is again reached. The Danysz phenomenon applies similarly to other antigen-antibody reactions, where the dissociation of antigen-antibody complexes is slow.

ABSORPTION REACTIONS

Sera from animals injected with whole microorganisms or from humans who have passed through several infections tend to react with a variety of related antigens. This raises the question whether the serum contains an antibody specific for a given antigen or merely a related antibody that cross-reacts. Such sera may be rendered specific for one antigen by removing related antibodies through absorption with specific antigens. This is done by mixing the serum with concentrated antigen (eg, a dense bacterial suspension), incubating to permit combination, and then centrifuging the precipitate or agglutinated material and removing the supernatant serum. It is now "absorbed" and should no longer contain antibodies specific for the absorbing antigen. Such absorptions may be performed with a series of antigens, finally leaving a serum that will react only with a single remaining antigen, for which it is

highly specific. This is valuable in "antigenic analysis" of bacteria and other biologic substances.

INHIBITION REACTIONS

In addition to various direct methods of demonstrating and measuring antigen-antibody reactions discussed above, some indirect methods exist that, in essence, use competition for an antibody combining site by 2 antigenic groups or competition for an antigenic group by 2 antibodies. They are especially useful when there is no visible evidence of direct reaction between antigen and antibody. *Examples:* Inhibition of precipitation by nonprecipitating antibody or by a fragment of digested antibody; inhibition of viral hemagglutination by antibody; inhibition of the Prausnitz-Küstner reaction by blocking antibody.

IMMUNOFLUORESCENCE
(Fluorescent Antibody Tests, FA)

Certain fluorescent dyes (eg, fluorescein isothiocyanate, rhodamine) can be covalently attached to globulin molecules and thus made visible by using ultraviolet light in the fluorescence microscope. If such fluorescent dyes are conjugated with antibody molecules and all excess is carefully eliminated, such "labeled" antibody may be used to locate and identify specific antigen because of the high specificity of the antigen-antibody bond. By means of such "direct immunofluorescence reactions," bacteria may be identified and viral or other antigens may be located inside cells. In bacteriologic diagnosis, specific direct immunofluorescence is valuable for the rapid identification of group A hemolytic streptococci, *Treponema pallidum,* and other organisms. In special laboratories, immunofluorescence has been applied to the rapid screening of enteric pathogens, *Yersinia,* bacteria causing childhood meningitis, and others.

The "indirect immunofluorescence reactions" involve 3 reagents: antigen + its antibody A + a fluorescent-labeled antibody to antibody A. Any one of the 3 reagents can be unknown. For example, in the serodiagnosis of syphilis, *T pallidum* antigen fixed to a slide is overlaid with the patient's unknown serum and then washed. Fluorescein-labeled antihuman globulin (made in an animal) is then placed on the preparation, which is examined by ultraviolet light. If the patient's serum contains specific antibodies to *T pallidum,* brightly fluorescent spirochetes are seen. If the spirochetes do not fluoresce, no specific antitreponemal antibodies are present. (See FTA-ABS Test in Chapter 27.)

Immunofluorescence can be used for the detection of viral and bacterial antigens or antibodies, tumor antigens, and many others. The indirect test is often more sensitive than the direct immunofluorescence test because more fluorescein-labeled antibodies adhere per antigenic site.

ELECTROPHORESIS METHODS

When an electric current passes through a solution of proteins, the proteins migrate with different velocity from anode to cathode (see p 174). This permits separation of different globulins on some supporting structure, eg, starch, cellulose acetate, paper, gels. This method can be quantitated to permit measurement of different serum proteins in a given sample.

Immunoelectrophoresis combines electrophoretic separation of proteins in a mixture with immune precipitation of the components by antibody. Small wells are cut in a layer of agar on a glass slide, and each is filled with an antigen or mixture of antigens (serum). After electrophoresis with direct current for several hours, a trough is cut in the agar and filled with antiserum. The serum is permitted to diffuse against the electrophoretically separated antigens on the slide. A precipitate arc forms where specific antigen-antibody reactions occur. It can be washed and stained for protein and compared to standards. This method permits (for example) detection of the absence of a specific immunoglobulin in serum, or the presence of an unusually sharp, high peak of an abnormal globulin, as in myeloma.

Counterimmunoelectrophoresis (CIE, double electroimmunodiffusion) is an extension of immunoelectrophoresis that relies on the movement of antigen toward the anode and of antibody toward the cathode during the passage of electric current through a gel. Antigen and antibody are each placed in a well in the gel. As they move toward each other, their meeting and precipitation at an intermediate point is greatly accelerated. Visible precipitin lines develop in 30–60 minutes, and the method is 10 times more sensitive than double diffusion without electric current. The method is limited to acidic antigens that carry a negative charge. It is most useful for the rapid detection of antigens in body fluids, eg, polysaccharides in cerebrospinal fluid of patients with meningitis caused by *Haemophilus,* pneumococcus, etc.

RADIOIMMUNOASSAY (RIA)

Radioimmunoassays are the most sensitive and versatile methods for the quantitation of substances that are antigens or haptens and can be radioactively labeled. Radioimmunoassay is particularly applicable to the measurement of serum levels of many hormones, drugs, and other biologic materials. The method is based on competition for specific antibody between the labeled (known) and the unlabeled (unknown) concentration of the material. The complexes that form between antigen (or hapten) and antibody can then be separated and the amount of radioactivity determined. The concentration of the unknown (unlabeled) antigen is determined by comparison with the effect of standards.

The radioallergosorbent test (RAST) is a specialized radioimmunoassay to measure the amount of serum IgE antibodies that react with a specific allergen.

ENZYME-LINKED IMMUNOASSAY

This technique is increasingly popular because it is very sensitive and does not require specialized equipment, as do immunofluorescence and radioimmunoassay. The method depends on conjugation of an enzyme to either an antigen or an antibody and use of the enzyme activity as a quantitative label. Many variations of the method can be constructed, depending on the nature of the enzyme employed and the antigen-antibody system to be measured. A widely employed variant is the **enzyme-linked immunosorbent assay** (ELISA), which can be used to measure either antigen or antibody. To measure antibody, the known antigen is fixed to a solid phase (eg, plastic cup or microplate), incubated with test serum dilutions, washed, and then incubated with anti-immunoglobulin labeled with an enzyme (eg, horseradish peroxidase). Enzyme activity is measured by adding the specific substrate: the color reaction is estimated colorimetrically. The enzyme activity is a direct function of the amount of antibody bound.

To measure antigen, a known specific antibody is fixed to the solid phase, the test material containing antigen is added and washed, and a second enzyme-labeled antibody is added. This test requires that the antigen have at least 2 determinants. After washing, substrate is added and enzyme activity is estimated colorimetrically and related to antigen concentration.

OTHER TYPES OF SEROLOGIC REACTIONS

Protection or Neutralization (Nt) Tests

These are widely employed in the determination of antiviral and a few antibacterial antibodies. They utilize the ability of antibody-containing sera to block the infectivity of these agents upon inoculation of the mixture into susceptible hosts or cells.

Detection of Immune Complexes

Immune complexes deposited in tissue can be made visible by staining with complement components that have been made fluorescent and that bind to the complex. Immune complexes in biologic fluids (eg, serum) can be detected by binding to C1q or to rheumatoid factor (see below); they can also be demonstrated by attachment to receptors on cultured Raji line lymphoblastoid cells and subsequent fixation of a radiolabeled anti-immunoglobulin antibody. The clinical usefulness of immune complex determinations is still uncertain.

Opsonophagocytic Tests

In these tests, phagocytic cells from the patient (especially polymorphonuclear neutrophils) are mixed with viable bacteria of certain species, or with yeasts, in the presence of serum to observe the rate of ingestion and (by subculture) the rate of intracellular killing. By means of such tests, defects in cellular immunity are studied (see Phagocytosis in Chapter 11). Polymorphonuclear cells from patients with specific deficiencies in phagocytosis and intracellular killing (eg, chronic granulomatous disease) also give abnormally depressed responses in the nitroblue tetrazolium dye test.

Ferritin-Labeled Antibody Technique

Electron-dense ferritin can be conjugated with antibody molecules that become visible in the electron microscope. This permits localization of antigen in cells and ultrathin sections examined by electron microscopy.

Hemagglutination Tests, Active & Passive

Red blood cells from various animal species may be clumped by certain viruses. This "active hemagglutination" can be specifically inhibited by antibody to virus, and the hemagglutination inhibition (HI) is a convenient serologic test. Red cells also present a convenient surface onto which many types of antigens can be adsorbed. Such coated cells will clump when mixed with antibodies to these specific antigens ("passive hemagglutination"). Other convenient particles such as latex or bentonite may substitute for red cells. An IgM in the serum of most patients with rheumatoid disease can be measured by agglutination of latex particles coated with human IgG. Human IgG will be clumped by this IgM "rheumatoid factor." Clinically applicable serologic tests for the diagnosis of infection are listed in Chapter 32.

THE COMPLEMENT SYSTEM

The term complement (C) denotes a complex system of proteins and other factors found in normal serum of vertebrates. Some genes controlling the production of complement components are located on human chromosome 6 in proximity to the HLA locus. Some components have enzymatic activity; others are enhancers or inhibitors. Activation of the complement sequence of reactions may occur by the "classic" pathway set off by antigen-antibody reactions or by the "alternative" pathway ("bypass"), which does not require antigen-antibody reactions. The sequence of reactions can lead to the production of biologically active factors (eg, chemotactic factors), to damage of cell membranes (eg, lysis of cells), or to various pathologic processes (eg, nephrotoxic nephritis).

The steps in the complement reaction sequence can most easily be illustrated by the events leading to cell lysis. In the sequence shown in Fig 12–9, E represents a cell membrane carrying an antigenic site (either an intrinsic or artificially attached antigen) and A represents an antibody (IgG, IgM) to that antigen.

Complement of guinea pigs and humans has been studied most extensively. At present, at least 11 distinct components of guinea pig complement are recognized. Complement must either be kept frozen or used in the form of fresh serum to avoid deterioration of some components. On heating at 56 °C, activity is lost completely in 30 minutes. Complement activity depends upon the ionic strength of the medium, pH (optimum, 7.2–7.4), volume (inverse relationship), temperature (optimum, 30–37 °C), and the presence of Ca^{2+} (see step 2) and Mg^{2+} (step 4).

Different animal sera contain different proportions of the various complement components. The component that is lowest in titer or activity in a given serum limits the hemolytic complement activity of that serum. C1 exists in serum as an aggregate of 3 proteins: C1q, C1r, and C1s. C1q can attach to antigen-antibody complexes or to certain aggregated immunoglobulins (eg, IgM, IgG-1) without any activation. All other components are converted one after another from inactive to activated forms. The final step in cytolysis requires only the production of a single membrane lesion induced by complement action.

Alternative Pathway of Complement Activation

While the "classic" pathway depends on starting the reaction sequence by C1q attaching to antigen-antibody complexes, another pathway exists for activating complement-mediated reactions. A variety of substances can bring about the formation of a C3 activator that cleaves C3 in a fashion analogous to that of C3 convertase in the classic pathway. This "alternative pathway" then proceeds C3–C9, as in the classic pathway shown in Fig 12–9. Polysaccharides, lipopolysaccharides, and some immunoglobulin aggregates (eg, IgA, IgE, IgG-4, which do *not* initiate the complement sequence via C1q) activate the **properdin** system as an alternative pathway of complement activation.

The properdin system consists of a unique serum protein (properdin), a glycine-rich β-glycoprotein (C3 proactivator), and other serum proteins. The activation of this system culminates in cleavage of C3. The reaction sequence then proceeds as in the classic pathway. The properdin system can enhance resistance to gram-negative infections, but it can also participate in the mediation of immunologic injury to tissue (eg, nephritis).

There are other activators of the alternative pathway. Proteolytic enzymes released from lysosomes of phagocytic cells can cleave C3; other proteolytic enzymes involved in the blood coagulation cascade or produced by bacteria can do likewise.

COMPLEMENT-MEDIATED REACTIONS

Immune Hemolysis & Cytolysis

The production of membrane injury of red blood cells by complement acting on antigen-antibody com-

(1) $E + A \longrightarrow EA$. (E represents a cell membrane carrying an antigenic site; A represents antibody to that antigen.)

(2) $EA + C\overline{1} \xrightarrow{Ca^{2+}} EAC\overline{1}$. ($C\overline{1}$ represents the activated form of C1 with enzyme activity; Ca^{2+} is required for the stability of the complex.)

(3) $EAC\overline{1} + C4 \longrightarrow EAC\overline{1,4}$. (The $C\overline{1}$ enzyme, an esterase, has cleaved C4 and C2, part of which attached to the activated complex or the cell membrane.)

(4) $EAC\overline{1,4}, + C2 \xrightarrow{Mg^{2+}} EAC\overline{1,4,2}$. ($Mg^{2+}$ is required for stability of the activated complex; the C4,2, moiety is an enzyme, C3 convertase, active in next step.)

Alternative
pathway

(5) $EAC\overline{1,4,2} + C3 \longrightarrow EAC\overline{1,4,2,3} + C3$ fragments with activity of anaphylatoxin and chemotaxis. (Cleavage of C3 occurs either by C3 convertase in the classic pathway or by C3 activator in the alternative pathway.)

(6) $EAC\overline{1,4,2,3} + C5,C6,C7 \longrightarrow EAC\overline{1,4,2,3,5,6,7} + C5$ fragments with anaphylatoxin activity. (The C5,6,7 complex on the cell membrane is chemotactic for polymorphonuclear leukocytes.)

(7) $EAC\overline{1,4,2,3,5,6,7} + C8,C9 \longrightarrow EAC\ \overline{1-9}$. (The final complex results in membrane damage ["holes"], cell damage, or lysis.)

Figure 12–9. Complement reaction sequence.

plexes on the membrane is the basis for a sensitive serologic test, the complement fixation (CF) test (see below). Many other types of cells (lymphocytes, tumor cells, etc) are also subject to immune cytolysis.

Some gram-negative bacteria and spirochetes coated with specific antibody go through the sequence of steps (1–7) shown above and exhibit bacteriolysis. It is not clear how often this reaction plays any role in host defenses. Cytolytic reactions may cause injury to normal tissues in allergic vasculitis or glomerulitis.

Chemotaxis

Complement bound by antigen-antibody complexes releases chemotactic factors and attracts leukocytes that in turn release lysosomal enzymes and thus cause damage to tissues.

Fragments of C3, C5, and the C5,6,7 complex also attract leukocytes. This may aid in the localization and inactivation of infectious agents or may enhance tissue injury. This chemotaxis is depressed by alcohol and in cirrhotic patients. Complement components are found attached to antigen-antibody complexes in "complex" diseases, eg, on synovial membranes in rheumatoid arthritis or on glomerular basement membranes in nephritis (see p 194).

Immune Adherence & Opsonization

Fragments of C3 and C5 promote the adherence of antigen-antibody complexes to leukocytes or platelets and the phagocytosis of opsonized (antibody-coated) microorganisms by leukocytes and macrophages.

Anaphylatoxin Effect

Fragments of C3 and C5 can produce degranulation of mast cells with the release of histamine and other mediators. This results in symptoms of vasodilatation, increased capillary permeability, bronchospasm, and other symptoms resembling anaphylaxis.

Hereditary Angioedema

Persons with this disorder are deficient in a normal C1 esterase inhibitor (a glycoprotein). Consequently, their serum intermittently has increased C1 activity that liberates a vasoactive kinin from C2. This kinin produces acute, transient local accumulations of edema fluid. C1 activation can be prevented by aminocaproic acid, tranexamic acid, or the steroid danazol.

Low Serum Complement Levels

Low serum complement levels—particularly low C3—are encountered in antigen-antibody complex diseases such as lupus erythematosus and acute glomerulonephritis and in cryoglobulinemia.

Hereditary Deficiencies

Hereditary deficiency of certain complement components (eg, C2, C3, C4, C6, C8) may lead to increased susceptibility to infection. *Neisseria* bacteremia occurs frequently in C5–C9 deficiency.

THE COMPLEMENT FIXATION TEST

Complement fixation (CF) tests depend upon 2 distinct reactions. The first involves antigen and antibody (of which one is known, the other unknown) plus a fixed amount of pretitrated complement. If antigen and antibody are specific for one another, they will combine; the combination will take up ("fix") the added complement. The second reaction involves testing for the presence of free (unattached) complement. This is done by the addition of red cells "sensitized" with specific hemolysin. If complement has been "fixed" by the antigen-antibody complex, then none will be available for lysis of the sensitized red cells. If the antigen and antibody are not specific for each other, or if one of them is lacking, then complement remains free to attach to the sensitized red cells and lyse them. Therefore, a positive CF test gives no hemolysis; a negative test gives hemolysis. This can be written schematically as follows:

I. Specific Ag X + Complement → Complement not bound
II. Specific Ab anti-X + Complement → Complement not bound
III. X + Anti-X + Complement → Complement bound ("fixed")

To detect whether complement is bound or not bound, a hemolytic system (see below) of red blood cells (RBC) + anti-RBC antibody (Ab) is added to each of the mixtures I, II, and III, with these results:

I + RBC + Ab → Lysis of RBC = Negative test
II + RBC + Ab → Lysis of RBC = Negative test
III + RBC + Ab → No lysis of RBC = Positive test

A positive test occurs only if X and anti-X have combined to bind available complement. If either antigen X alone or antibody anti-X alone (I or II) inactivates complement, it is unsatisfactory for the test and is called anticomplementary. Anticomplementary antigens or sera are detected by suitable controls in the test. Anticomplementary activity can sometimes be removed by heating or dilution.

For the practical performance of the test, it is necessary to control all reagents and environmental conditions carefully. In order to eliminate any complement that might be present in the serum used as source of antibody, all sera must be inactivated by heating for 30 minutes at 56 °C. To the antigen and the inactivated serum, a carefully titrated amount of complement is added (usually 1.2–2 units). The mixture is then left at 37 °C or in the refrigerator for a specified time to permit interaction of antigen and antibody and "fixation" of complement. Next, the "hemolytic system" is added; this consists of a suspension of sheep red cells "sensitized" by the addition of hemolysin (ie, anti-sheep rabbit serum). The mixture is then incubated at 37 °C for 30 minutes and read for hemolysis.

If properly controlled, the CF test is a sensitive method in the diagnostic laboratory. It is used for the identification of antibody and estimation of its titer (with known antigens) or the identification of antigens (with known antibody). The serologic diagnosis of many viral and fungal infections and of some immunologic disorders rests on CF tests (see Chapter 35).

RECOMMENDED ACTIVE IMMUNIZATION

Every individual—child or adult—should be adequately immunized against infectious diseases. The schedule of administration, dose, and recommended method of administration vary with each product and change often. Always consult the manufacturer's package insert and follow its recommendations.

ACTIVE IMMUNIZATION IN CHILDHOOD

A schedule for active immunizations in childhood is shown in Table 12–6. This is a composite and can be expected to change at intervals.

RECOMMENDED IMMUNIZATION OF ADULTS FOR TRAVEL

Every adult, whether traveling or not, must be immunized against tetanus, diphtheria, and poliomyelitis and receive booster doses at appropriate intervals. Every traveler must fulfill the immunization requirements of the health authorities of different countries. These are listed in Centers for Disease Control: *Health Information for International Travel, 1982*. Superintendent of Documents, US Government Printing Office, Washington, DC 20402; and also in *MMWR* 1983;**32(Suppl)**.

Tetanus
Booster injection of 0.5 mL tetanus toxoid, for adult use, every 7–10 years, assuming completion of primary immunization. (All countries.)

Diphtheria
Because diphtheria is still prevalent in many parts of the world, a booster injection of diphtheria toxoid for adult use is indicated. This is usually given in combination with tetanus toxoid (Td) purified, for adults.

Poliomyelitis
Adults who have previously been immunized against poliomyelitis should receive oral poliovaccine again. Only those who have never been immunized or are immunosuppressed or immunodeficient should be given inactivated trivalent vaccine (at least 3 doses) before travel into endemic areas.

Smallpox
As of 1980, smallpox has been eradicated from the world. Smallpox vaccination is no longer administered to civilians, and a vaccination certificate is no longer required of travelers. Military personnel, however, continue to be vaccinated in the USA and elsewhere, and occasional complications of vaccinia are still encountered.

Typhoid
Suspension of killed *Salmonella typhi* can provide effective immunity. Two doses are given 4 weeks or more apart, and a single booster dose is given once every 3 years for probable exposure. (All countries.)

Paratyphoid vaccines are probably ineffective and are not recommended at present.

Yellow Fever
Live attenuated yellow fever virus, 0.5 mL subcutaneously. WHO certificate requires registration of manufacturer and batch number of vaccine. Vaccina-

Table 12–6. Recommended schedule for active immunization of children.*

Normal Infants and Children[1]		Those Not Immunized in Infancy (7–18 Years)	
Age	Product Administered or Test Recommended	Schedule	Product Administered
2 months	DTP,[2] TOPV[3]	Initial	Td,[7] TOPV
4 months	DTP, TOPV	1 month later	Measles vaccine, mumps vaccine, rubella vaccine
6 months	DTP, TOPV[4]	2 months later	Td, TOPV
15–19 months	DTP, TOPV Measles vaccine, mumps vaccine, rubella vaccine;[5] tuberculin test[6]	6–12 months later	Td, TOPV
4–6 years (school entry)	DTP, TOPV; tuberculin test Haemophilus influenzae vaccine[8]	14–16 years of age	Td
Every 10 years thereafter	Td[7]	Every 10 years thereafter	Td

*Follow manufacturer's directions for dose and precautions. A physician may choose to obtain informed consent for immunizations.

[1]A child who experiences any type of seizure after immunization should receive only diphtheria-tetanus (DT) vaccine subsequently.

[2]**DTP:** Toxoids of diphtheria and tetanus, aluminum-precipitated or aluminum hydroxide-adsorbed, combined with pertussis bacterial antigen. Three doses intramuscularly at 4- to 8-week intervals. Fourth dose intramuscularly about 1 year later. Not suitable for children over 7 years old.

[3]**TOPV:** Trivalent (types I, II, and III) oral live poliomyelitis virus vaccine. Inactivated trivalent vaccine (Salk type) preferred for immunodeficient children, children with immunodeficient members of the household, and for those initially immunized after age 18, but not recommended for others.

[4]Optional dose, if exposure to wild poliomyelitis virus is anticipated.

[5]These are live vaccines of attenuated viruses grown in cell culture. They may be administered as a mixture or singly at 1-month intervals. Persons who received measles vaccine (inactivated) before 1968 or before age 15 months should be reimmunized with measles vaccine. Some physicians prefer to give rubella vaccine to prepubertal females (age 10–14 years). These live vaccines are not recommended for severely immunodeficient children.

[6]It is desirable to give a tuberculin test prior to measles vaccination and at intervals thereafter, depending on probable risk of exposure.

[7]**Td:** Tetanus toxoid and diphtheria toxoid, purified, suitable for adults. It should be given every 7–10 years.

[8]H influenzae polysaccharide vaccine available for children 2–6 years of age; optional.

References:

Centers for Disease Control: General recommendations on immunization. *MMWH* (Jan 14) 1983;**32**:1.

Cody CL et al: Nature and rates of adverse reactions associated with DTP and DT immunization in infants and children. *Pediatrics* 1981;**68**:650.

Committee on Control of Infectious Diseases: *Report,* 19th ed. American Academy of Pediatrics, 1982.

CDC Immunization Practices Advisory Committee: Polysaccharide vaccine for prevention of *Haemophilus influenzae* type b. disease. *MMWR* 1985 (April 19);**34**:201.

tion available in the USA only at approved centers. Vaccination must be repeated at intervals of 10 years or less. (Africa, South America.)

Cholera

Suspension of killed vibrios, including prevalent antigenic types. Two injections are given intramuscularly 4–6 weeks apart. This must be followed by booster injections every 6 months during periods of possible exposure. Protection depends largely on booster doses. WHO certificate is valid for 6 months only. (Middle Eastern countries, Asia, occasionally others.) Benefit doubtful.

Plague

Suspension of killed plague bacilli given intramuscularly, 3 injections 4 or more weeks apart. A single booster injection 6 months later is desirable. (Some areas in South America, Southeast Asia, occasionally others.)

Typhus

Suspensions of inactivated typhus rickettsiae can

give some protection. However, no approved vaccine is available in the USA or Canada in 1986.

Measles

Persons born since 1957 who have not had live measles vaccine (after age 15 months) and who do not have a convincing history of clinical measles should receive measles vaccine (see pp 394 and 481).

Hepatitis A

No active immunization available. Temporary passive immunity may be induced by the intramuscular injection of immune globulin USP, 0.02 mL/kg every 2–3 months, or 0.1 mL/kg every 6 months. Recommended for all parts of the world where environmental sanitation is poor and the risk of exposure to hepatitis A is high through contaminated food and water and contact with infected persons.

Hepatitis B

While not directly travel-related, postexposure prophylaxis against hepatitis is mentioned here. In 1982, an inactivated hepatitis B vaccine was licensed for use in persons at high risk who have no anti-HBs antibody. It might be considered for travelers to hyperendemic areas. (China, Southeast Asia.)

Pneumococcal Pneumonia

Elderly travelers or those with chronic respiratory insufficiency may be given the 23-type pneumococcal polysaccharide vaccine, which is licensed in the USA.

Meningococcal Meningitis

If travel is contemplated to an area where meningococcal meningitis is highly endemic or epidemic, polysaccharide vaccines from types A, C, W-135, and Y may be indicated. (Africa, South America, Nepal.)

Malaria

Take chloroquine phosphate, 500 mg once weekly, beginning 1 week prior to arrival in malaria-endemic area and continuing for 6 weeks after leaving it. Immunization not available. (In Southeast Asia, Africa, and South America, chloroquine-resistant *Plasmodium falciparum* may be present; pyrimethamine-sulfadoxine mixture may be required.)

Rabies

For travelers to areas where rabies is common in domestic animals (eg, India, parts of South America), preexposure prophylaxis with human diploid cell vaccine should be considered. It usually consists of 3 injections given 1 week apart, with a booster 3 weeks later (see Table 39–2). Only the vaccine manufactured by Merieux is accepted in the USA in 1986.

REFERENCES

Acute O, Reinherz EL: The human T-cell receptor: Structure and function. *N Engl J Med* 1985;**312**:1100.

CDC Immunization Practices Advisory Committee: Adult Immunization: Recommendations of the Immunization Practices Advisory Committee (ACIP). *MMWR* (Sept 28) 1984;**33 (Suppl 1)**:1.

Centers for Disease Control: General recommendations on immunization. *MMWR* (Jan 14) 1983;**32**:1.

Cline MJ et al: Monocytes and macrophages: Functions and diseases. *Ann Intern Med* 1978;**88**:78.

Colten HR et al: Genetics and biosynthesis of complement proteins. *N Engl J Med* 1981;**304**:653.

Cunningham-Rundles C et al: Efficacy of intravenous immunoglobulin in primary humoral immunodeficiency diseases. *Ann Intern Med* 1984;**101**:435.

Diamond B, Scharff MD: Monoclonal antibodies. *JAMA* 1982;**248**:3165.

Edelman GM: Antibody structure and molecular immunology. *Science* 1973;**180**:830.

Fearon DT, Austen KF: The alternative pathway of complement: A system for host resistance to microbial infection. *N Engl J Med* 1980;**303**:259.

Fulginiti VA (editor): *Immunization in Clinical Practice*. Lippincott, 1982.

Gallin JI: Abnormal phagocyte chemotaxis: Pathophysiology, clinical manifestations and management of patients. *Rev Infect Dis* 1981;**3**:1196.

Gigliotti F et al: Reproducible production of protective human monoclonal antibodies. *J Infect Dis* 1984;**149**:43.

Goldman JN, Goldman MB: The genetics of antibody production. *JAMA* 1984;**251**:774.

Goldstein IM, Marder SR: Infections and hypocomplementemia. *Annu Rev Med* 1983;**34**:47.

Hill HR, Matsen JM: Enzyme-linked immunosorbent assay and radioimmunoassay in the serologic diagnosis of infectious disease. *J Infect Dis* 1983;**147**:258.

Horwitz MA: Phagocytosis of microorganisms. *Rev Infect Dis* 1982;**4**:104.

Nusbacher J, Bove JR: Rh immunoprophylaxis. *N Engl J Med* 1980;**303**:935.

Oxelius VA: Immunoglobulin G subclasses and human disease. *Am J Med* 1984;**76**:183.

Pollack MS, Rich RR: The HLA complex and the pathogenesis of infectious diseases. *J Infect Dis* 1985;**151**:1.

Quie PG: Perturbation of the normal mechanisms of intraleukocytic killing of bacteria. *J Infect Dis* 1983;**148**:189.

Reinherz EL, Schlossman SF: Regulation of the immune response: Inducer and suppressor T-lymphocyte subsets in human beings. *N Engl J Med* 1980;**303**:370.

Robinson JE et al: Diffuse polyclonal B-cell lymphoma during primary infection with Epstein-Barr virus. *N Engl J Med* 1980;**302**:1293.

Roitt IM: *Essential Immunology*, 5th ed. Blackwell, 1984.

Rosen FS, Cooper MD, Wedgewood RJP: The primary immunodeficiencies. (2 parts.) *N Engl J Med* 1984;**311**:235, 300.

Rosenthal AS: Regulation of the immune response: Role of the macrophage. *N Engl J Med* 1980;**303**:1153.

Rowlands DT Jr, Daniele RP: Surface receptors in the immune response. *N Engl J Med* 1975;**293**:26.

Ruddy S et al: The complement system of man. *N Engl J Med* 1972;**287**:642.

Siegal FP: Suppressors in the network of immunity. *N Engl J Med* 1978;**298**:102.

Solomon A: Bence-Jones proteins and light chains of immunoglobulins. (2 parts.) *N Engl J Med* 1976;**294**:17, 91.

Stites DP et al (editors):*Basic and Clinical Immunology,* 5th ed. Lange, 1984.

Uhr JW et al: Organization of the immune response genes. *Science* 1979;**206**:292.

Unanue ER: Cooperation between mononuclear phagocytes and lymphocytes in immunity. *N Engl J Med* 1980;**303**: 977.

Yalow RS: Radio-immunoassay: A probe for the fine structure of biologic systems. *Science* 1978;**200**:1236.

Immunology:
II. Antibody-Mediated & Cell-Mediated (Hypersensitivity & Immunity) Reactions

13

ANTIBODY-MEDIATED HYPERSENSITIVITY

The principal mechanism in most antibody-mediated hypersensitivity reactions is the combination of antibody (Ab) with antigen (Ag) to form complexes that stimulate certain cells to release a variety of mediators. The main reactions in this category are of the anaphylaxis and serum sickness type. Interactions between antibodies and red blood cell or platelet antigens usually do not involve the release of mediators.

ANAPHYLAXIS

The experimental demonstration of anaphylaxis involves the following steps:

(1) Sensitization: An adequate sensitizing dose of antigen must be absorbed. In the guinea pig, as little as 0.1 μg of a soluble protein is sufficient.

(2) Waiting period: A waiting period of 2–3 weeks is required. During this period, cytotropic antibody (in guinea pigs, IgE and some IgG) attaches to mast cells and basophilic leukocytes.

(3) "Eliciting injection": The rapid intravenous injection of a massive dose (0.1–10 mg) of the same antigen as used for sensitization permits the antigen to combine with cell-bound antibody rapidly. The complex stimulates the prompt release of mediators that set off the symptoms of anaphylaxis (eg, bronchospasm) within 3–5 minutes.

(4) Passive transfer: If serum is taken after the waiting period (2) from the sensitized animal and injected into the skin of a normal animal, the injected site becomes sensitized in 24 hours (ie, homocytotropic antibodies attach to mast cells and basophils). When antigen is given intravenously to such an animal together with a dye (eg, Evans blue), a local anaphylactic reaction at the sensitized site results in a marked increase in capillary permeability that permits the dye to stain the sensitized area of skin. This **passive cutaneous anaphylaxis** is suitable for quantitation of some anaphylactic events.

Anaphylactic reactivity in humans manifests itself as systemic, generalized anaphylaxis or as local anaphylaxis involving skin or respiratory tract or other target organ or tissue.

Generalized anaphylaxis in humans begins within 5–30 minutes after administration of the inciting agent, with flush, urticaria, paroxysmal cough, dyspnea, wheezing, vomiting, cyanosis, circulatory collapse, and shock. Major causes of death are laryngeal and massive airway edema and cardiac arrhythmias. Major causes of generalized anaphylaxis in humans are drugs (eg, penicillins), biologicals (eg, animal sera), insect stings (eg, bee or wasp venom), and foods (eg, shellfish).

Local anaphylaxis in humans begins within a few minutes after contact (inhalation, ingestion) between the responsible antigen and the sensitive shock organ and manifests itself commonly as hay fever, asthma, urticaria, or vomiting. About 10% of the population are prone to become spontaneously sensitized to various environmental antigens (allergens), eg, pollens of ragweed, grasses, or trees; foods; and animal danders. These individuals develop allergic reactions **(atopy)** when exposed to the antigen. There is a marked familial predisposition to atopy, but each individual must become sensitized to the specific allergen before manifesting atopic reactions.

Cutaneous anaphylaxis is seen in the skin test for immediate type hypersensitivity. Two or 3 minutes after 0.1 mL of antigen is injected intracutaneously (often into the flexor surface of the forearm), itching begins at the site, followed by an elevated, blanched irregular wheal surrounded by a zone of erythema ("flare"). This hive (urticarial reaction) reaches a maximum in 10–15 minutes and subsides within less than 1 hour.

Mechanism of Anaphylaxis

As a result of the original sensitization with antigen, specialized, cytotropic antibody is formed that binds to mast cells and basophils, especially in skin, the respiratory tract, and vascular endothelium. In humans, the cytotropic antibody is IgE. When the same antigen is again absorbed, it reaches these cells and results in aggregation of IgE molecules bound to cell surfaces by their Fc fragment. This is the stimulus for the release of pharmacologically active chemical mediators from the cell (degranulation). Aggregated Fc fragments of IgE proteins can also elicit a cell release of mediators even without the presence of antigen. Large amounts of soluble antigen-antibody complexes that are capable of binding complement can also evoke anaphylaxis under special circumstances.

Pharmacologically Active Chemical Mediators

Pharmacologically active chemical mediators released during anaphylaxis include the following:

A. Histamine: Histamine (formed by decarboxylation of histidine) occurs in platelets and in granules of tissue mast cells and basophils, cells that—in humans—bind IgE through special sites of the Fc fragment. The histamine released as a result of anaphylaxis causes vasodilation, increased capillary permeability (edema), and smooth muscle contraction (bronchospasm). The relative amount of histamine and of other mediators released determines the efficacy of antihistamine drugs, which only block histamine receptor sites. Antihistamines are relatively effective in allergic rhinitis but relatively ineffective in asthma (in which much more SRS-A [see below] is released than histamine).

B. Slow-Reacting Substance of Anaphylaxis (SRS-A): SRS-A is a mixture of leukotrienes. It does not exist in a preformed state but is formed during type I anaphylactic reactions. Leukotrienes are formed from arachidonic acid by the lipoxygenase pathway and have potent biologic effects, including increased vascular permeability and smooth muscle contraction. They are principal mediators in the bronchoconstriction of asthma, and their synthesis is not inhibited by antihistamines.

C. Eosinophil Chemotactic Factor of Anaphylaxis (ECF-A): ECF-A is a peptide (MW 600) that exists preformed in mast cell granules. When released during anaphylaxis, it is chemotactic for human eosinophils that are prominent in immediate allergic reactions.

D. Serotonin: Serotonin (hydroxytryptamine) exists preformed in mast cells and especially in blood platelets and is released during anaphylaxis. It causes capillary dilation and increased vascular permeability, and smooth muscle constriction in some species, but appears to be of minor importance in human anaphylactic reactions.

E. Kinins: Kinins are basic peptides derived from plasma proteins. They are not primary mediators in anaphylactic reactions but contribute to the clinical features of such reactions through their secondary involvement. Factor XII (Hageman factor) in the blood clotting cascade may be activated in anaphylaxis. This may result in activation of plasmin, a fibrinolytic enzyme, and of kallikrein, which splits bradykinin from an α globulin. Bradykinin levels in blood are elevated during anaphylactic reactions, and bradykinin may participate in producing vasodilatation, increased vas-

cular permeability, and smooth muscle contraction. Other kinins also participate in anaphylactic reactions.

F. Prostaglandins and Thromboxanes: These compounds are related to leukotrienes and are derived from arachidonic acid via the cyclooxygenase pathway. Prostaglandins can produce dilatation and increased permeability of capillaries and constriction of bronchial smooth muscle. Thromboxanes aggregate platelets and act in conjunction with platelet-activating factors.

The chemical mediators are active for only a few minutes after release. Histamine, serotonin, bradykinin, and SRS-A are enzymatically inactivated. They are resynthesized at a slow rate. The manifestations of anaphylaxis vary among animal species because mediators are released at different rates and in different amounts, and different tissues ("shock organs") have different sensitivity to mediators. Whereas the respiratory tract (bronchospasm, laryngeal edema) is a principal shock organ in humans, the liver (hepatic veins) plays that role in the dog.

Desensitization

Major manifestations of anaphylaxis depend on the sudden release of large amounts of mediators, usually as a result of a massive dose of antigen suddenly combining with IgE on many mast cells. If, on the other hand, only very small amounts of antigen are administered at 15-minute intervals, complex formation occurs only on a small scale and not enough mediator is released at a given moment to produce a major reaction. This is the basis of **acute desensitization,** which makes it possible to administer a drug or foreign serum to a hypersensitive person. However, days or weeks later, hypersensitivity is restored.

Chronic desensitization (hyposensitization) relies on a different principle. When small amounts of an antigen (especially high-molecular-weight polymerized ragweed antigen) are administered at weekly intervals to a person hypersensitive to that antigen, IgG antibodies (**blocking antibodies**) appear in the serum. When a desensitized person is exposed to antigen, the blocking antibodies combine with the antigens and prevent their reaching IgE antibody on mast cells and basophils. Consequently, the blocking antibody can prevent allergic reactions.

Blocking antibodies differ from IgE cytotropic antibodies (reagins). Reagins bind to human skin, persist there for weeks, are heat-labile, and do not cross the placenta. Blocking antibodies are IgG, do not bind to human skin or persist there, are heat-stable, and cross the placenta.

Passive Transfer of Atopy

If the serum of a person with atopic hypersensitivity is injected into the skin of a normal person, IgE antibody binds to skin mast cells and sensitizes them during the next 20 hours. Injection of that sensitized skin site with the antigen produces an immediate type wheal-and-flare anaphylactic response of the skin site. In the normal person, that skin site maintains its ability to react to the antigen for several weeks. This **Prausnitz-Küstner (PK) reaction** is commonly used for the identification of important allergens in atopic patients who may show many positive direct skin tests.

Treatment of Anaphylactic Reactions

The purpose of treatment is to counteract the effects of released chemical mediators or to block their action. In systemic anaphylaxis, the main efforts are directed at maintaining ventilation and cardiac function. This implies maintenance of a patent airway, assisted ventilation if necessary, and epinephrine (1:1000 solution), 0.1–0.5 mL given in an intravenous infusion. A soluble corticosteroid may be administered for a later effect, and metaraminol may help to overcome the cardiovascular collapse.

Local anaphylactic reactions tend to respond to epinephrine or aminophylline (7 mg/kg), and their continued activity may be blocked by corticosteroids. Antihistamines are relatively effective in allergic rhinitis but ineffective in asthma (see above).

The release of mediators of allergic reaction from mast cell granules can be inhibited by the administration of cromolyn sodium, a substance that stabilizes lysosomal membranes. This may prevent or terminate an allergic reaction.

Anaphylactoid Reactions

These resemble anaphylaxis but are precipitated by injection of particle suspensions or colloids (barium sulfate, inulin, procaine, etc) that activate factor XII, plasmin, kallikrein, and the alternative pathway of the complement sequence. They are unrelated to antigen-antibody reactions or allergy.

Anaphylaxis in Isolated Tissues in Vitro

When an organ (eg, uterus, gut) from a sensitized animal is suspended in a salt solution, addition of the specific antigen results in prompt muscular contraction and liberation of mediators into the solution (**Schultz-Dale reaction**). This is due to the binding of antigen to cytotropic antibody on tissue mast cells.

Prevention of Anaphylaxis

Since anaphylaxis caused by drugs or biologic products may produce serious or life-threatening illness, a careful history of previous exposure or reaction must be taken before such substances are administered. Skin tests (see p 358) or conjunctival tests* can often predict the presence of hypersensitivity and therefore the real risk of a major, severe reaction.

ARTHUS REACTION

This antibody-mediated hypersensitivity reaction requires large amounts of antigen-antibody complexes that fix complement, attract polymorphonuclear leukocytes, and are phagocytosed by them. The cells release lysosomal enzymes that cause tissue damage,

typically with vasculitis of blood vessel walls. The lesions subside within several days.

Any class of complement-fixing immunoglobulin can mediate the Arthus reaction, but the higher the level of antibody the more intense the lesion; it requires at least 1000 times more antibody than anaphylaxis, and preformed antigen-antibody complexes can elicit it.

Whereas in anaphylaxis the structural changes in tissues are limited to vasodilation, edema, and a few polymorphonuclear leukocytes, the appearance of the Arthus reaction is much more intensive inflammation. It begins with thrombosis of small vessels surrounded by edema and intense infiltration with polymorphonuclear leukocytes; areas of necrosis then develop in the walls of blood vessels. Neutrophils degenerate, and the debris is taken up by mononuclear cells and eosinophils. The phagocytosed antigen-antibody complexes are broken down and eliminated, and the inflammation subsides. In humans, lesions corresponding to the Arthus reaction occur sometimes in serum sickness or in hypersensitivity pneumonitis ("farmer's lung") or allergic alveolitis.

SERUM SICKNESS

Persons who receive a large amount of a drug (eg, penicillin) or foreign protein (eg, antiserum) may tolerate these injections well but develop an illness 4–18 days later. Typical serum sickness consists of fever, widespread urticarial eruption, pain and swelling of joints, and enlargement of lymph nodes and spleen. These signs usually subside within a week.

During serum sickness, some tissues exhibit lesions of vasculitis (as in the Arthus reaction) but also vasodilatation, edema, and smooth muscle contraction (as in anaphylaxis). The mechanism is as follows: After a large amount of antigen is injected, its concentration gradually declines and at the same time antibody production starts. The simultaneous presence of antigen and antibody leads to the formation of soluble antigen-antibody complexes that set off the immune response, combining vasculitis with the release of chemical mediators. Serum sickness subsides when the antigen has been eliminated.

IMMUNE COMPLEX DISEASE

Several antibody-mediated hypersensitivity reactions can be elicited by preformed, soluble antigen-antibody complexes (see above). Immune complexes of intermediate size (less than 11S) are more likely to be deposited than either larger or smaller complexes. A number of disease entities are attributed to immune complex deposits initiating tissue disorders—al-

---

*One drop of dilute material is placed into the conjunctival sac. A positive reaction is indicated by itching, redness, and tearing in a few minutes.

though the antigen often is not established. Examples are glomerulonephritis and rheumatoid arthritis. In addition, circulating immune complexes can be detected (by radioimmunoassay or by binding to cultured Raji cells) in various disorders ranging from infective endocarditis and viral and parasitic infections to "autoimmune diseases," eg, systemic lupus erythematosus.

Glomerulonephritis in Different Diseases

Acute glomerulonephritis usually follows by several weeks the onset of a group A β-hemolytic *Streptococcus* infection. During acute glomerulonephritis, the levels of serum complement (especially C3) are usually low, suggesting an antigen-antibody reaction. By immunofluorescence, lumpy deposits of Ig and C3 are seen along basement membranes of renal glomeruli—suggesting the presence of antigen-antibody complexes. Although streptococcal antigens have been infrequently demonstrated in glomeruli, it is assumed that streptococcal antigen-antibody complexes filtered out in glomeruli initiated the reaction and fixed C3.

An analogous lesion with "lumpy" immunofluorescent deposits containing immunoglobulin and C3 occurs in serum sickness caused by a known foreign protein and in the glomerulonephritis associated with infective endocarditis or viral hepatitis.

In systemic lupus erythematosus (SLE), patients have circulating antibody to DNA. In the glomerulonephritis of SLE, the lumpy immunofluorescent deposits in glomeruli contain DNA as antigen, immunoglobulin (?antibody to DNA), and C3. In other patients with glomerulonephritis (eg, Goodpasture's syndrome), there is linear immunofluorescence along the basement membrane of glomeruli, caused by the combination of basement membrane antigen with antibody and complement.

At least in animals, viral infections can cause glomerulonephritis by an immune complex mechanism. In chronically infected mice, lymphocytic choriomeningitis antigen and its antiviral antibody form complexes that are deposited in glomeruli, bind complement, and initiate inflammatory lesions. The virus of Aleutian mink disease causes a similar immune complex disease with glomerulonephritis.

In penicillin-induced nephritis, the drug binds to tubular basement membrane protein, and antibody to this antigen is formed and deposited. Complement is bound to the complex, and polymorphonuclear leukocytes are attracted to produce the interstitial nephritis.

Rheumatoid Arthritis

Rheumatoid arthritis is a chronic inflammatory joint disease that is particularly common in young women. The synovial fluid contains high concentrations of immunoglobulin aggregates, complement, and polymorphonuclear leukocytes. The nature of the antigen is undetermined. The reaction between human immunoglobulins and rheumatoid factors (IgM and IgG molecules that bind to antigenic determinants on the Fc fragments of IgG) is employed diagnostically and might play a causative role.

Autoimmune Diseases

Antigen-antibody complexes have been demonstrated in various autoimmune diseases and may participate in their pathogenesis. Autoimmune diseases are discussed on pp 200–202.

DRUG HYPERSENSITIVITY

Drugs are now among the commonest causes of hypersensitivity reactions, and antibiotics are high on the list. Penicillin hypersensitivity has been studied extensively and is used as an example here.

To induce hypersensitivity, the drug—or a reactive metabolic derivative—must covalently bind to host protein in order to become antigenic. The subsequent allergic reaction is specific for the haptens rather than for the drug itself. Such compounds can induce antibody formation and immediate and delayed type hypersensitivity. The likelihood of any one individual developing hypersensitivity to a given drug is probably influenced by genetic predisposition; the route, duration, and amount of drug exposure; the level of antibody production; and other factors.

In the case of penicillin, some important reactive products are penicilloyl compounds and minor determinant groups. When covalently bound to protein, these can induce antibody-mediated hypersensitivity and local or generalized anaphylaxis.

In order to detect possible hypersensitivity to penicillin, skin tests can be performed with penicilloyl polylysine (which will not itself induce hypersensitivity), with alkaline degradation products (containing minor determinants) of penicillin, or with penicillin itself. An immediate type wheal-and-flare reaction suggests that IgE antibodies have become bound to mast cells and that such a reactive person may be subject to generalized anaphylaxis.

In view of the very large number of people who have been given penicillin—many of whom have developed IgE antibody—it is surprising that anaphylactic reactions are so rare. Two possible explanations might be considered: (1) Most persons who develop IgE antipenicilloyl antibody also develop IgG antibody of the same specificity, which may well act as blocking antibody. (2) Penicillin molecules themselves may be univalent for antipenicilloyl antibody and thus may inhibit rather than favor aggregation of IgE antibody. Persons who handle penicillins occupationally may develop contact dermatitis, a form of delayed type hypersensitivity with positive skin test (see below).

Penicilloyl antibody and the corresponding antigen are the basis for the serum sickness that may follow a single penicillin injection as a result of complex formation. Penicilloyl hapten bound to tubular basement membrane can be an inciting cause of interstitial nephritis, which is an immune complex disease.

Many different drugs have been incriminated in cytotoxic hypersensitivity reactions that often manifest themselves as hematologic disorders. Thus, hemolytic anemias may result from the attachment of penicillin, phenacetin, quinidine, and other drugs to surface proteins on red blood cells. Autoimmune antibodies form (mainly IgG), and antigen-antibody complex formation results in hemolysis of the attached cell.

Drugs like apronalide (Sedormid) or quinine attach as haptens to platelets, giving rise to autoantibodies that first clump and then lyse the platelets to produce thrombocytopenia with bleeding tendency. Other drugs, such as hydralazine, may modify host tissue and favor the production of autoantibodies directed against cell DNA. Such patients then have antinuclear factors similar to those found in systemic lupus erythematosus.

CELL-MEDIATED HYPERSENSITIVITY & IMMUNITY

The outstanding differences between antibody-mediated and cell-mediated hypersensitivity reactions are shown in Table 12–3. Cell-mediated hypersensitivity reactions begin several hours after contact with antigen and reach a peak 24–72 hours later. The reactivity can be transferred by lymphoid cells but *not* by serum and consists of inflammatory changes with heavy infiltrates of mononuclear cells. Cell-mediated hypersensitivity is closely related to cell-mediated immunity. For both, the central component is the immunologically committed T lymphocyte and its interactions and products. The prototype of cell-mediated hypersensitivity and of "delayed" type skin reactions is seen in tuberculin hypersensitivity.

TUBERCULIN HYPERSENSITIVITY

Koch's Phenomenon (See Chapter 26)

When a tuberculous guinea pig is injected subcutaneously with a suspension of tubercle bacilli, there is a massive inflammatory reaction at the injection site that tends to wall off the injected material and often leads to necrosis; this is called Koch's phenomenon. This reaction does not require living tubercle bacilli but occurs similarly with tuberculoprotein (PPD). These soluble preparations produce local inflammatory reactions, particularly edema, infiltration with lymphoid cells and macrophages, hemorrhage, and marked enlargement of the regional lymph nodes; and focal reactions, consisting of hemorrhagic inflammation and dense cellular infiltration within existing tuberculous lesions. Because focal reactions may "stir up" tuberculous activity, administration of excessive doses of tuberculoprotein to hypersensitive individuals during skin tests must be avoided.

Delayed Type Skin Reaction

The typical skin test of the delayed type is exemplified by the tuberculin test. There is no immediate reaction following the intracutaneous injection of tuberculoprotein. After a few hours, redness, edema, and induration develop and tend to increase for 48–72 hours. If the reaction is marked, there may be central blanching, hemorrhage, and necrosis. The redness and edema disappear quickly, but the induration of the skin reaction can be felt for days or weeks. Histologically, the lesion of the skin test is characterized by initial vasodilation, edema, and polymorphonuclear cell infiltration; this is followed soon afterward by marked and persistent focal accumulation and diffuse infiltration with lymphoid (mainly helper T cells) and mononuclear cells. The intensity of the tuberculin skin reaction in the hypersensitive individual bears no relationship to the level of antibodies that may be demonstrated. Transfer of lymphoid cells from a skin-test-positive person can transfer reactivity to a skin-test-negative person.

PASSIVE TRANSFER OF CELL-MEDIATED HYPERSENSITIVITY

It is not possible to transfer tuberculin or other cell-mediated hypersensitivity with serum. However, viable T lymphocytes taken from a reactive person and transferred to a nonreactive person will temporarily make the recipient reactive (eg, tuberculin-positive). In humans, it is also possible to transfer some reactivity of cell-mediated hypersensitivity by means of nonviable extracts from T lymphocytes. This material has been called "transfer factor."

Properties of "Transfer Factor"

Transfer factor is a stable dialyzable extract of immune lymphocytes with a molecular weight below 2000. It contains RNA and protein but no DNA. After injection of transfer factor, delayed type hypersensitivity begins in 2–7 days and may last for several months.

The mechanism of transfer factor activity remains uncertain. It can transfer specific delayed type hypersensitivity to tuberculin, streptococcal antigens, coccidioidin, allograft antigens, and others.

In some patients with defects in cell-mediated immunity, transfer factor may temporarily restore competent cell-mediated reactions. In about half of the patients with Wiskott-Aldrich syndrome, transfer factor has resulted in temporary improvement of clinical status.

Some patients with severe combined immune deficiency disease have also shown significant, albeit temporary, improvement. In chronic mycobacterial and fungal infections (eg, disseminated mucocutaneous candidiasis and coccidioidomycosis), transfer factor therapy, combined with antimicrobial drugs, has resulted in encouraging remissions. Improvement has been reported in the immunologic status of patients with various cancers (eg, osteosarcoma and melanoma), but the clinical efficacy of this adjuvant treatment remains to be established.

INDUCTION OF CELL-MEDIATED IMMUNITY & DELAYED HYPERSENSITIVITY

The development of delayed type hypersensitivity is favored by the introduction of small amounts of antigens on cell surfaces or in lipid mixtures called **adjuvants.** Thus, tuberculin sensitivity can be induced by infection with *Mycobacterium tuberculosis* but also by injection of small amounts of tuberculoprotein together with wax D (a peptidoglycolipid) or tuberculoprotein in Freund's complete adjuvant. If larger amounts of antigen are introduced, there is less cell-mediated hypersensitivity and more antibody response. Whereas very small antigenic determinants (eg, haptens) are effective in inducing antibody responses, cell-mediated responses seem to require larger and more complex structures as determinants of specificity. In other words, cell-mediated responses appear to be carrier-dependent.

The first step in the induction of cell-mediated responses may be the uptake of the antigen by macrophages and its subsequent presentation to the receptors on T lymphocytes. Once suitable lymphocytes have been contacted, these may be stimulated to proliferate and become "sensitized" lymphocytes (see below).

When a person carrying such "sensitized" T lymphocytes is again exposed to the antigen (eg, when a tuberculin skin test is applied), only a few sensitized T lymphocytes are necessary to initiate a cell-mediated hypersensitivity response. The few sensitized T lymphocytes can recruit large numbers of other lymphocytes and macrophages to produce the cellular infiltration characteristic of a cell-mediated reaction. They accomplish this and other effects through the release of mediators ("lymphokines") that include the following:

A. Mediators Affecting Macrophages:

1. Chemotactic factor attracts monocytes, which then become macrophages.

2. Aggregation factor clumps suspended macrophages in vitro.

3. Migration inhibitory factor (MIF) inhibits the migration of normal macrophages. It is probably an acidic glycoprotein with a molecular weight of 25,000–50,000. This may be the substance that "activates" macrophages (see p 164).

B. Mediators Affecting Polymorphonuclear Leukocytes (PMNs):

1. Leukocyte inhibitory factor inhibits migration of PMNs in a manner resembling that of MIF, although it is chemically different. It is a protein with a molecular weight of 68,000 and is inactivated by chymotrypsin.

2. Chemotactic factors for PMNs, basophils, and eosinophils selectively attract each type of cell. Factors that promote activity of eosinophil chemotaxis

have been extracted from trichina and schistosome larvae.

C. Mediators Affecting Lymphocytes:

1. Blastogenic or mitogenic factor causes some lymphocytes to differentiate into large, rapidly dividing blast cells with greatly increased synthesis of DNA.

2. Transfer factor (see above).

3. Interleukin-1 (see p 165) is produced by macrophages and is able to induce fever.

4. Interleukin-2 (T cell growth factor; see p 166).

D. Mediators Affecting Cells in Culture or Affecting Viruses:

1. Lymphotoxin can damage or lyse many types of cells.

2. Interferon can block virus replication in other cells.

These different "mediators" are named on the basis of their observed activity; there is no inference that they represent distinct chemical entities.

TESTS TO EVALUATE CELL-MEDIATED HYPERSENSITIVITY OR IMMUNITY

The assessment of cell-mediated reactivity is increasingly important as greater numbers of persons suffer from spontaneous or medically induced defects of cell-mediated immunity. Increasing numbers of children with congenital defects survive, and in increasing numbers of patients cell-mediated immunity is suppressed by disease (eg, AIDS) or by antitumor drugs, corticosteroids, or immunosuppressive drugs used for organ transplants. In the following tests, it is assumed that defects in cell-mediated reactivity probably indicate defects in cell-mediated immunity to infectious agents.

Skin Tests

Skin tests may be used to determine cell-mediated hypersensitivity to commonly encountered antigens in order to assess the competence of cell-mediated reactions. Most normal persons respond with delayed type reactions to skin test antigens of *Candida, Trichophyton,* mumps, streptokinase-streptodornase, or PPD.

Tests for Competence to Develop Cell-Mediated Hypersensitivity

Simple chemicals applied to human skin in lipid solvents induce cell-mediated hypersensitivity in normal persons. One percent 1-chloro-2,4-dinitrobenzene (dinitrochlorobenzene, DNCB) or dinitrofluorobenzene (DNFB) in acetone is applied to the skin and washed off 24 hours later. When a test dose of 0.03–0.1% of the same chemical is applied to the same area 7–14 days later, a delayed type reaction signifies the competence to develop cell-mediated reactions.

Skin Graft Rejection

A normal person will reject a skin graft from an unrelated individual in a predictable time sequence of reactions (see below). Inability to reject such a skin graft is strong evidence of impaired cell-mediated responses.

In Vitro Evaluation of Responses of Lymphoid Cells

A. Lymphocyte Blast Transformation: When sensitized T lymphocytes are exposed to a specific antigen, they transform into large blast cells (the number and proportion of blasts can be counted) with greatly increased DNA synthesis (the incorporation of tritiated thymidine into DNA can be measured). However, only a small number of cells undergo this *specific* blast transformation. A larger number of T lymphocytes undergo *nonspecific* blast transformation when exposed to mitogens such as phytohemagglutinin (a kidney bean extract), pokeweed mitogen, or concanavalin A (a jack bean extract). The measurements in nonspecific and specific blast transformations are the same.

B. Macrophage Migration Inhibitory Factor: Upon challenge by an antigen to which cultured lymphocytes are sensitive, they elaborate macrophage migration inhibitory factor (MIF). This will inhibit the migration of guinea pig peritoneal macrophages from a capillary tube.

C. Rosette Formation: When incubated with sheep red blood cells, most T lymphocytes form rosettes. Although the mechanism of this effect is not clear, it permits an estimate of the proportion of circulating lymphocytes that behave in this manner. There is good correlation between rosette-forming and MIF-producing T lymphocytes.

D. Enumeration of T and B Cells and Subpopulations: Largely because of current concern with AIDS (see p 198 and Chapter 47), lymphoid cell counts are performed and their ratios determined frequently. Specific monoclonal antibodies directed at T cell markers permit the enumeration of T cells, OKT4-reactive helper cells, OKT8-reactive suppressor cells, and the ratios of these cells. B cells can be counted by using fluorescent-labeled antibody against all immunoglobulin classes.

DELAYED HYPERSENSITIVITY SKIN TESTS AS DIAGNOSTIC TOOLS

Cell-mediated hypersensitivity develops with many types of infection. Delayed type skin reactivity can be a valuable aid in diagnosis if it is cautiously interpreted. A positive skin reaction indicates only that the individual has at some time in the past been infected with the specific agent. It provides information about the nature of a specific illness only if conversion from a negative to a positive skin test occurs during the course of the illness. Blood transfusion may passively transfer delayed hypersensitivity by means of sensitized lymphocytes. Furthermore, the general skin reactivity declines markedly in far-advanced stages of

many diseases **(anergy).** Similar anergy may be encountered during the childhood exanthems (measles, chickenpox); thus a tuberculin-positive child may temporarily give a tuberculin-negative reaction during one of these illnesses. Anergy is also a regular feature of sarcoidosis, Hodgkin's disease, and other advanced neoplasms, as well as uremia. Patients receiving large doses of corticosteroids or immunosuppressive drugs (eg, cancer chemotherapy, organ transplants) have marked depression of cell-mediated hypersensitivity and immunity.

Bacterial Infections

Skin tests may be useful to support a diagnosis of tuberculosis, tularemia, chancroid, and some other infections. In leprosy, the reaction to lepromin is more an indication of the immunologic state of the disease (ie, tuberculoid) than a help in diagnosis. Various types of skin tests are described in Chapter 32. Although specific purified protein derivatives are available, mycobacterial infections cross-react extensively. Many available skin test preparations are open to criticism, and their use has pitfalls for diagnosis.

Mycotic Infections

Delayed type skin reactions occur in virtually all deep mycoses. If adequate skin testing material is available and if the concentration used is sufficiently dilute to avoid cross-reactions, the skin tests may be helpful in the diagnosis of past infections such as coccidioidomycosis, histoplasmosis, blastomycosis, and others. Most normal adults give positive skin tests with *Candida* antigens, and a negative test suggests a defect in cell-mediated immunity. In some deep mycoses (eg, histoplasmosis), the skin test itself may result in a significant rise of specific antibodies and thus lead to misleading diagnostic serologic tests.

Helminthic Infections

In most protozoan and helminthic parasitic infections—including trichinosis, filariasis, and ascariasis—immediate type skin reactions occur with application of worm extracts. Some delayed type reactions may also occur, eg, in trichinosis, echinococcosis (with heated hydatid cyst fluid), and others. Skin tests are probably never as specific as refined serologic tests in these disorders.

Viral Infections

Cell-mediated hypersensitivity occurs in many viral infections, including herpes simplex, mumps, and vaccinia. However, serologic tests are preferred for assessment of immunity.

Combined "Immediate" & "Delayed" Reactions

Skin-testing preparations from many infectious agents may produce both antibody-mediated and cell-mediated responses. This is usually due to the presence of multiple antigens in such preparations—some eliciting one response and some another.

RELATIONSHIP OF CELL-MEDIATED REACTIONS & RESISTANCE TO INFECTION

Whereas antibodies provide protection against toxin-induced disorders and to a certain extent against virus infections, they play a limited role in host defenses against microbial infections, except in those whose virulence depends on polysaccharide capsules. Cell-mediated reactions are of paramount importance in maintaining resistance to most microbial infections. In some cell-mediated reactions, antibodies cooperate in processes of recovery; eg, opsonins facilitate phagocytosis and chemotactic fragments of complement enhance inflammatory reactions and localization of infection. One of the most important contributions of cell-mediated reactions to resistance to infection is the "activation" of macrophages (see p 164). Sensitized T lymphocytes act on normal macrophages and "activate" them to a high level of phagocytic activity and intracellular killing ability.

The role played by antibody-mediated and by cell-mediated reactions, respectively, can be estimated to some extent by noting the types of infection that develop in persons who have a specified immune defect. The absence of complement components (especially C5–C9) favors bloodstream dissemination of neisseriae. Persons with isolated B cell defects and lack of antibody responses may be unusually susceptible to pyogenic coccal (especially pneumococcal) infections but handle intracellular bacterial or fungal and many viral infections normally. Conversely, persons with isolated T cell defects and deficient cell-mediated reactions may be overwhelmed by opportunistic organisms (Nocardia, Pneumocystis, Candida, Aspergillus) and incapable of handling mycobacterial or fungal infections. T cell defects and impaired cell-mediated reactions also permit the widespread dissemination of many viral infections (eg, herpes zoster). An outstanding example of this type of disease is acquired immune deficiency syndrome (AIDS), which is discussed in Chapter 47.

Manifestations of hypersensitivity accompany many infectious processes. At times the hypersensitivity is incidental (eg, erythema nodosum in coccidioidomycosis), but at other times the cell-mediated hypersensitivity may significantly enhance the inflammatory reaction in foci of infection (eg, tuberculosis of the lung) and may lead to increased tissue destruction. In still other situations (Koch's phenomenon), the cell-mediated hypersensitivity reaction may favor localization of the infectious agent and limitation of its spread.

CONTACT ALLERGY TO DRUGS & SIMPLE CHEMICALS

Common allergic skin disorders in humans are attributable to sensitization by contact of skin with many simple chemicals (nickel, formaldehyde), drugs (sulfonamides), cosmetics, plant materials (catechols from poison ivy and poison oak), and others. Chlorogenic acid, a simple phenolic compound of low molecular weight, is a hapten contained in many different plants, eg, coffee beans, castor beans, fruits, and vegetables. It becomes a complete antigen by combining with host protein and can induce respiratory or skin allergy in heavily exposed humans (eg, coffee workers). Presumably, these materials form covalent bonds with proteins of skin. Induction of cell-mediated hypersensitivity is probably aided by skin lipids or lipid vehicles acting like adjuvants.

Upon skin contact with the offending agent, the sensitized person develops erythema and swelling, itching, vesication, or necrosis in 12–48 hours. Histologically, the reaction is an intense mononuclear cell infiltrate resembling the tuberculin test. Patch testing on a small area of skin reproduces the lesion and can identify the allergen.

ROLE OF LIPIDS, WAXES, & ADJUVANTS IN THE DEVELOPMENT OF CELL-MEDIATED REACTIONS

It has been mentioned above that tuberculoprotein stimulates the development of delayed hypersensitivity reactions only if it is administered together with wax from the tubercle bacillus. The same wax permits sensitization of animals with simple chemicals, such as picryl chloride, which does not elicit hypersensitivity if injected alone. It is conceivable that the strongly allergenic properties of substances applied to the skin (compared with other routes of administration) are aided by the many lipids available in the skin. In general, it appears that the delayed type of hypersensitivity develops best if the allergen is administered in such a fashion as to elicit a focal inflammatory response. Lipids often elicit focal granulomatous tissue lesions.

When weakly antigenic or allergenic materials are mixed with lipids (eg, lanolin or paraffin) and killed tubercle bacilli, they elicit a much greater antibody response and cell-mediated reactions than the antigens alone, and occasionally result in the production of "autoimmune" diseases. Such enhancing mixtures (often lanolin + paraffin oil + tubercle bacilli) are referred to as "adjuvants" (eg, Freund's adjuvant).

The main roles of the adjuvant appear to be the favoring of helper T cells and the maintenance of long-lasting antigen levels in tissue to be taken up by macrophages and presented to lymphocytes.

EXTRINSIC ALLERGIC ALVEOLITIS (Hypersensitivity Pneumonitis)

A large group of recurrent, debilitating pulmonary disorders is caused by hypersensitivity reactions to inhaled antigens in persons hypersensitive to these antigens. Patients usually have high titers of precipitating antibody against the offending antigen. The pathogenesis may involve immune complex disease as well as cell-mediated hypersensitivity: There is delayed onset of reaction, absence of bronchospasm, infiltration of interstitial tissue with mononuclear cells, and, at times, epithelioid cells and granulomas. Although the pathogenesis of the disorders appears to be the same, the inciting agent differs: in farmer's lung, it is *Micropolyspora* species from moldy hay; in mushroom worker's lung, *Thermoactinomyces vulgaris* from mushroom compost; in maple-bark disease of paper-mill workers, *Cryptostroma corticale* from moldy bark; in the hypersensitivity pneumonitis of office workers, thermophilic actinomycetes contaminating the air-conditioning system; and in sequoiosis of redwood mill workers, moldy dust from *Sequoia* trees. There are many more.

Opportunistic fungi sometimes establish themselves in the respiratory tract. *Aspergillus* species may grow on bronchial surfaces or in tuberculous cavities, but they may also invade pulmonary tissue and produce granulomas in which hypersensitivity probably plays a role. The lung lesions of schistosomiasis and some other parasitic infestations may be caused by cell-mediated hypersensitivity to the parasite's antigens.

INTERFERENCE WITH CELL-MEDIATED OR ANTIBODY-MEDIATED HYPERSENSITIVITY OR IMMUNITY

Interference by Antibody

A. Antilymphocyte Serum (ALS): Antiserum can be made in one animal species against thymus cells (T lymphocytes) of a second species. When such antiserum is injected into the second species, it selectively depresses cell-mediated reactions, including allograft rejection. The practical usefulness of ALS is limited by its being a foreign serum. Antilymphoblast globulin is better tolerated in humans.

B. Tumor-Enhancing Antibody: Certain antibodies to transplanted tumors interfere with their rejection by the host. This might be attributed to attachment of antibody or antigen-antibody complexes to important tumor cell antigens, thus blocking their recognition or rejection by T lymphocytes (see p 204).

C. Antibody Formation: Antibody present at the time of antigen administration tends to block antibody formation. A practical example is the administration of anti-Rh globulin to Rh-negative mothers immediately after delivery of an Rh-positive infant. The newborn's red blood cells entering the mother's circulation (when the placenta separates) tend to induce anti-Rh antibody formation. Such antibodies might cause fetal erythroblastosis in a subsequent Rh-positive infant. Administered Rh_0 (D) immune globulin rapidly attaches to Rh-positive cells so that they will not act as antigens.

However, in some circumstances, an antibody globulin and the corresponding antigen (eg, tetanus immune globulin and tetanus toxoid) administered simultaneously will not combine if they are given intramuscularly into widely separate areas. This explains the efficacy of emergency prophylaxis of tetanus or rabies.

Interference by Inhibitors of Inflammation or Lymphocyte Proliferation

Corticosteroids and a variety of "immunosuppressive" drugs (eg, azathioprine) given to prolong the survival of organ transplants suppress cell-mediated hypersensitivity and immunity. They are the principal reason for the marked increase in susceptibility of organ transplant recipients to bacterial, viral, mycotic, and protozoal infections, which are often progressive and lethal. Suppression of antibody formation usually is not important clinically.

Many drugs used in cancer chemotherapy have similar effects. Corticosteroids alone (in high dosage) in immunologic diseases (rheumatoid arthritis, systemic lupus erythematosus, etc) likewise suppress cell-mediated reactions and therefore open the way for the development of infectious ("opportunistic") complications.

Virus infection of effector T cells can result in a marked reduction in the number of these cells. Retrovirus HTLV III/LAV appears to infect and replicate in T lymphocytes, causing a fall in total lymphocyte counts and the particularly marked destruction of helper T cells that leads to the extreme susceptibility of AIDS patients to opportunistic infections and neoplasms.

Other Types of Interference

Lymphoreticular disorders (Hodgkin's disease, sarcoid, lymphosarcoma) or widely disseminated infections (tuberculosis, coccidioidomycosis, lepromatous leprosy) are typically associated with deficient cell-mediated reactions, including anergy to skin tests. Antibody levels are generally normal. If the infection is controlled by treatment, cell-mediated reactivity returns. Transfer factor can accomplish the same result in these disorders for a brief period.

Widespread neoplastic disease also leads to interference with cell-mediated responses. In this situation, cell-mediated skin reactivity has been restored by levamisole (tetrahydro-6-phenyl-imidazothiazole), an anthelmintic drug. The mechanism is not known. Intensive treatment with some interferons may similarly restore depressed cell-mediated immunity.

TOLERANCE

Interference by Antigens

Specific immunologic unresponsiveness is called tolerance. The following features may determine whether an antigen will induce tolerance rather than an immunologic response:

(1) Immunologic maturity of the host. *Examples:*
(a) Neonatal tolerance to allografts (see below).
(b) Vertical transmission of animal viruses: Some

tumor viruses and lymphocytic choriomeningitis virus are transmitted from mother to fetus. Viruses multiply in the fetus and persist after birth, but there is little or no antibody response or cell-mediated response. The offspring is tolerant and permits tumor development. On the other hand, if an uninfected mouse offspring matures and is then infected with viruses, it develops an immune response and resists tumor development.

(2) Structure and dose of antigen. *Example:* If very low or very high doses of an antigen are administered, there may be tolerance instead of an immune response. If purified polysaccharides or amino acid copolymers are injected intravenously in huge doses, there may be "immune paralysis"—a lack of response. This tolerance may terminate when much of the antigenic mass has been degraded or excreted or when a cross-reacting antigen is administered. T cells become tolerant more readily and remain tolerant longer than B cells. Intravenous administration of an antigen is more likely to establish tolerance than administration by other routes.

Some Hypotheses for the Induction of Tolerance

(1) Failure of macrophages to effectively present the antigen to T cells: Neonatal macrophages lack determinants needed for the antigen-presenting function. Deaggregated materials are not taken up well by macrophages for presentation.

(2) Under some circumstances, it is probable that suppressor T cells engage in inhibiting the reactivity in lymphocytic clones.

(3) Antigen administered in very low or very high doses may result in deletion of potentially reactive B cell clones or in deletion of both B cell and helper T cell clones.

Many alternatives or extensions of these hypotheses have been proposed.

Desensitization

Repeated doses of antigen in rapid succession may make the host "tolerant" temporarily in antibody-mediated reactions (through the mechanism shown in [3] above). Desensitization is rarely not successful in cell-mediated reactions (see p 192).

Tolerance to Tissue Allografts

(1) If animals of one strain are injected in utero with cells (lymphoid cells, bone marrow) from a second strain, the injected animal, upon maturing, will accept an allograft from the second strain.

(2) Tolerance is established more readily if the antigenic disparity between donor and recipient is slight rather than major.

(3) Tolerance is established best in the immunologically immature. The timing varies: Mice and rats in utero are immunologically immature; sheep amd humans in the third trimester in utero are immunologically mature.

(4) Tolerance in T cells is more effective than in B

cells (see above). It may be favored by enhanced activity of suppressor T cells.

(5) **Graft-versus-host (GVH) reactions:** When lymphoid cells are transferred from an immunologically competent donor to an immunodeficient recipient, the donor cells may establish themselves in the recipient but "reject" the host. This can result in growth retardation, runting, or death. GVH reactions are a serious problem in "immunologic reconstitution" by grafts of lymphoid cells, bone marrow, or thymus to immunodeficient children (see p 203).

AUTOIMMUNE DISEASES

Certain disease states are attributed to immune responses of a host to its own tissues. The mechanism of pathogenesis is speculative—often based on circumstantial evidence rather than definitive proof.

In general, the tissue antigens present during fetal and neonatal life are recognized as "self" and so are tolerated by the host. No antibodies or cell-mediated reactions are developed to them. On the other hand, antigens not present during fetal or neonatal life are rejected as "not self," and immune responses to them may develop. Very complex interactions are involved.

The differentiation of "self" from "not self" must be an important homeostatic function of the animal body. "Autoimmune disease" may be considered a failure of this homeostatic function, a disorder of immune regulation.

In certain specialized situations, tolerance may be lost and immunologic reaction to host antigens develops. Some possible mechanisms are as follows:

A. Release of Sequestered Antigen: Certain tissues are normally sequestered, so that their antigens have no access to antibody-forming cells. The lens and uveal tract of the eye, sperm, and central nervous system tissue are normally isolated from the circulation and are thus not recognized as "self." Entrance of these antigens into the circulation elicits relatively organ-specific antibodies and also T cell responses. When these antigens are administered with adjuvant, various disorders such as endophthalmitis, aspermatogenesis, thyroiditis, or encephalitis can be produced experimentally (see below).

B. Escape of Tolerance at the T Cell Level: Collaboration between helper T cells and B cells is required for most immune responses. Unresponsiveness to a "self" antigen may be maintained by self-tolerance at the helper T cell level even when B cells, which escape from tolerance faster, are no longer tolerant. While most antigen-antibody reactions are highly specific, cross reactions do occur. Termination of tolerance may occur when the host becomes immune to antigens that cross-react with tolerated ("self") antigens, eg, vegetable substances that cross-react with red blood cell antigens, streptococcal antigens that cross-react with human heart tissue antigens. Termination of tolerance can follow such immunization, and autoimmune responses result. Other possible examples of this postulated mechanism are the development of antinuclear (anti-DNA) antibodies after administration of hydralazine and the development of red cell antibodies resulting in hemolytic anemia after administration of methyldopa.

C. Diminished Suppressor T Cell Function: In general, immune responses are subject to complex regulation. It is likely that suppressor T cell activity enters into the lack of response to "self" antigens, ie, limits an immune response. A major loss of such suppressor T cell function may enhance and magnify immune responses to "self" antigens and thus lead to autoimmune diseases. For example, in a suitable genetic setting, antibodies to normal host antigens may be formed, eg, an antibody to normal IgG. This antibody (IgM or IgG) occurs in rheumatoid arthritis and may play a causative role in the formation of immune complexes in joints (see below). However, proof that diminished suppressor T cell function is an important mechanism in autoimmune disease is lacking.

The following are oversimplified examples of disorders that may involve "autoimmune" reactions.

Chronic Thyroiditis

If rabbits are repeatedly injected with extracts of homologous thyroid gland, they develop antibodies and cell-mediated immunity against thyroid antigens. These can be demonstrated by serologic techniques. At the same time, many of the animals develop chronic thyroiditis that histologically resembles Hashimoto's thyroiditis in humans. Patients suffering from chronic thyroiditis have in their serum specific antibodies against thyroid antigens, whereas persons not suffering from thyroid disease lack such antibodies. It is probable, therefore, that human thyroiditis develops as an "autoimmune" disease. Thyroid antigens are no longer recognized as "self" by the host; consequently, antibodies and cell-mediated reactions are formed against them. It is likely that lymphoid cells are sensitized to thyroid antigens and that these cells provoke the inflammatory process which, in turn, leads to fibrosis and loss of function of the gland. Antibodies to thyroglobulin may also play a role.

Allergic Encephalitis

When animal brain substance is mixed with adjuvants and injected into other members of the same animal species, many of these animals will develop encephalitis. The experiment can even be performed successfully by removing the frontal lobe from a monkey, mixing the ground brain material with adjuvant, and injecting it intramuscularly into the same monkey. Such an animal may develop demyelinating disease of the central nervous system with disseminated lesions in the brain and cord. Histologically, these lesions greatly resemble "postvaccinal" encephalomyelitis, which occurs in persons who have been repeatedly injected with animal brain material, as in older rabies vaccine.

Experimental allergic encephalitis cannot be transferred passively by serum but can be passively transferred with lymphoid cells. The severity of lesions bears no relationship to antibrain antibodies measured by CF, and such antibodies may even protect against lesions. The likelihood is great that the illness is based on cell-mediated reactions and that a protein of brain acts as allergen. One such encephalitogenic nonapeptide has been characterized and synthesized.

Diabetes, Myasthenia Gravis, & Hyperthyroidism

In patients with myasthenia gravis, a degenerative central nervous system disease, the serum contains an antibody to the acetylcholine receptors of neuromuscular junctions. Thus, it is possible that the pathogenesis of myasthenia gravis involves an antibody-mediated autoimmune attack on acetylcholine receptors of the neuromuscular junctions.

In at least 2 other disorders—Graves' disease and extreme insulin resistance in diabetes—autoantibodies to hormone receptors have been implicated. Some patients with insulin resistance have circulating antibodies to insulin receptors that interfere with insulin binding.

Some patients with Graves' disease (hyperthyroidism) have a circulating antibody to thyrotropin (TSH) receptors. Such an autoimmune antibody stimulates the cell and thus resembles the hormone in activity (stimulatory hypersensitivity).

It is possible that these are disorders of immune regulation in which the normally functioning suppressor T cells are not functioning. This may result in inappropriate B cell responses and antibody formation. Such immune regulation is controlled by immune response genes that are in close proximity to the major histocompatibility complex (HLA region) on chromosomes.

Rheumatic Fever

The development of rheumatic fever is regularly preceded by multiple infections with group A β-hemolytic streptococci. Cross-reactions occur between antigens of human heart and streptococci. Certain group A streptococci contain a cell membrane antigen that cross-reacts with human cardiac muscle fibers, especially the sarcolemma. Thus, antibodies to the streptococci might react with heart muscle. There is also cross-reactivity between structural glycoproteins of heart valves and streptococcal group-specific carbohydrate. The pathogenetic role of these cross-reacting antibodies is not established, but prompt elimination of streptococcal antigens prevents rheumatic fever.

Blood Diseases

Various forms of human hemolytic anemias, granulocytopenias, thrombocytopenias, and other blood disorders have been attributed either to the development of autoantibodies directed against antigens in red blood cells or platelets or to the attachment of antigen-antibody complexes to the cell surface. As a result of such antigen-antibody reactions, cells would be destroyed. The responsible antibodies have been demonstrated in a number of instances. For example, in the thrombocytopenic purpura caused by apronalide (Sedormid) or quinine, the sensitive person's serum contains antibody that can lyse platelets onto which the drug has been adsorbed.

Pernicious anemia may represent an "autoimmune" reaction to intrinsic factor, a special protein secreted by parietal cells into the stomach.

Systemic Lupus Erythematosus (SLE) & Other "Collagen Vascular Diseases"

This is a group of human diseases characterized by focal inflammatory lesions, vasculitis, and collagen degeneration. It includes systemic lupus erythematosus (SLE) and other rheumatoid disorders. The causes of these diseases are not known, but typical cases have followed sensitization by drugs, foreign serum, and other immune stimuli. In these diseases, and particularly in systemic lupus erythematosus, a variety of antibodies against various normal body constituents have been identified, including autoantibodies to red cell antigen, cellular DNA, clotting factors, etc. The typical LE cell is a granulocyte that has taken up an aggregate of DNA-anti-DNA complex; the intracellular DNA can be identified by immunofluorescence. The complement level in active systemic lupus erythematosus is low, indicating antigen-antibody reactions that bind complement. The nephritis of systemic lupus erythematosus appears to be an "immune complex disease."

There is a 3-fold predominance of black women among patients with systemic lupus erythematosus. A concordance in monozygotic twins emphasizes the role of immunoregulatory genes in the complex origin of these disorders. Alternatively, it may be that viruses play a role in the pathogenesis of systemic lupus erythematosus by combining with autoantigens to stimulate immune reactions.

In patients with rheumatoid arthritis, a "rheumatoid factor" can be regularly shown by hemagglutination, latex fixation, or precipitation tests. This is an IgM (*rarely* IgG) that reacts with normal human IgG and may be a true autoantibody to IgG. Rheumatoid arthritis may be an "immune complex disease" (see pp 193 and 201).

TRANSPLANTATION IMMUNITY

Blood groups of the ABO system are transplantation antigens, but they are carbohydrates (see Chapter 12). Most other transplantation antigens are glycoproteins of cell membranes.

It has long been known that an animal will accept a graft of its own tissue (eg, skin) but not that of another of the same species except an identical twin. An autograft is a graft of tissue from one animal onto itself, and it "takes" regularly and permanently. An isograft is a graft of tissue from one individual to another genetically identical individual, and it usually "takes" permanently. A heterograft (xenograft) is a graft from one species to another species. It is always rejected. An allograft (homograft) is a graft from one member of a noninbred species to another member, eg, from one human to another human. It is rejected by the **homograft reaction.** Initial vascularization and circulation of the graft are good, but after 11–14 days, marked reduction in circulation and infiltration of the bed of the graft with mononuclear cells occur, and the graft eventually becomes necrotic and sloughs. In the homograft rejection, a cell-mediated reaction with competent lymphoid cells is of primary importance, but antibodies can also participate in the reaction. If a second homograft from the same donor is applied to a recipient who has rejected the first graft, an accelerated ("second-set") rejection is observed in 5–6 days. Hyperacute— and perhaps acute— rejection of a vascularized graft is associated with antibodies to antigens on vascular endothelium. Allograft rejection includes contributions from many major elements of the immune system; it is helper T cell-dependent, because helper T cells activate cytotoxic T cells, macrophages, and B cells. The precise role of each cell type and of antibodies is still uncertain.

The problem of tissue transplantation resides in specific "transplantation (HLA) antigens" that exist in all mammalian cells. These antigens are of a great variety and are under the control of a number of different "histocompatibility (HLA) genes." In inbred strains of mice, at least 14 independently segregating genetic loci for transplantation antigens have been recognized. At each of these loci there exist multiple alleles, so that the number and variety of transplantation antigens are enormous. If inbred mice are cross-mated, the F1 offspring are tolerant of grafts from either parent but either parent rejects the F1 hybrid graft. In humans, the major histocompatibility complex includes at least 4 (or 5) closely linked genes designated *HLA-A, -B, -C, -D,* and *-DR*. These genetic loci determine strong transplantation antigens. Several other weaker transplantation antigens are determined by other genetic loci. Antigens determined by these several genetic loci are defined by their interaction with antisera in the lymphocytotoxicity test or by the mixed lymphocyte reaction. It appears that the newly recognized *DR* genes determine antigens that occur on B lymphocytes and macrophages. The tests by which the antigens are determined are described below. Potent antisera are empirically found in large-scale screening.

The major histocompatibility genetic loci occur on each member of a single chromosome pair (in humans, chromosome 6). For each histocompatibility locus, many alleles exist, controlling expression of specific antigens. Because of this polymorphism, each individual is likely to have at least 4 strong transplantation antigens on cells. The term "haplotype" denotes the products of the major histocompatibility complex in haploid form. Each individual has strong transplantation antigens arranged in pairs of haplotypes, with each haplotype being controlled by the major histocompatibility loci of one chromosome of a pair. Many antigens have now been identified, resulting in thousands of potential haplotypes. Consequently, the likelihood is very small that 2 random individuals would have completely or partly identical haplotypes. Within a family, on the other hand, only 4 haplotypes are involved (2 from each parent), which permits a reasonable opportunity of genetic matching of family members as donors or recipients of transplants. About 25% of siblings are identical at one haplotype. To characterize the haplotype present in a donor or recipient, both lymphocytotoxicity and mixed lymphocyte culture tests must be done with a broad range of reagents (lymphocytes and sera).

It is also considered essential that donor and recipient be compatible by matching of ABO blood groups. The following procedures are employed in determining the degree of histocompatibility for "matching" donor and recipient of transplants.

A. Mixed Lymphocyte Culture (MLC): This test applies only to living donors and requires 5 days to complete. At present, it is not applicable to cadaver organ transplants. For the test, lymphocytes from donor and recipient are separated from blood. Potential donor cells are treated with mitomycin or radiation to stop DNA replication. The untreated recipient cells are grown in culture with the donor cell antigens. Their response is assayed by the incorporation of tritium-labeled thymidine. The level of cellular radioactivity becomes an indicator of cellular stimulation as a result of exposure to antigens that are recognized as foreign. The greater the disparity of donor and recipient cells, the higher the stimulation of cell growth and of labeled thymidine incorporation into DNA. An ideal match would show similar responses in single or mixed cell cultures. The higher the percentage of relative response is in mixed cell culture (above that in the sum of single cell culture), the greater the antigenic disparity and the less suitable the match.

The mixed lymphocyte culture is particularly useful in selecting the best donor within a family of compatible serologically defined (HLA) types. Mixed lymphocyte culture compatibility takes precedence over the results of HLA typing in donor selection. A recent modification of the mixed lymphocyte culture test is the primed lymphocyte test (PLT), which can give similar results in less than 2 days.

B. Histocompatibility Antigen (HLA) Typing by Lymphocytotoxicity: Viable purified lymphocytes from blood of the tissue donor are added to a panel of standard sera and the recipient's serum. Complement is added, then dye (eosin or trypan blue) and formalin. Cell death occurs if an antigen + antibody + complement reaction takes place. Cell death is established by counting the number of viable cells that exclude the dye (dead cells are stained by dye). An alternative method is to preincubate lymphocytes with ^{51}Cr and determine the release of this isotope as an indication of cell death.

Results of Organ Transplants

If donor and recipient are well matched by mixed lymphocyte culture and histocompatibility antigen typing, the long-term survival of a transplanted organ or tissue is enhanced. In 1985, the 5-year survival rate of 2-haplotype-matched kidney transplants from related donors was near 95%; that of a one-haplotype-matched kidney was near 80%; and that of kidneys from cadaver donors was near 60%. However, the survival rate was higher if the graft recipient had several previous transfusions. The reason for this is much debated.

In one center, well-matched transplants of bone marrow from siblings established themselves in 33 of 37 patients with aplastic anemia, half of whom lived with functioning grafts. However, about 70% of patients with successful marrow grafts exhibited graft-versus-host (GVH) disease (see above). The grafted cells took over from the host in bone marrow transplants following the intensive irradiation and cyclophosphamide treatment for leukemia. The results of graft-versus-host reactions included skin lesions and malfunctions of liver and gut, so that less than one-third of patients with graft-versus-host reactions survived. It is possible that antithymocyte globulin may have some benefit in graft-versus-host disease.

To delay or diminish rejection of transplanted tissue or organs, attempts are made to suppress immunologic rejection mechanisms. At present this involves the administration of corticosteroids, immunosuppressive drugs such as azathioprine or cyclosporine, antilymphocytic serum, and radiation. Unfortunately, all of these immunosuppressive measures enhance the recipient's susceptibility to endogenous or exogenous infection. Opportunistic "nonpathogenic" microorganisms (bacteria, fungi, viruses, protozoa) may prove fatal to the immunosuppressed transplant recipient. Such disorders as cytomegalovirus pneumonia, *Pneumocystis carinii* pneumonia, or disseminated herpes zoster are prominent examples of endogenous infections that occur mainly in the immunosuppressed. In addition, there is a greatly enhanced susceptibility to the development and spread of neoplasms in such patients (see Chapter 11).

HLA & Disease

Histocompatibility antigens also appear to be genetic markers for a variety of diseases. Ankylosing spondylitis and Reiter's disease are associated with the antigen HLA-B27. HLA-B8 and HLA-DR3 have been associated with a high incidence of such "autoimmune" disorders as insulin-dependent (type 1) diabetes mellitus, systemic lupus erythematosus, Sjögren's syndrome, and others. Possible explanations have been suggested in Chapter 11.

The longer a tissue or organ graft survives in the recipient, the greater the chance that tolerance to the graft may be established under the cover of immunosuppressive measures. The establishment of tolerance by means of repeated administration of donor cells into recipients has been attempted only rarely. (See Chapter 12.)

TUMOR IMMUNITY

Animals carrying chemical-induced or virus-induced tumors develop a certain amount of resistance to that tumor which can be demonstrated experimentally, although it is usually insufficient to cause complete regression of the tumor.

In the course of neoplastic transformation of cells, new antigens develop at the cell surface that permit the host's immune responses to recognize such cells as "foreign." (Some tumors in adults contain antigen found in *fetal* but not in adult cells. Thus, a carcinoembryonic antigen [CEA] is found in the serum of patients with neoplasms of the gut.) Cell-mediated responses (see p 195) attack these "foreign" tumor cells and tend to limit their proliferation. It is probable that these cell-mediated responses are an effective surveillance system that can eliminate some newly arising clones of neoplastic cells ("forbidden clones"). Some of the cells able to kill and lyse tumor cells in the absence of antibody are "natural killer" (NK) cells. NK cells are of uncertain derivation, behave as "null" cells (ie, they cannot be identified as either T cells or B cells), and can be actively cytolytic in experimental systems. Other demonstrated responses to tumor cells are activation of macrophages and antibody-dependent cytolysis by T cells. The role, if any, of these cell-mediated responses in the control of tumors in humans has not been defined.

Tumor antigens also stimulate the development of specific antibodies. Some such antibodies may be cytotoxic. Others interfere with recognition and disposal of tumor cells by cell-mediated immune responses of the host, and such antitumor antibodies (or antigen-antibody complexes) thus produce an enhancement of tumor growth.

Some immunologic features of virus-induced tumors of animals are discussed in Chapter 46.

There is tentative evidence that spontaneously arising human tumors have new cell surface antigens against which the host develops both cytotoxic antibodies and cellular hypersensitivity. The possibility is under investigation that enhancement of such immune responses may permit containment of malignant neoplasms. Enhancement by the administration of bacille Calmette Guérin (BCG) into surface tumors (melanomas) has led to tumor regression. Interferon is receiving a trial as an immunomodulator in these same circumstances of tumor therapy (see p 199).

REFERENCES

Altman LC: Basic immune mechanisms in immediate hypersensitivity. *Med Clin North Am* 1981;**65**:941.

AMA Council on Scientific Affairs: The acquired immunodeficiency syndrome. *JAMA* 1984;**252**:2037.

Austen KF: Systemic anaphylaxis in the human being. *N Engl J Med* 1974;**291**:661.

Austen WG, Cosimi AB: Heart transplantation after 16 years. *N Engl J Med* 1984:**311**:1436.

Bach FH, van Rood JJ: The major histocompatibility complex: Genetics and biology. (3 parts.) *N Engl J Med* 1976; **295**:806, 872, 927.

Beaven MA: Histamine. *N Engl J Med* 1976;**294**:319.

Bleich HL, Moore MJ: Release of inflammatory mediators from stimulated neutrophils. *N Engl J Med* 1980;**303**:27.

Blume KG et al: Bone marrow ablation and allogeneic marrow transplantation in acute leukemia. *N Engl J Med* 1980; **302**:1041.

Butterworth AE, David JR: Eosinophil function. *N Engl J Med* 1981;**304**:154.

Catalona WJ et al: Dinitrochlorobenzene contact sensitization. *N Engl J Med* 1972;**286**:399.

Committee on Drugs of the American Academy of Pediatrics: Anaphylaxis. *Pediatrics* 1973;**51**:136.

Dale DC, Petersdorf RG: Corticosteroids and infectious diseases. *Med Clin North Am* 1973;**57**:1277.

David JR: Lymphocyte mediators and cellular hypersensitivity. *N Engl J Med* 1973;**288**:143.

Denman AM: Immunodeficiency and general medicine. *Br Med J* 1980;**281**:1376.

Dinarello CA: Interleukin-1. *Rev Infect Dis* 1984;**6**:51.

Flax MH: Drug-induced autoimmunity. *N Engl J Med* 1974; **291**:414.

Garraty G, Petz LD: Drug-induced hemolytic anemia. *Am J Med* 1975;**58**:398.

Gilliland BC: Serum sickness and immune complexes. *N Engl J Med* 1984;**311**:1435.

Goetzl EJ: Asthma: New mediators and old problems. *N Engl J Med* 1984;**311**:252.

Golden DBK et al: Regimens of hymenoptera venom immunotherapy. *Ann Intern Med* 1980;**92**:620.

Hunt KJ et al: A controlled trial of immunotherapy in insect hypersensitivity. *N Engl J Med* 1978;**299**:157.

Krown S et al: Preliminary observations on the effect of recombinant leukocyte A interferon in homosexual men with Kaposi's sarcoma. *N Engl J Med* 1983;**308**:1071.

Levin AS et al: Transfer factor therapy in immune deficiency states. *Annu Rev Med* 1973;**24**:175.

McDonald JC: The biologic implications of HLA. *Arch Intern Med* 1981;**141**:100.

Najarian JS et al: Seven years' experience with antilymphoblast globulin for renal transplantation. *Ann Surg* 1976;**184**:352.

Nathan CF et al: The macrophage as an effector cell. *N Engl J Med* 1980;**303**:622.

Ortho Multicenter Transplant Study Group: A randomized clinical trial of OKT3 monoclonal antibody for acute rejection of cadaveric renal transplants. *N Engl J Med* 1985;**313**:337.

Rapaport FT et al: Recent advances in clinical and experimental transplantation. *JAMA* 1977;**237**:2835.

Rose NR: HLA and disease. *Arch Intern Med* 1978;**138**:527.

Russell PS, Cosimi AB: Transplantation. *N Engl J Med* 1979; **301**:470.

Sampson HA, Jolie PL: Increased plasma histamine concentrations after food challenges in children with atopic dermatitis. *N Engl J Med* 1984;**311**:372.

Satoh J: Human monoclonal autoantibodies that react with multiple endocrine organs. *N Engl J Med* 1983;**309:**217.

Sbarbaro JA: Skin test antigens: An evaluation whose time has come. *Am Rev Respir Dis* 1978;**118:**1.

Schatz M et al: Immunologic lung disease. *N Engl J Med* 1979; **300:**1310.

Seligman M et al: AIDS: An immunologic reevaluation. *N Engl J Med* 1984;**311:**1286.

Shoenfeld Y, Schwartz RS: Immunologic and genetic factors in autoimmune diseases. *N Engl J Med* 1984;**311:**1019.

Stossel TP: Phagocytosis. (3 parts.) *N Engl J Med* 1974;**290:** 717,774,833.

Theofilopoulos AN et al: Isolation of circulating immune complexes using Raji cells. *J Clin Invest* 1978;**61:**1570.

VanArsdel PP Jr: Diagnosing drug allergy. *JAMA* 1983;**247:** 2576.

Waldmann TA et al: Disorders of suppressor immunoregulatory cells in the pathogenesis of immunodeficiency and autoimmunity. *Ann Intern Med* 1978;**88:**226.

Weissman G: The eicosanoids of asthma. *N Engl J Med* 1983; **308:**454.

Williams RC Jr: Immune complexes in human disease. *Annu Rev Med* 1981;**32:**13.

Gram-Positive Bacilli

AEROBIC SPOREFORMING BACILLI

ANTHRAX

The genus *Bacillus* includes large gram-positive rods occurring in chains. They form spores and are aerobes. Most members of this genus are saprophytic organisms prevalent in soil, water, and air and on vegetation, such as *Bacillus cereus* and *Bacillus subtilis*. Some are insect pathogens. *B cereus* can grow in foods and produce an enterotoxin that causes food poisoning (Table 18–4). Such organisms may occasionally produce disease in immunocompromised humans (eg, meningitis, endocarditis, endophthalmitis, conjunctivitis, or acute gastroenteritis). *Bacillus anthracis* is the principal pathogen of the genus.

Morphology & Identification

A. Typical Organisms: The typical cells, measuring $1 \times 3–4 \ \mu m$, have square ends and are arranged in long chains; spores are located in the center of the nonmotile bacilli.

B. Culture: Colonies are round and have a "cut glass" appearance in transmitted light. Hemolysis is uncommon with anthrax but common with the saprophytic bacilli. Gelatin is liquefied, and growth in gelatin stabs resembles an inverted fir tree.

C. Growth Characteristics: The saprophytic bacilli utilize simple sources of nitrogen and carbon for energy and growth. The spores are resistant to environmental changes, withstand dry heat and certain chemical disinfectants for moderate periods, and persist for years in dry earth. Animal products contaminated with anthrax spores (eg, hides, bristles, hair, wool, bone) can be sterilized only by autoclaving.

D. Variation: Variation occurs with respect to virulence, spore formation, and colony form. (In general, virulence is associated with rough colonies.) To minimize variation, living spore suspensions are employed to preserve unstable properties such as virulence.

Antigenic Structure

The capsular substance of *B anthracis*, which consists of a polypeptide of high molecular weight composed of D-glutamic acid, is a hapten. The bacterial bodies contain protein and a somatic polysaccharide, both of which are antigenic.

Pathogenesis

Anthrax is primarily a disease of sheep, cattle, horses, and many other animals; humans are affected only rarely. The infection is usually acquired by the entry of spores through injured skin or mucous membranes, rarely by inhalation of spores into the lung. In animals, the portal of entry is the mouth and the gastrointestinal tract. The spores from contaminated soil find easy access when ingested with spiny or irritating vegetation. In humans, scratches in the skin or inhalation (see below) leads to infection.

The spores germinate in the tissue at the site of entry, and growth of the vegetative organisms results in formation of a gelatinous edema and congestion. Bacilli spread via lymphatics to the bloodstream, and they multiply freely in the blood and tissues shortly before and after the death of the animal. In the plasma of animals dying from anthrax, a toxic factor has been demonstrated. This material kills mice or guinea pigs upon inoculation and is specifically neutralized by anthrax antiserum. Its nature is still uncertain.

The exudate in anthrax contains a polypeptide, identical with that in the capsule of the bacillus, which is able to evoke histologic reactions similar to those of

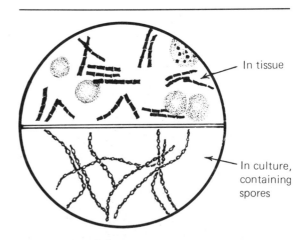

In tissue

In culture, containing spores

Figure 14–1. Anthrax bacilli in a smear from tissue or culture.

anthrax infection. Other proteins isolated from exudate stimulate solid immunity to anthrax upon injection into animals. From culture filtrates ("anthrax toxin"), 3 substances have been separated by glass filtration and chromatography: (1) "protective antigen" (a protein), (2) "edema factor," and (3) "toxic factor." Mixtures of (1), (2), and (3) are more toxic in animals and more immunogenic than single substances. Production of toxin is under genetic control of a plasmid, loss of which results in loss of toxin production.

Another type of anthrax is inhalation anthrax ("woolsorter's disease"). The inhalation of anthrax spores from the dust of wool, hair, or hides results in germination of the spores in the lungs or in tracheobronchial lymph nodes and the production of hemorrhagic mediastinitis, pneumonia, meningitis, and sepsis, which is usually rapidly fatal. In anthrax sepsis, the number of organisms in the blood exceeds 10^7/mL just prior to death.

Pathology

In susceptible animals, the organisms proliferate at the site of entry. The capsules remain intact, and the organisms are surrounded by a large amount of proteinaceous fluid containing few leukocytes from which they rapidly disseminate and reach the bloodstream.

In resistant animals, the organisms proliferate for a few hours, by which time there is massive accumulation of leukocytes. The capsules gradually disintegrate and disappear. The organisms remain localized.

Clinical Findings

In humans, anthrax gives rise to an infection of the skin (malignant pustule). A papule first develops within 12–36 hours after entry of the organisms or spores through a scratch. This papule rapidly changes into a vesicle, then a pustule, and finally a necrotic ulcer from which the infection may disseminate, giving rise to septicemia.

In inhalation anthrax, early manifestations may be mediastinitis, sepsis, meningitis, or hemorrhagic pulmonary edema. Hemorrhagic pneumonia with shock is a terminal event.

While animals often acquire anthrax through ingestion of spores and spread of the organisms from the intestinal tract, this is exceedingly rare in humans. Thus, abdominal pain, vomiting, and bloody diarrhea are rare clinical signs.

Diagnostic Laboratory Tests

A. Specimens: Fluid or pus from local lesion; blood, sputum.

B. Stained Smears: From the local lesion or blood of dead animals; chains of large gram-positive rods are often seen. Anthrax can be identified in dried smears by immunofluorescence staining techniques.

C. Culture: When grown on blood agar plates, the organisms produce nonhemolytic gray colonies with typical microscopic morphology. Carbohydrate fermentation is not useful. In semisolid medium, anthrax bacilli are always nonmotile, whereas related nonpathogenic organisms (eg, *B cereus*) exhibit motility by "swarming." Virulent anthrax cultures kill mice or guinea pigs upon intraperitoneal injection.

D. Ascoli Test: Extracts of infected tissues show a ring of precipitate when layered over immune serum.

E. Serologic Tests: Precipitating or hemagglutinating antibodies can be demonstrated in the serum of vaccinated or infected persons or animals.

Resistance & Immunity

Some animals (guinea pig) are highly susceptible, whereas others (rat) are very resistant to anthrax infection. This fact has been attributed to a variety of defense mechanisms: leukocytic activity, body temperature, and the bactericidal action of the blood. Certain basic polypeptides that kill anthrax bacilli have been isolated from animal tissues. A synthetic polylysine has a similar action.

Active immunity to anthrax can be induced in susceptible animals by vaccination with live attenuated bacilli, with spore suspensions, or with protective antigens from culture filtrates (see above). Immune serum is sometimes injected together with live bacilli into animals. Anthrax immunization is based on the classic experiments of Louis Pasteur, who in 1881 proved that cultures that had been grown in broth at 42–52 °C for several months lost much of their virulence and could be injected live into sheep and cattle without causing disease; subsequently, such animals proved to be immune. There are great variations in the efficacy of various vaccines.

Treatment

Many antibiotics are effective against anthrax in humans, but treatment must be started early. Penicillin is satisfactory treatment except in inhalation anthrax, in which the mortality rate remains high. Some other gram-positive bacilli may be resistant to penicillin by virtue of β-lactamase production. Tetracyclines, erythromycin, or clindamycin may be effective.

Epidemiology, Prevention, & Control

Soil is contaminated with anthrax spores from the carcasses of dead animals. These spores remain viable for decades. Perhaps spores can germinate in soil at pH 6.5 at proper temperature. Grazing animals infected through injured mucous membranes serve to perpetuate the chain of infection. Contact with infected animals or with their hides, hair, and bristles is the source of infection in humans. Control measures include (1) disposal of animal carcasses by burning or by deep burial in lime pits, (2) decontamination (usually by autoclaving) of animal products, (3) protective clothing and gloves for handling potentially infected materials, and (4) active immunization of domestic animals with live attenuated vaccines. Persons with high occupational risk should be immunized with a cell-free vaccine obtainable from the Centers for Disease Control, Atlanta 30333.

ANAEROBIC SPOREFORMING BACILLI

THE CLOSTRIDIA

The clostridia are anaerobic, gram-positive, motile rods that form spores. Many decompose proteins or form toxins, and some do both. Their natural habitat is the soil or the intestinal tract of animals and humans, where they live as saprophytes. Among the pathogens are the organisms causing botulism, tetanus, and gas gangrene.

Morphology & Identification

A. Typical Organisms: All species of clostridia are large gram-positive rods, and all can produce spores. The spores are usually wider than the diameter of the rods in which they are formed. In the various species, the spore is placed centrally, subterminally, or terminally. Most species of clostridia are motile and possess peritrichous flagella.

B. Culture: Clostridia grow only under anaerobic conditions, established by one of the following means:

1. Agar plates or culture tubes are placed in an airtight jar from which air is removed and replaced by nitrogen with 10% CO_2, or oxygen may be removed by other means (Gaspack).

2. Fluid media are put in deep tubes containing either fresh animal tissue (eg, chopped cooked meat) or 0.1% agar and a reducing agent such as thioglycolate. Such tubes can be handled like aerobic media, and growth will occur from the bottom up to within 15 mm of the surface exposed to air.

C. Colony Forms: Some organisms produce large raised colonies with entire margins (eg, *Clostridium perfringens*); others produce smaller colonies that extend in a meshwork of fine filaments (eg, *Clostridium tetani*). Many clostridia produce a zone of hemolysis on blood agar.

D. Growth Characteristics: The outstanding characteristic of anaerobic microorganisms is their inability to utilize oxygen as the final hydrogen acceptor. They lack cytochrome and cytochrome oxidase and are unable to break down hydrogen peroxide because they lack catalase and peroxidase. Therefore, H_2O_2 tends to accumulate to toxic concentrations in the presence of oxygen. Clostridia and other obligate anaerobes probably also lack superoxide dismutase and consequently permit the accumulation of the toxic free radical superoxide anion. Such anaerobes can carry out their metabolic reactions only at a negative oxidation-reduction potential (E_h), ie, in an environment that is strongly reducing.

Clostridia can ferment a variety of sugars; many can digest proteins. Milk is turned acid by some and digested by others and undergoes "stormy fermentation" (ie, clot torn by gas) with a third group (eg, *C perfringens*). Various enzymes are produced by different species (see below).

E. Antigenic Characteristics: Clostridia share some antigens but also possess specific soluble antigens that permit grouping by precipitin tests.

CLOSTRIDIUM BOTULINUM

This microorganism is worldwide in distribution; it is found in soil and occasionally in animal feces.

Types of *C botulinum* are distinguished by the antigenic type of toxin they produce. Spores of the organism are highly resistant to heat, withstanding 100 °C for at least 3–5 hours. Heat resistance is diminished at acid pH or high salt concentration.

Toxin

During the growth of *C botulinum* and during autolysis of the bacteria, toxin is liberated into the environment. Eight antigenic varieties of toxin (A–H) are known. Types A, B, and E are most commonly associated with human illness. Type C produces limberneck in fowl; type D, botulism in cattle. Types A, B, and E toxins have been purified and fractionated to yield a neurotoxic protein (MW 150,000). These are among the most highly toxic substances known: The lethal dose for a human is probably about 1–2 μg. The toxins are destroyed by heating for 20 minutes at 100 °C. Toxin production is under control of a viral gene. Some toxigenic *C botulinum* strains yield bacteriophages that may infect nontoxigenic strains and convert them to toxigenicity.

Pathogenesis

Although *C botulinum* types A and B have been implicated in rare cases of wound infection and botulism, the illness is not an infection. Botulism is an intoxication resulting from the ingestion of food in which *C botulinum* has grown and produced toxin. The most common offenders are spiced, smoked, vacuum-packed, or canned alkaline foods that are eaten with-

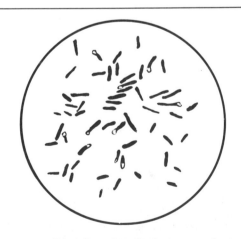

Figure 14–2. *C botulinum* from broth grown under anaerobic conditions.

out cooking. In such foods, spores of *C botulinum* germinate; under anaerobic conditions, vegetative forms grow and produce toxin.

The toxin acts by blocking release of acetylcholine at synapses and neuromuscular junctions. Flaccid paralysis results. The electromyogram and edrophonium (Tensilon) strength tests are typical.

Clinical Findings
(See also Table 18–4.)

Symptoms begin 18–96 hours after ingestion of the toxic food, with visual disturbances (incoordination of eye muscles, double vision), inability to swallow, and speech difficulty; signs of bulbar paralysis are progressive, and death occurs from respiratory paralysis or cardiac arrest. Gastrointestinal symptoms are not regularly prominent. There is no fever. The patient remains fully conscious until shortly before death. The mortality rate is high. Patients who recover do not develop antitoxin in the blood.

Occasionally, infants in the first months of life develop weakness, signs of paralysis, and electromyographic evidence of botulism. *C botulinum* and botulinus toxin are found in feces but not in serum. It is assumed that *C botulinum* grew in the gut and produced toxin. Most of these infants recover with supportive therapy alone. However, infant botulism may be one of the causes of sudden infant death syndrome. The feeding of honey has been implicated as a possible cause of infant botulism.

Diagnostic Laboratory Tests

Toxin can often be demonstrated in serum from the patient, and toxin may be found in leftover food. Mice injected intraperitoneally die rapidly. The antigenic type of toxin is identified by neutralization with specific antitoxin in mice. *C botulinum* may be grown from food remains and tested for toxin production, but this is rarely done and is of questionable significance. In infant botulism, *C botulinum* and toxin can be demonstrated in bowel contents but not in serum. Toxin may be demonstrated by passive hemagglutination or radioimmunoassay.

Treatment

Potent antitoxins to 3 types of botulinus toxins have been prepared in animals. Since the type responsible for an individual case is usually not known, trivalent (A, B, E) antitoxin (available from the Centers for Disease Control, Atlanta 30333; central telephone number [404] 329-3311) must be promptly administered intravenously with customary precautions. Adequate ventilation must be maintained by mechanical respirator, if necessary. Guanidine hydrochloride has been given experimentally with occasional benefit. These measures have reduced the mortality rate from 65% to below 25%.

Epidemiology, Prevention, & Control

Since spores of *C botulinum* are widely distributed in soil, they often contaminate vegetables,fruits, and other materials. A large restaurant-based outbreak in 1983 was associated with sauteed onions. When such foods are canned or otherwise preserved, they either must be sufficiently heated to ensure destruction of spores or must be boiled for 20 minutes before consumption. Strict regulation of commercial canning has largely overcome the danger of large outbreaks, but commercially canned mushrooms and vichyssoise have caused deaths. At present, the chief danger lies in home-canned foods, particularly string beans, corn, peppers, olives, peas, and smoked fish or vacuum-packed fresh fish in plastic bags. Toxic foods may be spoiled and rancid, and cans may "swell"; or the appearance may be innocuous. The risk from home-canned foods can be reduced if the food is boiled for more than 20 minutes before consumption. Toxoids are used for active immunization of cattle in South Africa.

CLOSTRIDIUM TETANI

C tetani is worldwide in distribution in the soil and in the feces of horses and other animals. Several types of *C tetani* can be distinguished by specific flagellar antigens. All share a common O (somatic) antigen, which may be masked, and all produce the same antigenic type of neurotoxin, tetanospasmin. L forms of *C tetani* also produce tetanospasmin.

Toxin

Vegetative cells of *C tetani* produce tetanospasmin and release it mainly when they lyse. Toxin production appears to be under control of a plasmid gene. The intracellular toxin is a polypeptide (MW 160,000) that proteolytic enzymes split into 2 fragments of increased toxicity. Purified toxin contains more than 2×10^7 mouse lethal doses per milligram. Tetanospasmin acts in several ways upon the central nervous system. It in-

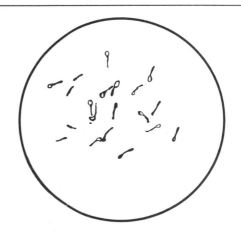

Figure 14–3. *C tetani* from blood agar grown under anaerobic conditions.

hibits release of acetylcholine, thus interfering with neuromuscular transmission. The most important action, however, is the inhibition of postsynaptic spinal neurons by blocking the release of an inhibitory mediator. This results in generalized muscular spasms, hyperreflexia, and seizures.

Pathogenesis

C tetani is not an invasive organism. The infection remains strictly localized in the area of devitalized tissue (wound, burn, injury, umbilical stump, surgical suture) into which the spores have been introduced. The volume of infected tissue is small, and the disease is almost entirely a toxemia. Germination of the spore and development of vegetative organisms that produce toxin are aided by (1) necrotic tissue, (2) calcium salts, and (3) associated pyogenic infections, all of which aid establishment of low oxidation-reduction potential.

The toxin released from vegetative cells may reach the central nervous system by retrograde axonal transport or via the bloodstream. In the central nervous system, the toxin rapidly becomes fixed to gangliosides in spinal cord and brain stem and exerts the actions described above.

Clinical Findings

The incubation period may range from 4–5 days to as many weeks. The disease is characterized by convulsive tonic contraction of voluntary muscles. Muscular spasms often involve first the area of injury and infection and then the muscles of the jaw (trismus, lockjaw), which contract so that the mouth cannot be opened. Gradually, other voluntary muscles become involved, resulting in tonic spasms. Any external stimulus may precipitate a tetanic seizure. The patient is fully conscious, and pain may be intense. Death usually results from interference with the mechanics of respiration. The mortality rate in generalized tetanus is approximately 50%.

Diagnostic Laboratory Tests

In clinical cases, diagnosis rests on the clinical picture and a history of injury. Anaerobic culture of tissues from contaminated wounds may yield *C tetani*, but neither preventive nor therapeutic use of antitoxin should ever be withheld pending such demonstration. Proof of isolation of *C tetani* must rest on production of toxin and its neutralization by specific antitoxin.

Prevention & Treatment

The results of treatment of tetanus are not satisfactory. Therefore, prevention is all-important. Prevention of tetanus depends upon (1) active immunization with toxoids; (2) proper care of wounds contaminated with soil, etc; (3) prophylactic use of antitoxin; and (4) administration of penicillin.

A. Antitoxin: Tetanus antitoxin, prepared in animals or humans, can neutralize the toxin, but only before it becomes fixed onto nervous tissue. One International Unit of antitoxin is defined as the activity contained in 0.03384 mg of the Second International Standard for Tetanus Antitoxin.

Because of the frequency of hypersensitivity reactions to foreign serum and because of the rapidity with which foreign serum is eliminated, the administration of human antitoxin is preferable. The intramuscular administration of 250–500 units of human antitoxin gives adequate systemic protection (0.01 unit or more per milliliter of serum) for 2–4 weeks. Tetanus immune globulin USP is universally available in the USA and widely available elsewhere. Only if human antitoxin is not available should heterologous (horse, sheep, rabbit) antitoxin be used in a prophylactic dose of 1500–6000 units. Whenever heterologous antitoxin is to be administered, tests for hypersensitivity to the foreign serum protein must be done. Active immunization with tetanus toxoid should always accompany antitoxin prophylaxis.

Patients who develop symptoms of tetanus always receive muscle relaxants, sedation, and assisted ventilation. Sometimes they are given very large doses of antitoxin (3000–10,000 units of tetanus immune globulin USP) intravenously in an effort to neutralize toxin that has not yet been bound to nervous tissue. However, the efficacy of antitoxin for treatment is doubtful except in neonatal tetanus, where it may be lifesaving. In neonatal tetanus, treatment with 10,000 units of equine antitoxin seems equivalent to treatment with 500 units of tetanus immune globulin USP.

B. Surgical Measures: Surgical debridement is vitally important because it removes the necrotic tissue that is essential for proliferation of the organisms. Hyperbaric oxygen has no proved effect.

C. Antibiotics: Penicillin strongly inhibits the growth of *C tetani* and stops further toxin production. Antibiotics may also control associated pyogenic infection.

D. "Booster" Shot: When a previously immunized individual sustains a potentially dangerous wound, an additional dose of toxoid should be injected to restimulate antitoxin production. This "recall" injection of toxoid may be accompanied by antitoxin injected into a different area of the body to provide immediately available antitoxin for the period during which antitoxin levels may be inadequate.

Control

Universal active immunization with tetanus toxoid should be mandatory. Tetanus toxoid is produced by detoxifying the toxin with formalin and then concentrating it. Aluminum-salt-adsorbed toxoids are employed. Three injections comprise the initial course of immunization, followed by another dose about 1 year later. Initial immunization should be carried out in all children during the first year of life. A "booster" injection of toxoid is given upon entry into school. Thereafter, "boosters" can be spaced 7–10 years apart to maintain serum levels of more than 0.01 unit antitoxin per milliliter. (Some authorities believe that the protective level of antitoxin is 0.1 Lf unit [see p 183] per milliliter of serum.) In young children, tetanus toxoid is often combined with diphtheria toxoid and pertussis vaccine. (For schedule of immunizations, see Table 12–6.)

Control measures are not possible because of the wide dissemination of the organism in the soil and the long survival of its spores. Narcotic addicts are a high-risk group.

CLOSTRIDIA THAT PRODUCE INVASIVE INFECTIONS

Many different toxin-producing clostridia can produce invasive infection (including myonecrosis and gas gangrene) if introduced into damaged tissue. About 30 species of clostridia may produce such an effect, but the commonest in invasive disease are *C perfringens* (90%) and some others. *Clostridium difficile* is an important cause of pseudomembranous enterocolitis. An enterotoxin of *C perfringens* is a common cause of food poisoning.

Toxins

The clostridia produce a large variety of toxins and enzymes that result in a spreading infection. Many of these toxins have lethal, necrotizing, and hemolytic properties. In some cases, these are different properties of a single substance; in other instances, they are due to different chemical entities. The alpha toxin of *C perfringens* type A is a lecithinase, and its lethal action is proportionate to the rate at which it splits lecithin (an important constituent of cell membranes) to phosphorylcholine and diglyceride. The theta toxin has similar hemolytic and necrotizing effects but is not a lecithinase. DNase and hyaluronidase, a collagenase that digests collagen of subcutaneous tissue and muscle, are also produced.

Some strains of *C perfringens* produce a powerful enterotoxin, especially when growing in meat dishes. When more than 10^8 vegetative cells are ingested and sporulate in the gut, enterotoxin is formed. The enterotoxin is a protein (MW 35,000) that appears identical with a component of the spore coat, is distinct from other clostridial toxins, and induces intense diarrhea in 6–18 hours. This illness tends to be self-limited.

Pathogenesis

Clostridial spores reach tissue either by contamination of traumatized areas (soil, feces) or from the intestinal tract. The spores germinate at low oxidation-reduction potential; vegetative cells multiply, ferment carbohydrates present in tissue, and produce gas. The distention of tissue and interference with blood supply, together with the secretion of necrotizing toxin and hyaluronidase, favor the spread of infection. Tissue necrosis extends, providing an opportunity for increased bacterial growth, hemolytic anemia, and, ultimately, severe toxemia and death.

In gas gangrene (clostridial myonecrosis), a mixed infection is the rule. In addition to the toxigenic clostridia, proteolytic clostridia and various cocci and gram-negative organisms are also usually present. *C perfringens* occurs in the genital tract of 5% of women. Clostridial uterine infections may follow instrumental abortions. Clostridial bacteremia is a frequent occurrence in patients with neoplasms. In New Guinea, *Clostridium perfringens* type C produces a necrotizing enteritis (pigbel) that can be highly fatal in children. Immunization with type C toxoid appears to have preventive value.

The action of *C perfringens* enterotoxin involves marked hypersecretion in the jejunum and ileum, with loss of fluids and electrolytes in diarrhea. The precise mechanism is not established, but it may not involve stimulation of adenylate cyclase or guanylate cyclase.

Clinical Findings
(See also Table 18–4.)

From a contaminated wound (eg, a compound fracture, postpartum uterus), the infection spreads in 1–3 days to produce crepitation in the subcutaneous tissue and muscle, foul-smelling discharge, rapidly progressing necrosis, fever, hemolysis, toxemia, shock, and death. Until the advent of specific therapy, early amputation was the only treatment. At times, the infection results only in anaerobic fasciitis or cellulitis. *C perfringens* food poisoning usually follows the ingestion of large numbers of clostridia that have grown in warmed meat dishes. The toxin forms when the organisms sporulate in the gut, with the onset of diarrhea—usually without vomiting or fever—in 6–18 hours. The illness lasts only 1–2 days.

Diagnostic Laboratory Tests
A. Specimens: Material from wounds, pus, tissue.

B. Smears: The presence of large gram-positive, sporeforming rods in Gram-stained smears suggests gas gangrene clostridia, but spores are not regularly present.

C. Culture: Material is inoculated into chopped meat–glucose medium and thioglycolate medium and

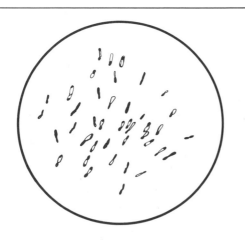

Figure 14–4. Gas gangrene bacilli.

onto blood agar plates incubated anaerobically. The growth from one of the media is transferred into milk. A clot torn by gas in 24 hours is suggestive of *C perfringens*. Once pure cultures have been obtained by selecting colonies from anaerobically incubated blood plates, they are identified by biochemical reactions (various sugars in thioglycolate, action on milk), hemolysis, and colony form. Lecithinase activity is evaluated by the precipitate formed around colonies on egg yolk media. Final identification rests on toxin production and neutralization by specific antitoxin.

Treatment

The most important aspect of treatment is prompt and extensive surgical debridement of the involved area and excision of all devitalized tissue, in which the organisms are prone to grow. Administration of antimicrobial drugs, particularly penicillin, is begun at the same time. Hyperbaric oxygen may be of help in the medical management of clostridial tissue infections. It is said to "detoxify" patients rapidly.

Antitoxins are available against the toxins of *C perfringens*, *Clostridium novyi*, *Clostridium histolyticum*, and *Clostridium septicum*, usually in the form of concentrated immune globulins. Polyvalent antitoxin (containing antibodies to several toxins) has been used. Although such antitoxin is sometimes administered to individuals with contaminated wounds containing much devitalized tissue, there is no evidence

for its efficacy. Food poisoning due to *C perfringens* enterotoxin usually requires only symptomatic care.

Prevention & Control

Early and adequate cleansing of contaminated wounds and surgical debridement, together with the administration of antimicrobial drugs directed against clostridia (eg, penicillin), are the best available preventive measures. Antitoxins should not be relied on. Although toxoids for active immunization have been prepared, they have not come into practical use.

CLOSTRIDIAL PSEUDOMEMBRANOUS COLITIS

Antibiotic-associated colitis occurs after the prolonged oral administration of clindamycin or other drugs. It has been attributed to the selection of drug-resistant *C difficile* that proliferates in the colon and produces a necrotizing toxin, a glycoprotein (MW 50,000). This toxin can be neutralized by antitoxins to several clostridial toxins, including that of *Clostridium sordellii*. Antibiotic-associated pseudomembranous colitis may have a high mortality rate unless the selecting drug is stopped and oral vancomycin (0.5 g every 6 hours) is given. Until now, all *C difficile* have been sensitive to vancomycin (see p 151).

REFERENCES

Arnon SS et al: Intestinal infection and toxin production by *Clostridium botulinum* as one cause of sudden infant death syndrome. *Lancet* 1978;**1**:1273.

Bartlett JG: *Clostridium difficile* and cytotoxin in feces of patients with antimicrobial agent–associated pseudomembranous colitis. *Infection* 1982;**10**:208.

Brachman PS: Inhalation anthrax. *Ann NY Acad Sci* 1980;**353**:83.

Caplan ES, Kluge RM: Gas gangrene: Review of 34 cases. *Arch Intern Med* 1976;**136**:788.

Davis JC et al: Hyperbaric medicine in the US Air Force. *JAMA* 1973;**224**:205.

Dowell VR: Botulism and tetanus: Selected epidemiologic and microbiologic aspects. *Rev Infect Dis* 1984;**6**:520.

Edmondson RS, Flowers MW: Intensive care in tetanus: Management, complications and mortality in 100 cases. *Br Med J* 1979;**1**:1401.

Finegold SM: *Anaerobic Bacteria in Human Disease*. Academic Press, 1977.

Hansen N, Tolo V: Wound botulism complicating an open fracture: A case report and review of the literature. *J Bone Joint Surg [Am]* 1979;**61**:312.

Laird WJ et al: Plasmid-associated toxigenicity in *Clostridium tetani*. *J Infect Dis* 1980;**142**:623.

Lamb R: A new look at infectious diseases: Anthrax. *Br Med J* 1973;**1**:157.

Merson MH et al: Botulism in the United States. *JAMA* 1974;**229**:1305.

Midura TF et al: Isolation of *Clostridium botulinum* from honey. *J Clin Microbiol* 1979;**9**:282.

Mikesell P et al: Evidence for plasmid-mediated toxin production in *Bacillus anthracis*. *Infect Immun* 1983;**39**:371.

Nathenson G, Zakzewski B: Current status of passive immunity to diphtheria and tetanus in the newborn. *J Infect Dis* 1976;**133**:199.

Simpson LL: The action of botulinal toxin. *Rev Infect Dis* 1979;**1**:656.

Stark RL: Biological characteristics of *Cl perfringens*. *Infect Immun* 1971;**4**:89.

Sugiyama H: *Clostridium botulinum* neurotoxicity. *Microbiol Rev* 1980;**44**:419.

Terranova W et al: Botulism type B: Epidemiologic aspects of an extensive outbreak. *Am J Epidemiol* 1978;**108**:150.

Thomas M et al: Hospital outbreak of *Clostridium perfringens* food poisoning. *Lancet* 1977;**1**:1046.

Thompson JA et al: Infant botulism: Clinical spectrum and epidemiology. *Pediatrics* 1980;**66**:939.

Tuazon CU et al: Serious infections from *Bacillus* species. *JAMA* 1979;**241**:1137.

Weinstein L: Tetanus. *N Engl J Med* 1973;**289**:1293.

Corynebacteria

15

Corynebacteria are gram-positive rods, nonmotile and nonsporeforming, that often possess club-shaped ends and irregularly staining granules. They are often in characteristic arrangements, resembling "Chinese characters" or palisades. Several species form part of the normal flora of the human respiratory tract, other mucous membranes, and skin. *Corynebacterium diphtheriae* produces a powerful exotoxin that causes diphtheria in humans.

Morphology & Identification

A. Typical Organisms: Corynebacteria are 0.5–1 μm in diameter and several micrometers long. Characteristically, they possess irregular swellings at one end that give them a "club-shaped" appearance. Irregularly distributed within the rod (often near the poles) are granules staining deeply with aniline dyes (metachromatic granules) that give the rod a beaded appearance.

Individual corynebacteria in stained smears tend to lie parallel or at acute angles to one another. True branching is rarely observed in cultures.

B. Culture: On Loeffler's coagulated serum medium, the colonies are small, granular, and gray, with irregular edges. On blood agar containing potassium tellurite, the colonies are gray to black because the tellurite is reduced intracellularly. The 3 types of *C diphtheriae* typically have the following appearance on such media: (1) var *gravis*—nonhemolytic, large, gray, irregular, striated colonies; (2) var *mitis*—hemolytic, small, black, glossy, convex colonies; (3) var *in-termedius*—nonhemolytic small colonies with characteristics between the 2 extremes. In broth, var *gravis* strains tend to form a pellicle, var *mitis* strains grow diffusely, and var *intermedius* strains settle as a granular sediment.

C. Growth Characteristics: Corynebacteria grow aerobically on most ordinary laboratory media. *Propionibacterium,* a "diphtheroid," is an anaerobe. On Loeffler's serum medium, corynebacteria grow much more readily than other respiratory pathogens, and the morphology of organisms is typical in smears. Acid, but not gas, is formed from some carbohydrates, as illustrated in Table 15–1.

D. Variation and Conversion: Corynebacteria tend to pleomorphism in microscopic and colonial morphology. Variation from smooth to rough forms has been described. Variants from toxigenic strains often are nontoxigenic. When some nontoxigenic diphtheria organisms are infected with bacteriophage from certain toxigenic diphtheria bacilli, the offspring of the exposed bacteria are lysogenic and toxigenic, and this trait is subsequently hereditary. (See Chapter 4, Genetics; and Chapter 9, Bacteriophage.) When toxigenic diphtheria bacilli are serially subcultured in specific antiserum against the temperate phage that they carry, they tend to become nontoxigenic. Thus, acquisition of phage leads to toxigenicity (lysogenic conversion). The actual production of toxin occurs perhaps only when the prophage of the lysogenic *C diphtheriae* becomes induced and lyses the cell. Whereas toxigenicity is under control of the phage gene, invasiveness is under control of bacterial genes.

Antigenic Structure

Serologic differences have been observed between types and within each type of *C diphtheriae*, but no satisfactory classification exists. Serologic tests are not usually employed in identification. Diphtheria toxin contains at least 4 antigenic determinants.

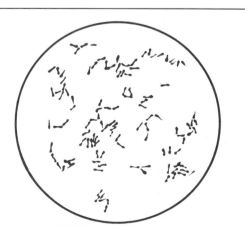

Figure 15–1. *C diphtheriae* from Loeffler's medium.

Table 15–1. Examples of metabolic reactions.

	Glucose*	Maltose*	Sucrose*	Urease
C diphtheriae	+	+	−	−
C xerosis	+	+	+	−
C pseudodiph-theriticum†	−	−	−	+
C pyogenes (C haemolyticum)	+	+	+	−

*Acid but no gas formed.
†Also called *C hofmannii*.

Pathogenesis

Some corynebacteria, notably *C pseudodiphtheriticum*, *C hofmannii*, *C xerosis*, *C pyogenes (C haemolyticum)*, *C ulcerans*, and group JK corynebacteria, are commonly called diphtheroids. They are normal inhabitants of the mucous membranes of the respiratory tract, urinary tract, and conjunctiva and rarely cause disease. A number of other diphtheroids cause infections in animals and, rarely, in humans. Anaerobic diphtheroids *(Propionibacterium acnes)* regularly reside in normal skin. They participate in the pathogenesis of acne. They produce lipases, which split off free fatty acids from skin lipids. These fatty acids can produce tissue inflammation and contribute to acne.

In immunosuppressed patients, various corynebacteria behave as opportunists and produce infection with bacteremia accompanied by a high mortality rate, especially during granulocytopenia.

The principal human pathogen of the group is *C diphtheriae*. In nature, *C diphtheriae* occurs in the respiratory tract, in wounds, or on the skin of infected persons or normal carriers. It is spread by droplets or by contact to susceptible individuals; virulent bacilli then grow on mucous membranes or in skin abrasions and start producing toxin.

All toxigenic *C diphtheriae* are capable of elaborating the same disease-producing exotoxin. In vitro production of this toxin depends largely on the concentration of iron. Toxin production is optimal at $0.14\ \mu g$ of iron per milliliter of medium but is virtually suppressed at $0.5\ \mu g/mL$. Other factors influencing the yield of toxin in vitro are osmotic pressure, amino acid concentration, pH, and availability of suitable carbon and nitrogen sources. The factors that control toxin production in vivo are not well understood.

Diphtheria toxin is a heat-labile polypeptide (MW 62,000) that can be lethal in a dose of $0.1\ \mu g/kg$. If disulfide bonds are broken, the molecule can be split into 2 fragments. Fragment B (MW $\sim 38,000$) has no independent activity but is required for the transport of fragment A into the cell. Fragment A inhibits polypeptide chain elongation—provided nicotinamide adenine dinucleotide (NAD) is present—by inactivating the elongation factor EF-2 (formerly called transferase II). This factor is required for translocation of polypeptidyl–transfer RNA from the acceptor to the donor site on the eukaryotic ribosome. Toxin fragment A inactivates EF-2 by catalyzing a reaction that yields free nicotinamide plus an inactive adenosine diphosphate–ribose–EF-2 complex. An exotoxin with a similar mode of action can be produced by strains of *Pseudomonas aeruginosa*. It is assumed that the abrupt arrest of protein synthesis is responsible for the necrotizing and neurotoxic effects of diphtheria toxin.

Corynebacterium minutissimum is the cause of erythrasma, a superficial infection of axillary and pubic skin. The organism produces bright pink fluorescence under ultraviolet light in skin lesions and when cultured in Mueller-Hinton agar.

Gardnerella vaginalis (formerly called *Corynebacterium vaginale* or *Haemophilus vaginalis*), a gram-negative rod, is a frequent member of the normal flora of the vagina. Alone or in combination with anaerobes, *G vaginalis* causes a vaginitis with a malodorous discharge.

Pathology

Diphtheria toxin is absorbed into the mucous membranes and causes destruction of epithelium and a superficial inflammatory response. The necrotic epithelium becomes embedded in exuding fibrin and red and white cells, so that a grayish "pseudomembrane" is formed—commonly over the tonsils, pharynx, or larynx. Any attempt to remove the pseudomembrane exposes and tears the capillaries and thus results in bleeding. The regional lymph nodes in the neck enlarge, and there may be marked edema of the entire neck. The diphtheria bacilli within the membrane continue to produce toxin actively. This is absorbed and results in distant toxic damage, particularly parenchymatous degeneration, fatty infiltration, and necrosis in heart muscle, liver, kidneys, and adrenals, sometimes accompanied by gross hemorrhage. The toxin also produces nerve damage, resulting often in paralysis of the soft palate, eye muscles, or extremities.

Wound or skin diphtheria occurs chiefly in the tropics. A membrane may form on an infected wound that fails to heal. However, absorption of toxin is usually slight and the systemic effects negligible. The "virulence" of diphtheria bacilli is due to their capacity for establishing infection, growing rapidly, and then quickly elaborating toxin that is effectively absorbed. *C diphtheriae* does not actively invade deep tissues and practically never enters the bloodstream.

Clinical Findings

When diphtheritic inflammation begins in the respiratory tract, sore throat and fever usually develop. Prostration and dyspnea soon follow because of the obstruction caused by the membrane. This obstruction may even cause suffocation if not promptly relieved by intubation or tracheostomy. Irregularities of cardiac rhythm indicate damage to the heart. Later, there may be difficulties with vision, speech, swallowing, or movement of the arms or legs. All of these manifestations tend to subside spontaneously.

In general, var *gravis* tends to produce more severe disease than var *mitis*, but similar illness can be produced by all types.

In some immunocompromised patients, various diphtheroids can cause pneumonia, endocarditis, and soft tissue and bone infections. When found in blood culture, they pose a problem in interpretation: Are they contaminants from normal skin flora or involved in a pathologic process?

Diagnostic Laboratory Tests

These serve to confirm the clinical impression and are of epidemiologic significance. *Note:* Specific treatment must never be delayed for laboratory reports if the clinical picture is strongly suggestive of diphtheria.

A. Specimens: Swabs from the nose, throat, or other suspected lesions must be obtained before antimicrobial drugs are administered.

B. Smears: Smears stained with alkaline methylene blue or Gram's stain show beaded rods in typical arrangement.

C. Culture: Inoculate a blood agar plate (to rule out hemolytic streptococci), a Loeffler slant, and a tellurite plate, and incubate all 3 at 37 °C. Unless the swab can be inoculated promptly, it should be kept moistened with sterile horse serum so the bacilli will remain viable. In 12–18 hours, the Loeffler slant may yield organisms of typical "diphtherialike" morphology. In 36–48 hours, the colonies on tellurite medium are sufficiently definite for recognition of the type of *C diphtheriae*.

Any diphtherialike organism cultured must be submitted to a "virulence" test before the bacteriologic diagnosis of diphtheria is definite. Such tests are really tests for toxigenicity of an isolated diphtherialike organism. They can be done in one of 3 ways as follows:

1. In vivo test–A culture is emulsified and 4 mL is injected subcutaneously into each of 2 guinea pigs, one of which has received 250 units of diphtheria antitoxin intraperitoneally 2 hours previously. The unprotected animal should die in 2–3 days, whereas the protected animal survives.

2. In vitro test–A strip of filter paper saturated with antitoxin is placed on an agar plate containing 20% horse serum. The cultures to be tested for toxigenicity are streaked across the plate at right angles to the filter paper. After 48 hours' incubation, the antitoxin diffusing from the paper strip has precipitated the toxin diffusing from toxigenic cultures and resulted in lines radiating from the intersection of the strip and the bacterial growth.

3. Tissue culture test–The toxigenicity of *C diphtheriae* can be shown by incorporation of bacteria into an agar overlay of cell culture monolayers. Toxin produced diffuses into cells below and kills them.

Resistance & Immunity

Since diphtheria is principally the result of the action of the toxin formed by the organism rather than invasion by the organism, resistance to the disease depends largely on the availability of specific neutralizing antitoxin in the bloodstream and tissues. It is generally true that diphtheria occurs only in persons who possess no antitoxin or less than 0.01 Lf unit/mL. Thus, the treatment of diphtheria rests largely on rapid suppression of toxin-producing bacteria by antimicrobial drugs and the early administration of specific antitoxin against the toxin formed by the organisms at their site of entry and multiplication. Antitoxic immunity to diphtheria may be active or passive. The relative amount of antitoxin that a person possesses at a given time can be estimated in one of 2 ways:

A. Titration of Serum for Antitoxin Content: (Too complex for routine use.) Serum is mixed with varying amounts of toxin and the mixture injected into susceptible animals. The greater the amount of toxin neutralized, the higher the concentration of antitoxin in the serum.

B. Schick Test: This test is based on the fact that diphtheria toxin is very irritating and results in a marked local reaction when injected intradermally unless it is neutralized by circulating antitoxin. One Schick test dose (amount of standard toxin that, when mixed with 0.001 unit of the US Standard diphtheria antitoxin and injected intradermally into a guinea pig, will induce a 10-mm erythematous reaction) is injected into the skin of one forearm and an identical amount of heated toxin is injected into the other forearm as a control. (Heating for 15 minutes at 60 °C destroys the effect of the toxin.) The test should be read at 24 and 48 hours and again in 6 days and interpreted as follows:

1. Positive reaction (susceptibility to diphtheria toxin, ie, absence of adequate amounts of neutralizing antitoxin; less than 0.01 Lf unit/mL)–Toxin produces redness and swelling that increase for several days and then slowly fade, leaving a brownish pigmented area. The control site shows no reaction.

2. Negative reaction (adequate amount of antitoxin present; usually in excess of 0.02 Lf unit/mL of serum)–Neither injection site shows any reaction.

3. Pseudoreaction–Schick test reactions may be complicated by hypersensitivity to materials other than the toxin contained in the injections. A pseudoreaction shows redness and swelling on both arms which disappear simultaneously on the second or third day. It constitutes a negative reaction.

4. Combined reaction–A combined reaction begins like a pseudoreaction, with redness and swelling at both injection sites; the toxin later continues to exert its effects, however, whereas the reaction at the control site subsides rapidly. This denotes hypersensitivity as well as relative susceptibility to toxin.

Treatment

Diphtheria antitoxin is produced in various animals (horses, sheep, goats, and rabbits) by the repeated injection of purified and concentrated toxoid. One International Unit of diphtheria antitoxin = 0.0628 mg of International Standard (Copenhagen). Treatment with antitoxin is mandatory when there is strong clinical suspicion of diphtheria. From 20,000 to 100,000 units are injected intramuscularly or intravenously after suitable precautions have been taken (skin or conjunctival test) to rule out hypersensitivity to the animal serum. The antitoxin should be given on the day the clinical diagnosis of diphtheria is made and need not be repeated. Intramuscular injection may be used in mild cases.

Antimicrobial drugs (penicillin, erythromycin) inhibit the growth of diphtheria bacilli. Although these drugs have virtually no effect on the disease process, they arrest toxin production. They also help to eliminate coexistent streptococci and *C diphtheriae* from the respiratory tracts of patients or carriers.

Antibiotic administration (tetracycline) in acne may inhibit the lipolytic action of anaerobic diphtheroids (*Propionibacterium acnes*); this reduces tissue inflammation. Variable benefit has been claimed for this treatment of acne.

Corynebacteria that produce bacteremia in immunocompromised patients or endocarditis on prosthetic valves are sometimes resistant to penicillins and erythromycin but may be susceptible to vancomycin. Treatment must be guided by antimicrobial drug susceptibility tests.

Epidemiology, Prevention, & Control

Before artificial immunization, diphtheria was mainly a disease of small children. The infection occurred either clinically or subclinically at an early age and resulted in the widespread production of antitoxin in the population. An asymptomatic infection during adolescence and adult life served as a stimulus for maintenance of high antitoxin levels. Thus, most members of the population, except children, were immune.

With the introduction of artificial active immunization, the situation has changed. After active immunization during the first few years of life, antitoxin levels are generally adequate until adulthood. Young adults should be given boosters of toxoid, because toxigenic diphtheria bacilli are not sufficiently prevalent in the population of many developed countries to provide the stimulus of subclinical infection with stimulation of resistance. Levels of antitoxin decline with time, and many older persons have insufficient amounts of circulating antitoxin to protect them against diphtheria.

The principal aim of prevention therefore must be to limit the distribution of toxigenic diphtheria bacilli in the population and to maintain as high a level of active immunization as possible.

A. Isolation: To limit contact with diphtheria bacilli to a minimum, patients with diphtheria must be isolated and every effort made to rid them of the organisms. Without treatment, a large percentage of in-fected persons continue to shed diphtheria bacilli for weeks or months after recovery (convalescent carriers). This danger may be greatly reduced by active early treatment with antibiotics. However, there are some healthy carriers from whom diphtheria bacilli cannot be readily eradicated with penicillin or erythromycin. Tonsillectomy is sometimes performed as a last resort.

B. Active Immunization: The following preparations have been employed:

1. Fluid toxoid—A filtrate of broth culture of a toxigenic strain is treated with 0.3% formalin and incubated at 37 °C until toxicity has disappeared. Toxoid is purified and standardized in flocculating units (Lf doses). Fluid toxoid itself is not often used for immunization now.

2. Toxoids for delayed absorption—Fluid toxoids prepared as above are adsorbed onto aluminum hydroxide or aluminum phosphate. This material remains longer in a depot after injection and is a better antigen. Such toxoids are commonly combined with tetanus toxoid and sometimes with pertussis vaccine as a single injection to be used in initial immunization of children (see Table 12–6). For booster injection of adults, only Td toxoids are used; these combine a full dose of tetanus toxoid with a 10-fold smaller dose of diphtheria toxoid in order to diminish the likelihood of adverse reactions.

All children must receive an initial course of immunizations and boosters as indicated in Table 12–6. Regular boosters with Td are particularly important for adults who travel to developing countries, where the incidence of clinical diphtheria may be 1000-fold higher than in developed countries where immunization is universal.

3. Toxin-antitoxin mixtures—These have been abandoned because of the danger of dissociation of the "neutral" mixture and the potential serious reactions to the free toxin.

REFERENCES

Bainton D et al: Immunity of children to diphtheria, tetanus and poliomyelitis. *Br Med J* 1979;**1**:854.

Collier RJ: Diphtheria toxin: Mode of action and structure. *Bacteriol Rev* 1975;**39**:54.

Hodes HL: Diphtheria. *Pediatr Clin North Am* 1979;**26**:445.

Josey WE et al: *Corynebacterium vaginale* in women with leukorrhea. *Am J Obstet Gynecol* 1976;**126**:574.

Kaplan K, Weinstein L: Diphtheroid infections of man. *Ann Intern Med* 1969;**70**:919.

Laird W, Groman N: Tissue culture test for toxigenicity of *C diphtheriae*. *Appl Microbiol* 1973;**25**:709.

Lipsky BA et al: Infections caused by non-diphtheria corynebacteria. *Rev Infect Dis* 1982;**4**:1220.

McCormack WM et al: Vaginal colonization with *Corynebacterium vaginale*. *J Infect Dis* 1977;**136**:740.

Nathenson G, Zakzewski B: Current status of passive immunity to diphtheria and tetanus in the newborn. *J Infect Dis* 1976;**133**:199.

Pearson TA et al: *Corynebacterium* sepsis in oncology patients. *JAMA* 1977;**238**:1737.

Rosenberg EW: Bacteriology of acne. *Annu Rev Med* 1969; **20**:201.

Stamm W et al: Infection due to *Corynebacterium* species in marrow transplant patients. *Ann Intern Med* 1979;**91**:167.

Thompson HL, Ellner PD: Rapid determination of *Corynebacterium diphtheriae* toxigenicity by counterimmunoelectrophoresis. *J Clin Microbiol* 1978;**7**:493.

Washington JA: Bacteriology, clinical spectrum of diseases, and therapeutic aspects in coryneform bacterial infection. Page 69 in: *Current Clinical Topics in Infectious Diseases*. Vol 2. Remington JS, Swartz MN (editors). McGraw-Hill, 1981.

Yocum RC et al: Septic arthritis caused by *Propionibacterium acnes*. *JAMA* 1982;**248**:1740.

The Staphylococci

The staphylococci are gram-positive spherical cells, usually arranged in grapelike irregular clusters. They grow readily on many types of media and are active metabolically, fermenting carbohydrates and producing pigments that vary from white to deep yellow. Some are members of the normal flora of the skin and mucous membranes of humans; others cause suppuration, abscess formation, a variety of pyogenic infections, and even fatal septicemia. The pathogenic staphylococci often hemolyze blood, coagulate plasma, and produce a variety of extracellular enzymes and toxins. A common type of food poisoning is caused by a heat-stable staphylococcal enterotoxin. Staphylococci rapidly develop resistance to many antimicrobial agents and present difficult therapeutic problems.

The genus *Staphylococcus* has at least 20 species. *Staphylococcus aureus* is coagulase-positive, is a major pathogen for humans, and is responsible for many severe infections. The coagulase-negative staphylococci are normal human flora: *Staphylococcus epidermidis* sometimes causes infection of prosthetic devices, and *Staphylococcus saprophyticus* can cause urinary tract infections in young women. Some other species are important in veterinary medicine.

Morphology & Identification

A. Typical Organisms: Spherical cells about 1 μm in diameter arranged in irregular clusters (Fig 16–1). Single cocci, pairs, tetrads, and chains are also seen in liquid cultures. Young cocci stain strongly gram-positive; on aging, many cells become gram-negative. Staphylococci are nonmotile and do not form spores. Under the influence of certain chemicals (eg, penicillin), staphylococci are lysed or changed into L forms, but they are not affected by bile salts or optochin.

Micrococcus species often resemble staphylococci. They are found free-living in the environment and form regular packets of 4 or 8 cocci. Their colonies can be yellow, red, or orange.

B. Culture: Staphylococci grow readily on most bacteriologic media under aerobic or microaerophilic conditions. They grow most rapidly at 37 °C but form pigment best at room temperature (20–25 °C). Colonies on solid media are round, smooth, raised, and glistening. *S aureus* forms gray to deep golden yellow colonies. *S epidermidis* colonies are gray to white on primary isolation; many colonies develop pigment only upon prolonged incubation. No pigment is produced anaerobically or in broth. Various degrees of hemolysis are produced by *S aureus* and occasionally by other species. *Peptococcus* species, which are anaerobic cocci, resemble staphylococci in morphology.

C. Growth Characteristics: The staphylococci produce catalase, which differentiates them from the streptococci. Staphylococci slowly ferment many carbohydrates, producing lactic acid but not gas. Proteolytic activity varies greatly from one strain to another. Pathogenic staphylococci produce many extracellular substances, which are discussed below.

Staphylococci are relatively resistant to drying, heat (they withstand 50 °C for 30 minutes), and 9% sodium chloride but are readily inhibited by certain chemicals, eg, 3% hexachlorophene.

Staphylococci are variably sensitive to many antimicrobial drugs. Resistance falls into several classes: (1) β-lactamase production is common, is under plasmid control, and makes the organisms resistant to many penicillins (penicillin G, ampicillin, ticarcillin, and similar drugs). The plasmids are transmitted by transduction and perhaps also by conjugation. (2) Resistance to nafcillin (and to methicillin and oxacillin) is independent of β-lactamase production. The genes probably reside on the chromosome and are variably expressed. The mechanism of nafcillin resistance is

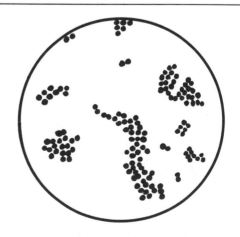

Figure 16–1. Gram stain appearance of staphylococci from broth culture.

probably related to the lack of or inaccessibility of certain penicillin-binding proteins (PBPs) in the organisms. (3) "Tolerance" implies that staphylococci are inhibited by a drug but not killed by it, ie, there is a very large difference between minimal inhibitory and minimal lethal concentrations of an antimicrobial drug. Tolerance can at times be attributed to a lack of activation of autolytic enzymes in the cell wall. (4) Plasmids can also carry genes for resistance to tetracyclines, erythromycins, and aminoglycosides. Staphylococci have remained susceptible to vancomycin.

D. Variation: A culture of staphylococci contains some bacteria that differ from the bulk of the population in expression of colony characteristics (colony size, pigment, hemolysis), in enzyme elaboration, in drug resistance, and in pathogenicity. In vitro, the expression of such characteristics is influenced by growth conditions: when nafcillin-resistant *S aureus* is incubated at 37 °C on blood agar, one in 10^7 organisms expresses nafcillin resistance; when it is incubated at 30 °C on agar containing 2–5% sodium chloride, one in 10^3 organisms expresses nafcillin resistance.

Antigenic Structure

Staphylococci contain antigenic polysaccharides and proteins as well as other substances important in cell wall structure (Fig 16–2). Peptidoglycan, a polysaccharide polymer containing linked subunits, provides the rigid exoskeleton of the cell wall. Peptidoglycan is destroyed by strong acid or exposure to lysozyme. It is important in the pathogenesis of infection: it elicits production of interleukin-1 (endogenous pyrogen) and opsonic antibodies by monocytes; and it can be a chemoattractant for polymorphonuclear

leukocytes, have endotoxinlike activity, produce a localized Shwartzman phenomenon, and activate complement.

Teichoic acids, which are polymers of glycerol or ribitol phosphate, are linked to the peptidoglycan and can be antigenic. Antiteichoic antibodies detectable by gel diffusion may be found in patients with active endocarditis due to *S aureus*.

Protein A is a cell wall component of many *S aureus* strains that binds to the Fc portion of IgG molecules except IgG3. The Fab portion of IgG bound to protein A is free to combine with a specific antigen. Protein A has become an important reagent in immunology and diagnostic technology; for example, protein A with attached IgG molecules directed against a specific bacterial antigen will agglutinate bacteria that have that antigen ("coagglutination").

Some *S aureus* strains have capsules, which inhibit phagocytosis by polymorphonuclear leukocytes unless specific antibodies are present. Most strains of *S aureus* have coagulase, or clumping factor, on the cell wall surface; coagulase binds nonenzymatically to fibrinogen, yielding aggregation of the bacteria.

Serologic tests have limited usefulness in identifying staphylococci. Phage typing is sometimes used for epidemiologic studies, but this is done only in reference laboratories. Phage typing is based on the lysis of *S aureus* by one or a series of specific bacteriophages. Such bacteriophage susceptibility (phage type) is a stable genetic characteristic based on staphylococcal surface receptors.

Toxins & Enzymes

Staphylococci can produce disease both through

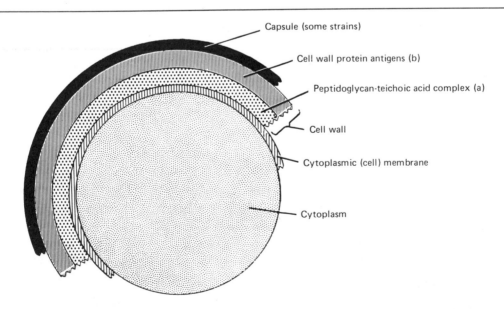

Figure 16–2. Antigenic structure of staphylococci. *(a)* Site of bacteriophage attachment. Species antigens present (antigenic determinant is N-acetylglucosamine linked to polyribitol phosphate). *(b)* Multiple antigens; several widely distributed.

Labels in figure:
- Capsule (some strains)
- Cell wall protein antigens (b)
- Peptidoglycan-teichoic acid complex (a)
- Cell wall
- Cytoplasmic (cell) membrane
- Cytoplasm

their ability to multiply and spread widely in tissues and through their production of many extracellular substances. Some of these substances are enzymes; others are considered to be toxins, although they may function as enzymes. Many of the toxins are under the genetic control of plasmids; some may be under both chromosomal and extrachromosomal control; and for others the mechanism of genetic control is not well defined.

A. Catalase: Staphylococci produce catalase, which converts hydrogen peroxide into water and oxygen.

B. Coagulase: *S aureus* produces coagulase, an enzymelike protein that clots oxalated or citrated plasma in the presence of a factor contained in many sera. The serum factor reacts with coagulase to generate both esterase and clotting activities, in a manner similar to the activation of prothrombin to thrombin. The action of coagulase circumvents the normal plasma clotting cascade. Coagulase may deposit fibrin on the surface of staphylococci, perhaps altering their ingestion by phagocytic cells or their destruction within such cells. Coagulase production is considered synonymous with invasive pathogenic potential.

C. Other Enzymes: Other enzymes produced by staphylococci include a hyaluronidase, or spreading factor; a staphylokinase resulting in fibrinolysis but acting much more slowly than streptokinase; proteinases; lipases; and β-lactamases.

D. Exotoxins: These include several toxins that are lethal for animals on injection, cause necrosis in skin, and contain soluble hemolysins which can be separated by electrophoresis. The alpha toxin (hemolysin) is a heterogeneous protein that can lyse erythrocytes and damage platelets and is probably identical with the lethal and dermonecrotic factors of exotoxin. Alpha toxin also has a powerful action on vascular smooth muscle. Beta toxin degrades sphingomyelin and is toxic for many kinds of cells, including human red blood cells. These toxins and 2 others, the gamma and delta toxins, are antigenically distinct and bear no relationship to streptococcal lysins. Exotoxin treated with formalin gives a nonpoisonous but antigenic toxoid, but this is not clinically useful.

E. Leukocidin: This toxin can kill exposed white blood cells of many animals. Its role in pathogenesis is uncertain, because pathogenic staphylococci may not kill white blood cells and may be phagocytosed as effectively as nonpathogenic varieties. However, they are capable of very active intracellular multiplication, whereas the nonpathogenic organisms tend to die inside the cell. Antibodies to leukocidin may play a role in resistance to recurrent staphylococcal infections.

F. Exfoliative Toxin: This toxin includes at least 2 proteins that yield the generalized desquamation of the staphylococcal scalded skin syndrome. Specific antibodies protect against the exfoliative action of the toxin.

G. Toxic Shock Syndrome Toxin: Most *S aureus* strains isolated from patients with toxic shock syndrome produce a toxin called toxic shock syndrome toxin 1 (TSST-1), which is the same as enterotoxin F and pyrogenic exotoxin C. In humans, the toxin is associated with fever, shock, and multisystem involvement, including a desquamative skin rash; there is no direct evidence that the toxin is the sole cause of toxic shock syndrome. In rabbits, TSST-1 produces fever, enhanced susceptibility to the effects of bacterial lipopolysaccharides, and other biologic effects similar to toxic shock syndrome but the skin rash and desquamation do not occur.

H. Enterotoxins: These are 6 (A–F) soluble toxins produced by nearly 50% of *S aureus* strains. The enterotoxins are heat-stable (they resist boiling for 30 minutes) and resistant to the action of gut enzymes. An important cause of food poisoning, enterotoxins are produced when *S aureus* grows in carbohydrate and protein foods. The gene for enterotoxin production may be on the chromosome, but a plasmid may carry a protein that regulates active toxin production. Ingestion of 25 μg of enterotoxin B by humans or monkeys results in vomiting and diarrhea. The emetic effect of enterotoxin is probably the result of central nervous system stimulation (vomiting center) after the toxin acts on neural receptors in the gut. Enterotoxins can be assayed by precipitin tests (gel diffusion).

Pathogenesis

Staphylococci, particularly *S epidermidis*, are members of the normal flora of the human skin and respiratory and gastrointestinal tracts. Nasal carriage of *S aureus* occurs in 40–50% of humans. Staphylococci are also found regularly on clothing, bed linens, and other fomites of human environments.

The pathogenic capacity of a given strain of *S aureus* is the combined effect of extracellular factors and toxins together with the invasive properties of the strain. At one end of the disease spectrum is staphylococcal food poisoning, attributable solely to the ingestion of preformed enterotoxin; at the other end are staphylococcal bacteremia and disseminated abscesses in all organs. The potential contribution of the various extracellular substances in pathogenesis is evident from the nature of their individual actions.

Pathogenic, invasive *S aureus* tend to produce coagulase and yellow pigment and to be hemolytic. Nonpathogenic, noninvasive staphylococci such as *S epidermidis* tend to be coagulase-negative and nonhemolytic. Such organisms rarely produce suppuration but may infect orthopedic or cardiovascular prostheses. *S saprophyticus* is typically nonpigmented, novobiocin-resistant, and nonhemolytic; it causes urinary tract infections in young women.

Pathology

The prototype of a staphylococcal lesion is the furuncle or other localized abscess. Groups of *S aureus* established in a hair follicle lead to tissue necrosis (dermonecrotic factor). Coagulase is produced and coagulates fibrin around the lesion and within the lymphatics, resulting in formation of a wall that limits the process and is reinforced by the accumulation of inflammatory cells and, later, fibrous tissue. Within the center of the lesion, liquefaction of the necrotic tissue occurs (enhanced by delayed hypersensitivity), and the abscess "points" in the direction of least resistance. Drainage of the liquid central necrotic tissue is followed by slow filling of the cavity with granulation tissue and eventual healing.

Focal suppuration (abscess) is typical of staphylococcal infection. From any one focus, organisms may spread via the lymphatics and bloodstream to other parts of the body. Suppuration within veins, associated with thrombosis, is a common feature of such dissemination. In osteomyelitis, the primary focus of *S aureus* growth is typically in a terminal blood vessel of the metaphysis of a long bone, leading to necrosis of bone and chronic suppuration. *S aureus* may cause pneumonia, meningitis, empyema, endocarditis, or sepsis with suppuration in any organ. Staphylococci of low invasiveness are involved in many skin infections (eg, acne, impetigo). Anaerobic cocci *(Peptococcus)* participate in mixed anaerobic infections.

Staphylococci also cause disease through the elaboration of toxins, without apparent invasive infection. Bullous exfoliation, the scalded skin syndrome, is caused by the production of exfoliative toxin. Toxic shock syndrome is associated with toxic shock syndrome toxin 1 (TSST-1).

Clinical Findings

A localized staphylococcal infection appears as a "pimple," hair follicle infection, or abscess. There is usually an intense, localized, painful inflammatory reaction that undergoes central suppuration and heals quickly when the pus is drained. The wall of fibrin and cells around the core of the abscess tends to prevent spread of the organisms and should not be broken down by manipulation or trauma.

S aureus infection can also result from direct contamination of a wound, eg, postoperative staphylococcal wound infection or infection following trauma (chronic osteomyelitis subsequent to an open fracture, meningitis following skull fracture).

If *S aureus* disseminates and bacteremia ensues, endocarditis, acute hematogenous osteomyelitis, meningitis, or pulmonary infection can result. The clinical presentations resemble those seen with other bloodstream infections. Secondary localization within an organ or system is accompanied by the symptoms and signs of organ dysfunction and intense focal suppuration.

Food poisoning due to staphylococcal enterotoxin is characterized by a short incubation period (1–8 hours); violent nausea, vomiting, and diarrhea; and rapid convalescence (Table 18–4). There is no fever.

Toxic shock syndrome (TSS) has an abrupt onset of high fever, vomiting, diarrhea, myalgias, a scarlatiniform rash, and hypotension with cardiac and renal failure in the most severe cases. TSS often occurs within 5 days of the onset of menses in young women who use tampons, but it also occurs in children or in men with staphylococcal wound infections. The syndrome can recur. TSS-associated *S aureus* can be found in the vagina, on tampons, in wounds or other localized infections, or in the throat but virtually never in the bloodstream.

Diagnostic Laboratory Tests

A. Specimens: Surface swab, pus, blood, tracheal aspirate, or spinal fluid for culture, depending upon the localization of the process. Antibody determinations in serum are rarely of value.

B. Smears: Typical staphylococci are seen in stained smears of pus or sputum. It is not possible to distinguish saprophytic *(S epidermidis)* from pathogenic *(S aureus)* organisms.

C. Culture: Specimens planted on blood agar plates give rise to typical colonies in 18 hours at 37 °C, but hemolysis and pigment production may not occur until several days later and are optimal at room temperature. Specimens contaminated with a mixed flora can be cultured on media containing 7.5% NaCl; the salt inhibits most other normal flora but not *S aureus*.

D. Catalase Test: A drop of hydrogen peroxide solution is placed on a slide, and a small amount of the bacterial growth is placed in the solution. The formation of bubbles (the release of oxygen) indicates a positive test. The test can also be performed by pouring hydrogen peroxide solution over a heavy growth of the bacteria on an agar slant and observing for the appearance of bubbles.

E. Coagulase Test: Citrated rabbit (or human) plasma diluted 1:5 is mixed with an equal volume of broth culture and incubated at 37 °C. A tube of plasma mixed with sterile broth is included as a control. If clots form in 1–4 hours, the test is positive.

All coagulase-positive staphylococci are considered pathogenic for humans. Infections of prosthetic devices can be caused by coagulase-negative *S epidermidis*.

F. Serologic and Typing Tests: Antibodies to teichoic acid can be detected in prolonged, deep infections (eg, staphylococcal endocarditis) and sometimes distinguish them from staphylococcal bacteremia. These serologic tests have little practical value.

Antibiotic susceptibility patterns are helpful in tracing *S aureus* infections and in determining if multiple *S epidermidis* isolates from blood cultures represent bacteremia due to the same strain, seeded by a nidus of infection.

Phage typing is used for epidemiologic tracing of infection only in severe outbreaks of *S aureus* infections, as might occur in a hospital.

Treatment

Most persons harbor staphylococci on the skin and in the nose or throat. Even if the skin can be cleared of staphylococci (eg, in eczema), reinfection by droplets will occur almost immediately. Because pathogenic organisms are commonly spread from one lesion (eg, a furuncle) to other areas of the skin by fingers and clothing, scrupulous local antisepsis is important to control recurrent furunculosis.

Serious multiple skin infections (acne, furunculosis) occur most often in adolescents. Similar skin infections occur in patients receiving prolonged courses of corticosteroids, implying a role for hormones in the pathogenesis of staphylococcal skin infections. In acne, lipases of staphylococci and corynebacteria liberate fatty acids from lipids and thus cause tissue irritation. Tetracyclines are used for long-term treatment.

Abscesses and other closed suppurating lesions are treated by drainage, which is essential, and antimicrobial therapy. Many antimicrobial drugs have some effect against staphylococci in vitro. However, it is difficult to eradicate pathogenic staphylococci from infected persons, because the organisms rapidly develop resistance to many antimicrobial drugs and the drugs cannot act in the central necrotic part of a suppurative lesion. It is also very difficult to eradicate the *S aureus* carrier state.

Acute hematogenous osteomyelitis responds well to antimicrobial drugs. In chronic osteomyelitis, surgical drainage and removal of dead bone is accompanied by long-term administration of appropriate drugs, but eradication of the infecting staphylococci is difficult. Hyperbaric oxygen and the application of vascularized myocutaneous flaps have aided healing in chronic osteomyelitis.

Bacteremia, endocarditis, pneumonia, and other severe infections due to *S aureus* require prolonged intravenous therapy with a β-lactamase–resistant penicillin. Vancomycin is often reserved for use with nafcillin-resistant staphylococci. If the infection is found to be due to non–β-lactamase–producing *S aureus*, penicillin G is the drug of choice, but only a small percentage of *S aureus* strains are susceptible to penicillin G.

S epidermidis infections are difficult to cure because they occur in prosthetic devices where the bacteria can sequester themselves from the circulation and thus from antimicrobial drugs. *S epidermidis* is more often resistant to antimicrobial drugs than is *S aureus*; approximately 60% of *S epidermidis* strains are nafcillin-resistant.

Because of the frequency of drug-resistant strains, meaningful staphylococcal isolates should usually be tested for antimicrobial susceptibility to help in the choice of systemic drugs. Resistance to drugs of the erythromycin group tends to emerge so rapidly that these drugs should not be used singly for treatment of chronic infection. Drug resistance (to penicillins, tetracyclines, aminoglycosides, erythromycins, etc) determined by plasmids can be transmitted among staphylococci by transduction and perhaps by conjugation.

Penicillin G–resistant *S aureus* strains from clinical infections always produce penicillinase. They now constitute 70–90% of *S aureus* isolates in communities in the USA. They are often susceptible to β-lactamase–resistant penicillins, cephalosporins, or vancomycin. Nafcillin resistance is independent of β-lactamase production, and its clinical incidence varies greatly in different countries and at different times. The selection pressure of β-lactamase–resistant antimicrobial drugs may not be the sole determinant for resistance to these drugs: For example, in Denmark, nafcillin-resistant *S aureus* comprised 40% of isolates in 1970 and only 10% in 1980, without notable changes in the use of nafcillin or similar drugs. In the USA, nafcillin-resistant *S aureus* accounted for only 0.1% of isolates in 1970 but in the mid-1980s constituted 10–30% of isolates from nosocomial infections in some hospitals.

In view of the rapid emergence of drug resistance among staphylococci, hospitals have sometimes restricted the use of an antistaphylococcal drug to the treatment of seriously ill patients. Such restriction could prolong the useful period of a new drug. Vancomycin remains the most widely effective drug against staphylococci.

Epidemiology & Control

Staphylococci are ubiquitous human parasites. The chief sources of infection are shedding human lesions, fomites contaminated from such lesions, and the human respiratory tract and skin. Contact spread of infection has assumed added importance in hospitals, where a large proportion of the staff and patients carry antibiotic-resistant staphylococci in the nose or on the skin. Although cleanliness, hygiene, and aseptic management of lesions can control the spread of staphylococci from lesions, few methods are available to prevent the wide dissemination of staphylococci from carriers. Aerosols (eg, glycols) and ultraviolet irradiation of air have little effect.

In hospitals, the areas at highest risk for severe staphylococcal infections are the newborn nursery, intensive care units, operating rooms, and cancer chemotherapy wards. Massive introduction of "epidemic" pathogenic *S aureus* into these areas may lead to serious clinical disease. Personnel with active staphylococcal lesions and carriers may have to be excluded from these areas. In such individuals, the application of topical antiseptics (eg, chlorhexidine or bacitracin cream) to nasal or perineal carriage sites may diminish shedding of dangerous organisms. Rifampin coupled with a second oral antistaphylococcal drug sometimes provides long-term suppression and possibly cure of nasal carriage; this form of therapy is usually reserved for major problems of staphylococcal carriage, because staphylococci can rapidly develop resistance to rifampin. Antiseptics such as hexachlorophene used on the skin of newborns diminish colonization by staphylococci, but toxicity prevents their widespread use.

REFERENCES

Archer GL, Tenenbaum MJ: Antibiotic-resistant *Staphylococcus epidermidis* in patients undergoing cardiac surgery. *Antimicrob Agents Chemother* 1980;**17**:269.

Bergdoll MS et al: A new staphylococcal enterotoxin, enterotoxin F, associated with toxic-shock-syndrome *Staphylococcus aureus* isolates. *Lancet* 1981;**1**:1017.

Breckinridge JC, Bergdoll MS: Outbreak of food-borne gastroenteritis due to a coagulase-negative enterotoxin-producing staphylococcus. *N Engl J Med* 1971;**284**:541.

Effersoe P, Kjerulf K: Clinical aspects of outbreak of staphylococcal food poisoning during air travel. *Lancet* 1975;**2**:599.

Fekety FR Jr: The epidemiology and prevention of staphylococcal infection. *Medicine* 1964;**43**:593.

Haley RW et al: The emergence of methicillin-resistant *Staphylococcus aureus* infections in United States hospitals. *Ann Intern Med* 1982;**97**:297.

Hyams PJ et al: Staphylococcal bacteremia and hexachlorophene bathing: Epidemic in a newborn nursery. *Am J Dis Child* 1975;**129**:595.

Maki DG et al: Infection control in intravenous therapy. *Ann Intern Med* 1973;**79**:867.

Mandell GL: Catalase, superoxide dismutase, and virulence of *Staphylococcus aureus:* In vitro and in vivo studies with emphasis on staphylococcal-leukocyte interaction. *J Clin Invest* 1975;**55**:561.

Melish ME et al: The staphylococcal scalded skin syndrome: Isolation and partial characterization of the exfoliative toxin. *J Infect Dis* 1972;**125**:129.

Musher DM et al: Infections due to *Staphylococcus aureus*. *Medicine* 1977;**56**:383.

Nolan SM, Beaty HN: *Staphylococcus aureus* bacteremia: Current clinical patterns. *Am J Med* 1976;**60**:495.

Peacock JE et al: Methicillin-resistant *Staphylococcus aureus*: Introduction and spread within a hospital. *Ann Intern Med* 1980;**93**:526.

Sabath LD: Mechanisms of resistance to beta-lactam antibiotic in strains of *Staphylococcus aureus*. *Ann Intern Med* 1982; **97**:339.

Schliefer KH, Kandler O: Peptidoglycan types of bacterial cell walls and their taxonomic implications. *Bacteriol Rev* 1972; **36**:407.

Schlievert PM et al: Identification and characterization of an exotoxin from *Staphylococcus aureus* associated with toxic-shock syndrome. *J Infect Dis* 1981;**143**:509.

Shands KN et al: Toxic-shock syndrome in menstruating women. *N Engl J Med* 1980;**303**:1436.

Thornsberry C, McDougal LK: Successful use of broth microdilution in susceptibility tests for methicillin-resistant (heteroresistant) staphylococci. *J Clin Microbiol* 1983;**18**:1084.

Waldvogel FA, Vasey V: Osteomyelitis: The past decade. *N Engl J Med* 1980;**303**:360.

Watanakunakorn C, Baird IM: *Staphylococcus aureus* bacteremia and endocarditis associated with a removable infected intravenous device. *Am J Med* 1977;**63**:253.

Wheat LJ et al: Antibody response to peptidoglycan during staphylococcal infections. *J Infect Dis* 1983;**147**:16.

The Streptococci

17

The streptococci are gram-positive spherical bacteria that characteristically form pairs or chains during growth. They are widely distributed in nature. Some are members of the normal human flora; others are associated with important human diseases attributable in part to infection by streptococci, in part to sensitization to them. Streptococci elaborate a variety of extracellular substances and enzymes.

Streptococci are a heterogeneous group of bacteria, and no one system suffices to classify them. Twenty species, including *Streptococcus pyogenes* (group A), *Streptococcus agalactiae* (group B), and the enterococci (group D), are characterized by combinations of features: colony growth characteristics, hemolysis patterns on blood agar (alpha hemolysis, beta hemolysis, or no hemolysis), antigenic composition of group-specific cell wall substances, and biochemical reactions. *Streptococcus pneumoniae* (pneumococcus) types are further classified by the antigenic composition of the capsular polysaccharides (see p 230).

Morphology & Identification

A. Typical Organisms: Individual cocci are spherical or ovoid and are arranged in chains (Fig 17–1). The cocci divide in a plane perpendicular to the long axis of the chain. The members of the chain often have a striking diplococcal appearance, and rodlike forms are occasionally seen. The lengths of the chains vary widely and are conditioned by environmental factors. Streptococci are gram-positive. However, as a culture ages and the bacteria die, they lose their gram-positivity and appear to be gram-negative; this can occur after overnight incubation.

Some streptococci elaborate a capsular polysaccharide comparable to that of pneumococci. Most group A, B, and C strains (see p 225) produce capsules composed of hyaluronic acid. The capsules are most noticeable in very young cultures. They impede phagocytosis. The streptococcal cell wall contains proteins (M, T, R, antigens), carbohydrates (group-specific), and peptidoglycans (Fig 17–2). Hairlike pili project through the capsule of group A streptococci. The pili consist partly of M protein and are covered with lipoteichoic acid. The latter is important in the attachment of streptococci to epithelial cells.

B. Culture: Most streptococci grow in solid media as discoid colonies, usually 1–2 mm in diameter. Group A strains that produce capsular material often give rise to mucoid colonies. Matt and glossy colonies

of group A strains are discussed below. *Peptostreptococcus* is an obligate anaerobe.

C. Growth Characteristics: Energy is obtained principally from the utilization of sugars. Growth of streptococci tends to be poor on solid media or in broth unless enriched with blood or tissue fluids. Nutritive requirements vary widely among different species. The human pathogens are most exacting, requiring a variety of growth factors. Growth and hemolysis are aided by incubation in 10% CO_2.

Whereas most pathogenic hemolytic streptococci grow best at 37 °C, group D enterococci grow well between 15 °C and 45 °C. Enterococci also grow in high (6.5%) sodium chloride concentrations, in 0.1% methylene blue, and in bile-esculin agar. Most streptococci are facultative anaerobes. Other characteristics are discussed below.

D. Variation: Variants of the same *Streptococcus* strain may show different colony forms. This is particularly marked among group A strains, giving rise to either matt or glossy colonies. Matt colonies consist of organisms that produce much M protein. Such organisms tend to be virulent and relatively insusceptible to phagocytosis by human leukocytes. Glossy colonies tend to produce little M protein and are often nonvirulent.

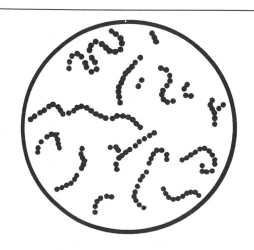

Figure 17–1. Gram stain appearance of streptococci from broth culture.

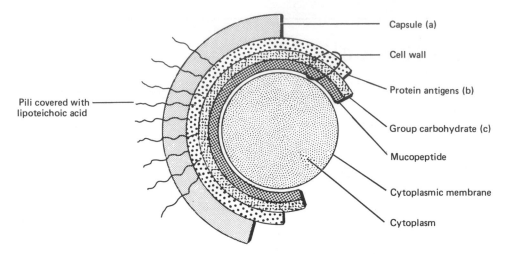

Figure 17–2. Antigen structure of group A streptococcal cell. **(a)** Capsule is hyaluronic acid. **(b)** Cell wall protein antigens M, T, and R. **(c)** Group-specific carbohydrate of group A streptococci is rhamnose-N-acetylglucosamine.

Antigenic Structure

Hemolytic streptococci can be divided into serologic groups (A–U), and certain groups can be subdivided into types. Several antigenic substances are found:

(1) Group-specific cell wall antigen: This carbohydrate is contained in the cell wall of many streptococci and forms the basis of serologic grouping (Lancefield groups A–U). Extracts of group-specific antigen for grouping streptococci may be prepared by extraction of centrifuged culture with hot hydrochloric acid, nitrous acid, or formamide; by enzymatic lysis of streptococcal cells (eg, with pepsin or trypsin); or by autoclaving of cell suspensions at 15 lb pressure for 15 minutes. The serologic specificity of the group-specific carbohydrate is determined by an amino sugar. For group A streptococci, this is rhamnose-N-acetylglucosamine; for group B, rhamnose-glucosamine polysaccharide; for group C, rhamnose-N-acetylgalactosamine; for group D, glycerol teichoic acid containing D-alanine and glucose; for group F, glucopyranosyl-N-acetylgalactosamine.

(2) M protein: This substance is closely associated with virulence of group A streptococci and occurs chiefly in organisms producing matt or mucoid colonies. Repeated passage on artificial media may lead to loss of M protein production, which may be restored by rapidly repeated animal passage. M protein interferes with the ingestion of virulent streptococci by phagocytic cells.

M protein determines the type specificity of group A streptococci, as demonstrated by agglutination or precipitation reactions with M type-specific sera. There are more than 60 types in group A. Types are assigned Arabic numbers. In humans, antibodies to an M protein protect against infection with this specific M type of group A *Streptococcus*. Group G streptococci have surface virulence-associated proteins that are similar to the M proteins of group A streptococci.

(3) T substance: This antigen has no relationship to virulence of streptococci. Unlike M protein, T substance is acid-labile and heat-labile. It is obtained from streptococci by proteolytic digestion, which rapidly destroys M proteins. T substance permits differentiation of certain types of streptococci by agglutination with specific antisera, while other types share the same T substance. Yet another surface antigen has been called **R protein.**

(4) Nucleoproteins: Extraction of streptococci with weak alkali yields mixtures of proteins and other substances of little serologic specificity, called **P substances,** which probably make up most of the streptococcal cell body.

Toxins & Enzymes

More than 20 extracellular products that are antigenic are elaborated by group A streptococci, including the following:

(1) Streptokinase (fibrinolysin) is produced by many strains of beta-hemolytic streptococci. It transforms the plasminogen of human plasma into plasmin, an active proteolytic enzyme that digests fibrin and other proteins. This process of digestion may be interfered with by nonspecific serum inhibitors and by a specific antibody, antistreptokinase. Streptokinase has been given intravenously for treatment of pulmonary emboli and venous thromboses.

(2) Streptodornase (streptococcal deoxyribonuclease) depolymerizes DNA. The enzymatic activity can be measured by the decrease in viscosity of known DNA solutions. Purulent exudates owe their viscosity largely to deoxyribonucleoprotein. Mixtures of streptodornase and streptokinase are used in "enzymatic debridement." They help to liquefy exudates and facilitate removal of pus and necrotic tissue; antimicrobial drugs thus gain better access, and infected surfaces recover more quickly. An antibody to DNase develops after streptococcal infections (normal limit = 100 units), especially after skin infections with pyoderma.

(3) Hyaluronidase splits hyaluronic acid, an important component of the ground substance of connective tissue. Thus, hyaluronidase aids in spreading infecting microorganisms (spreading factor). Hyaluronidases are antigenic and specific for each bacterial or tissue source. Following infection with hyaluronidase-producing organisms, specific antibodies are found in the serum.

(4) Erythrogenic toxin is soluble and is destroyed by boiling for 1 hour. It causes the rash that occurs in scarlet fever. Only strains elaborating this toxin can cause scarlet fever. Erythrogenic toxin is elaborated only by lysogenic streptococci. Strains devoid of the temperate phage genome do not produce toxin. A nontoxigenic *Streptococcus,* after lysogenic conversion (see Chapter 9), will produce erythrogenic toxin. Erythrogenic toxin is antigenic.

(5) Some streptococci elaborate a **diphosphopyridine nucleotidase** into the environment. This enzyme may be related to the organism's ability to kill leukocytes. Proteinases and amylase are produced by some strains.

(6) Hemolysins: Many streptococci are able to hemolyze red blood cells in vitro in varying degrees. Complete disruption of erythrocytes with release of hemoglobin is called **beta hemolysis.** Incomplete lysis of erythrocytes with the formation of green pigment is called **alpha hemolysis.**

Beta-hemolytic group A streptococci elaborate 2 hemolysins (streptolysins):

Streptolysin O is a protein (MW 60,000) that is hemolytically active in the reduced state (available –SH groups) but rapidly inactivated in the presence of oxygen. It combines quantitatively with antistreptolysin O, an antibody that appears in humans following infection with any streptococci that produce streptolysin O. This antibody blocks hemolysis by streptolysin O. This phenomenon forms the basis of a quantitative test for the antibody. An antistreptolysin O (ASO) serum titer in excess of 160–200 units is considered abnormally high and suggests either recent infection with streptococci or persistently high antibody levels due to an exaggerated immune response to an earlier exposure in a hypersensitive person.

Streptolysin S is the agent responsible for the hemolytic zones around streptococcal colonies on blood agar plates. It is not antigenic, but it may be inhibited by a nonspecific inhibitor that is frequently present in the sera of humans and animals and is independent of past experience with streptococci.

Classification of Streptococci

A practical arrangement of streptococci into major categories is based on (1) colony morphology and hemolysis on blood agar; (2) biochemical reactions and resistance to physical and chemical factors; (3) serologic specificity of group-specific substance and other cell wall or capsular antigens; and (4) ecologic features. Combinations of the above permit the following arrangement for the sake of convenience:

I. Beta-Hemolytic Streptococci: In general, these produce soluble hemolysins that can be recognized readily on culture. They elaborate group-specific carbohydrates. Acid extracts containing these carbohydrates, the group-specific substances, give precipitin reactions with specific antisera that permit arrangement into groups A–H and K–U. The following are of particular medical relevance and are sometimes referred to by specific names:

Group A–*Streptococcus pyogenes* is the main human pathogen associated with local or systemic invasion and poststreptococcal immunologic disorders. Group A streptococci are usually bacitracin-sensitive. On sheep blood agar, they typically produce large zones of beta hemolysis.

Group B–*Streptococcus agalactiae* is a member of the normal flora of the female genital tract and an important cause of neonatal sepsis and meningitis. On sheep blood agar, group B streptococci typically produce small zones of beta hemolysis. They hydrolyze sodium hippurate, are rarely bacitracin-sensitive, and give a positive response to the so-called CAMP test (from *C*hristie, *A*tkins, *M*unch-*P*etersen; see *Austr J Exp Biol Med* 1944;**22:**197).

Groups C and G occur sometimes in the pharynx; may cause sinusitis, bacteremia, or endocarditis; and may be mistaken for group A organisms. Most group C and G streptococci produce beta hemolysis on sheep blood agar.

Group D includes enterococci (eg, *Streptococcus faecalis, Streptococcus faecium*) and nonenterococci (eg, *Streptococcus bovis, Streptococcus equinus*). On sheep blood agar, most group D streptococci are alpha-hemolytic or nonhemolytic; they may be beta-hemolytic on rabbit or horse blood agar. **Enterococci** typically grow in the presence of 6.5% NaCl or 40% bile, are inhibited but not killed by penicillins, occur in normal enteric flora, and are found in urinary tract or cardiovascular infections or in meningitis. **Nonenterococcal group D streptococci** are inhibited by 6.5% NaCl or 40% bile and are readily killed by penicillin. They may cause urinary tract infections or endocarditis.

Groups E, F, H, and K–U—with the exceptions noted below—occur primarily in animals other than humans.

II. Non-Beta-Hemolytic Streptococci: These usually show alpha hemolysis or no hemolysis on blood agar. The principal members are as follows:

Streptococcus pneumoniae (pneumococci) are bile-soluble, and their growth is inhibited by optochin (ethylhydrocupreine hydrochloride) disks. Their role in disease is discussed separately below.

Viridans streptococci, including *Streptococcus salivarius* (group K), *Streptococcus mitis, Streptococcus mutans, Streptococcus sanguis* (group H), and others, are not bile-soluble, and their growth is not inhibited by optochin disks. They are the most prevalent members of the normal flora in the human upper respiratory tract and are important for the healthy state of the mucous membranes there. They may reach the bloodstream as a result of trauma and are a principal cause of infective endocarditis when they settle on abnormal heart valves. Some viridans streptococci (eg, *S mutans*) synthesize large polysaccharides such as dextrans or levans from sucrose and contribute importantly to the genesis of dental caries.

Group N streptococci have variable hemolytic activity. They are rarely found in human disease states but produce normal coagulation ("souring") of milk; they are also called lactic streptococci.

III. Peptostreptococci: These grow only under anaerobic or microaerophilic conditions and produce variable hemolysis. They often participate in mixed anaerobic infections in the abdomen, pelvis, lung, or brain. They are members of the normal flora of the gut and female genital tract.

Pathogenesis & Clinical Findings

A variety of distinct disease processes are associated with streptococcal infections. The biologic properties of the infecting organisms, the nature of the host response, and the portal of entry of the infection all greatly influence the pathologic picture. Infections can be divided into several categories.

A. Diseases Attributable to Invasion by Beta-Hemolytic Group A Streptococci *(Streptococcus pyogenes):* The portal of entry determines the principal clinical picture. In each case, however, there is a diffuse and rapidly spreading infection that involves the tissues and extends along lymphatic pathways with only minimal local suppuration. From the lymphatics, the infection can extend to the bloodstream.

1. Erysipelas–If the portal of entry is the skin, erysipelas results, with massive brawny edema and a rapidly advancing margin of infection.

2. Puerperal fever–If the streptococci enter the uterus after delivery, puerperal fever develops, which is essentially a septicemia originating in the infected wound (endometritis).

3. Sepsis–Infection of traumatic or surgical wounds with streptococci results in sepsis or surgical scarlet fever.

B. Diseases Attributable to Local Infection With Beta-Hemolytic Group A Streptococci and Their Products:

1. Streptococcal sore throat–The commonest infection due to beta-hemolytic streptococci is streptococcal sore throat. Virulent group A streptococci adhere to the pharyngeal epithelium by means of lipoteichoic acid covering surface pili. The glycoprotein fibronectin (MW 440,000) on epithelial cells probably serves as lipoteichoic acid ligand. In infants and small children, the sore throat occurs as a subacute nasopharyngitis with a thin serous discharge and little fever but with a tendency of the infection to extend to the middle ear, the mastoid, and the meninges. The cervical lymph nodes are usually enlarged. The illness may persist for weeks. In older children and adults, the disease is more acute and is characterized by intense nasopharyngitis, tonsillitis, and intense redness and edema of the mucous membranes, with purulent exudate; enlarged, tender cervical lymph nodes; and (usually) a high fever. Twenty percent of infections are asymptomatic. A similar clinical picture can occur with infectious mononucleosis, diphtheria, gonococcal infection, and adenovirus infection. If the infecting streptococci produce erythrogenic toxin and the patient has no antitoxic immunity, **scarlet fever rash** occurs. Antitoxin to the erythrogenic toxin prevents the rash but does not interfere with the streptococcal infection. With the most intense inflammation, tissues may break down and form peritonsillar abscesses (quinsy) or Ludwig's angina, where massive swelling of the floor of the mouth blocks air passages.

Streptococcal infection of the upper respiratory tract does not usually involve the lungs. Pneumonia due to beta-hemolytic streptococci is rapidly progressive and severe and is most commonly a sequela to viral infections, eg, influenza or measles, which seem to enhance susceptibility greatly.

2. Streptococcal pyoderma–Local infection of superficial layers, especially in children, is called impetigo. It consists of superficial blisters that break down and eroded areas whose denuded surface is covered with pus or crusts. It spreads by continuity and is highly communicable in children, especially in hot, humid climates. More widespread infection occurs in eczematous or wounded skin or in burns and may progress to cellulitis. Group A streptococcal skin infections are often attributable to M types 49, 57, and 59–61 and may precede glomerulonephritis but do not often lead to rheumatic fever.

C. Infective Endocarditis:

1. Acute endocarditis–In the course of bacteremia, beta-hemolytic streptococci, pneumococci, or other bacteria may settle on normal or previously deformed heart valves, producing acute endocarditis. Rapid destruction of the valves frequently leads to fatal cardiac failure in days or weeks unless a prosthesis can be inserted during antimicrobial therapy. *Staphylococcus aureus* and gram-negative bacilli are encountered occasionally in this disease, particularly in narcotics users. Patients with prosthetic heart valves are at special risk.

2. Subacute endocarditis–Subacute endocarditis often involves abnormal valves (congenital deformities and rheumatic or atherosclerotic lesions). Although any organism reaching the bloodstream may establish itself on thrombotic lesions that develop on endothelium injured as a result of circulatory stresses, subacute endocarditis is most frequently due to members of the normal flora of the respiratory or intestinal tract that have accidentally reached the blood. After dental extraction, at least 30% of patients have viridans streptococcal bacteremia. These streptococci, ordinarily the most prevalent members of the upper respiratory flora, are also the most frequent cause of subacute bacterial endocarditis. About 5–10% of cases are due to enterococci originating in the gut or urinary tract. The lesion is slowly progressive, and a certain amount of healing accompanies the active inflammation; vegetations consist of fibrin, platelets, blood cells, and bacteria adherent to the valve leaflets. The clinical course is gradual, but the disease is invariably fatal in untreated cases. The typical clinical picture includes fever, anemia, weakness, a heart murmur, embolic phenomena, an enlarged spleen, and renal lesions.

D. Other Infections: Various streptococci, particularly enterococci, can cause urinary tract infections. Anaerobic streptococci (*Peptostreptococcus*) occur in the normal female genital tract, the mouth, and the intestine. They may give rise to suppurative lesions, either alone or in association with other anaerobes, particularly *Bacteroides*. Such infections may occur in wounds, in the breast, in postpartum endometritis, following rupture of an abdominal viscus, or in chronic suppuration of the lung. The pus usually has a foul odor. A variety of other streptococci (groups C–L and O) that are usually found in other animals may also occasionally produce infections in humans.

Group B streptococci are part of the normal vaginal flora in 5–25% of women and may affect the newborn. Group B streptococcal infection during the first month of life may present as fulminant sepsis, meningitis, or respiratory distress syndrome. Intrapartum intravenous ampicillin appears to prevent colonization of infants whose mothers carry group B streptococci. Although group B streptococci appear sensitive to penicillin, they may be "tolerant" (see Chapter 10) and difficult to eradicate from neonatal infection unless an aminoglycoside is also given.

E. Poststreptococcal Diseases (Rheumatic Fever, Glomerulonephritis): Following an acute group A streptococcal infection, there is a latent period of 1–4 weeks, after which nephritis or rheumatic fever occasionally develops. The latent period suggests that these poststreptococcal diseases are not attributable to the direct effect of disseminated bacteria but represent instead a hypersensitivity response. Nephritis is more commonly preceded by infection of the skin; rheumatic fever, by infection of the respiratory tract.

1. Acute glomerulonephritis–This sometimes develops 3 weeks after streptococcal infection, particularly with types 12, 4, 2, and 49. Some strains are particularly nephritogenic. In one study, 23% of children with a skin infection with a type 49 strain developed nephritis or hematuria. Other nephritogenic types are 59–61. After random streptococcal infections, the incidence of nephritis is less than 0.5%.

Glomerulonephritis may be initiated by antigen-antibody complexes on the glomerular basement membrane. The most important antigen is probably in the streptococcal protoplast membrane. In acute nephritis, there is blood and protein in the urine, edema, high blood pressure, and urea nitrogen retention; serum complement levels are low. A few patients die; some develop chronic glomerulonephritis with ultimate kidney failure; the majority recover completely.

2. Rheumatic fever–This is the most serious sequela to hemolytic streptococcal infection because it results in damage to heart muscle and valves. Certain strains of group A streptococci contain cell membrane antigens that cross-react with human heart tissue antigens. Sera from patients with rheumatic fever contain antibodies to these antigens.

The onset of rheumatic fever is often preceded by a group A *Streptococcus* infection 1–4 weeks earlier, although the infection may be mild and may not be detected. Untreated streptococcal infections were followed by rheumatic fever in up to 3% of military personnel and 0.3% of civilian children in the 1950s. In the 1980s, rheumatic fever has become very rare in the USA (< 0.05% of streptococcal infections), but it occurs up to 100 times more frequently in tropical countries, eg, Egypt. In general, patients with more severe streptococcal sore throats have a greater chance of developing rheumatic fever.

Typical symptoms and signs of rheumatic fever include fever, malaise, a migratory nonsuppurative polyarthritis, and evidence of inflammation of all parts of the heart (endocardium, myocardium, pericardium). The carditis characteristically leads to thickened and deformed valves and to small perivascular granulomas in the myocardium (Aschoff bodies) that are finally replaced by scar tissue. Erythrocyte sedimentation rates, serum transaminase levels, electrocardiograms, and other tests are used to estimate rheumatic activity.

Rheumatic fever has a marked tendency to be reactivated by recurrent streptococcal infections, whereas nephritis does not. The first attack of rheumatic fever usually produces only slight cardiac damage, which, however, increases with each subsequent attack. It is therefore important to protect such patients from recurrent hemolytic group A streptococcal infections by prophylactic penicillin administration.

Diagnostic Laboratory Tests

A. Specimens: Specimens to be obtained depend upon the nature of the streptococcal infection. A throat swab, pus, or blood is obtained for culture. Serum is obtained for antibody determinations.

B. Smears: Smears from pus often show single cocci or pairs rather than definite chains. Cocci are sometimes gram-negative. If smears of pus show streptococci but cultures fail to grow, anaerobic organisms must be suspected. Smears of throat swabs are rarely contributory, because streptococci (viridans) are always present and have the same appearance as group A streptococci on stained smears.

C. Culture: Specimens suspected of containing streptococci are cultured on blood agar plates. If anaerobes are suspected, suitable anaerobic media must also be inoculated. Incubation in 10% CO_2 often speeds hemolysis. Slicing the inoculum into the blood agar has a similar effect, because oxygen does not readily diffuse through the medium to the deeply embedded organisms, and it is oxygen that inactivates streptolysin O.

Blood cultures will grow hemolytic group A streptococci (eg, in sepsis) within hours or a few days. Certain alpha-hemolytic streptococci and enterococci may grow very slowly, so blood cultures in cases of suspected endocarditis may have to be incubated for 2 weeks (rather than the standard 1 week) before being discarded as negative.

The degree and kind of hemolysis (and colonial appearance) may help place an organism in a definite group. Group A streptococci can be rapidly identified by a fluorescent antibody test. Serologic grouping and typing by means of precipitin tests or coagglutination should be performed when needed for definitive classification and for epidemiologic reasons. Streptococci belonging to group A may be presumptively identified by inhibition of growth by bacitracin. A bacitracin disk containing 0.04 unit strongly inhibits growth of more than 95% of group A streptococci but rarely streptococci of other groups. The bacitracin test for identification of group A streptococci should be used only when more definitive tests are not available.

D. Serologic Tests: Several commercial kits are available for rapid detection of group A streptococcal antigen from throat swabs. These kits use enzymatic or chemical methods to extract the antigen from the swab, then use enzyme-linked immunosorbent assay (ELISA) or agglutination tests to demonstrate the presence of the antigen. The tests can be completed 1–4 hours after the specimen is obtained. They are 90–95% sensitive and 98–99% specific when compared to culture methods. Although kit tests are rapid, they are more expensive than cultures for individual determinations.

A rise in the titer of antibodies to many group A streptococcal antigens can be estimated: such antibodies include antistreptolysin O (ASO), particularly in respiratory disease; anti-DNase and antihyaluronidase, particularly in skin infections; antistreptokinase; anti-M type-specific antibodies; and others. Of these, the anti-ASO titer is most widely used.

Antibodies to several streptococcal antigens and enzymes are measured by the streptozyme test, which is performed by many diagnostic laboratories. The antigens are adsorbed onto sheep red blood cells on a slide, and agglutination by antibodies occurs within a few minutes.

Immunity

Resistance against streptococcal diseases is type-specific. Thus, a host who has recovered from infection by one group A streptococcal M type is relatively insusceptible to reinfection by the same type but fully susceptible to infection by another M type. Anti-M type-specific antibodies can be demonstrated in a test that exploits the fact that streptococci are rapidly killed after phagocytosis. M protein interferes with phagocytosis, but in the presence of type-specific antibody to M protein, streptococci are killed by human leukocytes.

Immunity against erythrogenic toxin is due to antitoxin in the blood. This antitoxic immunity protects against the rash of scarlet fever but has no effect on infection with streptococci.

Antibody to streptolysin O (antistreptolysin O, ASO) develops following infection; it blocks hemolysis by streptolysin O but does not indicate immunity. High titers (> 250 units) indicate recent or repeated infections and are found more often in rheumatic individuals than in those with uncomplicated streptococcal infections.

Treatment

All beta-hemolytic group A streptococci are sensitive to penicillin G, and most are sensitive to erythromycin. Some are resistant to tetracyclines. Alpha-hemolytic streptococci and enterococci vary in their susceptibility to antimicrobial agents. Particularly in bacterial endocarditis, antibiotic sensitivity tests are useful to determine which drugs may be used for optimal therapy. In these cases, laboratory tests should include determinations of both inhibitory and killing power of drugs or drug combinations. Aminoglycosides often enhance the rate of bactericidal action of penicillin on streptococci, particularly enterococci.

Antimicrobial drugs have no effect on established glomerulonephritis and rheumatic fever. However, in acute streptococcal infections, every effort must be made to rapidly eradicate streptococci from the patient, eliminate the antigenic stimulus (before day 8), and thus prevent poststreptococcal disease. Doses of penicillin or erythromycin that result in effective tissue levels for 10 days usually accomplish this. Antimicrobial drugs are also very useful in preventing reinfection with beta-hemolytic group A streptococci in rheumatic subjects.

Epidemiology, Prevention, & Control

Many streptococci (viridans streptococci, enterococci, etc) are members of the normal flora of the human body. They produce disease only when established in parts of the body where they do not normally occur (eg, heart valves). To prevent such accidents, particularly in the course of surgical procedures on the respiratory, gastrointestinal, and urinary tracts that result in temporary bacteremia, antimicrobial agents are often administered prophylactically to persons with known heart valve deformity and to those with prosthetic valves or joints.

The ultimate source of group A streptococci is a person harboring these organisms. The individual may have a clinical or subclinical infection or may be a carrier distributing streptococci directly to other persons via droplets from the respiratory tract or skin. The nasal discharges of a person harboring beta-hemolytic streptococci are the most dangerous source for spread of these organisms. The role of contaminated bedding, utensils, or clothing is doubtful. The infected udder of a cow yields milk that may cause epidemic spread of hemolytic streptococci. Immunologic grouping and typing of streptococci are valuable tools for epidemiologic tracing of the transmission chain.

Control procedures are directed mainly at the human source: (1) Detection and early antimicrobial therapy of respiratory and skin infections with group A streptococci. This requires maintenance of adequate penicillin levels in tissues for 10 days (eg, benzathine penicillin G, 1.2 million units given once intramuscularly). Erythromycin is an alternative drug of choice. Prompt eradication of streptococci from early infections can effectively prevent the development of poststreptococcal disease. (2) Antistreptococcal chemoprophylaxis in persons who have suffered an attack of rheumatic fever. This involves giving one injection of benzathine penicillin G, 1.2 million units intramuscularly, every 3–4 weeks or daily oral penicillin or oral sulfonamide. The first attack of rheumatic fever infrequently causes major heart damage. However, such persons are particularly susceptible to reinfections with streptococci that precipitate relapses of rheumatic activity and give rise to cardiac damage. Chemoprophylaxis in such individuals, especially children, must be continued for years. Chemoprophylaxis is not used in glomerulonephritis because of the small number of nephritogenic types of streptococci. An exception may be family groups with a high rate of poststreptococcal nephritis. (3) Eradication of group A streptococci from carriers. This is especially important when carriers are in areas such as obstetric delivery rooms, operating rooms, classrooms, or nurseries. Unfortunately, it is often difficult to eradicate hemolytic streptococci from permanent carriers, and individuals may occasionally have to be shifted away from "sensitive" areas for some time. (4) Dust control, ventilation, air filtration, ultraviolet light, and aerosol mists are all of doubtful efficacy in the control of streptococcal transmission. Milk should always be pasteurized. (5) Group B streptococci account for most cases of neonatal sepsis at present. They are derived from the mother's genital tract, where carriage is asymptomatic. Neonatal illness may be favored by deficiency of maternal antibody. Drug prophylaxis in mother and child has not been unequivocally successful. (6) Vaccines against groups A and B streptococci are under investigation.

STREPTOCOCCUS PNEUMONIAE (Pneumococcus)

The pneumococci (Streptococcus pneumoniae) are gram-positive diplococci, often lancet-shaped or arranged in chains, possessing a capsule of polysaccharide that permits typing with specific antisera. Pneumococci are readily lysed by surface-active agents such as bile salts. Surface-active agents probably remove or inactivate the inhibitors of cell wall autolysins. Pneumococci are normal inhabitants of the upper respiratory tract of humans and can cause pneumonia, sinusitis, otitis, bronchitis, bacteremia, meningitis, and other infectious processes.

Morphology & Identification

A. Typical Organisms: The typical gram-positive, lancet-shaped diplococci (Figs 17–3, 17–4, 17–5) are often seen in specimens of young cultures. In sputum or pus, single cocci or chains are also seen. With age, the organisms rapidly become gram-negative and tend to lyse spontaneously.

Autolysis of pneumococci is greatly enhanced by surface-active agents. Lysis of pneumococci occurs in a few minutes when ox bile (10%) or sodium deoxycholate (2%) is added to a broth culture or suspension of organisms at neutral pH. Viridans streptococci do not lyse and are thus easily differentiated from pneumococci. On solid media, the growth of pneumococci is inhibited around a disk of optochin; viridans streptococci are not inhibited by optochin.

Other identifying points include almost uniform virulence for mice when injected intraperitoneally and the "capsule swelling test," or quellung reaction (see below).

B. Culture: Pneumococci form a small round colony, at first dome-shaped and later developing a central plateau with an elevated rim and alpha hemolysis on blood agar. Growth is enhanced by 5–10% CO_2.

C. Growth Characteristics: Most energy is obtained from fermentation of glucose; this is accompanied by the rapid production of lactic acid, which limits growth. Neutralization of broth cultures with alkali at intervals results in massive growth.

D. Variation: A culture of pneumococci contains a few organisms that are unable to produce capsular polysaccharide and thus give rise to rough colonies; most of the organisms are polysaccharide-producing and give rise to smooth colonies. Rough forms predominate if the culture is grown in type-specific antipolysaccharide serum.

E. Transformation: When pneumococci of a type that does not make polysaccharide capsules are grown in the presence of DNA extracted from a pneumococcus type that does produce capsular polysaccharide, encapsulated pneumococci of the latter type are formed. Similar transformation reactions have been performed that involve changes in drug resistance.

Antigenic Structure

A. Component Structures: The capsular poly-

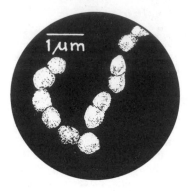

Figure 17–3. Drawing from electron micrograph of pneumococci.

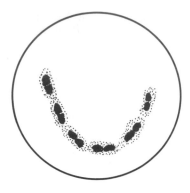

Figure 17–4. Pneumococci in a stained smear.

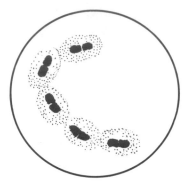

Figure 17–5. Pneumococci mixed with type-specific antiserum yielding capsular swelling (quellung reaction).

saccharide (SSS = specific soluble substance) is immunologically distinct for each of the more than 85 types. The polysaccharide is an antigen that primarily elicits a B cell response (see Chapter 12).

The somatic portion of the pneumococcus contains an M protein that is characteristic for each type and a group-specific carbohydrate that is common to all pneumococci. The carbohydrate can be precipitated by C-reactive protein, a substance found in the serum of certain patients.

B. Quellung Reaction: When pneumococci of a certain type are mixed with specific antipolysaccharide serum of the same type—or with polyvalent antiserum—on a microscope slide, the capsule swells markedly (Fig 17–5). This reaction is useful for rapid identification and for typing of the organisms, either in sputum or in cultures. The polyvalent antiserum, which contains antibody to more than 80 types ("omniserum"), is a good reagent for rapid microscopic determination of whether pneumococci are present in fresh sputum.

Pathogenesis

A. Types of Pneumococci: In adults, types 1–8 are responsible for about 75% of cases of pneumococcal pneumonia and for more than half of all fatalities in pneumococcal bacteremia; in children, types 6, 14, 19, and 23 are frequent causes.

B. Production of Disease: Pneumococci produce disease through their ability to multiply in the tissues. They produce no toxins of significance. The virulence of the organism is a function of its capsule, which prevents or delays ingestion of encapsulated cells by phagocytes. A serum that contains antibodies against the type-specific polysaccharide protects against infection. If such a serum is absorbed with the type-specific polysaccharide, it loses its protective power. Animals or humans immunized with a given type of pneumococcal polysaccharide are subsequently immune to that type of pneumococcus and possess precipitating and opsonizing antibodies for that type of polysaccharide.

C. Loss of Natural Resistance: Since 40–70% of humans are at some time carriers of virulent pneumococci, the normal respiratory mucosa must possess great natural resistance to the pneumococcus. Among the factors that probably lower this resistance and thus predispose to pneumococcal infection are the following:

1. Abnormalities of the respiratory tract–Viral and other infections that damage surface cells; abnormal accumulations of mucus (eg, allergy), which protect pneumococci from phagocytosis; bronchial obstruction (eg, atelectasis); and respiratory tract injury due to irritants disturbing its mucociliary function.

2. Alcohol or drug intoxication, which depresses phagocytic activity, depresses the cough reflex, and facilitates aspiration of foreign material.

3. Abnormal circulatory dynamics (eg, pulmonary congestion, heart failure).

4. Malnutrition, general debility, sickle cell anemia, hyposplenism, nephrosis, or complement deficiency.

Pathology

Pneumococcal infection causes an outpouring of fibrinous edema fluid into the alveoli, followed by red cells and leukocytes, which results in consolidation of portions of the lung. Many pneumococci are found throughout this exudate, and they may reach the bloodstream via the lymphatic drainage of the lungs. The alveolar walls remain normally intact during the infection. Later, mononuclear cells actively phagocytose the debris, and this liquid phase is gradually reabsorbed. The pneumococci are taken up by phagocytes and digested intracellularly.

Clinical Findings

The onset of pneumococcal pneumonia is usually sudden, with fever, chills, and sharp pleural pain. The sputum is similar to the alveolar exudate, being characteristically bloody or rusty. Early in the disease, when the fever is high, bacteremia is present in 10–20% of cases. Before the days of chemotherapy, recovery from the disease began between the fifth and tenth days and was associated with the development of type-specific antibodies. The mortality rate was as high as 30%, depending on age and underlying illness. Bacteremic pneumonia always has the highest mortality rate. With antimicrobial therapy, the illness is usually terminated promptly; if drugs are given early, the development of consolidation is interrupted.

Pneumococcal pneumonia must be differentiated from pulmonary infarction, atelectasis, neoplasm, congestive heart failure, and pneumonia caused by many other bacteria. Empyema (pus in the pleural space) is a significant complication and requires aspiration and drainage.

From the respiratory tract, pneumococci may reach other sites. The sinuses and middle ear are most frequently involved. Infection sometimes extends from the mastoid to the meninges. Bacteremia from pneumonia has a triad of severe complications: meningitis, endocarditis, and septic arthritis. With the early use of chemotherapy, acute pneumococcal endocarditis and arthritis have become rare.

Diagnostic Laboratory Tests

Blood is drawn for culture, and sputum is collected for demonstration of pneumococci by smear and culture. Serum antibody tests are impractical. Sputum may be examined in several ways.

(1) Stained smears: A Gram-stained film of rusty-red sputum shows typical organisms, many polymorphonuclear neutrophils, and many red cells.

(2) Capsule swelling tests: Fresh emulsified sputum mixed with antiserum gives capsule swelling (the quellung reaction; Fig 17–5) for identification of pneumococci and possible typing. Peritoneal exudate can also be used for capsule swelling tests.

(3) Culture: Sputum cultured on blood agar and incubated in CO_2 or a candle jar. Blood culture.

(4) Intraperitoneal injection of sputum into laboratory mice: Animals die in 18–48 hours; heart blood gives pure culture of pneumococci. This form of culture for pneumococci is very sensitive but seldom used because of the need to maintain a mouse colony.

(5) Pneumococcal meningitis should be diagnosed by prompt examination and culture of cerebrospinal fluid.

Immunity

Immunity to infection with pneumococci is type-specific and depends both on antibodies to capsular polysaccharide and on intact phagocytic function. Vaccines can induce production of antibodies to capsular polysaccharides (see below).

Treatment

Since pneumococci are sensitive to many antimicrobial drugs, early treatment usually results in rapid recovery, and antibody response seems to play a much diminished role. The penicillins are the drugs of choice. Recently, some drug resistance has appeared; pneumococci resistant to tetracyclines, erythromycin, and lincomycin have been isolated from patients. Pneumococci of greatly increased resistance to penicillin (minimum inhibitory concentration, 4 units/mL) have appeared in New Guinea and elsewhere and have produced hospital-centered outbreaks in South Africa. Some of these pneumococci are resistant to multiple drugs, but no plasmids or β-lactamase production has been identified. Penicillin-resistant pneumococci present little difficulty in pneumonia, but in meningitis, where limited amounts of the drug reach the central nervous system, they are a severe management problem.

Epidemiology, Prevention, & Control

Pneumococcal pneumonia accounts for about 60–80% of all bacterial pneumonias. It is an endemic disease with a high incidence of carriers. In the development of illness, predisposing factors (see above) are more important than exposure to the infectious agent, and the healthy carrier is more important in disseminating pneumococci than the sick patient.

It is possible to immunize individuals with type-specific polysaccharides. Such vaccines can probably provide 90% protection against bacteremic pneumonia. Among workers in South African gold mines, vaccines containing 12 polysaccharide types have given good antibody response and good protection against disease. A vaccine containing 14 pneumococcal types was beneficial in patients with sickle cell disease or after splenectomy. In 1983, an expanded polysaccharide vaccine containing 23 types was licensed in the USA. Such vaccines are used especially in children but may also be appropriate for elderly, debilitated, or immunosuppressed individuals. Pneumococcal vaccines have greatly reduced immunogenicity in children under 2 years of age and in patients with lymphomas; in such high-risk patients, penicillin prophylaxis must accompany vaccination.

In addition, it is desirable to avoid predisposing factors, to establish the diagnosis promptly, and to begin adequate chemotherapy early. At present, most fatalities from pneumococcal pneumonia occur in persons over 50 years of age; persons with impaired natural resistance, eg, those with sickle cell disease or asplenia; and those with bacteremia.

REFERENCES

AHA Committee Report: Prevention of rheumatic fever. *Circulation* 1977;**55**:S1.

Anthony BF, Okada DM: The emergence of group B strepto-

cocci infections of the newborn infant. *Annu Rev Med* 1977; **28**:355.

Aukenthaler R et al: Group G streptococcal bacteremia: Clinical study and review of the literature. *Rev Infect Dis* 1983;**5**:196.

Baker CJ, Kasper DL: Correlation of maternal antibody deficiency with susceptibility to neonatal group B streptococcal infection. *N Engl J Med* 1976;**294**:753.

Beachey EH, Ofek I: Epithelial cell binding of group A streptococci by lipoteichoic acid on fimbriae denuded of M protein. *J Exp Med* 1976;**143**:759.

Blair DC, Martin DB: Beta hemolytic streptococcal endocarditis: Predominance of non–group A organisms. *Am J Med Sci* 1978;**276**:269.

Breese BB: Streptococcal pharyngitis and scarlet fever. *Am J Dis Child* 1978;**132**:612.

Broome CV et al: Epidemiology of clinically significant isolates of *Streptococcus pneumoniae* in the United States. *Rev Infect Dis* 1981;**3**:277.

Colman G, Ball LC: Identification of streptococci in a medical laboratory. *J Appl Bacteriol* 1984;**57**:1.

Deibel RH: The group D streptococci. *Bacteriol Rev* 1964; **28**:330.

Dillon HC: Poststreptococcal glomerulonephritis following pyoderma. *Rev Infect Dis* 1979;**1**:935.

Facklam RR: Physiological differentiation of viridans streptococci. *J Clin Microbiol* 1977;**5**:184.

Ferrieri P et al: Natural history of impetigo. 1. Site sequence of acquisition and familial patterns of spread of cutaneous streptococci. *J Clin Invest* 1972;**51**:2851.

Howard JB, McCracken GH Jr: The spectrum of group B streptococcal infections in infancy. *Am J Dis Child* 1974;**128**:815.

Kaplan EL et al: The role of the carrier in treatment failures after antibiotic therapy for group A streptococci in the upper respiratory tract. *J Lab Clin Med* 1981;**98**:326.

Kaplan MH: Rheumatic fever, rheumatic heart disease, and the streptococcal connection: The role of streptococcal antigens cross-reactive with heart tissue. *Rev Infect Dis* 1979;**1**:988.

Klein JO: The epidemiology of pneumococcal disease in infants and children. *Rev Infect Dis* 1981;**3**:246.

Klein RS et al: Association of *Streptococcus bovis* with carcinoma of the colon. *N Engl J Med* 1977;**296**:800.

Lancefield RC: A serologic differentiation of human and other groups of hemolytic streptococci. *J Exp Med* 1933;**57**:571.

Moellering RC et al: Endocarditis due to group D streptococci: Comparison of disease caused by *Streptococcus bovis* with that produced by the enterococci. *Am J Med* 1974;**57**:239.

Nelson KE et al: The epidemiology and natural history of streptococcal pyoderma: An endemic disease of the rural Southern United States. *Am J Epidemiol* 1976;**103**:270.

Patterson MJ, Hafeez AEB: Group B streptococci in human disease. *Bacteriol Rev* 1976;**40**:774.

Robbins JB et al: Considerations for formulating the second-generation pneumococcal capsular polysaccharide vaccine with emphasis on the cross-reactive types within groups. *J Infect Dis* 1983;**148**:1136.

Roberts RB et al: Viridans streptococcal endocarditis: The role of various species, including pyridoxal-dependent streptococci. *Rev Infect Dis* 1979;**1**:955.

Stamm WE et al: Wound infections due to group A *Streptococcus* traced to a vaginal carrier. *J Infect Dis* 1978;**138**:287.

Wannamaker LW: Changes and changing concepts in the biology of group A streptococci and in epidemiology of streptococcal infections. *Rev Infect Dis* 1979;**1**:967.

Ward J: Antibiotic-resistant *Streptococcus pneumoniae:* Clinical and epidemiological aspects. *Rev Infect Dis* 1981;**3**:254.

Enteric Gram-Negative Rods (*Enterobacteriaceae*)

18

The *Enterobacteriaceae* are a large, heterogeneous group of gram-negative rods whose natural habitat is the intestinal tract of humans and animals. The family includes many genera (eg, *Escherichia, Shigella, Salmonella, Enterobacter, Klebsiella, Serratia,* and *Proteus*). Some enteric organisms, eg, *Escherichia coli,* are part of the normal flora and incidentally cause disease, while others, the salmonellae and shigellae, are regularly pathogenic for humans. The *Enterobacteriaceae* are facultative anaerobes or aerobes, ferment a wide range of carbohydrates, possess a complex antigenic structure, and produce a variety of toxins and other virulence factors. *Enterobacteriaceae*, enteric gram-negative rods, and enteric bacteria are the terms used in this chapter, but these bacteria may also be called coliforms.

Classification

The taxonomy of the *Enterobacteriaceae* is complex and is rapidly changing as further DNA homology studies are performed. More than 20 genera and 100 species have been defined. In this chapter, taxonomy will be minimized and the names employed in the medical literature will generally be used. A comprehensive approach to the identification of *Enterobacteriaceae* is presented by Kelly, Brenner, and Farmer in *Manual of Clinical Microbiology,* 4th ed, Lennette EH (editor), American Society for Microbiology, 1985.

The family *Enterobacteriaceae* is characterized biochemically by the ability to reduce nitrates to nitrites and to ferment glucose with the production of acid or acid and gas. The *Enterobacteriaceae* do not require increased amounts of sodium chloride for growth and are oxidase-negative. Many biochemical tests are used to differentiate species of *Enterobacteriaceae* (Table 18–1); in laboratories in the USA, commercially prepared kits are used to a large extent for this purpose.

The major groups of *Enterobacteriaceae* are described and discussed briefly in the following paragraphs. Specific characteristics of salmonellae, shigellae, and the other medically important enteric gram-negative rods and the diseases they cause are discussed separately later in this chapter.

Morphology & Identification

A. Typical Organisms: The *Enterobacteriaceae* are short gram-negative rods that may form chains. Typical morphology is seen in growth on solid media in vitro, but morphology is highly variable in

Table 18–1. Biochemical reaction patterns in primary tests for the common clinically significant *Enterobacteriaceae*.*

	Citrobacter	*Enterobacter*	*Escherichia*	*Klebsiella*	*Morganella*	*Proteus*	*Providencia*	*Salmonella*	*Serratia*	*Shigella*
Arginine	±	±	−	−	−	−	−	±	−	−
Citrate	+	+	−	+	−	±	+	±	+	−
DNase	−	−	−	−	−	−	−	−	+	−
Gas	+	+	+	±	±	±	±	±	±	−
Glucose	+	+	+	+	+	+	+	+	+	+
H$_2$S	±	−	−	−	−	+	−	±	−	−
Indole	±	−	+	±	+	±	+	−	−	±
Lysine	−	±	+	+	−	−	−	+	+	−
Motility	+	+	±	−	+	+	+	+	+	−
Ornithine	±	+	±	−	+	±	−	+	+	±
Phenylalanine	−	−	−	−	+	+	+	−	−	−
Sucrose	±	+	±	+	−	±	±	−	+	−
Urease	−	−	−	±	+	+	±	−	−	−
VP†	−	+	−	+	−	−	−	−	+	−
TSI‡ slant	Alk (A)	A	A (Alk)	A	Alk	Alk	Alk	Alk	Alk (A)	Alk
butt	AG	AG	AG	AG	AG	AG	AG	A;G±	A	A

*Results for common clinical isolates: ± = variable; + = most (usually ≥ 90%) of strains positive; − = few (usually ≤ 10%) of strains positive; A = acid (yellow); G = gas; Alk = alkaline. (**Note:** There are exceptions to nearly all of the results listed.)
†VP = Voges-Proskauer reaction.
‡TSI = Triple sugar iron agar.

clinical specimens. Capsules are large and regular in *Klebsiella,* less so in *Enterobacter,* and uncommon in the other species.

B. Culture: *E coli* and most of the other enteric bacteria form circular, convex, smooth colonies with distinct edges. *Enterobacter* colonies are similar but somewhat more mucoid. *Klebsiella* colonies are large and very mucoid and tend to coalesce with prolonged incubation. The salmonellae and shigellae produce colonies similar to *E coli* but do not ferment lactose. Some strains of *E coli* produce hemolysis on blood agar.

C. Growth Characteristics: Carbohydrate fermentation patterns and the activity of amino acid decarboxylases and other enzymes are commonly used in biochemical differentiation (Table 18–1). Some tests, eg, the production of indole from tryptophan, are commonly used in rapid identification systems while others, eg, the Voges-Proskauer reaction (production of acetylmethylcarbinol from dextrose) are used less commonly. Culture on "differential" media that contain special dyes and carbohydrates (eg, eosin–methylene blue [EMB], MacConkey's, or deoxycholate medium) distinguishes lactose-fermenting (colored) from non-lactose-fermenting colonies (nonpigmented) and may allow rapid presumptive identification of enteric bacteria (Table 18–2).

Many complex media have been devised to help in identification of the enteric bacteria. One such medium is triple sugar iron agar, which is often used to differentiate salmonellae and shigellae from other enteric gram-negative rods in stool cultures. The medium contains 0.1% glucose, 1% sucrose, 1% lactose, ferrous sulfate (for detection of H_2S production), tissue extracts (protein growth substrate), and a pH indicator (phenol red). It is poured in a test tube to produce a slant with a deep butt and is inoculated by stabbing bacterial growth into the butt. If only glucose is fermented, the slant and the butt initially turn yellow from the small amount of acid produced; as the fermentation products are subsequently oxidized to CO_2 and H_2O and released from the slant and as oxidative decarboxylation of proteins continues with formation of amines, the slant turns alkaline (red). If lactose or sucrose is fermented, so much acid is produced that the slant and butt remain yellow (acid). Salmonellae and shigellae typically yield an alkaline slant and an acid butt with no gas production (Table 18–1). Although *Proteus, Providencia,* and *Morganella* produce an alkaline slant, they can be identified by their rapid formation of red color in Christensen's urea medium. Organisms producing acid on the slant and acid and gas (bubbles) in the butt are other enteric bacteria.

1. *Escherichia–E coli* typically produces positive tests for indole, lysine decarboxylase, and mannitol fermentation and produces gas from glucose. An isolate from urine can be quickly identified as *E coli* by its hemolysis on blood agar, typical colonial morphology with an iridescent "sheen" on differential media such as EMB agar (see p 81), and a positive spot indole test.

2. *Klebsiella-Enterobacter-Serratia* group– *Klebsiella* species exhibit mucoid growth, large polysaccharide capsules, and lack of motility and usually give positive tests for lysine decarboxylase and citrate. Most *Enterobacter* species give positive tests for motility, citrate, and ornithine decarboxylase and produce gas from glucose. *Enterobacter aerogenes* has small capsules. *Serratia* produces DNase, lipase, and gelatinase. *Klebsiella, Enterobacter,* and *Serratia* usually give positive Voges-Proskauer reactions.

3. *Proteus-Morganella-Providencia* group– The members of this group deaminate phenylalanine, are motile, grow on potassium cyanide medium (KCN), and ferment xylose. *Proteus* species move very actively by means of peritrichous flagella, resulting in "swarming" on solid media unless the swarming is inhibited by chemicals, eg, phenylethyl alcohol or CLED (cystine-lactose-electrolyte-deficient) medium. *Proteus* species and *Morganella morganii* are urease-positive, while *Providencia* species usually are urease-negative. The *Proteus-Providencia* group ferment lactose very slowly or not at all. *Proteus mirabilis* is more susceptible to antimicrobial drugs, including penicillins, than other members of the group.

4. *Citrobacter–*These bacteria typically are citrate-positive and differ from the salmonellae in that they do not decarboxylate lysine. They ferment lactose very slowly if at all.

5. The salmonellae (see p 241)–Salmonellae are motile rods that characteristically ferment glucose and mannose without producing gas but do not ferment lactose or sucrose. Most salmonellae produce

Table 18–2. Rapid, presumptive identification of gram-negative enteric bacteria.

Lactose Fermented Rapidly	Lactose Fermented Slowly	Lactose Not Fermented
Escherichia coli: Metallic sheen on differential media; motile; flat, nonviscous colonies.		*Shigella* species: Nonmotile; no gas from dextrose.
Enterobacter aerogenes: Raised colonies, no metallic sheen; often motile; more viscous growth.	*Edwardsiella, Serratia, Citrobacter, Arizona, Providencia, Erwinia*	*Salmonella* species: Motile; acid and usually gas from dextrose. *Proteus* species: "Swarming" on agar; urea rapidly hydrolyzed (smell of ammonia).
Klebsiella pneumoniae: Very viscous, mucoid growth; nonmotile.		*Pseudomonas* species (see Chapter 19): Soluble pigments, blue-green and fluorescing; sweetish smell.

H₂S. They are often pathogenic for humans or animals when ingested. *Arizona* is included in the *Salmonella* group.

6. The shigellae (see p 243)—Shigellae are nonmotile and usually do not ferment lactose but do ferment other carbohydrates, producing acid but not gas. They do not produce H₂S. The 4 *Shigella* species are closely related to *E coli*. Many share common antigens with one another and with other enteric bacteria.

**7. Other *Enterobacteriaceae*—*Yersinia* species are discussed in Chapter 20. Other genera occasionally found in human infections include *Edwardsiella* and *Ewingella*. Rarely, *Hafnia*, *Cedecea*, and *Kluyvera* cause disease.

D. Variation: All cultures contain variants and stable mutants with respect to colonial morphology (rough or smooth), antigenic characteristics, biochemical behavior, and virus resistance. Extensive studies have been made of the plasmid biology, genetics, and sexual recombination of inherited characteristics of *E coli* strain K12.

Antigenic Structure

Enterobacteriaceae have a complex antigenic structure. They are classified by more than 150 different heat-stable somatic O (lipopolysaccharide) antigens, more than 100 heat-labile K (capsular) antigens, and more than 50 H (flagellar) antigens (Figure 18–1). In *Salmonella typhi* the capsular antigens are called Vi antigens.

O antigens are the most external part of the cell wall lipopolysaccharide and consist of repeating units of polysaccharide. Some O-specific polysaccharides contain unique sugars. O antigens are resistant to heat and alcohol and usually are detected by bacterial agglutination. Antibodies to O antigens are predominantly IgM.

While each genus of *Enterobacteriaceae* is associated with specific O groups, a single organism may carry several O antigens. Thus, most shigellae share

one or more O antigens with *E coli*. *E coli* may cross-react with some *Providencia*, *Klebsiella*, and *Salmonella* species. Occasionally, O antigens may be associated with specific human diseases, eg, specific O types of *E coli* are found in diarrhea and in urinary tract infections (see p 239).

K antigens are external to O antigens on some but not all *Enterobacteriaceae*. Some are polysaccharides, including the K antigens of *E coli;* others are proteins. K antigens may interfere with agglutination by O antisera, and they may be associated with virulence (eg, *E coli* strains producing K1 antigen are prominent in neonatal meningitis, and K antigens of *E coli* cause attachment of the bacteria to epithelial cells prior to gastrointestinal or urinary tract invasion).

Klebsiellae form large capsules consisting of polysaccharides (K antigens) covering the somatic (O or H) antigens and can be identified by capsular swelling tests with specific antisera. Human infections of the respiratory tract are caused particularly by capsular types 1 and 2; those of the urinary tract, by types 8, 9, 10, and 24.

H antigens are located on flagella and are denatured or removed by heat or alcohol. They are preserved by treating motile bacterial variants with formalin. Such H antigens agglutinate with anti-H antibodies, mainly IgG. The determinants in H antigens are a function of the amino acid sequence in flagellar protein (flagellin). Within a single serotype, flagellar antigens may be present in either or both of 2 forms, called phase 1 (conventionally designated by lower-case letters) and phase 2 (conventionally designated by arabic numerals) (Table 18–5). The organism tends to change from one phase to the other; this is called phase variation. H antigens on the bacterial surface may interfere with agglutination by anti-O antibody.

There are many examples of overlapping antigenic structures between *Enterobacteriaceae* and other bacteria. Most *Enterobacteriaceae* share the O14 antigen of *E coli*. The type 2 capsular polysaccharide of klebsiellae is very similar to the polysaccharide of type 2 pneumococci. Some K antigens cross-react with capsular polysaccharides of *Haemophilus influenzae* or *Neisseria meningitidis*. Thus, *E coli* O75:K100:H5 can induce antibodies that react with *H influenzae* type b.

The antigenic classification of *Enterobacteriaceae* often indicates the presence of each specific antigen. Thus, the antigenic formula of an *E coli* may be O55:K5:H21; that of *Salmonella schottmülleri* is O1,4,5,12:Hb:1,2.

Colicins (Bacteriocins)

Many gram-negative organisms produce bacteriocins. These viruslike bactericidal substances are produced by certain strains of bacteria active against some other strains of the same or closely related species. Their production is controlled by plasmids. Colicins are produced by *E coli*, marcescins by *Serratia*, and pyocins by *Pseudomonas*. Bacteriocin-producing

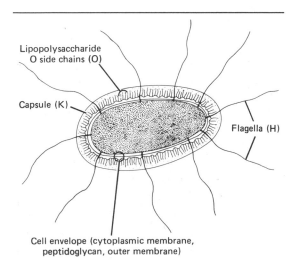

Figure 18–1. Antigenic structure of *Enterobacteriaceae*.

strains are resistant to their own bacteriocin; thus, bacteriocins can be used for "typing" of organisms.

Toxins & Enzymes

Most gram-negative bacteria possess complex lipopolysaccharides in their cell walls. These substances, endotoxins, have a variety of pathophysiologic effects that are summarized below. Many gram-negative enteric bacteria also produce exotoxins of clinical importance. Some specific toxins are discussed in subsequent sections.

Endotoxins of Gram-Negative Bacteria

The endotoxins of gram-negative bacteria are complex lipopolysaccharides derived from bacterial cell walls and often liberated when the bacteria lyse. The substances are heat-stable, have molecular weights variously estimated to be between 100,000 and 900,000, and can be extracted (eg, with phenol-water). They have 3 main regions (Table 18–3).

A. Pathophysiologic Effects: The pathophysiologic effects of endotoxins are similar regardless of their bacterial origin (except for those of *Bacteroides* species; see Chapter 24). The administration of endotoxin to animals or humans results in a series of events in which the endotoxin is taken up by reticuloendothelial or endothelial cells, degraded, or neutralized. The following are prominently observed clinically or experimentally: fever, leukopenia and hypoglycemia, hypotension and shock, impaired perfusion of essential organs, activation of C3 and the complement cascade, intravascular coagulation, and death.

1. Fever–(See p 165.) Normal body temperature is maintained within narrow limits by a balance between heat production and heat loss governed by thermoregulatory centers in the hypothalamus. Infections (bacteria, viruses, fungi), antigen-antibody complexes, delayed type hypersensitivity reactions, certain steroids, and endotoxins can result in fever production. These insults act on various cells (monocytes and probably others) and result in the release of interleukin-1 (endogenous pyrogen), which acts on the thermoregulatory center to "set" it at a higher level.

Injection of endotoxin gives fever after 60–90 minutes, the time needed to release interleukin-1. Injection of interleukin-1 gives fever within 30 minutes. Repeated injection of interleukin-1 gives the same fever response each time, but repeated injection of endotoxin gives less and less fever response ("tolerance"

—due in part to reticuloendothelial blockade and in part to IgM antibodies to lipopolysaccharide).

2. Leukopenia–Bacteremia with gram-negative organisms is often accompanied by early leukopenia. Injection of endotoxin produces early leukopenia. In both instances, a secondary leukocytosis occurs later. The early leukopenia coincides with the temperature rise resulting from liberation of interleukin-1. Endotoxin enhances glycolysis in many cell types and leads to hypoglycemia.

3. Hypotension–Early in gram-negative bacteremia, there may be widespread arteriolar and venular constriction (chill) followed by peripheral vascular dilatation, increased vascular permeability, decrease in venous return, lowered cardiac output, stagnation in the microcirculation, peripheral vasoconstriction, shock, and impaired organ perfusion and its consequences (see below). Injection of endotoxins can also produce this complex sequence. Endotoxins can activate the release of vasoactive substances—eg, serotonin, kallikrein, and kinins—to initiate the sequence. Disseminated intravascular coagulation (DIC; see below) contributes to these vascular changes. However, vascular changes leading to shock also may occur in infections with gram-positive bacteria and viruses that contain no lipopolysaccharides.

4. Impaired organ perfusion and acidosis–As a result of vascular reactions, hypotension, and shock, vital organs (kidneys, heart, lungs, and brain) become anoxic and perform inadequately. This in turn may aggravate the vascular problems. Poor perfusion of tissues also results in accumulation of organic acids and metabolic (especially lactic) acidosis.

5. Activation of C3 and complement cascade–Endotoxins are among the many different agents that can activate the "alternative pathway" of the complement cascade. C3 can be activated by endotoxins in the absence of preceding activation of C1, 4, 2, precipitating a variety of complement-mediated reactions (anaphylatoxins, chemotactic responses, membrane damage, etc) and a drop in serum complement components (C3, 5–9).

6. Disseminated intravascular coagulation (DIC)–DIC is a frequent complication of gram-negative bacteremia, although it also can occur in other infections. Endotoxin activates factor XII (Hageman factor)—the first step of the intrinsic clotting system—and thus the "coagulation cascade" is set into motion, culminating in the conversion of fibrinogen to fibrin.

Table 18–3. Composition of lipopolysaccharide "endotoxins" in the cell walls of gram-negative bacteria.

Chemistry	Common Name
(a) Repeating oligosaccharide (eg, man-rha-gal) combinations make up type-specific haptenic determinants (outermost on cell wall).	(a) O-specific polysaccharide; "somatic antigen" of "smooth" colonies. Induce specific immunity.
(b) (N-Acetylglucosamine, glucose, galactose, heptose.) Same in all gram-negative bacteria.	(b) Common core polysaccharide ("rough" colony antigen). Induce some nonspecific resistance to gram-negative sepsis.
(c) Backbone of alternating heptose and phosphate groups linked through KDO (2-keto-3-deoxy-octonic acid) to lipid. Lipid is linked to peptidoglycan (by glycoside bonds). (See Fig 2–17.)	(c) Lipid A with KDO responsible for primary toxicity.

At the same time, plasminogen can be activated by endotoxin to plasmin (a proteolytic enzyme), which can attack fibrin with the formation of fibrin split products. Reduction in platelets and fibrinogen and detection of fibrin split products are evidence of DIC.

The presence of endotoxin leads to platelets sticking to vascular endothelium and occlusion of small blood vessels. That, in turn, causes ischemic or hemorrhagic necrosis in various organs. Heparin can sometimes prevent lesions of DIC.

Shwartzman phenomenon. This phenomenon is probably a specialized model for DIC precipitated by endotoxin. If an animal is injected intradermally with endotoxin and injected intravenously with endotoxin the following day, necrosis of the prepared skin site occurs in a few hours. If endotoxin is given intravenously on 2 successive days, DIC occurs and resembles histologically the DIC seen in gram-negative bacteremias. It has been suggested that the first dose of endotoxin "blocks" the reticuloendothelial system, so that it is unable to efficiently remove the second endotoxin dose. The reticuloendothelial system can be "blocked" by carbon particles or corticosteroids instead of by the first endotoxin dose.

7. Death—Death may occur as a result of massive organ dysfunction, shock, and DIC. It is not directly related to the amount of endotoxin that can be found circulating in the bloodstream.

Endotoxin levels can be assayed by the *"Limulus test"*: a lysate of amebocytes from the horseshoe crab *(Limulus)* gels or coagulates in the presence of 0.0001 μg/mL of endotoxin. This test is not entirely specific and has no prognostic value at present.

8. Other biologic actions of endotoxins— Endotoxin stimulates the secretion of opioid peptides (endorphins) into the blood. Administration of opiate antagonists (eg, naloxone) during endotoxin-induced hypotension can result in a rise in blood pressure. This occurs in experimental animals but has not been proved for clinical cases of gram-negative sepsis.

In pregnant animals, endotoxin can produce decidual hemorrhage, premature labor, and abortions. Pregnant women with active urinary tract infections caused by gram-negative bacteria may have premature labor and consequently a high neonatal mortality rate.

B. Immunologic Features of Reactions to Endotoxins: From birth, humans constantly encounter lipopolysaccharides on the surfaces of gram-negative bacteria that form the normal gut flora. As a result, antibodies are continually being produced to the many antigenic determinants of lipopolysaccharides, and delayed type hypersensitivity is being established. Immunologic responses occur to the O-specific polysaccharides and the core polysaccharides (linked to proteins).

It is known (from studies on cesarean piglets completely free of antibodies) that true "primary toxicity" of endotoxins exists. In humans, this "primary toxicity" is inseparable from immunologic responses.

1. Immediate type—Endotoxins combine with antibodies. The antigen-antibody complexes together with complement can trigger the same type of reactions as attributed to "primary toxicity" of endotoxins: interleukin-1 (endogenous pyrogen) release, coagulopathy, vasoactive substance release, vascular necrosis, etc.

2. Delayed type—Cellular hypersensitivity to endotoxin antigens exists. Delayed hypersensitivity can induce reactions attributable to "primary toxicity" of endotoxins: fever, inflammatory lesions, vascular necrosis, etc.

The immune responses can also have a protective role.

3. Tolerance—IgM antibodies to endotoxin can enhance endotoxin uptake and degradation by reticuloendothelial cells. This is one form of "tolerance." IgM antibodies also may prevent DIC.

4. Antibodies—When humans are repeatedly injected with killed suspensions of certain *E coli* mutants, antiserum is produced with a high titer of antibodies to the lipopolysaccharide core (glycolipid). Injection of such human antiserum into patients suffering from gram-negative septic shock substantially reduces shock and lowers the mortality rate.

Exotoxins of Gram-Negative Enteric Bacteria

Many bacteria produce exotoxins of considerable medical importance, in addition to endotoxins. Outstanding features of some of these exotoxins are listed in Table 18–4. (*Note:* In Table 18–4, some of the bacteria are gram-negative and some are gram-positive; some of the diarrheas are caused by toxins and others are due to bacterial invasion.) *E coli* enterotoxins are discussed below and *Shigella dysenteriae* exotoxin is discussed on p 244.

Enterotoxins are also produced by some strains of *Yersinia enterocolitica* (see Chapter 20), *Vibrio parahaemolyticus* (see Chapter 21), *Aeromonas* species (see Chapter 19), and other bacteria, but their role in pathogenesis is not yet defined.

DISEASES DUE TO *ENTEROBACTERIACEAE* OTHER THAN *SALMONELLA* & *SHIGELLA*

Causative Organisms

E coli and many of the other enteric bacteria (*E aerogenes, Proteus, Morganella, Providencia,* and *Citrobacter*) are members of the normal intestinal flora. In the intestine, they generally do not cause disease and may even contribute to normal function and nutrition. The bacteria become pathogenic only when they reach tissues outside the intestinal tract, particularly the urinary and biliary tracts, lungs, peritoneum, and meninges, causing inflammation at these sites. *Klebsiella pneumoniae* is a respiratory pathogen that is also present in the respiratory tract and feces of about 5% of normal individuals. Other klebsiellae are encountered in hospital-acquired infections and in inflammatory conditions of the upper respiratory tract. *Serratia marcescens,* ordinarily free-living, is an op-

Table 18–4. Acute bacterial diarrheas and "food poisoning."

Organism	Incubation Period (Hours)	Vomiting	Diarrhea	Fever	Epidemiology	Pathogenesis	Clinical Features
Staphylococcus	1–8 (rarely, up to 18)	+++	+	–	Staphylococci grow in meats, dairy and bakery products and produce enterotoxin.	Enterotoxin acts on receptors in gut that transmit impulse to medullary centers.	Abrupt onset, intense vomiting for up to 24 hours, regular recovery in 24–48 hours. Occurs in persons eating the same food. No treatment usually necessary except to restore fluids and electrolytes.
Bacillus cereus	2–16	+++	++	–	Reheated fried rice causes vomiting or diarrhea.	Enterotoxins formed in food or in gut from growth of *B cereus*.	With incubation period of 2–8 hours, mainly vomiting. With incubation period of 8–16 hours, mainly diarrhea.
Clostridium perfringens	8–16	±	+++	–	Clostridia grow in rewarmed meat dishes. Huge numbers ingested.	Enterotoxin produced during sporulation in gut, causes hypersecretion.	Abrupt onset of profuse diarrhea; vomiting occasionally. Recovery usual without treatment in 1–4 days. Many clostridia in cultures of food and feces of patients.
Clostridium botulinum	24–96	±	Rare	–	Clostridia grow in anaerobic foods and produce toxin.	Toxin absorbed from gut blocks acetylcholine at neuromuscular junction.	Diplopia, dysphagia, dysphonia, respiratory embarrassment. Treatment requires clear airway, ventilation, and intravenous polyvalent antitoxin (see p 219). Toxin present in food and serum. Mortality rate high.
Escherichia coli (some strains)	24–72	±	++	–	Organisms grow in gut and produce toxin. May also invade superficial epithelium.	Toxin* causes hypersecretion in small intestine ("traveler's diarrhea").†	Usually abrupt onset of diarrhea; vomiting rare. A serious infection in newborns. In adults, "traveler's diarrhea" is usually self-limited in 1–3 days. Use diphenoxylate (Lomotil) but no antimicrobials.
Vibrio parahaemolyticus	6–96	+	++	±	Organisms grow in seafood and in gut and produce toxin, or invade.	Toxin causes hypersecretion; vibrios invade epithelium; stools may be bloody.	Abrupt onset of diarrhea in groups consuming the same food, especially crabs and other seafood. Recovery is usually complete in 1–3 days. Food and stool cultures are positive.
Vibrio cholerae (mild cases)	24–72	+	+++	–	Organisms grow in gut and produce toxin.	Toxin* causes hypersecretion in small intestine. Infective dose >10^7 vibrios.	Abrupt onset of liquid diarrhea in endemic area. Needs prompt replacement of fluids and electrolytes IV or orally. Tetracyclines shorten excretion of vibrios. Stool cultures positive.
Shigella sp (mild cases)	24–72	±	++	+	Organisms grow in superficial gut epithelium. *S dysenteriae* produces toxin.	Organisms invade epithelial cells, blood, mucus, and PMNs in stools. Infective dose <10^3 organisms.	Abrupt onset of diarrhea, often with blood and pus in stools, cramps, tenesmus, and lethargy. Stool cultures are positive. Give trimethoprim-sulfamethoxazole or ampicillin or chloramphenicol in severe cases. Do not give opiates. Often mild and self-limited. Restore fluids.
Salmonella sp	8–48	±	++	+	Organisms grow in gut. Do not produce toxin.	Superficial infection of gut, little invasion. Infective dose >10^5 organisms.	Gradual or abrupt onset of diarrhea and low-grade fever. No antimicrobials unless systemic dissemination is suspected. Stool cultures are positive. Prolonged carriage is frequent.
Clostridium difficile	?	–	+++	+	Antibiotic-associated colitis.	Toxin causes epithelial necrosis in colon; pseudomembranous colitis.	Especially after abdominal surgery, abrupt bloody diarrhea and fever. Toxin in stool. Oral vancomycin useful in therapy.
Campylobacter jejuni	2–10 days	–	+++	++	Infection via oral route from foods, pets. Organism grows in small intestine.	Invasion of mucous membrane. Toxin production uncertain.	Fever, diarrhea; PMNs and fresh blood in stool, especially in children. Usually self-limited. Special media needed for culture at 43 °C. Erythromycin in severe cases with invasion. Usual recovery in 5–8 days.
Yersinia enterocolitica	?	±	++	+	Fecal-oral transmission. Food-borne. Animals infected.	Gastroenteritis or mesenteric adenitis. Occasional bacteremia. Toxin produced occasionally.	Severe abdominal pain, diarrhea, fever; PMNs and blood in stool; polyarthritis, erythema nodosum, especially in children. If severe, treat with gentamicin. Keep stool specimen at 4 °C before culture.

* Toxin stimulates adenylate cyclase activity and increases cAMP concentration in gut; this increases secretion of chloride and water and reduces reabsorption of sodium.

† Heat-stable toxin activates guanylate cyclase and results in hypersecretion.

portunistic pathogen. When normal host defenses are inadequate, particularly in early infancy and old age, in the terminal stages of other diseases, after immunosuppression, or with indwelling venous or urethral catheters, the bacteria may reach the bloodstream and cause sepsis. In the neonatal period, high susceptibility to *E coli* sepsis may be caused by the absence of bactericidal IgM antibodies.

Pathogenesis & Clinical Findings

The clinical manifestations of infections with *E coli* and the other enteric bacteria depend on the site of the infection and cannot be differentiated by symptoms or signs from processes caused by other bacteria.

A. E coli:

1. Urinary tract infection–*E coli* is the most common cause of urinary tract infection and accounts for approximately 90% of first urinary tract infections in young women. The symptoms and signs include urinary frequency, dysuria, hematuria, and sometimes pyuria. Flank pain is associated with upper tract infection. None of these symptoms or signs is specific for *E coli* infection. Urinary tract infection can result in bacteremia with clinical signs of sepsis.

Nephropathogenic *E coli* typically produce hemolysin and ferment dulcitol. Most of the infections are caused by *E coli* with O antigen types 4, 7, and 75, although it is not known whether there is a direct pathogenic role for the types or they are common causes of urinary tract infection because they are prevalent. K antigen appears to be important in the pathogenesis of upper tract infection. Pyelonephritis is associated with a specific type of pilus, P pilus, which binds to the P blood group substance.

2. Traveler's diarrhea–Enterotoxigenic *E coli* are a common cause of "traveler's diarrhea," which may occur by several mechanisms. Some strains of *E coli* produce a heat-labile exotoxin (LT)(MW 80,000) that is under the genetic control of a transmissible plasmid. Its subunit B attaches to the G_{M1} ganglioside at the brush border of epithelial cells of the small intestine and facilitates the entry of subunit A (MW 26,000) into the cell, where the latter activates adenylate cyclase. This markedly increases the local concentration of cyclic adenosine monophosphate (cAMP), which results in intense and prolonged hypersecretion of water and chlorides and inhibits the reabsorption of sodium. The gut lumen is distended with fluid, and hypermotility and diarrhea ensue, lasting for several days.

LT is antigenic and cross-reacts with the enterotoxin of *Vibrio cholerae*. LT stimulates the production of neutralizing antibodies in the serum (and perhaps on the gut surface) of persons previously infected with enterotoxigenic *E coli*. Persons residing in areas where such organisms are highly prevalent (eg, in some developing countries) are likely to possess antibodies and are less prone to develop diarrhea on reexposure to enterotoxigenic *E coli*. A single antitoxin to LT appears to bind LT from different strains of *E coli* and also from *V cholerae*. Assays for LT include the

following: (1) fluid accumulation in the intestine of laboratory animals; (2) typical cytologic changes in cultured cell lines of Chinese hamster ovary or other cells; (3) stimulation of steroid production in cultured adrenal tumor cells; and (4) binding and immunologic assays with standardized antisera to LT. These assays are done only in reference laboratories.

Some strains of *E coli* produce a heat-stable enterotoxin (ST)(MW 5000) that is under the genetic control of a heterogeneous group of plasmids. ST activates guanylate cyclase in enteric epithelial cells and stimulates fluid secretion. Many ST-positive strains also produce LT, and these may produce more severe diarrhea.

The plasmids carrying the genes for enterotoxins (LT, ST) also may carry genes for colonization factors that facilitate the attachment of *E coli* strains to intestinal epithelium. Recognized colonization factors occur with particular frequency in some serotypes (eg, O78:H11; 06:H16). Certain serotypes of enterotoxigenic *E coli* (eg, O78:H12) occur worldwide; others have a limited recognized distribution (eg, O159:H[variable] in Japan; O139:H28 in Brazil). It is possible that virtually any *E coli* may acquire a plasmid encoding for enterotoxins. There is no definite association of enterotoxigenic *E coli* with the enteropathogenic strains causing outbreaks of diarrhea in nurseries. Likewise, there is no association between enterotoxigenic strains and those able to invade intestinal epithelial cells.

3. Sepsis–When normal host defenses are inadequate, *E coli* may reach the bloodstream and cause sepsis. Newborns may be highly susceptible to *E coli* sepsis because they lack IgM antibodies. Sepsis may occur secondary to urinary tract infection.

4. Meningitis–*E coli* and group B streptococci are the leading causes of meningitis in infants. *E coli* causes about 40% of cases of neonatal meningitis, and approximately 75% of *E coli* from meningitis cases have the K1 antigen. This antigen cross-reacts with the group B capsular polysaccharide of *N meningitidis*. The mechanism of virulence associated with the K1 antigen is not understood.

B. Klebsiella-Enterobacter-Serratia; Proteus-Morganella-Providencia; and Citrobacter: The pathogenesis of disease due to these groups of enteric gram-negative rods is similar to that of the nonspecific factors in disease due to *E coli*.

1. Klebsiellae–*K pneumoniae* is present in the respiratory tract and feces of about 5% of normal individuals. It causes a small proportion (about 3%) of bacterial pneumonias. *K pneumoniae* can produce extensive hemorrhagic necrotizing consolidation of the lung. It occasionally produces urinary tract infection and bacteremia with focal lesions in debilitated patients. Other enterics also may produce pneumonia. *K pneumoniae* and *Klebsiella oxytoca* cause hospital-acquired infections. Two other klebsiellae are associated with inflammatory conditions of the upper respiratory tract: *Klebsiella ozaenae* has been isolated from the nasal mucosa in ozena, a fetid, progressive atrophy of mucous membranes; and *Klebsiella rhinoscleromatis* from rhinoscleroma, a destructive granuloma of the nose and pharynx.

2. Enterobacter aerogenes–This organism has small capsules, may be found free-living as well as in the intestinal tract, and causes urinary tract infections and sepsis.

3. Serratia–*S marcescens* is a common opportunistic pathogen in hospitalized patients. *Serratia* (usually nonpigmented) causes pneumonia, bacteremia, and endocarditis—especially in narcotics addicts and hospitalized patients. *S marcescens* is often multiply resistant to aminoglycosides and penicillins; infections can be treated with third-generation cephalosporins.

4. Proteus–*Proteus* species produce infections in humans only when the bacteria leave the intestinal tract. They are found in urinary tract infections and produce bacteremia, pneumonia, and focal lesions in debilitated patients or those receiving intravenous infusions. *P mirabilis* causes urinary tract infections and occasionally other infections. *Proteus vulgaris* and *Morganella morganii* are important nosocomial pathogens.

Proteus species produce urease, resulting in rapid hydrolysis of urea with liberation of ammonia. Thus, in urinary tract infections with *Proteus,* the urine becomes alkaline, promoting stone formation and making acidification virtually impossible. The rapid motility of *Proteus* may contribute to its invasion of the urinary tract.

Motile strains of *Proteus* contain H antigen in addition to the somatic O antigen. Certain strains share specific polysaccharides with some rickettsiae and are agglutinated by sera from patients with rickettsial diseases (the now obsolete Weil-Felix test).

Strains of *Proteus* vary greatly in antibiotic sensitivity. *P mirabilis* is often inhibited by penicillins; the most active antibiotics for other members of the group are aminoglycosides and cephalosporins.

5. Providencia–*Providencia* species (*Providencia rettgeri, Providencia alcalifaciens,* and *Providencia stuartii*) are members of the normal intestinal flora. All cause urinary tract infections and are often resistant to antimicrobial therapy.

6. Citrobacter–*Citrobacter* can cause urinary tract infections and sepsis.

Diagnostic Laboratory Tests

A. Specimens: Urine, blood, pus, spinal fluid, sputum, or other material, as indicated by the localization of the disease process.

B. Smears: The *Enterobacteriaceae* resemble each other morphologically. The presence of large capsules is suggestive of *Klebsiella;* direct capsule swelling tests can be performed on klebsiellae visible in fresh specimens.

C. Culture: Specimens are plated on both blood agar and differential media. With differential media, rapid preliminary identification of gram-negative enteric bacteria is often possible (see p 234).

Immunity

Specific antibodies develop in systemic infections, but it is uncertain whether significant immunity to the organisms follows. Antibodies against the core glycolipid of *Enterobacteriaceae* are associated with protection against the hemodynamic sequelae of bacteremia due to gram-negative rods and also reduce the fever response and augment intravascular clearance of certain organisms.

Treatment

No single specific therapy is available. The sulfonamides, ampicillin, cephalosporins, chloramphenicol, tetracyclines, and aminoglycosides have marked antibacterial effects against the enterics, but variation in susceptibility is great, and laboratory tests for antibiotic sensitivity are essential. Multiple drug resistance is common and is under the control of transmissible plasmids.

Certain conditions predisposing to infection by these organisms require surgical correction, eg, relief of urinary tract obstruction, closure of a perforation in an abdominal organ, or resection of a bronchiectatic portion of lung.

Treatment of gram-negative bacteremia and impending septic shock requires restoration of fluid and electrolyte balance and treatment of disseminated intravascular coagulation in addition to administration of antimicrobial drugs. Administration of antiglycolipid antibody is experimental but can prevent shock and death.

Various means have been proposed for the prevention of traveler's diarrhea, including daily ingestion of bismuth subsalicylate suspension (bismuth subsalicylate can inactivate *E coli* enterotoxin in vitro) and regular doses of tetracyclines or other antimicrobial drugs for limited periods. Because none of these methods are entirely successful or lacking in adverse effects, it is widely recommended that caution be observed in regard to food and drink in areas where environmental sanitation is poor and that early and brief treatment (eg, with trimethoprim-sulfamethoxazole) be substituted for prophylaxis.

Epidemiology, Prevention, & Control

The enteric bacteria establish themselves in the normal intestinal tract within a few days after birth and from then on constitute a main portion of the normal aerobic (facultative anaerobic) microbial flora. *E coli* is the prototype. Enterics found in water or milk are accepted as proof of fecal contamination from sewage or other sources.

Control measures are not feasible as far as the normal endogenous flora is concerned. Enteropathogenic *E coli* serotypes should be controlled like salmonellae (see below). Some of the enterics constitute a major problem in hospital infection. It is particularly important to recognize that many enteric bacteria are "opportunists" which cause illness when they are introduced into debilitated patients. Within hospitals or other institutions, these bacteria commonly are transmitted by personnel, instruments, or parenteral medications. Their control depends on hand washing, rigorous asepsis, sterilization of equipment, disinfection, restraint in intravenous therapy, and strict precautions in keeping the urinary tract sterile (ie, closed drainage).

THE *SALMONELLA-ARIZONA* GROUP

Salmonellae are often pathogenic for humans or animals when acquired by the oral route. They are transmitted from animals and animal products to humans, where they cause enteritis, systemic infection, and enteric fever.

Morphology & Identification

Salmonellae vary in length. Most species except *Salmonella pullorum-gallinarum* are motile with peritrichous flagella. Salmonellae grow readily on simple media, but they almost never ferment lactose or sucrose. They form acid and sometimes gas from glucose and mannose. They usually produce H_2S. They survive freezing in water for long periods. Salmonellae are resistant to certain chemicals (eg, brilliant green, sodium tetrathionate, sodium deoxycholate) that inhibit other enteric bacteria; such compounds are therefore useful for inclusion in media to isolate salmonellae from feces.

Antigenic Structure

While salmonellae are initially detected by their biochemical characteristics, groups and species are identified by antigenic analysis. Like other *Enterobacteriaceae*, salmonellae possess several O antigens (from a total of more than 60) and different H antigens in one or both of 2 phases. Some salmonellae have capsular (K) antigens, referred to as Vi, which may interfere with agglutination by O antisera and are associated with invasiveness. Agglutination tests with absorbed antisera for different O and H antigens form the basis for serologic classification of the salmonellae.

Classification

The classification of salmonellae is complex. Prior to 1983, a classification with 3 primary species was used: *Salmonella typhi* (1 serotype), *Salmonella choleraesuis* (1 serotype), and *Salmonella enteritidis* (more than 1500 serotypes). Since 1983, on the basis of DNA hybridization studies, one species, *S choleraesuis*, with 6 subspecies has been designated for the *Salmonella-Arizona* group. In practice, however, the species and subspecies names are not used; laboratory reports typically list a specific serogroup, eg, *Salmonella* species serogroup C1. Reports from reference laboratories that serotype isolates include the serotype name, eg, *Salmonella* serotype *typhimurium*, which is often shortened to *S typhimurium* (as if it were a genus-species designation). Three salmonellae should be identified routinely because of their clinical significance: *S typhi, S choleraesuis,* and *Salmonella paratyphi A*. These 3 salmonellae can be identified by biochemical tests and serogrouping, with follow-up serotyping confirmation. Table 18–5 lists examples of a few named salmonellae and their antigenic formulas.

Variation

Organisms may lose H antigens and become nonmotile. Loss of O antigen is associated with a change from smooth to rough colony form. Vi antigen may be lost partially or completely. Antigens may be acquired (or lost) in the process of transduction.

Pathogenesis & Clinical Findings

S typhi and perhaps *S paratyphi A* and *Salmonella schottmülleri* (formerly *Salmonella paratyphi B*) are primarily infective for humans, and infection with these organisms implies acquisition from a human source. The vast majority of salmonellae, however, are chiefly pathogenic in animals that constitute the reservoir for human infection: poultry, pigs, rodents, cattle, pets (from turtles to parrots), and many others.

The organisms almost always enter via the oral route, usually with contaminated food or drink. The mean infective dose to produce clinical or subclinical infection in humans is $10^5–10^8$ salmonellae (but perhaps as few as 10^3 *S typhi* organisms). Among the host factors that contribute to resistance to *Salmonella* infection are gastric acidity, normal intestinal microbial flora, and local intestinal immunity (see below).

Salmonellae produce 3 main types of disease in humans, but mixed forms are frequent (Table 18–6).

A. The "Enteric Fevers" (Typhoid Fever): This syndrome is produced mainly by *S typhi, S paratyphi A,* and *S schottmülleri*. The ingested salmonellae reach the small intestine, from which they enter the lymphatics and then the bloodstream. They are carried by the blood to many organs, including the intestine. The organisms multiply in intestinal lymphoid tissue and are excreted in stools.

After an incubation period of 10–14 days, fever, malaise, headache, constipation, bradycardia, and myalgia occur. The fever rises to a high plateau, and the spleen and liver become enlarged. Rose spots are seen briefly in rare cases. The white blood cell count is normal or low. In the preantibiotic era, the chief complications of enteric fever were intestinal hemorrhage and perforation, and the mortality rate was 10–15%. Treatment with chloramphenicol or ampicillin has reduced the mortality rate to less than 1%. Occasional *S*

Table 18–5. Representative antigenic formulas of salmonellae.

O Group	Serotype	Antigenic Formula*
D	*S typhi*	**9, 12**, (Vi):d:–
A	*S paratyphi A*	**1, 2, 12**:a:–
C₁	*S choleraesuis*	**6, 7**:c:1, 5
B	*S typhimurium*	**1, 4, 5, 12**:i:1, 2
D	*S enteritidis*	**1, 9, 12**:g, m:–

*O antigens: boldface numerals.
(Vi): Vi antigen if present.
Phase 1 H antigen: lower-case letter.
Phase 2 H antigen: numeral.

Table 18–6. Clinical diseases induced by salmonellae.

	Enteric Fevers	Septicemias	Enterocolitis
Incubation period	7–20 days	Variable	8–48 hours
Onset	Insidious	Abrupt	Abrupt
Fever	Gradual, then high plateau, with "typhoidal" state	Rapid rise, then spiking "septic" temperature	Usually low
Duration of disease	Several weeks	Variable	2–5 days
Gastrointestinal symptoms	Often early constipation; later, bloody diarrhea	Often none	Nausea, vomiting, diarrhea at onset
Blood cultures	Positive in 1st–2nd week of disease	Positive during high fever	Negative
Stool cultures	Positive from 2nd week on; negative earlier in disease	Infrequently positive	Positive soon after onset

typhi strains resistant to these drugs have responded to trimethoprim-sulfamethoxazole.

The principal lesions are hyperplasia and necrosis of lymphoid tissue (eg, Peyer's patches), hepatitis, focal necrosis of the liver, and inflammation of the gallbladder, periosteum, lungs, and other organs.

B. Bacteremia With Focal Lesions: This is associated commonly with *S choleraesuis* but may be caused by any *Salmonella* serotype. Following oral infection, there is early invasion of the bloodstream (with possible focal lesions in lungs, bones, meninges, etc), but intestinal manifestations are often absent. Blood cultures are positive.

C. Enterocolitis (Formerly "Gastroenteritis"): This is the most common manifestation of *Salmonella* infection. Eight to 48 hours after ingestion of salmonellae (in the USA, *S typhimurium* is prominent), there is nausea, headache, vomiting, and profuse diarrhea, with few leukocytes in the stools. Low-grade fever is common, but the episode usually resolves in 2–3 days.

Inflammatory lesions of the small and large intestine are present. Bacteremia is rare (2–4%) except in immunodeficient persons. Blood cultures are usually negative, but stool cultures are positive for salmonellae and may remain positive for several weeks after clinical recovery.

Diagnostic Laboratory Tests

A. Specimens: Blood for culture must be taken repeatedly. In enteric fevers and septicemias, blood cultures are often positive in the first week of the disease. Bone marrow cultures may be useful. Urine cultures may be positive after the second week.

Stool specimens also must be taken repeatedly. In enteric fevers, the stools yield positive results from the second or third week on; in enterocolitis, during the first week.

Duodenal drainage establishes the presence of salmonellae in the biliary tract in carriers.

B. Bacteriologic Methods for Isolation of Salmonellae:

1. Enrichment cultures–The specimen (usually stool) is put into selenite F or tetrathionate broth, both of which inhibit replication of normal intestinal bacteria and permit multiplication of salmonellae. After incubation for 1–2 days, this is plated on differential and selective media or examined by direct immunofluorescence.

2. Selective medium cultures–The specimen is plated on *Salmonella-Shigella* (SS) agar or deoxycholate-citrate agar, both of which favor growth of salmonellae and shigellae over other *Enterobacteriaceae*.

3. Differential medium cultures–EMB, MacConkey's, or deoxycholate medium permits rapid detection of lactose nonfermenters (not only salmonellae and shigellae but also *Proteus, Serratia, Pseudomonas,* etc). Gram-positive organisms are somewhat inhibited. Bismuth sulfite medium permits rapid detection of *S typhi,* which forms black colonies because of H_2S production.

4. Final identification–Suspect colonies from solid media are identified by biochemical reaction patterns (Table 18–1) and slide agglutination tests with specific sera.

C. Serologic Methods: Serologic techniques are used to identify unknown cultures with known sera (see below) and may also be used to determine antibody titers in patients with unknown illness, although the latter is not very useful in diagnosis of *Salmonella* infections.

1. Rapid slide agglutination test–In this test, known sera and unknown culture are mixed on a slide and the mixture observed under the low-power objective. Clumping, when it occurs, can be observed within a few minutes. This test is particularly useful for rapid preliminary identification of cultures.

2. Tube dilution agglutination test (Widal test)–Serum agglutinins rise sharply during the second and third weeks of *Salmonella* infection. At least 2 serum specimens, obtained at intervals of 7–10 days, are needed to prove a rise in antibody titer. Serial (2-fold) dilutions of unknown serum are tested against antigens from representative salmonellae. The results are interpreted as follows: (1) High or rising titer of O ($\geq$ 1:160) suggests that active infection is present. (2) High titer of H ($\geq$ 1:160) suggests past immunization or past infection. (3) High titer of antibody to the Vi antigen occurs in some carriers.

Immunity

Infection with *S typhi, S paratyphi,* and *S schottmülleri* usually confers a certain degree of immunity. Reinfection may occur but is often milder than the first infection. Circulating antibodies to O and Vi are related to resistance to infection and disease. However, relapses may occur in 2–3 weeks after recovery in spite of antibodies. Secretory IgA antibodies may prevent attachment of salmonellae to intestinal epithelium.

Persons with S/S hemoglobin (sickle cell disease) are exceedingly susceptible to *Salmonella* infections, particularly osteomyelitis. Persons with A/S hemoglobin (sickle cell trait) may be more susceptible than normal individuals (those with A/A hemoglobin).

Treatment

While enteric fevers and bacteremias with focal lesions require antimicrobial treatment, the vast majority of cases of enterocolitis do not. In enterocolitis, clinical symptoms and excretion of the salmonellae may be prolonged by antimicrobial therapy. In severe diarrhea, replacement of fluids and electrolytes is essential.

Antimicrobial therapy is with chloramphenicol, ampicillin, or trimethoprim-sulfamethoxazole. Multiple drug resistance transmitted genetically by plasmids among enteric bacteria is a problem in *Salmonella* infections. As many as 25% of salmonellae are resistant to ampicillin and 5% are resistant to chloramphenicol; resistance to trimethoprim-sulfamethoxazole is also increasing.

In most carriers, the organisms persist in the gallbladder (particularly if gallstones are present) and in the biliary tract. Some chronic carriers have been cured by ampicillin alone, but in most cases cholecystectomy must be combined with drug treatment.

Epidemiology

The feces of persons who have unsuspected subclinical disease or are carriers are a more important source of contamination than frank clinical cases that are promptly isolated, eg, when carriers working as food handlers are "shedding" organisms. Many animals, including cattle, rodents, and fowl, are naturally infected with a variety of salmonellae and have the bacteria in their tissues (meat), excreta, or eggs. The incidence of typhoid fever has decreased, but the incidence of other *Salmonella* infections has increased markedly in the USA. The problem is aggravated by the widespread use of animal feeds containing antimicrobial drugs that favor the proliferation of drug-resistant salmonellae and their potential transmission to humans.

A. Carriers: After manifest or subclinical infection, some individuals continue to harbor salmonellae in their tissues for variable lengths of time (convalescent carriers or healthy permanent carriers). Three percent of survivors of typhoid become permanent carriers, harboring the organisms in the gallbladder, biliary tract, or, rarely, the intestine or urinary tract.

B. Sources of Infection: The sources of infection are food and drink that have been contaminated with salmonellae. The following sources are important:

1. Water–Contamination with feces often results in explosive epidemics.

2. Milk and other dairy products (ice cream, cheese, custard)–Contamination with feces is due to inadequate pasteurization or improper handling. Limited outbreaks are traceable to the source of supply.

3. Shellfish–From contaminated water.

4. Dried or frozen eggs–From infected fowl or contaminated during processing.

5. Meats and meat products–From infected animals (poultry) or contaminated with feces by rodents or humans.

6. "Recreational" drugs–Marihuana and other drugs.

7. Animal dyes–Dyes (eg, carmine) used in drugs, foods, and cosmetics.

8. Household pets–Turtles, dogs, cats, etc.

Prevention & Control

Sanitary measures must be taken to prevent contamination of food and water by rodents or other animals that excrete salmonellae. Infected poultry, meats, and eggs must be thoroughly cooked. Carriers must not be allowed to work as food handlers and should observe strict hygienic precautions.

Two injections of acetone-killed bacterial suspensions of *S typhi,* followed by a booster injection some months later, give partial resistance to small infectious inocula of typhoid bacilli but not to large ones. Oral administration of a live avirulent mutant strain of *S typhi* has given significant protection in areas of high endemicity. Vaccines against other salmonellae give less protection and are not recommended.

THE SHIGELLAE

The natural habitat of shigellae is limited to the intestinal tracts of humans and other primates, where they produce bacillary dysentery.

Morphology & Identification

A. Typical Organisms: Shigellae are slender gram-negative rods; coccobacillary forms occur in young cultures.

B. Culture: Shigellae are facultative anaerobes but grow best aerobically. Convex, circular, transparent colonies with intact edges reach a diameter of about 2 mm in 24 hours.

C. Growth Characteristics: All shigellae ferment glucose. With the exception of *Shigella sonnei,* they do not ferment lactose. The inability to ferment lactose distinguishes shigellae on differential media: Shigellae form acid from carbohydrates but rarely produce gas. They may also be divided into those that ferment mannitol and those that do not (Table 18–7).

D. Variation: Mutants with different biochemi-

Table 18–7. Pathogenic species of *Shigella*.

Present Designation	Group and Type	Mannitol	Ornithine Decarboxylase	Earlier Designation
S dysenteriae	A (1–10)	–	–	S shigae, Shiga's bacillus
S flexneri	B (1–6)	+	–	S paradysenteriae, Flexner subgroup
S boydii	C (1–15)	+	–	S paradysenteriae, Boyd subgroup
S sonnei	D 1	+	+	Sonne bacillus

cal, antigenic, and pathogenic properties often emerge from parent strains. Variation from smooth (S) to rough (R) colony form is associated with loss of invasiveness.

Antigenic Structure

Shigellae have a complex antigenic pattern. There is great overlapping in the serologic behavior of different species, and most of them share O antigens with other enteric bacilli.

The somatic O antigens of shigellae are lipopolysaccharides. Their serologic specificity depends on the polysaccharide. There are more than 40 serotypes. The classification of shigellae relies on biochemical and antigenic characteristics. The principal pathogenic species are shown in Table 18–7.

Pathogenesis & Pathology

Shigella infections are almost always limited to the gastrointestinal tract; bloodstream invasion is quite rare. Shigellae are highly communicable: the infective dose is less than 10^3 organisms (whereas it is 10^5–10^8 for salmonellae and vibrios). The essential pathologic process is invasion of the mucosal epithelium; microabscesses in the wall of the large intestine and terminal ileum lead to necrosis of the mucous membrane, superficial ulceration, bleeding, and formation of a "pseudomembrane" on the ulcerated area. This consists of fibrin, leukocytes, cell debris, a necrotic mucous membrane, and bacteria. As the process subsides, granulation tissue fills the ulcers and scar tissue forms.

Toxins

A. Endotoxin: Upon autolysis, all shigellae release their toxic lipopolysaccharide. This endotoxin probably contributes to the irritation of the bowel wall.

B. *Shigella dysenteriae* Exotoxin: *S dysenteriae* type 1 (Shiga bacillus) produces a heat-labile exotoxin that affects both the gut and the central nervous system. The exotoxin is a protein that is antigenic (stimulating production of antitoxin) and lethal for experimental animals. Acting as an enterotoxin, it produces diarrhea as does the heat-labile *E coli* enterotoxin, perhaps by the same mechanism (see p 239). In humans, the exotoxin also inhibits sugar and amino acid absorption in the small intestine. Acting as a "neurotoxin," this material may contribute to the extreme severity and fatal nature of *S dysenteriae* infections and to the central nervous system reactions (meningismus, coma) observed in them. Patients with *Shigella flexneri* or *Shigella sonnei* infections develop

antitoxin that neutralizes *S dysenteriae* exotoxin in vitro. The toxic activity is distinct from the invasive property of shigellae in dysentery. The 2 may act in sequence, the toxin producing an early nonbloody, voluminous diarrhea and the invasion of the large intestine resulting in later dysentery with blood and pus in stools.

Clinical Findings

After a short incubation period (1–2 days), there is a sudden onset of abdominal pain, fever, and watery diarrhea. The diarrhea has been attributed to an exotoxin acting in the small intestine (see above). A day or so later, as the infection involves the ileum and colon, the number of stools increase; they are less liquid but often contain mucus and blood. Each bowel movement is accompanied by straining and tenesmus (rectal spasms), with resulting lower abdominal pain. In more than half of adult cases, fever and diarrhea subside spontaneously in 2–5 days. However, in children and the elderly, loss of water and electrolytes may lead to dehydration, acidosis, and even death. The illness due to *S dysenteriae* may be particularly severe.

On recovery, most persons shed dysentery bacilli for only a short period, but a few remain chronic intestinal carriers and may have recurrent bouts of the disease. Upon recovery from the infection, most persons develop circulating antibodies to shigellae, but these do not protect against reinfection.

Diagnostic Laboratory Tests

A. Specimens: Fresh stool, mucus flecks, and rectal swabs for culture. Large numbers of fecal leukocytes and some red blood cells may often be seen microscopically. Serum specimens, if desired, must be taken 10 days apart to demonstrate a rise in titer of agglutinating antibodies.

B. Culture: The materials are streaked on differential selective media (eg, MacConkey's or EMB agar) and on thiosulfate-citrate-bile agar, which suppress other *Enterobacteriaceae* and gram-positive organisms. Colorless (lactose-negative) colonies are inoculated into triple sugar iron agar (see p 234). Organisms that fail to produce H_2S, that produce acid but not gas in the butt and an alkaline slant in triple sugar iron agar medium, and that are nonmotile should be subjected to slide agglutination by specific *Shigella* antisera.

C. Serology: Normal persons often have agglutinins against several *Shigella* species. However, serial determinations of antibody titers may show a rise in specific antibody.

Immunity

Infection is followed by a type-specific antibody response. Injection of killed shigellae stimulates production of antibodies in serum but fails to protect humans against infection. IgA antibodies in the gut may be important in limiting reinfection; these may be stimulated by live attenuated strains given orally as experimental vaccines. Serum antibodies to somatic *Shigella* antigens are IgM.

Treatment

A potent specific antitoxin against *S dysenteriae* exotoxin is available, but convincing proof of its clinical efficacy is lacking. Chloramphenicol, ampicillin, tetracycline, and trimethoprim-sulfamethoxazole are most commonly inhibitory for *Shigella* isolates and can suppress acute clinical attacks of dysentery. They often fail to eradicate the organisms from the intestinal tract, however, and permit establishment of the carrier state. Multiple drug resistance can be transmitted by plasmids, and resistant infection is widespread. It is claimed that a single dose of tetracycline hydrochlo-ride, 2.5 g orally, or ampicillin, 100 mg/kg orally, is effective therapy for acute dysentery in adults. It is probable that many such cases are self-limited. Opiates should be avoided in *Shigella* dysentery.

Epidemiology, Prevention, & Control

Shigellae are transmitted by "food, fingers, feces, and flies" from person to person. Most cases of *Shigella* infection occur in children under 10 years of age. *S dysenteriae* has spread widely in Central and South America. In 1969 in Guatemala, there were 110,000 cases, with 8000 deaths. Mass chemoprophylaxis for limited periods of time (eg, in military personnel) has been tried, but resistant strains of shigellae tend to emerge rapidly. Since humans are the main recognized host of pathogenic shigellae, control efforts must be directed at eliminating the organisms from this reservoir by (1) sanitary control of water, food, and milk; sewage disposal; and fly control; (2) isolation of patients and disinfection of excreta; and (3) detection of subclinical cases and carriers, particularly food handlers.

REFERENCES

Blaser MJ, Newman LS: A review of human salmonellosis: 1. Infective dose. *Rev Infect Dis* 1982;**4:**1096.

Carpenter CCJ: Mechanisms of bacterial diarrheas. *Am J Med* 1980;**68:**313.

Carr DB et al: Endotoxin-stimulated opioid peptide secretion: Two secretory pools and feedback control in vivo. *Science* 1982;**217:**845.

Cherubin CE et al: Septicemia with non-typhoid *Salmonella*. *Medicine* 1974;**53:**365.

Dinarella CA, Wolff SM: Molecular basis of fever in humans. *Am J Med* 1982;**72:**799.

Edelman R, Levine MM: Summary of a workshop on enteropathogenic *Escherichia coli*. *J Infect Dis* 1983;**147:**1108.

Edwards PR, Ewing WH: *Identification of Enterobacteriaceae,* 3rd ed. Burgess, 1972.

Elin RJ, Wolff SM: Nonspecificity of *Limulus* amebocyte lysate test: Positive reactions with polynucleotides and proteins. *J Infect Dis* 1973;**128:**349.

Farmer JJ III et al: Biochemical identification of new species and biogroups of *Enterobacteriaceae* isolated from clinical specimens. *J Clin Microbiol* 1985;**21:**46.

Farmer JJ III et al: The *Salmonella-Arizona* group of *Enterobacteriaceae:* Nomenclature, classification, and reporting. *Clin Microbiol Newsletter* 1984:**6:**63.

Gendrel D et al: *Salmonella* infections and hemoglobin S. *J Pediatr* 1982;**101:**68.

Goldschmidt MC, Dupont HL: Enteropathogenic *Escherichia coli:* Lack of correlation of serotype with pathogenicity. *J Infect Dis* 1976;**133:**153.

Gorbach SL: Travellers' diarrhea. (Editorial.) *N Engl J Med* 1982;**307:**881.

Hornick RB et al: Typhoid fever: Pathogenesis and immunologic control. (2 parts.) *N Engl J Med* 1970;**283:**686, 739.

Jann K, Jann B: The K antigens of *Escherichia coli. Prog Allergy* 1983;**33:**53.

Johnson RH et al: *Arizona hinshawii* infections: New cases, antimicrobial sensitivities, and literature review. *Ann Intern Med* 1976;**85:**587.

Karmali MA et al: *Escherichia coli* cytotoxin, hemolytic-uraemic syndrome, and haemorrhagic colitis. *Lancet* 1983;**2:**1299.

Levine MM: Bacillary dysentery: Mechanisms and treatment. *Med Clin North Am* 1982;**66:**623.

Lipsky BA et al: *Citrobacter* infections in humans: Experience at the Seattle Veterans Administration Medical Center and a review of the literature. *Rev Infect Dis* 1980;**2:**746.

Low D et al: Gene clusters governing the production of hemolysin and mannose-resistance hemagglutination are closely linked in *E coli* serotype 04 and 04 isolates from urinary tract infections. *Infect Immun* 1984;**43:**353.

Luderitz O et al: Lipid A: Chemical structure and biologic activity. *J Infect Dis* 1973;**128(Suppl):**S17.

Mandell GL, Douglas RG Jr, Bennett JE (editors): *Principles and Practice of Infectious Disease,* 2nd ed. Wiley, 1985.

McCabe WR et al: Humoral immunity to type-specific and cross-reactive antigens of gram-negative bacilli. *J Infect Dis* 1973;**128(Suppl):**S284.

Meals RA: Paratyphoid fever: Report of 62 cases with several unusual findings and a review of the literature. *Arch Intern Med* 1976;**136:**1422.

Montgomerie JZ, Ota JK: *Klebsiella* bacteremia. *Arch Intern Med* 1980;**140:**525.

O'Brien TF et al: Molecular epidemiology of antibiotic resistance in *Salmonella* from animals and human beings in the United States. *N Engl J Med* 1982;**307:**1.

Parsons R et al: Salmonella infections of the abdominal aorta. *Rev Infect Dis* 1983;**5:**227.

Riley LW et al: Hemorrhagic colitis associated with a rare *Escherichia coli* serotype. *N Engl J Med* 1983;**308:**681.

Taylor DN et al: Salmonellosis associated with marijuana: A multistate outbreak traced by plasmid fingerprinting. *N Engl J Med* 1982;**306:**1249.

Taylor DN et al: Typhoid in the United States and the risk to the international traveler. *J Infect Dis* 1983;**148:**599.

Thomas FE et al: Sequential hospitalwide outbreaks of resistant *Serratia* and *Klebsiella* infections. *Arch Intern Med* 1977;

137:581.

Tulloch EF et al: Invasive *Escherichia coli* dysentery. *Ann Intern Med* 1973;**79**:13.

Wahdan MH et al: A controlled field trial of live *Salmonella typhi* strain Ty 21a oral vaccine against typhoid: Three year results. *J Infect Dis* 1982;**145**:292.

Warren JW, Hornick RB: Immunization against typhoid fever. *Annu Rev Med* 1979;**30**:457.

Wenzel RP et al: *Providencia stuartii:* Hospital pathogen. *Am J Epidemiol* 1976;**104**:170.

Wilfert CM: *E coli* meningitis: K1 antigen and virulence. *Annu Rev Med* 1978;**29**:129.

Winston DJ et al: Infectious complications of human bone marrow transplantation. *Medicine* 1979;**58**:1.

Woodward TE, Woodward WE: A new oral vaccine against typhoid fever. *J Infect Dis* 1982;**145**:289.

Young LS et al: Gram-negative rod bacteremia: Microbiologic, immunologic, and therapeutic considerations. *Ann Intern Med* 1977;**86**:456.

Yu VL: *Serratia marcescens:* Historical perspective and clinical review. *N Engl J Med* 1979;**300**:887.

Ziegler EJ et al: Treatment of gram-negative bacteremia and shock with human antiserum to a mutant *Escherichia coli*. *N Engl J Med* 1982;**307**:1225.

Pseudomonas, Acinetobacter, Aeromonas, & Plesiomonas

19

The *Pseudomonas, Acinetobacter, Aeromonas,* and *Plesiomonas* species are widely distributed in soil and water. *Pseudomonas aeruginosa* sometimes colonizes humans and is the major human pathogen of the group. *P aeruginosa* is invasive and toxigenic, produces infections in patients with abnormal host defenses, and is an important nosocomial pathogen.

THE *PSEUDOMONAS* GROUP

The *Pseudomonas* group are gram-negative, motile, aerobic rods some of which produce water-soluble pigments. Pseudomonads occur widely in soil, water, plants, and animals. *P aeruginosa* is frequently present in small numbers in the normal intestinal flora and on the skin of humans. Other *Pseudomonas* species infrequently cause disease. The medically important pseudomonads are listed in Table 19–1.

1. *PSEUDOMONAS AERUGINOSA*

P aeruginosa is widely distributed in nature and is commonly present in moist environments in hospitals. It can colonize normal humans, in whom it is a saprophyte. It causes disease in humans with abnormal host defenses.

Morphology & Identification

A. Typical Organisms: *P aeruginosa* is motile and rod-shaped, measuring about 0.6×2 μm. It is gram-negative and occurs as single bacteria, in pairs, and occasionally in short chains.

Table 19–1. Pseudomonads isolated from specimens from humans.

Group	Genus and Species
Fluorescent group	P aeruginosa P fluorescens P putida
Pseudomallei group	P mallei P pseudomallei P cepacia
Others	P maltophilia P pseudoalcaligenes P putrefaciens P stutzeri

B. Culture: *P aeruginosa* is an obligate aerobe that grows readily on many types of culture media, sometimes producing a sweet or grapelike odor. Some strains hemolyze blood. *P aeruginosa* forms smooth round colonies with a fluorescent greenish color. It often produces the nonfluorescent bluish pigment pyocyanin, which diffuses into the agar. Other *Pseudomonas* species do not produce pyocyanin. Many strains of *P aeruginosa* also produce the fluorescent pigment pyoverdin, which gives a greenish color to the agar. Some strains produce the dark red pigment pyorubin or the black pigment pyomelanin.

P aeruginosa in a culture can produce multiple colony types, giving the impression of a culture of mixed species of bacteria. *P aeruginosa* from different colony types may also have different biochemical and enzymatic activities and different antimicrobial susceptibility patterns. Cultures from patients with cystic fibrosis often yield *P aeruginosa* organisms that form very mucoid colonies.

C. Growth Characteristics: *P aeruginosa* grows well at 37–42 °C; its growth at 42 °C helps differentiate it from other *Pseudomonas* species. It is oxidase-positive. It does not ferment carbohydrates, but many strains oxidize glucose. Identification is usually based on colonial morphology, oxidase positivity, the presence of characteristic pigments, and growth at 42 °C. Differentiation of *P aeruginosa* from other pseudomonads on the basis of biochemical activity requires testing with a large battery of substrates.

Antigenic Structure & Toxins

Pili (fimbrae) extend from the cell surface and promote attachment to host epithelial cells. Polysaccharide capsules are responsible for the mucoid colonies seen in cultures from patients with cystic fibrosis. The lipopolysaccharide, which exists in multiple immunotypes, is responsible for many of the endotoxic properties of the organism (see Chapter 18). *P aeruginosa* can be typed by lipopolysaccharide immunotype and by pyocin (bacteriocin) susceptibility. Most *P aeruginosa* isolates from clinical infections produce extracellular enzymes, including elastases, proteases, and 2 hemolysins: a heat-labile phospholipase C and a heat-stable glycolipid.

Many strains of *P aeruginosa* produce exotoxin A, which causes tissue necrosis and is lethal for animals when injected in purified form. The toxin blocks protein synthesis by a mechanism of action identical to that of diphtheria toxin (see p 214), although the structures of the 2 toxins are not identical. Antitoxins to exotoxin A are found in some human sera, including those of patients who have recovered from serious *P aeruginosa* infections.

Pathogenesis

P aeruginosa is pathogenic only when introduced into areas devoid of normal defenses, eg, when mucous membranes and skin are disrupted by direct tissue damage; when intravenous or urinary catheters are used; or when neutropenia is present, as in cancer chemotherapy. The bacterium attaches to and colonizes the mucous membranes or skin, invades locally, and produces systemic disease. These processes are promoted by the pili, enzymes, and toxins described above. Lipopolysaccharide plays a direct role in causing fever, shock, oliguria, leukocytosis and leukopenia, disseminated intravascular coagulation, and adult respiratory distress syndrome (see Chapter 18).

P aeruginosa (and other species, eg, *Pseudomonas cepacia, Pseudomonas putida, Pseudomonas maltophilia*) is resistant to many antimicrobial agents and therefore becomes dominant and important when more susceptible bacteria of the normal flora are suppressed.

Clinical Findings

P aeruginosa produces infection of wounds and burns, giving rise to blue-green pus; meningitis, when introduced by lumbar puncture; and urinary tract infection, when introduced by catheters and instruments or in irrigating solutions. Involvement of the respiratory tract, especially from contaminated respirators, results in necrotizing pneumonia. The bacterium is often found in mild otitis externa in swimmers. It may cause invasive (malignant) otitis externa in diabetic patients. Infection of the eye, which may lead to rapid destruction of the eye, occurs most commonly after injury or surgical procedures. In infants or debilitated persons, *P aeruginosa* may invade the bloodstream and result in fatal sepsis; this occurs commonly in patients with leukemia or lymphoma who have received antineoplastic drugs or radiation therapy and in patients with severe burns. In most *P aeruginosa* infections, the symptoms and signs are nonspecific and are related to the organ involved. Occasionally, verdoglobin (a breakdown product of hemoglobin) or fluorescent pigment can be detected in wounds, burns, or urine by ultraviolet fluorescence. Hemorrhagic necrosis of skin occurs often in sepsis due to *P aeruginosa;* the lesions, called ecthyma gangrenosum, are surrounded by erythema and often do not contain pus. *P aeruginosa* can be seen on Gram-stained specimens from ecthyma lesions, and cultures are positive. Ecthyma gangrenosum is very uncommon in bacteremia due to organisms other than *P aeruginosa*.

Diagnostic Laboratory Tests

A. Specimens: Specimens from skin lesions, pus, urine, blood, spinal fluid, sputum, and other material should be obtained as indicated by the type of infection.

B. Smears: Gram-negative rods are often seen in smears. There are no specific morphologic characteristics that differentiate pseudomonads in specimens from enteric or other gram-negative rods.

C. Culture: Specimens are plated on blood agar and the differential media commonly used to grow the enteric gram-negative rods. Pseudomonads grow readily on most of these media, but they may grow more slowly than the enterics. *P aeruginosa* does not ferment lactose and is easily differentiated from the lactose-fermenting bacteria. Culture is the specific test for diagnosis of *P aeruginosa* infection (see p 247).

Treatment

Clinically significant infections with *P aeruginosa* should not be treated with single-drug therapy, because the success rate is low with such therapy and because the bacteria can rapidly develop resistance when single drugs are employed. One of the penicillins most useful against *P aeruginosa*—ticarcillin, mezlocillin, and piperacillin—should be used in combination with an aminoglycoside, usually gentamicin, tobramycin, or amikacin. Other drugs active against *P aeruginosa* include aztreonam; imipenem; the newer quinolones, including ciprofloxacin; and the newer cephalosporins, including cefoperazone, ceftriaxone, and cefsulodin. The susceptibility patterns of *P aeruginosa* vary geographically, and susceptibility tests should be done as an adjunct to selection of antimicrobial therapy.

Epidemiology & Control

P aeruginosa is primarily a nosocomial pathogen, and the methods for control of infection are similar to those for other nosocomial pathogens. Since *Pseudomonas* thrives in moist environments, special attention should be paid to sinks, water baths, showers, hot tubs, and other wet areas. For epidemiologic purposes, strains can be typed by pyocins and by lipopolysaccharide immunotypes. Vaccine from appropriate types administered to high-risk patients provides some protection against *Pseudomonas* sepsis. Such treatment has been used experimentally in patients with leukemia, burns, cystic fibrosis, and immunosuppression.

2. PSEUDOMONAS PSEUDOMALLEI

P pseudomallei, a small, motile, aerobic, gram-negative rod that resembles other nonpigmented pseudomonads but is antigenically distinct, causes melioidosis. Melioidosis occurs in Burma, Vietnam, Guam, the Philippines, and perhaps also in the western hemisphere. The organism is present in soil, water, and plants and may produce infection in rodents and other animals. Human infection probably originates from any of these sources, by contamination of skin abrasions and possibly by ingestion or inhalation. The epidemiology of this disorder is uncertain.

Melioidosis may manifest itself as an acute or chronic lung disease, may produce abscesses and septicemia, and has a high mortality rate if untreated. A positive serologic test is diagnostically helpful and constitutes evidence of past infection. Sometimes latent infection is reactivated as a result of immunosuppression. *P pseudomallei* should be tested for antibiotic susceptibility in vitro to guide treatment. Chloramphenicol, 2–3 g/d, plus an aminoglycoside or a tetracycline may be the treatment of choice. Trimethoprim-sulfamethoxazole may be effective. Drug resistance emerges frequently.

3. PSEUDOMONAS MALLEI

P mallei is a small, nonmotile, nonpigmented, aerobic, gram-negative rod that grows readily on most bacteriologic media. It causes glanders, a disease of horses transmissible to humans. In horses, the disease has prominent pulmonary involvement, subcutaneous ulcerative lesions, and lymphatic thickening with nodules; systemic disease also occurs. Human infection, which can be fatal, usually begins as an ulcer of the skin or mucous membranes followed by lymphangitis and sepsis. Inhalation of the organisms may lead to primary pneumonia.

The diagnosis is based on rising agglutinin titers and culture of the organism from local lesions of humans or horses. Human cases can be treated effectively with a tetracycline plus an aminoglycoside.

The disease has been controlled by slaughter of infected horses and mules and at present is very rare. In some countries, laboratory infections are the only source of the disease.

4. OTHER PSEUDOMONADS

Some of the many *Pseudomonas* species are listed in Table 19–1; occasionally these pseudomonads are opportunistic pathogens. *Pseudomonas cepacia* is sometimes cultured from patients with cystic fibrosis. *Pseudomonas maltophilia* can infect many organs. The diagnosis of infections caused by these pseudomonads is made by culturing the bacteria and identifying them by differential reactions on a complex set of biochemical substrates. Many of these pseudomonads have antimicrobial susceptibility patterns different from *P aeruginosa*.

ACINETOBACTER

Acinetobacter calcoaceticus is a species of aerobic gram-negative bacteria that are widely distributed in soil and water and can occasionally be cultured from skin, mucous membranes, and secretions.

There are 2 subspecies of *A calcoaceticus, lwoffi* and *anitratus*. These were previously called by a number of different names, including *Mima polymorpha* and *Herellea vaginicola*. Subspecies *anitratus* is the more common subspecies. The bacteria are usually coccobacillary or coccal in appearance; they resemble neisseriae on smears, because diplococcal forms predominate in body fluids and on solid media. Rod-shaped forms occur, and occasionally the bacteria appear to be gram-positive. *Acinetobacter* grows well on most types of media used to culture specimens from patients. *Acinetobacter* recovered from meningitis and sepsis has been mistaken for *Neisseria meningitidis;* similarly, *Acinetobacter* recovered from the female genital tract has been mistaken for *Neisseria gonorrhoeae*. However, the neisseriae produce oxidase and *Acinetobacter* does not.

Acinetobacter is usually a commensal and only occasionally causes nosocomial infection. The organisms have been isolated from blood, sputum, skin, pleural fluid, and urine, but their pathogenic role is not clearly established. *Acinetobacter* encountered in nosocomial pneumonias often originates in the water of room humidifiers or vaporizers. In patients with *Acinetobacter* bacteremia, intravenous catheters are almost always the source of infection. In patients with burns or with immune deficiencies, *Acinetobacter* acts as an opportunistic pathogen and can produce sepsis. *Acinetobacter* strains are often resistant to antimicrobial agents, and therapy of infection can be difficult. Susceptibility testing should be done to help select the best antimicrobial drugs for therapy. *Acinetobacter* strains respond most commonly to gentamicin, amikacin, or tobramycin and to carbenicillin.

AEROMONAS

Aeromonas species are free-living gram-negative rods found especially in water. Occasionally, they cause diarrhea or other primary infections or nosocomial infections.

Aeromonas hydrophila is a motile rod commonly isolated from water, soil, or food and occasionally from the human intestinal tract. *Aeromonas sobria* is similar but less commonly pathogenic for humans. *A hydrophila* can be found in the blood in persons with seriously impaired host defenses or endocarditis. It can cause freshwater wound infections. It is occasionally isolated from the feces of patients with diarrhea. *A hydrophila* cultured from stool specimens grows readily on the differential media used to culture enteric gram-negative rods and can easily be confused with the enteric bacteria. However, *Aeromonas* is oxidase-positive, so colonies which look like those of enteric gram-negative rods with areas of hemolysis on blood agar can be tested for oxidase activity and oxidase-positive colonies subjected to further testing. Most *Aeromonas* strains are susceptible to tetracyclines, aminoglycosides, and cephalosporins.

PLESIOMONAS

Plesiomonas shigelloides is a facultatively anaerobic gram-negative rod with polar flagella. The bacterium is most common in tropical and subtropical areas. It has been isolated from freshwater fish and many other animals. Most isolates from humans have been from stool cultures of patients with diarrhea. *Plesiomonas* grows on the differential media used to isolate *Salmonella* and *Shigella* from stool specimens (see Chapter 18). Some *Plesiomonas* strains share antigens with *Shigella sonnei,* and cross-reactions with *Shigella* A and C antisera occur. *Plesiomonas* can be distinguished from shigellae in diarrheal stools by the oxidase test: *Plesiomonas* is oxidase-positive and shigellae are not.

REFERENCES

Bodey GP et al: Infections caused by *Pseudomonas aeruginosa.* Rev Infect Dis 1983;**5:**279.

Burke V et al: The microbiology of childhood gastroenteritis: *Aeromonas* species and other infective agents. *J Infect Dis* 1983;**148:**68.

Davis WA II et al: Human *Aeromonas* infections: A review of the literature and a case report of endocarditis. *Medicine* 1978;**57:**267.

Doroghazi RM et al: Invasive external otitis: Report of 21 cases and review of the literature. *Am J Med* 1981;**71:**603.

Flick MR, Cluff LE: *Pseudomonas* bacteremia: Review of 108 cases. *Am J Med* 1976;**60:**501.

Glew RH et al: Infections with *Acinetobacter calcoaceticus* (*Herellea vaginicola*): Clinical and laboratory studies. *Medicine* 1977;**56:**79.

Gracey M et al: *Aeromonas*-associated gastroenteritis. *Lancet* 1982;**2:**1304.

Jones RJ et al: Controlled trial of *Pseudomonas* immunoglobulin and vaccine in burn patients. *Lancet* 1980;**2:**1263.

Millership SE et al: Faecal carriage rate of *Aeromonas hydrophila. J Clin Pathol* 1983;**36:**920.

Pathak A et al: Neonatal septicemia and meningitis due to *Plesiomonas shigelloides. Pediatrics* 1983;**71:**389.

Pier GB: Pulmonary disease associated with *Pseudomonas aeruginosa* in cystic fibrosis: Current status of the host-bacterium interaction. *J Infect Dis* 1985;**151:**575.

Piggott JA, Hochholzer L: Human melioidosis: A histopathologic study of acute and chronic melioidosis. *Arch Pathol* 1970;**90:**101.

Pollack M: The role of exotoxin A in *Pseudomonas* disease and immunity. *Rev Infect Dis* 1983;**Suppl 5:**S979.

Raz R et al: Nosocomial bacteremia due to *Acinetobacter calcoaceticus. Infection* 1982;**10:**168.

Retailliau HF et al: *Acinetobacter calcoaceticus:* A nosocomial pathogen with an unusual seasonal pattern. *J Infect Dis* 1979;**139:**371.

Wolff RL et al: *Aeromonas hydrophila* bacteremia in ambulatory immunocompromised hosts. *Am J Med* 1980;**68:**238.

Yersinia, Francisella, & Pasteurella

20

These organisms are short, pleomorphic, gram-negative rods that can exhibit bipolar staining. They do not form spores and are catalase-positive, oxidase-negative, and microaerophilic or facultatively anaerobic. Most have animals as their natural hosts, but they can produce serious disease in humans.

The genus *Yersinia* includes *Yersinia pestis*, the cause of plague; *Yersinia pseudotuberculosis* and *Yersinia enterocolitica*, important causes of human diarrheal diseases; and others. *Francisella tularensis* has vertebrate and invertebrate animal reservoirs and occasionally results in septic infections in humans. Several species of *Pasteurella* are primarily animal pathogens but can also produce human disease.

YERSINIA PESTIS & PLAGUE

Plague is an infection of wild rodents, transmitted from one rodent to another and occasionally from rodents to humans by the bites of fleas. Serious infection often results, which in previous centuries produced pandemics of "black death" with millions of fatalities.

Morphology & Identification

Y pestis is a plump gram-negative rod that exhibits striking bipolar staining with special stains (Fig 20–1). It is nonmotile. It grows as a facultative anaerobe on

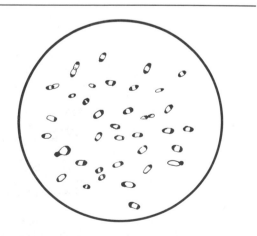

Figure 20–1. Typical organisms of *Y pestis* from smear of lymph node.

many bacteriologic media. Growth is more rapid in media containing blood or tissue fluids and fastest at 30 °C. In cultures on blood agar at 37 °C, colonies may be very small at 24 hours. A virulent inoculum, derived from infected tissue, produces gray and viscous colonies, but after passage in the laboratory, the colonies become irregular and rough. The organism has little biochemical activity, and this is somewhat variable.

Antigenic Structure

All yersiniae possess lipopolysaccharides that have endotoxic activity when released. The organisms produce many antigens and toxins that act as virulence factors. The envelope contains a protein (fraction I) that is produced mainly at 37 °C, confers antiphagocytic properties, and activates complement. Virulent, wild-type *Y pestis* carries V-W antigens, which are encoded by genes on plasmids. A 72-kilobase plasmid is essential for virulence; avirulent strains lack this plasmid. Some stable, avirulent strains (eg, EV76) have served as live vaccines.

Y pestis produces a coagulase at 28 °C (the normal temperature of the flea, which becomes "blocked" as a result of its action) but not at 35 °C (transmission via fleas is low or absent in very hot weather).

Among several exotoxins produced, one is lethal for mice in amounts of 1 μg. This homogeneous protein (MW 74,000) produces beta-adrenergic blockade and is cardiotoxic in animals. Its role in human infection is unknown.

Y pestis also produces a bacteriocin (pesticin); the enzyme isocitrate lyase, which is said to be distinctive; and other products. Some antigens of *Y pestis* cross-react with other yersiniae; bacteriophages of *Y pestis* may lyse other yersiniae.

Pathogenesis & Pathology

When a flea feeds on a rodent infected with *Y pestis,* the ingested organisms multiply in the gut of the flea and, helped by the coagulase, block its proventriculus so that no food can pass through. Subsequently, the "blocked," hungry flea bites ferociously, and the aspirated blood, contaminated with *Y pestis* from the flea, is regurgitated into the bite wound. The inoculated organisms may be phagocytosed, but they can multiply intracellularly or extracellularly. They rapidly reach the lymphatics, and an intense hemorrhagic inflammation develops in the enlarged lymph nodes, which may undergo necrosis and become fluctuant. While the invasion may stop there, *Y pestis* often reach the bloodstream and become widely disseminated. Hemorrhagic and necrotic lesions may develop in all organs; meningitis, pneumonia, and serosanguinous pleuropericarditis are prominent.

Primary pneumonic plague results from inhalation of infective droplets (usually from a coughing patient), with hemorrhagic consolidation, sepsis, and death.

Clinical Findings

After an incubation period of 2–7 days, there is high fever and painful lymphadenopathy, commonly with greatly enlarged, tender nodes ("buboes") in the groin or axilla. Vomiting and diarrhea may develop with early sepsis. Later, disseminated intravascular coagulation leads to hypotension, altered mental status, and renal and cardiac failure. Terminally, signs of pneumonia and meningitis can appear, and *Y pestis* multiplies intravascularly and can be seen in blood smears.

Diagnostic Laboratory Tests

Plague should be suspected in febrile patients who have been exposed to rodents in known endemic areas. Rapid recognition and laboratory confirmation of the disease are essential in order to institute lifesaving therapy.

A. Specimens: Blood is taken for culture and aspirates of enlarged lymph nodes for smear and culture. Acute and convalescent sera may be examined for antibody levels. In pneumonia, sputum is cultured; in possible meningitis, cerebrospinal fluid is taken for smear and culture.

B. Smears: Material from needle aspiration is examined after staining with Giemsa's stain and with specific immunofluorescent stains. With Wayson's stain, *Y pestis* may show a striking bipolar appearance. Spinal fluid and sputum smears should also be stained.

C. Culture: All materials are cultured on blood agar and MacConkey's agar plates and in infusion broth. Growth on solid media may be slow, but blood cultures are often positive in 24 hours. Cultures can be tentatively identified by biochemical reactions. Definite identification of cultures is best done by immunofluorescence (available at Centers for Disease Control, Plague Control Branch, Fort Collins, CO 80422; telephone number [303] 482-0213).

All cultures are highly infectious and must be handled with extreme caution.

D. Serology: In patients who have not been previously vaccinated, a convalescent serum antibody titer of 1:16 or greater is presumptive evidence of *Y pestis* infection. A titer rise in 2 sequential specimens confirms the serologic diagnosis.

Treatment

Unless promptly treated, plague may have a mortality rate of nearly 50%; pneumonic plague, nearly 100%. The drug of choice is streptomycin, 30 mg/kg/d intramuscularly in 2 equal doses, continued for 7–10 days. Tetracycline, 30–40 mg/kg/d orally, is an alternative drug and is sometimes given in combination with streptomycin. Drug resistance has not been noted in *Y pestis*.

Epidemiology & Control

Plague is an infection of wild rodents (field mice, gerbils, moles, skunks, and other animals) that occurs in many parts of the world. The chief enzootic areas are India, Southeast Asia (especially Vietnam), Africa, and North and South America. The western states of the USA and Mexico always contain reservoirs of infection. Epizootics with high mortality rates occur intermittently; at such times, the infection can spread to domestic rodents (eg, rats) and other animals (eg, cats), and humans can be infected by flea bites or by contact. The commonest vector of plague is the rat flea *(Xenopsylla cheopis),* but other fleas may also transmit the infection.

The control of plague requires surveys of infected animals, vectors, and human contacts (in the USA, this is done by the Plague Control Branch of Centers for Disease Control) and destruction of plague-infected animals. If a human case is diagnosed, health authorities must be notified promptly. All patients with suspected plague should be isolated, particularly if pulmonary involvement has not been ruled out. All specimens must be treated with extreme caution. Contacts of patients with suspected plague pneumonia should receive tetracycline, 0.5 g/d for 5 days, as chemoprophylaxis.

A formalin-killed vaccine (plague vaccine USP) is available for travelers to hyperendemic areas and for persons at special high risk.

YERSINIA ENTEROCOLITICA & YERSINIA PSEUDOTUBERCULOSIS

These are non-lactose-fermenting gram-negative rods that are urease-positive and oxidase-negative. They grow best at 25 °C and are motile at 25 °C but nonmotile at 37 °C. They are found in the intestinal tract of a variety of animals, in which they may cause disease, and are transmissible to humans, in whom they can produce a variety of clinical syndromes.

Y enterocolitica exists in more than 50 serotypes; most isolates from human disease belong to serotypes O3, O8, and O9. There are striking geographic differences in the distribution of *Y enterocolitica* serotypes. *Y pseudotuberculosis* exists in at least 6 serotypes, but serotype O1 accounts for most human infections. *Y enterocolitica* can produce a heat-stable enterotoxin, but the role of this toxin in diarrhea associated with infection is not well defined.

Y enterocolitica has been isolated from rodents and domestic animals (eg, sheep, cattle, swine, dogs, and cats) and waters contaminated by them. Transmission to humans probably occurs by contamination of food, drink, or fomites. *Y pseudotuberculosis* occurs in domestic and farm animals and birds, which excrete the organisms in feces. Human infection probably results from ingestion of materials contaminated with animal feces. Person-to-person transmission with either of these organisms is probably rare.

Pathogenesis & Clinical Findings

An inoculum of 10^8-10^9 yersiniae must enter the alimentary tract to produce infection. During the incubation period of 5–10 days, yersiniae multiply in the gut mucosa, particularly the ileum. This leads to inflammation and ulceration, and leukocytes appear in feces. The process may extend to mesenteric lymph nodes and, rarely, to bacteremia.

Early symptoms include fever, abdominal pain, and diarrhea. Diarrhea may be due to an enterotoxin or to the invasion of the mucosa, and it ranges from watery to bloody. At times, the abdominal pain is severe and located in the right lower quadrant, suggesting appendicitis. One to 2 weeks after onset some patients develop arthralgia, arthritis, and erythema nodosum, suggesting an immunologic reaction to the infection. Very rarely, *Yersinia* infection produces pneumonia, meningitis, or sepsis; in most cases, it is self-limited.

Diagnostic Laboratory Tests

A. Specimens: Specimens may be stool, blood, or material obtained at surgical exploration.

B. Smears: Stained smears are not contributory.

C. Culture: The number of yersiniae in stool may be small and can be increased by "cold enrichment": a small amount of feces or a rectal swab is placed in buffered saline, pH 7.6, and kept at 4 °C for 2–4 weeks; many fecal organisms do not survive, but *Y enterocolitica* will multiply. Subcultures made at intervals on MacConkey agar may yield yersiniae.

D. Serology: In paired serum specimens taken 2 or more weeks apart, a rise in agglutinating antibodies can be shown; however, cross reactions between yersiniae and other organisms (vibrios, salmonellae, brucellae) may confuse the results.

Treatment

Most *Yersinia* infections with diarrhea tend to be self-limited, and the possible benefits of antimicrobial drugs are unknown. Gentamicin, 5 mg/kg/d intravenously in divided doses, or chloramphenicol, 50 mg/kg/d orally, has been given if the illness seems very severe. Proven *Yersinia* sepsis or meningitis has a mortality rate of more than 50% in spite of such treatment, but these occur mainly in immunocompromised patients. In cases where the clinical manifestations strongly point to either appendicitis or mesenteric adenitis, surgical exploration has been the rule unless several simultaneous cases indicate *Yersinia* infection is likely.

Prevention & Control

Contact with farm and domestic animals, their feces, or materials contaminated by them probably accounts for most human infections. Meat and dairy products have occasionally been indicated as sources of infection, and group outbreaks have been traced to contaminated food or drink. Conventional sanitary precautions are probably helpful. There are no specific preventive measures.

FRANCISELLA TULARENSIS & TULAREMIA

Francisella tularensis is widely found in animal reservoirs and is transmissible to humans by biting arthropods, direct contact with infected animal tissue, inhalation of aerosols, or ingestion of contaminated food or water. The resulting disease, tularemia, is rare in the USA, and its clinical presentation depends on the route of infection.

Morphology & Identification

A. Typical Organisms: *F tularensis* is a small, gram-negative, pleomorphic rod. It is rarely seen in smears of tissue.

B. Specimens: Blood is taken for serologic tests.

C. Culture: Growth does not occur in most ordinary bacteriologic media, but small colonies appear in 1–3 days on glucose cysteine blood agar or glucose blood agar incubated at 37 °C under aerobic conditions. The organism is usually identified by its growth requirements and immunofluorescence staining or agglutination by specific antisera. *Caution:* In order to avoid laboratory-acquired infection, *Francisella* should not be cultured in ordinary clinical laboratory facilities; this should be undertaken only with proper isolation facilities.

D. Serology: All isolates are serologically identical, possessing a polysaccharide antigen and one or more protein antigens that cross-react with brucellae. However, there are 2 biological categories of strains, called Jellison type A and type B. Type A occurs only in North America, is lethal for rabbits, produces severe illness in humans, ferments glycerol, and contains citrulline ureidase. Type B lacks these biochemical features, is not lethal for rabbits, produces milder disease in humans, and is isolated often from rodents or from water in Europe, Asia, and North America.

The usual antibody response consists of agglutinins developing 7–10 days after onset of illness. A skin test using an antigen derived by ether extraction of the organism gives a delayed-type positive test before antibodies appear.

Pathogenesis & Clinical Findings

F tularensis is highly infectious: penetration of the skin or mucous membranes or inhalation of 50 organisms can result in infection. Most commonly, organisms enter through skin abrasions. In 2–6 days, an inflammatory, ulcerating papule develops. Regional lymph nodes enlarge and may become necrotic, sometimes draining for weeks. Inhalation of an infective aerosol results in peribronchial inflammation and localized pneumonitis. Oculoglandular tularemia can develop when an infected finger or droplet touches the conjunctiva. Yellowish granulomatous lesions on the lids may be accompanied by preauricular adenopathy. In all cases, there is fever, malaise, headache, and pain in the involved region and regional lymph nodes.

Diagnostic Laboratory Tests

In general, smears and cultures are not contributory, and the diagnosis rests on serologic studies. Paired serum samples collected 2 weeks apart can show a rise in agglutination titer. A single serum titer of 1:160 is highly suggestive if the history and physical findings are compatible with the diagnosis. Because antibodies reactive in the agglutination test for tularemia also react in the test for brucellosis, both tests should be done for positive sera; the titer for the disease affecting the patient is usually 4-fold greater than that for the other disease. A skin test (availability of the antigen is limited) may give a tuberculinlike response in the first week of illness, often before the agglutination titer rises.

Treatment

Streptomycin, 30 mg/kg/d intramuscularly, or gentamicin, 5 mg/kg/d intramuscularly, given in divided doses for 10 days produces almost uniform rapid improvement. Tetracycline, 50 mg/kg/d orally or parenterally, may be equally effective, but relapses occur more frequently.

Prevention & Control

Humans acquire tularemia from handling infected rabbits or muskrats or from bites by an infected tick or deerfly. Less often, the source is contaminated water or food or contact with a dog or cat that has caught an infected wild animal. Avoidance is the key to prevention. The infection in wild animals cannot be controlled.

Persons at exceedingly high risk, particularly laboratory personnel, may be immunized by the administration of a live attenuated strain of *F tularensis* available from the US Army Medical Research Institute of Infectious Diseases, Frederick, MD 21701. The vaccine is administered by multiple puncture through the skin. While not completely protective, it provides partial immunity. A similar live vaccine has been administered in Russia on a large scale.

PASTEURELLAE

Pasteurella species are primarily animal pathogens, but they can produce a range of human diseases. The generic term pasteurellae formerly included all yersiniae and *Francisella* as well as the pasteurellae discussed below.

Pasteurellae are nonmotile gram-negative coccobacilli with a bipolar appearance on stained smears. They are aerobes or facultative anaerobes that grow readily on ordinary bacteriologic media at 37 °C. They are all oxidase-positive and catalase-positive but diverge in other biochemical reactions.

Pasteurella multocida occurs worldwide in the respiratory and gastrointestinal tracts of many domestic and wild animals. It is perhaps the commonest organism in human wounds inflicted by bites from cats and dogs. It is one of the common causes of hemorrhagic septicemia in a variety of animals, including rabbits, rats, horses, sheep, fowl, cats, and swine. It can also produce human infections in many systems and may at times be part of normal human flora.

Pasteurella hemolytica occurs in the upper respiratory tract of cattle, sheep, swine, horses, and fowl. It is a prominent cause of epizootic pneumonia in cattle and sheep and of fowl cholera in chickens and turkeys, causing major economic losses. Human infection appears to be rare.

Pasteurella pneumotropica is a normal inhabitant of the respiratory tract and gut of mice and rats and can cause pneumonia or sepsis when the host-parasite balance is disturbed. A few human infections have followed animal bites.

Pasteurella ureae has rarely been found in animals but occurs as part of a mixed flora in human chronic respiratory disease or other suppurative infections.

Clinical Findings

The commonest presentation is an animal bite, with acute onset of redness, swelling, and pain within hours of the bite. Regional lymphadenopathy is variable, and fever is often low-grade. Sometimes *Pasteurella* infections present as bacteremia or chronic respiratory infection without an evident connection with animals.

REFERENCES

Black RE et al: Epidemic *Yersinia enterocolitica* infection due to contaminated chocolate milk. *N Engl J Med* 1978;**298**:76.

Buchanan TM et al: The tularemia skin test: 325 skin tests in 210 persons—serologic correlation and review of the literature. *Ann Intern Med* 1971;**74**:336.

Butler T et al: *Yersinia pestis* infection in Vietnam. *J Infect Dis* 1976;**133**:493.

Evans ME et al: Tularemia and the tomcat. *JAMA* 1981; **246**:1343.

Guerrant RL et al: Tickborne oculoglandular tularemia: Case report and review of seasonal and vectorial associations in 106 cases. *Arch Intern Med* 1976;**136**:811.

Isberg RR, Falkow S: A single genetic locus encoded by *Yersinia pseudotuberculosis* permits invasion of cultured animal cells by *Escherichia coli* K12. *Nature* 1985;**317**:262.

Johnson RH, Rumans LW: Unusual infections caused by *Pasteurella multocida*. *JAMA* 1977;**237**:146.

Klock LE et al: Tularemia epidemic associated with the deerfly.

JAMA 1973;**226**:149.

Mann JM et al: Peripatetic plague. *JAMA* 1982;**247**:47.

Martone WJ et al: Tularemia pneumonia in Washington, DC. *JAMA* 1979;**242**:4315.

Mason WL et al: Treatment of tularemia, including pulmonary tularemia, with gentamicin. *Am Rev Respir Dis* 1980;**121**:39.

Okamoto K et al: Partial characterization of heat-stable enterotoxin produced by *Yersinia enterocolitica*. *Infect Immun* 1981;**31**:554.

Polt SS et al: Human brucellosis caused by *Brucella canis*. *Ann Intern Med* 1982;**97**:717.

Portnoy DA, Falkow S: Virulence-associated plasmids from *Yersinia enterocolitica* and *Yersinia pestis*. *J Bacteriol* 1981;**148**:877.

Portnoy DA et al: Genetic analysis of essential plasmid determinants of pathogenicity in *Yersinia pestis*. *J Infect Dis* 1983;**148**:297.

Rabson AR et al: Generalized *Yersinia enterocolitica* infection. *J Infect Dis* 1975;**131**:447.

Sheperd AJ et al: Isolation of *Pasteurella pneumotropica* from rodents in South Africa. *J Hygiene* 1982;**89**:79.

Vantrappen G et al: *Yersinia* enteritis. *Med Clin North Am* 1982;**66**:639.

von Reyn CF et al: Epidemiologic and clinical features of an outbreak of bubonic plague in New Mexico. *J Infect Dis* 1977;**136**:489.

Welty TK et al: Nineteen cases of plague in Arizona. *West J Med* 1985;**142**:641.

Williams JE, Cavanaugh DC: Measuring the efficacy of vaccination in affording protection against plague. *Bull WHO* 1979;**57**:309.

21

Vibrios & Campylobacters

Vibrio and *Campylobacter* species are gram-negative rods. Vibrios are widely distributed in marine environments and campylobacters in animals and birds. They are important causes of enteritis. Some strains of *Vibrio cholerae* produce an enterotoxin that causes cholera, a profuse watery diarrhea that can rapidly lead to dehydration and death. *Campylobacter jejuni* is one of the common causes of enteritis in humans.

THE VIBRIOS

Vibrios are among the most common bacteria in surface waters worldwide. They are curved, gram-negative, aerobic rods and are motile, possessing a polar flagellum. They do not form spores. *Vibrio cholerae* serogroup O1 and related vibrios cause cholera in humans, while other vibrios may cause sepsis or enteritis. The vibrios are members of the family *Enterobacteriaceae* (see Chapter 18). The medically important vibrios are listed in Table 21–1.

1. VIBRIO CHOLERAE

V cholerae is a waterborne organism that causes cholera. The epidemiology of cholera (see below) closely parallels the recognition of its transmission in water and the development of sanitary water systems.

Morphology & Identification
A. Typical Organisms: Upon first isolation, *V cholerae* is a comma-shaped, curved rod 2–4 μm long (Fig 21–1). It is actively motile by means of a polar

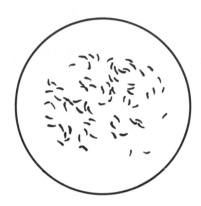

Figure 21–1. Typical organisms of *V cholerae* from broth.

flagellum. On prolonged cultivation, vibrios may become straight rods that resemble the gram-negative enteric bacteria.

B. Culture: *V cholerae* produces convex, smooth, round colonies that are opaque and granular in transmitted light. *V cholerae* and most other vibrios grow well at 37 °C on many kinds of media, including defined media containing mineral salts and asparagine as sources of carbon and nitrogen. *V cholerae* grows well on thiosulfate-citrate-bile-sucrose (TCBS) agar, on which it produces yellow colonies. Vibrios are oxidase-positive, which differentiates them from enteric gram-negative bacteria grown on blood agar. Characteristically, vibrios grow at a very high pH (8.5–9.5) and are rapidly killed by acid. Cultures containing fermentable carbohydrates therefore quickly become sterile.

In areas where cholera is endemic, direct cultures on selective media such as TCBS and enrichment cultures in alkaline peptone water are appropriate. However, routine stool cultures on special media such as TCBS generally are not necessary or cost-effective in areas where cholera is rare.

C. Growth Characteristics: *V cholerae* regularly ferments sucrose and mannose but not arabinose. When grown in a peptone medium containing adequate amounts of tryptophan and nitrate, it produces indole and reduces nitrate. Upon addition of sulfuric acid, a red color develops (nitroso-indole reaction, "cholera red test"). Glucose inhibits this reaction. A positive oxidase test is a key step in the preliminary identification of *V cholerae* and other vibrios.

Table 21–1. The medically important vibrios.

	Human Disease
V cholerae serogroup O1	Epidemic and pandemic cholera.
V cholerae serogroup non-O1	Choleralike diarrhea; mild diarrhea; rarely, extraintestinal infection.
V parahaemolyticus	Gastroenteritis, possibly extraintestinal infection.
Others (*V mimicus, V vulnificus, V hollisae, V fluvialis, V damsela, V alginolyticus, V metschnikovii*)	Ear, wound, soft tissue, and other extraintestinal infections, all uncommon.

Antigenic Structure & Biologic Classification

Many vibrios share a single heat-labile flagellar H antigen. Antibodies to the H antigen are probably not involved in the protection of susceptible hosts.

V cholerae has O lipopolysaccharides that confer serologic specificity. There are more than 100 O antigen groups, depending upon the classification scheme. *V cholerae* strains of O group 1 cause classic cholera; occasionally non-O1 *V cholerae* cause choleralike disease. Antibodies to the O antigens tend to protect laboratory animals against infections with *V cholerae*.

The group O1 antigen has 3 determinants, which occur in combinations and are termed the Inaba, Ogawa, and Hikojima serotypes. The "classical" and El Tor biotypes are distinguished on the basis of hemolysis and antimicrobial susceptibility patterns. Serotype and biotype identifications are used for epidemiologic studies.

Vibrio cholerae Enterotoxin

V cholerae and related vibrios produce a heat-labile enterotoxin with a molecular weight of about 80,000, consisting of subunits A (MW 28,000) and B. Ganglioside G_{M1} serves as the mucosal receptor for subunit B, which promotes entry of subunit A into the cell. Subunit A activates adenylate cyclase and results in prolonged hypersecretion of water and electrolytes—as much as 20 L daily—leading to severe dehydration, shock, acidosis, and death. The genes for *V cholerae* enterotoxin are on the bacterial chromosome. Cholera enterotoxin is antigenically related to LT of *Escherichia coli* and can stimulate the production of neutralizing antibodies. However, the precise role of antitoxic and antibacterial antibodies in protection against cholera is not clear.

Some strains of *V cholerae* (eg, El Tor) produce soluble hemolysins. Others digest red blood cells without liberating a soluble hemolysin. They remove myxovirus receptors from the red cell surface by means of a receptor-destroying enzyme, neuraminidase.

Pathogenesis & Pathology

Under natural conditions, *V cholerae* is pathogenic only for humans. A person may have to ingest 10^8–10^{10} organisms to become infected and develop disease, in contrast to salmonellosis or shigellosis, in which ingestion of 10^2–10^5 organisms can induce infection.

Cholera is not an invasive infection. The organisms do not reach the bloodstream but remain localized within the intestinal tract. There they multiply, invade superficial epithelium, and liberate cholera toxin and perhaps mucinases and endotoxin. Cholera toxin is adsorbed onto epithelial cell gangliosides and stimulates hypersecretion of water and chloride in all parts of the small intestine while inhibiting absorption of sodium. As a result, there is an outpouring of fluid and electrolytes, with resulting diarrhea, dehydration, acidosis, shock, and death.

Clinical Findings

After an incubation period of 1–4 days, there is a sudden onset of nausea and vomiting and profuse diarrhea with abdominal cramps. The stools resemble "rice water" and contain mucus, epithelial cells, and large numbers of vibrios. There is rapid loss of fluid and electrolytes, which leads to profound dehydration, circulatory collapse, and anuria. The mortality rate without treatment is between 25% and 50%. The diagnosis of a full-blown case of cholera presents no problem in the presence of an epidemic. However, sporadic or mild cases are not readily differentiated from other diarrheal diseases. The El Tor biotype tends to cause milder disease than the "classical" biotype.

Diagnostic Laboratory Tests

A. Specimens: Specimens for culture consist of mucus flecks from stools.

B. Smears: The microscopic appearance of smears made from stool samples is not distinctive. Darkfield or phase contrast microscopy may show the rapidly motile vibrios.

C. Culture: Growth is rapid in peptone agar, on blood agar with a pH near 9.0, or on TCBS agar, and typical colonies can be picked in 18 hours. For enrichment, a few drops of stool can be incubated for 6–8 hours in taurocholate-peptone broth (pH 8.0–9.0); organisms from this culture can be stained or subcultured.

D. Specific Tests: *V cholerae* organisms are further identified by slide agglutination tests using anti-O group 1 antiserum and by biochemical reaction patterns.

Immunity

Gastric acid provides some protection against cholera vibrios ingested in small numbers.

An attack of cholera is followed by immunity to reinfection, but the duration and degree of immunity are not known. In experimental animals, specific IgA antibodies occur in the lumen of the intestine. Similar antibodies in serum develop after infection but last only a few months. The relative roles of vibriocidal and antitoxic antibodies in the circulation and in the gut are not established.

Treatment

The most important part of therapy consists of water and electrolyte replacement to correct the severe dehydration and salt depletion. Many antimicrobial agents are effective against *V cholerae*. Oral tetracycline tends to reduce stool output in cholera and shortens the period of excretion of vibrios. In some endemic areas, tetracycline resistance of *V cholerae* has emerged, carried by transmissible plasmids.

Epidemiology, Prevention, & Control

Worldwide epidemics of cholera occurred in the 1800s and early 1900s. The "classical" biotype was prevalent through the early 1960s; the El Tor biotype, discovered in 1905, became prevalent in the late 1960s and has caused pandemic disease in Asia, the Middle East, and Africa. The disease has been rare in North America since the mid 1800s, but an endemic focus may exist on the Gulf Coast of Louisiana and Texas.

Cholera is endemic in India and Southeast Asia. From these centers, it is carried along shipping lanes, trade routes, and pilgrim migration routes. The disease is spread by individuals with mild or early illness and by water, food, flies, and person-to-person contact. In many instances, only 1–5% of exposed susceptible persons develop disease. The carrier state seldom exceeds 3–4 weeks, and true chronic carriers are rare. Vibrios survive in water for up to 3 weeks.

Control rests on education and on improvement of sanitation, particularly of food and water. Patients should be isolated, their excreta disinfected, and contacts followed up. Chemoprophylaxis with antimicrobial drugs may have a place. Repeated injection of a vaccine containing either lipopolysaccharides extracted from vibrios or dense *Vibrio* suspensions can confer limited protection to heavily exposed persons (eg, family contacts) but is not effective as an epidemic control measure. Very few countries require that travelers arriving from endemic areas have proof of immunization with these vaccines. The WHO vaccination certificate for cholera is only valid for 6 months.

2. *VIBRIO PARAHAEMOLYTICUS & OTHER VIBRIOS*

Vibrio parahaemolyticus is a halophilic bacterium that causes acute gastroenteritis following ingestion of contaminated seafood such as raw fish or shellfish. After an incubation period of 12–24 hours, nausea and vomiting, abdominal cramps, fever, and watery to bloody diarrhea occur. The mechanism of illness is not yet clear; fecal leukocytes are often observed. The enteritis tends to subside spontaneously in 1–4 days with no treatment other than restoration of water and electrolyte balance. No enterotoxin has yet been isolated from this organism. The disease occurs worldwide, with highest incidence in areas where people eat raw seafood. *V parahaemolyticus* does not grow well on some of the differential media used to grow salmonellae and shigellae, but it does grow well on blood agar. It also grows well on TCBS, where it yields green colonies. *V parahaemolyticus* is usually identified by its oxidase-positive growth on blood agar.

Vibrio vulnificus is also a halophilic *Vibrio* from seawater. It can cause intense skin lesions in persons who have handled shellfish or other marine animals and can occasionally produce enteritis, bacteremia, and death in elderly or debilitated persons.

Several other vibrios also cause disease in humans: *V mimicus* causes diarrhea after ingestion of uncooked seafood, particularly raw oysters. *V hollisae* and *V fluvialis* also cause diarrhea. *V alginolyticus* causes eye, ear, or wound infection after exposure to seawa-ter. *V damsela* also causes wound infections. Other vibrios are very uncommon causes of disease in humans.

THE CAMPYLOBACTERS

These organisms were formerly grouped with vibrios and were known mainly as pathogens for various animals, in whom they caused sepsis, abortion, or enteritis. The widespread use of selective media since the 1970s has greatly increased the recognition of *Campylobacter jejuni* as a common cause of diarrhea in humans. The medically important campylobacters are listed in Table 21–2.

1. *CAMPYLOBACTER JEJUNI*

C jejuni has emerged as a common human pathogen, causing mainly enteritis and occasionally systemic invasion. The bacterium is at least as common as salmonellae and shigellae as a cause of diarrhea; an estimated 2 million cases occur in the USA each year.

Morphology & Identification

A. Typical Organisms: *C jejuni* and the other campylobacters are gram-negative rods with comma, S, or "gull-wing" shapes. They are motile, with a single polar flagellum, and do not form spores.

B. Culture: The culture characteristics are most important in the isolation and identification of *C jejuni* and the other campylobacters. Selective media are needed, and incubation must be in an atmosphere with reduced O_2 (5% O_2) with added CO_2 (10% CO_2). A relatively simple way to produce the incubation atmosphere is to place the plates in an anaerobe incubation jar without the catalyst and to produce the gas with a commercially available gas-generating pack or by gas exchange. Incubation of primary plates should be at 42–43 °C. Although *C jejuni* grows well at 36–37 °C, incubation at 42 °C prohibits growth of most of the other bacteria present in feces, thus simplifying the identification of *C jejuni*. Several selective media are in widespread use: Skirrow's medium incorporates

Table 21–2. The medically important *Campylobacter* species.

	Reservoir	Human Disease
C jejuni	Many animals and birds.	Diarrhea (common).
C fetus subspecies *fetus*	Cattle and sheep.	Septicemia in debilitated and immunocompromised patients.
C coli	Pigs.	Diarrhea.
C laridis	Animals and birds.	Diarrhea.
C cinaedi, C hyo-intestinalis, and *C fennelliae*		Infections in homosexual men.

vancomycin, polymyxin B, and trimethoprim; Campy BAP medium includes cephalothin as well. Both media are suitable for isolation of *C jejuni* at 42 °C; when incubated at 36–37 °C, Skirrow's medium is helpful in isolating other campylobacters but Campy BAP medium is not, since many of the other campylobacters are susceptible to cephalothin. The colonies tend to be colorless or gray. They may be watery and spreading or round and convex, and both colony types may appear on one agar plate.

C. Growth Characteristics: Because of the selective media and incubation conditions for growth, an abbreviated set of tests is usually all that is necessary for identification. *C jejuni* and the other campylobacters pathogenic for humans are oxidase- and catalase-positive. Campylobacters do not oxidize or ferment carbohydrates. Gram-stained smears show typical morphology. Nitrate reduction, hydrogen sulfide production, hippurate tests, and antimicrobial susceptibilities can be used for further identification of species.

Antigenic Structure & Toxins

The campylobacters have lipopolysaccharides with endotoxic activity. Cytopathic extracellular toxins and enterotoxins have been found, but the significance of the toxins in human disease is not well understood.

Pathogenesis & Pathology

The infection is acquired by the oral route from food, drink, contact with infected animals, or anal-genital-oral sexual activity. *C jejuni* is susceptible to gastric acid, and ingestion of about 10^4 organisms is usually necessary to produce infection. This inoculum is similar to that required for *Salmonella* and *Shigella* infection but less than that for *Vibrio* infection. The organisms multiply in the small intestine, invade the epithelium, and produce inflammation that results in the appearance of red and white blood cells in the stools. Occasionally, the bloodstream is invaded and a clinical picture of enteric fever develops. Localized tissue invasion coupled with the toxic activity appears to be responsible for the enteritis.

Clinical Findings

Clinical manifestations are acute onset of crampy abdominal pain, profuse diarrhea that may be grossly bloody, headache, malaise, and fever. Usually the illness is self-limited to a period of 5–8 days, but occasionally it continues longer. *C jejuni* isolates are usually susceptible to erythromycin, and therapy shortens the duration of fecal shedding of bacteria. Most cases resolve without antimicrobial therapy.

Diagnostic Laboratory Tests

A. Specimens: Diarrheal stool is the usual specimen. Campylobacters from other types of specimens are usually incidental findings or are found in the setting of known outbreaks of disease.

B. Smears: Gram-stained smears of stool may show the typical "gull-wing"-shaped rods. Darkfield or phase contrast microscopy may show the typical darting motility of the organisms.

C. Culture: Culture on the selective media described above is the definitive test to diagnose *C jejuni* enteritis. If another species of *Campylobacter* is suspected, medium without cephalothin should be used and incubated at 36–37 °C.

Epidemiology & Control

Campylobacter enteritis resembles other acute bacterial diarrheas, particularly *Shigella* dysentery. The source of infection may be food (eg, milk), contact with infected animals or humans and their excreta, or oral-anal sexual contact. Outbreaks arising from a common source, eg, unpasteurized milk, may require public health control measures. Human carriers exist, but their role in transmission is unknown.

2. OTHER *CAMPYLOBACTER* SPECIES

Campylobacter species other than *C jejuni* are encountered infrequently. This is partially due to the standard methods used for isolation of campylobacters from stool specimens. *C coli* occasionally causes diarrhea. *C fetus* subspecies *fetus* sometimes causes systemic infection in debilitated patients. *C laridis* is often found in sea gulls and occasionally causes diarrhea in humans. A group of *Campylobacter*-like organisms (CLO) have been isolated from stool cultures from homosexual men and have been given species names (Table 21–2).

REFERENCES

Barker WH Jr, Gangarosa EJ: Food poisoning due to *Vibrio parahaemolyticus*. *Annu Rev Med* 1974;**25**:75.

Blake PA et al: Disease caused by a marine vibrio: Clinical characteristics and epidemiology. *N Engl J Med* 1979;**300**:1.

Blake PA et al: Disease of humans (other than cholera) caused by vibrios. *Annu Rev Microbiol* 1980;**34**:341.

Blaser MJ, Reller LB: *Campylobacter* enteritis. *N Engl J Med* 1981;**305**:1444.

Blaser MJ et al: *Campylobacter* enteritis in the United States: A multicenter study. *Ann Intern Med* 1983;**98**:360.

Blaser MJ et al: Reservoirs for human campylobacteriosis. *J Infect Dis* 1980;**141**:665.

Cash RA et al: Response of man to infection with *Vibrio cholerae*. 1. Clinical, serologic, and bacteriologic responses to a known inoculum. *J Infect Dis* 1974;**129**:45.

Colwell RR: Polyphasic taxonomy of the genus *Vibrio:* Numerical taxonomy of *Vibrio cholerae*, *Vibrio parahaemolyticus*, and related *Vibrio* species. *J Bacteriol* 1970;**104**:410.

Fennell CL et al: Characterization of *Campylobacter*-like organisms isolated from homosexual men. *J Infect Dis* 1984;**149**:58.

Field M: Modes of action of enterotoxins from *Vibrio cholerae* and *Escherichia coli*. *Rev Infect Dis* 1979;**1**:918.

Guerrant RL et al: Campylobacteriosis in man: Pathogenic mechanisms and review of 91 blood stream infections. *Am J Med* 1978;**65**:584.

Hornick RB et al: The Broad Street pump revisited: Response of volunteers to ingested cholera vibrios. *Bull NY Acad Med* 1971;**47**:1192.

Klipstein FA, Engert RF: Properties of crude *Campylobacter jejuni* heat-labile enterotoxin. *Infect Immun* 1984;**45**:314.

Morris JG et al: Non-O group 1 *Vibrio cholerae* gastroenteritis in the United States: Clinical, epidemiological, and laboratory characteristics of sporadic cases. *Ann Intern Med* 1981;**94**:656.

Pai CH et al: Erythromycin in treatment of *Campylobacter* enteritis in children. *Am J Dis Child* 1983;**137**:286.

Rodrick GE et al: Human *Vibrio* gastroenteritis. *Med Clin North Am* 1982;**66**:665.

Ruiz-Palacios GM et al: Cholera-like enterotoxin produced by *Campylobacter jejuni*. *Lancet* 1983;**2**:250.

Samadi AR et al: Classical *Vibrio cholerae* biotype displaces El Tor in Bangladesh. *Lancet* 1983;**1**:805.

Skirrow MB: *Campylobacter* enteritis: A "new" disease. *Br Med J* 1977;**2**:9.

Sommer A et al: Efficacy of cholera vaccination. *Lancet* 1973;**1**:230.

Haemophilus, Bordetella, & Brucella

22

THE *HAEMOPHILUS* SPECIES

This is a group of small, gram-negative, pleomorphic bacteria that require enriched media, usually containing blood or its derivatives, for isolation. *Haemophilus influenzae* type b is an important human pathogen; *Haemophilus ducreyi,* a sexually transmitted pathogen, causes chancroid; others are among the normal flora of mucous membranes.

1. *HAEMOPHILUS INFLUENZAE*

H influenzae is found on the mucous membranes of the upper respiratory tract in humans. It is an important cause of meningitis in children and occasionally causes respiratory tract infections in children and adults.

Morphology & Identification

A. Typical Organisms: In specimens from acute infections, the organisms are short ($1.5 \mu m$) coccoid bacilli, sometimes occurring in short chains. In cultures, the morphology depends both on age and on the medium. At 6–8 hours in rich medium, coccobacillary forms predominate. Later there are longer rods, lysed bacteria, and very pleomorphic forms.

Organisms in young cultures (6–18 hours) on rich medium have a definite capsule. Capsule swelling tests are used for "typing" *H influenzae* (see below).

B. Culture: On brain-heart infusion agar with blood, small, round, convex colonies with a strong iridescence develop in 24 hours. The colonies on "chocolate" (heated blood) agar take 36–48 hours to develop diameters of 1 mm. Isovitalex in media enhances growth. There is no hemolysis. Around staphylococcal (or other) colonies, the colonies of *H influenzae* grow much larger ("satellite phenomenon").

C. Growth Characteristics: Identification of organisms of the *Haemophilus* group depends in part upon demonstrating the need for certain growth factors called X and V. Factor X acts physiologically as hemin; factor V can be replaced by nicotinamide adenine nucleotide (NAD) or other coenzymes. The requirements for X and V factors of various *Haemophilus* species are listed in Table 22–1. Carbohydrates are fermented poorly and irregularly.

D. Variation: In addition to morphologic variation, *H influenzae* has a marked tendency to lose its capsule and the associated type specificity. Nonencapsulated variant colonies lack iridescence.

E. Transformation: Under proper experimental circumstances, the DNA extracted from a given type of *H influenzae* is capable of transferring that type specificity to other cells (transformation). Resistance to ampicillin and chloramphenicol is controlled by genes on transmissible plasmids.

Antigenic Structure

Encapsulated *H influenzae* contains capsular polysaccharides (MW > 150,000) of one of 6 types (a–f). The capsular antigen of type b is a polyribose-ribitol phosphate (PRP). Encapsulated *H influenzae* can be typed by a capsule swelling test with specific antiserum; this test is analogous to the "quellung test" for pneumococci. Comparable typing can be done by immunofluorescence as well. Most *H influenzae* organisms in the normal flora of the upper respiratory tract are not encapsulated.

The somatic antigen of *H influenzae* consists of at least 2 proteins: the P substance constitutes much of the bacterial body, whereas the M substance is a labile surface antigen. Typical endotoxic lipopolysaccharides can be derived from many fluid cultures of *H influenzae,* but their antigenic nature is not clear.

Pathogenesis

H influenzae produces no exotoxin, and the role of its toxic somatic antigen in natural disease is not clearly understood. The nonencapsulated organism is a regular member of the normal respiratory flora of humans. The encapsulated forms of *H influenzae,* partic-

Table 22–1. Characteristics and growth requirements of some hemophilic bacteria.

Organism	Hemolysis	Requires		Capsule
		X	V	
H influenzae	–	+	+	+
H parainfluenzae	–	–	+	+
H haemolyticus	+	+	+	–
H suis	–	+	+	+
H haemoglobinophilus	–	+	–	–
B pertussis	+	–	–	+

ularly type b, produce suppurative respiratory infections (sinusitis, laryngotracheitis, epiglottitis, otitis) and, in young children, meningitis. The blood of many persons over age 3–5 years is bactericidal for *H influenzae,* and clinical infections are less frequent in such individuals. Recently, however, bactericidal antibodies have been absent from 25% of adults in the USA, and clinical infections are occurring more often in adults.

In human influenza of the pandemic type, *H influenzae* was probably a secondary invader producing pneumonitis in respiratory tracts already damaged by influenza virus. On the other hand, *Haemophilus suis* is an essential component in the pathogenesis of swine influenza. Swine influenza is caused by a virus related to influenza type A but requires in addition the presence of *H suis* for the development of clinical symptoms. *H influenzae* is not pathogenic for laboratory animals.

Clinical Findings

H influenzae type b enters by way of the respiratory tract in small children and produces a nasopharyngitis, often with fever. Other types rarely produce disease. There may be local extension with involvement of the sinuses or the middle ear. *H influenzae* type b and pneumococci are the 2 commonest etiologic agents of bacterial otitis media and acute sinusitis. The organisms may reach the bloodstream and be carried to the meninges or, less frequently, may establish themselves in the joints to produce septic arthritis. *H influenzae* is now the commonest cause of bacterial meningitis in children age 5 months to 5 years in the USA. Clinically, it resembles other forms of childhood meningitis, and diagnosis rests on bacteriologic demonstration of the organism.

Occasionally, a fulminating obstructive laryngotracheitis with swollen, cherry-red epiglottis develops in infants and requires prompt tracheostomy or intubation as a lifesaving procedure. Pneumonitis and epiglottitis due to *H influenzae* may follow upper respiratory tract infections in small children and old or debilitated people.

Diagnostic Laboratory Tests

A. Specimens: Specimens consist of nasopharyngeal swabs, pus, blood, and spinal fluid for smears and cultures.

B. Direct Identification: When organisms are present in large numbers in specimens, they may be identified by immunofluorescence or mixed directly with specific rabbit antiserum (tybe b) for a capsule swelling test. Commercial kits are available for immunologic detection of *H influenzae* antigens in spinal fluid. A positive test indicates the fluid contains high concentrations of specific polysaccharide from *H influenzae* type b.

C. Culture: Specimens are grown on Isovitalex-enriched chocolate agar until typical colonies can be identified with the capsule swelling test (36–48 hours). *H influenzae* is differentiated from related gram-negative bacilli by its requirements for X and V factors, its lack of hemolysis on blood agar (Table 22–1), and by immunologic means.

Immunity

Infants under age 3 months may have serum antibodies transmitted from the mother. During this time *H influenzae* infection is rare, but subsequently the antibodies are lost. Children often acquire *H influenzae* infections, which are usually asymptomatic but may be in the form of respiratory disease or meningitis (*H influenzae* is the most common cause of bacterial meningitis in children from 5 months to 5 years of age). By age 3–5 years, many children have anti-PRP antibodies that promote complement-dependent phagocytosis. Injection of PRP into children over 2 years of age induces the same antibodies, but in children under age 2 years, the present preparations are poorly immunogenic. The same antibodies can also be induced by cross-reacting *E coli* O75:K100:H5 carried in the gut.

There is a correlation between the presence of bactericidal antibodies and resistance to major *H influenzae* type b infections. However, it is not known whether these antibodies alone account for immunity. Pneumonia or arthritis due to *H influenzae* can develop in adults with such antibodies.

Treatment

The mortality rate of untreated *H influenzae* meningitis may be up to 90%. Many strains of *H influenzae* type b are susceptible to ampicillin, but up to 25% produce β-lactamase under control of a transmissible plasmid and are resistant. Most strains are susceptible to chloramphenicol, and essentially all strains are susceptible to the newer cephalosporins. Cefotaxime, 150–200 mg/kg/d intravenously, may give excellent results; it or similar drugs may become the treatment of choice. Prompt diagnosis and antimicrobial therapy are essential to minimize late neurologic and intellectual impairment. Prominent among late complications of influenzal meningitis is the development of a localized subdural accumulation of fluid that requires surgical drainage.

Epidemiology, Prevention, & Control

Encapsulated *H influenzae* type b is transmitted from person to person by the respiratory route. The patient with influenzal meningitis is not an important source of infection. Because an increasing number of adults lack bactericidal antibody and are susceptible to systemic *Haemophilus* infections, immunization with capsular polysaccharides (PRP vaccine) is now proposed for mothers at high risk who lack antibody; it should also be given to all children over age 2 years and to those between 18 and 23 months of age who are at high risk (eg, children who attend day care centers and those with asplenia). Children under age 2 may require a second vaccine dose later.

Contact with patients suffering from *H influenzae* clinical infection poses little risk for **adults but** presents a definite risk for siblings and close contacts under age 4 years. Prophylaxis with rifampin, 20 mg/kg/d for 4 days, is recommended for such children.

2. HAEMOPHILUS AEGYPTIUS

This organism was formerly called the Koch-Weeks bacillus; it is sometimes called *H influenzae* biotype III. It resembles *H influenzae* closely and has been associated with a highly communicable form of conjunctivitis.

3. HAEMOPHILUS APHROPHILUS

This organism is sometimes encountered in infective endocarditis and pneumonia. It is present in the normal oral and respiratory tract flora. It is related to *Actinobacillus (Haemophilus) actinomycetemcomitans* and is occasionally mistaken for *Actinomyces*.

4. HAEMOPHILUS DUCREYI

H ducreyi causes chancroid (soft chancre), a sexually transmitted disease. Chancroid consists of a ragged ulcer on the genitalia, with marked swelling and tenderness. The regional lymph nodes are enlarged and painful. The disease must be differentiated from syphilis, herpes simplex infection, and lymphogranuloma venereum.

The small gram-negative rods occur in strands in the lesions, usually in association with other pyogenic microorganisms. *H ducreyi* requires X factor but not V factor. It is grown best from scrapings of the ulcer base on chocolate agar containing 1% Isovitalex and vancomycin, 3 μg/mL, and incubated in 10% CO_2 at 35 °C. There is no permanent immunity following chancroid infection. Treatment with oral trimethoprim-sulfamethoxazole or oral erythromycin often results in healing in 2 weeks.

5. OTHER HAEMOPHILUS SPECIES

Haemophilus haemoglobinophilus requires X factor but not V factor and has been found in dogs but not in human disease. *Haemophilus haemolyticus* is the most markedly hemolytic organism of the group in vitro; it occurs both in the normal nasopharynx and in association with rare upper respiratory tract infections of moderate severity in childhood. *Haemophilus parainfluenzae* resembles *H influenzae* and is a normal inhabitant of the human respiratory tract; it has been encountered occasionally in infective endocarditis and in urethritis. *Haemophilus suis* resembles *H influenzae* bacteriologically and acts synergistically with swine influenza virus to produce the disease in hogs.

THE BORDETELLAE

There are 3 species of bordetellae. *Bordetella pertussis,* a highly communicable and important pathogen of humans, causes whooping cough (pertussis). *Bordetella parapertussis* and *Bordetella bronchiseptica* are much less common causes of disease.

1. BORDETELLA PERTUSSIS

Morphology & Identification
A. Typical Organisms: The organisms are short, gram-negative coccobacilli resembling *H influenzae*. With toluidine blue stain, bipolar metachromatic granules can be demonstrated. A capsule is present.

B. Culture: Primary isolation of *B pertussis* requires enriched media. Bordet-Gengou medium (potato-blood-glycerol agar) that contains penicillin G, 0.5 μg/mL, is used; a charcoal-containing medium similar to that used for *Legionella pneumophila* is also suitable. When the plates are incubated at 35–37 °C for 3–7 days in a moist environment (eg, a sealed plastic bag), "mercury drop" or "pearl" colonies form. The small, faintly gram-negative rods are identified by immunofluorescence staining.

C. Growth Characteristics: The organism is a strict aerobe and forms acid but not gas from glucose and lactose. It does not require X and V factors on subculture. Hemolysis of blood-containing medium is associated with virulent *B pertussis*.

D. Variation: When isolated from patients and cultured on enriched media, *B pertussis* is in the smooth, encapsulated, virulent phase I. Phase IV is the designation for the form that does not produce toxin and lacks other virulence factors. Phases II and III are intermediates.

Antigenic Structure & Biologically Active Substances
B pertussis is serotyped on the basis of K agglutinogens and contains type 1 and at least one other, most commonly type 3. The cell wall also contains lipopolysaccharide.

There are several biologically active substances. Pertussis toxin, the major virulence factor, is an exotoxin and elicits prolonged immunity; it has histamine-sensitizing and islet cell–activating properties and is responsible for the paroxysmal coughing characteristic of the disease. Phase I variants contain pertussis toxin while phase IV variants do not. The biologically active substances important to the virulence of phase I *B pertussis* are under genetic control of a single gene. There are 2 hemagglutinins, a fimbrial hemagglutinin and a leukocytosis-promoting factor, which promotes marked lymphocytosis in the host. Adenylate cyclase complexes impair normal phagocytic cell function. A heat-labile toxin and several other antigens are found in the protoplasm upon disruption of the cell.

Pathogenesis & Pathology

B pertussis survives for only brief periods outside the human host. There are no vectors. Transmission is largely by the respiratory route from early cases and possibly via carriers. The organism adheres to and multiplies rapidly on the epithelial surface of the trachea and bronchi and interferes with ciliary action. The blood is not invaded. The bacteria liberate toxins and substances that irritate surface cells, causing coughing and marked lymphocytosis. Later, there may be necrosis of parts of the epithelium and polymorphonuclear infiltration, with peribronchial inflammation and interstitial pneumonia. Secondary invaders like staphylococci or *H influenzae* may give rise to bacterial pneumonia. Obstruction of the smaller bronchioles by mucous plugs results in atelectasis and diminished oxygenation of the blood. This probably contributes to the frequency of convulsions.

Clinical Findings

After an incubation period of about 2 weeks, the "catarrhal stage" develops, with mild coughing and sneezing. During this stage, large numbers of organisms are sprayed in droplets, and the patient is highly infectious but not very ill. During the "paroxysmal" stage, the cough develops its explosive character and the characteristic "whoop" upon inhalation. This leads to rapid exhaustion and may be associated with vomiting, cyanosis, and convulsions. The "whoop" and major complications occur predominantly in infants; paroxysmal coughing predominates in older children and adults. The white blood count is high (16,000–30,000/μL), with an absolute lymphocytosis. Convalescence is slow. Rarely, whooping cough is followed by the serious and potentially fatal complication of encephalitis. Several types of adenovirus and *Chlamydia trachomatis* can produce a clinical picture resembling that caused by *B pertussis*.

Diagnostic Laboratory Tests

Specimens consist of nasopharyngeal swabs or cough droplets expelled onto a "cough plate" held in front of the patient's mouth during a paroxysm.

A. Direct Fluorescent Antibody (FA) Test: The FA reagent can be used to examine nasopharyngeal swab specimens. However, false-positive and false-negative results may occur. The FA test is most useful in identifying *B pertussis* after culture on solid media.

B. Culture: Collected mucus or droplets are cultured on modified Bordet-Gengou or blood-charcoal agar (see above). The antibiotics in the media tend to inhibit other respiratory flora but permit growth of *B pertussis*. The iridescent 1- to 2-mm colonies may be surrounded by a narrow zone of hemolysis. Organisms are identified by immunofluorescence staining or by slide agglutination with specific antiserum.

C. Serology: Serologic tests on patients are of little diagnostic help, because a rise in agglutinating or precipitating antibodies does not occur until the third week of illness.

Immunity

Recovery from whooping cough or adequate vaccination is followed by immunity. Second infections may occur but are mild; reinfections occurring years later in adults may be severe. It is probable that the first defense against *B pertussis* infection is the antibody that prevents attachment of the bacteria to the cilia of the respiratory epithelium. Toxin-producing phase I cells are necessary to make pertussis vaccine.

Treatment

B pertussis is susceptible to several antimicrobial drugs in vitro. Administration of erythromycin during the catarrhal stage of disease promotes elimination of the organisms and may have prophylactic value. Treatment after onset of the paroxysmal phase rarely alters the clinical course. Oxygen inhalation and sedation may prevent anoxic damage to the brain.

Prevention

During the first year of life, every infant should receive 3 injections of killed phase I *B pertussis* organisms. This crude suspension of bacteria, in proper concentration, is usually administered in combination with toxoids of diphtheria and tetanus (DTP; see Table 12–6). The *B pertussis* component is an effective immunogen but can lead to neurologic reactions similar to the encephalitis seen with pertussis. Should this happen, DTP should not be given again; instead, DT should be substituted. Vaccine quality and acceptance of the preparation are variable. When pertussis vaccination was discontinued in some areas, the number of clinical cases increased markedly. It is hoped that a purer antigen may be developed for universal use in the future.

Prophylactic administration of erythromycin for 5 days may also benefit unimmunized infants or heavily exposed adults.

Epidemiology & Control

Whooping cough is endemic in most densely populated areas worldwide and also occurs intermittently in epidemics. The source of infection is usually a patient in the early catarrhal stage of the disease. Communicability is high, ranging from 30 to 90%. Most cases occur in children under age 5 years; most deaths occur in the first year of life.

Control of whooping cough rests mainly on adequate active immunization of all infants.

2. BORDETELLA BRONCHISEPTICA

B bronchiseptica is a small gram-negative bacillus that inhabits the respiratory tracts of canines, in which it may cause "kennel cough" and pneumonitis. It grows on blood agar medium.

3. *BORDETELLA PARAPERTUSSIS*

This organism may produce a disease similar to whooping cough. The infection is often subclinical. *B parapertussis* grows more rapidly than typical *B pertussis* and produces larger colonies. It also grows on blood agar.

THE BRUCELLAE

The brucellae are obligate parasites of animals and humans and are characteristically located intracellularly. They are relatively inactive metabolically. *Brucella melitensis* typically infects goats; *Brucella suis,* swine; *Brucella abortus,* cattle; and *Brucella canis,* dogs. The disease in humans, brucellosis (undulant fever, Malta fever), is characterized by an acute bacteremic phase followed by a chronic stage that may extend over many years and may involve many tissues.

Morphology & Identification

A. Typical Organisms: The appearance in young cultures varies from cocci to rods 1.2 μm in length, with short coccobacillary forms predominating. They are gram-negative but often stain irregularly, and are aerobic, nonmotile, and nonsporeforming. Capsules can be demonstrated on smooth and mucoid variants.

B. Culture: Small, convex, smooth colonies appear on enriched media in 2–5 days.

C. Growth Characteristics: Brucellae are adapted to an intracellular habitat, and their nutritional requirements are complex. Some strains have been cultivated on defined media containing amino acids, vitamins, salts, and glucose. Fresh specimens from animal or human sources are usually inoculated on trypticase-soy agar or blood culture media. *B abortus* requires 5–10% CO_2 for growth, whereas the other 3 species grow in air.

Brucellae utilize carbohydrates but produce neither acid nor gas in amounts sufficient for classification. Catalase and oxidase are produced by some strains. Hydrogen sulfide is produced by many strains, and nitrates are reduced to nitrites.

Brucellae are moderately sensitive to heat and acidity. They are killed in milk by pasteurization.

D. Variation: Smooth, mucoid, and rough variants are recognized by colonial appearance and virulence. The typical virulent organism forms a smooth,

transparent colony; upon culture, it tends to mutate to the rough form, which is avirulent.

The serum of susceptible animals contains a globulin and a lipoprotein that suppress growth of nonsmooth, avirulent types and favor the growth of virulent types. Resistant animal species lack these factors, so that rapid mutation to avirulence can occur. D-Alanine has a similar effect in vitro.

Antigenic Structure

Different species of brucellae cannot be differentiated by agglutination tests but can be distinguished by agglutinin absorption reactions. It is probable that 2 antigens, A and M, are present in different proportions in the 4 species. In addition, a superficial L antigen has been demonstrated that resembles the Vi antigen of salmonellae.

Species differentiation among the 4 *Brucella* species is made possible by their characteristic sensitivity to dyes and their production of H_2S (Table 22–2).

Pathogenesis & Pathology

Although each species of *Brucella* has a preferred host, all can infect a wide range of animals, including humans.

The common routes of infection in humans are the intestinal tract (ingestion of infected milk), mucous membranes (droplets), and skin (contact with infected tissues of animals). The organisms progress from the portal of entry, via lymphatic channels and regional lymph nodes, to the thoracic duct and the bloodstream, which distributes them to the parenchymatous organs. Granulomatous nodules that may develop into abscesses form in lymphatic tissue, liver, spleen, bone marrow, and other parts of the reticuloendothelial system. In such lesions, the brucellae are principally intracellular. Osteomyelitis, meningitis, or cholecystitis also occasionally occurs. The main histologic reaction in brucellosis consists of proliferation of mononuclear cells, exudation of fibrin, coagulation necrosis, and fibrosis. The granulomas consist of epithelioid and giant cells, with central necrosis and peripheral fibrosis.

The 4 brucellae that infect humans have apparent differences in pathogenicity. *B abortus* usually causes mild disease without suppurative complications; noncaseating granulomas of the reticuloendothelial system are found. *B canis* also causes mild disease. *B suis* infection tends to be chronic with suppurative lesions; caseating granulomas may be present. *B melitensis* infection is more acute and severe.

Table 22–2. Characteristics of brucellae.

Organism	Preferred Host	CO₂ Requirement	H₂S Production	Growth in Presence of	
				Thionine (1:25,000)	Basic Fuchsin (1:50,000)
B abortus	Cattle	+	++	–	+
B melitensis	Goats, sheep	–	–	–	+
B suis	Swine	–	+	+	–
B canis	Dogs	–	–	+	–

Persons with active brucellosis react more markedly (fever, myalgia) than normal persons to injected *Brucella* endotoxin. Sensitivity to endotoxin thus may play a role in pathogenesis.

Placentas and fetal membranes of cattle, swine, sheep, and goats contain erythritol, a growth factor for brucellae. The proliferation of organisms in pregnant animals leads to placentitis and abortion in these species. There is no erythritol in human placentas, and abortion is not part of *Brucella* infection of humans.

Clinical Findings

The incubation period is 1–6 weeks. The onset is insidious, with malaise, fever, weakness, aches, and sweats. The fever usually rises in the afternoon; its fall during the night is accompanied by drenching sweat. There may be gastrointestinal and nervous symptoms. Lymph nodes enlarge, and the spleen becomes palpable. Hepatitis may be accompanied by jaundice. Deep pain and disturbances of motion, particularly in vertebral bodies, suggest osteomyelitis. These symptoms of generalized *Brucella* infection generally subside in weeks or months, although localized lesions and symptoms may continue.

Following the initial infection, a chronic stage may develop, characterized by weakness, aches and pains, low-grade fever, nervousness, and other nonspecific manifestations compatible with psychoneurotic symptoms. Brucellae cannot be isolated from the patient at this stage, but the agglutinin titer may be high. The diagnosis of "chronic brucellosis" is difficult to establish with certainty unless local lesions are present.

Diagnostic Laboratory Tests

A. Specimens: Blood should be taken for culture, biopsy material for culture (lymph nodes, bone, etc), and serum for serologic tests.

B. Culture: Blood or tissues are incubated in trypticase-soy broth and on thionine-tryptose agar. At intervals of several days, subcultures are made on solid media of similar composition. All cultures are incubated in 10% CO_2 and should be observed and subcultured for at least 3 weeks before being discarded as negative.

If organisms resembling brucellae are isolated, they are typed by H_2S production, dye inhibition, and agglutination by absorbed sera. As a rule, brucellae can be cultivated from patients only during the acute phase of the illness or during recurrence of activity.

C. Serology: IgM antibodies appear early in the disease. Somewhat later, IgG and blocking antibodies appear. Whereas IgM antibody may persist after recovery (ie, when active infection is terminated spontaneously or by treatment), the finding of a substantial IgG antibody titer indicates active infection and active disease. Usual agglutination tests may fail to detect infection with *B canis*.

1. Agglutination test–To be reliable, agglutination tests must be performed with standardized heat-killed, phenolized, smooth *Brucella* antigens available from brucellosis centers and should be incubated at 37 °C for 24 hours. IgG agglutinin titers above 1:80 indicate active infection. Individuals injected with cholera vaccine may develop agglutination titers to brucellae. If the serum agglutination test is negative in patients with strong clinical evidence of *Brucella* infection, tests must be made for the presence of "blocking" antibodies. These can be detected by adding antihuman globulin to the antigen-serum mixture. Brucellosis agglutinins are cross-reactive with tularemia agglutinins, and tests for both diseases should be done on positive sera; usually, the titer for one disease will be much higher than that for the other.

2. 2-Mercaptoethanol test–The addition of 2-mercaptoethanol destroys IgM and leaves IgG for agglutination reactions. The test is not as sensitive as the standard agglutination test, but the results correlate better with chronic active disease.

3. Blocking antibodies–These are IgA antibodies that interfere with agglutination by IgG and IgM and cause a serologic test to be negative in low serum dilutions (prozone) although positive in higher dilutions. These antibodies appear during the subacute stage of infection, tend to persist for many years independently of activity of infection, and are detected by the Coombs antiglobulin method.

D. Skin Test: When Brucellergen or a protein *Brucella* extract is injected intradermally, erythema, edema, and induration develop within 24 hours in some infected individuals. The skin test is unreliable and is rarely used. Application of the skin test may stimulate the agglutinin titer.

Immunity

An antibody response occurs with infection, and it is probable that some resistance to subsequent attacks is produced. Immunogenic fractions from *Brucella* cell walls have a high phospholipid content, lysine predominates among 8 amino acids, and there is no heptose (thus distinguishing the fractions from endotoxin).

Treatment

Brucellae may be susceptible to tetracyclines or ampicillin. Symptomatic relief may occur within a few days after treatment with these drugs is begun. However, because of their intracellular location, the organisms are not readily eradicated completely from the host. For best results, treatment must be prolonged. Combined treatment with streptomycin and a tetracycline may be considered.

Epidemiology, Prevention, & Control

Brucellae are animal pathogens transmitted to humans by accidental contact with infected animal feces, urine, milk, and tissues. The common sources of infection for humans are unpasteurized milk, milk products, and cheese and occupational contact (eg, farmers, veterinarians, slaughterhouse workers) with infected animals. Occasionally the airborne route may be important. Because of occupational contact, *Bru-*

cella infection is much more frequent in men. The majority of infections remain asymptomatic (latent).

Infection rates vary greatly with different animals and in different countries. In the USA, about 4% of cattle are infected, about 15% of cattle herds contain infected animals, and infection in hogs is common. In other countries, infection is much more prevalent. Eradication of brucellosis in cattle can be attempted by test and slaughter, active immunization of heifers with avirulent live strain 19, or combined testing, segregation, and immunization. Cattle are examined by means of agglutination tests.

Active immunization of humans against *Brucella* infection is still experimental. Control rests on limitation of spread and possible eradication of animal infection, pasteurization of milk and milk products, and reduction of occupational hazards wherever possible.

REFERENCES

Barkin RM, Pichichero ME: Diphtheria-pertussis-tetanus vaccine: Reactogenicity of commercial products. *Pediatrics* 1979;**63**:256.

Brooks GF, Buchanan TM: Tularemia in the United States: Epidemiologic aspects in the 1960s and follow-up of the outbreak of tularemia in Vermont. *J Infect Dis* 1970;**121**:1357.

Buchanan TM et al: Brucellosis in the United States, 1960–1972: An abbatoir-associated disease. 1. Clinical features and therapy. 2. Diagnostic aspects. 3. Epidemiology and evidence for acquired immunity. *Medicine* 1974;**53**:403, 415, 427.

Cox F et al: Rifampin prophylaxis for contacts of *Haemophilus influenzae* type b disease. *JAMA* 1981;**245**:1043.

Hall WH, Manion RE, Zinneman HH: Blocking serum lysis of *Brucella abortus* by hyperimmune rabbit immunoglobulin A. *J Immunol* 1971;**107**:41.

Hammond GW et al: Epidemiologic, clinical, laboratory, and therapeutic features of an urban outbreak of chancroid in North America. *Rev Infect Dis* 1980;**2**:867.

Hirschmann JV, Everett ED: *Haemophilus influenzae* infections in adults: Report of nine cases and a review of the literature. *Medicine* 1979;**58**:80.

Honig PJ et al: *H influenzae* pneumonia in infants and children. *J Pediatr* 1973;**83**:215.

Kendrick PL: Can whooping cough be eradicated? *J Infect Dis* 1975;**132**:707.

Koplan JP et al: Pertussis vaccine: An analysis of benefits, risks and costs. *N Engl J Med* 1979;**301**:906.

Kraus SJ et al: Chancroid therapy: A review of cases confirmed by culture. *Rev Infect Dis* 1982;**4(Suppl)**:S848.

Linnemann CC Jr, Perry EB: *Bordetella parapertussis:* Recent experience and a review of the literature. *Am J Dis Child* 1977;**131**:560.

Linnemann CC Jr et al: Use of pertussis vaccine in an epidemic involving hospital staff. *Lancet* 1975;**2**:540.

Medeiros AA, O'Brien TF: Ampicillin-resistant *Haemophilus influenzae* type B possessing a TEM-type beta-lactamase but little permeability barrier to ampicillin. *Lancet* 1975;**1**:716.

Peltola H et al: *Haemophilus influenzae* type b capsular polysaccharide vaccine in children: A double-blind field study of 100,000 vaccinees 3 months to 5 years of age in Finland. *Pediatrics* 1977;**60**:730.

Philpott-Howard J, Williams JD: Increase in antibiotic resistance of *Haemophilus influenzae* in the United Kingdom since 1977. *Br Med J* 1982;**2**:1597.

Pittman M: The concept of pertussis as a toxin-mediated disease. *Pediatr Infect Dis* 1984;**3**:467.

Polt SS et al: Human brucellosis caused by *Brucella canis*. *Ann Intern Med* 1982;**97**:717.

Swensen RM et al: Human infection with *Brucella canis*. *Ann Intern Med* 1972;**76**:435.

Wise RI: Brucellosis in the United States: Past, present, and future. *JAMA* 1980;**244**:2318.

Young EJ: Human brucellosis. *Rev Infect Dis* 1983;**5**:821.

Young LS et al: Tularemia epidemic: Vermont, 1968. Forty-seven cases linked to contact with muskrats. *N Engl J Med* 1969;**280**:1253.

The Neisseriae

The family *Neisseriaceae* includes *Neisseria* species and *Branhamella catarrhalis* as well as *Acinetobacter* (see Chapter 19) and *Kingella* and *Moraxella* species (see Chapter 24). The neisseriae are gram-negative cocci that usually occur in pairs. *Neisseria gonorrhoeae* (gonococci) and *Neisseria meningitidis* (meningococci) are pathogenic for humans and typically are found associated with or inside polymorphonuclear cells. Some neisseriae are normal inhabitants of the human respiratory tract, rarely if ever cause disease, and occur extracellularly. Members of the group are listed in Table 23–1.

Gonococci and meningococci are closely related, with 70% DNA homology, and are differentiated by a few laboratory tests and specific characteristics: meningococci have polysaccharide capsules while gonococci do not, and meningococci rarely have plasmids while most gonococci do. Most importantly, the 2 species are differentiated by the usual clinical presentations of the diseases they cause: meningococci typically are found in the upper respiratory tract and cause meningitis, while gonococci cause genital infections. The clinical spectra of the diseases caused by gonococci and meningococci overlap, however. Study of the pathogenic neisseriae, especially the gonococci, has contributed greatly to our knowledge about the molecular basis of diseases due to mucosal pathogens.

Morphology & Identification

A. Typical Organisms: The typical *Neisseria* is a gram-negative, nonmotile diplococcus, approximately 0.8 μm in diameter (Fig 23–1). Individual cocci are kidney-shaped; when the organisms occur in pairs, the flat or concave sides are adjacent.

B. Culture: In 48 hours on enriched media (eg, Mueller-Hinton, modified Thayer-Martin), gonococci and meningococci form convex, glistening, elevated, mucoid colonies 1–5 mm in diameter. Colonies are transparent or opaque, nonpigmented, and nonhemolytic. *Neisseria flavescens*, *Neisseria subflava*, and *Neisseria lactamica* have a yellow pigmentation. *Neisseria sicca* produces opaque, brittle, wrinkled colonies. *B catarrhalis* produces nonpigmented or gray opaque colonies.

C. Growth Characteristics: The neisseriae are strict aerobes with complex growth requirements. Most neisseriae ferment carbohydrates, producing acid but not gas, and their carbohydrate fermentation patterns are a means of distinguishing them (Table 23–1). The neisseriae produce oxidase and give positive oxidase reactions; the oxidase test is a key test for identifying them. When bacteria are spotted on a filter paper soaked with tetramethylparaphenylenediamine hydrochloride, the neisseriae rapidly turn dark purple.

Meningococci and gonococci grow best on media containing complex organic substances such as heated blood, hemin, and animal proteins and in an atmosphere containing 5% CO_2 (eg, candle jar). Growth is inhibited by some toxic constituents of the medium, eg, fatty acids or salts. The organisms are rapidly killed by drying, sunlight, moist heat, and many disinfectants. They produce autolytic enzymes that result in

Table 23–1. Biochemical reactions of the neisseriae.

	Growth on MTM, ML, or NYC Medium*	Acid Formed From				DNase
		Glucose	Maltose	Lactose	Sucrose or Fructose	
N gonorrhoeae	+	+	−	−	−	−
N meningitidis	+	+	+	−	−	−
N lactamica	+	+	+	+	−	−
N sicca	−	+	+	−	+	−
N subflava	−	+	+	−	±	−
N mucosa	−	+	+	−	+	−
N flavescens	−	−	−	−	−	−
N cinerea	±	−	−	−	−	−
B catarrhalis	−	−	−	−	−	+

*MTM = modified Thayer-Martin medium, ML = Martin-Lewis medium, NYC = New York City medium.

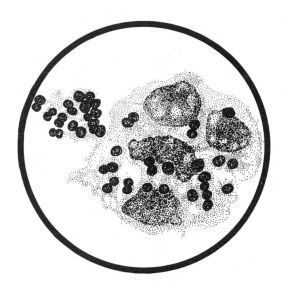

Figure 23–1. Gonococci associated with and within a polymorphonuclear leukocyte in urethral exudate from a man with urethritis. A stain of purulent cerebrospinal fluid from a patient with meningococcal meningitis would have a similar appearance.

rapid swelling and lysis in vitro at 25 °C and at an alkaline pH.

NEISSERIA GONORRHOEAE (Gonococcus)

Gonococci ferment only glucose and differ antigenically from the other neisseriae. Gonococci usually produce smaller colonies than those of the other neisseriae. Gonococci that require arginine, hypoxanthine, and uracil (Arg^-, Hyx^-, Ura^- auxotype) tend to grow most slowly on primary culture. Gonococci isolated from clinical specimens or maintained by selective subculture have typical small colonies containing piliated bacteria; these colonies are designated types 1 and 2, or types P^+ and P^{++}. On nonselective subculture, larger colonies containing nonpiliated gonococci are also formed; these are designated types 3 and 4, or P^-. Opaque and transparent variants of both the small and large colony types also occur; the opaque colonies are associated with the presence of a surface-exposed protein, protein II.

Antigenic Structure

N gonorrhoeae is antigenically heterogeneous and capable of changing its surface structures in vitro—and presumably in vivo—to avoid host defenses. Surface structures include the following:

A. Pili: Pili are the hairlike appendages that extend up to several micrometers from the gonococcal surface. They enhance attachment to host cells and resistance to phagocytosis. They are made up of stacked pilin proteins (MW 17,000–21,000). The N terminus of the pilin molecule, which contains a high percentage of hydrophobic amino acids, is conserved. The amino acid sequence near the mid portion of the molecule also is conserved; this portion of the molecule serves in attachment to host cells and is less prominent in the immune response. The amino acid sequence near the carboxy terminus is highly variable; this portion of the molecule is most prominent in the immune response. The pilins of almost all strains of *N gonorrhoeae* are antigenically different, and a single strain can make several antigenically distinct forms of pilin.

B. Protein I: Protein I extends through the gonococcal cell membrane. It occurs in trimers to form pores in the surface through which some nutrients enter the cell. The molecular weight of protein I varies from 34,000 to 37,000. Each strain of gonococcus expresses only one type of protein I, but the protein I of different strains is antigenically different. Serologic typing of protein I by agglutination reactions with monoclonal antibodies has distinguished 18 serovars of type IA and 28 serovars of type IB. (Serotyping is done only in reference laboratories.)

C. Protein II: This protein functions in adhesion of gonococci within colonies and in attachment of gonococci to host cells. One portion of the protein II molecule is in the gonococcal outer membrane, and the rest is exposed on the surface. The molecular weight of protein II ranges from 24,000 to 32,000. A strain of gonococcus can express 0–2 or occasionally 3 types of protein II. Protein II is present in gonococci from opaque colonies but may or may not be present in those from transparent colonies.

D. Protein III: This protein (MW ~ 33,000) is antigenically conserved in all gonococci. Protein III associates with protein I in the formation of pores in the cell surface.

E. Lipopolysaccharide (LPS): In contrast to that of the enteric gram-negative rods (see Chapter 18), gonococcal LPS does not have long O-antigenic side chains. Its molecular weight is 3000–7000. Gonococci can express more than one antigenically different LPS chain simultaneously. Toxicity in gonococcal infections is largely due to the endotoxic effects of LPS.

F. Other Proteins: Several antigenically constant proteins of gonococci have poorly defined roles in pathogenesis. **H8** is a surface-exposed protein that is heat modifiable like protein II. The **outer membrane–macromolecular complex** is a high-molecular-weight material. An **iron-regulated protein,** similar in molecular weight to protein I, is expressed when the available iron supply is limited, eg, in human infection. Gonococci elaborate an **IgA1 protease** that splits and inactivates IgA1, a major mucosal immunoglobulin of humans. Meningococci also elaborate a similar IgA1 protease.

Pathogenesis, Pathology, & Clinical Findings

Gonococci exhibit several morphologic types of colonies (see above), but only piliated bacteria from colony types 1 and 2 appear to be virulent. Gonococci that form opaque colonies and express protein II are isolated from men with symptomatic urethritis and from uterine cervical cultures at mid cycle. Gonococci that form transparent colonies are frequently isolated from men with asymptomatic urethral infection, from menstruating women, and from invasive forms of gonorrhea, including salpingitis and disseminated infection. In women, the colony type formed by a single strain of gonococcus changes during the menstrual cycle.

Gonococci contain several plasmids; 95% of strains have a small, "cryptic" plasmid (MW 2.4×10^6) of unknown function. Two other plasmids (MW 3.4×10^6 and 4.7×10^6) contain genes that code for β-lactamase production, which causes resistance to penicillin. These plasmids are transmissible by conjugation among gonococci; they are similar to a plasmid found in penicillinase-producing *Haemophilus* and may have been acquired from *Haemophilus* or other gram-negative organisms. Five to 20% of gonococci contain a plasmid (MW 24×10^6) with the genes that code for conjugation; the incidence is highest in geographic areas where penicillinase-producing gonococci are most common.

Gonococci attack mucous membranes of the genitourinary tract, eye, rectum, and throat, producing acute suppuration that may lead to tissue invasion; this is followed by chronic inflammation and fibrosis. In males, there is usually urethritis, with yellow, creamy pus and painful urination. The process may extend to the epididymis. As suppuration subsides in untreated infection, fibrosis occurs, sometimes leading to urethral strictures. Urethral infection in men can be asymptomatic. In females, the primary infection is in the endocervix and extends to the urethra and vagina, giving rise to mucopurulent discharge. It may then progress to the uterine tubes, causing salpingitis, fibrosis, and obliteration of the tubes. Infertility occurs in 20% of women with gonococcal salpingitis. Chronic gonococcal cervicitis or proctitis is often asymptomatic.

Gonococcal bacteremia leads to skin lesions (especially hemorrhagic papules and pustules) on the hands, forearms, feet, and legs and to tenosynovitis and suppurative arthritis, usually of the knees, ankles, and wrists. Gonococci can be cultured from only 30% of patients with gonococcal arthritis. Gonococcal endocarditis is an uncommon but severe infection. Gonococci sometimes cause meningitis and eye infections in adults; these have manifestations similar to those due to meningococci.

Gonococcal ophthalmia neonatorum, an infection of the eye of the newborn, is acquired during passage through an infected birth canal. The initial conjunctivitis rapidly progresses and, if untreated, results in blindness. To prevent gonococcal ophthalmia neonatorum, instillation of tetracycline, erythromycin, or silver nitrate into the conjunctival sac of the newborn is compulsory in the USA.

Gonococci that produce localized infection are often serum-sensitive but relatively resistant to antimicrobial drugs. In contrast, gonococci that enter the bloodstream and produce disseminated infection are usually serum-resistant but quite susceptible to penicillin and other antimicrobial drugs and are of the auxotype that requires arginine, hypoxanthine, and uracil for growth.

Diagnostic Laboratory Tests

A. Specimens: Pus and secretions are taken from the urethra, cervix, rectum, conjunctiva, throat, or synovial fluid for culture and smear. Blood culture is necessary in systemic illness, but a special culture system is helpful, since gonococci (and meningococci) are susceptible to the polyanethol sulfonate present in standard blood culture media.

B. Smears: Gram-stained smears of urethral or endocervical exudate reveal many diplococci within pus cells. These give a presumptive diagnosis. Stained smears of the urethral exudate from men have a sensitivity of about 90% and a specificity of 98–99%. Stained smears of endocervical exudates have a sensitivity of about 50% and a specificity of about 95% when examined by an experienced microscopist. Cultures of urethral exudate from men are not necessary when the stain is positive, but cultures should be done for women. Stained smears of conjunctival exudates can also be diagnostic, but those of specimens from the throat or rectum are generally not helpful.

C. Culture: Immediately after collection, pus or mucus is streaked on enriched selective medium (eg, modified Thayer-Martin medium—*Public Health Rep* 1966;**81**:559) and incubated in an atmosphere containing 5% CO_2 (candle extinction jar) at 37 °C. To avoid overgrowth by contaminants, the culture medium should contain antimicrobial drugs (eg, vancomycin, 3 μg/mL; colistin, 7.5 μg/mL; amphotericin B, 1 μg/mL; and trimethoprim, 3 μg/mL). If immediate incubation is not possible, the specimen should be placed in a JEMBEC or similar transport-culture system. Forty-eight hours after culture, the organisms can be quickly identified by their appearance on a Gram-stained smear, by oxidase positivity, and by coagglutination, immunofluorescence staining, or other laboratory tests. The species of subcultured bacteria may be determined by fermentation reactions (Table 23–1). The species of bacteria isolated from anatomic sites other than the genital tract should be identified.

D. Serology: Serum and genital fluid contain IgG and IgA antibodies against gonococcal pili, outer membrane proteins, and LPS. Some IgM of human sera is bactericidal for gonococci in vitro.

In infected individuals, antibodies to gonococcal pili and outer membrane proteins can be detected by immunoblotting, radioimmunoassay, and ELISA (enzyme-linked immunosorbent assay) tests. However, these tests are not useful as diagnostic aids for several reasons: gonococcal antigenic heterogeneity; the delay in development of antibodies in acute infection; and a high background level of antibodies in the sexually active population.

Immunity

Repeated gonococcal infections are common. Protective immunity to reinfection does not appear to develop as part of the disease process, because of the antigenic variety of gonococci. While antibodies can be demonstrated, including the IgA and IgG on mucosal surfaces, they either are highly strain-specific or have little protective ability.

Treatment

Since the development and widespread use of penicillin, gonococcal resistance to penicillin has gradually risen, owing to the selection of chromosomal mutants, so that many strains now require 2 or more units of penicillin G per milliliter for inhibition. This has led to a gradual rise in the recommended dose: 4.8 million units of aqueous procaine penicillin G intramuscularly plus 1 g of probenecid orally is now recommended for acute genital infections. Single-dose therapy with amoxicillin, 3 g orally, or ampicillin, 3.5 g orally, either drug combined with 1 g of probenecid orally, is also effective for acute genital infections. Tetracycline hydrochloride, 500 mg orally 4 times a day for 7 days, or doxycycline, 100 mg orally twice a day for 7 days, should also be given, since these regimens are effective in treating coexistent *Chlamydia trachomatis* infections.

Tetracycline or aqueous procaine penicillin G is the drug of choice for pharyngeal gonococcal infection.

Penicillinase-producing *N gonorrhoeae* (PPNG) first appeared in 1976. These totally penicillin-resistant gonococcal strains have appeared in many parts of the world, with the highest incidence in special populations, eg, 50% in prostitutes in the Philippines. Other areas with a high incidence of PPNG include Singapore and parts of sub-Sahara Africa. Focal outbreaks of disease due to PPNG have occurred in many areas of the USA and elsewhere, and endemic foci are being established. Such infections require spectinomycin therapy or, for pharyngitis, trimethoprim-sulfamethoxazole in large doses for 5 days. Spectinomycin-resistant PPNG have been encountered since 1981. Cefoxitin, cefuroxime, cefotaxime, and other newer cephalosporins are effective against PPNG.

Most cases of severe disseminated gonorrhea are still caused by penicillin-susceptible strains, and penicillin G, 10 million units daily for 3–5 days, followed by amoxicillin, 500 mg orally, or ampicillin, 500 mg orally, to complete a 7-day course of treatment is acceptable therapy. For disseminated gonococcal infection, give a single dose of amoxicillin, 3 g orally, or ampicillin, 3.5 g orally, on the first day of treatment followed by 500 mg of the drug 4 times a day for the next 6 days. In chronic salpingitis, prostatitis, and other long-established infections, longer courses of treatment are suggested.

In urethritis in men, if clinical cure is apparent after treatment, it is not necessary to prove cure by culture. In other forms of gonococcal infection, cure should be established by follow-up, including cultures from the involved sites. Since other sexually transmitted diseases may have been acquired at the same time, steps must also be taken to diagnose and treat these diseases (see discussions of chlamydiae, syphilis, etc).

Epidemiology, Prevention, & Control

Gonorrhea is worldwide in distribution, and its incidence has risen steadily since 1955. It is almost exclusively transmitted by sexual contact, often by women and men with asymptomatic infections. The infectivity of the organism is such that the chance of acquiring infection from a single exposure to an infected sexual partner is 20–30% for men and even greater for women. The infection rate can be reduced by avoiding multiple sexual partners, rapidly eradicating gonococci from infected individuals by means of early diagnosis and treatment, and finding cases and contacts through education and screening of populations at high risk. Mechanical prophylaxis (condoms) provides partial protection. Chemoprophylaxis is of limited value because of the rise in antibiotic resistance of the gonococcus.

Gonococcal ophthalmia neonatorum is prevented by local application of 0.5% erythromycin ophthalmic ointment or 1% tetracycline ointment to the conjunctiva of newborns. Although instillation of silver nitrate solution is also effective and is the classic method for preventing ophthalmia neonatorum, silver nitrate is difficult to store and causes conjunctival irritation; its use is gradually being replaced by use of erythromycin or tetracycline ointment.

NEISSERIA MENINGITIDIS (Meningococcus)

Antigenic Structure

At least 13 serogroups of meningococci (A, B, C, D, X, Y, Z, W-135, 29E, H, I, K, and L) have been identified by immunologic specificity of capsular polysaccharides. The group A polysaccharide is a polymer of N-acetylmannosamine phosphate, and that of group C is a polymer of N-acetyl-O-acetylneuraminic acid. Meningococcal antigens are found in blood and cerebrospinal fluid of patients with active disease. Outbreaks and sporadic cases in the western hemisphere in the last decade have been caused mainly by groups B, C, W-135, and Y; outbreaks in southern Finland and Sao Paulo, Brazil, were due to groups A and C; those in Africa were due mainly to group A. Group C and, especially, group A are associated with epidemic disease.

The outer membrane proteins of meningococci have been divided into 5 classes on the basis of molecular weight. All strains have either class 2 or class 3 proteins; these are analogous to the protein I porins of gonococci and are responsible for the serotype specificity of meningococci. As many as 20 serotypes have been defined; serotypes 2 and 15 have been associated with epidemic disease. The class 5 protein is comparable to protein II of the gonococci. Meningococci are piliated, but unlike gonococci, they do not form distinctive colony types indicating piliated bacteria. Meningococcal LPS is responsible for many of the toxic effects found in meningococcal disease.

Pathogenesis, Pathology, & Clinical Findings

Humans are the only natural hosts for whom meningococci are pathogenic. The nasopharynx is the portal of entry. There, the organisms attach to epithelial cells with the aid of pili; they may form part of the transient flora without producing symptoms. From the nasopharynx, organisms may reach the bloodstream, producing bacteremia; the symptoms may be like an upper respiratory tract infection. Fulminant meningococcemia is more severe, with high fever and hemorrhagic rash; there may be disseminated intravascular coagulation and circulatory collapse (Waterhouse-Friderichsen syndrome).

Meningitis is the most common complication of meningococcemia. It usually begins suddenly, with intense headache, vomiting, and stiff neck, and progresses to coma within a few hours.

During meningococcemia, there is thrombosis of many small blood vessels in many organs, with perivascular infiltration and petechial hemorrhages. There may be interstitial myocarditis, arthritis, and skin lesions. In meningitis, the meninges are acutely inflamed, with thrombosis of blood vessels and exudation of polymorphonuclear leukocytes, so that the surface of the brain is covered with a thick purulent exudate.

It is not known what transforms an asymptomatic infection of the nasopharynx into meningococcemia and meningitis, but this can be prevented by specific bactericidal serum antibodies against the infecting serotype. *Neisseria* bacteremia is favored by the absence of bactericidal antibody (IgG), inhibition of serum bactericidal action by a blocking IgA antibody, or a complement deficiency (C5, C6, C7, or C8). Meningococci are readily phagocytosed in the presence of a specific opsonin.

Diagnostic Laboratory Tests

A. Specimens: Specimens of blood are taken for culture, and specimens of spinal fluid are taken for smear, culture, and chemical determinations. Nasopharyngeal swab cultures are suitable for carrier surveys. Puncture material from petechiae may be taken for smear and culture.

B. Smears: Gram-stained smears of the sediment of centrifuged spinal fluid or of petechial aspirate often show typical neisseriae within polymorphonuclear leukocytes or extracellularly.

C. Culture: Culture media without sodium polyanethol sulfonate are helpful in culturing blood specimens. Cerebrospinal fluid specimens are plated on heated blood agar ("chocolate" agar) and incubated at 37 °C in an atmosphere of 5% CO_2 (candle jar). Freshly drawn spinal fluid can be directly incubated at 37 °C if agar culture media are not immediately available. A modified Thayer-Martin medium with antibiotics (VCN: vancomycin, colistin, nystatin) favors the growth of neisseriae, inhibits many other bacteria, and is used for nasopharyngeal cultures. Colonies of neisseriae on solid media, particularly in mixed culture, can be identified by the oxidase test. Spinal fluid and blood generally yield pure cultures that can be further identified by carbohydrate fermentation reactions (Table 23–1) and agglutination with type-specific or polyvalent serum.

D. Serology: Antibodies to meningococcal polysaccharides can be measured by latex agglutination or hemagglutination tests or by their bactericidal activity. These tests are done only in reference laboratories.

Immunity

Immunity to meningococcal infection is associated with the presence of specific, complement-dependent, bactericidal antibodies in the serum. These antibodies develop after subclinical infections with different strains or injection of antigens and are group-specific. The immunizing antigens for groups A and C are the capsular polysaccharides. For group B, the immunizing antigen is less well defined and may include membrane proteins. Infants may have passive immunity through IgG antibodies transferred from the mother. Children under the age of 2 years do not reliably produce antibodies when immunized with meningococcal or other bacterial polysaccharides.

Treatment

Penicillin G is the drug of choice for treating meningococcal disease. Chloramphenicol is used in persons allergic to penicillins.

Epidemiology, Prevention, & Control

Meningococcal meningitis occurs in epidemic waves (eg, in military installations; in Brazil, there were more than 15,000 cases in 1974) and a smaller number of sporadic interepidemic cases. Five to 30% of the normal population may harbor meningococci (often nontypable isolates) in the nasopharynx during interepidemic periods. During epidemics, the carrier rate goes up to 70 or 80%. A rise in the number of cases is preceded by an increased number of respiratory carriers. Treatment with oral penicillin does not eradicate the carrier state. Rifampin, 600 mg orally twice daily for 2 days (or minocycline, 100 mg every 12 hours), can often eradicate the carrier state and serve as chemoprophylaxis for household and other close contacts. Since the appearance of many sulfonamide-resistant meningococci, chemoprophylaxis with sulfonamides is no longer reliable.

Clinical cases of meningitis present only a negligible source of infection, and therefore isolation has only limited usefulness. More important is the reduction of personal contacts in a population with a high carrier rate. This is accomplished by avoidance of crowding. Specific polysaccharides of groups A, C, Y, and W-135 can stimulate antibody response and protect susceptible persons against infection. Such vaccines are currently used in selected populations (eg, the military; civilian epidemics).

OTHER NEISSERIAE

N lactamica very rarely causes disease but is important because it grows in the selective media (eg, modified Thayer-Martin medium) used for cultures of gonococci and meningococci from clinical specimens. *N lactamica* can be cultured from 3–40% of persons and most often is found in children. Unlike the other neisseriae, it ferments lactose.

N sicca, N subflava, N cinerea, N mucosa, and *N flavescens* are also members of the normal flora of the respiratory tract, particularly the nasopharynx, and very rarely produce disease.

B catarrhalis is also a member of the normal flora of the upper respiratory tract; it occasionally causes pneumonia or other forms of disease. Most strains of *B catarrhalis* from clinically significant infections produce β-lactamase. *B catarrhalis* can be differentiated from the other neisseriae by its lack of carbohydrate fermentation and its production of DNase. In tests used to detect DNase production by gram-negative bacilli, *B catarrhalis* yields positive results.

REFERENCES

Britigan BE et al: Gonococcal infection: A model of molecular pathogenesis. *N Engl J Med* 1985;**312**:1683.

Brooks GF, Donegan EA: *Gonococcal Infection.* Edward Arnold, 1985.

Brooks GF et al (editors): *Immunobiology of* Neisseria gonorrhoeae: *Proceedings of a Conference Held in San Francisco, CA, 18–20 Jan 1978.* American Society for Microbiology, 1978.

Centers for Disease Control: 1985 STD treatment guidelines. *MMWR* (Oct 18) 1985;**34(Suppl 4)**:75S.

DeVoe IW: The meningococcus and mechanisms of pathogenicity. *Microbiol Rev* 1982;**46**:162.

Doern GV et al: *Branhamella (Neisseria) catarrhalis* systemic disease in humans. *Arch Intern Med* 1981;**141**:1690.

Frasch CE et al: Serotype antigens of *Neisseria meningitidis* and a proposed scheme for designation of serotypes. *Rev Infect Dis* 1985;**7**:504.

Goldschneider I et al: Human immunity to the meningococcus. 1. The role of humoral antibodies. *J Exp Med* 1969;**129**:1307.

Hook ED III, Homes KK: Gonococcal infections. *Ann Intern Med* 1985;**102**:229.

Knapp JS et al: Serologic classification of *Neisseria gonorrhoeae* with use of monoclonal antibodies to gonococcal outer membrane protein I. *J Infect Dis* 1984;**150**:44.

Koomey JM et al: Genetic and biochemical analysis of gonococcal IgA1 protease: Cloning in *Escherichia coli* and construction of mutants of gonococci that fail to produce the activity. *Proc Natl Acad Sci USA* 1982;**79**:7881.

Kornfeld SJ et al: Secretory immunity and the bacterial IgA proteases. *Rev Infect Dis* 1981;**3**:521.

McGee ZA et al: Mechanisms of mucosal invasion by pathogenic *Neisseria. Rev Infect Dis* 1983;**5(Suppl 4)**:S708.

Meyer TF et al: Pilus expression in *Neisseria gonorrhoeae* involves chromosomal rearrangement. *Cell* 1982;**30**:45.

Peltola H: Meningococcal disease: Still with us. *Rev Infect Dis* 1983;**5**:71.

Petersen BH et al: *Neisseria meningitidis* and *Neisseria gonorrhoeae* bacteremia associated with C6, C7, or C8 deficiency. *Ann Intern Med* 1979;**90**:917.

Rothbard JB et al: Antibodies to peptides corresponding to a conserved sequence of gonococcal pilins block bacterial adhesion. *Proc Natl Acad Sci USA* 1985;**82**:915.

Schoolnik GK et al: Gonococcal pili: Primary structure and receptor binding domain. *J Exp Med* 1984;**159**:1351.

Schoolnik GK et al (editors): *The Pathogenic Neisseria: Proceedings of the Fourth International Symposium, Asilomar, CA, Oct. 1984.* American Society for Microbiology, 1985.

Stern A et al: Opacity determinants of *Neisseria gonorrhoeae:* Gene expression and chromosomal linkage to the gonococcal pilus gene. *Cell* 1984;**37**:447.

Young LS et al: A simultaneous outbreak of meningococcal and influenza infections. *N Engl J Med* 1972;**287**:5.

24

Miscellaneous Pathogenic Bacteria

LEGIONELLA PNEUMOPHILA & OTHER LEGIONELLAE

A widely publicized outbreak of pneumonia in persons attending an American Legion convention in Philadelphia in 1976 prompted investigations that defined *Legionella pneumophila* and the legionellae. Other outbreaks of respiratory illness caused by related organisms since 1947 have been diagnosed retrospectively. At least 20 species of *Legionella* exist, some with multiple serotypes. *Legionella pneumophila* is the major cause of disease in humans; *Legionella micdadei* sometimes causes pneumonia. The other legionellae are rarely isolated from patients or have been isolated only from the environment.

Morphology & Identification

Legionella pneumophila is the prototype bacterium of the group.

A. Typical Organisms: Legionellae are fastidious, aerobic gram-negative bacteria that are 0.5–1 μm wide and 2–50 μm long. They often stain poorly by Gram's method and are not seen in stains of clinical specimens. Gram-stained smears should be made for suspect *Legionella* growth on agar media. Basic fuchsin (0.1%) should be used as the counterstain, because safranin stains the bacteria very poorly.

B. Culture: Legionellae can be grown on complex media such as buffered charcoal–yeast extract agar (BCYE) with α-ketoglutarate, at pH 6.9, temperature 35 °C, and 90% humidity. Antibiotics can be added to make the medium selective for *Legionella*. A biphasic BCYE medium can be used for blood cultures.

Legionella grow slowly; visible colonies are usually present after 3 days of incubation. Colonies that appear after overnight incubation are not *Legionella*. Colonies are round or flat with entire edges. They vary in color from colorless to iridescent pink or blue and are translucent or speckled. Variation in colony morphology is common, and the colonies may rapidly lose their color and speckles. Many other genera of bacteria grow on BCYE medium and must be differentiated from *Legionella* by Gram-staining and other tests.

Legionella in blood cultures usually require 2 weeks or more to grow. Colonies can be seen on the agar surface of the biphasic medium.

C. Growth Characteristics: The legionellae are

catalase-positive. *L pneumophila* is oxidase-positive; the other legionellae are variable in oxidase activity. *L pneumophila* hydrolyzes hippurate; the other legionellae do not. Most legionellae produce gelatinase and beta-lactamase; *L micdadei* produces neither gelatinase nor beta-lactamase.

Antigens & Cell Products

Antigenic specificity of *L pneumophila* is thought to be due to complex antigenic structures. There are at least 10 serogroups of *L pneumophila*; serogroup 1 was the cause of the 1976 outbreak of Legionnaires' disease and remains the most common serogroup isolated from humans. *Legionella* species cannot be identified by serogrouping alone, because there is cross-reactive antigenicity among different *Legionella* species. Occasionally, *Bacteroides* and some *Pseudomonas* species also cross-react with *L pneumophila* antisera.

The legionellae produce distinctive 14- to 17-carbon branched-chain fatty acids. Gas-liquid chromatography is used to help characterize and determine the species of legionellae.

The legionellae make proteases, phosphatase, lipase, DNase, and RNase. A hemolysin and cytotoxin have been described. The toxins and their mechanism of action are not well characterized.

Pathogenesis & Pathology

The legionellae are ubiquitous in warm moist environments. Infection of debilitated or immunosuppressed humans commonly follows inhalation of the bacteria from aerosols generated from contaminated air-conditioning systems, shower heads, and similar sources. Once in the lung, the bacteria multiply, producing pneumonia that varies from patchy involvement to severe, often bilateral, multilobar consolidation. Small abscesses and pleural effusions are common. On microscopic examination, polymorphonuclear cells, macrophages, red blood cells, and proteinaceous material are seen in the alveolar spaces. The epithelium lining the alveoli is lost. The *Legionella* are intracellular.

Clinical Findings

Asymptomatic infection is common in all age groups, as shown by elevated titers of specific antibodies. The incidence of clinically significant disease is highest in men over age 55 years. Factors associated with high risk include smoking, chronic bronchitis and emphysema, steroid and other immunosuppressive treatment (as in renal transplantation), cancer chemotherapy, and diabetes mellitus. When pneumonia occurs in patients with these risk factors, *Legionella* should be investigated as the cause.

Infection may result in nondescript febrile illness of short duration or in a severe, rapidly progressive illness with high fever, chills, malaise, nonproductive cough, hypoxia, diarrhea, and delirium. Chest x-rays reveal patchy, often multilobar consolidation. There may be leukocytosis, hyponatremia, hematuria (and even renal failure), or abnormal liver function. During some outbreaks, the mortality rate has reached 10%. The diagnosis is based on the clinical picture and exclusion of other causes of pneumonia by laboratory tests. Demonstration of *Legionella* in clinical specimens can rapidly yield a specific diagnosis. The diagnosis can also be made by culture for *Legionella* or by serologic tests, but results of these tests are often delayed beyond the time when specific therapy must be started.

Legionella pneumophila also produces a disease called "Pontiac fever," after the clinical syndrome that occurred in an outbreak in Pontiac, Michigan. The syndrome is characterized by fever and chills, myalgia, malaise, and headache that develop over 6–12 hours. Dizziness, photophobia, neck stiffness, and confusion also occur. Respiratory symptoms are much less prominent in Pontiac fever than in Legionnaires' disease and include mild cough and sore throat.

Diagnostic Laboratory Tests

A. Specimens: In human infections, the organisms can be recovered from bronchial washings, pleural fluid, lung biopsy specimens, or blood. Isolation of *Legionella* from sputum is more difficult because of the predominance of bacteria of the normal flora. *Legionella* is rarely recovered from other anatomic sites.

B. Smears: Legionellae are not demonstrable in Gram-stained smears of clinical specimens. Direct fluorescent antibody tests of specimens can be diagnostic, but multiple antisera must be used. The direct fluorescent antibody test has low sensitivity compared to culture. Silver stains are sometimes used on tissue specimens.

C. Culture: Specimens are cultured on BCYE agar (see above). Cultured organisms can be rapidly identified by immunofluorescence staining.

D. Specific Tests: Sometimes *Legionella* antigens can be demonstrated in the patient's urine by immunologic methods. However, these tests are not commercially available.

E. Serologic Tests: Levels of antibodies to legionellae rise slowly during the illness. Serologic tests have a sensitivity of 60–80% and a specificity of 95–99%. Since less than 10% of all cases of pneumonia are due to *Legionella*, the predictive value of a positive serologic test in sporadic cases is low (40–70%).

Serologic tests are most useful in obtaining a retrospective diagnosis in outbreaks of *Legionella* infections.

Immunity

Infected patients make antibodies against *Legionella*, but the peak antibody response may not occur until 4–8 weeks after infection. There is a lymphocyte response as measured by blastogenesis assays. The role of these immune responses in protection from disease is unknown.

Treatment

Legionellae are susceptible to erythromycin and some other drugs. The treatment of choice is erythromycin, 500 mg intravenously every 4–6 hours; this has been effective even in certain immunocompromised patients. Rifampin, 10–20 mg/kg/d, has been used in patients whose response to treatment was delayed. Assisted ventilation may be necessary, and management of shock is essential.

Epidemiology & Control

The legionellae are ubiquitous in the environment and worldwide in distribution. They commonly occur in soil and in freshwater lakes and streams and have been found in high numbers in air-conditioning systems and washing facilities, eg, shower stalls. The latter sources have been responsible for outbreaks of human disease, especially in hospitals. Chlorination and heating of water and cleaning can help control the multiplication of *Legionella* in water and air-conditioning systems. Legionellae are not communicable from infected patients to others.

LISTERIA MONOCYTOGENES

Listeria monocytogenes is a short, gram-positive, nonsporeforming rod. It has a tumbling end-over-end motility at 22 °C but not at 37 °C; the motility test rapidly differentiates *Listeria* from diphtheroids that are members of the normal flora of skin. Growth on simple media is enhanced by the presence of blood, ascitic fluid, or glucose. Isolation can be enhanced if the tissue is kept at 4 °C for some days before inoculation into bacteriologic media. The organism is a facultative anaerobe and is catalase-positive. Most strains produce hemolysis on blood agar plates. *Listeria* produces acid but not gas in a variety of carbohydrates. There are several antigenic types.

Spontaneous infection occurs in many domestic and wild animals and in humans. In smaller animals (rabbits, chickens) there is a septicemia with focal abscesses in liver and heart muscle and marked monocytosis. A glyceride extracted from *Listeria* can likewise induce monocytosis in rabbits. This cellular reaction, however, is not related to human infectious mononucleosis. *Listeria* infection leads to the production of cold agglutinins for human and sheep red cells as well as specific agglutinating antibodies.

In humans and in ruminants (eg, sheep) *Listeria* may cause meningoencephalitis with or without bacteremia. Listeriosis in adults may be superimposed on lymphoma or immunodeficiency. The diagnosis rests on isolation of the organism in cultures of blood and spinal fluid. Perinatal human listeriosis (**granulomatosis infantiseptica**) may be an intrauterine infection. The early-onset syndrome results in intrauterine sepsis and death before or after delivery. It tends to be caused by serotypes Ia, Ib, or IVb. The late-onset syndrome causes the development of meningitis between birth and the third week of life; it is often caused by serotype IVb and has a significant mortality rate.

Adults can develop *Listeria* sepsis and meningoencephalitis (and, rarely, focal infections). These infections occur most commonly in immunosuppressed patients, in whom *Listeria* is one of the most common causes of meningitis. The clinical presentation of *Listeria* meningitis in these patients varies from insidious to fulminant and is nonspecific. The route of infection for adults is uncertain. *Listeria* may colonize the gut when raw vegetables that have been contaminated from soil or contaminated milk or cheese is ingested.

Many antimicrobial drugs inhibit *Listeria* in vitro. Clinical cures have been obtained with ampicillin or penicillin plus an aminoglycoside and with erythromycin.

ERYSIPELOTHRIX RHUSIOPATHIAE (Erysipelothrix insidiosa)

Erysipelothrix resembles *Listeria* but is nonmotile and produces an entirely different disease. In its smooth form, it grows as clear, minute colonies in which short, nonsporeforming rods are arranged in short chains; in its rough form, long filaments predominate. Growth is aided by blood and glucose in the medium. On blood agar, only slight hemolysis is produced. Carbohydrates are fermented irregularly, and catalase is not produced. The antigenic pattern is not established.

Infection with *E rhusiopathiae* occurs in worldwide distribution in a variety of animals, especially swine. In swine, it causes the disease swine erysipelas, which is very different from erysipelas of humans; the latter is caused by group A beta-hemolytic streptococci. *E rhusiopathiae* infection in humans is through skin abrasions and follows contact with fish, shellfish, meat, or poultry. The infection, called erysipeloid, is limited to the skin. There are pain, edema, and purplish erythema with sharp margins that extends peripherally but clears centrally. Relapses and extension of the lesions to distant areas are common, but there is usually no fever. Rarely, endocarditis occurs. There is no permanent immunity following an attack. The diagnosis rests on isolation of the organism in cultures from a skin biopsy. The fragments should be incubated in glucose broth for 24 hours, then subcultured on blood agar plates. Typical clinical appearance

in a person with occupational exposure is highly suggestive of infection due to this organism.

Penicillin appears to be the antibiotic of choice.

ANAEROBES

Bacteroides

This is a large group of nonsporeforming, nonmotile, strictly anaerobic, usually gram-negative bacteria that are very pleomorphic. They may appear as slender rods, branching forms, or round bodies. They grow most readily on complex media, eg, brain-heart infusion agar, in an anaerobic atmosphere containing 10% CO_2.

The capsular polysaccharides of *Bacteroides* are important virulence factors. During infection with *Bacteroides fragilis*, patients develop antibodies to these capsular polysaccharides. *B fragilis* produces a superoxide dismutase and can survive in the presence of oxygen for days. *Bacteroides* apparently lack the lipopolysaccharide structures with endotoxic activity that other gram-negative bacteria possess.

Bacteroides are normal inhabitants of the upper respiratory, intestinal, and female genital tracts. Normal stools contain 10^{11} organisms per gram. Most commonly isolated are the *B fragilis* group (5 species), particularly from the large intestine, and the *Bacteroides melaninogenicus* group (7 species), particularly from the oropharynx, gut, and vagina. *Bacteroides bivius* and *Bacteroides disiens* occur in the female genital tract. Classification is based on colonial and biochemical features and characteristic appearance in gas chromatography.

In anaerobic infections (lung, brain, peritoneum, pelvis), *Bacteroides* are often associated with other anaerobic organisms, particularly anaerobic streptococci (*Peptostreptococcus*), anaerobic staphylococci (*Peptococcus*), anaerobic gram-positive rods (*Clostridium* and *Eubacterium* species), and fusiform bacteria (*Fusobacterium* species; see p 299), as well as gram-positive and gram-negative facultative anaerobes that are part of the normal flora.

Bacteroides are found in abdominal, lung, and brain abscesses and in empyema; they may cause suppuration in surgical infection such as peritonitis following injury to the bowel; and they may participate in pelvic inflammatory disease. In such anaerobic infections, the pus is often foul-smelling. Bacteremia is common, and endocarditis may develop.

Organisms of the *B fragilis* group are relatively resistant to penicillins owing to their production of beta-lactamases but are susceptible to clindamycin, metronidazole, and chloramphenicol. About two-thirds of the organisms of the *B melaninogenicus* group produce beta-lactamase, but infections with these organisms can usually be treated with penicillin. *Bacteroides* organisms from infections of the female genital tract usually produce beta-lactamase and are clearly resistant to penicillin. Cefoxitin and the newer cephalosporins tend to be effective in *Bacteroides* infections.

Fusobacteria

The fusobacteria are pleomorphic gram-negative rods. Most species produce butyric acid and convert threonine to propionic acid. The *Fusobacterium* group includes several species frequently isolated from mixed bacterial infections caused by normal mucosal flora. Occasionally, a *Fusobacterium* will be the only species in an infection (eg, osteomyelitis).

Veillonellae

Veillonellae are small, anaerobic, gram-negative cocci that are part of the normal flora of the mouth. They ferment sugars and probably are not pathogenic.

Anaerobic Gram-Positive Rods

Four of the many species in the genus *Clostridium* are of major importance because they cause toxin-mediated diseases (see Chapter 14): *Clostridium tetani* causes tetanus, *Clostridium botulinum* causes botulism, *Clostridium perfringens* causes gas gangrene and food poisoning, and *Clostridium difficile* causes pseudomembranous colitis. The other *Clostridium* species are sometimes isolated from mixed flora infections, usually with bowel flora.

The *Actinomyces* group includes several species that cause actinomycosis (see p 334).

Eubacterium species are found in mixed flora infections associated with oropharyngeal or bowel flora.

Lactobacillus species are major members of the normal flora of the vagina. They very rarely cause disease.

Propionibacterium species are members of the normal flora of the skin and cause disease when they infect plastic shunts and appliances. They participate in the genesis of acne.

PEPTOCOCCI & PEPTOSTREPTOCOCCI

Peptococcus and *Peptostreptococcus* species are found on the skin and as part of the normal flora of mucous membranes. There are many species. Usually, they are found in mixed infections due to normal flora. Occasionally, cultures from breast, brain, or pulmonary infections will be positive for only one of these gram-positive cocci.

UNCOMMON GRAM-NEGATIVE BACTERIA

Achromobacter

Achromobacter xylosoxidans is an oxidase-positive gram-negative rod that has been isolated from many body sites but is very uncommon as a sole cause of infection.

Actinobacillus

*Actinobacillus (Haemophilus) actinomycetemcom-*itans is a small, gram-negative, coccobacillary organism that grows slowly. As its name implies, it is often found in actinomycosis. It also causes severe periodontal disease in adolescents, endocarditis, abscesses, osteomyelitis, and other infections. It is treatable with tetracycline or chloramphenicol and sometimes with penicillin G, ampicillin, or erythromycin.

Alcaligenes

The *Alcaligenes* group includes 4 species of oxidase-positive gram-negative rods. They have peritrichous flagella and are motile, which differentiates them from the pseudomonads. They alkalinize citrate medium and oxidation-fermentation medium containing glucose and are urease-negative. They may be part of the normal human bacterial flora and have been isolated from respirators, nebulizers, and renal dialysis systems. They are occasionally isolated from urine, blood, spinal fluid, wounds, and abscesses.

Capnocytophaga

The *Capnocytophaga* species are fastidious gram-negative gliding bacteria that are members of the normal oral flora of humans. They are fusiform and fermentative and are facultative anaerobes that require CO_2 for aerobic growth. They occasionally cause bacteremia and systemic disease in immunocompromised patients.

Cardiobacterium

Cardiobacterium hominis, another bacterium with a descriptive name, is a facultatively anaerobic, pleomorphic gram-negative rod that is part of the normal flora of the upper respiratory tract and bowel and occasionally causes endocarditis. Since it grows slowly in blood culture media, it may be necessary to observe the cultures for several weeks in order to diagnose infection.

Chromobacteria

Chromobacterium violaceum and other species of chromobacteria are gram-negative pigmented rods resembling pseudomonads. They occur in subtropical climates in soil and water and may infect animals and humans through breaks in the skin or via the gut. This may result in abscesses, diarrhea, and sepsis, with many deaths. Chromobacteria are often susceptible to chloramphenicol, tetracyclines, and aminoglycosides.

DF-2 Bacteria

The DF-2 group of gram-negative bacteria are oxidase-positive and catalase-positive. They are so named because they are **dysgonic fermenters;** they do not show their fermentation patterns on routine media. They are members of the normal oral flora of dogs; when transmitted to humans, they occasionally cause fulminant infection in asplenic patients, alcoholics, and, rarely, in healthy people.

Eikenella corrodens

E corrodens is a small, fastidious, capnophilic

gram-negative rod that is part of the gingival and bowel flora of 40–70% of humans. About 50% of isolates form pits in agar during the several days of incubation required for growth. *Eikenella* is oxidase-positive and does not ferment carbohydrates. It is found in mixed flora infections associated with contamination by oral mucosal or bowel flora; it is often present with streptococci. It occurs frequently in infections from human bites. *Eikenella* is uniformly resistant to clindamycin, which can be used to make a selective agar medium. *Eikenella* is susceptible to ampicillin and the newer penicillins and cephalosporins.

Flavobacterium

The *Flavobacterium* group includes at least 5 species. The organisms are long, thin, nonmotile gram-negative rods that are oxidase-positive, proteolytic, and weakly fermentative. They often form distinctive yellow colonies. The flavobacteria are commonly found in sink drains, faucets, and on medical equipment that has been exposed to contaminated water sources and not sterilized. The flavobacteria occasionally colonize the respiratory tract and rarely cause meningitis. They are often resistant to many antimicrobial drugs.

Kingella

The *Kingella* group includes 3 species, of which *Kingella kingae* is the most common. *Kingella kingae*, previously known as a member of the genus *Moraxella*, is an oxidase-positive, nonmotile organism that is hemolytic when grown on blood agar. It is a gram-negative rod, but coccobacillary and diplococcal forms are common. It is part of the normal oral flora and occasionally causes infections of bone, joints, and tendons. The organism probably enters the circulation with minor oral trauma such as tooth brushing. It is susceptible to penicillin, ampicillin, erythromycin, and other antimicrobial drugs.

Moraxella

The *Moraxella* group includes 6 species. They are nonmotile, nonfermentative, and oxidase-positive. On staining, they appear as small gram-negative bacilli, coccobacilli, or cocci. They are members of the normal flora of the upper respiratory tract and occasionally cause bacteremia, endocarditis, conjunctivitis, meningitis, or other infections. They are uniformly susceptible to penicillin and other antimicrobial drugs.

BACTERIA THAT CAUSE VAGINOSIS

Gardnerella vaginalis

G vaginalis (previously called *Corynebacterium vaginale* and *Haemophilus vaginalis*) is a serologically distinct organism isolated from the normal female genitourinary tract and also associated with vaginitis. In wet smears, this "nonspecific" vaginitis, or bacterial vaginosis, yields "clue cells," which are vaginal epithelial cells covered with many tiny rods, and there is an absence of other common causes of vaginitis such as *Trichomonas* or yeasts. Vaginal discharge often has a distinct "fishy" odor and contains many anaerobes in addition to *G vaginalis*. The vaginitis attributed to this organism is suppressed by metronidazole, suggesting an association with anaerobes. Oral metronidazole, 750 mg–1 g daily for 1 week, is generally curative.

Mobiluncus

This genus comprises motile, curved, gram-negative, anaerobic rods isolated from "bacterial vaginosis," which may be a clinical variant of "nonspecific vaginitis" associated with *G vaginalis*. It is possible that *Mobiluncus* may be part of the normal vaginal anaerobic flora in women, and it is likely that it is part of the anaerobic flora in bacterial vaginosis. The organisms are most commonly detected in Gram-stained smears of vaginal secretions, but they grow with difficulty in anaerobic cultures. They may well be the same organisms described by Curtis in 1913 in smears of secretions from vaginitis.

STREPTOBACILLUS MONILIFORMIS

Streptobacillus moniliformis is an aerobic, gram-negative, highly pleomorphic organism that forms irregular chains of bacilli interspersed with fusiform enlargements and large round bodies. It grows best at 37 °C in media containing serum protein, egg yolk, or starch but ceases to grow at 22 °C. L forms can easily be demonstrated in most cultures of the organism. Subculture of pure colonies of L forms in liquid media often yields the streptobacilli again. All strains of streptobacilli appear to be antigenically identical.

S moniliformis is a normal inhabitant of the throats of rats, and humans can be infected by rat bites. The human disease (rat-bite fever) is characterized by septic fever, blotchy and petechial rashes, and polyarthritis. Diagnosis rests on cultures of blood, joint fluid, or pus; on mouse inoculation; and on serum agglutination tests.

This organism can also produce infection after being ingested in milk—the disease is called Haverhill fever and has occurred in epidemics.

Penicillin and perhaps other antibiotics are therapeutically effective.

Rat-bite fever of somewhat different clinical appearance (sodoku) is caused by *Spirillum minor* (see Chapter 27).

BARTONELLA BACILLIFORMIS

Bartonella is a gram-negative, very pleomorphic, motile organism that causes bartonellosis in humans. There are 2 stages of bartonellosis: the initial stage is **Oroya fever**, a serious infectious anemia; the eruptive stage, **verruga peruana**, commonly begins 2–8 weeks later, although verruga may also appear in the absence of Oroya fever. The infection is limited to the mountainous areas of the American Andes in tropical Peru, Colombia, and Ecuador and is transmitted by sandflies (*Phlebotomus* and *Lutzomyia*).

Bartonella grows in semisolid nutrient agar containing 10% rabbit serum and 0.5% hemoglobin. After about 10 days' incubation at 28 °C, some turbidity develops in the medium and rod-shaped and granular organisms can be seen in Giemsa-stained smears.

Oroya fever is characterized by the rapid development of severe anemia due to blood destruction, enlargement of the spleen and liver, and hemorrhage into the lymph nodes. Masses of bartonellae fill the cytoplasm of cells lining the blood vessels, and endothelial swelling may lead to vascular occlusion and thrombosis. The mortality rate of untreated Oroya fever is about 40%. The diagnosis is made by examining stained blood smears and blood cultures in semisolid medium.

Verruga peruana consists of vascular, granulomatous skin lesions that occur in successive crops; it lasts for about 1 year and produces little systemic reaction and no fatalities. Bartonellae can be seen in the granuloma; blood cultures are often positive, but there is no anemia.

Penicillin, streptomycin, and chloramphenicol are dramatically effective in Oroya fever and greatly reduce the mortality rate, particularly when blood transfusions are also given. Control of the disease depends upon elimination of the sandfly vectors: Insecticides, insect repellents, and elimination of sandfly breeding areas are of value. Prevention with antibiotics may be useful.

CALYMMATOBACTERIUM (DONOVANIA) GRANULOMATIS

C granulomatis, related to the klebsiellae, causes granuloma inguinale, an uncommon sexually transmitted disease. The organism grows with difficulty on media containing egg yolk. Ampicillin or tetracycline is effective treatment.

CAT-SCRATCH DISEASE

This is usually a benign, self-limited illness with fever and lymphadenopathy that develops about 2 weeks after contact with a cat (usually a scratch, lick, or bite). A primary skin lesion (papule or pustule) develops at the site 3–10 days after the contact. The patient usually appears well but may have low-grade fever and occasionally headache, sore throat, or conjunctivitis. The regional lymph nodes are markedly enlarged and sometimes tender, and they may not subside for several weeks or even months. They may suppurate and discharge pus.

The causative agent appears to be a small, pleomorphic, rod-shaped bacterium present mainly in the walls of capillaries near follicular hyperplasia or within microabscesses. The organisms are seen best in tissue sections stained with Warthin-Starry silver impregnation stain; they may also be detected with an immunofluorescence test using convalescent antiserum. They appear to be gram-variable and have not been grown in culture with certainty.

The diagnosis is based on (1) a suggestive history and physical findings; (2) aspiration of pus from lymph nodes that contains no pyogenic bacteria; (3) a positive skin test; and (4) representative histopathology, including bacteria seen on silver-impregnated stains.

Skin test material is obtained by aspirating pus aseptically from a typical case and heat-treating it to ensure freedom from infectious agents. The skin test is of the delayed hypersensitivity type and appears to be both reliable and specific. The material has been available from Dr. A.M. Margileth, Department of Pediatrics, Uniformed Services University of the Health Sciences, Bethesda, Md.

Treatment is mainly supportive: reassurance, hot moist soaks, and analgesics. Antimicrobial drugs do not appear to influence the course of the illness. Aspiration of pus or surgical removal of an excessively large lymph node may ameliorate symptoms.

REFERENCES

Barresi JA: *Listeria monocytogenes*: A cause of premature labor and neonatal sepsis. *Am J Obstet Gynecol* 1980;**136**:410.

Brooks GF et al: *Eikenella corrodens*. A recently recognized pathogen: Infections in medical-surgical patients and in association with methylphenidate abuse. *Medicine* 1974;**53**:325.

Cordes LG et al: Legionnaires' disease outbreak at an Atlanta, Georgia, country club: Evidence for spread from an evaporative condenser. *Am J Epidemiol* 1980;**111**:425.

Dorff GJ et al: Infections with *Eikenella corrodens*: A newly recognized human pathogen. *Ann Intern Med* 1974;**80**:305.

Eickhoff TC: Epidemiology of Legionnaires' disease. *Ann Intern Med* 1979;**90**:499.

Ellis ME, Mandal BK: Hyperbaric oxygen treatment: 10 years' experience of a regional infectious disease unit. *J Infect* 1983;**6**:17.

Finegold SM: *Anaerobic Bacteria in Human Disease*. Academic Press, 1977.

Geraci JE et al: *Cardiobacterium hominis* endocarditis: Four cases with clinical and laboratory observations. *Mayo Clin Proc* 1978;**53**:49.

Gerber MA et al: The aetiological agent of cat scratch disease. *Lancet* 1985;**1**:1236.

Goldstein EJC et al: Isolation of *Eikenella corrodens* from pulmonary infections. *Am Rev Respir Dis* 1979;**119**:55.

Goldstein EJC et al: Susceptibility of *Eikenella corrodens* to newer beta-lactam antibiotics. *Antimicrob Agents Chemother* 1980;**18**:832.

Gorbach SL, Bartlett JG: Anaerobic infections. *N Engl J Med* 1974;**290**:1177.

Kasper DL et al: Surface antigens as virulence factors in infection with *Bacteroides fragilis*. *Rev Infect Dis* 1979;**1**:278.

Kirby BD et al: Legionnaires' disease: Report of sixty-five nosocomially acquired cases and review of the literature. *Medicine* 1980;**59**:188.

Kuberski T: Granuloma inguinale (donovanosis). *Sex Transm Dis* 1980;**7**:29.

Mardh P-A, Taylor-Robinson D (editors): *Bacterial Vaginosis*. Almqvist & Wiksell, 1984.

Meyer RD: *Legionella* infections: A review of five years of research. *Rev Infect Dis* 1983;**5**:258.

Nieman RE, Lorber B: Listeriosis in adults. A changing pattern: Report of eight cases and review of the literature, 1968–1978. *Rev Infect Dis* 1980;**2**:207.

Redfield DC et al: Bacteria, arthritis, and skin lesions due to *Kingella kingae*. *Arch Dis Child* 1980;**55**:411.

Roberts MC et al: Comparison of gram stain, DNA probe and culture for identification of species of *Mobiluncus* in female genital specimens. *J Infect Dis* 1985;**152**:74.

Sanford JP: Legionnaires' disease: The first thousand days. *N Engl J Med* 1979;**300**:654.

Stamm WE et al: Indwelling arterial catheters as a source of nosocomial bacteremia: An outbreak caused by *Flavobacterium* species. *N Engl J Med* 1975;**292**:1099.

Visintine AM et al: *Listeria monocytogenes* infection in infants and children. *Am J Dis Child* 1977;**131**:393.

Wear DJ et al: Cat scratch disease: A bacterial infection. *Science* 1983;**221**:1403.

Zaleznik DF, Kasper DL: The role of anaerobic bacteria in abscess formation. *Annu Rev Med* 1982;**33**:217.

Mycoplasmas (Mollicutes) & Cell Wall–Defective Bacteria

25

Mycoplasmas are a group of organisms with the following characteristics: (1) The smallest reproductive units have a size of 125–250 nm. (2) Mycoplasmas are highy pleomorphic because they lack a rigid cell wall and instead are bounded by a triple-layered "unit membrane" that contains a sterol (mycoplasmas require sterols for growth). (3) They are completely resistant to penicillin because they lack the cell wall structures where penicillin acts, but they are inhibited by tetracycline or erythromycin. (4) They can reproduce in cell-free media; on agar, the center of the whole colony is characteristically embedded beneath the surface. (5) Growth is inhibited by specific antibody. (6) Mycoplasmas do not revert to, or originate from, bacterial parental forms. (7) Mycoplasmas have an affinity for mammalian cell membranes. Mycoplasmas were formerly called PPLO (pleuropneumonia-like organisms).

L phase variants (L forms) are wall-defective microbial forms (WDMFs) that can replicate serially as nonrigid cells and produce colonies on solid media. Some L phase variants are stable; others are unstable and revert to bacterial parental forms. WDMFs are not genetically related to mycoplasmas. WDMFs can result from spontaneous mutation or from the effects of chemicals. Treatment of eubacteria with cell wall–inhibiting drugs or lysozyme can produce WDMFs. **Protoplasts** are WDMFs usually derived from gram-positive organisms; they are osmotically fragile, with external surfaces free of cell wall constituents. **Spheroplasts** are WDMFs usually derived from gram-negative bacteria; they retain some outer membrane material (see p 20).

Morphology & Identification

A. Typical Organisms: Mycoplasmas cannot be studied by the usual bacteriologic methods because of the small size of their colonies, the plasticity and delicacy of their individual cells (owing to the lack of a rigid cell wall), and their poor staining with aniline dyes. The morphology appears different according to the method of examination (eg, darkfield, immunofluorescence, Giemsa-stained films from solid or liquid media, agar fixation).

Growth in fluid media gives rise to many different forms, including rings, bacillary and spiral bodies, filaments, and granules. Growth on solid media consists principally of plastic protoplasmic masses of indefinite shape that are easily distorted. These structures vary greatly in size, ranging from 50 to 300 nm in diameter.

B. Culture: Many strains of mycoplasmas grow in heart infusion peptone broth with 2% agar (pH 7.8) to which about 30% human ascitic fluid or animal serum (horse, rabbit) has been added. Following incubation at 37 °C for 48–96 hours, there may be no turbidity; but Giemsa stains of the centrifuged sediment show the characteristic pleomorphic structures, and subculture on solid media yields minute colonies.

After 2–6 days on special agar medium incubated in a Petri dish that has been sealed to prevent evaporation, isolated colonies measuring 20–500 μm can be detected with a hand lens. These colonies are round, with a granular surface and a dark center typically buried in the agar. They can be subcultured by cutting out a small square of agar containing one or more colonies and streaking this material on a fresh plate or dropping it into liquid medium. The organisms can be stained for microscopic study by placing a similar square on a slide and covering the colony with a coverglass onto which an alcoholic solution of methylene blue and azure has been poured and then evaporated (agar fixation). Such slides can also be stained with specific fluorescent antibody.

C. Growth Characteristics: Mycoplasmas are unique in microbiology because of (1) their extremely small size and (2) their growth on complex but cell-free media.

Mycoplasmas pass through filters with 450-nm pore size and thus are comparable to chlamydiae or large viruses. However, parasitic mycoplasmas grow on cell-free media that contain lipoprotein and sterol. The sterol requirement for growth and membrane synthesis is unique. Mycoplasmas are resistant to thallium acetate in a concentration of 1:10,000, which can be used to inhibit bacteria.

Many mycoplasmas use glucose as a source of energy; ureaplasmas require urea.

Some human mycoplasmas produce peroxides and hemolyze red blood cells. In cell cultures and in vivo, mycoplasmas develop predominantly at cell surfaces. Many established animal and human cell culture lines carry mycoplasmas as contaminants.

D. Variation: The extreme pleomorphism of mycoplasmas is one of their principal characteristics. There is no genetic relationship between mycoplasmas and WDMFs or their parent bacteria. The characteristics of WDMFs are similar to those of mycoplasmas, but by definition, mycoplasmas do not revert to parental bacterial forms or originate from them. WDMFs continue to synthesize some antigens that are normally located in the cell wall of the parent bacteria (eg, streptococcal L forms produce M protein and capsular polysaccharide). Reversion of L forms to the parental bacterial form is enhanced by growth in the presence of 15–30% gelatin or 2.5% agar. Reversion is inhibited by inhibitors of protein synthesis.

Antigenic Structure

Many antigenically distinct species of mycoplasmas have been isolated from animals (eg, mice, chickens, turkeys). In humans, at least 11 species can be identified, including *Mycoplasma hominis, Mycoplasma salivarium, Mycoplasma orale, Mycoplasma fermentans, Mycoplasma pneumoniae, Ureaplasma urealyticum,* and others. The last 2 species are of pathogenic significance.

The species are classified by biochemical and serologic features. The CF antigens of mycoplasmas are glycolipids. Antigens for ELISA tests are proteins. Some species have more than one serotype.

Diseases Due to Mycoplasmas

It is uncertain whether WDMFs cause tissue reactions resulting in disease. They may be important for the persistence of microorganisms in tissue and recurrence of infection after antimicrobial treatment, as in rare cases of endocarditis.

The parasitic mycoplasmas appear to be strictly host-specific, being communicable and potentially pathogenic only within a single host species. In animals, mycoplasmas appear to be intracellular parasites with a predilection for mesothelial cells (pleura, peritoneum, synovia of joints). Several extracellular products can be elaborated (eg, hemolysins).

A. Diseases of Animals: Bovine pleuropneumonia is a contagious disease of cattle producing pneumonia and pleural effusion, with occasional deaths. The disease probably has an airborne spread. Mycoplasmas are found in inflammatory exudates.

Agalactia of sheep and goats in the Mediterranean area is a generalized infection with local lesions in the skin, eyes, joints, udder, and scrotum; it leads to atrophy of lactating glands in females. Mycoplasmas are present in blood early; in milk and exudates later.

In poultry, several economically important respiratory diseases are caused by mycoplasmas. The organisms can be transmitted from hen to egg to chick. Swine, dogs, rats, mice, and other species harbor mycoplasmas that can produce infection involving particularly the pleura, peritoneum, joints, respiratory tract, and eye. In mice, a *Mycoplasma* of spiral shape *(Spiroplasma)* can induce cataracts.

B. Diseases of Humans: Mycoplasmas have been cultivated from human mucous membranes and tissues, particularly from the genital, urinary, and respiratory tracts and from the mouth. Some mycoplas-

mas are normal inhabitants of the genitourinary tract, particularly in females. In pregnant women, carriage of mycoplasmas on the cervix has been associated with chorioamnionitis and low birth weight of infants. *U urealyticum* (formerly called T strain mycoplasma), which requires 10% urea for growth, is found in the urethra of some men with nongonococcal urethritis. Such infection may play a role in male infertility. *M hominis* has been associated infrequently with pelvic inflammatory disease. *U urealyticum* and *M hominis* are suppressed by tetracyclines or erythromycin. However, a majority of cases of nongonococcal urethritis are caused by *Chlamydia trachomatis* (see p 311).

Infrequently, mycoplasmas have been isolated from brain abscesses and pleural joint effusions. Mycoplasmas are part of the normal flora of the mouth and can be grown from normal saliva, oral mucous membranes, sputum, or tonsillar tissue.

M hominis and *M salivarium* can be recovered from the oral cavity of many healthy adults, but an association with clinical disease is uncertain. Over half of normal adults have specific antibodies to *M hominis*.

M pneumoniae is a principal cause of nonbacterial pneumonia. In humans, the effects of infection with *M pneumoniae* range from inapparent infection to mild or severe upper respiratory disease, ear involvement (myringitis), and pneumonia (see p 283).

C. Diseases of Plants: Aster yellows, corn stunt, and other plant disease appear to be caused by mycoplasmas. They are transmitted by insects and can be suppressed by tetracyclines.

Diagnostic Laboratory Tests

A. Specimens: Specimens consist of throat swab, sputum, inflammatory exudates, and respiratory, urethral, or genital secretions.

B. Microscopic Examination: Direct examination of a specimen for mycoplasmas is useless. Cultures are examined as described above.

C. Cultures: The material is inoculated onto special solid media (see above) and incubated for 3–10 days at 37 °C with 5% CO_2 (under microaerophilic conditions), or into special broth (see above) and incubated aerobically. One or 2 transfers of media may be necessary before growth appears that is suitable for microscopic examination by staining or immunofluorescence. Colonies may have a "fried egg" appearance on agar.

D. Serology: Antibodies develop in humans infected with mycoplasmas and can be demonstrated by several methods. CF tests can be performed with glycolipid antigens extracted with chloroform-methanol from cultured mycoplasmas. HI tests can be applied to tanned red cells with adsorbed *Mycoplasma* antigens. Indirect immunofluorescence may be used. The test that measures growth inhibition by antibody is quite specific. When counterimmunoelectrophoresis is used, antigens and antibody migrate toward each other, and precipitin lines appear in 1 hour. With all these serologic techniques, there is adequate specificity for different human *Mycoplasma* species, but a rising antibody titer is required for diagnostic significance because of the high incidence of positive serologic tests in normal individuals.

Treatment

Many strains of mycoplasmas are inhibited by a variety of antimicrobial drugs, but most strains are resistant to penicillins, cephalosporins, and vancomycin. Tetracyclines and erythromycins are effective both in vitro and in vivo and are, at present, the drugs of choice in mycoplasmal pneumonia.

Epidemiology, Prevention, & Control

Isolation of infected livestock will control the highly contagious pleuropneumonia and agalactia in limited areas. No vaccines are available. Mycoplasmal pneumonia behaves like a communicable viral respiratory disease (see below).

Mycoplasmal Pneumonia & Nonbacterial Pneumonias

A. Causative Organisms: Acute nonbacterial pneumonitis may be due to many different infectious agents, including adenoviruses, influenza viruses, respiratory syncytial virus, parainfluenza type 3 virus, chlamydiae, and *Coxiella burnetii* (the cause of Q fever). However, the single most prominent causative agent, especially for persons between ages 5 and 15 years, is *M pneumoniae*. Mycoplasmal pneumonia appears to be much more common in military recruits than in college populations of comparable age.

B. Clinical Findings: The first step in *M pneumoniae* infection is the attachment of the tip of the organism to a receptor on the surface of respiratory epithelial cells. The clinical spectrum of *M pneumoniae* infection ranges from asymptomatic infection to serious pneumonitis, with occasional neurologic and hematologic (ie, hemolytic anemia) involvement and a variety of possible skin lesions. Bullous myringitis occurs in spontaneous cases and in experimentally inoculated volunteers.

The incubation period varies from 1 to 3 weeks. The onset is usually insidious, with lassitude, fever, headache, sore throat, and cough. Initially, the cough is nonproductive, but it is occasionally paroxysmal. Later there may be blood-streaked sputum and chest pain. Early in the course, the patient appears only moderately ill, and physical signs of pulmonary consolidation are often negligible compared to the striking consolidation seen on x-rays. Later, when the infiltration is at a peak, the illness may be severe. Resolution of pulmonary infiltration and clinical improvement occur slowly over 1–4 weeks. Although the course of the illness is exceedingly variable, death is very rare and is usually attributable to cardiac failure. Complications are uncommon, but hemolytic anemia may occur. The most common pathologic findings are interstitial and peribronchial pneumonitis and necrotizing bronchiolitis. On rare occasions, central nervous system involvement has accompanied or followed mycoplasmal pneumonia.

C. Laboratory Findings: The following laboratory findings apply to *M pneumoniae* pneumonia: The white and differential counts are within normal limits. The causative *Mycoplasma* can be recovered by culture, early in the disease, from the pharynx and from sputum. There is a rise in specific antibodies to *M pneumoniae* that is demonstrable by CF, immunofluorescence, passive hemagglutination, and growth inhibition tests.

A variety of nonspecific reactions can be observed. Cold hemagglutinins for group O human erythrocytes appear in about 50% of untreated patients, in rising titer, with the maximum reached in the third or fourth week after onset. A titer of 1:64 or more supports the diagnosis of *M pneumoniae* infection.

D. Treatment: Tetracyclines or erythromycins in full systemic doses (2 g daily for adults) can produce clinical improvement but do not eradicate the mycoplasmas.

E. Epidemiology, Prevention, & Control: *M pneumoniae* infections are endemic all over the world. In populations of children and young adults where close contact prevails, and in families, the infection rate may be high (50–90%), but the incidence of pneumonitis is variable (3–30%). For every case of frank pneumonitis, there exist several cases of milder respiratory illness. *M pneumoniae* is apparently transmitted mainly by direct contact involving respiratory secretions. Second attacks are infrequent. The presence of antibodies to *M pneumoniae* has been associated with resistance to infection but may not be responsible for it. Cell-mediated immune reactions occur. The pneumonic process may be attributed in part to an immunologic response rather than only to infection by mycoplasmas. Experimental vaccines have been prepared from agar-grown *M pneumoniae*. Several such killed vaccines have aggravated subsequent disease; a degree of protection has been claimed with the use of other vaccines, but none are available for clinical use.

REFERENCES

Cassell GH, Cole BC: Mycoplasmas as agents of human disease. *N Engl J Med* 1981;**304**:80.

Edwards EA et al: A longitudinal study of *Mycoplasma pneumoniae*: Infections in Navy recruits by isolation and seroepidemiology. *Am J Epidemiol* 1976; **104**:556.

Goldschmidt BL et al: Rapid detection of *Mycoplasma* anti-

body. *J Immunol* 1976;**117**:1054.

Kundsin RB et al: *Ureaplasma urealyticum* incriminated in perinatal morbidity and mortality. *Science* 1981;**213**:474.

Platt R et al: Infection with *Mycoplasma hominis* in postpartum fever. *Lancet* 1980;**2**:1217.

Taylor-Robinson D, McCormack WM: The genital mycoplasmas. (2 parts.) *N Engl J Med* 1980;**302:** 1003, 1063.

Thompson SE III et al: The microbiology and therapy of acute pelvic inflammatory disease in hospitalized patients. *Am J Obstet Gynecol* 1980;**136:**179.

Ti TY et al: Isolation of *Mycoplasma hominis* from the blood of men with multiple trauma and fever. *JAMA* 1982;**247:**60.

Toth A et al: Subsequent pregnancies among 161 couples treated for T-mycoplasma genital-tract infection. *N Engl J Med* 1983;**308:**505.

Wenzel RP et al: Field trial of an inactivated *Mycoplasma pneumoniae* vaccine. 1. Vaccine efficacy. *J Infect Dis* 1976;**134:**571.

Mycobacteria

26

The mycobacteria are rod-shaped, nonsporeforming, aerobic bacteria that do not stain readily but, once stained, resist decolorization by acid or alcohol and are therefore called "acid-fast" bacilli. In addition to many saprophytic forms, the group includes pathogenic organisms (eg, *Mycobacterium tuberculosis*, *Mycobacterium leprae*) that cause chronic diseases producing lesions of the infectious granuloma type. The importance of atypical mycobacteria as opportunistic pathogens in immunocompromised persons is increasing.

MYCOBACTERIUM TUBERCULOSIS

Morphology & Identification:

A. Typical Organisms: In animal tissues, tubercle bacilli are thin straight rods measuring about 0.4 × 3 μm. On artificial media, coccoid and filamentous forms are seen. Mycobacteria cannot be classified as either gram-positive or gram-negative. Once stained by basic dyes they cannot be decolorized by alcohol, regardless of treatment with iodine. True tubercle bacilli are characterized by "acid-fastness," eg, 95% ethyl alcohol containing 3% hydrochloric acid (acid-alcohol) quickly decolorizes all bacteria except the mycobacteria. Acid-fastness depends on the integrity of the structure of the waxy envelope. The Ziehl-Neelsen technique of staining is employed for identification of acid-fast bacteria. In sputum or sections of tissue, mycobacteria can be demonstrated by yellow-orange fluorescence after staining with fluorochrome stains (eg, auramine, rhodamine).

B. Culture: Three types of media are employed.

1. Simple synthetic media—Large inocula grow on simple synthetic media in several weeks. Small inocula fail to grow in such media because of the presence of minute amounts of toxic fatty acids. The toxic effect of fatty acids can be neutralized by animal serum or albumin, and the fatty acids may then actually promote growth. Activated charcoal aids growth.

2. Oleic acid–albumin media—These media may support the proliferation of small inocula, particularly if Tweens (water-soluble esters of fatty acids) are present (eg, Dubos' medium). Ordinarily, mycobacteria grow in clumps or masses because of the hydrophobic character of the cell surface. Tweens wet the surface and thus permit dispersed growth in liquid media. Growth is often more rapid than on complex media.

3. Complex organic media—Small inocula, eg, specimens from patients, are grown on media containing complex organic substances, eg, egg yolk, animal serum, tissue extracts. These media often contain penicillin or malachite green (eg, Löwenstein-Jensen medium) to inhibit other bacteria.

C. Growth Characteristics: Mycobacteria are obligate aerobes and derive energy from the oxidation of many simple carbon compounds. Increased CO_2 tension enhances growth. Biochemical activities are not characteristic, and the growth rate is much slower than that of most bacteria. The doubling time of tubercle bacilli is about 18 hours. Saprophytic forms tend to grow more rapidly, proliferate well at 22 °C, produce more pigment, and be less acid-fast than pathogenic forms.

D. Reaction to Physical and Chemical Agents: Mycobacteria tend to be more resistant to chemical agents than other bacteria because of the hydrophobic nature of the cell surface and their clumped growth. Dyes (eg, malachite green) or antibacterial agents (eg, penicillin) that are bacteriostatic to other bacteria can be incorporated into media without inhibiting the growth of tubercle bacilli. Acids and alkalies permit the survival of some exposed tubercle bacilli and are used for "concentration" of clinical specimens and partial elimination of contaminating organisms. Tubercle bacilli are resistant to drying and survive for long periods in dried sputum.

E. Variation: Variation can occur in colony appearance, pigmentation, cord factor production, virulence, optimal growth temperature, and many other cellular or growth characteristics.

F. Pathogenicity of Mycobacteria: There are marked differences in the ability of different mycobacteria to cause lesions in various host species. Examples are shown in Table 26–1.

M tuberculosis and *Mycobacterium bovis* are equally pathogenic for humans. The route of infection (respiratory versus intestinal) determines the pattern of lesions. In developed countries, *M bovis* has become very rare. Some "atypical" mycobacteria (eg, *Mycobacterium kansasii*) produce human disease indistinguishable from tuberculosis; others (eg, *Mycobacterium fortuitum*) cause only surface lesions or act as opportunists.

Constituents of Tubercle Bacilli

The constituents listed below are found largely in cell walls. Mycobacterial cell walls can induce de-

Table 26–1. Pathogenicity of mycobacteria.

Species	Human	Guinea Pig	Fowl	Cattle
M tuberculosis	+++	+++	–	–
M bovis	+++	+++	–	+++
M kansasii	+++	–	–	–
M avium-intracellulare*	+	–	+++	–
M fortuitum-chelonei*	+	–	–	–
M leprae	++	–	–	–

*Complex

layed hypersensitivity, induce some resistance to infection, and replace whole mycobacterial cells in Freund's adjuvant. Mycobacterial cell contents only elicit delayed hypersensitivity reactions in previously sensitized animals.

A. Lipids: Mycobacteria are rich in lipids, including fatty acids and waxes. In the cell, the lipids are largely bound to proteins and polysaccharides. Lipids are probably responsible for most of the cellular tissue reactions to tubercle bacilli. Phosphatide fractions can produce tuberclelike cellular responses and caseation necrosis. Lipids are to some extent responsible for acid-fastness. Bound lipids are removed by hot acid, which destroys acid-fastness. Acid-fastness is also lost after sonic disruption of normal cells. It appears to depend on both the integrity of the cell wall and the presence of certain lipids. Analysis of lipids by gas chromatography reveals patterns that aid in classification of different species.

Virulent strains of tubercle bacilli form microscopic "serpentine cords" in which acid-fast bacilli are arranged in parallel chains. Cord formation is correlated with virulence. A "cord factor" (trehalose-6,6'-dimycolate) has been extracted from virulent bacilli with petroleum ether. It inhibits migration of leukocytes, causes chronic granulomas, and can serve as an immunologic "adjuvant" (see Chapter 13).

B. Proteins: Each type of mycobacterium contains several proteins that elicit the tuberculin reaction. Proteins bound to a wax fraction can, upon injection, induce tuberculin sensitivity. They can also elicit the formation of a variety of antibodies.

C. Polysaccharides: Mycobacteria contain a variety of polysaccharides. Their role in the pathogenesis of disease is uncertain. They can induce the immediate type of hypersensitivity and can interfere with some antigen-antibody reactions in vitro.

Pathogenesis

Mycobacteria produce no recognized toxins. Organisms in droplets of 1–5 μm are inhaled and reach alveoli. The disease results from establishment and proliferation of virulent organisms and interactions with the host. Injected avirulent bacilli (eg, BCG) survive only for months or years in the normal host. Resistance and hypersensitivity of the host greatly influence the development of the disease.

Pathology

The production and development of lesions and their healing or progression are determined chiefly by (1) the number of mycobacteria in the inoculum and their subsequent multiplication, and (2) the resistance and hypersensitivity of the host.

A. Two Principal Lesions:

1. Exudative type–This consists of an acute inflammatory reaction, with edema fluid, polymorphonuclear leukocytes, and, later, monocytes around the tubercle bacilli. This type is seen particularly in lung tissue, where it resembles bacterial pneumonia. It may heal by resolution, so that the entire exudate becomes absorbed; it may lead to massive necrosis of tissue; or it may develop into the second (productive) type of lesion. During the exudative phase, the tuberculin test becomes positive.

2. Productive type–When fully developed, this lesion, a chronic granuloma, consists of 3 zones: (1) a central area of large, multinucleated giant cells containing tubercle bacilli; (2) a mid zone of pale epithelioid cells, often arranged radially; and (3) a peripheral zone of fibroblasts, lymphocytes, and monocytes. Later, peripheral fibrous tissue develops and the central area undergoes caseation necrosis. Such a lesion is called a tubercle. A caseous tubercle may break into a bronchus, empty its contents there, and form a cavity. It may subsequently heal by fibrosis or calcification.

B. Spread of Organisms in the Host: Tubercle bacilli spread in the host by direct extension, through the lymphatic channels and bloodstream, and via the bronchi and gastrointestinal tract.

In the first infection, tubercle bacilli always spread from the initial site via the lymphatics to the regional lymph nodes. The bacilli may spread farther and reach the bloodstream, which in turn disseminates bacilli to all organs (miliary distribution). The bloodstream can be invaded also by erosion of a vein by a caseating tubercle or lymph node. If a caseating lesion discharges its contents into a bronchus, they are aspirated and distributed to other parts of the lungs or are swallowed and passed into the stomach and intestines.

C. Intracellular Site of Growth: Once mycobacteria establish themselves in tissue, they reside principally intracellularly in monocytes, reticuloendothelial cells, and giant cells. The intracellular location is one of the features that makes chemotherapy difficult and favors microbial persistence. Within the cells of immune animals, multiplication of tubercle bacilli is greatly inhibited.

Primary Infection & Reactivation Types of Tuberculosis

When a host has first contact with tubercle bacilli, the following features are usually observed: (1) An acute exudative lesion develops and rapidly spreads to the lymphatics and regional lymph nodes. The "Ghon complex" is the primary tissue lesion (usually in the lung) together with the involved lymph nodes. The exudative lesion in tissue often heals rapidly. (2) The lymph node undergoes massive caseation, which usually calcifies. (3) The tuberculin test becomes positive.

This primary infection type occurred in the past usually in childhood but now is seen frequently in adults who have remained free from infection and therefore tuberculin-negative in early life. In primary infections, the involvement may be in any part of the lung but is most often at the base.

The reactivation type is usually caused by tubercle bacilli that have survived in the primary lesion. Reactivation tuberculosis is characterized by chronic tissue lesions, the formation of tubercles, caseation, and fibrosis. Regional lymph nodes are only slightly involved, and they do not caseate. The reactivation type almost always begins at the apex of the lung, where the oxygen tension (P_{O_2}) is highest.

The contrast between primary infection and reinfection is shown experimentally in **Koch's phenomenon.** When a guinea pig is injected subcutaneously with virulent tubercle bacilli, the puncture wound heals quickly, but a nodule forms at the site of injection in 2 weeks. This nodule ulcerates, and the ulcer does not heal. The regional lymph nodes develop tubercles and caseate massively. When the same animal is later injected with tubercle bacilli in another part of the body, the sequence of events is quite different: there is rapid necrosis of skin and tissue at the site of injection, but the ulcer heals rapidly. Regional lymph nodes either do not become infected at all or do so only after a delay.

These differences between primary infection and reinfection or reactivation are attributed to (1) resistance and (2) hypersensitivity induced by the first infection of the host with tubercle bacilli. It is not clear to what extent each of these components participates in the modified response in reactivation tuberculosis.

Immunity & Hypersensitivity

Unless a host dies during the first infection with tubercle bacilli, a certain resistance is acquired (see Koch's phenomenon, above), and there is an increased capacity to localize tubercle bacilli, retard their multiplication, limit their spread, and reduce lymphatic dissemination. This can be largely attributed to the ability of mononuclear cells to limit the multiplication of ingested organisms and perhaps to destroy them. Mononuclear cells acquire this "cellular immunity" in the course of initial infection of the host.

Antibodies form against a variety of the cellular constituents of the tubercle bacilli. The presence of antibodies can be determined by precipitation, CF, passive hemagglutination, and ELISA (enzyme-linked immunosorbent assay) tests. None of these serologic reactions bears any unequivocal relation to the immune state of the host, but high titers of IgG antibody to PPD, detectable by the ELISA test, are believed to exist in many patients with active pulmonary tuberculosis.

In the course of primary infection, the host also acquires hypersensitivity to the tubercle bacilli. This is made evident by the development of a positive tuberculin reaction (see below). Tuberculin sensitivity can be induced by whole tubercle bacilli or by tuberculo-protein in combination with the chloroform-soluble wax of the tubercle bacillus, but not by tuberculoprotein alone. Hypersensitivity and resistance appear to be distinct aspects of related cell-mediated reactions.

Tuberculin Test

A. Material: Old tuberculin (OT) is a concentrated filtrate of broth in which tubercle bacilli have grown for 6 weeks. In addition to the reactive tuberculoproteins, this material contains a variety of other constituents of tubercle bacilli and of growth medium. A purified protein derivative (PPD) can be obtained by chemical fractionation of OT and is the preferred material for skin testing. PPD is standardized in terms of its biologic reactivity as "tuberculin units" (TU). By international agreement, the TU is defined as the activity contained in a specified weight of Seibert's PPD Lot # 49608 in a specified buffer. This is PPD-S, the standard for tuberculin against which the potency of all products must be established by biologic assay— ie, by reaction size in humans. First strength tuberculin has 1 TU; intermediate strength has 5 TU; and second strength has 250 TU. Bioequivalency of PPD products is not based on weight of the material but on comparative activity.

B. Dose of Tuberculin: A large amount of tuberculin injected into a hypersensitive host may give rise to severe local reactions and a flare-up of inflammation and necrosis at the main sites of infection (focal reactions). For this reason, tuberculin tests in surveys employ 5 TU; in persons suspected of extreme hypersensitivity, skin testing is begun with 1 TU. More concentrated material (250 TU) is administered only if the reaction to 5 TU is negative. The volume is usually 0.1 mL injected intracutaneously. The PPD preparation must be stabilized with polysorbate-80 to prevent adsorption to glass.

C. Reactions to Tuberculin: In an individual who has not had contact with mycobacteria, there is no reaction to PPD-S. An individual who has had a primary infection with tubercle bacilli develops induration, edema, erythema in 24–48 hours, and, with very intense reactions, even central necrosis. The skin test should be read in 48 or 72 hours. It is considered positive if the injection of 5 TU is followed by induration 10 mm or more in diameter. Positive tests tend to persist for several days. Weak reactions may disappear more rapidly.

The tuberculin test becomes positive within 4–6 weeks after infection (or injection of avirulent bacilli). It may be negative in the presence of tuberculous infection when "anergy" develops due to overwhelming tuberculosis, measles, Hodgkin's disease, sarcoidosis, or immunosuppression. A positive tuberculin test may occasionally revert to negative upon isoniazid treatment of a recent converter. After BCG vaccination, a positive test may last for only 3–7 years. Only the elimination of viable tubercle bacilli results in reversion of the tuberculin test to negative. However, persons who had been PPD-positive years ago and are healthy may fail to give a positive skin test. When such persons are retested 2 weeks later, their PPD skin test—"boosted" by the recent antigen injection—will give a positive size of induration again. The reactivity to tuberculin can be transferred only by cells—not by serum—from a tuberculin-positive to a tuberculin-negative person.

D. Interpretation of Tuberculin Test: A positive tuberculin test indicates that an individual has been infected in the past and continues to carry viable mycobacteria in some tissue. It does not imply that active disease or immunity to disease is present. Tuberculin-positive persons are at risk of developing disease from reactivation of the primary infection, whereas tuberculin-negative persons who have never been infected are not subject to that risk, although they may become infected from an external source.

PPDs from other mycobacteria have been prepared. They exhibit some species specificity in low concentrations and marked cross-reaction in higher concentrations (see Other Mycobacteria, below).

Clinical Findings

Since the tubercle bacillus can involve every organ system, its clinical manifestations are protean. Fatigue, weakness, weight loss, and fever may be signs of tuberculous disease. Pulmonary involvement giving rise to chronic cough and spitting of blood usually is associated with far-advanced lesions. Meningitis or urinary tract involvement can occur in the absence of other signs of tuberculosis. Bloodstream dissemination leads to miliary tuberculosis with lesions in many organs and a high mortality rate.

Diagnostic Laboratory Tests

Neither the tuberculin test nor any now available serologic test can prove the presence of active disease due to tubercle bacilli. Only isolation of tubercle bacilli gives such proof.

A. Specimens: Specimens consist of fresh sputum, gastric washings, urine, pleural fluid, spinal fluid, joint fluid, biopsy material, or other suspected material.

B. Smears: Sputum, or sediment from gastric washings, urine, exudates, or other material, is examined for acid-fast bacilli by Ziehl-Neelsen staining, by a comparable method, or by fluorescence microscopy with auramine-rhodamine stain. If such organisms are found, this is presumptive evidence of mycobacterial infection.

C. Concentration for Stained Smear: If a direct smear is negative, sputum may be liquefied by addition of 20% Clorox (1% hypochlorite solution) and then centrifuged, and the sediment stained and examined microscopically. This "digested material" is unsuitable for culture.

D. Culture: Urine, spinal fluid, and materials not contaminated with other bacteria may be cultured directly. Sputum is first treated with 2% sodium hydroxide or other agents bactericidal for contaminating microorganisms but less so for tubercle bacilli (see Table

26–2). The liquefied sputum is then neutralized and centrifuged and the sediment inoculated into appropriate media. Incubation of the inoculated media is continued for up to 8 weeks.

Isolated mycobacteria should be identified and tested for drug susceptibility.

E. Animal Inoculation: Part of the cultured material may be inoculated subcutaneously into guinea pigs, which are tuberculin tested after 3–4 weeks and autopsied after 6 weeks to search for evidence of tuberculosis. This is now rarely done, because culture methods are adequately sensitive.

F. Serology: No known serologic test is of value in diagnosis.

Treatment

Physical and mental rest, nutritional buildup, and various forms of collapse therapy were used in the past but have been supplanted by specific chemotherapy. The most widely used antituberculosis drugs at present are isoniazid (INH; see Chapter 10), ethambutol, rifampin, and streptomycin. Unfortunately, resistant variants of tubercle bacilli against each of these drugs emerge rapidly. Treatment is most successful when the drugs are used concomitantly (eg, INH + rifampin; INH + ethambutol; etc), thus delaying the emergence of resistant forms. Occasionally, primary infection occurs with tubercle bacilli resistant to one or more drugs. (In the USA, 3–13% of primary infections are caused by INH-resistant *M tuberculosis;* among Asian immigrants, that percentage may be 60%. This influences treatment choices.) Other drugs (eg, ethionamide, pyrazinamide, viomycin, cycloserine) are less frequently employed because of their more pronounced side effects. The available chemotherapeutic drugs result in suppression of tuberculous activity and eradication of most—but not all—tubercle bacilli. Clinical cure can usually be achieved in 6–12 months. Host factors are important in control of the residual organisms. The sputum-positive patient becomes noninfective within 2–3 weeks after beginning effective chemotherapy.

The following explanations have been advanced for the slow response of chronic tuberculosis to drug therapy: (1) Most bacilli are intracellular. (2) The caseous material in lesions, although it is itself inimical to bacterial proliferation, interferes with drug action. (3) In chronic lesions, tubercle bacilli are nonproliferating, metabolically inactive "persisters" that are not susceptible to drug action.

Epidemiology

The most frequent source of infection is the human who excretes, particularly from the respiratory tract, large numbers of tubercle bacilli. Close contact (eg, in the family) and massive exposure (eg, in medical personnel) make transmission by droplet nuclei most likely. The milk of tuberculous cows is a source of infection where bovine tuberculosis is not well controlled and where milk is not pasteurized.

Susceptibility to tuberculosis is a function of 2

Table 26–2. Culture and preliminary identification of pathogenic acid-fast organisms in sputum specimens.[*][†]

I. To sputum specimen, add equal volume of fresh mixture of N-acetyl-L-cysteine, sodium hydroxide, and trisodium citrate.

II. Mix mechanically; let stand at room temperature 15 minutes; then add phosphate buffer of pH 6.8 to make 50 mL.

III. Centrifuge at 3000 g for 15 minutes; discard supernatant; and add 2 mL of 0.2% bovine albumin fraction V. Shake to resuspend, and inoculate 0.1 mL onto a selective medium (eg, 7H10) and Löwenstein-Jensen medium.

IV. Incubate in CO_2 at 35–37 °C; inspect cultures once weekly. When growth is visible, make smears and acid-fast stains. If acid-fast organisms are present, proceed as follows:

    A. Growth in less than 7 days (rapid growers):

        1. Positive arylsulfatase test (3 days), growth on MacConkey agar–

           a. Nitrate reduction positive–*M fortuitum.*

           b. Nitrate reduction negative–*M chelonei.*

        2. Negative arylsulfatase test–Various nonpathogenic *Mycobacterium* species.

    B. Growth in more than 7 days (slow growers): (If nonpigmented, expose to light for 2–5 hours, then reincubate for 18 hours.)

        1. Nonpigmented growth–

           a. Niacin test positive, nitrate reduction positive–*M tuberculosis.*

           b. Niacin test negative, nitrate reduction variable–*Mycobacterium* other than *M tuberculosis,* eg, *M avium-intracellulare.*

        2. Pigmented growth–

           a. Pigmented when grown in light, nonpigmented in dark–Photochromogen, eg, *M kansasii.*

           b. Pigmented when grown in light or dark–Scotochromogen, eg, *M scrofulaceum.*

[*]Sommers HM, McClatchy JK: *Cumitech 16: Laboratory Diagnosis of the Mycobacterioses.* Morello JA (editor). American Society for Microbiology, 1983.
[†]Strong BE, Kubica GP: Isolation and identification of *Mycobacterium tuberculosis.* US Department of Health and Human Services Publication No. (CDC) 81-8390, 1981.

risks: the risk of acquiring the infection and the risk of clinical disease after infection has occurred. For the tuberculin-negative person, the risk of acquiring tubercle bacilli depends on exposure to sources of infectious bacilli—principally sputum-positive patients. This risk is proportionate to the rate of active infection in the population, crowding, socioeconomic disadvantage, and inadequacy of medical care. These factors, rather than genetic ones, probably account for the significantly higher rate of tuberculosis in American Indians, Eskimos, and blacks.

The second risk—the development of clinical disease after infection—has a genetic component (proved in animals and suggested in black Americans by a higher incidence of disease in those with HLA-Bw15 histocompatibility antigen). It is influenced by age (high risk in infancy and at age 16–21), by undernutrition, and by immunologic status, coexisting diseases (eg, silicosis, diabetes), and individual host resistance factors discussed below.

Infection occurs at an earlier age in urban than in rural populations. Disease occurs only in a small proportion of infected individuals. In the USA at present, active disease represents mainly endogenous reactivation tuberculosis and occurs most commonly among elderly malnourished or alcoholic poor males. Nevertheless, primary infection can occur in elderly persons of rural origin exposed to an infectious source, eg, an active case in a nursing home.

Prevention & Control

(1) Public health measures designed for early detection of cases and sources of infection (tuberculin test, x-ray) and for their prompt treatment until patients are noninfectious.

(2) Eradication of tuberculosis in cattle ("test and slaughter") and pasteurization of milk.

(3) Drug treatment of asymptomatic tuberculin

"converters" in the age groups most prone to develop complications (eg, children) and in tuberculin-positive persons who must receive immunosuppressive drugs.

(4) Immunization: Various living avirulent tubercle bacilli, particularly BCG (bacille Calmette Guérin, an attenuated bovine organism), have been used to induce a certain amount of resistance in those heavily exposed to infection. Vaccination with these organisms is a substitute for primary infection with virulent tubercle bacilli, without the danger inherent in the latter. The available vaccines are inadequate from many technical and biologic standpoints. Nevertheless, in 1984 in London, most tuberculin-negative 12-year-olds were given BCG. In Sweden, most 1-year-olds received it. In the USA, the use of BCG is suggested only for tuberculin-negative persons who are heavily exposed (members of tuberculous families, medical personnel). Statistical evidence indicates that an increased resistance for a limited period follows BCG vaccination.

The possible immunizing value of nonliving bacterial fractions is still under investigation.

(5) Individual host resistance: Nonspecific factors may reduce host resistance, thus favoring the conversion of asymptomatic infection into disease. Among such "activators" of tuberculosis are starvation, gastrectomy, and administration of high doses of corticosteroids or immunosuppressive drugs. Such patients may receive INH "prophylaxis" at any age.

OTHER MYCOBACTERIA

In addition to tubercle bacilli *(M tuberculosis, M bovis),* other mycobacteria of varying degrees of pathogenicity have been grown from human sources in past decades. These "atypical" mycobacteria were initially grouped according to speed of growth at various temperatures and production of pigments. Photochromogens produced pigment in light but not in darkness; scotochromogens developed pigment when growing in the dark; and nonphotochromogens developed various degrees of pigmentation unrelated to exposure to light (Runyon, *Med Clin North Am* 1959;**43**:273; examples in Table 26–2). More recently, individual species or complexes are defined by additional laboratory characteristics (eg, reduction of nitrate, production of urease or catalase) and certain antigenic features. Most of them occur in the environment, are not readily transmitted from person to person, and are opportunistic.

A few species or complexes that are significant in medicine are outlined below.

A. Mycobacterium kansasii: *M kansasii* is a "photochromogen" that requires complex media for growth at 37 °C. It can produce pulmonary and systemic disease indistinguishable from tuberculosis, especially in patients with impaired immune responses. Sensitive to rifampin, it is often treated with rifampin + ethambutol + INH with good clinical response. The source of infection is uncertain, and communicability is low or absent.

B. Mycobacterium avium-intracellulare Complex: The members of this group grow optimally at 41 °C and produce smooth, soft colonies with little color. Able to infect birds, they cause human disease infrequently. Infection with *M intracellulare,* however, is common in the southeastern USA, where the organism occurs in soil and water and results in skin test reactions to PPD. Overt pulmonary disease occurs mainly in immunocompromised persons, including AIDS patients. Resistance to antituberculosis drugs is common, and disease due to this organism requires treatment with up to 5 antimycobacterial drugs.

C. Mycobacterium scrofulaceum: This is a scotochromogen occasionally found in water and as a saprophyte in adults with chronic lung disease. It is a common cause of chronic cervical lymphadenitis in small children and rarely causes other granulomatous disease. Surgical excision of involved cervical lymph nodes may be curative, and resistance to antituberculosis drugs is common. Occasionally, infection responds to combined treatment with INH + rifampin + streptomycin or cycloserine. (*Mycobacterium shulgai* and *Mycobacterium xenopi* are similar.)

D. Mycobacterium marinum and Mycobacterium ulcerans: These organisms occur in water, grow best at low temperature (31 °C), may infect fish, and can produce superficial skin lesions (ulcers, "swimming pool granulomas") in humans. Surgical excision, tetracyclines, and antituberculosis drugs may be tried in therapy.

E. Mycobacterium fortuitum-chelonei Complex: These are saprophytes found in soil and water that grow rapidly (3–6 days) in culture and form no pigment. They can produce superficial and systemic disease in humans on rare occasions. *M chelonei* has contaminated porcine valves used as prostheses in human cardiac surgery. The organisms are often resistant to commonly used drugs but may be susceptible to amikacin, doxycycline, erythromycin, or rifampin.

Saprophytic Mycobacteria Not Associated With Human Illness

Mycobacterium phlei is frequently found on plants, in soil, or in water. *Mycobacterium gordonae* is similar. *Mycobacterium smegmatis* occurs regularly in human sebaceous secretions, and it might be confused with pathogenic acid-fast organisms. *Mycobacterium paratuberculosis* produces a chronic enteritis in cattle but presumably does not infect humans.

Extracts and PPD prepared from many of these mycobacteria may cross-react with PPD-S from *M tuberculosis,* resulting in positive skin tests in persons who are tuberculin-negative. This is a particular problem if a high proportion of the population becomes hypersensitive to mycobacteria acquired from the environment. For example, about half of people in the southeastern USA have contact with *M avium-intracellulare* but have not been infected with *M tuberculosis*. Nevertheless, they are PPD-positive due to cross-reactions.

MYCOBACTERIUM LEPRAE

Although this organism was described by Hansen in 1873 (9 years before Koch's discovery of the tubercle bacillus), it has not been cultivated on nonliving bacteriologic media. It causes leprosy. There are more than 10 million cases of leprosy, mainly in Asia.

Typical acid-fast bacilli—singly, in parallel bundles, or in globular masses—are regularly found in scrapings from skin or mucous membranes (particularly the nasal septum) in lepromatous leprosy. The bacilli are often found within the endothelial cells of blood vessels or in mononuclear cells. The organisms have not been grown on artificial media. When bacilli from human leprosy (ground tissue, nasal scrapings) are inoculated into foot pads of mice, local granulomatous lesions develop with limited multiplication of bacilli. Inoculated armadillos develop extensive lepromatous leprosy, and armadillos spontaneously infected with leprosy have been found in Texas. *M leprae* from armadillo or human tissue contains a unique *o*-diphenoloxidase, perhaps an enzyme characteristic of leprosy bacilli.

Clinical Findings

The onset of leprosy is insidious. The lesions involve the cooler tissues of the body: skin, superficial nerves, nose, pharynx, larynx, eyes, and testicles. The skin lesions may occur as pale, anesthetic macular lesions 1–10 cm in diameter; diffuse or discrete erythematous, infiltrated nodules 1–5 cm in diameter; or a diffuse skin infiltration. Neurologic disturbances are manifested by nerve infiltration and thickening, with resultant anesthesia, neuritis, paresthesia, trophic ulcers, and bone reabsorption and shortening of digits. The disfiguration due to the skin infiltration and nerve involvement in untreated cases may be extreme.

The disease is divided into 2 major types, lepromatous and tuberculoid, with several intermediate stages. In the lepromatous type, the course is progressive and malign, with nodular skin lesions; slow, symmetric nerve involvement; abundant acid-fast bacilli in the skin lesions; continuous bacteremia; and a negative lepromin (extract of lepromatous tissue) skin test. In lepromatous leprosy, cell-mediated immunity is markedly deficient and the skin is infiltrated with suppressor T cells. In the tuberculoid type, the course is benign and nonprogressive, with macular skin lesions, severe asymmetric nerve involvement of sudden onset with few bacilli present in the lesions, and a positive lepromin skin test. In tuberculoid leprosy, cell-mediated immunity is intact and the skin is infiltrated with helper T cells.

Systemic manifestations of anemia and lymphadenopathy may also occur. Eye involvement is common. Amyloidosis may develop.

Diagnosis

Scrapings with a scalpel blade from skin or nasal mucosa or from a biopsy of earlobe skin are smeared on a slide and stained by the Ziehl-Neelsen technique. Biopsy of skin or of a thickened nerve gives a typical histologic picture. No serologic tests are of value. Nontreponemal serologic tests for syphilis frequently yield false-positive results in leprosy.

Treatment

Several specialized sulfones (eg, dapsone, DDS; see Chapter 10) and rifampin suppress the growth of *M leprae* and the clinical manifestations of leprosy if given for many months. Sulfone resistance is beginning to emerge in leprosy. For this reason, initial treatment with a combination of sulfone + rifampin is being explored. Clofazimine is an oral drug (100–300 mg/d) used in sulfone-resistant leprosy.

Epidemiology

Transmission of leprosy is most likely to occur when small children are exposed for prolonged periods to heavy shedders of bacilli. Nasal secretions are the most likely infectious material for family contacts. The incubation period is probably 2–10 years. Without prophylaxis, about 10% of exposed children may acquire the disease. Treatment tends to reduce and abolish the infectivity of patients. Spontaneously infected armadillos have been found in Texas, but they play no role in transmission of leprosy to humans.

Prevention & Control

Identification and treatment of patients with leprosy is the key to control. Children of presumably contagious parents are given chemoprophylactic drugs until treatment of the parents has made them noninfectious. If any member of a living group has lepromatous leprosy, such prophylaxis is required for children in the group. Experimental BCG vaccination and an *M leprae* vaccine are also being explored for family contacts and possibly for community contacts in endemic areas.

REFERENCES

Alvarez S, McCabe WR: Extrapulmonary tuberculosis revisited. *Medicine* 1984;**63**:25.

Centers for Disease Control: Guidelines for short-course tuberculosis chemotherapy. *MMWR* 1980;**29**:97.

Comstock GW et al. The prognosis of a positive tuberculin reaction in childhood and adolescence. *Am J Epidemiol* 1974;**99**:131.

Dutt AK, Stead WW: Present chemotherapy for tuberculosis. *J Infect Dis* 1982;**146**:698.

Eickhoff TC: The current status of BCG immunization against tuberculosis. *Annu Rev Med* 1977;**28**:411.

Grove DI, Warren KS, Mahmoud AA. Algorithms in the diagnosis and management of exotic diseases. 15. Leprosy. *J Infect Dis* 1976;**134**:205.

Gunnels JJ, Bates JH, Swindoll H: Infectivity of sputum-positive tuberculous patients on chemotherapy. *Am Rev Respir Dis* 1974;**109**:323.

Hill JD, Stevenson DK: Tuberculosis in unvaccinated children, adolescents, and young adults: A city epidemic. *Br Med J* 1983;**286**:1471.

Kalish SB et al: Use of an enzyme-linked immunosorbent assay technique in the differential diagnosis of active pulmonary tuberculosis in humans. *J Infect Dis* 1983;**147**:523.

Lai KK et al: Mycobacterial cervical lymphadenopathy: Relation of etiologic agents to age. *JAMA* 1984;**251**:1286.

Lester TW: Drug-resistant and atypical mycobacterial disease: Bacteriology and treatment. *Arch Intern Med* 1979;**139**:1399.

Lipsky BA et al: Factors affecting the clinical value of microscopy for acid-fast bacilli. *Rev Infect Dis* 1984;**6**:214.

Mackaness GB: The immunology of antituberculous immunity. *Am Rev Respir Dis* 1968;**97**:337.

Molavi A, LeFrock JL: Tuberculosis meningitis. *Med Clin North Am* 1985;**69**:315.

Ortbals DW, Marr JJ: A comparative study of tuberculosis and other mycobacterial infections and their association with malignancy. *Am Rev Respir Dis* 1978;**117**:39.

PHS Advisory Committee on Immunization Practices: BCG vaccines. *MMWR* 1979;**28**:241.

Pitchenik AE et al: The prevalence of tuberculosis and drug resistance among Haitians. *N Engl J Med* 1982;**307**:162.

Runyon EH et al: *Mycobacterium.* In: *Manual of Clinical Microbiology*, 2nd ed. Lennette EH, Spaulding EH, Truant JP (editors). American Society for Microbiology, 1974.

Sbarbaro JA: Tuberculosis. *Med Clin North Am* 1980;**64**:417.

Shepard CC: Leprosy today. *N Engl J Med* 1982;**307**:1640.

Snider DE: The tuberculin skin test. *Am Rev Respir Dis* 1982;**125**:108.

Stead WW et al: Tuberculosis as an endemic and nosocomial infection among the elderly in nursing homes. *N Engl J Med* 1985;**312**:1483.

Thompson NJ et al: The booster phenomenon in serial tuberculin testing. *Am Rev Respir Dis* 1979;**119:**587.

Van Voorhis WC et al: The cutaneous infiltrates of leprosy: Cellular characteristics and the predominant T-cell phenotypes. *N Engl J Med* 1982;**307:**1593.

Wallace RJ et al: Spectrum of disease due to rapidly growing mycobacteria. *Rev Infect Dis 1983;* **5:**657.

Wolinsky E: Nontuberculous mycobacteria and associated diseases. *Am Rev Respir Dis* 1979;**119:**107.

Yawalkar SJ et al: Once monthly rifampin plus daily dapsone in initial treatment of lepromatous leprosy. *Lancet* 1982;**1:**1199.

Zakowski P et al: Disseminated *Mycobacterium avium-intracellulare* infection in homosexual men dying of acquired immunodeficiency. *JAMA* 1982;**248:**2980.

Spirochetes & Other Spiral Microorganisms

27

The spirochetes are a large, heterogeneous group of spiral, motile organisms. (See Chapter 3 for general morphologic characteristics.)

One family *(Spirochaetaceae)* of the order *Spirochaetales* includes 3 genera of free-living, large spiral organisms. The other *(Treponemataceae)* includes 3 genera pathogenic for humans: (1) *Treponema,* which causes syphilis, bejel, yaws, and pinta; (2) *Borrelia,* which causes relapsing fever and Lyme disease; and (3) *Leptospira,* which causes systemic infections with fever, jaundice, and meningitis.

TREPONEMA PALLIDUM

Morphology & Identification

A. Typical Organisms: Slender spirals measuring about 0.2 μm in width and 5–15 μm in length. The spiral coils are regularly spaced at a distance of 1 μm from each other. The organisms are actively motile, rotating steadily around their central axial filaments even after attaching to cells by their tapered ends. The long axis of the spiral is ordinarily straight but may sometimes bend, so that the organism forms a complete circle for moments at a time, returning then to its normal straight position.

The spirals are so thin that they are not readily seen unless darkfield illumination or immunofluorescent stain is employed. They do not stain well with aniline dyes, but they do reduce silver nitrate to metallic silver that is deposited on the surface, so that treponemes can be seen in tissues (Levaditi silver impregnation).

Treponemes ordinarily reproduce by transverse fission, and divided organisms may adhere to one another for some time.

B. Culture: *Treponema pallidum* pathogenic for humans has never been cultured with certainty on artificial media, in fertile eggs, or in tissue culture. Nonpathogenic treponemes (eg, Reiter strain) can be cultured anaerobically in vitro. They are saprophytes antigenically related to *T pallidum.*

C. Growth Characteristics: Because *T pallidum* cannot be grown, no studies of its physiology have been made. A saprophytic strain (Reiter) grows on a defined medium of 11 amino acids, vitamins, salts, minerals, and serum albumin.

In proper suspending fluids and in the presence of reducing substances, *T pallidum* may remain motile for 3–6 days at 25 °C. In whole blood or plasma stored at 4 °C, organisms remain viable for at least 24 hours, which is of potential importance in blood transfusions.

D. Reactions to Physical and Chemical Agents: Drying kills the spirochete rapidly, as does elevation of the temperature to 42 °C also. Treponemes are rapidly immobilized and killed by trivalent arsenicals, mercury, and bismuth. This killing effect is accelerated by high temperatures and can be partially reversed and the organisms reactivated by compounds containing $-$SH (eg, cysteine, BAL [dimercaprol]). Penicillin is treponemicidal in minute concentrations, but the rate of killing is slow, presumably because of the metabolic inactivity and slow multiplication rate of the organism (estimated division time is 30 hours). Resistance to penicillin has not been demonstrated in syphilis.

E. Variation: A life cycle has been postulated for *T pallidum,* including granular stages and cystlike spherical bodies in addition to the spirochetal form. The occasional ability of *T pallidum* to pass through bacteriologic filters has been attributed to the filtrability of the granular stage.

Antigenic Structure

The antigens of *T pallidum* have not been defined. In the human host, the spirochete stimulates the development of antibodies capable of staining *T pallidum*

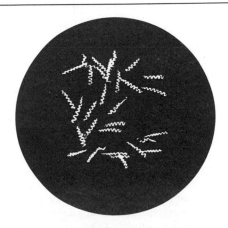

Figure 27–1. Typical organisms of *Treponema pallidum* from tissue fluid in dark field.

by indirect immunofluorescence, immobilizing and killing live motile *T pallidum,* and fixing complement in the presence of suspensions of *T pallidum* or related spirochetes. The spirochetes also cause the development of a distinct antibodylike substance, reagin, which gives positive CF and flocculation tests with aqueous suspensions of lipids extracted from normal mammalian tissues. Both reagin and antitreponemal antibody can be used for the serologic diagnosis of syphilis.

Pathogenesis, Pathology, & Clinical Findings

A. Acquired Syphilis: Natural infection with *T pallidum* is limited to the human host. Human infection is usually transmitted by sexual contact, and the infectious lesion is on the skin or mucous membranes of genitalia. In 10–20% of cases, however, the primary lesion is intrarectal, perianal, or oral. It may be anywhere on the body. *T pallidum* can probably penetrate intact mucous membranes, or it may enter through a break in the epidermis.

Spirochetes multiply locally at the site of entry, and some spread to nearby lymph nodes and then reach the bloodstream. In 2–10 weeks after infection, a papule develops at the site of infection and breaks down to form an ulcer with a clean, hard base ("hard chancre"). The inflammation is characterized by a predominance of lymphocytes and plasma cells. This "primary lesion" always heals spontaneously, but 2–10 weeks later the "secondary" lesions appear. These consist of a red maculopapular rash anywhere on the body and moist, pale papules (condylomas) in the anogenital region, axillas, and mouth. There may also be syphilitic meningitis, chorioretinitis, hepatitis, nephritis (immune complex type), or periostitis. The secondary lesions also subside spontaneously. Both primary and secondary lesions are rich in spirochetes and highly infectious. Contagious lesions may recur within 3–5 years after infection, but thereafter the individual is not infectious. Syphilitic infection may remain subclinical, and the patient may pass through the primary or secondary stage (or both) without symptoms or signs yet develop tertiary lesions.

In about 30% of cases, early syphilitic infection progresses spontaneously to complete cure without treatment. In another 30%, the untreated infection remains latent (principally evident by positive serologic tests). In the remainder, the disease progresses to the "tertiary stage," characterized by the development of granulomatous lesions (gummas) in skin, bones, and liver; degenerative changes in the central nervous system (meningovascular syphilis, paresis, tabes); or cardiovascular lesions (aortitis, aortic aneurysm, aortic valve insufficiency). In all tertiary lesions, treponemes are very rare, and the exaggerated tissue response must be attributed to hypersensitivity to the organisms. However, treponemes can occasionally be found in the eye or central nervous system in late syphilis.

B. Congenital Syphilis: A pregnant syphilitic woman can transmit *T pallidum* to the fetus through the placenta beginning in the 10th to 15th week of gestation. Some of the infected fetuses die and miscarriages result; others are stillborn at term. Others are born live but develop the signs of congenital syphilis in childhood: interstitial keratitis, Hutchinson's teeth, saddle nose, periostitis, and a variety of central nervous system anomalies. Adequate treatment of the mother during pregnancy prevents congenital syphilis. The reagin titer in the blood of the child rises with active infection but falls with time if antibody was passively transmitted from the mother. In congenital infection, the child makes IgM antitreponemal antibody.

C. Experimental Disease: Rabbits can be experimentally infected in the skin, testis, and eye with human *T pallidum*. The animal develops a chancre rich in spirochetes, and organisms persist in lymph nodes, spleen, and bone marrow for the entire life of the animal, although there is no progressive disease.

Diagnostic Laboratory Tests

A. Specimens: Tissue fluid expressed from early surface lesions for demonstration of spirochetes; blood serum for serologic tests.

B. Darkfield Examination: A drop of tissue fluid or exudate is placed on a slide and a coverslip pressed over it to make a thin layer. The preparation is then examined under oil immersion with darkfield illumination for typical motile spirochetes.

Treponemes disappear from lesions within a few hours after the beginning of antibiotic treatment.

C. Immunofluorescence: Tissue fluid or exudate is spread on a glass slide, air dried, and mailed to the laboratory. It is fixed, stained with a fluorescein-labeled antitreponeme serum, and examined by means of immunofluorescence microscopy for typical fluorescent spirochetes.

D. Serologic Tests for Syphilis (STS): These use either treponemal or nontreponemal antigens.

1. Nontreponemal antigen tests–The antigens employed are lipids extracted from normal mammalian tissue. The purified cardiolipin from beef heart is a diphosphatidylglycerol. It requires the addition of lecithin and cholesterol or other "sensitizers" to react with syphilitic "reagin." "Reagin" is a mixture of IgM and IgA antibodies directed against some antigens widely distributed in normal tissues. Reagin is found in patients' serum after 2–3 weeks of untreated syphilitic infection and in spinal fluid after 4–8 weeks of infection. Two types of tests determine the presence of reagin.

a. Flocculation tests (VDRL [Venereal Disease Research Laboratories]; RPR [Rapid plasma reagin])–These tests are based on the fact that the particles of the lipid antigen (beef heart cardiolipin) remain dispersed with normal serum but form visible clumps when combining with reagin. Results develop within a few minutes, particularly if the suspension is agitated, and the tests lend themselves to automation and to use for surveys because of their low cost. Positive VDRL or RPR tests revert to negative in 6–18 months after effective treatment of syphilis.

b. Complement fixation (CF) tests (Wassermann, Kolmer)–CF tests are based on the fact that reagin-containing sera fix complement in the presence of cardiolipin "antigen." It is necessary to ascertain that the serum is not "anticomplementary" (ie, that it does not destroy complement in the absence of antigen).

Both (a) and (b) can give quantitative results. An estimate of the amount of reagin present in serum can be made by performing (a) or (b) with 2-fold dilutions of serum and expressing the titer as the highest dilution that gives a positive result. Quantitative results are valuable in establishing a diagnosis and in evaluating the effect of treatment.

Nontreponemal tests are subject to false-positive results. These either are due to technical difficulties of the test or are "biologic" false positives attributable to the occurrence of "reagins" in a variety of human disorders. Prominent among the latter are other infections (malaria, leprosy, measles, infectious mononucleosis, etc), vaccinations, collagen-vascular diseases (systemic lupus erythematosus, polyarteritis nodosa, rheumatic disorders), and other conditions. Nontreponemal antibody tests may become negative spontaneously in progressive tertiary syphilis; thus, a negative VDRL does not rule out such disease activity.

2. Treponemal antibody tests–

a. Fluorescent treponemal antibody (FTA-ABS) test–A test employing indirect immunofluorescence (killed *T pallidum* + patient's serum + labeled antihuman gamma globulin) shows excellent specificity and sensitivity for syphilis antibodies if the patient's serum has been absorbed with sonicated Reiter spirochetes prior to the FTA test. The FTA-ABS test is the first to become positive in early syphilis, and it usually remains positive many years after effective treatment of early syphilis. The test cannot be used to judge the efficacy of treatment. The presence of IgM FTA in the blood of newborns is good evidence of in utero infection (congenital syphilis).

b. TPI test–Demonstration of *T pallidum* immobilization (TPI) by specific antibodies in the patient's serum after the second week of infection. Dilutions of serum are mixed with complement and with live, actively motile *T pallidum* extracted from the testicular chancre of a rabbit, and the mixture is observed microscopically. If specific antibodies are present, spirochetes are immobilized; in normal serum, active motion continues. This test requires live treponemes from infected animals, is difficult to perform, and is now done rarely.

c. *T pallidum* complement fixation test–Spirochetes extracted from syphilomas of rabbits form specific antigens for CF tests that probably measure the same antibody as the TPI test, above. Such spirochetal suspensions are difficult to prepare. Antigens prepared from cultured Reiter spirochetes are occasionally employed in the Reiter complement fixation test.

d. *T pallidum* hemagglutination (TPHA) test–Red blood cells are treated to adsorb treponemes on their surface. When mixed with serum containing antitreponemal antibodies, the cells become clumped. This test is similar to the FTA-ABS test in specificity and sensitivity, but it becomes positive somewhat later in the course of infection.

VDRL and FTA-ABS tests can also be performed on spinal fluid. Antibodies do not reach the cerebrospinal fluid from the bloodstream but are probably formed in the central nervous system in response to syphilitic infection.

Immunity

A person with active or latent syphilis or yaws appears to be resistant to superinfection with *T pallidum*. However, if early syphilis or yaws is treated adequately and the infection is eradicated, the individual again becomes fully susceptible. The various immune responses usually fail to eradicate the infection or arrest its progression.

Treatment

Penicillin in concentrations of 0.003 unit/mL has definite treponemicidal activity, and penicillin is the treatment of choice. In syphilis of less than 1 year's duration, penicillin levels are maintained for 2 weeks by a single injection of benzathine penicillin G, 2.4 million units intramuscularly. In older or latent syphilis, benzathine penicillin G, 2.4 million units intramuscularly, is given 3 times at weekly intervals. In neurosyphilis, the same therapy is acceptable, but larger amounts of penicillin (eg, aqueous penicillin G, 20 million units intravenously daily for 2–3 weeks) are sometimes recommended. Other antibiotics, eg, tetracyclines or erythromycin, can occasionally be substituted. Prolonged follow-up is essential. In neurosyphilis, treponemes occasionally survive such treatment. A typical Jarisch-Herxheimer reaction may occur within hours after treatment is begun. It is due to the release of toxic products (?endotoxin) from dying or killed spirochetes.

Epidemiology, Prevention, & Control

At present, the incidence of syphilis (and other sexually transmitted diseases) is rising in most parts of the world. With the exceptions of congenital syphilis and the rare occupational exposure of medical personnel, syphilis is acquired through sexual exposure. Its incidence is particularly high among homosexual males, and reinfection in treated persons is common. An infected person may remain contagious for 3–5 years during "early" syphilis. "Late" syphilis, of more than 5 years' duration, is usually not contagious. Consequently, control measures depend on (1) prompt and adequate treatment of all discovered cases; (2) followup on sources of infection and contacts so they can be treated; (3) sex hygiene; and (4) prophylaxis at the time of exposure. Both mechanical prophylaxis (condoms) and chemoprophylaxis (eg, penicillin after exposure) have great limitations. Several venereal diseases can be transmitted simultaneously. Therefore, it is important to consider the possibility of syphilis when any one sexually transmitted disease has been found.

DISEASES RELATED TO SYPHILIS

These diseases are all caused by treponemes indistinguishable from *T pallidum*. All give positive treponemal and nontreponemal serologic tests for syphilis, and some cross-immunity can be demonstrated in experimental animals and perhaps in humans. All are nonvenereal diseases and are commonly transmitted by direct contact. None of the causative organisms have been cultured on artificial media.

Bejel
Bejel occurs chiefly in Africa but also in the Middle East, in Southeast Asia, and elsewhere, particularly among children, and produces highly infectious skin lesions; late visceral complications are rare. Penicillin is the drug of choice.

Yaws (Frambesia)
Yaws is endemic, particularly among children, in many humid, hot tropical countries. It is caused by *Treponema pertenue*. The primary lesion, an ulcerating papule, occurs usually on the arms or legs. Transmission is by person-to-person contact in children under age 15. Transplacental, congenital infection does not occur. Scar formation of skin lesions and bone destruction are common, but visceral or nervous system complications are very rare. It has been debated whether yaws represents a variant of syphilis adapted to nonvenereal transmission in hot climates. There appears to be cross-immunity between yaws and syphilis. Diagnostic procedures and therapy are similar to those for syphilis. The response to penicillin treatment is dramatic.

Pinta
Pinta is caused by *Treponema carateum* and occurs endemically in all age groups in Mexico, Central and South America, the Philippines, and some areas of the Pacific. The disease appears to be restricted to dark-skinned races. The primary lesion, a nonulcerating papule, occurs on exposed areas. Some months later, flat, hyperpigmented lesions appear on the skin; depigmentation and hyperkeratosis take place years afterward. Late cardiovascular and nervous system involvement occurs very rarely. Transmission is nonvenereal, either by direct contact or through the agency of flies or gnats. Diagnosis and treatment are the same as for syphilis.

Rabbit Syphilis
Rabbit syphilis *(Treponema cuniculi)* is a natural venereal infection of rabbits producing minor lesions of the genitalia. The causative organism is morphologically indistinguishable from *T pallidum* and may lead to confusion in experimental work.

OTHER SPIROCHETAL ORGANISMS

BORRELIA RECURRENTIS

Morphology & Identification
A. Typical Organisms: *Borrelia recurrentis* is an irregular spiral 10–30 μm long and 0.3 μm wide. The distance between turns varies from 2 to 4 μm. The organisms are highly flexible and move both by rotation and by twisting. *B recurrentis* stains readily with bacteriologic dyes as well as with blood stains such as Giemsa's or Wright's stain.

B. Culture: The organism can be cultured in fluid media containing blood, serum, or tissue; but it rapidly loses its pathogenicity for animals when transferred repeatedly in vitro. Multiplication is rapid in chick embryos when blood from patients is inoculated into the chorioallantoic membrane.

C. Growth Characteristics: Virtually nothing is known of the metabolic requirements or activity of borreliae. At 4 °C, the organisms survive for several months in infected blood or in culture. In some ticks (but not in lice), spirochetes are passed from generation to generation.

D. Variation: The only significant variation of *Borrelia* is with respect to its antigenic structure.

Antigenic Structure
Isolates of *Borrelia* from different parts of the world, from different hosts, and from different vectors (ticks or lice) either have been given different species names or have been designated strains of *B recurrentis*. Biologic differences between these strains or species do not appear to be stable.

Agglutinins, CF antibodies, and lytic antibodies develop in high titer after infection with borreliae. Apparently the antigenic structure of the organisms

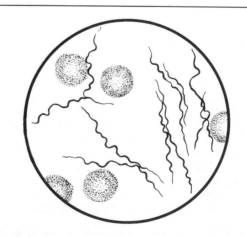

Figure 27–2. *Borrelia recurrentis* in blood smear.

changes in the course of a single infection. The antibodies produced initially may act as a selective factor that permits the survival only of antigenically distinct variants. The relapsing course of the disease appears to be due to the multiplication of such antigenic variants, against which the host must then develop new antibodies. Ultimate recovery (after 3–10 relapses) is associated with the presence of antibodies against several antigenic variants.

Pathology

Fatal cases show spirochetes in great numbers in the spleen and liver, necrotic foci in other parenchymatous organs, and hemorrhagic lesions in the kidneys and the gastrointestinal tract. Spirochetes have been occasionally demonstrated in the spinal fluid and brains of persons who have had meningitis. In experimental animals (guinea pigs, rats), the brain may serve as a reservoir of borreliae after they have disappeared from the blood.

Pathogenesis & Clinical Findings

The incubation period is 3–10 days. The onset is sudden, with chills and an abrupt rise of temperature. During this time, spirochetes abound in the blood. The fever persists for 3–5 days and then declines, leaving the patient weak but not ill. The afebrile period lasts 4–10 days and is followed by a second attack of chills, fever, intense headache, and malaise. There are from 3 to 10 such recurrences, generally of diminishing severity. During the febrile stages (especially when the temperature is rising), organisms are present in the blood; during the afebrile periods, they are absent. Borreliae are not often found in the urine.

Antibodies against the spirochetes appear during the febrile stage, and the attack is probably terminated by their agglutinating and lytic effects. These antibodies may select out antigenically distinct variants that multiply and cause a relapse. Several distinct antigenic varieties of borreliae may be isolated from a single patient's several relapses, even following experimental inoculation with a single organism.

Diagnostic Laboratory Tests

A. Specimens: Blood obtained during the rise in fever, for smears and animal inoculation.

B. Smears: Thin or thick blood smears stained with Wright's Giemsa's stain reveal large, loosely coiled spirochetes among the red cells.

C. Animal Inoculation: White mice or young rats are inoculated intraperitoneally with blood. Stained films of tail blood are examined for spirochetes 2–4 days later.

D. Serology: Spirochetes grown in culture can serve as antigens for CF tests, but the preparation of satisfactory antigens is difficult. Patients suffering from epidemic (louse-borne) relapsing fever may develop agglutinins for *Proteus* OXK and also a positive VDRL.

Immunity

Immunity following infection is usually of short duration.

Treatment

The great variability of the spontaneous remissions of relapsing fever makes evaluation of chemotherapeutic effectiveness difficult. Tetracyclines, erythromycin, and penicillin are all believed to be effective. Treatment for a single day may be sufficient to terminate an individual attack.

Epidemiology, Prevention, & Control

Relapsing fever is endemic in many parts of the world. Its main reservoir is the rodent population, which serves as a source of infection for ticks of the genus *Ornithodorus*. The distribution of endemic foci and the seasonal incidence of the disease are largely determined by the ecology of the ticks in different areas. In the USA, infected ticks are found throughout the West, especially in mountainous areas, but clinical cases are rare. In the tick, *Borrelia* may be transmitted transovarially from generation to generation.

Spirochetes are present in all tissues of the tick and may be transmitted by the bite or by crushing the tick. The tick-borne disease is not epidemic. However, when an infected individual harbors lice, the lice become infected by sucking blood; 4–5 days later, they may serve as a source of infection for other individuals. The infection of lice is not transmitted to the next generation, and the disease is the result of rubbing crushed lice into bite wounds. Severe epidemics may occur in louse-infested populations, and transmission is favored by crowding, malnutrition, and cold climate.

In endemic areas, human infection may occasionally result from contact with the blood and tissues of infected rodents. The mortality rate of the endemic disease is low, but in epidemics it may reach 30%.

Prevention is based on avoidance of exposure to ticks and lice and on delousing (cleanliness, insecticides). No vaccines are available.

LYME DISEASE

This illness is named after the town of Lyme, Connecticut. Most cases have been clustered on the northeastern seaboard of the USA, but the disease occurs elsewhere in the USA and also in Europe and Australia. It typically occurs in the summer. It presents with a unique expanding, annular skin lesion (erythema chronicum migrans). Often there is headache, stiff neck, fever, myalgia, arthralgia, or lymphadenopathy. Weeks or months later, some patients develop neurologic symptoms and frank arthritis that may recur for several years.

The disease is transmitted by small ixodid ticks, often *Ixodes dammini*, which carry spirochetes (*Borrelia burgdorferi*). The same spirochetes have been found in blood and cerebrospinal fluid of patients. Such persons also develop IgM antibodies to these spirochetes 3–6 weeks after onset of the illness. The serum levels of IgM correlate with disease activity. It is probable that deposition of antigen-antibody complexes is responsible for the recurrent arthritis or neurologic difficulties which occur in some patients.

Treatment with penicillin or tetracycline early in the acute illness results in prompt recovery and prevents late arthritis and other complications.

LEPTOSPIRAE

Morphology & Identification

A. Typical Organisms: Tightly coiled, thin, flexible spirochetes 5–15 μm long, with very fine spirals 0.1–0.2 μm wide. One end of the organism is often bent, forming a hook. There is active rotational motion, but no flagella have been discovered. Electron micrographs show a thin axial filament and a delicate membrane. The spirochete is so delicate that in the dark field it may appear only as a chain of minute cocci. It does not stain readily but can be impregnated with silver.

B. Culture: Leptospirae grow best under aerobic conditions at 28–30 °C in protein-rich semisolid media (Fletcher, others), where they produce round colonies 1–3 mm in diameter in 6–10 days. Leptospirae also grow on chorioallantoic membranes of embryonated eggs.

C. Growth Requirements: Leptospirae derive energy from oxidation of long-chain fatty acids and cannot use amino acids or carbohydrates as major energy sources. Ammonium salts are a main source of nitrogen. Leptospirae can survive for weeks in water, particularly at alkaline pH.

Antigenic Structure

The main strains ("serovars") of *Leptospira inter-* *rogans* isolated from humans or animals in different parts of the world (Table 27–1) are all serologically related and exhibit marked cross-reactivity in serologic tests. This indicates considerable overlapping in antigenic structure, and quantitative tests and antibody absorption studies are necessary for a specific serologic diagnosis. A serologically reactive lipopolysaccharide with group reactivity has been extracted from leptospirae.

Pathogenesis & Clinical Findings

Human infection results usually from ingestion of water or food contaminated with leptospirae. More rarely, the organisms may enter through mucous membranes or breaks in the skin. After an incubation period of 1–2 weeks, there is a variable febrile onset during which spirochetes are present in the bloodstream. They then establish themselves in the parenchymatous organs (particularly liver and kidneys), producing hemorrhage and necrosis of tissue and resulting in dysfunction of those organs (jaundice, hemorrhage, nitrogen retention). The illness is often biphasic. After an initial improvement, the second phase develops when the IgM antibody titer rises. It manifests itself often as "aseptic meningitis" with intense headache, stiff neck, and pleocytosis in the cerebrospinal fluid. Nephritis and hepatitis may also recur, and there may be skin, muscle, and eye lesions. During World War II, pretibial fever occurred at Fort Bragg, a US Army base, with patchy erythema on the lower legs or a generalized rash. The degree and distribution of organ involvement vary in the different diseases produced by different leptospirae in various parts of the world (Table 27–1). Many infections are mild or subclinical. Hepatitis is frequent in patients with leptospirosis. It is often associated with elevation of serum creatine phosphokinase, whereas that enzyme is present in normal concentrations in viral hepatitis.

Table 27–1. Principal leptospiral diseases.

Leptospira interrogans serovar*	Source of Infection	Disease in Humans	Clinical Findings	Distribution
autumnalis	?	Pretibial fever or Ft. Bragg fever	Fever, rash over tibia	USA, Japan
ballum	Mice	–	Fever, rash, jaundice	USA, Europe, Israel
bovis	Cattle, voles	–	Fever, prostration	USA, Israel, Australia
canicola	Dog urine	Infectious jaundice	Influenzalike illness, aseptic meningitis	Worldwide
grippotyphosa	Rodents, water	Marsh fever	Fever, prostration, aseptic meningitis	Europe, USA, Africa
hebdomadis	Rats, mice	Seven-day fever	Fever, jaundice	Japan, Europe
icterohaemorrhagiae	Rat urine, water	Weil's disease	Jaundice, hemorrhages, aseptic meningitis	Worldwide
mitis	Swine	Swineherd's disease	Aseptic meningitis	Australia
pomona	Swine, cattle	Swineherd's disease	Fever, prostration, aseptic meningitis	Europe, USA, Australia

*Formerly called species.

Kidney involvement in many animal species is chronic and results in the elimination of large numbers of leptospirae in the urine; this is probably the main source of contamination and infection of humans. Human urine also may contain spirochetes in the second and third weeks of disease.

Agglutinating, CF, and lytic antibodies develop during the infection. Serum from convalescent patients protects experimental animals against an otherwise fatal infection. The immunity resulting from infection in humans and animals appears to be serovar-specific. Dogs have been artificially immunized with killed cultures of leptospirae.

Diagnostic Laboratory Tests

A. Specimens: Specimens consist of blood for microscopic examination, culture, and inoculation of young hamsters or guinea pigs; and serum for agglutination tests.

B. Microscopic Examination: Darkfield examination or thick smears stained by Giemsa's technique occasionally show leptospirae in fresh blood from early infections. Darkfield examination of centrifuged urine may also be positive.

C. Culture: Whole fresh blood or urine can be cultured in Fletcher's semisolid or Tween 80 albumin medium. Growth is slow, and cultures should be kept for several weeks.

D. Animal Inoculation: A sensitive technique for the isolation of leptospirae consists of the intraperitoneal inoculation of young hamsters or guinea pigs with fresh plasma or urine. Within a few days, spirochetes become demonstrable in the peritoneal cavity; on the death of the animal (8–14 days), hemorrhagic lesions with spirochetes are found in many organs.

E. Serology: Agglutinating antibodies attaining very high titers (1:10,000 or higher) develop slowly in leptospiral infection, reaching a peak 5–8 weeks after infection. Leptospiral antibody can be detected by macroscopic slide agglutination tests using killed leptospirae or by microscopic agglutination of live organisms. Cross-absorption of sera may permit identification of a serovar-specific antibody response. Agglutination of live suspensions is most specific for the serovar and may be followed by lysis. Passive hemagglutination of red blood cells with adsorbed leptospirae is sometimes used.

Immunity

A solid serovar-specific immunity follows infection, but reinfection with different serovars may occur.

Treatment

In very early infection, antibiotics (penicillin, tetracyclines) have some therapeutic effect but do not eradicate the infection. Doxycycline has marked prophylactic efficacy.

Epidemiology, Prevention, & Control

The leptospiroses are essentially animal infections; human infection is only accidental, following contact with water or other materials contaminated with the excreta of animal hosts. Rats, mice, wild rodents, dogs, swine, and cattle are the principal sources of human infection. They excrete leptospirae in urine and feces both during the active illness and during the asymptomatic carrier state. Leptospirae remain viable in stagnant water for several weeks; drinking, swimming, bathing, or food contamination may lead to human infection. Persons most likely to come in contact with water contaminated by rats (eg, miners, sewer workers, farmers, fishermen) run the greatest risk of infection. Children acquire the infection from dogs more frequently than do adults. Control consists of preventing exposure to potentially contaminated water and reducing contamination by rodent control. Doxycycline, 200 mg orally once weekly during heavy exposure, is effective prophylaxis. Dogs can receive distemper-hepatitis-leptospirosis vaccinations.

SPIRILLUM MINOR
(Spirillum morsus muris)

Spirillum minor causes one form of rat-bite fever (sodoku). This very small (3–5 μm) and rigid spiral organism is carried by rats all over the world. The organism is inoculated into humans through the bite of a rat and results in a local lesion, regional gland swelling, skin rashes, and fever of the relapsing type. The frequency of this illness depends upon the degree of contact between humans and rats. The *Spirillum* can be isolated by inoculation of guinea pigs or mice with material from enlarged lymph nodes or blood but has not been grown in bacteriologic media. In the USA and Europe, this disease has been recognized only infrequently. Several other motile gram-negative spiral aerobic organisms can produce spirillum fever (Kowal J: *N Engl J Med* 1961;**264:**123).

SPIROCHETES OF THE NORMAL MOUTH & MUCOUS MEMBRANES

A number of spirochetes occur in every normal mouth. Some of them have been named (eg, *Borrelia buccalis*), but neither their morphology nor their physiologic activity permits definitive classification. On normal genitalia, a spirochete called *Borrelia refringens* is occasionally found that may be confused with *T pallidum*. These organisms are harmless saprophytes under ordinary conditions. Most of them are strict anaerobes that can be grown in petrolatum-sealed meat infusion broth tubes with tissue added.

FUSOSPIROCHETAL DISEASE

Under certain circumstances, particularly injury to mucous membranes, nutritional deficiency, or concomitant infection (eg, with herpes simplex virus) of the epithelium, the normal spirochetes of the mouth, together with cigar-shaped, banded, anaerobic fusiform bacilli (fusobacteria), find suitable conditions for vast increase in numbers. This occurs in ulcerative gingivostomatitis (trench mouth), often called Vincent's stomatitis. When this type of process produces ulcerative tonsillitis and massive tissue involvement, it may be called Vincent's angina. It also occurs in lung abscesses where pyogenic microorganisms and *Bacteroides* species have broken down tissue; in bronchiectasis, where anatomic and physiologic disturbances interfere with normal drainage; in leg ("tropical") ulcers with mixed infection and venous stasis; and in bite wounds and similar situations.

In all of these instances, necrotic tissue provides the anaerobic environment required by the fusospirochetal flora. The anaerobic conditions in turn prevent rapid healing and may contribute to tissue breakdown. Fusiform bacilli (fusobacteria) coexist with other anaerobes (*Bacteroides, Peptostreptococcus;* see Chapter 24). The fusospirochetal flora is readily inhibited by antibiotics. Antibiotic therapy may thus control gingivostomatitis or angina. However, the fusospirochetal organisms are not primary pathogens. Effective treatment must direct itself against the initial cause of tissue breakdown.

Fusospirochetal disease is generally not transmissible through direct contact, since everyone carries the organisms in the mouth. However, outbreaks occur occasionally in children or young adults. This is attributed to the transmission of a viral agent (eg, herpes simplex virus) in a susceptible population group or to nutritional deficiency and poor oral hygiene ("trench mouth").

REFERENCES

Andrew ED, Marrocco GR: Leptospirosis in New England. *JAMA* 1977;**238:**2027.

Burke JP et al (editors): International symposium on yaws and other endemic treponematoses. *Rev Infect Dis* 1985;**7:**S217.

Butler T et al: *Borrelia recurrentis* infection. *J Infect Dis* 1978;**137:**573.

Centers for Disease Control: Sexually transmitted diseases: Treatment guidelines 1982. *MMWR* (Aug 20) 1982;**31:**35S.

Clark EG, Danbolt N: The Oslo study of the natural course of untreated syphilis. *Med Clin North Am* 1964;**48:**613.

Fitzgerald TJ: Pathogenesis and immunology of *Treponema pallidum. Annu Rev Microbiol* 1981;**35:**29.

Fiumara NJ: Treatment of primary and secondary syphilis: Serological response. *JAMA* 1980;**243:**2500.

Hardin JA et al: Immune complexes and the evolution of Lyme arthritis. *N Engl J Med* 1979;**301:**1358.

Harter CA. Benirschke K: Fetal syphilis in the first trimester. *Am J Obstet Gynecol* 1976;**124:**705.

Hopkins DR: Yaws in the Americas, 1950–1975. *J Infect Dis* 1977;**136:**548.

Johnson RC: The spirochetes. *Annu Rev Microbiol* 1977;**31:**89.

Kampmeier RH: Syphilis therapy: An historical perspective. *J Am Vener Dis Assoc* 1976;**3:**99.

Lee TJ, Sparling F: Syphilis: An algorithm. *JAMA* 1979; **242:**1187.

Malison MD: Relapsing fever. *JAMA* 1979;**241:**2819.

Martone WJ, Kaufmann AF: Leptospirosis in humans in the United States 1974–1978. *J Infect Dis* 1979;**140:**1020.

Meyerhoff J: Lyme disease. *Am J Med* 1983;**75:**663.

Moffat EM et al: Cellular immune findings in Lyme disease: Correlation with serum IgM and disease activity. *Am J Med* 1984;**77:**625.

Pace JL, Czonka GW: Endemic non-venereal syphilis (bejel) in Saudi Arabia. *Br J Vener Dis* 1984;**60:**293.

Pavia CS et al: Cell-mediated immunity during syphilis. *Br J Vener Dis* 1978;**54:**144.

Steere AC et al: Neurologic abnormalities of Lyme disease. *Ann Intern Med* 1983;**99:**767.

Steere AC et al: The spirochetal etiology of Lyme disease. *N Engl J Med* 1983;**308:**733.

Takafuji ET et al: An efficacy trial of doxycycline chemoprophylaxis against leptospirosis. *N Engl J Med* 1984;**310:**497.

Tramont EC: Persistence of *T pallidum* following penicillin G therapy. *JAMA* 1976;**236:**2206.

Wong M et al: Leptospirosis: Childhood disease. *J Pediatr* 1977;**90:**532.

Young EJ et al: Studies on the pathogenesis of the Jarisch-Herxheimer reaction. *J Infect Dis* 1982;**146:**606.

Rickettsial Diseases

28

Rickettsiae are small bacteria that are obligate intracellular parasites and—except for Q fever—are transmitted to humans by arthropods. At least 4 rickettsiae *(Rickettsia rickettsii, Rickettsia conorii, Rickettsia tsutsugamushi, Rickettsia akari)*—and perhaps others—are transmitted transovarially in the arthropod, which serves as both vector and reservoir. Rickettsial diseases (except Q fever) typically exhibit fever, rashes, and vasculitis. They are grouped on the basis of clinical features, epidemiologic aspects, and immunologic characteristics (Table 28–1).

Properties of Rickettsiae

Rickettsiae are pleomorphic, appearing either as short rods, 600 × 300 nm in size, or as cocci, and they occur singly, in pairs, in short chains, or in filaments. When stained, they are readily visible under the optical microscope. With Giemsa's stain they stain blue; with Macchiavello's stain they stain red and contrast with the blue-staining cytoplasm in which they appear.

A wide range of animals are susceptible to infection with rickettsial organisms. Rickettsiae grow readily in the yolk sac of the embryonated egg (yolk sac suspensions contain up to 10^9 rickettsial particles per milliliter). Pure preparations of rickettsiae can be obtained by differential centrifugation of yolk sac suspensions. Many rickettsial strains also grow in cell culture.

Purified rickettsiae contain both RNA and DNA in a ratio of 3.5:1 (similar to the ratio in bacteria). Rickettsiae have cell walls that are made up of peptidoglycans containing muramic acid and diaminopimelic acid and thus resemble the cell walls of gram-negative bacteria. They divide like bacteria. In cell culture, the generation time is 8–10 hours at 34 °C.

Purified rickettsiae contain various enzymes concerned with metabolism. Thus they oxidize intermediate metabolites like pyruvic, succinic, and glutamic acids and can convert glutamic acid into aspartic acid. Rickettsiae lose their biologic activities when they are

Table 28–1. Rickettsial diseases.

Disease	Rickettsia	Geographic Area of Prevalence	Insect Vector	Mammalian Reservoir	Weil-Felix Agglutination		
					OX19	OX2	OXK
Typhus group							
Epidemic typhus	*Rickettsia prowazekii*	South America, Africa, Asia, ?North America	Louse	Humans	++	±	−
Murine typhus	*Rickettsia typhi*	Worldwide; small foci	Flea	Rodents	++	−	−
Scrub typhus	*Rickettsia tsutsugamushi*	Southeast Asia, Japan	Mite*	Rodents	−	−	++
Spotted fever group							
Rocky Mountain spotted fever (RMSF)	*Rickettsia rickettsii*	Western hemisphere	Tick*	Rodents, dogs	+	+	−
Fièvre boutonneuse Kenya tick typhus South African tick fever Indian tick typhus	*Rickettsia conorii*	Africa, India, Mediterranean countries	Tick*	Rodents, dogs	+	+	−
Queensland tick typhus	*Rickettsia australis*	Australia	Tick*	Rodents, marsupials	+	+	−
North Asian tick typhus	*Rickettsia sibirica*	Siberia, Mongolia	Tick*	Rodents	+	+	−
Rickettsialpox	*Rickettsia akari*	USA, Korea, USSR	Mite*	Mice	−	−	−
RMSF-like	*Rickettsia canada*	North America	Tick*	Rodents	?	?	−
Other							
Q fever	*Coxiella burnetii*	Worldwide	None†	Cattle, sheep, goats	−	−	−
Trench fever	*Rochalimaea quintana*	Rare	Louse	Humans	?	?	?

*Also serve as arthropod reservoir, by maintaining the rickettsiae through transovarian transmission.
†Human infection results from inhalation of dust.

stored at 0 °C; this is due to the progressive loss of nicotinamide adenine dinucleotide (NAD). All of these properties can be restored by subsequent incubation with NAD. They may also lose their biologic activity if they are starved by incubation for several hours at 36 °C. This loss can be prevented by the addition of glutamate, pyruvate, or adenosine triphosphate (ATP). Subsequent incubation of the starved organism with glutamate at 30 °C leads to recovery of activity.

Rickettsiae grow in different parts of the cell. Those of the typhus group are usually found in the cytoplasm; those of the spotted fever group, in the nucleus. Coxiellae grow only in cytoplasmic vacuoles. Thus far, one agent grouped with the rickettsiae, *Rochalimaea quintana,* has been grown on cell-free media. It has been suggested that rickettsiae grow best when the metabolism of the host cells is low. Thus, their growth is enhanced when the temperature of infected chick embryos is lowered to 32 °C. If the embryos are held at 40 °C, rickettsial multiplication is poor. Conditions that influence the metabolism of the host can alter its susceptibility to rickettsial infection.

Rickettsial growth is enhanced in the presence of sulfonamides, and rickettsial diseases are made more severe by these drugs. Para-aminobenzoic acid (PABA), the structural analog of the sulfonamides, inhibits the growth of rickettsial organisms. Tetracyclines or chloramphenicol inhibits the growth of rickettsiae and can be therapeutically effective.

In general, rickettsiae are quickly destroyed by heat, drying, and bactericidal chemicals. Although rickettsiae are usually killed by storage at room temperature, dried feces of infected lice may remain infective for months at room temperature.

The organism of Q fever is the rickettsial agent most resistant to drying. This organism may survive pasteurization at 60 °C for 30 minutes and can survive for months in dried feces or milk. This may be due to the formation of endosporelike structures by *Coxiella burnetii.*

Rickettsial Antigens & Antibodies

A variety of rickettsial antibodies are known; all of them participate in the reactions discussed below. The antibodies that develop in humans after vaccination generally are more type-specific than the antibodies developing after natural infection.

A. Agglutination of *Proteus vulgaris* (Weil-Felix Reaction): The Weil-Felix reaction is commonly used in diagnostic work. Rickettsiae and *Proteus* organisms share certain antigens. Thus, during the course of rickettsial infections, patients develop antibodies that agglutinate certain strains of *P vulgaris.* For example, the *Proteus* strain OX19 is agglutinated strongly by sera from persons infected with epidemic or endemic typhus; weakly by sera from those infected with Rocky Mountain spotted fever; and not at all by those infected with Q fever. Convalescent sera from scrub typhus patients react most strongly with the *Proteus* strain OXK (Table 28–1).

B. Agglutination of Rickettsiae: Rickettsiae are agglutinated by specific antibodies. This reaction is very sensitive and can be diagnostically useful when heavy rickettsial suspensions are available for microagglutination tests.

C. CF With Rickettsial Antigens: CF antibodies are commonly used in diagnostic laboratories. A 4-fold or greater antibody titer rise is usually required as laboratory support for the diagnosis of acute rickettsial infection. Convalescent titers often exceed 1:64. Group-reactive soluble antigens are available for the typhus group, the spotted fever group, and Q fever. They originate in the cell wall. Some insoluble antigens may give species-specific reactions. ELISA (enzyme-linked immunosorbent assay) tests have been performed with rickettsial antigens.

D. Immunofluorescence Test With Rickettsial Antigens: Suspensions of rickettsiae can be partially purified from infected yolk sac material and used as antigens in indirect immunofluorescence tests with patient's serum and a fluorescein-labeled antihuman globulin. The results indicate the presence of partly species-specific antibodies, but some cross-reactions are observed. Antibodies after vaccination are IgG; early after infection, IgM.

E. Passive Hemagglutination Test: Treated red blood cells adsorb soluble rickettsial antigens and can then be agglutinated by antibody.

F. Neutralization of Rickettsial Toxins: Rickettsiae contain toxins that produce death in animals within a few hours after injection. Toxin-neutralizing antibodies appear during infection, and these are specific for the toxins of the typhus group, the spotted fever group, and scrub typhus rickettsiae. Toxins exist only in viable rickettsiae—inactivated rickettsiae are nontoxic.

Pathology

Rickettsiae multiply in endothelial cells of small blood vessels and produce vasculitis. The cells become swollen and necrotic; there is thrombosis of the vessel, leading to rupture and necrosis. Vascular lesions are prominent in the skin, but vasculitis occurs in many organs and appears to be the basis of hemostatic disturbances. In the brain, aggregations of lymphocytes, polymorphonuclear leukocytes, and macrophages are associated with the blood vessels of the gray matter; these are called typhus nodules. The heart shows similar lesions of the small blood vessels. Other organs may also be involved.

Immunity

In cell cultures of macrophages, rickettsiae are phagocytosed and replicate intracellularly even in the presence of antibody. The addition of lymphocytes from immune animals stops this multiplication in vitro. Infection in humans is followed by partial immunity to reinfection from external sources, but relapses occur (see Brill's disease, below).

Clinical Findings

Except for Q fever, in which there is no skin lesion,

rickettsial infections are characterized by fever, headache, malaise, prostration, skin rash, and enlargement of the spleen and liver.

A. Typhus Group:

1. Epidemic typhus—In epidemic typhus, systemic infection and prostration are severe, and fever lasts for about 2 weeks. The disease is more severe and is more often fatal in patients over 40 years of age. During epidemics, the case-fatality rate has been 6–30%.

2. Endemic typhus—The clinical picture of endemic typhus has many features in common with that of epidemic typhus, but the disease is milder and is rarely fatal except in elderly patients.

B. Spotted Fever Group: The spotted fever group resembles typhus clinically; however, unlike the rash in other rickettsial diseases, the rash of the spotted fever group usually appears first on the extremities, moves centripetally, and involves the palms and soles. Some, like Brazilian spotted fever, may produce severe infections; others, like Mediterranean fever, are mild. The case-fatality rate varies greatly. In untreated Rocky Mountain spotted fever, it is usually much greater in older age groups (up to 60%) than in younger adults or children.

Rickettsialpox is a mild disease with a rash resembling that of varicella. About a week before onset of fever, a firm red papule appears at the site of the mite bite and develops into a deep-seated vesicle that in turn forms a black eschar (see below).

C. Scrub Typhus: This disease resembles epidemic typhus clinically. One feature is the eschar, the punched-out ulcer covered with a blackened scab that indicates the location of the mite bite. Generalized lymphadenopathy and lymphocytosis are common. Localized eschars may also be present in the spotted fever group.

D. Q Fever: This disease resembles influenza, nonbacterial pneumonia, hepatitis, or encephalopathy rather than typhus. There is no rash or local lesion. Rarely, infective endocarditis develops. The Weil-Felix test is negative, but there is a rise in the titer of specific antibodies (eg, microimmunofluorescence) to *C burnetii,* phase 2. Transmission results from inhalation of dust contaminated with rickettsiae from dried feces, urine, or milk or from aerosols in slaughterhouses.

E. Trench Fever: The disease is characterized by headache, exhaustion, pain, sweating, coldness of the extremities, and fever associated with a roseolar rash. Relapses occur. Trench fever has been known mainly in armies during wars in central Europe.

Laboratory Findings

Isolation of rickettsiae is technically quite difficult and so is of only limited usefulness in diagnosis. Whole blood (or emulsified blood clot) is inoculated into guinea pigs, mice, or eggs. Rickettsiae are recovered most frequently from blood drawn soon after onset, but they have been found as late as the 12th day of the disease.

If the guinea pigs fail to show disease (fever, scrotal swellings, hemorrhagic necrosis, death), serum is collected for antibody tests to determine if the animal has had an inapparent infection.

Some rickettsiae can infect mice, and rickettsiae are seen in smears of peritoneal exudate. In Rocky Mountain spotted fever, skin biopsies taken from patients between the fourth and eighth days of illness may reveal rickettsiae by immunofluorescence stain.

The most sensitive and specific serologic tests are microimmunofluorescence, microagglutination, and CF. An antibody rise should be demonstrated during the course of the illness.

Treatment

Tetracyclines and chloramphenicol are effective provided treatment is started early. Tetracycline, 2–3 g, or chloramphenicol, 1.5–2 g, is given daily orally and continued for 3–4 days after defervescence. In severely ill patients, the initial doses can be given intravenously.

Sulfonamides enhance the disease and are contraindicated.

The antibiotics do not free the body of rickettsiae, but they do suppress their growth. Recovery depends in part upon the immune mechanisms of the patient.

Epidemiology

A variety of arthropods, especially ticks and mites, harbor *Rickettsia*-like organisms in the cells that line the alimentary tract. Many such organisms are not evidently pathogenic for humans.

The life cycles of different rickettsiae vary:

(1) *Rickettsia prowazekii* has a life cycle limited to humans and to the human louse *(Pediculus humanus corporis* and *Pediculus humanus capitis).* The louse obtains the organism by biting infected human beings and transmits the agent by fecal excretion on the surface of the skin of another person. Whenever a louse bites, it defecates at the same time. The scratching of the area of the bite allows the rickettsiae excreted in the feces to penetrate the skin. As a result of the infection the louse dies, but the organisms remain viable for some time in the dried feces of the louse. Rickettsiae are not transmitted from one generation of lice to another. Typhus epidemics have been controlled by delousing large proportions of the population with insecticides.

Brill's disease is a recrudescence of an old typhus infection. The rickettsiae can persist for many years in the lymph nodes of an individual without any symptoms being manifest. The rickettsiae isolated from such cases behave like classic *R prowazekii;* this suggests that humans themselves are the reservoir of the rickettsiae of epidemic typhus. Epidemic typhus epidemics have been associated with war and the lowering of standards of personal hygiene, which in turn have increased the opportunities for human lice to flourish. If this occurs at the time of recrudescence of an old typhus infection, an epidemic may be set off. Brill's disease occurs in local populations of typhus areas as well as in persons who migrate from such areas to places where the disease does not exist. Serologic characteristics readily distinguish Brill's disease from primary epidemic typhus. Antibodies arise earlier and are IgG rather than the IgM detected after primary infection. They reach a maximum by the tenth day of disease. The Weil-Felix reaction is usually negative. This early IgG antibody response and the mild course of the disease suggest that partial immunity is still present from the primary infection.

In the USA, *R prowazekii* has an extrahuman reservoir in the southern flying squirrel. In areas where southern flying squirrels are indigenous, human infections have occurred after bites by ectoparasites of this rodent.

(2) *Rickettsia typhi* has its reservoir in the rat, in which the infection is inapparent and long-lasting. Rat fleas carry the rickettsiae from rat to rat and sometimes from rat to humans, who develop endemic typhus. Cat fleas can serve as vectors. In endemic typhus, the flea cannot transmit the rickettsiae transovarially.

(3) *Rickettsia tsutsugamushi* has its true reservoir in the mites that infest rodents. Rickettsiae can persist in rats for over a year after infection. Mites transmit the infection transovarially. Occasionally, infected mites or rat fleas bite humans, and scrub typhus results. The rickettsiae persist in the mite-rat-mite cycle in the scrub or secondary jungle vegetation that has replaced virgin jungle in areas of partial cultivation. Such areas may become infested with rats and trombiculid mites.

(4) *Rickettsia rickettsii* may be found in healthy wood ticks *(Dermacentor andersoni)* and is passed transovarially. Vertebrates such as rodents, deer, and humans are occasionally bitten by infected ticks in the western USA. In order to be infectious, the tick carrying the rickettsiae must be engorged with blood, for this increases the number of rickettsiae in the tick. Thus, there is a delay of 45–90 minutes between the time of the attachment of the tick and its becoming infective. In the eastern USA, Rocky Mountain spotted fever is transmitted by the dog tick *Dermacentor variabilis.* Dogs are hosts to dog ticks and may serve as a reservoir for tick infection. Small rodents are another reservoir. Most cases of Rocky Mountain spotted fever in the USA now occur in the eastern and southeastern regions.

(5) *Rickettsia akari* has its vector in bloodsucking mites of the species *Allodermanyssus sanguineus.* These mites may be found on the mice *(Mus musculus)* trapped in apartment houses in the USA where rickettsialpox has occurred. Transovarial transmission of the rickettsiae occurs in the mite. Thus the mite may act as a true reservoir as well as a vector. *R akari* has also been isolated in Korea.

(6) *Rochalimaea quintana* is the causative agent of trench fever; it is found in lice and in humans, and its life cycle is like that of *R prowazekii.* The disease has been limited to fighting armies. This organism can be grown on blood agar in 10% CO_2.

(7) *Coxiella burnetii* is found in ticks, which transmit the agent to sheep, goats, and cattle. Workers in slaughterhouses and in plants that process wool and cattle hides have contracted the disease as a result of handling infected animal tissues. *C burnetii* is transmitted by the respiratory pathway rather than through the skin. There may be a chronic infection of the udder of the cow. In such cases the rickettsiae are excreted in the milk and occasionally may be transmitted to humans by ingestion or inhalation.

Infected sheep may excrete *C burnetii* in the feces and urine and heavily contaminate their skin and woolen coat. The placentas of infected cows and sheep contain the rickettsiae, and parturition creates infectious aerosols. The soil may be heavily contaminated from one of the above sources, and the inhalation of infected dust leads to infection of humans and livestock. It has been proposed that endospores formed by *C burnetii* contribute to its persistence amd dissemination. *Coxiella* infection is now widespread among sheep and cattle in the USA. *Coxiella* can cause endocarditis (with a rise in the titer of antibodies to *C burnetii,* phase 1) in addition to pneumonitis and hepatitis.

Rickettsia canada has been isolated from ticks. Its role in human disease is uncertain.

Geographic Occurrence

A. Epidemic Typhus: Potentially worldwide, it has disappeared from the USA, Britain, and Scandinavia. It is still present in the Balkans, Asia, Africa, Mexico, and the Andes. In view of its long duration in humans as a latent infection (Brill's disease), it can flourish quickly under proper environmental conditions, as it did in Europe during World War II as a result of the deterioration of community hygiene.

B. Endemic, Murine Typhus: Worldwide, especially in areas of high rat infestation. It may exist in the same areas as—and may be confused with—epidemic typhus or scrub typhus.

C. Scrub Typhus: Far East, especially Burma, India, Ceylon, New Guinea, Japan, and Taiwan. The larval stage (chigger) of various trombiculid mites serves both as a reservoir, through transovarian transmission, and as a vector for infecting humans and rodents.

D. Spotted Fever Group: These infections occur around the globe, exhibiting as a rule some epidemiologic and immunologic differences in different areas. Transmission by a tick of the *Ixodidae* family is common to the group. The diseases that are grouped together include Rocky Mountain spotted fever (western and eastern RMSF), Colombian, Brazilian, and Mexican spotted fevers; Mediterranean (boutonneuse), South African tick, and Kenya fevers; North Queensland tick typhus; and North Asian tickborne rickettsiosis.

E. Rickettsialpox: The human disease has been found among inhabitants of apartment houses in the northern USA. However, the infection also occurs in Russia, Africa, and Korea.

F. Q Fever: The disease is recognized around the world and occurs mainly in persons associated with goats, sheep, or dairy cattle. It has attracted attention because of outbreaks in veterinary and medical centers where large numbers of people were exposed to animals shedding *Coxiella*.

Seasonal Occurrence

Epidemic typhus is more common in cool climates, reaching its peak in winter and waning in the spring. This is probably a reflection of crowding, lack of fuel, and low standards of personal hygiene, which favor louse infestation.

Rickettsial infections that must be transmitted to the human host by vector reach their peak incidence at the time the vector is most prevalent—the summer and fall months.

Control

Control is achieved by breaking the infection chain or by immunizing and treating with antibiotics. Patients with rickettsial disease who are free from ectoparasites are not contagious and do not transmit the infection.

A. Prevention of Transmission by Breaking the Chain of Infection:

1. Epidemic typhus–Delousing with insecticide.

2. Murine typhus–Rat-proofing buildings and using rat poisons.

3. Scrub typhus–Clearing from campsites the secondary jungle vegetation in which rats and mites live.

4. Spotted fever–Similar measures for the spotted fevers may be used; clearing of infested land; per-

sonal prophylaxis in the form of protective clothing such as high boots, socks worn over trousers; tick repellents; and frequent removal of attached ticks.

5. Rickettsialpox–Elimination of rodents and their parasites from human domiciles.

B. Prevention of Transmission of Q Fever by Adequate Pasteurization of Milk: The presently recommended conditions of "high-temperature, short-time" pasteurization at 71.5 °C (161 °F) for 15 seconds are adequate to destroy viable *Coxiella*.

C. Prevention by Vaccination: Active immunization may be carried out using formalinized antigens prepared from the yolk sacs of infected chick embryos or from cell cultures. Such vaccines have been prepared for epidemic typhus *(R prowazekii)*, Rocky Mountain spotted fever *(R rickettsii),* and Q fever *(C burnetii)*. The *Coxiella* vaccine (formalinized phase 1) has benefited occupationally exposed abattoir workers in Australia. However, commercially produced vaccines are not available in the USA in 1986. Cell-culture-grown, inactivated suspensions of rickettsiae are under study as vaccines. A live vaccine (strain E) for epidemic typhus is effective and used experimentally but produces a self-limited disease.

D. Chemoprophylaxis: Chloramphenicol has been used as a chemoprophylactic agent against scrub typhus in endemic areas. Oral administration of 3-g doses at weekly intervals controls infection so that no disease occurs even though rickettsiae appear in the blood. The antibiotic must be continued for a month after the initiation of infection to keep the person well. Tetracyclines may be equally effective.

REFERENCES

Berman SJ, Kundin WD: Scrub typhus in South Vietnam. *Ann Intern Med* 1973;**79**:26.

Bradford WD, Hackett DB: Myocardial involvement in Rocky Mountain spotted fever. *Arch Pathol Lab Med* 1978;**102**:357.

Bretman LR et al : Rickettsialpox: Report of an outbreak and a contemporary review. *Medicine* 1981;**60**:363.

Caughey JE: Pleuropericardial lesion in Q fever. *Br Med J* 1977;**1**:1447.

Clements ML et al: Reactogenicity, immunogenicity and efficacy of a chick embryo–cell derived vaccine for Rocky Mountain spotted fever. *J Infect Dis* 1983;**148**: 922.

Donohue JF: Lower respiratory tract involvement in Rocky Mountain spotted fever. *Arch Intern Med* 1980;**140**:223.

Duma RJ et al : Epidemic typhus in the United States associated with flying squirrels. *JAMA* 1981;**245**: 2318.

Gordon JC et al : Rocky Mountain spotted fever in dogs associated with human patients in Ohio. *J Infect Dis* 1983;**148**: 1123.

Hackstadt T, Williams JC: Biochemical stratagem for obligate parasitism of eukaryotic cells by *Coxiella burnetii*. *Proc Natl Acad Sci USA* 1981;**78**:3240.

Hechemy KE: Laboratory diagnosis of Rocky Mountain spotted fever. *N Engl J Med* 1979;**300**:859.

Hinrichs DJ, Jerrels TR: In vitro evaluation of immunity to *Coxiella burnetii*. *J Immunol* 1976;**117**:996.

Janigan DT et al: An inflammatory pseudotumor of the lung in Q fever pneumonia. *N Engl J Med* 1983;**308**:86.

Marmion BP et al: Vaccine prophylaxis of abbatoir-associated Q fever. *Lancet* 1985;**2**:1411.

Phillip RN et al: Comparison of serologic methods for diagnosis of Rocky Mountain spotted fever. *Am J Epidemiol* 1977; **105**:56.

Sheehy TW et al: Scrub typhus: Comparison of chloramphenicol and tetracycline. *Arch Intern Med* 1973;**132**:77.

Tobin MJ et al: Q fever endocarditis. *Am J Med* 1982;**72**:396.

Wells GM et al: Rocky Mountain spotted fever caused by blood transfusion. *JAMA* 1978;**239**:2763.

Wisseman CL, Waddell AD: In vitro studies of rickettsia-host cell interactions. *Infect Immun* 1975;**11**:1391.

Woodward TE: A historical account of the rickettsial diseases. *J Infect Dis* 1973;**127**:583.

Chlamydiae

Chlamydiae are a large group of obligate intracellular parasites closely related to gram-negative bacteria. They are divided into 2 species, *Chlamydia psittaci* and *Chlamydia trachomatis,* on the basis of antigenic composition, intracellular inclusions, sulfonamide susceptibility, and disease production (see below). All chlamydiae exhibit similar morphologic features, share a common group antigen, and multiply in the cytoplasm of their host cells by a distinctive developmental cycle.

Because of their obligate intracellular parasitism, chlamydiae were once considered viruses. Chlamydiae differ from viruses in the following important characteristics:

(1) Like bacteria, they possess both RNA and DNA.

(2) They multiply by binary fission; viruses never do.

(3) They have a rigid cell wall that resembles a bacterial type cell wall but lacks muramic acid and is not susceptible to lysozyme action.

(4) They possess ribosomes; viruses never do.

(5) They have a variety of metabolically active enzymes, eg, they can liberate CO_2 from glucose. Some can synthesize folates.

(6) Their growth can be inhibited by many antimicrobial drugs.

Chlamydiae can be viewed as gram-negative bacteria that lack mechanisms for the production of metabolic energy and cannot synthesize ATP. This defect restricts them to an intracellular existence, where the host cell furnishes energy-rich intermediates.

Developmental Cycle

All chlamydiae share a general sequence of events in their reproduction. The infectious particle is a small cell ("elementary body") about 0.3 μm in diameter with an electron-dense nucleoid. It is taken into the host cell by phagocytosis. A vacuole, derived from the host cell surface membranes, forms around the small particle. This small particle is reorganized into a large one (reticulate body, initial body), measuring about 0.5–1 μm and devoid of an electron-dense nucleoid. Within the membrane-bound vacuole, the reticulate

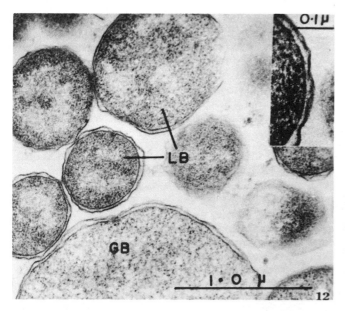
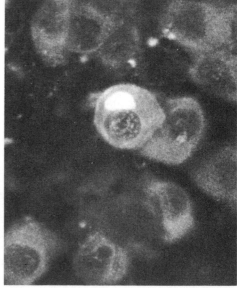

Figure 29–1. Chlamydiae. *Left:* Chlamydiae in various stages of intracellular development. LB = "elementary body" particles with cell walls. GB = "reticulate large body," "initial body." *Right:* Fluorescent inclusion body of *C trachomatic* in epithelial cell (conjunctival scraping) stained with specific fluorescein-labeled antiserum.

body grows in size and divides repeatedly by binary fission. Eventually the entire vacuole becomes filled with small particles derived by binary fission from reticulate bodies to form an "inclusion" in the host cell cytoplasm. The newly formed small particles may be liberated from the host cell to infect new cells. The developmental cycle takes 24–48 hours.

Structure & Chemical Composition

Examination of highly purified suspensions of chlamydiae, washed free of host cell materials, indicates the following: the outer **cell wall** resembles the cell wall of gram-negative bacteria. It has a relatively high lipid content. It is rigid but does not contain a typical bacterial peptidoglycan; perhaps it contains a tetrapeptide-linked matrix. Penicillin-binding proteins occur in chlamydiae, and chlamydial cell wall formation is inhibited by penicillins and cycloserine, substances that inhibit transpeptidation of bacterial peptidoglycans. Lysozyme has no effect on chlamydial cell walls. N-Acetyl-muramic acid appears to be absent from chlamydial cell walls. Both DNA and RNA are present in both small and large particles. In small particles, most DNA is concentrated in the electron-dense central nucleoid. In large particles, the DNA is distributed irregularly throughout the cytoplasm. Most RNA probably exists in ribosomes, in the cytoplasm. The large particles contain about 4 times as much RNA as DNA, whereas the small, infective particles contain about equal amounts of RNA and DNA.

The circular genome of chlamydiae (MW 7×10^8) is similar to bacterial chromosomes. Chlamydiae contain large amounts of **lipids,** especially phospholipids, which are well characterized.

A toxic principle is intimately associated with infectious chlamydiae. It kills mice after the intravenous administration of more than 10^8 particles. Toxicity is destroyed by heat but not by ultraviolet light.

Staining Properties

Chlamydiae have distinctive staining properties (similar to those of rickettsiae) that differ somewhat at different stages of development. Single mature particles (elementary bodies) stain purple with Giemsa's stain and red with Macchiavello's stain, in contrast to the blue of host cell cytoplasm. The larger, noninfective bodies (initial bodies) stain blue with Giemsa's stain. The Gram reaction of chlamydiae is negative or variable, and Gram's stain is not useful in the identification of the agents.

Fully formed, mature intracellular inclusions of *C trachomatis* are compact masses near the nucleus which are dark purple when stained with Giemsa's stain because of the densely packed mature particles. If stained with dilute Lugol's iodine solution, some of these inclusions appear brown because of the glycogenlike matrix that surrounds the particles. Inclusions of *C psittaci* are diffuse intracytoplasmic aggregates without glycogen.

Antigens

Chlamydiae possess 2 types of antigens. Both are probably located in the cell wall. **Group antigens** are shared by all chlamydiae. These are heat-stable lipoprotein-carbohydrate complexes, with 2-keto-3-deoxy-octonic acid as an immunodominant component. Antibody to these group antigens can be detected by CF and immunofluorescence. **Specific antigens** (species-specific or immunotype-specific) remain attached to cell walls after group antigens have been largely removed by treatment with fluorocarbon or deoxycholate. Some specific antigens are membrane proteins that have been purified by immunoadsorption. Specific antigens can best be detected by immunofluorescence, particularly using monoclonal antibodies. Specific antigens are shared by only a limited number of chlamydiae, but a given organism may contain several specific antigens. Fifteen **immunotypes** (serotypes, serovars) of *C trachomatis* have been identified (A, B, Ba, C–K, Ll–L3), and the last 3 are LGV immunotypes. The toxic effects of chlamydiae are associated with antigens. Specific neutralization of these toxic effects by antiserum permits similar antigenic grouping of organisms.

A very unstable hemagglutinin capable of clumping some chicken and mouse erythrocytes is present in chlamydiae. This hemagglutination is blocked by group antibody.

Growth & Metabolism

Chlamydiae require an intracellular habitat, because they are unable to synthesize ATP and depend on the host cell for energy requirements. All types of chlamydiae proliferate in embryonated eggs, particularly in the yolk sac. Some also grow in cell cultures and in various animal tissues. Cells have attachment sites for chlamydiae. Removal of these sites prevents easy uptake of chlamydiae.

Chlamydiae appear to have an endogenous metabolism similar to that of some bacteria but participate only to a limited extent in potentially energy-yielding processes. They can liberate CO_2 from glucose, pyruvate, and glutamate; they also contain dehydrogenases. Nevertheless, they require energy-rich intermediates from the host cell to carry out their biosynthetic activities.

Reactions to Physical & Chemical Agents

Chlamydiae are rapidly inactivated by heat. They lose infectivity completely after 10 minutes at 60 °C. They maintain infectivity for years at −50 °C to −70 °C. During the process of freeze-drying, much of the infectivity is lost. Some air-dried chlamydiae may remain infective for long periods.

Chlamydiae are rapidly inactivated by ether (in 30 minutes) or by phenol (0.5% for 24 hours).

The replication of chlamydiae can be inhibited by many antibacterial drugs. Cell wall inhibitors such as penicillins and cycloserine result in the production of morphologically defective forms but are not effective in clinical diseases. Inhibitors of protein synthesis (tetracyclines, erythromycins) are effective in most clinical infections. Some chlamydiae synthesize folates and are susceptible to inhibition by sulfonamides. Aminoglycosides have little inhibitory activity for chlamydiae.

Characteristics of Host-Parasite Relationship

The outstanding biologic feature of infection by chlamydiae is the balance that is often reached between host and parasite, resulting in prolonged, often lifetime persistence. Subclinical infection is the rule—and overt disease the exception—in the natural hosts of these agents. Spread from one species (eg, birds) to another (eg, humans) more frequently leads to disease. Antibodies to several antigens of chlamydiae are regularly produced by the infected host. These antibodies have little protective effect. The infectious agent commonly persists in the presence of high antibody titers. Treatment with effective antimicrobial drugs (eg, tetracyclines) for prolonged periods may eliminate the chlamydiae from the infected host. Very early, intensive treatment may suppress antibody formation. Late treatment with antimicrobial drugs in moderate doses may suppress disease but permit persistence of the infecting agent in tissues.

The immunization of susceptible animals with various inactivated or living vaccines tends to induce protection against death from the toxic effect of living challenge organisms. However, such immunization in animals or humans has been singularly unsuccessful in protecting against reinfection. Prior infection or immunization at most tends to result in milder disease upon reinfection, but at times, the accompanying hypersensitization aggravates inflammation and scarring (eg, in trachoma).

Classification

Historically, chlamydiae were arranged according to their pathogenic potential and their host range. Antigenic differences were defined by antigen-antibody reactions studied by immunofluorescence, toxin neutralization, and other methods. At present, 2 species are accepted:

(1) *C psittaci:* This species produces diffuse intracytoplasmic inclusions that lack glycogen; it is usually resistant to sulfonamides. It includes agents of psittacosis in humans, ornithosis in birds, meningopneumonitis, feline pneumonitis, and many other animal pathogens.

(2) *C trachomatis:* This species produces compact intracytoplasmic inclusions that contain glycogen; it is usually inhibited by sulfonamides. It includes agents of mouse pneumonitis and several human disorders such as trachoma, inclusion conjunctivitis, nongonococcal urethritis, salpingitis, cervicitis, pneumonitis of infants, and lymphogranuloma venereum.

In nucleic acid hybridization experiments, the 2 species appear not to be closely related.

PSITTACOSIS (Ornithosis)

Psittacosis is a disease of birds that may be transferred to humans. In humans, the agent, *C psittaci,* produces a spectrum of clinical manifestations ranging from severe pneumonia and sepsis with a high mortality rate to a mild inapparent infection.

Properties of the Agent

A. Size and Staining Properties: Similar to other members of the group (see above).

B. Animal Susceptibility and Growth of Agent: Psittacosis agent can be propagated in embryonated eggs, in mice and other animals, and in some cell cultures. In all these host systems, growth can be inhibited by tetracyclines and, to a limited extent, by penicillins. In intact animals and in humans, tetracyclines can suppress illness but may not be able to eliminate the infectious agent or end the carrier state.

C. Antigenic Properties: The heat-stable group-reactive CF antigen resists proteolytic enzymes but is destroyed by potassium periodate. It is probably a lipopolysaccharide.

Infected tissue contains a toxic principle, intimately associated with the agent, that rapidly kills mice upon intravenous or intraperitoneal infection. This toxic principle is active only in particles that are infective.

Specific serotypes characteristic for certain mammalian and avian species may be demonstrated by cross-neutralization tests of toxic effect. Neutralization of infectivity of the agent by specific antibody or cross-protection of immunized animals can also be used for serotyping, and the results parallel those of immunofluorescence typing.

D. Cell Wall Antigens: Walls of the infecting agent have been prepared by treatment with deoxycholate followed by trypsin. The deoxycholate extracts contained group-reactive CF antigens, while the cell walls retained the species-specific antigens. The cell wall antigens were also associated with toxin neutralization and infectivity neutralization.

Pathogenesis & Pathology

The agent enters through the respiratory tract, is found in the blood during the first 2 weeks of the disease, and may be found in the sputum at the time the lung is involved.

Psittacosis causes a patchy inflammation of the lungs in which consolidated areas are sharply demarcated. The exudate is predominantly mononuclear. Only minor changes occur in the large bronchioles and bronchi. The lesions are similar to those found in pneumonitis caused by some viruses and mycoplasmas. Liver, spleen, heart, and kidney are often enlarged and congested.

Clinical Findings

A sudden onset of illness taking the form of influenza or nonbacterial pneumonia in a person exposed to birds is suggestive of psittacosis. The incubation period averages 10 days. The onset is usually sudden, with malaise, fever, anorexia, sore throat, photophobia, and severe headache. The disease may progress no further and the patient may improve in a few days. In severe cases, the signs and symptoms of bronchial pneumonia appear at the end of the first week of the disease. The clinical picture often resembles that of influenza, nonbacterial pneumonia, or typhoid fever. The mortality rate may be as high as 20% in untreated cases, especially in the elderly.

Laboratory Diagnosis

A. Recovery of Agent: The psittacosis agent can be isolated from blood or sputum of patients or from lung tissue in fatal cases. This is infrequently accomplished because it requires specialized facilities. Specimens are inoculated intra-abdominally into mice, into the yolk sacs of embryonated eggs, and into cell cultures. Infection in the test systems is confirmed by the serial transmission of the infectious agent, its microscopic demonstration, and serologic identification of the recovered agent.

B. Serology: A variety of antibodies may develop in the course of infection. In humans, CF with group antigen is the most widely used diagnostic test. A single titer of 1:32 or higher in an illness compatible with this diagnosis is presumptive evidence of chlamydial pneumonia. For definitive diagnosis, acute and later phase sera should be run in the same test in order to establish an antibody rise. In birds, the indirect CF test may provide additional diagnostic information. Although antibodies usually develop within 10 days, the use of antibiotics may delay their development for 20–40 days or suppress it altogether.

Sera of patients with other chlamydial infections may fix complement in high titer with psittacosis antigen. In patients with psittacosis, the high titer persists for months, and in carriers, even for years. Infection of live birds is suggested by a positive CF test and an enlarged spleen or liver. This can be confirmed by demonstration of particles in smears or sections of organs and by passage of the agent in mice and eggs.

Immunity

Immunity in animals and humans is incomplete. A carrier state in humans can persist for 10 years after recovery. During this period, the agent may continue to be excreted in the sputum.

Skin tests with group antigen are positive soon after infection with any member of the group. However, skin tests are not usually employed in diagnosis.

Live or inactivated vaccines induce only partial resistance in animals. They have not been used in humans.

Treatment

Tetracyclines are the drugs of choice and should be continued for 10 days after defervescence to prevent relapse. Psittacosis agents are not sensitive to aminoglycosides, and most strains are not susceptible to sulfonamides. Although antibiotic treatment may control the clinical evidence of disease, it may not free the patient from the agent, ie, the patient may become a carrier. Intensive antibiotic treatment may also delay the normal course of antibody development. Strains may become drug-resistant.

With the introduction of antibiotic therapy, the mortality rate has dropped from 20% to 2%. Death occurs most frequently in patients over 40 years of age.

Epidemiology

The term psittacosis is applied to the human disease acquired from contact with birds and also the infection of psittacine birds (parrots, parakeets, cockatoos, etc). The term ornithosis is applied to infection with similar agents in all types of domestic birds (pigeons, chickens, ducks, geese, turkeys, etc) and free-living birds (gulls, egrets, petrels, etc). Outbreaks of human disease can occur whenever there is close and continued contact between humans and infected birds that excrete or shed large amounts of infectious agent. Birds often acquire infection as fledglings in the nest; may develop diarrheal illness or no illness; and often carry the infectious agent for their normal life span. When subjected to stress (eg, malnutrition, shipping), birds may become sick and die. The agent is present in tissues (eg, spleen) and is often excreted in feces by healthy birds. The inhalation of infected dried bird feces is a common method of human infection. Another source of infection is the handling of infected tissues (eg, in poultry rendering plants) and inhalation of an infected aerosol.

Birds kept as pets have been an important source of human infection. Foremost among these were the many psittacine birds imported from South America, Australia, and the Far East and kept in aviaries in the USA. Latent infections often flared up in these birds during transport and crowding, and sick birds excreted exceedingly large quantities of infectious agent. Control of bird shipment, quarantine, testing of imported birds for psittacosis infection, and prophylactic tetracyclines in bird feed help to control this source. Pigeons kept for racing or as pets or raised for squab meat have been important sources of infection. Pigeons populating civic buildings and thoroughfares in many cities are not infrequently infected but shed relatively small quantities of agent.

Among the personnel of poultry farms involved in the dressing, packing, and shipping of ducks, geese, turkeys, and chickens, subclinical or clinical infection is relatively frequent. Outbreaks of disease among birds have at times resulted in heavy economic losses and have been followed by outbreaks in humans.

Persons who develop psittacosis may become infectious for other persons if the evolving pneumonia results in expectoration of large quantities of infectious sputum. This has been a rare occupational risk for hospital personnel.

Control

Shipments of psittacine birds should be held in

quarantine to ensure that there are no obviously sick birds in the lot. A proportion of each shipment should be tested for antibodies and examined for agent. An intradermal test has been recommended for detecting ornithosis in turkey flocks. The incorporation of tetracyclines into bird feed has been used to reduce the number of carriers. The source of human infection should be traced, if possible, and infected birds should be killed.

OCULAR, GENITAL, & RESPIRATORY INFECTIONS DUE TO *CHLAMYDIA TRACHOMATIS*

TRACHOMA

Trachoma is an ancient eye disease, well described in the Ebers Papyrus, which was written in Egypt 3800 years ago. It is a chronic keratoconjunctivitis that begins with acute inflammatory changes in the conjunctiva and cornea and progresses to scarring and blindness.

Properties of *C trachomatis*

A. Size and Staining Properties: Similar to other chlamydiae (see above).

B. Animal Susceptibility and Growth: Humans are the natural host for *C trachomatis*. Monkeys and chimpanzees can be infected in the eye and genital tract. All chlamydiae multiply in the yolk sacs of embryonated hens' eggs and cause death of the embryo when the number of particles becomes sufficiently high. *C trachomatis* also replicates in various cell lines, particularly when cells are treated with cycloheximide, cytochalasin B, or idoxuridine. *C trachomatis* of different immunotypes replicates differently. Isolates from trachoma do not grow as well as those from LGV or genital infections. Intracytoplasmic replication results in a developmental cycle (see p 306) that leads to formation of compact inclusions with a glycogen matrix in which particles are embedded.

A toxic factor is associated with *C trachomatis* provided the particles are viable. Neutralization of this toxic factor by immunotype-specific antisera permits typing of isolates that gives results analogous to those achieved by typing by immunofluorescence. The immunotypes specifically associated with endemic trachoma are A, B, Ba, and C.

Clinical Findings

In experimental infections, the incubation period is 3–10 days. In endemic areas, initial infection occurs in early childhood and the onset is insidious. Chlamydial infection is often mixed with bacterial conjunctivitis in endemic areas, and the 2 together produce the clinical picture. The earliest symptoms of trachoma are

lacrimation, mucopurulent discharge, conjunctival hyperemia, and follicular hypertrophy. Biomicroscopic examination of the cornea reveals epithelial keratitis, subepithelial infiltrates, and extension of limbal vessels into the cornea (pannus).

As the pannus extends downward across the cornea, there is scarring of conjunctiva, lid deformities (entropion, trichiasis), and added insult caused by eyelashes sweeping across the cornea. With secondary bacterial infection, loss of vision progresses over a period of years. There are, however, no systemic symptoms or signs of infection.

Laboratory Diagnosis

A. Recovery of *C trachomatis*: Typical cytoplasmic inclusions are found in epithelial cells of conjunctival scrapings stained with fluorescent antibody or by Giemsa's method. These occur most frequently in the early stages of the disease and on the upper tarsal conjunctiva.

Inoculation of conjunctival scrapings into embryonated eggs or cycloheximide-treated cell cultures permits growth of *C trachomatis* if the number of viable infectious particles is sufficiently large. Centrifugation of the inoculum into treated cells increases the sensitivity of the method. The diagnosis can sometimes be made in the first passage by looking for inclusions after 2–3 days of incubation by immunofluorescence or staining with iodine or Giemsa's stain.

B. Serology: Infected individuals often develop both group antibodies and immunotype-specific antibodies in serum and in eye secretions. Immunofluorescence is the most sensitive method for their detection. Neither ocular nor serum antibodies confer significant resistance to reinfection.

Treatment

In endemic areas, sulfonamides, erythromycins, and tetracyclines have been used to suppress chlamydiae and bacteria that cause eye infections. Periodic topical application of these drugs to the conjunctivas of all members of the community is sometimes supplemented with oral doses; the dosage and frequency of administration vary with the geographic area and the severity of endemic trachoma. Drug-resistant *C trachomatis* has not been definitely identified except in laboratory experiments. Even a single monthly dose of 300 mg of doxycycline can result in significant clinical improvement, reducing the danger of blindness. Topical application of corticosteroids is not indicated and may reactivate latent trachoma. Chlamydiae can persist during and after drug treatment, and recurrence of activity is common.

Epidemiology & Control

It is believed that over 400 million people throughout the world are infected with trachoma and that 20 million are blinded by it. The disease is most prevalent in Africa, Asia, and the Mediterranean basin, where hygienic conditions are poor and water is scarce. In such hyperendemic areas, childhood infection may be universal, and severe, blinding disease (resulting from frequent bacterial superinfections) is common. In the USA, trachoma occurs sporadically in some areas, and endemic foci persist on Indian reservations.

Control of trachoma depends mainly upon improvement of hygienic standards and drug treatment. When socioeconomic levels rise in an area, trachoma becomes milder and eventually may disappear. Experimental trachoma vaccines have not given encouraging results. Surgical correction of lid deformities may be necessary in advanced cases.

GENITAL CHLAMYDIAL INFECTIONS & INCLUSION CONJUNCTIVITIS

C trachomatis, immunotypes D–K, is a common cause of sexually transmitted diseases that may also produce infection of the eye (inclusion conjunctivitis). In sexually active adults, particularly in the USA and western Europe—and especially in higher socioeconomic groups — *C trachomatis* is a prominent cause of nongonococcal urethritis and, rarely, epididymitis in males. In females, *C trachomatis* causes urethritis, cervicitis, salpingitis, and pelvic inflammatory disease. Any of these anatomic sites of infection may give rise to symptoms and signs, or the infection may remain asymptomatic but communicable to sex partners. Up to 50% of nongonococcal or postgonococcal urethritis or the urethral syndrome is attributed to chlamydiae and produces dysuria, nonpurulent discharge, and frequency of urination.

This enormous reservoir of infectious chlamydiae in adults can be manifested by symptomatic genital tract illness in adults or by an ocular infection that closely resembles trachoma. In adults, this inclusion conjunctivitis results from self-inoculation of genital secretions and was formerly thought to be "swimming pool conjunctivitis."

The newborn acquires the infection during passage through an infected birth canal. Inclusion conjunctivitis of the newborn begins as a mucopurulent conjunctivitis 7–12 days after delivery. It tends to subside with erythromycin or tetracycline treatment, or spontaneously after weeks or months. Occasionally, inclusion conjunctivitis persists as a chronic chlamydial infection with a clinical picture indistinguishable from subacute or chronic childhood trachoma in nonendemic areas and usually not associated with bacterial conjunctivitis.

Laboratory Diagnosis
A. Recovery of *C trachomatis:* Scrapings of epithelial cells from urethra, cervix, vagina, or conjunctiva and biopsy specimens from salpinx or epididymis can be inoculated into chemically treated cell cultures for growth of *C trachomatis* (see above). Isolates can be typed by microimmunofluorescence with specific sera. The same genital tract specimens can also be examined directly by immunofluorescence for chlamydial particles. In neonatal—and sometimes

adult—inclusion conjunctivitis, the cytoplasmic inclusions in epithelial cells are so dense that they are readily detected in conjunctival exudate and scrapings examined by immunofluorescence or stained by Giemsa's method.

B. Serologic Tests: Because of the relatively great antigenic mass of chlamydiae in genital tract infections, serum antibodies occur much more commonly than in trachoma and are of higher titer. A titer rise occurs during and after acute chlamydial infection.

In genital secretions (eg, cervical), antibody can be detected during active infection and is directed against the infecting immunotype.

Treatment
It is essential that chlamydial infections be treated simultaneously in both sex partners and in offspring to prevent reinfection.

Tetracyclines (eg, doxycycline, 100 mg/d by mouth for 10–20 days) are commonly used in nongonococcal or postgonococcal urethritis and in nonpregnant infected females. Erythromycin, 250 mg 4–6 times daily for 2 weeks, is given to pregnant women. Topical tetracycline or erythromycin is used for inclusion conjunctivitis, sometimes in combination with a systemic drug.

Epidemiology & Control
Genital chlamydial infection and inclusion conjunctivitis are sexually transmitted diseases that are spread by indiscriminate contact with multiple sex partners. Neonatal inclusion conjunctivitis originates in the mother's infected genital tract. Prevention of neonatal eye disease depends upon diagnosis and treatment of the pregnant woman and her sex partner. As in all sexually transmitted diseases, the presence of multiple etiologic agents (gonococci, treponemes, *Trichomonas,* herpes, mycoplasmas, etc) must be considered. Instillation of 1% silver nitrate into the newborn's eyes does not prevent development of chlamydial conjunctivitis. The ultimate control of this—and all—sexually transmitted disease depends on reduction in promiscuity, use of condoms, and early diagnosis and treatment of the infected reservoir.

RESPIRATORY TRACT INVOLVEMENT WITH *C TRACHOMATIS*

Adults with inclusion conjunctivitis often manifest upper respiratory tract symptoms (eg, otalgia, otitis, nasal obstruction, pharyngitis), presumably resulting from drainage of infectious chlamydiae through the nasolacrimal duct. Pneumonitis is infrequent in adults unless they are immunocompromised.

Newborns infected by the mother may develop respiratory tract involvement 2–12 weeks after birth, culminating in pneumonia. There is striking tachypnea, paroxysmal cough, absence of fever, and eosinophilia. Consolidation of lungs and hyperinflation can be seen by x-ray. Diagnosis can be established by isolation of *C trachomatis* from respiratory secretions and can be suspected if pneumonitis develops in a newborn who has inclusion conjunctivitis. In such neonatal pneumonia, an IgM antibody titer to *C trachomatis* of 1:32 or more is considered diagnostic. Systemic erythromycin (40 mg/kg/d) is effective treatment in severe cases.

LYMPHOGRANULOMA VENEREUM (LGV)

LGV is a sexually transmitted disease characterized by suppurative inguinal adenitis; it is more common in tropical climates. The causative agent is *C trachomatis* of immunotypes L1–L3.

Properties of the Agent
A. Size and Staining Properties: See above.

B. Animal Susceptibility and Growth of Agent: The agent can be transmitted to monkeys and mice and can be propagated in tissue cultures or in chick embryos. Most strains grow in cell cultures; their infectivity for cells is not enhanced by pretreatment with DEAE-dextran.

C. Antigenic Properties: The particles contain CF heat-stable chlamydial group antigens that are shared with all other chlamydiae. They also contain one of 3 specific antigens (L1–L3), which can be defined by immunofluorescence. Infective particles contain a toxic principle.

Clinical Findings
Several days to several weeks after exposure, a small, evanescent papule or vesicle develops on any part of the external genitalia, anus, rectum, or elsewhere. The lesion may ulcerate, but usually it remains unnoticed and heals in a few days. Soon thereafter, the regional lymph nodes enlarge and tend to become matted and often painful. In males, inguinal nodes are most commonly involved both above and below Poupart's ligament, and the overlying skin often turns purplish as the nodes suppurate and eventually discharge pus through multiple sinus tracts. In females and in homosexual males, the perirectal nodes are prominently involved, with proctitis and a bloody mucopurulent anal discharge. Lymphadenitis may be most marked in the cervical chains.

During the stage of active lymphadenitis, there are often marked systemic symptoms including fever, headaches, meningismus, conjunctivitis, skin rashes, nausea and vomiting, and arthralgias. Meningitis, arthritis, and pericarditis occur rarely. Unless effective antimicrobial drug treatment is given at that stage, the chronic inflammatory process progresses to fibrosis, lymphatic obstruction, and rectal strictures. The lymphatic obstruction may lead to elephantiasis of the penis, scrotum, or vulva. The chronic proctitis of women or homosexual males may lead to progressive rectal strictures, rectosigmoid obstruction, and fistula formation.

Laboratory Diagnosis
A. Smears: Pus, buboes, or biopsy material may be stained, but particles are rarely recognized.

B. Isolation of Agent: Suspected material is inoculated into yolk sacs of embryonated eggs, cell cultures, or the brains of mice. The inoculum can be treated with an aminoglycoside (but not with penicillin or ether) to lessen bacterial contamination. The agent is identified by morphology and serologic tests.

C. Serologic Tests: Antibodies are commonly demonstrated by the CF reaction. The test becomes positive 2–4 weeks after onset of illness, at which time skin hypersensitivity can sometimes also be demonstrated. In a clinically compatible case, a rising antibody level or a single titer of more than 1:64 is good evidence of active infection. If treatment has eradicated the LGV infection, the CF titer falls. Serologic diagnosis of LGV can employ immunofluorescence, but the antibody is broadly reactive with many chlamydial antigens.

D. Frei Test: Intradermal injection of heat-inactivated egg-grown LGV (0.1 mL) is compared to control material prepared from noninfected yolk sac. The skin test is read in 48–72 hours. An inflammatory nodule more than 6 mm in diameter at the test (but not the control) site constitutes a positive reaction. This can occur with different chlamydiae that share the group antigen. Thus, the Frei test lacks diagnostic specificity, and no licensed Frei test antigens are available in the USA at present.

Immunity
Untreated infections tend to be chronic, with persistence of the agent for many years. Little is known about active immunity. The coexistence of latent infection, antibodies, and cell-mediated reactions is typical of many chlamydial infections.

Treatment
The sulfonamides amd tetracyclines have been used with good results, especially in the early stages. In some drug-treated persons there is a marked decline in complement-fixing antibodies, which may indicate that the infective agent has been eliminated from the body. Late stages require surgery.

Epidemiology
The disease is most often spread by sexual contact, but not exclusively so. The portal of entry may sometimes be the eye (conjunctivitis with an oculoglandular syndrome). The genital tracts and rectums of chronically infected (but at times asymptomatic) persons serve as reservoirs of infection.

Although the highest incidence of LGV has been reported from subtropical and tropical areas, the infection occurs all over the world.

Laboratory personnel exposed to aerosols of *C trachomatis* immunotypes L1–L3 can develop a chlamydial pneumonitis with mediastinal and hilar adenopathy. If the infection is recognized, treatment with tetracyclines or erythromycin is effective.

Control

The measures used for the control of other sexually transmitted diseases apply also to the control of LGV. Case-finding and early treatment and control of infected persons are essential.

OTHER AGENTS OF THE GROUP

Many mammals are subject to chlamydial infections, mainly with *C psittaci*. Common animal disease entities are pneumonitis, arthritis, enteritis, and abortion, but infection is often latent. Some of these agents may also be transmitted to humans and cause disease in them.

Chlamydiae have been isolated from Reiter's disease in humans, both from the involved joints and from the urethra. The causative role of these agents remains uncertain.

REFERENCES

Abrams AJ: Lymphogranuloma venereum. *JAMA* 1968;**205**:59.

Beem MO et al: Treatment of chlamydial pneumonia of infancy. *Pediatrics* 1979;**63**:198.

Bernstein DI et al: Mediastinal and supraclavicular lymphadenitis and pneumonitis due to *Chlamydia trachomatis*, serovars L₁ and L₂. *N Engl J Med* 1984;**311**:1543.

Bolan RK et al: Lymphogranuloma venerum and acute ulcerative proctitis. *Am J Med* 1982;**72**:703.

Bowie WR et al: Etiology of nongonococcal urethritis: Evidence for *Chlamydia trachomatis* and *Ureaplasma urealyticum*. *J Clin Invest* 1977;**59**:735.

Bowie WR et al: Tetracycline in nongonococcal urethritis. *Br J Vener Dis* 1980;**58**:332.

Caldwell HD, Hitchcock PJ: Monoclonal antibody against a genus-specific antigen of *Chlamydia:* Location of epitope on chlamydial lipopolysaccharide. *Infect Immun* 1984;**44**:306.

Caldwell HD, Kuo CC: Purification of a *Chlamydia trachomatis* antigen by immunoadsorption with monospecific antibody. *J Immunol* 1977;**118**:437.

Centers for Disease Control: Sexually transmitted diseases: Treatment guidelines 1982. *Rev Infect Dis* 1982;**4(Suppl)**:S729.

Clyde WA, Genny GE, Schachter J: *Cumitech 19: Laboratory Diagnosis of Chlamydial and Mycoplasmal Infections.* American Society for Microbiology, 1984.

Hanna L et al: Immune responses to chlamydial antigens in humans. *Med Microbiol Immunol* 1982;**171**:1.

Jawetz E: Chemotherapy of chlamydial infections. *Adv Pharmacol Chemother* 1969;**7**:253.

Komaroff AL et al: Serologic evidence of chlamydial and mycoplasmal pharyngitis in adults. *Science* 1983;**222**:927.

Mardh PA et al: *Chlamydia trachomatis* infection in patients with acute salpingitis. *N Engl J Med* 1977;**296**:1377.

Mordhorst CH et al: Childhood trachoma in a nonendemic area. *JAMA* 1978;**239**:1765.

Oriel JD, Ridgeway GL: Comparison of erythromycin and tetracycline in the treatment of cervical infection by *Chlamydia trachomatis*. *J Infect* 1980;**2**:259.

Paavonen J et al: Treatment of nongonococcal urethritis with trimethoprim-sulphadiazine. *Br J Vener Dis* 1980;**56**:101.

Podgore JK et al: Asymptomatic urethral infections due to *Chlamydia trachomatis* in male US military personnel. *J Infect Dis* 1982;**146**:828.

Quinn TC et al: *Chlamydia trachomatis* proctitis. *N Engl J Med* 1981;**305**:195.

Saikku P et al: An epidemic of mild pneumonia due to an unusual strain of *Chlamydia psittaci*. *J Infect Dis* 1985;**151**:832.

Schaad UB, Rossi E: Infantile chlamydial pneumonia: A review based on 115 cases. *Eur J Pediatr* 1982;**146**:530.

Schachter J, Grossman M: Chlamydial infections. *Annu Rev Med* 1981;**32**:45.

Schachter J, Grossman M, Azimi PH: Serology of *Chlamydia trachomatis* in infants. *J Infect Dis* 1982;**146**:530.

Schachter J et al: Infection with *Chlamydia trachomatis:* Involvement of multiple anatomic sites in neonates. *J Infect Dis* 1979;**139**:232.

Schaffner W et al: The clinical spectrum of endemic psittacosis. *Arch Intern Med* 1967;**119**:433.

Stamm WE et al: Causes of the acute urethral syndrome in women. *N Engl J Med* 1980;**303**:409.

Stamm WE et al: Effect of treatment regimens for *Neisseria gonorrheae* on simultaneous infection with *Chlamydia trachomatis*. *N Engl J Med* 1984;**310**:545.

Normal Microbial Flora of the Human Body

The term "normal microbial flora" refers to the population of microbial associates that inhabit the internal and external surfaces of healthy normal humans and animals. It is doubtful whether a normal viral flora exists in humans.

The skin and mucous membranes always harbor a variety of microorganisms that can be arranged into 2 groups: (1) The resident flora consists of relatively fixed types of microorganisms regularly found in a given area at a given age; if disturbed, it promptly reestablishes itself. (2) The transient flora consists of nonpathogenic or potentially pathogenic microorganisms that inhabit the skin or mucous membranes for hours, days, or weeks; it is derived from the environment, does not produce disease, and does not establish itself permanently on the surface. Members of the transient flora are generally of little significance so long as the normal resident flora remains intact. However, if the resident flora is disturbed, transient microorganisms may colonize, proliferate, and produce disease.

Organisms frequently encountered in specimens obtained from various areas of the human body—and considered normal flora—are listed in Table 32–5.

ROLE OF THE RESIDENT FLORA

The microorganisms that are constantly present on body surfaces are commensals. Their flourishing in a given area depends upon physiologic factors of temperature, moisture, and the presence of certain nutrients and inhibitory substances. Their presence is not essential to life, because "germ-free" animals can be reared in the complete absence of a normal microbial flora. Yet the resident flora of certain areas plays a definite role in maintaining health and normal function. Members of the resident flora in the intestinal tract synthesize vitamin K and aid in the absorption of nutrients. On mucous membranes and skin, the resident flora may prevent colonization by pathogens and possible disease through "bacterial interference." The mechanism of bacterial interference is not clear. It may involve competition for receptors or binding sites on host cells, competition for nutrients, mutual inhibition by metabolic or toxic products, mutual inhibition by antibiotic materials or bacteriocins, or other mechanisms. Suppression of the normal flora clearly creates a partial local void that tends to be filled by organisms from the environment or from other parts of the body. Such organisms behave as opportunists and may become pathogens.

On the other hand, members of the normal flora may themselves produce disease under certain circumstances. These organisms are adapted to the noninvasive mode of life defined by the limitations of the environment. If forcefully removed from the restrictions of that environment and introduced into the bloodstream or tissues, these organisms may become pathogenic. For example, streptococci of the viridans group are the commonest resident organisms of the upper respiratory tract. If large numbers of them are introduced into the bloodstream (eg, following tooth extraction or tonsillectomy), they may settle on deformed or prosthetic heart valves and produce infective endocarditis. Small numbers occur transiently in the bloodstream with minor trauma (eg, dental scaling or vigorous toothbrushing). *Bacteroides* are the commonest resident bacteria of the large intestine and are quite harmless in that location. If introduced into the free peritoneal cavity or into pelvic tissues along with other bacteria as a result of trauma, they cause suppuration and bacteremia. Spirochetes, fusobacteria (fusiform bacilli), and *Bacteroides melaninogenicus* are resident in every normal mouth. In the presence of tissue damage through trauma, nutritional deficiency, or infection, they proliferate vastly in the necrotic tissue, producing "fusospirochetal" disease. There are many other examples, but the important point is that microbes of the normal resident flora are harmless and may be beneficial in their normal location in the host and in the absence of coincident abnormalities. They may produce disease if introduced into foreign locations in large numbers and if predisposing factors are present. For these reasons, members of the resident flora found in disease may be called "opportunists."

NORMAL FLORA OF THE SKIN

Because of its constant exposure to and contact with the environment, the skin is particularly apt to contain transient microorganisms. Nevertheless, there is a constant and well-defined resident flora, modified in different anatomic areas by secretions, habitual wearing of clothing, or proximity to mucous membranes (mouth, nose, and perineal areas).

The predominant resident microorganisms of the skin are aerobic and anaerobic diphtheroid bacilli (eg, *Corynebacterium, Propionibacterium*); nonhemolytic aerobic and anaerobic staphylococci (*Staphylococcus epidermidis*, occasionally *Staphylococcus aureus, Peptococcus*); gram-positive, aerobic, sporeforming bacilli that are ubiquitous in air, water, and soil; alpha-hemolytic streptococci *(Streptococcus viridans)* and enterococci *(Streptococcus faecalis)*; and gram-negative coliform bacilli and *Acinetobacter*. Fungi and yeasts are often present in skin folds; acid-fast, nonpathogenic mycobacteria occur in areas rich in sebaceous secretions (genitalia, external ear).

Among the factors that may be important in eliminating nonresident microorganisms from the skin are the low pH, the fatty acids in sebaceous secretions, and the presence of lysozyme. Neither profuse sweating nor washing and bathing can eliminate or significantly modify the normal resident flora. The number of superficial microorganisms may be diminished by vigorous daily scrubbing with soap containing hexachlorophene or other disinfectants, but the flora is rapidly replenished from sebaceous and sweat glands even when contact with other skin areas or with the environment is completely excluded. Placement of an occlusive dressing on skin tends to result in a large increase in the total microbial population and may also produce qualitative alterations in the flora.

NORMAL FLORA OF THE MOUTH & UPPER RESPIRATORY TRACT

The mucous membranes of the mouth and pharynx are often sterile at birth but may be contaminated by passage through the birth canal. Within 4–12 hours after birth, viridans streptococci become established as the most prominent members of the resident flora and remain so for life. They probably originate in the respiratory tracts of the mother and attendants. Early in life, aerobic and anaerobic staphylococci, gram-negative diplococci (neisseriae, *Branhamella*), diphtheroids, and occasional lactobacilli are added. When teeth begin to erupt, the anaerobic spirochetes, *Bacteroides* (especially *B melaninogenicus*), *Fusobacterium* species, *Rothia* and *Capnocytophaga* species (see p 316), and some anaerobic vibrios and lactobacilli establish themselves. *Actinomyces* species are normally present in tonsillar tissue and on the gingivae in adults, and various protozoa may also be present. Yeasts (*Candida* species) occur in the mouth.

In the pharynx and trachea, a similar flora establishes itself, whereas few bacteria are found in normal bronchi. Small bronchi and alveoli are normally sterile. The predominant organisms in the upper respiratory tract, particularly the pharynx, are nonhemolytic and alpha-hemolytic streptococci and neisseriae. Staphylococci, diphtheroids, *Haemophilus*, pneumococci, *Mycoplasma*, and *Bacteroides* are also encountered.

The flora of the nose consists of prominent corynebacteria, staphylococci *(S aureus, S epidermidis)*, and streptococci.

The Role of the Normal Mouth Flora in Dental Caries

Caries is a disintegration of the teeth beginning at the surface and progressing inward. First the surface enamel, which is entirely noncellular, is demineralized. This has been attributed to the effect of acid products of bacterial fermentation. Subsequent decomposition of the dentin and cement involves bacterial digestion of the protein matrix.

An essential first step in caries production appears to be the formation of plaque on the hard, smooth enamel surface. The plaque consists mainly of gelatinous deposits of high-molecular-weight glucans in which acid-producing bacteria adhere to the enamel. The carbohydrate polymers (glucans) are produced mainly by streptococci (*Streptococcus mutans*, peptostreptococci), perhaps in association with actinomycetes. There appears to be a strong correlation between the presence of *S mutans* and caries on specific enamel areas. The essential second step in caries production appears to be the formation of large amounts of acid (pH < 5.0) from carbohydrates by streptococci and lactobacilli in the plaque. High concentrations of acid demineralize the adjoining enamel and initiate caries.

In experimental "germ-free" animals, cariogenic streptococci can induce the formation of plaque and of caries. Adherence to smooth surfaces requires both the synthesis of water-insoluble glucan polymers by glucosyltransferases and the participation of binding sites on the surface of microbial cells. (Perhaps carbohydrate polymers also aid the attachment of some streptococci to endocardial surfaces.) Other members of the oral microflora, eg, *Veillonella*, may complex with glucosyltransferase of *Streptococcus salivarius* in saliva and then synthesize water-insoluble carbohydrate polymers to adhere to tooth surfaces. Adherence may be initiated by salivary IgA antibody to *S mutans*. Certain diphtheroids and streptococci that produce levans can induce specific soft tissue damage and bone resorption typical of periodontal disease. Proteolytic organisms, including actinomycetes and bacilli, play a role in the microbial action on dentin that follows damage to the enamel. The development of caries also depends on genetic, hormonal, nutritional, and many other factors. Control of caries involves physical removal of plaque, limitation of sucrose intake, good nutrition with adequate protein intake, and reduction of acid production in the mouth by limitation of available carbohydrates and frequent cleansing. The application of fluoride to teeth or its ingestion in water results in enhancement of acid resistance of the enamel. Control of periodontal disease requires removal of calculus (calcified deposit) and good mouth hygiene.

Periodontal pockets in the gingiva are particularly rich sources of organisms that are rarely encountered elsewhere. While they may participate in periodontal disease and tissue destruction, attention is drawn to them when they are implanted elsewhere, eg, producing infective endocarditis or bacteremia in a granulopenic host. Examples are *Capnocytophaga* species and *Rothia dentocariosa.* *Capnocytophaga* are fusiform, gram-negative, gliding anaerobes; *Rothia* are pleomorphic, aerobic, gram-positive rods. Both probably participate in the complex microbial flora of periodontal disease with prominent bone destruction. In granulopenic immunodeficient patients, they can lead to serious opportunistic lesions in other organs.

NORMAL FLORA OF THE INTESTINAL TRACT

At birth the intestine is sterile, but organisms are soon introduced with food. In breast-fed children, the intestine contains large numbers of lactic acid streptococci and lactobacilli. These aerobic and anaerobic, gram-positive, nonmotile organisms (eg, *Bifidobacterium*) produce acid from carbohydrates and tolerate pH 5.0. In bottle-fed children, a more mixed flora exists in the bowel, and lactobacilli are less prominent. As food habits develop toward the adult pattern, the bowel flora changes. Diet has a marked influence on the relative composition of the intestinal and fecal flora. Bowels of newborns in intensive care nurseries tend to be colonized by abnormal organisms, eg, *Klebsiella, Citrobacter, Enterobacter.*

In the normal adult, the esophagus contains microorganisms arriving with saliva and food. The stomach's acidity keeps the number of microorganisms at a minimum (10^3–10^5/g of contents) unless obstruction at the pylorus favors the proliferation of gram-positive cocci and bacilli. The normal acid pH of the stomach markedly protects against infection with some enteric pathogens, eg, cholera. Administration of cimetidine in peptic ulcer leads to a great increase in microbial flora of the stomach, including many organisms usually prevalent in feces. As the pH of intestinal contents becomes alkaline, the resident flora gradually increases. In the adult duodenum, there are 10^3–10^6 bacteria per gram of contents; in the jejunum and ileum, 10^5–10^8 bacteria per gram; and in the cecum and transverse colon, 10^8–10^{10} bacteria per gram. In the upper intestine, lactobacilli and enterococci predominate, but in the lower ileum and cecum, the flora is fecal. In the sigmoid colon and rectum, there are about 10^{11} bacteria per gram of contents, constituting 10–30% of the fecal mass. In diarrhea, the bacterial content may diminish greatly, whereas in intestinal stasis the count rises.

In the normal adult colon, 96–99% of the resident bacterial flora consists of anaerobes: *Bacteroides,* especially *Bacteroides fragilis; Fusobacterium* species; anaerobic lactobacilli, eg, *Bifidobacterium;* clostridia (*Clostridium perfringens,* 10^3–10^5/g); and anaerobic streptococci (*Peptostreptococcus* species). Only 1–4% are aerobes (gram-negative coliform bacteria, enterococci, and small numbers of *Proteus, Pseu-*

domonas, lactobacilli, *Candida,* and other organisms). More than 100 distinct types of organisms occur regularly in normal fecal flora. Minor trauma (eg, sigmoidoscopy, barium enema) may induce transient bacteremia in about 10% of procedures.

Intestinal bacteria are important in synthesis of vitamin K, conversion of bile pigments and bile acids, absorption of nutrients and breakdown products, and antagonism to microbial pathogens. The intestinal flora produces ammonia and other breakdown products that are absorbed and can contribute to hepatic coma. Among aerobic coliform bacteria, only a few serotypes persist in the colon for prolonged periods, and most serotypes of *Escherichia coli* are present only over a period of a few days.

Antimicrobial drugs taken orally can, in humans, temporarily suppress the drug-susceptible components of the fecal flora. This is commonly done by the preoperative oral administration of insoluble drugs. For example, neomycin plus erythromycin can in 1–2 days suppress part of the bowel flora, especially aerobes. Metronidazole accomplishes that for anaerobes. When surgery on the lower bowel is performed when the counts are at their lowest, some protection against infection by accidental spill can be achieved. However, soon thereafter the counts of fecal flora rise again to normal or higher than normal levels, principally of organisms selected out because of relative resistance to the drugs employed. The drug-susceptible microorganisms are replaced by drug-resistant ones, particularly staphylococci, *Enterobacter,* enterococci, *Proteus, Pseudomonas, Clostridium difficile,* and yeasts.

The feeding of large quantities of *Lactobacillus acidophilus* may result in the temporary establishment of this organism in the gut and the concomitant partial suppression of other gut microflora.

Growth of young chickens, turkeys, and pigs is greatly accelerated by admixture of antibiotics to the feed. The nature of this phenomenon is not clear; it probably does not occur in humans or ruminants. Antibiotic-fed animals have a predominantly drug-resistant intestinal flora, which may be transmitted to human contacts. Such animals are also a source of drug-resistant salmonellae and other enteric pathogens that can be transmitted to humans.

NORMAL FLORA OF THE URETHRA

The anterior urethra of both sexes contains small numbers of the same types of organisms found on the skin and perineum. These organisms regularly appear in normal voided urine in numbers of 10^2–10^4/mL.

NORMAL FLORA OF THE VAGINA

Soon after birth, aerobic lactobacilli (Döderlein's bacilli) appear in the vagina and persist as long as the pH remains acid (several weeks). When the pH becomes neutral (remaining so until puberty), a mixed flora of cocci and bacilli is present. At puberty, aerobic and anaerobic lactobacilli reappear in large numbers and contribute to the maintenance of acid pH through the production of acid from carbohydrates, particularly glycogen. This appears to be an important mechanism in preventing the establishment of other, possibly harmful microorganisms in the vagina. If lactobacilli are suppressed by the administration of antimicrobial drugs, yeasts or various bacteria increase in numbers and cause irritation and inflammation. After the menopause, lactobacilli again diminish in numbers and a mixed flora returns. The normal vaginal flora often includes also group B hemolytic streptococci, anaerobic streptococci (peptostreptococci), *Bacteroides* species, clostridia, *Gardnerella (Haemophilus) vaginalis, Ureaplasma urealyticum,* and sometimes *Listeria* or *Mobiluncus* species (see p 278). The cervical mucus has antibacterial activity and contains lysozyme. In some women, the vaginal introitus contains a heavy flora resembling that of the perineum and perianal area. This may be a predisposing factor in recurrent urinary tract infections. Vaginal organisms present at time of delivery may infect the newborn (eg, group B streptococci).

NORMAL FLORA OF THE EYE (CONJUNCTIVA)

The predominant organisms of the conjunctiva are diphtheroids (*Corynebacterium xerosis*), neisseriae, and gram-negative bacilli resembling *Haemophilus* (Morax-Axenfeld bacillus, *Moraxella* species). Staphylococci and nonhemolytic streptococci are also frequently present. The conjunctival flora is normally held in check by the flow of tears, which contain antibacterial lysozyme.

REFERENCES

Aly R et al: Correlation of human in vivo and in vitro cutaneous antimicrobial factors. *J Infect Dis* 1975;**131**:579.

Barksdale L: Identifying *Rothia dentocariosa*. *Ann Intern Med* 1979;**91**:786.

Bartlett JB, Polk BF: Bacterial flora of the vagina. *Rev Infect Dis* 1984;**6**:S67.

Bentley DW et al: The microflora of the human ileum and colon. *J Lab Clin Med* 1972;**79**:421.

Drude RB Jr, Hines C Jr: The pathophysiology of intestinal bacterial overgrowth syndromes. *Arch Intern Med* 1980;**140**:1349.

Fainstein V et al: Patterns of oropharyngeal and fecal flora in patients with acute leukemia. *J Infect Dis* 1981;**144**:10.

Glickman I: Periodontal disease. *N Engl J Med* 1971;**284**:1071.

Goldmann DA et al: Bacterial colonization of neonates admitted to an intensive care environment. *J Pediatr* 1978;**93**:288.

Gorbach SL, Bartlett JG: Anaerobic infections. *N Engl J Med* 1974;**290**:1177.

Hess J et al: Penicillin prophylaxis in children with cardiac disease: Post-extraction bacteremia and penicillin-resistant strains of viridans streptococci. *J Infect Dis* 1983;**147**:133.

Leyden JJ et al: Age-related changes in the resident bacterial flora of the human face. *J Invest Dermatol* 1975;**65**:379.

Levy SB et al: Changes in intestinal flora of farm personnel after introduction of a tetracycline-supplemented feed on a farm. *N Engl J Med* 1976;**295**:583.

Mackowiak PA: The normal microbial flora. *N Engl J Med* 1982;**307**:83.

McCormack WM et al: Sexually transmitted conditions among women college students. *Am J Obstet Gynecol* 1981;**139**:130.

Parenti DM, Snydman DR: *Capnocytophaga* species: Infections in nonimmunocompromised and immunocompromised hosts. *J Infect Dis* 1985;**151**:140.

Roberts MC et al: Comparison of gram stain, DNA probe, and culture for the identification of species of *Mobiluncus* in female genital specimens. *J Infect Dis* 1985;**152**:74.

Scherp HW: Dental caries. *Science* 1971;**173**:1199.

Shooter RA et al: *E coli* serotypes in the faeces of healthy adults over a period of several months. *J Hyg* 1977;**78**:95.

Simon GL, Gorbach SL: Intestinal microflora. *Med Clin North Am* 1982;**66**:557.

Slade HD: Cell surface antigenic polymers of *Streptococcus mutans* and their role in adherence of the microorganisms in vitro. Page 411 in: *Microbiology 1977.* Schlessinger D (editor). American Society for Microbiology, 1977.

Thadepalli H et al: Anaerobic infections of the female genital tract. *Am J Obstet Gynecol* 1973;**117**:1034.

Wolinsky E: When is an infection disease? *Rev Infect Dis* 1981;**3**:1025.

31

Medical Mycology

Many fungi cause plant diseases, but only about 100 of the thousands of known species of yeasts and molds cause disease in humans or animals. Only the dermatophytes and *Candida* are commonly transmitted from one human to another.

For convenience, human mycotic infections may be grouped into superficial, subcutaneous, and deep (or systemic) mycoses. Superficial fungal infections of skin, hair, and nails may be chronic and resistant to treatment but rarely affect the general health of the patient. Deep mycoses, on the other hand, may produce systemic involvement and are sometimes fatal. The actinomycetes are not fungi but filamentous branching bacteria. However, since they produce disease pictures resembling fungal infections, they are discussed in this section.

The deep mycoses are caused by organisms that live free in nature in soil or on decaying organic material and are frequently limited to certain geographic areas. In such areas, many people acquire the fungal infection. A majority develop only minor symptoms or none at all, and only a small minority of infections progress to full-blown serious or fatal disease. The host's cell-mediated immune reactions are of paramount importance in determining the outcome of such infections.

Pathogenic fungi generally produce no toxins. In the host, they regularly induce hypersensitivity to their chemical constituents. In systemic mycoses, the typical tissue reaction is a chronic granuloma with varying degrees of necrosis and abscess formation.

The general morphology of fungi has been described in Chapter 1. Some typical structures of pathogenic fungi are mentioned below; others are given with the descriptions of specific disease entities.

STRUCTURES OF FUNGI

When grown on suitable media, many fungi produce long, branching filaments. These fungi are commonly called **molds.** Each filament is called a **hypha**. Hyphae may become divided into a chain of cells by the formation of transverse walls, or septa. These are called septate hyphae. As the hyphae continue to grow and branch, a mat of growth called a **mycelium** develops. The part of the growth that projects above the surface of the substrate is called an **aerial** mycelium; the part that penetrates the substrate and absorbs food is known as the **vegetative** mycelium.

Most fungi reproduce by forming spores through mitosis, during which the chromosome number remains the same. Fungi with only asexual spore formation (or no spore formation) are called **fungi imperfecti.** In the past, most fungi pathogenic for humans were known only in the imperfect (asexual) state. In recent decades, however, the sexual forms of many fungi were discovered and were given new names. Microbiology laboratories and clinicians continue to use the older names (representing asexual replication), but at times the name of the sexual form will also be mentioned here. Fungi are called **dimorphic** if the tissue form and the free-living form differ markedly.

The following types of sexual spores occur in fungi of medical interest, as a result of mating:

(1) Zygospores: In certain zygomycetes, the tips of approximating hyphae fuse, meiosis occurs, and large, thick-walled zygospores develop.

(2) Ascospores: Usually 4–8 spores form within a specialized cell called an ascus, in which meiosis has taken place (Fig 31–1).

(3) Basidiospores: Following meiosis, 4 spores usually form on the surface of a specialized cell called a basidium.

Asexual Reproduction

Conidia are asexual propagules seen in most colonies of fungi of medical interest (Figs 31–1 through 31–3 and 31–5 through 31–9). When no sexual stage is known, classification is based on the morphologic development of conidia. They may form on specialized conidiophores, on the sides or ends of nonspecialized hyphae, or from a hyphal cell (see p 2). Specialized names have been given to each developmental form of conidia. When more than one kind of conidium is produced within a given colony, the small, single-celled conidia are called microconidia, and the large, often multicellular conidia are called macroconidia. The following "spores" represent 3 of the more common types of conidia.

A. Blastospores (Blastoconidia): A simple structure develops by budding, with subsequent separation of the bud from the parent cell (eg, in yeasts) (Fig 31–1).

B. Chlamydospores (Chlamydoconidia): Terminal or intercalary cells in a hypha enlarge and develop thick walls. These structures are resistant to unfavorable environmental conditions and germinate when conditions become more favorable for vegetative growth (Fig 31–2).

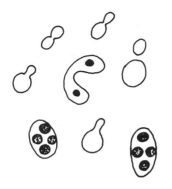

Figure 31–1. *Saccharomyces.* Budding blastospores. Conjugating blastospores. Ascus containing ascospores.

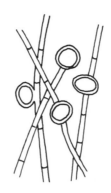

Figure 31–2. Terminal and intercalary chlamydospores.

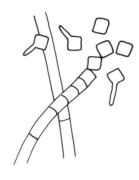

Figure 31–3. *Geotrichum.* Arthrospore formation. Germinating arthrospores.

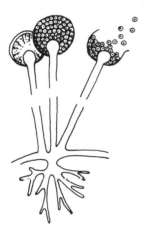

Figure 31–4. *Rhizopus.* Developing sporangiophores. Sporangiospores released. Rhizoid.

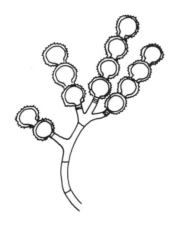

Figure 31–5. *Scopulariopsis.* Conidiophore shows spore scars. Terminal conidium is oldest.

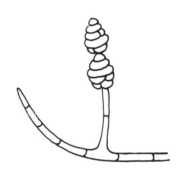

Figure 31–6. *Alternaria.* Black, multicellular conidia in chains. Terminal conidium is youngest.

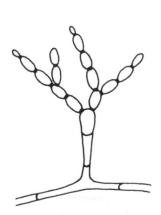

Figure 31–7. *Cladosporium.* Chains of conidia. Terminal conidium is youngest and has budded from subterminal conidium.

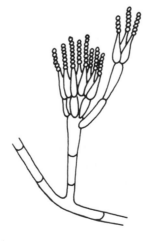

Figure 31–8. *Penicillium.* Conidia form within a phialide. Terminal conidium is oldest.

×1000

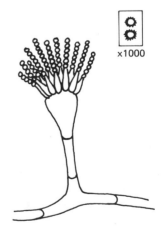

Figure 31–9. *Aspergillus fumigatus.* Phialides form on top of swollen vesicle. Terminal conidium is oldest. Mature conidia have rough walls.

C. Arthrospores (Arthroconidia): Structures result from a hypha fragmenting into individual cells (eg, in *Coccidioides*) (Fig 31–15).

SUPERFICIAL MYCOSES

The superficial mycoses are caused by fungi that invade only superficial keratinized tissue (skin, hair, and nails) but do not invade deeper tissues. The most important of these are the **dermatophytes,** a group of closely related fungi classified into 3 genera: *Epidermophyton, Microsporum,* and *Trichophyton.* In nonviable keratinized tissue, these form only hyphae and arthrospores. In culture, they develop characteristic colonies and conidia, by means of which they can be divided into species. Sexual spores of some species have been found. Some species are found only in soil and never produce infection. Other soil species may produce disease in humans. Others have evolved to complete parasitism, are communicable, and are not found in soil.

Most dermatophytes are worldwide in distribution, but some species show a higher incidence in certain regions than in others (eg, *Trichophyton schoenleinii* in the Mediterranean, *Trichophyton rubrum* in tropical climates). Many domestic and other animals have infections caused by dermatophytes and may transmit them to humans (eg, *Microsporum canis* from cats and dogs).

Morphology & Identification

Representative colonies form on Sabouraud's agar at room temperature. Conidia formation may be observed by means of slide cultures.

A. Trichophyton (Arthroderma): Microconidia are the predominant spore form. Smooth-walled, pencil-shaped macroconidia with blunt ends are rarer. Each species varies in colony morphology and pigmentation. Conidia formation may also vary according to the species under observation (Fig 31–10). The medium on which the fungi grow greatly influences these characteristics. The use of different nutritional media is sometimes needed in order to differentiate among the species.

In culture, colonies of *Trichophyton mentagrophytes* range from granular to powdery, and they usually display abundant grapelike clusters of subspherical microconidia on terminal branches. Some cottony strains develop only rare teardrop-shaped microconidia along the sides of the hyphae. Coiled hyphae are frequent. *T rubrum* usually has some teardrop-shaped microconidia along the sides of the hyphae; in some strains these may be abundant. Colonies often develop a red color on the reverse side. The larger microconidia of *Trichophyton tonsurans* are usually numerous and clavate and may be borne on short branches. Colonies are usually powdery.

B. Microsporum (Nannizzia): Macroconidia are the predominant conidial form (Fig. 31–11). They are large, rough-walled, multicellular, and spindle-shaped, and they form on the ends of hyphae. Microconidia are not used as a means of differentiating species. *Microsporum* species usually infect skin and hair but rarely the nails.

M canis forms numerous thick-walled, 8- to 15-celled macroconidia that frequently have curved or hooked spiny tips. A yellow-orange pigment usually develops on the reverse side of the colony. Infected hairs fluoresce a bright green under Wood's light. *Microsporum gypseum* has abundant thinner-walled, 4- to 6-celled macroconidia in buff to brownish-colored colonies. *Microsporum audouini* rarely forms conidia in the colony, but many thick-walled chlamydospores may be present. This fungus grows poorly on sterile rice grains, whereas other *Microsporum* species show rapid growth. Infected hairs fluoresce.

C. Epidermophyton floccosum: In this monotypic genus, only 1- to 5-celled, club-shaped macroconidia (Fig 31–11) are formed in the greenish-yellow

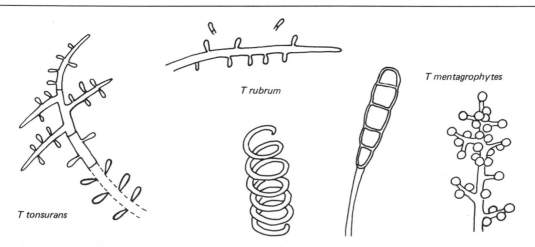

Figure 31–10. *Trichophyton* species. Microconidia and typical macroconidium.

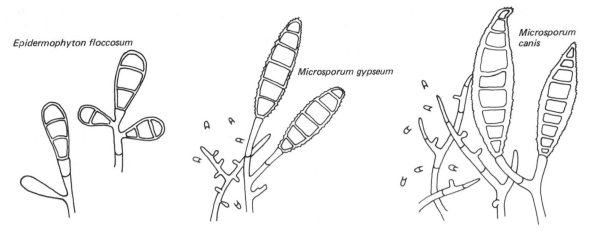

Epidermophyton floccosum

Microsporum gypseum

Microsporum canis

Figure 31–11. Macroconidia and microconidia.

colony, which mutates readily to form a sterile white overgrowth. This fungus invades skin and nails but never hair.

Antigenic Structure

Trichophytin, a crude extract from dermatophytes, produces a positive tuberculinlike response in most adults. A galactomannan peptide is the reactive component. The carbohydrate portion is related to an immediate response, whereas the peptide moiety is associated with the delayed response and is believed also to be associated with immunity. Patients without the delayed type reaction or with an immediate type reaction are more susceptible to chronic dermatophytosis. Resistance to infection, both partial and local, may be acquired after the primary infection. This resistance varies in duration and degree depending on the host, site, and species of fungus causing the infection.

Clinical Findings
(Table 31–1.)

A. Tinea Pedis (Athlete's Foot): This is the most prevalent of all dermatophytoses. The toe webs are infected with a *Trichophyton* species or with *E floccosum*. Initially there is itching between the toes and the development of small vesicles that rupture and discharge a thin fluid. The skin of the toe webs becomes macerated and peels, whereupon cracks appear that are prone to secondary bacterial infection. When secondary infection does occur, lymphangitis and lymphadenitis develop. When the fungal infection becomes chronic, peeling and cracking of the skin are the principal manifestations. Nail infection (**tinea unguium, onychomycosis**) follows prolonged tinea pedis. Nails become yellow, brittle, thickened, or crumbling.

In the course of dermatophytosis, the individual

Table 31–1. Some clinical features of dermatophyte infection.

Skin Disease	Location of Lesions	Clinical Appearance	Fungi Most Frequently Responsible
Tinea corporis (ringworm)	Nonhairy, smooth skin.	Circular patches with advancing red, vesiculated border and central scaling. Pruritic.	*Microsporum canis, Trichophyton mentagrophytes*
Tinea pedis* (athlete's foot)	Interdigital spaces on feet of persons wearing shoes.	Acute: itching, red vesicular. Chronic: itching, scaling, fissures.	*T rubrum, T mentagrophytes, Epidermophyton floccosum*
Tinea cruris (jock itch)	Groin.	Erythematous scaling lesion in intertriginous area. Pruritic.	*T rubrum, T mentagrophytes, E floccosum*
Tinea capitis	Scalp hair. Endothrix: fungus inside hair shaft. Ectothrix: fungus on surface of hair.	Circular bald patches with short hair stubs or broken hair within hair follicles. Kerion rare. *Microsporum*-infected hairs fluoresce.	*M canis, T tonsurans*
Tinea barbae	Beard hair.	Edematous, erythematous lesion.	*T rubrum, T mentagrophytes*
Tinea unguium (onychomycosis)	Nail.	Nails thickened or crumbling distally; discolored; lusterless. Usually associated with tinea pedis.	*T rubrum, T mentagrophytes, E floccosum*
Dermatophytid (id reaction)	Usually sides and flexor aspects of fingers. Palm. Any site on body.	Pruritic vesicular to bullous lesions. Most commonly associated with tinea pedis.	No fungi present in lesion. May become secondarily infected with bacteria.

*May be associated with lesions of hands and nails (onychomycosis).

may become hypersensitive to constituents or products of the fungus and may develop allergic manifestations, called dermatophytids (usually vesicles), elsewhere on the body (most often on the hands). The trichophytin skin test is markedly positive in such persons.

B. Tinea Corporis, Tinea Cruris (Ringworm): This is a dermatophytosis of the nonhairy skin of the body that gives rise commonly to the annular lesions of ringworm, with a clearing, scaly center surrounded by a red advancing border that often contains vesicles.

Dermatophytes grow only within dead, keratinized tissue. Fungal metabolic products diffuse through the malpighian layer to cause erythema, vesicle formation, and pruritus. The role of antibody activity is not understood at present. As hyphae age and break up into arthrospores, the cells containing them are shed. This partly accounts for the central clearing of the "ringworm" lesion. Active hyphal growth is into the peripheral "ring" of uninfected stratum corneum. Continuing growth downward into the newly forming stratum corneum of the thicker plantar and palmar surfaces accounts for the persistent infections at those sites.

C. Tinea Capitis (Ringworm of the Scalp): *Microsporum* infection occurs in childhood and usually heals spontaneously by puberty. Untreated *Trichophyton* infections may persist into adulthood. Infection begins on the skin of the scalp, with subsequent growth of the dermatophyte down the keratinized wall of the hair follicle. Infection of the hair takes place just above the hair root. The fungus continues to grow downward on the upward-growing hair shaft. *Microsporum* species grow primarily as a sheath around the hair (ectothrix), whereas *Trichophyton* species vary in their growth patterns. Some invade the hair shaft (endothrix), making it so fragile that it breaks off within or at the surface of the hair follicle (black-dot ringworm). In infections with other species, the hair breaks a short distance above the scalp, leaving short stubs in a balding, usually circular patch. Redness, edema, scaling, and vesicle formation may be seen. In some patients, a pronounced inflammation called **kerion** may occur around the area of infection and may even resemble pyogenic infection. *T schoenleinii* forms cuplike crusts (scutula) around infected follicles.

Infection with *Trichophyton* species may involve the bearded region of humans (tinea barbae); the highly inflammatory reaction they cause closely resembles pyogenic infections of that area. Rarely, dermatophytes not only colonize a human but produce systemic manifestations of infection. This occurs only in immunocompromised persons.

Diagnostic Laboratory Tests

A. Specimens: Specimens consist of scrapings of both skin and nails, and hairs plucked from involved areas. *Microsporum*-infected hairs fluoresce under Wood's light in a darkened room.

B. Microscopic Examination: Specimens are placed on a slide in a drop of 10–20% potassium hydroxide, covered with a coverslip, and examined immediately and then again after 20 minutes. In skin or nails, branching hyphae or chains of arthrospores are seen (Fig 31–12). In hairs, *Microsporum* species form dense sheaths of spores in a mosaic pattern around the hair; *Trichophyton* species form parallel rows of spores outside (ectothrix) or inside (endothrix) the hair shaft.

C. Culture: All final identification of dermatophytes rests on cultures. Specimens are inoculated onto Sabouraud's agar slants, incubated for 1–3 weeks at room temperature, and further examined in slide cultures if necessary.

Treatment

Therapy consists of thorough removal of infected and dead epithelial structures and application of a topical antifungal chemical. Overtreatment often causes dermatophytids. Attempts must be made to prevent reinfection. In widespread involvement, oral administration of griseofulvin (see Chapter 10) for 1–4 weeks has been effective. Nail infections require months of griseofulvin treatment and sometimes surgical removal of the nail.

A. Scalp Infections: In scalp infections, hairs can be plucked manually, clipped, or otherwise epilated. Griseofulvin, 0.125–0.5 g/d orally, may be given for 1–2 weeks. Frequent shampoos and miconazole cream, 2%, or other antifungal agents may be effective if used for weeks.

B. Body Infections: Use miconazole cream, 2%; undecylenic acid cream, 5%; salicylic acid, 3%; or benzoic acid, 5%. In tinea versicolor, selenium sulfide is also effective.

C. Foot Infections:

1. Acute phase—Soak in potassium permanganate 1:5000 until the acute inflammation subsides; then apply antifungal chemicals as described above.

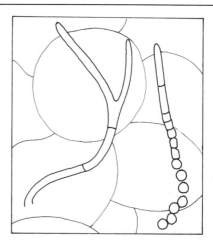

Figure 31–12. Dermatophyte in potassium hydroxide mount of skin or nail scraping. Branching hyphae. Arthrospore formation.

2. Chronic phase—Apply antifungal chemicals as creams at night (as powders during the day) as outlined above. Higher concentrations may be tolerated.

Epidemiology & Control

Infection arises from contact of uninfected skin or hair with infected skin scales or hair stubs. Hyphae then grow into the stratum corneum. Sporadic cases of ringworm infection are acquired from cats or dogs (*M canis*). Epidemics of tinea capitis have been traced to the use of shared barbershop clippers, transfer of infected hairs on seats, and person-to-person contact. Control depends on cleanliness, sterilization of instruments (using hot mineral oil), effective treatment of cases, and reduced contact with infectious materials.

Athlete's foot is found only in people who wear shoes. Infection spreads through the use of common showers and dressing rooms, where infected, desquamated skin serves as a source of infection. No really effective control measures (other than proper hygiene and the use of talc to keep interdigital spaces dry) are available. In many persons, chronic athlete's foot is asymptomatic and becomes activated only in excessive heat or moisture or with unsuitable footwear. Open-toed shoes or sandals are best for general wear.

OTHER SUPERFICIAL MYCOSES

Tinea Versicolor

Growth within the stratum corneum of clusters of spherical, thick-walled budding cells and short bent hyphae of *Malassezia furfur* usually causes no other pathologic signs than fine to brawny scales. Lesions appear principally on the chest, back, abdomen, neck, and upper arms. The lesions range from depigmented to brownish-red and are only of cosmetic importance.

Treatment consists of 1% selenium sulfide applied every other day for 15 minutes, then washed off.

Tinea Nigra

Light brown to blackish macular areas appear most commonly on the palmar or plantar stratum corneum. These are filled with brownish, branched, septate hyphae and budding cells of *Exophiala werneckii*. No scaling or other reaction develops.

Treatment consists of removing the infected stratum corneum mechanically or chemically.

Piedra

Hard black nodules are formed around the scalp hair by *Piedraia hortae*. Softer, white to light brown nodules caused by *Trichosporon cutaneum* form on axillary, pubic, beard, and scalp hair.

SUBCUTANEOUS MYCOSES

The fungi causing the subcutaneous mycoses grow in soil or on decaying vegetation. They must be introduced into the subcutaneous tissue in order to produce disease. In general, lesions spread slowly from the area of implantation. Extension via lymphatics draining the lesion is slow except for sporotrichosis. Each of these fungi has developed a unique morphologic form as a pathogen, except for *Basidiobolus haptosporus* and *Entomophthora coronata*, zygomycetes that grow as branching hyphae within subcutaneous lesions.

1. *SPOROTHRIX SCHENCKII*

Sporothrix schenckii is a fungus that lives on plants or wood and causes sporotrichosis, a chronic granulomatous infection, when traumatically introduced into the skin. There is often a characteristic spread along lymphatics draining the area. The fungus is dimorphic.

Morphology & Identification

The organisms are only rarely seen in pus and tissues from human infections; they may appear as small, round to cigar-shaped, gram-positive budding cells. In cultures at room temperature on Sabouraud's agar, cream-colored to black, folded, leathery colonies develop within 3–5 days. (Pigment formation of different strains of *S schenckii* is variable.) Simple, ovoid conidia are borne in clusters at the tip of long, slender conidiophores (resembling a daisy; see Fig 31–13) as well as along the sides of the thin hyphae. Culture at 37 °C produces spherical to ovoid budding cells.

Antigenic Structure

Heat-killed saline suspensions of cultures (or carbohydrate fractions from them) give positive delayed skin tests in infected humans or animals. A variety of antibodies are found in infected patients and sometimes also in normal individuals.

Pathogenesis & Clinical Findings

The fungus is introduced into the skin of the ex-

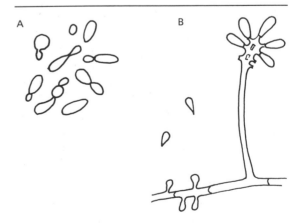

Figure 31–13. *Sporothrix schenckii.* **A:** Blastospores seen in tissue or 37 °C culture. **B:** Conidia formation in 20 °C culture.

tremities through trauma. A local lesion develops as a pustule, abscess, or ulcer, and the lymphatics leading from it become thickened and cordlike. Multiple subcutaneous nodules and abscesses occur along the lymphatics. Usually there is little systemic illness associated with these lesions, but dissemination of the infection—especially to joints—sometimes occurs, especially in debilitated patients. Rarely, primary infection in humans occurs through the lung. A variety of animals (rats, dogs, mules, and horses) are found naturally infected.

Histologically, the lesions show both chronic inflammation and granulomas that undergo necrosis.

Organisms in tissue can be identified by specific immunofluorescence. Around rare organisms, an eosinophilic antibody complex ("asteroid") may be seen in hematoxylin-eosin stains.

Diagnostic Laboratory Tests

A. Specimens: Specimens consist of pus or biopsy from lesions.

B. Microscopic Examination: In human lesions, organisms are seen infrequently, whereas budding cells are abundant in laboratory infections of mice.

C. Culture: On Sabouraud's agar, typical colonies with clusters of conidia are diagnostic. They should convert to yeast morphology during incubation at 37 °C.

D. Serology: Agglutination of yeast cell suspensions or of latex particles coated with antigen occurs in high titer with sera of infected patients but is not diagnostic.

Treatment

In a majority of cases, the infection is self-limited although chronic. Potassium iodide administered orally for weeks has some therapeutic benefit in the cutaneous-lymphatic form. In systemic involvement, amphotericin B is given intravenously. Oral ketoconazole may be beneficial.

Epidemiology & Control

S schenckii occurs worldwide in nature on plants (particularly sphagnum moss in the USA), thorns, and decaying wood; in soil; and on infected animals. Occupational exposure of gardeners, nursery workers, miners, and others in contact with plants and wood accounts for most cases. Prevention of trauma in these occupations is effective, since the organism must be passively introduced subcutaneously in order to cause disease.

2. CHROMOMYCOSIS

Chromomycosis is a slowly progressive granulomatous infection of skin caused by several species of black molds. *Phialophora verrucosa, Phialophora (Fonsecaea) pedrosoi,* and *Cladosporium carrionii* have been isolated most frequently.

Morphology & Identification

In exudates and tissues, these fungi produce dark-brown, thick-walled, rounded cells 5–15 μm in diameter that divide by septation. Septation in different planes with delayed separation may give rise to a cluster of 4–8 cells (Fig 31–14). Cells within superficial crusts of pus may germinate into brown, branching hyphae. Colonies vary in pigmentation from olive-gray to brown to black. The surface is generally velvety over a black, dense mat of mycelium.

A. *P verrucosa:* Conidia are primarily produced by vase-shaped phialides.

B. *P pedrosoi:* Most conidia form in short branching chains with the terminal cell budding to form a new conidium. Conidia may also form without chains directly on the top and sides of a conidiophore. Phialides are rare.

C. *C carrionii:* Only long, branching chains of conidia form on elongated conidiophores.

Pathogenesis & Clinical Findings

The fungi are introduced by trauma into the skin, often of the legs or feet. Slowly, over months or years, wartlike growths extend along the lymphatics of the affected area. Cauliflowerlike nodules with crusting abscesses eventually cover the area, and elephantiasis may result from secondary infection, obstruction, and fibrosis of lymph channels. Dissemination to other parts of the body is very rare.

Histologically, the lesions are granulomas; within leukocytes or giant cells, the dark-brown, round fungus cells may be seen.

Diagnostic Laboratory Tests

A. Specimens: Specimens consist of scrapings or biopsy from lesions.

B. Microscopic Examination: Scrapings are placed in 10% potassium hydroxide and examined microscopically for dark, round fungus cells. Tissue sections show granulomas and organisms.

C. Culture: Specimens should be cultured on Sabouraud's agar in order that the characteristic conidial structures and arrangement described above may be detected. Pathogenic species are distinguished

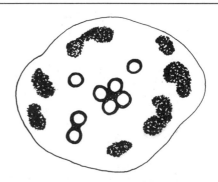

Figure 31–14. Chromomycosis. Pigmented fungal cells seen in giant cell.

from similar saprophytic black molds by the inability of the former to digest gelatin.

Treatment

Flucytosine, 150 mg/kg/d orally, or thiabendazole, 25 mg/kg/d orally, is occasionally effective. Locally applied heat over 40 °C is beneficial. Surgical removal of lesions and skin grafting may be required.

Epidemiology

Chromomycosis occurs mainly in the tropics. The fungi are saprophytic in nature, probably occurring on vegetation and in soil. The disease occurs chiefly on the legs of barefoot farm workers, presumably following traumatic introduction of the fungus. The disease is not communicable. Shoes and protection of legs probably would prevent infection.

3. MYCETOMA

Mycetoma is a localized, swollen lesion with granules that are compact colonies of the causative agent draining from sinuses. It is caused by a variety of fungi and actinomycetes (filamentous bacteria). Mycetoma develops when these soil organisms are implanted by trauma into subcutaneous tissue. The term maduromycosis is often used for those infections caused by fungi, but the clinical disease resembles actinomycotic mycetoma, although therapy is different. Mycetoma occurs worldwide but is primarily a disease occurring in people who do not wear shoes. It is particularly prevalent in tropical Africa.

Morphology & Identification

White, yellow, red, or black granules are extruded in pus. The granules due to fungi consist of intertwined, septate hyphae (3–5 μm), and depending on the species, they may have larger, thick-walled cells at the periphery . The actinomycete granule consists only of filamentous hyphae (1 μm in diameter). *Petriellidium (Allescheria) boydii* is among the more common fungal causes of mycetoma. The gray colony produces abundant ovoid conidia and occasionally ascospores within brown cleistotheca. *P boydii* may also cause opportunistic disease of the lungs and other organs in compromised hosts. Some other fungi causing mycetoma are *Madurella* species, *Phialophora* species, and *Acremonium* species. Each has its own characteristic colonial and microscopic morphology.

The most common causes of "actinomycotic" mycetoma are *Nocardia brasiliensis* and *Actinomadura madurae*. *N brasiliensis* may be acid-fast. These and other pathogenic actinomycetes are differentiated by biochemical tests and chromatographic analysis of cell wall components (see pp 334–336).

Pathogenesis & Clinical Findings

After one of the causative microorganisms has been introduced into the subcutaneous tissue (usually foot, hand, or back) by trauma, abscesses form that may extend through muscle and even into bone, eventually draining through chronic sinuses. The organism can be seen as a compact granule in the pus. Untreated lesions persist for years and extend deeper and peripherally, causing deformity and loss of function.

Histologically, the lesions resemble those of actinomycosis, with prominent abscess formation, granulation tissue, necrotic foci, and fibrosis. Within the abscess, the granule may be surrounded by an eosinophilic matrix of host material and immune complexes.

Very rarely, *P boydii* disseminates in an immunocompromised host or produces infection of a foreign body (eg, a cardiac pacemaker).

Diagnostic Laboratory Tests

Some granules have a characteristic morphology as well as color that aids in identification when cultures cannot be made. The diagnosis of mycetoma should never be made unless granules are seen.

Treatment

The actinomycotic mycetomas respond well to sulfonamides and sulfones if therapy is begun early before extensive deformity has occurred. Surgical drainage assists in healing. There is no established therapy for fungal mycetoma. Surgical excision of early lesions may prevent spread.

Epidemiology & Control

The organisms producing mycetoma occur in soil and on vegetation. Barefoot farm laborers are therefore most exposed. Properly cleaning wounds and wearing shoes are reasonable control measures.

SYSTEMIC MYCOSES

The systemic mycoses are caused by soil fungi. Infection is acquired by inhalation, and most infections are asymptomatic. In symptomatic disease, dissemination of infection may occur to any organ, although each fungus typically tends to attack certain organs. These fungi appear to cause disease in specific persons, in whom disseminated, often fatal infection may develop. The genetic features that predispose to disseminated disease are not clearly understood. All these fungi are dimorphic in that they have a unique morphologic adaptation to existence in tissue or to growth at 37 °C.

1. *COCCIDIOIDES IMMITIS*

Coccidioides immitis is a soil fungus that causes coccidioidomycosis. The infection is endemic in some arid regions of the southwestern USA and Latin America. Infection is usually self-limited; dissemination is rare but may be fatal.

Morphology & Identification

In histologic sections of tissue, in pus, or in sputum, *C immitis* appears as a spherule 15–60 μm in diameter, with a thick, doubly refractile wall (Fig 31–15). Endospores form within the spherule and fill it. Upon rupture of the wall, they are released into surrounding tissue, where they enlarge to form new spherules.

When grown on bacteriologic media or on Sabouraud's agar, a white to tan cottony colony develops. The aerial hyphae form alternating arthrospores (arthroconidia) and empty cells. Hyphae fragment easily and release the spores. The arthrospores are light, float in air, and are highly infectious. When they are inoculated into animals or inhaled by humans, these infectious spores develop into tissue spherules. Spherules can also be produced in the laboratory by cultivation of *C immitis* using specialized methods.

Antigenic Structure

Coccidioidin is a sterile filtrate from broth in which *C immitis* mycelium was grown. Spherulin is a sterile filtrate from broth in which spherules were grown. These materials give positive skin tests (in dilutions up to 1:10,000) in infected persons and serve as antigens in immunodiffusion (precipitin), latex agglutination, CF, and other tests. In low dilutions (1:10), these antigens cross-react with antigens of other fungi *(Histoplasma, Paracoccidioides)*. Some antisera give highly specific immunofluorescence tests with spherules in tissue.

Pathogenesis & Clinical Findings

Infection is acquired through the inhalation of airborne arthrospores. A respiratory infection follows that may be asymptomatic and may be evident only by the development of precipitating antibodies and a positive skin test in 2–3 weeks; on the other hand, an influenzalike illness, with fever, malaise, cough, and aches, may occur. About 5–10% of individuals in this latter category develop hypersensitivity reactions 1–2 weeks later in the form of erythema nodosum or erythema multiforme. This symptom complex is called "valley fever" or "desert rheumatism" and is self-limited. Some radiologic changes occur in the lungs in more than half of cases, occasionally taking the form of thin-walled cavities. The latter may heal or become chronic.

In fewer than 1% of persons who have been infected with *Coccidioides* does the disease progress to the disseminated, highly fatal form. This occurs much more frequently in some races (eg, Filipinos, blacks, or Mexicans) and also in pregnant women. The immunologic basis of racial susceptibility is not understood; general lowering of cell-mediated reactions may be responsible for enhanced susceptibility. In addition, the elevated levels of estradiol and progesterone in pregnancy can enhance the growth of *C immitis*. Spontaneous dissemination, if it occurs, usually develops within 1 year of initial infection, either by direct extension of a lesion or by hematogenous spread; meningitis and bone lesions are common. Dissemination denotes some defect in the individual's ability to localize and control *C immitis* infection. Most persons can be considered immune to reinfection after their skin tests have become positive. However, if such individuals are immunosuppressed by drugs or disease, dissemination can occur many years after primary *Coccidioides* infection.

Disseminated coccidioidomycosis is comparable to tuberculosis, with lesions in many organs, bones, and the central nervous system. Histologically, these are typical granulomas with interspersed suppuration. The histologic diagnosis depends on the detection of typical spherules filled with endospores. The clinical course often includes remissions and exacerbations.

Diagnostic Laboratory Tests

A. Specimens: Specimens consist of sputum, pus, spinal fluid, biopsy specimens, and blood for serologic diagnosis.

B. Microscopic Examination: Materials should be examined fresh (after centrifuging, if necessary) for typical spherules.

C. Cultures: Cultures can be grown on blood agar at 37 °C and on Sabouraud's agar at 20 °C. *Use extreme caution—arthrospores from cultures are highly infectious.*

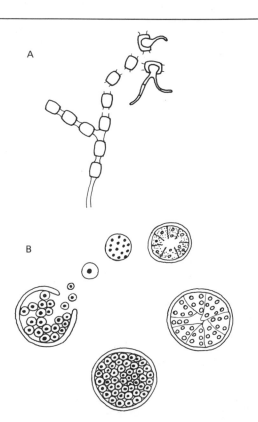

Figure 31–15. *Coccidioides immitis. A:* In soil. Arthrospore formation and germination. *B:* In tissue. Spherule formation with endospores.

D. Animal Inoculation: Mice injected intraperitoneally develop progressive lesions from which *Coccidioides* can be grown.

E. Serology: IgM and IgG precipitating antibodies to coccidioidin develop within 2–4 weeks after infection and can be detected readily by immunodiffusion and latex agglutination tests. These titers decline within a few months. CF antibodies rise at about the same time and persist in lower titer for 6–8 months but are sometimes undetectable in self-limited infection. By contrast, if dissemination occurs the CF antibody titer continues to rise. Such high CF titers are a poor prognostic sign. Their fall during treatment suggests improvement. In coccidioidal meningitis, the CF antibody titer may be high in cerebrospinal fluid and low in serum.

Patients with active disease or recent infection usually have high levels of IgE and circulating immune complexes. However, IgE levels do not permit differentiation of active pulmonary coccidioidomycosis from general dissemination.

F. Skin Test: (See Antigenic Structure, above.) The coccidioidin skin test reaches maximum induration (more than 5 mm in diameter) between 24 and 48 hours after injection of 0.1 mL of 1:100 dilution. It is often negative in disseminated disease. Cross-reactions with other fungi occur at a dilution of 1:10. Spherulin is more sensitive and as specific as coccidioidin in detecting reactors. Reactions to skin tests tend to diminish in size and intensity some years after primary infection in residents of endemic areas, but skin testing exerts a "booster" effect (see p 288).

Immunity

Following recovery from primary infection with *C immitis*, there usually is immunity to reinfection.

Treatment

In most persons, primary infection is self-limited and requires only supportive treatment. In disseminated coccidioidomycosis, intravenous amphotericin B, 0.4–0.8 mg/kg/d—or double the dose 3 times weekly—continued for months, may result in remissions. Systemic miconazole and ketoconazole have been moderately effective in treatment of chronic pulmonary coccidioidomycosis but have had very limited effect on disseminated disease. In meningeal involvement, oral doses of ketoconazole, 800 mg/d, combined with intravenous administration of amphotericin B have given some encouraging results. In coccidioidal meningitis, amphotericin B is also given intrathecally, but the long-term results are often poor.

Epidemiology & Control

The endemic area of *C immitis* in the USA includes the arid regions ("lower sonoran life zone") of the southwestern states, particularly the San Joaquin and Sacramento valleys of California, areas around Tucson and Phoenix in Arizona, and west Texas. *C immitis* also occurs in some arid areas of Central and South America. In these areas, the fungus is found in the soil and in rodents, and many humans have been infected, as shown by positive skin tests. The infection rate is highest during the dry months of summer and autumn, when dust is most prevalent. The dust storms in the winter of 1977, following a severe drought in the western USA, were followed by primary infections in previously *Coccidioides*-free areas near San Francisco.

The disease is not communicable from person to person, and there is no evidence that infected rodents contribute to its spread. A certain amount of control can be achieved by reducing dust, paving roads and airfields, planting grass or crops, and using oil sprays. Experimental vaccines are being tested.

2. HISTOPLASMA CAPSULATUM

Histoplasma capsulatum is a dimorphic soil fungus occurring in many parts of the world. It causes histoplasmosis, an intracellular mycosis of the reticuloendothelial system. The ascomycetous, sexual stage of the fungus is called *Emmonsiella capsulata*.

Morphology & Identification

H capsulatum forms oval, uninucleate budding cells measuring 2–4 μm in phagocytic cells and on glucose-cysteine blood agar slants or in tissue culture incubated at 37 °C (Fig 31–16). The bud arises at the smaller end of the yeast on a narrow bud base. On Sabouraud's agar incubated at room temperature, white to tan, cottony colonies develop, with either large (8–14 μm), thick-walled, spherical conidia that usually have fingerlike projections (tuberculate conidia) or small (2–4 μm) microconidia, or both (Fig 31–17).

Antigenic Structure

After initial infection with *Histoplasma*, persons have positive responses to skin tests with histoplasmin, a filtrate of broth in which *H capsulatum* has been grown. The reaction is delayed and tuberculinlike. Polysaccharides with precipitating and CF activity can be isolated from the yeast phase or mycelium. Cross-reactions with blastomycin are significant.

Pathogenesis & Clinical Findings

Infection with *H capsulatum* occurs via the respiratory tract. Inhaled conidia are engulfed by alveolar macrophages and eventually develop into budding

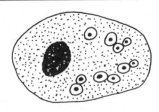

Figure 31–16. *Histoplasma capsulatum.* Macrophage containing blastospores.

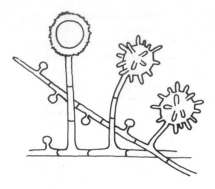

Figure 31–17. *Histoplasma capsulatum.* Macro- and microconidia in culture at 20 °C.

cells. Although organisms are soon spread throughout the body, most infections are asymptomatic. The small inflammatory or granulomatous foci in the lungs and spleen heal with calcification. With heavy respiratory exposure, clinical pneumonia may develop. Chronic cavitary histoplasmosis occurs most often in adult males. Severe, disseminated histoplasmosis develops in a small minority of infected individuals, particularly infants and aged or immunosuppressed individuals. The reticuloendothelial system is particularly involved, with lymphadenopathy, enlarged spleen and liver, high fever, anemia, and a high mortality rate. Ulcers of the nose, mouth, tongue, and intestine can occur. In such individuals, the histologic lesion shows focal areas of necrosis in small granulomas in many organs. Phagocytic cells (mononuclear or polymorphonuclear leukocytes of the blood, fixed reticuloendothelial cells of liver, spleen, and bone marrow) contain the small, oval yeast cells.

Many animals, including dogs and rodents, are spontaneously infected in endemic areas. Many laboratory animals can be infected with cultures.

Diagnostic Laboratory Tests

A. Specimens: Specimens consist of sputum, urine, scrapings from lesions, or buffy coat blood cells for culture; biopsies from bone marrow, skin, or lymph nodes for histology; and blood for serology.

B. Microscopic Examination: The small, ovoid cells may be detected intracellularly in histologic sections or in Giemsa-stained smears of bone marrow or blood. Specific immunofluorescence can identify *Histoplasma* cells in sections or smears.

C. Culture: Specimens are cultured at 37 °C on glucose-cysteine blood agar and on Sabouraud's agar at room temperature. Cultures must be kept for 3 weeks or more. Injection of organisms into mice may yield *Histoplasma* in lesions of spleen and liver upon culture.

D. Serology: Latex agglutination, precipitation, and immunodiffusion tests become positive within 2–5 weeks after infection. CF titers rise later in the disease; they fall to very low levels if the disease is inactive. With progressive disease, the CF test remains positive in high titer (1:32 or more). CF antibody cross-reacts with other fungal antigens. In immunodiffusion tests, 2 precipitin bands can be diagnostic: one (H) often connotes active histoplasmosis; the other (M) may arise from repeated skin testing or past contact.

E. Skin Test: The histoplasmin skin test (1:100) becomes positive soon after infection and remains positive for years. It may be negative in disseminated progressive disease. Repeated skin testing stimulates serum antibodies and thus interferes with diagnosis.

Immunity

Following initial infection with *Histoplasma*, most persons appear to develop some degree of immunity. Immunosuppression may lead to dissemination.

Treatment

Supportive therapy and rest enable most persons with symptomatic primary pulmonary histoplasmosis to recover. In disseminated disease, systemic treatment with amphotericin B, 0.6 mg/kg/d, has arrested and, at times, cured the disease, and ketoconazole has shown some limited benefits.

Epidemiology & Control

Histoplasmosis occurs in many parts of the world. In the USA, areas endemic for *H capsulatum* include the central and eastern states. The fungus has been recovered from the soil where human or animal outbreaks of infection have occurred. *Histoplasma* grows abundantly in soil mixed with bird feces (eg, chicken houses) or bat guano (caves). Exposure in such places may result in massive infection (eg, cave disease). Birds themselves are not affected.

In endemic areas, small infective inocula are spread by dust. A large proportion of inhabitants apparently become infected early in life but without symptoms. They develop positive histoplasmin skin tests and occasionally have miliary calcifications in the lungs. In the USA, midwestern cities have experienced large urban outbreaks of histoplasmosis following windstorms carrying dust. Clinical histoplasmosis infection in such outbreaks occurred somewhat more frequently in black than in white residents. The disease is not communicable from person to person. Spraying of formaldehyde on infected soil may destroy *Histoplasma*.

3. BLASTOMYCES DERMATITIDIS

Blastomyces dermatitidis is a dimorphic fungus that grows in mammalian tissues as a budding cell and in culture at 20 °C as a mold (Fig 31–18). It causes blastomycosis, a chronic granulomatous disease. Until recently it was recognized only in Canada, the USA, and Mexico and was referred to as "North American blastomycosis." However, it also occurs in Central America and Africa.

The ascomycetous sexual stage is called *Ajellomyces dermatitidis*.

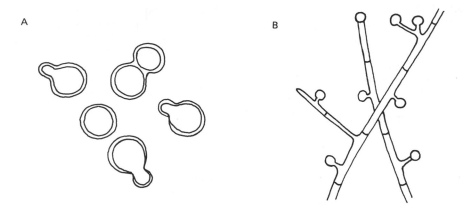

Figure 31–18. *Blastomyces dermatitidis.* ***A:*** In tissue or culture at 37 °C. ***B:*** In culture at 20 °C on Sabouraud's agar.

Morphology & Identification

In tissue, pus, or exudates, *B dermatitidis* appears as a round, multinucleate, budding cell (8–15 μm) with a doubly refractile wall. Each cell usually has only *one* bud with a broad base. Colonies on blood agar at 37 °C are wrinkled, waxy, and soft, and the cells are morphologically similar to the tissue stage, although short hyphal segments may also be present. When grown on Sabouraud's agar at room temperature, a white or brownish colony develops, with branching hyphae bearing round or ovoid conidia 2–10 μm in diameter on slender terminal or lateral conidiophores.

Antigenic Structure

Extracts of culture filtrates of *Blastomyces* contain blastomycin, probably a mixture of antigens. Blastomycin as a skin test gives positive delayed reactions in some patients but lacks specificity. Cross-reactions with histoplasmin are common. In CF tests, blastomycin is an unreliable antigen, giving cross-reactions with other fungal infections but also reacting to high titer in persons with widespread blastomycosis. Specific animal sera permit the demonstration of budding *Blastomyces* cells in tissues by means of immunofluorescence.

Pathogenesis & Clinical Findings

Human infection probably occurs most commonly via the respiratory tract. Mild and self-limited cases are recognized infrequently. When dissemination occurs, skin lesions on exposed surfaces are most common. They may evolve into ulcerated verrucous granulomas with an advancing border and central scarring. The border is filled with microabscesses and has a sharp, sloping edge. Lesions of bone, prostate, epididymis, and testis occur; other sites are less frequently involved.

Diagnostic Laboratory Tests

A. Specimens: Specimens consist of sputum, pus, exudates, urine, and biopsies from lesions.

B. Microscopic Examination: Wet mounts of specimens may show broadly attached buds on thick-walled cells. These may also be apparent in histologic sections and are most helpful in diagnosis.

C. Culture: Initial growth is best on Sabouraud's or enriched blood agar at 30 °C; cellular morphology is most typical at 37 °C.

D. Animal Inoculation: Massive doses of blastospore cultures injected intravenously or intraperitoneally into mice, guinea pigs, or rabbits are fatal in 5–20 days.

E. Serology: Blastospore antigens may give positive results in CF and immunodiffusion tests. A titer rise in successive sera may have diagnostic significance, but cross-reactions with other fungal antigens are common. Results of serologic tests contribute little to diagnosis.

Treatment

Although some benefit has been derived in disseminated cases from treatment with aromatic diamidines (eg, dihydroxystilbamidine), ketoconazole in doses of 400 mg/d or amphotericin B in doses up to 50 mg/d is the current drug of choice. Adjuvant surgical management of lesions is helpful. Relapses are not rare.

Epidemiology

Blastomycosis is a relatively common finding in dogs and some other animals in endemic areas. It is not communicable from animals or humans. It is assumed that both animals and humans are infected by inhaling conidia from *Blastomyces* growing in soil. Direct isolation from soil has been occasionally successful, especially from beaver dams with organically rich soil.

4. PARACOCCIDIOIDES BRASILIENSIS (Blastomyces brasiliensis)

Paracoccidioides brasiliensis is a dimorphic fungus that causes paracoccidioidomycosis, the predominant systemic mycosis in Latin America.

Morphology & Identification

P brasiliensis resembles *B dermatitidis*. The principal difference is that in tissue and in culture at 37 °C, *P brasiliensis* forms thick-walled yeast cells (10–60 μm in tissue) that characteristically have *multiple* buds (Fig 31–19). At room temperature, cultures are mycelial, with small conidia.

Pathogenesis & Clinical Findings

The infective organism is inhaled, and early lesions occur in the lung. Dissemination occurs later, primarily to the spleen, liver, mucous membranes, and skin. Asymptomatic lung infections may be followed by dissemination, with frequent and severe oral mucous membrane lesions. Lymph node enlargement or gastrointestinal disturbances may be the presenting symptom. Histologically, there is either a granuloma with central caseation or microabscess formation. Organisms are frequently seen in giant cells or in pus and are always characterized by their multiple budding.

Skin tests can be performed using "paracoccidioidin," a sterile filtrate of old broth cultures of the organism or extracts of the yeast phase. Some cross-reactions may occur with histoplasmin and blastomycin.

Diagnostic Laboratory Tests

In sputum, exudates, pus, or other material from lesions, the organism is often seen microscopically. Cultures on Sabouraud's or yeast extract agar are incubated at room temperature. Serology is most useful for diagnosis. Paracoccidioidin is used as an antigen in serologic tests. The sera of healthy persons living in endemic areas fail to react in CF or precipitin tests. A significant serum antibody titer denotes tissue involvement with the disease, and CF titers of 1:2048 or more occur in active disease. In immunodiffusion tests, 2 well-defined precipitin lines are said to be diagnostic of paracoccidioidomycosis. In such persons, the skin test is also positive, but it is not diagnostic.

Treatment

In paracoccidioidomycosis of mild or moderate severity, oral administration of sulfonamides may produce striking remissions. Ketoconazole is effective in the management of cases that fail to respond to sulfonamides and of more severe paracoccidioidomycosis. Amphotericin B is currently a drug of last resort only.

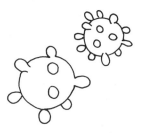

Figure 31–19. *Paracoccidioides brasiliensis.* In tissue or culture at 37 °C; multiple budding.

Epidemiology

Paracoccidioidomycosis occurs mainly in rural areas of Latin America, particularly among farmers. The disease manifestations are much more frequent in males than females, but infection occurs equally in both sexes. The fungus has been isolated from soil. The disease is not communicable.

OPPORTUNISTIC MYCOSES

Fungi that usually do not induce disease may do so in persons who have altered host defense mechanisms. Such opportunists may infect any or all organs of the body. The underlying predisposing condition may allow only certain opportunistic fungi or actinomycetes to infect the host. Often there are several organisms infecting a severely immunocompromised patient. *Candida* and other yeasts may be acquired from an endogenous source. Conidia of other fungi are commonly found in the air. Additional opportunists are *Fusarium, Penicillium, Geotrichum, Paecilomyces, Scopulariopsis,* and a number of black molds. Disease caused by known pathogenic fungi is often accelerated by impaired host defense mechanisms.

1. *CANDIDA* & RELATED YEASTS

Candida albicans is an oval, budding yeast that produces a pseudomycelium both in culture and in tissues and exudates. It is a member of the normal flora of the mucous membranes in the respiratory, gastrointestinal, and female genital tracts. In such locations, it may gain dominance and be associated with pathologic conditions. Sometimes it produces progressive systemic disease in debilitated or immunosuppressed patients, especially if cell-mediated immunity is impaired. *Candida* may produce bloodstream invasion, thrombophlebitis, endocarditis, or infection of the eyes and other organs when introduced intravenously (tubing, needles, hyperalimentation, narcotic abuse, etc).

Morphology & Identification

In smears of exudates, *Candida* appears as a gram-positive, oval, budding yeast, measuring 2–3 × 4–6 μm, and gram-positive, elongated budding cells resembling hyphae (pseudohyphae) (Fig 31–20). On Sabouraud's agar incubated at room temperature, soft, cream-colored colonies with a yeasty odor develop. The surface growth consists of oval budding cells. The submerged growth consists of pseudomycelium. This is composed of pseudohyphae that form blastospores at the nodes and sometimes chlamydospores terminally. *C albicans* ferments glucose and maltose, producing both acid and gas; produces acid from sucrose; and does not attack lactose. These carbohydrate fermentations, together with colonial and morphologic characteristics, differentiate *C albicans* from the other

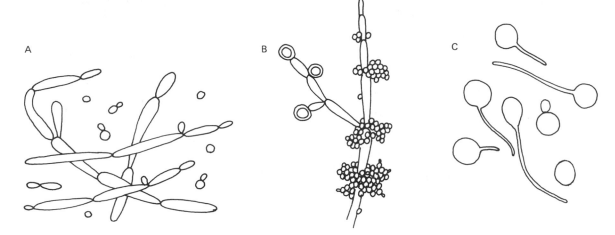

Figure 31–20. *Candida albicans. A:* Blastospores and pseudohyphae in exudate. *B:* Blastospores, pseudohyphae, and chlamydospores (conidia) in culture at 20° C. *C:* Young culture forms germ tubes when placed in serum for 3 hours at 37 °C.

species of *Candida (C krusei, C parapsilosis, C stellatoidea, C tropicalis, C pseudotropicalis, C guilliermondii,* and *C [Torulopsis] glabrata),* which live in soil, at times occur in normal human flora, and occasionally are implicated in human disease. Only the budding cells of 24-hour-old cultures of *C albicans* and *C stellatoidea*—not of other species—will form germ tubes in 2–3 hours when placed in serum at 37 °C.

Antigenic Structure

Agglutination tests with absorbed sera show that all *C albicans* strains fall into 2 groups: A and B. Group A appears to be antigenically identical with *C tropicalis;* group B, with *C stellatoidea. Candida* extracts for serologic and skin tests appear to consist of mixtures of antigens. They can be detected by precipitation, immunodiffusion, counterimmunoelectrophoresis, latex agglutination, and other tests. In disseminated candidiasis, there are often circulating mannan antigens of *Candida,* and sometimes precipitating antibodies to nonmannan antigens can be detected.

Pathogenesis & Pathology

Upon intravenous injection into mice or rabbits, dense suspensions of *C albicans* result in widespread abscesses, particularly in the kidney, and death in less than 1 week.

Histologically, the various skin lesions in humans show inflammatory changes. Some resemble abscess formation; others resemble chronic granuloma. Large numbers of *Candida* are sometimes found in the intestinal tract following administration of oral antibiotics, eg, tetracyclines, but this usually causes no symptoms. *Candida* may be carried by the bloodstream to many organs, including the meninges, but usually cannot establish itself and cause miliary abscess formation except in a grossly debilitated host. Dissemina-

tion and sepsis may occur in patients with compromised cellular immunity, eg, those undergoing cancer chemotherapy or those with lymphoma, AIDS (see Chapter 47), or other conditions. Temporary improvement can follow administration of transfer factor and other immunomodulators or chemotherapy.

Clinical Findings

Among the principal predisposing factors to *C albicans* infection are the following: diabetes mellitus, general debility, immunosuppression, indwelling urinary or intravenous catheters, intravenous narcotic abuse, administration of antimicrobials (which alter the normal bacterial flora), and corticosteroids.

A. Mouth: Infection of the mouth (thrush) occurs, mainly in infants, on the buccal mucous membranes and appears as white adherent patches consisting largely of pseudomycelium and desquamated epithelium, with only minimal erosion of the membrane. Growth of *Candida* in saliva is enhanced by glucose, antibiotics, and corticosteroids.

B. Female Genitalia: Vulvovaginitis resembles thrush but produces irritation, intense itching, and discharge. Loss of an acid pH in the vagina predisposes to candidal vulvovaginitis. Acid pH is normally maintained by the bacterial flora in the vagina. Diabetes, pregnancy, progesterone, and antibiotic therapy predispose to disease.

C. Skin: Infection of the skin occurs principally in moist, warm parts of the body, such as the axilla, intergluteal folds, groin, or inframammary folds; it is most common in obese and diabetic individuals. These areas become red and weeping and may develop vesicles.

Candida infection of the interdigital webs of the hands is seen most frequently following repeated prolonged immersion in water; it is most common in homemakers, cooks, vegetable and fish handlers, etc.

D. Nails: Painful, reddened swelling of the nail fold, resembling a pyogenic paronychia, may lead to thickening and transverse grooving of the nails and eventual loss of the nail.

E. Lungs and Other Organs: *Candida* infection may be a secondary invader of lungs, kidneys, and other organs where a preexisting disease is present (eg, tuberculosis or cancer). In uncontrolled leukemia and in immunosuppressed or surgical patients, candidal lesions may occur in many organs. *Candida* endocarditis (often due to *C parapsilosis)* occurs particularly in narcotic addicts or on prosthetic valves. Candiduria sometimes develops after urinary catheterization, but it tends to subside spontaneously.

F. Chronic Mucocutaneous Candidiasis: This disorder is a sign of deficiency of cellular immunity in children.

Diagnostic Laboratory Tests

A. Specimens: Specimens consist of swabs and scrapings from surface lesions, sputum, exudates, and material from removed intravenous catheters.

B. Microscopic Examination: Sputum, exudates, thrombi, etc, may be examined in Gram-stained smears for pseudohyphae and budding cells. Skin or nail scrapings are first placed in a drop of 10% potassium hydroxide.

C. Culture: All specimens are cultured on Sabouraud's agar at room temperature and at 37 °C; typical colonies are examined for cells and budding pseudomycelia. Chlamydospore (conidia) production by *C albicans* on corn meal agar or other conidia-enhancing media is an important differential test.

D. Serology: A carbohydrate extract of group A *Candida* gives positive precipitin reactions with sera of 50% of normal persons and 70% of persons with mucocutaneous candidiasis. In systemic candidiasis, a rise in the titer of antibodies to *Candida* may be detected by various tests. The interpretation of serologic test results remains controversial.

E. Skin Test: A *Candida* test is almost universally positive in normal adults. It is therefore used as an indicator of competent cellular immunity.

Immunity

Animals can be immunized actively and are then resistant to disseminated candidiasis. Human sera often contain IgG antibody that clumps *Candida* in vitro and may be candidacidal. The basis of resistance to candidiasis is complex and incompletely understood.

Treatment

Orally administered nystatin is not absorbed, remains in the gut, and has no effect on systemic *Candida* infections. Ketoconazole, 200–600 mg/d orally, has produced striking therapeutic response in some systemic *Candida* infections, especially in mucocutaneous candidiasis. Amphotericin B, 0.4–0.8 mg/kg/d injected intravenously, is an effective treatment of last resort. Amphotericin B is sometimes given in combi-

nation with flucytosine, 150 mg/kg/d orally, for enhanced effect in disseminated candidiasis.

Mucocutaneous candidiasis occurs mainly in immunodeficient children and occasionally responds to the administration of transfer factor obtained from persons with active cell-mediated reactions to *Candida*.

Local lesions are best treated by removing the cause, ie, avoiding moisture; keeping areas cool, powdered, and dry; and withdrawing antibiotics. There is no evidence to support vaccine therapy. Various chemicals have been employed topically with more or less success, eg, 1% gentian violet for thrush; and parahydroxybenzoic acid esters, sodium propionate, candicidin, or 2% miconazole for vaginitis. Nystatin suppresses intestinal and vaginal candidiasis.

Epidemiology & Control

The most important preventive measure is to avoid interfering with the normal balance of microbial flora and with normal host defenses. *Candida* infection is not communicable, since virtually all persons normally harbor the organism.

2. *CRYPTOCOCCUS NEOFORMANS*

Cryptococcus neoformans is a yeast characterized by a wide carbohydrate capsule both in culture and in tissue fluids. It occurs widely in nature and is found in very large numbers in dry pigeon feces. Human disease is usually opportunistic.

Morphology & Identification

In spinal fluid or tissue, the organism is round or ovoid, 4–12 μm in diameter, often budding, and surrounded by a wide capsule (Fig 31–21). On Sabouraud's agar at room temperature, the cream-colored colonies are shiny and mucoid. Cultures do not ferment carbohydrates but assimilate glucose, maltose, sucrose, and galactose (but not lactose). Urea is hydrolyzed. In contrast to nonpathogenic cryptococci, *C neoformans* grows well at 37 °C on most laboratory media provided they do not contain cycloheximide. Mating of serotypes A and D or B and C gives rise to mycelia and basidiospores of *Filobasidiella neoformans* or *Filobasidiella bacillispora*.

Antigenic Structure

Four serologic types of capsular polysaccharides—

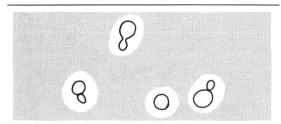

Figure 31–21. *Cryptococcus neoformans.* India ink preparation of spinal fluid.

A, B, C, and D—have been identified. The capsular antigen may be dissolved in spinal fluid, serum, or urine and can be detected with specific antisera to the carbohydrate by latex agglutination (particles coated with antibody) and other tests. The detection of cryptococcal capsular antigen is diagnostically reliable. Several serologic tests also can detect antipolysaccharide antibodies. The presence of these antibodies does not denote increased resistance to recurrence.

Pathogenesis

Infection in humans occurs via the respiratory tract and is either asymptomatic or associated with nonspecific pulmonary signs and symptoms. Very massive inhalation of cells may result in progressive systemic disease in a normal person. Usually, however, cryptococcosis is an opportunistic infection. In immunodeficient or immunosuppressed persons, the pulmonary infection may disseminate systemically and establish itself in the central nervous system and other organs.

Histologically, the reaction varies from mild inflammation to formation of typical granulomas.

Clinical Findings

Infection with *C neoformans* may remain subclinical. The commonest clinical manifestation is a slowly developing chronic meningitis with spontaneous remissions and exacerbations. The meningitis may resemble a brain tumor, brain abscess, degenerative central nervous system disease, or any mycobacterial or fungal meningitis. Cerebrospinal fluid pressure and protein content may be greatly increased and the cell count elevated, whereas the sugar content is normal or low. In addition, there may be lesions of skin, lungs, or other organs.

The course of cryptococcal meningitis may fluctuate over long periods, but ultimately all untreated cases are fatal. The disease is particularly common in immunocompromised persons, eg, AIDS patients. It is not communicable.

Diagnostic Laboratory Tests

A. Specimens: Specimens consist of spinal fluid, exudates, sputum, urine, and serum.

B. Microscopic Examination: Specimens are examined in wet mount, both directly and after mixing with India ink (which makes the large capsule stand out around the budding cell). Immunofluorescent stain is applied to dried smears. Filtration of cerebrospinal fluid through Millipore filters may reveal the organism.

C. Culture: Growth is rapid at 20–37 °C on Sabouraud's agar and other laboratory media provided they do not contain cycloheximide. Urea is hydrolyzed. *C neoformans* colonies produce brown pigment on media that contain substrate for phenol oxidase. Cultured cells should be injected into mice to determine their pathogenicity.

D. Serology: Tests for both antigen and antibody can be performed on cerebrospinal fluid and serum.

Latex slide agglutination or immunoelectrophoresis reveals antigen. Detection of antigen is diagnostically significant. With effective treatment, the antigen titer drops. Antibody agglutinates cryptococcal yeast cells or antigen-coated particles.

Treatment

Flucytosine, 150 mg/kg/d orally, is effective against many strains of *Cryptococcus,* but resistant mutants may emerge. Amphotericin B, 0.4–0.8 mg/kg/d intravenously, can also be effective but has many toxic side effects. The combination of the 2 drugs is given for meningitis for several months, often resulting in prolonged remission. Orally administered ketoconazole does not appear to be a drug of choice in cryptococcal meningitis.

Epidemiology & Control

Bird droppings containing *C neoformans* are the major source of infection for animals and humans. The organism grows luxuriantly in pigeon excreta, but the birds are not infected. One method of control is reduction of the pigeon population and site decontamination with alkali.

3. ASPERGILLOSIS

Broadly defined, aspergillosis is a group of mycoses with diverse causes and pathogenesis. *Aspergillus fumigatus* is a ubiquitous mold found on decaying vegetation. It may colonize and then invade tissues in the traumatized cornea, burns, wounds, or external ear (otitis externa). It and other *Aspergillus* species become opportunistic invaders in immunodeficient persons (eg, in patients with chronic granulomatous disease—but *not* in AIDS patients) or individuals with anatomic abnormalities of the respiratory tract (pulmonary aspergillosis). Various species of *Aspergillus* produce aflatoxins in foods.

In tissues, exudates, or sputum, *Aspergillus* species occur as filamentous, septate structures that usually branch dichotomously. Cultures on Sabouraud's agar incubated at 37–40 °C grow as gray-green colonies with a central dome of conidiophores. The latter support characteristic radiating chains of conidia (Fig 31–9). Extracts of cultures, particularly carbohydrates, are used as antigens in various serologic tests. Different forms of aspergillosis produce different serologic results, and rising antibody titers are of limited diagnostic help.

Pulmonary aspergillosis may occur in distinct forms. One is a "fungus ball" growing in a preexisting cavity (eg, tuberculous cavity, paranasal sinus, bronchiectasis) in which the *Aspergillus* does not invade tissue. Such patients usually require only treatment for the underlying disorder. They may give significant antibody responses to *Aspergillus* antigens.

A second form is an actively invasive granuloma with *Aspergillus* spreading in the lung, giving rise to necrotizing pneumonia, hemoptysis, and secondary dissemination to other organs. This occurs mainly in immunodeficient or immunosuppressed persons and requires active antifungal drug therapy with flucytosine and amphotericin B. A third form is allergic pulmonary aspergillosis, with asthma, eosinophilia, high serum IgE, and only minimal tissue invasion but abnormal bronchograms. *Aspergillus* antibodies may be demonstrable but have little diagnostic value. It has been claimed that the demonstration of galactomannan antigens in the circulating blood is evidence for invasive aspergillosis.

Diagnosis of aspergillosis rests most securely on demonstration of hyphal fragments in tissue biopsies by methenamine-silver stain. Treatment of invasive aspergillosis in immunosuppressed patients is only marginally successful. The same applies to the rare postsurgical *Aspergillus* endophthalmitis that usually leads to rapid loss of the infected eye.

Other fungi that may invade tissues in an immunoincompetent host and produce hyphae that resemble *Aspergillus* species include *Petriellidium, Fusarium,* and *Curvularia,* among others. These may produce disease states resembling the several forms of aspergillosis.

4. ZYGOMYCOSIS
(Mucormycosis, Phycomycosis)

Saprophytic zygomycetes (eg, *Mucor, Rhizopus*) are occasionally found in the tissues of compromised hosts. In persons suffering from diabetes mellitus (particularly with acidosis), extensive burns, leukemia, lymphoma, or other chronic illness or immunosuppression, *Rhizopus* species, *Mucor* species, and other zygomycetes invade and proliferate in the walls of blood vessels, producing thrombosis. This occurs commonly in paranasal sinuses, the lungs, and the gastrointestinal tract and results in ischemic necrosis of surrounding tissue with an intense polymorphonuclear infiltrate.

The organisms are rarely cultured during life but are seen in histologic preparations of tissues as broad, *nonseptate*, irregular hyphae in thrombosed vessels or sinuses with surrounding leukocytic and giant cell response.

In zygomycosis diagnosed during life, intense therapy of the underlying disorder accompanied by systemic amphotericin B therapy and in some cases surgical removal of infected tissue has resulted in remissions and occasional cure.

ACTINOMYCETES

The actinomycetes are a heterogeneous group of filamentous bacteria related to corynebacteria and mycobacteria and superficially resembling fungi. Characteristically, they grow as gram-positive, branching organisms that tend to fragment into bacterialike pieces. Some actinomycetes are acid-fast. Most are free-living, particularly in soil. The anaerobic species are part of the normal flora of the mouth. Some of the aerobic species found in soil (*Nocardia, Streptomyces*) may cause disease in humans and animals.

1. ACTINOMYCOSIS

Actinomycosis is a chronic suppurative disease that spreads by direct extension, forms draining sinus tracts, and is caused by *Actinomyces israelii* and related anaerobic filamentous bacteria, including *Arachnia* species. These form part of the normal flora of the oral cavity, and it is not clear what transforms carriage of the organisms into invasive disease. When they invade tissues, *Actinomyces* species are often associated with other oral bacteria. *Actinomyces bovis* causes "lumpy jaw" in cattle.

Morphology & Identification

In tissue, *Actinomyces* species occur as branching filaments surrounded by suppurating, fibrosing inflammation. The typical finding is a "sulfur granule" in pus (Fig 31–22). It consists of a colony of gram-positive mycelial filaments surrounded by eosinophilic "clubs." The latter may be antigen-antibody complexes.

A. Typical Organism: When a sulfur granule in pus is washed and crushed, it reveals a tangled mass of filaments that readily breaks up into coccoid or bacillary forms which are gram-positive and non-acid-fast and show characteristic V or Y branching.

B. Culture: "Sulfur granules" or other pus containing *Actinomyces* can be washed and inoculated into thioglycolate liquid medium, streaked onto brain-heart infusion agar, and incubated anaerobically at 37 °C. In thioglycolate, *A israelii* grows as fluffy balls near the bottom of the tube, whereas *A bovis* produces general turbidity. On solid media, *A israelii* produces small "spidery" colonies in 2–3 days that become white, heaped-up, irregular, or sometimes smooth, larger colonies in 10 days. Other species may have different colony forms.

C. Growth Characteristics: Of the 3 species most commonly responsible for actinomycosis, *A israelii* does not hydrolyze starch but ferments xylose and mannitol, whereas *A bovis* hydrolyzes starch but does not ferment these sugars. *Arachnia propionica* yields large amounts of propionic acid. Most *Actinomyces* species are nonhemolytic, nonproteolytic, and catalase-negative.

Antigenic Structure

Gel diffusion methods or immunofluorescence can differentiate *A israelii* from other actinomycete species and from other filamentous anaerobes that may produce granules in tissues. Species-specific antigens (mainly polysaccharides from the cell wall) occur in acetone extracts of culture supernate. There are at least 2 serotypes of *A israelii*.

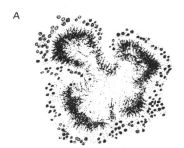
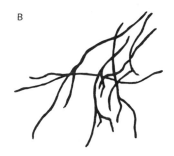
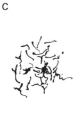

Figure 31–22. *Actinomyces israelii.* **A:** Sulfur granule in pus. **B:** In broth culture. **C:** Diphtheroidlike and branching in agar culture.

Pathogenesis & Pathology

Typical *A israelii* can be found on teeth and in tonsillar crypts of most normal persons. It is likely that trauma (eg, tooth extraction), pyogenic or necrotizing bacterial infection, or aspiration precipitates clinical actinomycosis.

The typical lesion consists of an abscess with central necrosis, surrounded by granulation tissue and fibrous tissue; the pus often contains "sulfur granules" and may drain to the outside through sinuses. Histologically, the lesions are not typical unless sulfur granules can be found or *Actinomyces* cultured. In early lesions a mixed bacterial flora is often seen.

Clinical Findings

The characteristic appearance of actinomycosis is a hard, red, relatively nontender swelling that usually develops slowly. It becomes fluctuant, points to a surface, and eventually drains, forming a chronic sinus tract with little tendency to heal. Lesions extend by contiguity. Dissemination via the bloodstream is very rare.

In about half of cases of actinomycosis, the initial lesion is cervicofacial, involving the face, neck, tongue, or mandible. About one-fifth of cases show predominant involvement of lungs (thoracic actinomycosis), with abscesses or empyema. In a similar number, the primary lesion is in the cecum, appendix, or pelvic organs and may develop multiple draining fistulas (abdominal actinomycosis). Pelvic actinomycosis has occurred particularly in women wearing intrauterine contraceptive devices (IUDs). *A israelii, A propionica,* and other species may cause similar disease.

Diagnostic Laboratory Tests

Animal inoculation, skin tests, and serologic tests are not useful.

A. Specimens: Specimens consist of pus from lesions, sinus tracts, or fistulas and sputum or tissue biopsy material.

B. Microscopic Examination: Every effort must be made to find "sulfur granules." These are rinsed, crushed, examined, and cultured. The appearance in wet mount of the central mycelium and peripheral clubs is characteristic (Fig 31–22). If no granules are found, stained smears of gram-positive branching rods and filaments are suggestive.

C. Culture: Material inoculated into thioglycolate medium and streaked onto brain-heart infusion blood agar plates must be incubated anaerobically for at least 2 weeks. The cultures are examined intermittently for characteristic morphology.

Immunity

Actinomyces are part of the normal body flora. It is uncertain whether antibodies or cell-mediated reactions are produced until tissue invasion occurs. Eosinophilic clubs are not present on granules found in tonsillar crypts; these eosinophilic reactions in tissue granules may denote an antigen-antibody complex.

Treatment

Prolonged administration of penicillin, 5–10 million units daily, is effective in many cases. However, drugs may penetrate the abscesses poorly, and some of the tissue destruction may be irreversible. Surgical drainage and surgical removal are accepted forms of treatment.

Epidemiology

Because of the many free-living actinomycetes and the occurrence of "lumpy jaw" in cattle, it was at one time believed that actinomycosis in humans was acquired from grasses, straws, etc, which acted by traumatizing the mucous membranes and introducing the causative organism. However, it is now established that potentially pathogenic *A israelii* is a common inhabitant of mucous membranes in the mouth, so that no introduction from the outside need be postulated. The disease is never communicable.

Most isolates from human sources are *A israelii;* most isolates from bovine sources are *A bovis.*

2. NOCARDIOSIS

Nocardia species and *Streptomyces* species are aerobic organisms that occur in soil. *Nocardia asteroides* and *Nocardia brasiliensis* are the main causes of nocardiosis, an opportunistic human pulmonary disease that may spread to other parts of the body. These organisms may also produce mycetoma (see p 325).

Morphology & Identification

N asteroides has thin, gram-positive, branching filaments that may fragment into bacillary or coccoid forms. Many isolates are acid-fast when decolorized with 1% sulfuric acid. Bacillary and filamentous forms may be seen in tissue exudates or in pus. Granules similar to those in actinomycosis or mycetoma are never seen, although filamentous clusters and colonies may occur. *Streptomyces* are not acid-fast and do not fragment into bacillary forms.

Nocardia species grow aerobically on many simple media. Growth is variable and slow. Colonies are waxy, with pigmentation varying from yellow to orange or red. White aerial hyphae may form over the surface of the colony. Sporulation occurs by fragmentation into arthrospores. *N asteroides* will not grow in gelatin media and is unable to digest casein or ferment carbohydrates. *N brasiliensis* gives positive results in these tests. All nocardiae are urease-positive. Chromatographic identification of cell wall constituents is used to differentiate species.

Antigenic Structure

Diagnostic and prognostic serologic tests have not yet been developed. Filtrates from *Nocardia* growth in broth can serve as antigen in various serologic tests. Antibodies occur in disease, but false-positive reactions occur in mycobacterial infections. Nocardiae and mycobacteria evidently share antigens.

Pathogenesis & Clinical Findings

Nocardiosis begins as a pulmonary infection that may be subclinical or produce pneumonia. The localized lesion may remain chronic as an enlarging abscess, sinus tract, or cavity. There is a predilection for brain abscess formation by hematogenous spread. Kidney lesions may also develop and extend through the cortex to the medulla. Disease caused by these organisms is most commonly seen in patients immunosuppressed by disease (eg, leukemia, lymphoma, AIDS) or drugs.

Diagnostic Laboratory Tests

A. Specimens: Specimens consist of sputum, pus, spinal fluid, and biopsy material. Serologic tests are unreliable at present. Sonicated extracts of *Nocardia* species may give precipitin lines with sera of infected persons in immunodiffusion tests.

B. Microscopic Examination: Gram-stained smears show coccal and bacillary forms or tangled masses of branching rods. Some strains are partially acid-fast.

C. Culture: *Nocardia* species grow on most laboratory media but may be inhibited by the presence of antibacterial quantities of antibiotics in the media. Guinea pigs, mice, and rabbits are susceptible to experimental infection.

D. Tissue Sections: Nocardiae are stained by methenamine-silver stain.

Treatment

The sulfonamides are the drugs of choice; trimethoprim-sulfamethoxazole may be slightly better, and minocycline is also effective. Surgical drainage or resection may be required. Treatment of the underlying disorder should be attempted.

Epidemiology

Potentially pathogenic nocardiae are ubiquitous in soil and probably enter the body by the respiratory route or through breaks in the skin. Infections in dogs, other pets, and farm animals are fairly common. Mastitis in dairy cattle is at times widespread. Nocardiosis is not communicable.

HYPERSENSITIVITY TO FUNGI

In the course of many fungal infections, delayed type hypersensitivity develops to one or more antigens of the fungus. This is true whether the organism grows as a saprophyte (see *Aspergillus*) or as an invasive opportunist and whether it grows on surfaces, in cavities, or in tissues. The inhalation of actinomycetes or molds growing in the environment may cause an allergic pneumonitis (see Chapter 13). Hypersensitivity evidenced by positive skin tests with fungal extracts may be helpful in diagnosis, but such skin tests are often negative in persons with disseminated systemic involvement. The return of a positive skin test reaction may be a sign of effective chemotherapy and of improved prognosis.

MYCOTOXINS

Many fungi produce poisonous substances called mycotoxins that can cause acute or chronic intoxication and damage. Ingestion of poisonous mushrooms (eg, *Amanita phalloides*) may cause severe damage to liver, kidney, or bone marrow. Chronic damage or neoplasms may be induced in animals or humans following ingestion of small quantities of toxin on contaminated food (eg, aflatoxin from *Aspergillus flavus*). Derivatives of fungal products (eg, LSD) may cause profound mental derangement.

REFERENCES

Aisner J et al: Treatment of invasive aspergillosis: Relation of early diagnosis and treatment to response. *Ann Intern Med* 1977;**86**:539.

Bennett JE: Chemotherapy of systemic mycoses. (2 parts.) *N Engl J Med* 1974;**290**:30, 320.

Bennett JE et al: A comparison of amphotericin B alone and combined with flucytosine in the treatment of cryptococcal meningitis. *N Engl J Med* 1979;**301**:126.

Bouza E et al: Coccidioidal meningitis: An analysis of 31 cases and review of the literature. *Medicine* 1981;**60**:139.

Craven PC et al: High-dose ketoconazole for treatment of fungal infections of the central nervous system. *Ann Intern Med* 1983;**98**:160.

Curry WA: Human nocardiosis: A clinical review with selected case reports. *Arch Intern Med* 1980;**140**:818.

Davies SF et al: Disseminated histoplasmosis in immunologically suppressed patients in a non-endemic area. *Am J Med* 1978;**64**:94.

Davis WA et al: Disseminated *Petriellidium boydii* and pacemaker endocarditis. *Am J Med* 1980;**69**:929.

Dismukes WE et al: Treatment of systemic mycoses with ketoconazole. *Ann Intern Med* 1983;**98**:13.

Drutz DJ, Catanzaro A: Coccidioidomycosis. (2 parts.) *Am Rev Respir Dis* 1978;**117**:559, 727.

Emmons CW et al: *Medical Mycology*, 3rd ed. Lea & Febiger, 1977.

Fisher BD et al: Invasive aspergillosis. *Am J Med* 1981;**71**:571.

Flynn NM et al: An unusual outbreak of windborne coccidioidomycosis. *N Engl J Med* 1979;**301**:358.

Fujita NK et al: Cryptococcal intracerebral mass lesions. *Ann Intern Med* 1981;**94**:382.

Goodwin RA, DesPrez RM: Histoplasmosis. *Am Rev Respir Dis* 1978;**117**:929.

Gordon MA, Gwinn DD: Summary of a workshop on serodiagnosis of systemic mycoses. *J Infect Dis* 1982;**146**:570.

Haupt HM et al: Colonization and infection with *Trichosporon* sp in the immunosuppressed host. *J Infect Dis* 1983;**147**:199.

Holmberg K, Berdischewsky M, Young LS: Serologic immunodiagnosis of invasive aspergillosis. *J Infect Dis* 1980;**141**:656.

Keebler C et al: Actinomycosis infection associated with intrauterine contraceptive devices. *Am J Obstet Gynecol* 1983;**145**:596.

Kobayashi RH et al: *Candida* esophagitis and laryngitis in chronic mucocutaneous candidiasis. *Pediatrics* 1980;**66**:380.

Laude TA et al: Tinea capitis in Brooklyn. *Am J Dis Child* 1982;**136**:1047.

Medoff G, Kobayashi GS: Strategies in the treatment of systemic fungal infections. *N Engl J Med* 1980;**302**:145.

Palmer DL et al: Diagnostic and therapeutic considerations in *Nocardia asteroides* infection. *Medicine* 1974;**53**:391.

Penn RL et al: Invasive fungal infections: The use of serologic tests in diagnosis and management. *Arch Intern Med* 1983;**143**:1215.

Pennington JE: *Aspergillus* lung disease. *Med Clin North Am* 1980;**64**:475.

Perfect JR et al: Cryptococcemia. *Medicine* 1983;**62**:98.

Restrepo A, Stevens DA, Utz JP (editors): Symposium on ketoconazole. *Rev Infect Dis* 1980;**2**:519.

Restrepo A et al: The gamut of paracoccidioidomycosis. *Am J Med* 1976;**61**:33.

Rinaldi MG: Invasive aspergillosis. *Rev Infect Dis* 1983;**5**:1061.

Sarosi GA, Davies SF: Blastomycosis. *Am Rev Respir Dis* 1979;**120**:911.

Smego RA: Combined therapy with amphotericin B and flucytosine for *Candida* meningitis. *Rev Infect Dis* 1984;**6**:791.

Smego RA, Gallis HA: The clinical spectrum of *Nocardia brasiliensis* infection in the United States. *Rev Infect Dis* 1984;**6**:164.

Varkey B, Rose HD: Pulmonary aspergilloma. *Am J Med* 1976;**61**:626.

Weese WC, Smith IM: Study of 57 cases of actinomycosis over a 36-year period. *Arch Intern Med* 1975;**135**:1562.

Wheat LJ et al: Cavitary histoplasmosis during two large urban outbreaks. *Medicine* 1984;**63**:201.

Wheat LJ et al: A large urban outbreak of histoplasmosis: Clinical features. *Ann Intern Med* 1981;**94**:331.

Yoshinoya S et al: Circulating immune complexes in coccidioidomycosis. *J Clin Invest* 1980;**66**:655.

32

Diagnostic medical microbiology is concerned with (1) the etiologic diagnosis of infectious disease by means of the isolation and identification of infectious agents and the demonstration of immunologic responses (antibody, skin reactivity) in the patient; and (2) the rational selection of antimicrobial drugs and dosage based on laboratory test results.

In the field of infectious diseases, the results of laboratory tests depend largely on the quality of the specimen, the timing and the care with which it is collected, and the technical proficiency and experience of laboratory personnel. Although general physicians should be competent to perform a few simple, crucial microbiologic tests—make and stain a smear, examine it microscopically, and streak a culture plate—the technical details of the more involved procedures are usually left to the bacteriologist or virologist and the technicians on the staff. Physicians who deal with infectious processes must know when and how to take specimens, what laboratory examinations to request, and how to interpret the results.

COMMUNICATION BETWEEN PHYSICIAN & LABORATORY

Diagnostic microbiology encompasses the characterization of thousands of agents that cause or are associated with infectious diseases. The techniques used to characterize infectious agents vary greatly depending upon the clinical syndrome and the type of agent being considered: virus, bacterium, fungus, or other parasite. Because no single test will permit isolation or characterization of all potential pathogens, clinical information is much more important for diagnostic microbiology than it is for clinical chemistry or hematology. The clinician must make a tentative diagnosis rather than wait until laboratory results are available. When tests are requested, the physician should inform the laboratory staff of the tentative diagnosis (type of infection or infectious agent suspected). Proper labeling of specimens includes such clinical data as well as the requesting physician's name, address, and telephone number.

Many pathogenic microorganisms grow slowly, and days or even weeks may elapse before they are isolated and identified. Treatment cannot be deferred until this process is complete. After obtaining the proper specimens and informing the laboratory of the tenta-

tive clinical diagnosis, the physician should begin treatment with drugs aimed at the organism thought to be responsible for the patient's illness. As the laboratory staff begins to obtain results, they inform the physician, who can then reevaluate the diagnosis and the clinical course of the patient and perhaps make changes in the therapeutic program. This "feedback" information from the laboratory will consist of preliminary reports of the results of individual steps in the isolation and identification of the causative agent.

SPECIMENS

The results of many diagnostic tests for infectious diseases depend largely upon the selection, timing, and method of collection of specimens. These factors are often more crucial for microbiologic specimens than for those designed to yield chemical or hematologic data. Microbial agents grow and die, are susceptible to many chemicals, and can be found at different anatomic sites and in different body fluids and tissues during the course of infectious diseases. Because the isolation of an infectious agent is very important in the formulation of a diagnosis, the specimen must be obtained from the site most likely to yield the agent at that particular stage of illness and must be handled in such a way as to favor survival and growth of the agent. For each type of specimen, suggestions for optimal handling are given in the following paragraphs.

Recovery of an infectious agent is most significant if the agent is isolated from a site normally devoid of microorganisms (a normally sterile area). Any type of microorganism cultured from blood, cerebrospinal fluid, joint fluid, or the pleural cavity is a significant diagnostic finding. Conversely, many parts of the body have a normal microbial flora that may be altered by endogenous or exogenous influences. The recovery of potential pathogens from the respiratory, gastrointestinal, or genitourinary tracts; from wounds; or from the skin must be considered in the context of the normal flora of each particular site. Microbiologic data must be correlated with clinical information to arrive at a meaningful interpretation of the results.

A few general rules apply to all specimens:

(1) The quantity of material must be adequate.

(2) The sample should be representative of the infectious process (eg, sputum, not saliva; pus from the underlying lesion, not from its sinus tract; a swab from the depth of the wound, not from its surface).

(3) Contamination of the specimen must be avoided by using only sterile equipment and aseptic precautions.

(4) The specimen must be taken to the laboratory and examined promptly. Special transport media may be helpful.

(5) Meaningful specimens must be secured before antimicrobial drugs are administered. If antimicrobial drugs are given before specimens are taken for microbiologic study, drug therapy may have to be stopped and repeat specimens obtained several days later.

The type of specimen to be examined is determined by the presenting clinical picture. If symptoms or signs point to involvement of one organ system, specimens are obtained from that source. In the absence of localizing signs or symptoms, repeated blood samples for culturing are taken first, and specimens from other sites are then considered in sequence, depending in part upon the likelihood of involvement of a given organ system in a given patient and in part upon the ease of obtaining specimens.

The above comments apply particularly to specimens intended for the isolation of bacterial or fungal agents. The isolation of viruses or chlamydiae is usually performed only in specialized laboratories. The requirements for collection of specimens for culture of viruses are different from those for collection of specimens for culture of bacteria or fungi. Specimens for culture of viruses need not be from the anatomic site that is most obviously involved in infection. Nasopharyngeal washings or stool specimens can be used to culture many viruses. Specimens for culture of viruses should be obtained as soon as possible after the onset of illness. Specimens for culture of chlamydiae should be from the site of infection: eye, sputum, urethra, or cervix. Specimens for culture of viruses or chlamydiae should be placed in antibiotic-containing transport media and rapidly transported to the laboratory. If necessary, the specimens can be held refrigerated or transported on wet ice for up to 24 (perhaps 48) hours before processing. If prolonged storage and shipment is required, the specimens should be frozen at $-70\ °C$ or placed in well-stoppered containers packed in dry ice.

Very few laboratories perform cultures for rickettsiae and mycoplasmas. If cultures for these agents are to be done, the laboratory staff can provide information on the best methods for specimen collection and transport.

SELECTION OF SPECIFIC LABORATORY INVESTIGATIONS

Tests specifically diagnostic for infectious diseases fall into 3 classes:

(1) Demonstration of an infectious agent (bacterial, mycotic, viral, protozoal, or helminthic) in specimens obtained from the patient.

(2) Demonstration of a meaningful antibody response in the patient. This frequently involves proof of a rise in specific antibody titer and therefore requires 2 serum specimens usually obtained at an interval of 10–20 days or longer.

(3) Demonstration of meaningful cell-mediated responses or skin tests to antigens associated with a particular infectious agent.

In the following paragraphs, some important applications of these specific classes of tests will be described.

DEMONSTRATION OF AN INFECTIOUS AGENT

Laboratory examinations usually include microscopic study of fresh unstained and stained materials and preparation of cultures with conditions suitable for growth of a wide variety of microorganisms, including the type of organism that is most suspect on clinical grounds. If a microorganism is isolated, complete identification may then be pursued. Isolated microorganisms may be tested for susceptibility to antimicrobial drugs. In certain types of diseases, assay of antimicrobial activity in the patient's serum or urine during treatment may be more informative than in vitro drug susceptibility tests (see Chapter 10). When significant pathogens are isolated before treatment, follow-up laboratory examinations during and after treatment may be appropriate.

Microscopy & Stains

Microscopic examination of stained or unstained specimens is a relatively simple and inexpensive but much less sensitive method than culture for detection of small numbers of bacteria. A specimen must contain at least 10^5 organisms/mL before it is likely that organisms will be seen on a smear. Liquid medium containing 10^5 organisms/mL does not appear turbid to the eye. Specimens containing 10^2–10^3 organisms/mL produce growth on solid media, and those containing 10 or fewer bacteria/mL may produce growth in liquid media.

Gram staining is the single most useful procedure in diagnostic microbiology. Most specimens submitted when bacterial infection is suspected should be smeared on glass slides, Gram-stained, and examined microscopically. The materials and method for Gram staining are outlined in Table 32–1. On microscopic examination, the Gram reaction (purple-blue indicates gram-positive organisms; red, gram-negative) and morphology (shape: cocci, rods, fusiform, or other; see Chapter 2) of bacteria should be noted. The appearance of bacteria on Gram-stained smears does not permit identification of species. Reports of gram-positive cocci in chains are suggestive of, but not definitive for, streptococcal species; gram-positive cocci in clusters suggest a staphylococcal species. Gram-negative rods can be large, small, or even coccobacillary. Some nonviable gram-positive bacteria can stain gram-negatively. Typically, bacterial morphology has been defined using organisms grown on agar. However, bacteria in body fluids or tissue can have highly variable morphology.

Specimens submitted for examination for mycobacteria should be stained for acid-fast organisms, using either Ziehl-Neelsen stain or Kinyoun stain (Table 32–1). An alternative stain for mycobacteria, auramine-rhodamine stain, is more sensitive than the acid-fast stains but requires fluorescence microscopy, and, if results are positive, confirmation with an acid-fast stain (see Chapter 26).

Fluorescent antibody (FA) staining is useful in the identification of many microorganisms. Such procedures are more specific than other staining techniques but also more cumbersome to perform. The fluorescein-labeled antibodies in common use are made from antisera produced by injecting animals with whole organisms or complex antigen mixtures. The resultant **polyclonal antibodies** may react with multiple antigens on the organism that was injected and may also cross-react with antigens of other microorganisms or possibly with human cells in the specimen. Quality control is important to minimize nonspecific FA staining. Use of **monoclonal antibodies** may circumvent the problem of nonspecific staining. FA staining is most useful in confirming the presence of specific organisms such as *Bordetella pertussis* or *Legionella pneumophila* in colonies isolated on culture media and in the identification of viruses after they have been grown in cell culture. The use of direct FA staining on

specimens from patients is more difficult and less specific.

Stains such as periodic acid-Schiff (PAS) and methenamine silver nitrate are used for tissues and other specimens in which fungi or other parasites may be present. Such stains are not specific for given microorganisms, but they may define structure so that morphologic criteria can be used for identification. *Pneumocystis carinii* cysts are identified morphologically in silver-stained specimens. After primary isolation of fungi, stains such as lactophenol cotton blue are used to distinguish fungal growth to identify organisms by their morphology.

Specimens to be examined for fungi, protozoa, and helminths can be examined unstained. Specimens to be examined for fungi are often treated with a solution of 10% potassium hydroxide, which breaks down the tissue surrounding the fungal mycelia to allow a better view of the hyphal forms. Unstained specimens or "wet mounts" are used for routine examination of stools and many other specimens for parasites. Phase contrast microscopy is sometimes useful in unstained specimens. Darkfield microscopy is used to detect *Treponema pallidum* in material from primary or secondary syphilitic lesions.

Culture Systems

For diagnostic bacteriology, it is necessary to use several types of media for routine culture, particularly when the possible organisms include aerobic, facultatively anaerobic, and obligately anaerobic bacteria. The specimens and culture media used to diagnose the more common bacterial infections are listed in Table 32–2. The standard medium for specimens is blood agar, usually made with 5% sheep blood. Most aerobic and facultatively anaerobic organisms will grow on blood agar. Chocolate agar, a medium containing heated blood with or without supplements, is a second necessary medium: some organisms that do not grow on blood agar, including pathogenic *Neisseria* and *Haemophilus*, will grow on chocolate agar. A selective medium for enteric gram-negative rods (either MacConkey agar or eosin methylene blue [EMB] agar) is a third type of medium used routinely. Specimens to be cultured for obligate anaerobes must be plated on at least 2 additional types of media, including a highly supplemented agar such as *Brucella* agar with hemin and vitamin K and a selective medium containing substances that inhibit the growth of enteric gram-negative rods and facultatively anaerobic or anaerobic gram-positive cocci.

Many other specialized media are used in diagnostic bacteriology; choices depend on the clinical diagnosis and the organism under consideration. The laboratory staff selects the specific media on the basis of the information in the culture request. Thus, freshly made Bordet-Gengou medium is used to culture for *B pertussis* in the diagnosis of whooping cough, and other special media are used to culture for *Vibrio cholerae*, *Corynebacterium diphtheriae*, and *Neisseria gonorrhoeae*. For culture of mycobacteria,

Table 32–1. Gram and acid-fast staining methods.

Gram stain (Hucker modification)
(1) Fix smear by heat.
(2) Cover with crystal violet for 1 minute.
(3) Wash with water. Do not blot.
(4) Cover with Gram's iodine for 1 minute.
(5) Wash with water. Do not blot.
(6) Decolorize for 10–30 seconds with gentle agitation in acetone (30 mL) and alcohol (70 mL).
(7) Wash with water. Do not blot.
(8) Cover for 10–30 seconds with safranin (2.5% solution in 95% alcohol).
(9) Wash with water and let dry.

Ziehl-Neelsen acid-fast stain
(1) Fix smear by heat.
(2) Cover with carbolfuchsin, steam gently for 5 minutes over direct flame (or for 20 minutes over a water bath).
(3) Wash with water.
(4) Decolorize in acid-alcohol until only a faint pink color remains.
(5) Wash with water.
(6) Counterstain for 10–30 seconds with Loeffler's methylene blue.
(7) Wash with water and let dry.

Kinyoun carbolfuchsin acid-fast stain
(1) Formula: Basic fuchsin, 4; phenol crystals, 8; alcohol (95%), 20; distilled water, 100.
(2) Stain fixed smear for 3 minutes (no heat necessary) and continue as with Ziehl-Neelsen stain.

Löwenstein-Jensen or other specialized medium is commonly used. These media usually contain inspissated egg and may contain inhibitors of other bacteria. Because many mycobacteria grow slowly, the cultures must be incubated and examined periodically for 6–8 weeks (see Chapter 26).

Broth cultures in highly enriched media are important for back-up cultures of biopsy tissues and body fluids such as cerebrospinal fluid. The broth cultures may give positive results when there is no growth on solid media because of the small number of bacteria present in the inoculum (see above).

Many yeasts will grow on blood agar. Biphasic and mycelial phase fungi often grow better on media designed specifically for fungi, eg, Sabouraud's dextrose agar and fungal media containing antimicrobial drugs. Cultures for fungi are commonly done in paired sets, with one set incubated at 25–30 °C and the other at 37 °C. Table 32–3 outlines specimens, culture media, and other tests to be used for diagnosis of fungal infections.

Viruses are grown in cell culture systems, in animals such as suckling mice, or in embryonated chicken eggs. Most cultures for viruses employ several different cell lines, including one primary, one diploid, and one heteroploid cell line for each specimen. The specific cell lines chosen depend on the tentative diagnosis. Table 32–4 lists common viral syndromes and the appropriate specimens and cell lines for culture of the viruses. Diagnostic techniques for viral disease are discussed in Chapter 34.

Protozoal and helminthic infections are usually diagnosed by microscopic examination of feces or some other specimen; cultures are rarely used. Medical parasitology is discussed in Chapter 48.

Antigen Detection

Immunologic systems designed to detect antigens of microorganisms can be used in the diagnosis of specific infections. Most such systems employ an antibody and either a colorimetric reaction (eg, enzyme-linked immunosorbent assay [ELISA]) or latex particle agglutination (see Chapter 12). These tests have replaced detection of antigen by counterimmunoelectrophoresis for the diagnosis of disease due to *Haemophilus influenzae*, *Neisseria meningitidis*, and *Streptococcus pneumoniae* and meningitis due to group B streptococci.

Monoclonal antibodies. Monoclonal antibody technology has opened many possibilities for diagnostic microbiology. Monoclonal antibodies are in widespread use in diagnostic laboratories as reagents for the identification of specific antigens that are markers of types, species, or classes of infectious agents (eg, herpes simplex types I and II, group A streptococcal carbohydrate) and cells or other markers (eg, T cell antigens). Monoclonal antibodies are antigen-specific. Consequently, the development of antibody mixtures that are cross-reactive with multiple antigens of bacterial species has been difficult, and polyclonal (rabbit, goat, etc) antibodies are used for many tests.

DNA hybridization. In DNA hybridization techniques, DNA encoding for specific genes is isolated and used as the probe. The use of such probes offers great opportunity to identify infectious agents that do not grow rapidly and to diagnose infections where the organisms are not easily cultured. Using DNA hybridization technique, it is possible to identify enterotoxin-producing *Escherichia coli* in a stool specimen without going through laborious subculturing and toxin assays. Similarly, it may be possible to identify organisms such as *T pallidum* and *Mycobacterium leprae* in clinical specimens. However, very few diagnostic microbiology laboratories are set up to use the radioisotopes required for many DNA probes. The application of nonisotopic techniques is likely to expand the use of DNA probes to the point where they can be applied routinely to the diagnosis of infections.

THE IMPORTANCE OF NORMAL MICROBIAL FLORA

Organisms such as *Mycobacterium tuberculosis*, *Salmonella typhi*, and *Brucella* species are considered pathogens whenever they are found in patients. However, many infections are caused by organisms that are permanent or transient members of the normal flora. For example, *E coli* is part of the normal gastrointestinal flora and is also the most common cause of urinary tract infection. Similarly, the vast majority of mixed bacterial infections with anaerobes are caused by organisms that are members of the normal flora.

The relative numbers of specific organisms found in a culture are important when members of the normal flora are the cause of infection. When numerous gram-negative rods of species such as *Klebsiella pneumoniae* are found mixed with a few normal nasopharyngeal bacteria in a sputum culture, the gram-negative rods are strongly suspect as the cause of pneumonia, because large numbers of gram-negative rods are not normally found in sputum or the nasopharyngeal flora; the organisms should be identified and reported. In contrast, abdominal abscesses commonly contain a normal distribution of aerobic, facultatively anaerobic, and obligately anaerobic organisms representative of the gastrointestinal flora. In such cases, identification of all species present is not warranted; instead, it is appropriate to report "normal gastrointestinal flora."

Yeasts in small numbers are commonly part of the normal microbial flora. However, other fungi are not normally present and therefore should be identified and reported. Viruses usually are not part of the normal flora as detected in diagnostic microbiology laboratories. However, some latent viruses, eg, herpes simplex, or live vaccine viruses such as poliovirus occasionally appear in cultures for viruses. In some parts of the world, stool specimens commonly yield evidence of parasitic infection. In such cases, it is the relative number of parasites correlated with the clinical

Table 32–2. Common localized bacterial infections: Agents, specimens, and diagnostic tests.

Disease	Specimen	Common Causative Agents	Usual Microscopic Findings	Culture Media	Comments
Cellulitis of skin	Swab	Group A β-hemolytic streptococci, *Staphylococcus aureus*, or both.	Occasionally gram-positive cocci.	Blood agar.	Aspirate from leading edge of infection may yield the organism.
Impetigo	Swab	As for cellulitis (above); rarely, *Corynebacterium diphtheriae*.	As for cellulitis (above) and pharyngitis (below).		
Skin ulcers	Swab	Mixed flora.	Mixed flora.	Blood, MacConkey, or EMB agar; anaerobic conditions.	Skin ulcers below the waist often contain aerobes and anaerobes like gastrointestinal flora.
Meningitis	CSF	*Neisseria meningitidis*.	Gram-negative intracellular or cell-associated diplococci.	Chocolate agar* and blood agar for CSF cultures.	Capsular swelling (quellung) reaction with type-specific serum helps in identification.
		Haemophilus influenzae.	Small gram-negative coccobacilli.	Chocolate agar.*	Quellung reaction with type b antiserum may be helpful.
		Streptococcus pneumoniae.	Gram-positive cocci in pairs.	Blood agar.	Quellung reaction with pneumococcal omniserum.
		Group B streptococci.	Gram-positive cocci in pairs and chains.	Blood agar.	Mainly in newborns; β-hemolytic.
		E coli and other *Enterobacteriaceae*.	Gram-negative rods.	Blood agar.	Mainly in newborns; no need for selective media in CSF culture.
		Listeria monocytogenes.	Gram-positive rods.	Blood agar.	β-Hemolytic and motile.
Brain abscess	Pus	Mixed infection: anaerobic gram-positive and gram-negative cocci and rods, aerobic gram-positive cocci.	Gram-positive cocci or mixed flora.	Blood agar, chocolate agar,* anaerobe media.	Specimen must be obtained surgically and transported under strict anaerobic conditions.
Perioral abscess	Pus	Mixed flora of mouth and pharynx.	Mixed flora.	Blood, MacConkey, or EMB agar; anaerobic conditions.	Usually mixed bacterial infection; rarely, actinomycosis.
Pharyngitis	Swab	Group A streptococci.	Not recommended.	Blood agar or selective medium.	β-Hemolytic.
		Corynebacterium diphtheriae.	Not recommended.	Loeffler or Pai's medium, then cysteine-tellurite or Tinsdale's medium.	Granular rods in "Chinese character" patterns in smears from culture. Toxicity testing required.
Whooping cough (pertussis)	Swab or "cough plate"	*Bordetella pertussis*.	Not recommended.	Fresh Bordet-Gengou medium or *Bordetella* charcoal agar.	Fluorescent antibody test identifies organisms from culture but rarely from direct smears.
Epiglottitis	Swab	*Haemophilus influenzae*.	Usually not helpful.	Chocolate agar* (also use blood agar).	*H influenzae* is part of normal flora in nasopharynx.

*A chemical supplement such as Isovitalex enhances growth of *Haemophilus* and *Neisseria* species.

Table 32–2 (cont'd). Common localized bacterial infections: Agents, specimens, and diagnostic tests.

Disease	Specimen	Common Causative Agents	Usual Microscopic Findings	Culture Media	Comments
Pneumonia	Sputum	*Streptococcus pneumoniae*.	Many PMNs, gram-positive cocci in pairs or chains. Capsule swelling with omniserum.	Blood agar; also MacConkey, EMB, and chocolate agar.	*S pneumoniae* are part of normal flora in naso-pharynx. Blood cultures specific (positive) in 10–20%.
		Staphylococcus au-reus.	Gram-positive cocci in pairs, tetrads, and clusters.	Blood agar; also MacConkey, EMB, and chocolate agar.	Uncommon cause of pneumonia. Usually β-hemolytic, coagulase-positive.
		Enterobacteriaceae and other gram-negative rods.	Gram-negative rods.	Blood agar; Mac-Conkey or EMB agar.	Uncommon causes of pneumonia.
		Mixed anaerobes and aerobes.	Mixed respiratory tract flora; some-times many PMNs.	Blood, MacConkey, or EMB agar; anaer-obic conditions.	Specimens must be ob-tained by bronchoscopy or transtracheal aspiration; expectorated sputum is unsatisfactory for anaer-obes.
Chest em-pyema	Pus	Same as pneumonia, or mixed flora infec-tion.	Mixed flora.	Boold, MacConkey, or EMB agar; anaer-obic conditions.	Usually pneumonia; mixed aerobic and anaerobic flora derived from oropharynx.
Liver abscess	Pus	*Escherichia coli; Bacteroides fragilis;* mixed aerobic or anaerobic flora.	Gram-negative rods and mixed flora.	Blood, MacConkey, or EMB agar; anaer-obic conditions.	Commonly enteric gram-negative aerobes and anaerobes; consider *Enta-moeba histolytica* infec-tion.
Cholecystitis	Bile	Gram-negative en-teric aerobes, also *Bacillus fragilis*.	Gram-negative rods.	Blood, MacConkey, or EMB agar; anaer-obic conditions.	Usually gram-negative rods from gastrointestinal tract.
Abdominal or perirectal abscess	Pus	Gastrointestinal flora.	Mixed flora.	Blood, MacConkey, or EMB agar; anaer-obic conditions.	Aerobic and anaerobic bowel flora; often more than 5 species grown.
Enteric fever, typhoid	Blood, feces, urine	*Salmonella typhi*.	Not recommended.	MacConkey, Hek-toen, bismuth sulfite agars; others.	Multiple specimens should be cultured; lactose-nega-tive. H_2S produced.
Enteritis, en-terocolitis, bacterial di-arrheas, "gastroen-teritis" (see p 241).	Feces	*Salmonella* species other than *S typhi*.	Gram stain or methylene blue stain may show PMNs.	MacConkey, Hek-toen, bismuth sulfite agars; others.	Non-lactose-fermenting colonies onto TSI[†] slants: Non-typhoid salmonellae produce acid and gas in butt, alkaline slant, and H_2S.
		Shigella species.	Gram stain or methylene blue stain may show PMNs.	MacConkey, Hek-toen, bismuth sulfite agars; others.	Non-lactose-fermenting colonies onto TSI[†] slants: Shigellae produce alkaline slant, acid butt without gas.
		Campylobacter je-juni.	"Gull-wing-shaped" gram-negative rods and often PMNs.	Skirrow's or similar medium.	Incubate at 42 °C; colonies oxidase-positive; smear shows "gull-wing-shaped" rods.
		Vibrio cholerae.	Not recommended.	Thiosulfate citrate bile salts sucrose agar; others. Tauro-cholate-peptone broth for enrich-ment.	Oxidase-positive colonies to Kligler iron agar slant: alkaline slant, acid butt without gas, no H_2S. Serologic tests needed.

†TSI, triple sugar iron agar.

Table 32–2 (cont'd). Common localized bacterial infections: Agents, specimens, and diagnostic tests.

Disease	Specimen	Common Causative Agents	Usual Microscopic Findings	Culture Media	Comments
Enteritis, enterocolitis, bacterial diarrheas, "gastroenteritis" (see p 241). (cont'd)	Feces	Other vibrios.	Not recommended.	As for *V cholerae*.	Differentiate from *V cholerae* by biochemical and culture tests.
		Yersinia enterocolitica.	Not recommended.	MacConkey, EMB, *Salmonella-Shigella* agar.	Enrichment at 4 °C helpful; incubate cultures at 25 °C.
Urinary tract infection	Urine (clean-catch midstream specimen or one obtained by bladder catheterization or suprapubic aspiration)	*Escherichia coli; Enterobacteriaceae;* other gram-negative rods.	Gram-negative rods seen on stained smear of uncentrifuged urine indicate more than 10^5 organisms/mL.	Blood agar; MacConkey or EMB agar.	Gray colonies that are β-hemolytic and give a positive spot indole test are *E coli;* others require further biochemical tests.
Urethritis/ cervicitis	Swab	*Neisseria gonorrhoeae*.	Gram-negative diplococci in or on PMNs. Specific for urethral discharge in men; less reliable in women.	Thayer-Martin or similar antibiotic-containing selective medium.	Positive stained smear diagnostic in men. Culture needed in women. Gonococci are oxidase-positive.
		Chlamydia trachomatis.	PMNs with no associated gram-negative diplococci.	Culture in McCoy cells treated with cycloheximide.	Crescent-shaped inclusions in epithelial cells by stains or immunofluorescence. Direct fluorescent antibody test can be helpful.
Genital ulcers	Swab	*Haemophilus ducreyi* (chancroid).	Mixed flora.	Chocolate agar with Isovitalex and vancomycin.	Differential diagnosis of genital ulcers includes herpes simplex infection.
		Treponema pallidum (syphilis).	Darkfield or fluorescent antibody examination shows spirochetes.	None.	
	Pus aspirated from suppurating lymph nodes	*Chlamydia trachomatis* (lymphogranuloma venereum).	PMNs with no associated gram-negative diplococci.	Culture pus in cell culture (as for urethritis).	
Pelvic inflammatory disease	Cervical swab	*Neisseria gonorrhoeae*.	PMNs with no associated gram-negative diplococci; mixed flora may be present.	Thayer-Martin or similar antibiotic-containing selective medium.	Causative organisms may be gonococci, anaerobes, others. Anaerobes always present in endocervix; thus, endocervical specimen not suitable for culture.
		Chlamydia trachomatis.	See above.	Cell culture (as for urethritis).	
	Aspirate from cul de sac or by laparoscope	*Neisseria gonorrhoeae*.	Gram-negative diplococci in or on PMNs. Specific for urethral discharge in men; unreliable in women.	Modified Thayer-Martin medium.	
		Chlamydia trachomatis.	See above.	Cell culture (as for urethritis).	
		Mixed flora.	Mixed flora.	Blood, MacConkey, or EMB agar; anaerobic conditions.	Usually mixed anaerobic and aerobic bacteria.

Table 32–2 (cont'd). Common localized bacterial infections: Agents, specimens, and diagnostic tests.

Disease	Specimen	Common Causative Agents	Usual Microscopic Findings	Culture Media	Comments
Arthritis	Joint aspirate, blood	*Staphylococcus aureus*.	Gram-positive diplococci in pairs, tetrads, and clusters.	Blood agar; chocolate agar.*	Occurs in both children and adults; coagulase-positive; usually β-hemolytic.
		Neisseria gonorrhoeae.	Gram-negative diplococci in or on PMNs. Specific for urethral discharge in men, less reliable in women.	Modified Thayer-Martin medium.	
		Others.	Morphology depends upon organisms.	Blood agar, chocolate agar*; anaerobic conditions.	Includes streptococci, gram-negative rods, and anaerobes.
Osteomyelitis	Pus or bone specimen obtained by aspiration or surgery	Multiple; often *Staphylococcus aureus*.	Morphology depends upon organisms.	Blood, MacConkey, EMB agar; anaerobic conditions.	Usually aerobic organisms; *S aureus* is most common; gram-negative rods frequent; anaerobes less common.

*A chemical supplement such as Isovitalex enhances growth of *Haemophilus* and *Neisseria* species.

presentation that is important. The presence of a few ova in a specimen should be noted but in itself does not mandate further diagnostic and therapeutic measures.

The organisms that comprise the normal flora of the human body are discussed more extensively in Chapter 30. Members of the normal flora that are most commonly present in patient specimens and that may be reported as "normal flora" are listed in Table 32–5.

THE DIAGNOSIS OF INFECTION BY ANATOMIC SITE

Blood

Since bacteremia frequently portends life-threatening illness, its early detection is essential. Blood culture is the single most important procedure to detect systemic infection due to bacteria. It provides valuable information for the management of febrile, acutely ill patients with or without localizing symptoms and signs and is essential in any patient in whom infective endocarditis is suspected even if the patient does not appear acutely or severely ill. In addition to its diagnostic significance, recovery of an infectious agent from the blood provides invaluable aid in determining antimicrobial therapy. Every effort should therefore be made to isolate the causative organisms in bacteremia.

In healthy persons, properly obtained blood specimens are sterile. Although microorganisms from the normal respiratory and gastrointestinal flora occasionally enter the blood, they are rapidly removed by the reticuloendothelial system. These transients rarely affect the interpretation of blood culture results. If a blood culture yields microorganisms, this fact is of great clinical significance provided that contamination

can be excluded. Contamination of blood cultures with normal skin flora is most commonly due to errors in the blood collection procedure. Therefore, proper technique in performing a blood culture is essential.

The following rules, rigidly applied, yield reliable results:

(1) Use only sterile equipment and strict aseptic technique.

(2) Apply a tourniquet and locate a fixed vein by touch.

(3) Prepare the skin by applying 2% tincture of iodine in widening circles, beginning with the site of proposed skin puncture. Remove iodine with 70% alcohol. After the skin has been prepared, do not touch it except with sterile gloves.

(4) Perform venipuncture and (for adults) withdraw approximately 20 mL of blood.

(5) Add the blood to aerobic and anaerobic blood culture bottles.

(6) Take specimens to the laboratory promptly, or place them in an incubator at 37 °C.

Several factors determine whether blood cultures will yield positive results: the volume of blood cultured, the dilution of blood in the culture medium, the use of both aerobic and anaerobic culture media, and the duration of incubation. For adults, a 20-mL blood sample is usually obtained, and half is placed in an aerobic blood culture bottle and half in an anaerobic one, with one pair of bottles comprising a single blood culture. However, different volumes of blood may be required for the many different blood culture systems that exist. An optimal dilution of blood in a liquid culture medium is 1:150–1:300; this minimizes the effects of the antibody, complement, and white blood cell antibacterial systems that are present. Because such large dilutions are impractical in blood cultures,

Table 32–3. Common fungal infections: Agents, specimens, and diagnostic tests.

	Specimen	Culture Media*	Serologic and Other Tests	Comments
Invasive (deep-seated) mycoses				
Aspergillosis: *Aspergillus fumigatus,* other *Aspergillus* species				
Pulmonary	Respiratory secretions.	SDA, BHIA, BHIA with antibiotics (blood agar).	Immunodiffusion tests available; interpretation of results controversial.	Serology seldom useful.
Disseminated	Biopsy specimen, blood.	As above.		*Aspergillus* is difficult to grow from blood of patients with disseminated infection.
Blastomycosis: *Blastomyces dermatiditis*				
Pulmonary	Respiratory secretions.	SDA, BHIA, BHIA with antibiotics and cyclophosphamide, others.	CF.	CF test usually negative and therefore not very useful. Culture is the best diagnostic test; serology seldom done.
Oral and cutaneous ulcers	Biopsy or swab specimen.	As above.	CF.	
Bone	Bone biopsy.	As above.	CF.	
Coccidioidomycosis: *Coccidioides immitis*				
Pulmonary	Respiratory secretions.	SDA, BHIA, BHIA with antibiotics and cyclophosphamide, others.	CF, immunodiffusion, precipitation, latex agglutination, skin test with coccidioidin or spherulin.	*C immitis* will grow on routine blood agar cultures; positive cultures pose a serious hazard for laboratory workers. Serology often more useful than culture. Skin test does not alter results of serology. Skin test result may have prognostic implications.
Disseminated	Biopsy specimen from site of infection, eg, skin, bone, etc.	As above.	As above except that skin test with coccidioidin may be negative.	
Histoplasmosis: *Histoplasma capsulatum*				
Pulmonary	Respiratory secretions	Smith's medium, SDA, BHIA, BHIA with antibiotics and cyclophosphamide.	CF, immunodiffusion, skin test.	Serology very useful. Skin test can "boost" antibody titer and should not be done as a diagnostic test.
Disseminated	Bone marrow, blood, biopsy specimen from site of infection.	As above plus biphasic blood culture medium.	As above.	
Nocardiosis: *Nocardia asteroides*				
Pulmonary	Respiratory secretions.	SDA, BHIA, blood agar or other bacteriologic media.	Modified acid-fast stain.	*Nocardia* are bacteria that clinically behave like fungi. Weakly acid-fast, branching, filamentous gram-positive rods are *Nocardia*. Serology seldom used.
Subcutaneous	Aspirate or biopsy of abscess.	As above.	Immunodiffusion.	
Brain	Material from brain abscess.	As above.		
Paracoccidioidomycosis (South American blastomycosis): *Paracoccidioides brasiliensis*				
	Biopsy specimen from lesion.	SDA, BHIA, BHIA with antibiotics and cyclophosphamide, others.	Immunodiffusion, CF, skin test (paracoccidioidin).	Immunodiffusion test 95% sensitive and specific; CF test and skin test cross-react with histoplasmin. Positive skin test is of prognostic value.
Sporotrichosis: *Sporothrix schenckii*				
Skin and subcutaneous nodules	Biopsy specimen.	SDA, BHIA, BHIA + AC.	Agglutination.	
Disseminated	Biopsy specimen from infected site.	As above.	As above.	

*SDA, Sabouraud's dextrose agar; BHIA, brain-heart infusion agar.

Table 32–3 (cont'd). Common fungal infections: Agents, specimens, and diagnostic tests.

	Specimen	Culture Media*	Serologic and Other Tests	Comments
Zygomycosis (phycomycosis, mucormycosis): *Rhizopus* species, *Mucor* species, others				
Nasal-ocular-cerebral	Nasal-orbital tissue.	SDA, BHIA.	None.	Nonseptate hyphae seen in microscopic sections.
Pulmonary and disseminated	Respiratory secretions, biopsy specimens.	As above.	None.	
Yeast infections				
Candidiasis: *Candida albicans* and similar yeasts *(Candida tropicalis, Candida parapsilosis,* other *Candida* species, *Torulopsis glabrata)*				
Mucous membrane	Secretions.	Blood agar, most other noninhibitory media for fungi and bacteria.	KOH wet mount useful for microscopy in localized infection.	
Skin	Swab specimen.			
Systemic	Blood, biopsy specimen, urine.	As above plus biphasic blood culture medium.	Immunodiffusion, skin test.	Serology seldom helpful. Skin test used to screen for energy, not to diagnose infection.
Cryptococcosis: *Cryptococcus neoformans*				
Pulmonary	Respiratory secretions.	SDA, BHIA.	Cryptococcal antigen rarely detected.	Antibodies to *C neoformans* rarely found.
Meningitis	CSF.	SDA, BHIA.	India ink preparation for microscopy; latex agglutination for cryptococcal antigen.	Repeated examination of CSF may be necessary to diagnose meningitis.
Disseminated	Bone marrow, bone, blood, other.	As above plus biphasic blood culture medium.	Latex agglutination for cryptococcal antigen.	
Primary skin infections				
Dermatophytosis: *Microsporum* species, *Epidermophyton* species, *Trichophyton* species				
	Hair, skin, nails from infected sites.	SDA with cycloheximide and chloramphenicol.	None.	

*SDA, Sabouraud's dextrose agar; BHIA, brain-heart infusion agar.

most such media contain 0.05% sodium polyanethol sulfonate (SPS), which inhibits the antibacterial systems. However, SPS also inhibits growth of neisseriae, some anaerobic gram-positive cocci, and *Gardnerella vaginalis*. If any of these organisms are suspected, alternative blood culture systems without SPS should be used.

The blood culture bottles are examined 2–3 times a day for the first 2 days and daily thereafter for 1 week. The laboratory should be informed if an infection with a slow-growing organism is suspected so that the blood culture bottles can be incubated longer. Most laboratories routinely Gram stain and subculture the contents of both aerobic and anaerobic blood culture bottles after the first 18–24 hours of incubation; thereafter, they detect positive blood cultures by observing turbidity due to growth in the medium. Some laboratories use blood culture media containing radiolabeled metabolic substrates; the gases in the culture bottles are monitored by automation to detect $^{14}CO_2$, a metabolic by-product that indicates growth.

The number of blood specimens that should be drawn for cultures and the period of time over which this is done depends in part upon the severity of the clinical illness. In hyperacute infections, eg, gram-negative sepsis with shock or staphylococcal sepsis, it is appropriate to culture 2 blood specimens obtained from different anatomic sites over a period of 10 minutes. In other bacteremic infections, eg, subacute endocarditis, 3 blood specimens should be obtained over 24 hours. A total of 3 blood cultures yields the infecting bacteria in more than 95% of bacteremic patients. If the initial 3 cultures are negative and occult abscess, fever of unknown origin, or some other obscure infection is suspected, additional blood specimens should be cultured before antimicrobial therapy is started.

It is necessary to determine the significance of a positive blood culture. The following criteria may be helpful in differentiating "true positives" from contaminated specimens:

(1) Growth of the same organism in repeated cultures obtained at different times from separate anatomic sites strongly suggests true bacteremia.

(2) Growth of different organisms in different culture bottles suggests contamination but occasionally may follow clinical problems such as enterovascular fistulas.

(3) Growth of normal skin flora, eg, *Staphylococcus epidermidis*, diphtheroids (corynebacteria and propionibacteria), or anaerobic gram-positive cocci,

Table 32–4. Viral infections: Agents, specimens, and diagnostic tests (see also Table 34–2).

Syndrome and Virus	Specimen	Detection System*†	Serologic Tests†	Comments†
Respiratory diseases				
Influenza viruses	Nasopharyngeal washings or swab.	Cell culture (PMK), embryonated eggs.	CF, HI.	Virus detected by hemadsorption of guinea pig erythrocytes in 2–4 days. HI or FA used to identify virus.
Parainfluenza viruses	Nasopharyngeal washings or swab.	Cell culture (PMK).	CF, HI.	Virus detected by hemadsorption of guinea pig erythrocytes in 4–7 days. HI, FA, and HAI used to identify virus.
Respiratory syncytial virus	Nasopharyngeal washings or swab.	Cell culture (HEL, HEp-2).	CF, IFA.	CPE usually visible in 1–7 days.
Adenovirus	Nasopharyngeal washings or swab, feces, conjunctival swab.	Cell culture (HEp-2, HEK).	CF, HI.	CPE usually visible in 3–7 days. FA used to identify virus.
Enteroviruses	Nasopharyngeal washing or swab, feces.	Cell culture (PMK, HEL), suckling mice.	Neutralization.	Serologic tests are best done with virus isolated from patients; coxsackievirus A rarely grows in tissue culture.
Febrile diseases				
Dengue, other arboviruses	Serum, CSF, autopsy specimens, vector (*Aedes* mosquito).	Suckling mice, cell culture (Vero).	CF, HI, neutralization.	Many viruses in this group are highly infectious and easily transmissible to laboratory personnel. Some should only be studied in self-contained laboratories with controlled access.
Hemorrhagic fevers				
See Chapter 36.	Serum, blood.	Suckling mice, cell culture (Vero).	CF, HI, neutralization.	See comment for Febrile Diseases.
Lymphocytic choriomeningitis (LCM)				
LCM virus	Blood, CSF.	Cell culture (Vero, BHK), suckling mice.	IFA.	FA and neutralization in mice used for identification of virus.
Lassa Fever				
Lassa virus	Blood, nasopharyngeal swab, exudates.	Cell culture (Vero, BHK).	IFA, CF.	Lassa virus isolation is restricted to self-contained laboratories with controlled access.
Encephalitis				
Arboviruses	Serum, CSF, nasopharyngeal swab.	Suckling mice, cell culture (Vero).	CF, HI, neutralization.	See comment for Febrile Diseases.
Enteroviruses	Feces.	Cell culture (PMK, HEL).	Neutralization.	
Rabies virus	Saliva, brain biopsy.	Suckling mice, direct FA.	Neutralization, IFA.	Direct FA is preferable because speed of diagnosis is important for effective treatment.
Herpesvirus	Brain biopsy.	Cell culture (HEL, HEp-2), direct FA.	CF.	CPE usually visible in 24–72 hours.
Meningitis				
Enterovirus	Feces, CSF.	Cell culture (PMK, HEL).	Neutralization.	
Mumps virus	CSF, nasopharyngeal swab.	Cell culture (PMK).	CF, HI.	Virus detected by hemadsorption of guinea pig erythrocytes in 4–7 days. HAI and FA used to identify virus in culture.
Infectious mononucleosis				
Epstein-Barr (EB) virus	Blood, nasopharyngeal swab.	Lymphoid cell culture.	IFA, heterophil agglutination.	Culture of EB virus not performed routinely in clinical virology laboratories.
Cytomegalovirus	Blood, urine.	Cell culture (HEL).	IFA, CF.	Tissue culture tubes should be held 4 weeks.

*AGMK, African green monkey kidney; BHK, baby hampster kidney; HEK, human embryonic kidney; HEL, human embryonic lung; HEp-2, human epithelial cell; PMK, primary monkey kidney.

†CF, complement fixation; CPE, cytopathic effect; ELISA, enzyme-linked immunosorbent assay; FA, fluorescent antibody; HAI, hemadsorption inhibition; HI, hemagglutination inhibition; IFA, indirect fluorescent antibody; RIA, radioimmunoassay.

Table 32–4 (cont'd). Viral infections: Agents, specimens, and diagnostic tests (see also Table 34–2).

Syndrome and Virus	Specimen	Detection System*†	Serologic Tests†	Comments†
Hepatitis (See Chapter 38 for available and indicated tests.)				
Hepatitis A virus	Serum.	None.	ELISA, RIA.	
Hepatitis B virus	Serum.	ELISA, RIA.	ELISA, RIA.	
Hepatitis non-A, non-B virus	Liver biopsy.	Histology.	None.	Diagnose clinically by ruling out other causes of hepatitis.
Enteritis				
Rotavirus	Feces.	ELISA.	None.	
Norwalk agent	Feces.	Immune electron microscopy.	None.	
Echovirus	Feces.	Cell culture (HEL, PMK).	Neutralization.	Neutralization rarely done; usually requires paired sera and virus isolate from patient.
Exanthems				
Varicella virus	Vesicles.	Cell culture (HEK).	CF, IFA.	CPE usually visible in 4 days–2 weeks.
Measles (rubeola) virus	Nasopharyngeal swab, blood, urine, feces.	Cell culture (PMK).	CF, HI.	Usually CPE visible in 2–3 weeks.
Mumps virus	Nasopharyngeal swab.	Cell culture (PMK).	CF, HI.	See comment for Meningitis, above.
Rubella virus	Nasopharyngeal swab, blood.	Cell culture (AGMK).	ELISA, HI, CF.	Pass to new cell culture system after 2 weeks, and challenge second passage with echovirus to determine infection with rubella virus. Rubella virus cultures may not be routine procedures in many laboratories.
Monkeypox, cowpox, vaccinia, and tana-viruses	Vesicles.	Embryonated eggs, electron microscopy.	CF, neutralization.	
Herpes simplex	Vesicles, usually oral, labial, or genital.	Cell culture (HEK).	CF, neutralization.	Cultures usually become positive in 24–72 hours; direct FA is rapid.

*AGMK, African green monkey kidney; BHK, baby hampster kidney; HEK, human embryonic kidney; HEL, human embryonic lung; HEp-2, human epithelial cell; PMK, primary monkey kidney.

†CF, complement fixation; CPE, cytopathic effect; ELISA, enzyme-linked immunosorbent assay; FA, fluorescent antibody; HAI, hemadsorption inhibition; HI, hemagglutination inhibition; IFA, indirect fluorescent antibody; RIA, radioimmunoassay.

in only one of several cultures suggests contamination. Growth of such organisms in more than one culture or from specimens from a patient with a vascular prosthesis enhances the likelihood that clinically significant bacteremia exists.

(4) Organisms such as viridans streptococci or enterococci are likely to grow in blood cultures from patients suspected to have endocarditis, and gram-negative rods such as *E coli* in blood cultures from patients with clinical gram-negative sepsis; therefore, when such "expected" organisms are found, they are more apt to be etiologically significant.

Virtually every species of bacteria has been grown in blood cultures at some time. The following are most commonly found: staphylococci, including *Staphylococcus aureus*; viridans streptococci; enterococci, including *Streptococcus faecalis*; gram-negative enteric bacteria, including *E coli, K pneumoniae*, and *Pseudomonas aeruginosa*; pneumococci; and *H influenzae*. *Candida* species, other yeasts, and some biphasic fungi such as *Histoplasma capsulatum* grow in blood cultures, but many fungi are rarely, if ever, isolated from blood. Cytomegalovirus and herpes simplex virus can occasionally be cultured from blood, but most viruses and rickettsiae and chlamydiae are not cultured from blood. Parasitic protozoa and helminths usually do not grow in routine blood cultures.

In most types of bacteremia, examination of direct blood smears is not useful. Diligent examination of Gram-stained smears of the buffy coat from anticoagulated blood will occasionally show bacteria in patients with *S aureus* infection, clostridial sepsis, or relapsing fever. In some microbial infections (eg, anthrax, plague, relapsing fever, rickettsioses, leptospirosis, spirillosis, psittacosis), inoculation of blood into experimental animals may give positive results more readily than does culture.

Urine

Bacteriologic examination of the urine is done mainly when signs or symptoms point to urinary tract infection, renal insufficiency, or hypertension. It

Table 32–5. Normal bacteria flora (see Chapter 30).

Skin

1. *Staphylococcus epidermidis.*
2. *Staphylococcus aureus* (in small numbers).
3. *Micrococcus* species.
4. Nonpathogenic *Neisseria* species.
5. Alpha-hemolytic and nonhemolytic streptococci.
6. *Propionibacterium* species.
7. *Peptococcus* species.
8. Small numbers of other organisms (*Candida* species, *Acinetobacter* species, etc).

Nasopharynx

1. Any amount of the following: Diphtheroids, nonpathogenic *Neisseria* species, α-hemolytic streptococci; *Staphylococcus epidermidis*, nonhemolytic streptococci, anaerobes (too many species to list; varying amounts of *Bacteroides* species, anaerobic cocci, diphtheroids, *Fusobacterium* species, etc).
2. Lesser amounts of the following when accompanied by organisms listed above: yeasts, *Haemophilus* species, pneumococci, *Staphylococcus aureus*, gram-negative rods, *Neisseria meningitidis.*

Gastrointestinal tract and rectum

1. Various *Enterobacteriaceae* except *Salmonella, Shigella, Yersinia, Vibrio,* and *Campylobacter* species.
2. Non–dextrose-fermenting gram-negative rods.
3. Enterococci.
4. *Staphylococcus epidermidis.*
5. Alpha-hemolytic and nonhemolytic streptococci.
6. Diphtheroids.
7. *Staphylococcus aureus* in small numbers.
8. Yeasts in small numbers.
9. Anaerobes in large numbers (too many species to list).

Genitalia

1. Any amount of the following: *Corynebacterium* species, *Lactobacillus* species, α-hemolytic and nonhemolytic streptococci, nonpathogenic *Neisseria* species.
2. The following when mixed and not predominant: enterococci, *Enterobacteriaceae* and other gram-negative rods, *Staphylococcus epidermidis, Candida albicans* and other yeasts.
3. Anaerobes (too many species to list); the following may be important when in pure growth or clearly predominant: *Bacteroides, Clostridium, Peptostreptococcus,* and *Peptococcus* species.

should always be done in persons with suspected systemic infection or fever of unknown origin. It is desirable for every woman in the first trimester of pregnancy.

Urine secreted in the kidney is sterile unless the kidney is infected. Uncontaminated bladder urine is also normally sterile. The urethra, however, contains a normal flora, so that normal voided urine contains small numbers of bacteria. Because it is necessary to distinguish contaminating organisms from etiologically important organisms, only *quantitative* urine examination can yield meaningful results.

The following steps are essential in proper urine examination:

A. Proper Collection of Specimen: Proper collection of the specimen is the single most important step in a urine culture. Satisfactory specimens from males can usually be obtained by cleansing the meatus with soap and water and collecting midstream urine in a sterile container. Satisfactory midstream specimens from females can be obtained after spreading the labia and cleansing the vulva. Catheterization carries a risk of introducing microorganisms into the bladder, but it is sometimes unavoidable. Separate specimens from the right and left kidneys and ureters can be obtained by the urologist using a catheter at cystoscopy. When an indwelling catheter and closed collection system are in place, urine should be obtained by sterile aspiration of the catheter with needle and syringe, not from the collection bag. To resolve diagnostic problems, urine can be aspirated aseptically directly from the full bladder by means of suprapubic puncture of the abdominal wall.

For most examinations, 0.5 mL of ureteral urine or 5 mL of voided urine is sufficient. Because many types of microorganisms multiply rapidly in urine at room or body temperature, urine specimens must be delivered to the laboratory rapidly or refrigerated not longer than overnight.

B. Microscopic Examination: Much can be learned from simple microscopic examination of urine. A drop of fresh uncentrifuged urine placed on a slide, covered with a coverglass, and examined with restricted light intensity under the high-dry objective of an ordinary clinical microscope can reveal leukocytes, epithelial cells, and bacteria if more than 10^5/mL are present. Finding 10^5 organisms/mL in a properly collected and examined urine specimen is strong evidence of active urinary tract infection. A Gram-stained smear of uncentrifuged midstream urine that shows gram-negative rods is diagnostic of urinary tract infection.

Brief centrifugation of urine readily sediments pus cells, which may carry along bacteria and thus may help in microscopic diagnosis of infection. The presence of other formed elements in the sediment—or the presence of proteinuria—is of little direct aid in the specific identification of active urinary tract infection. Pus cells may be present without bacteria, and, conversely, bacteriuria may be present without pyuria. The presence of many squamous epithelial cells, lactobacilli, or mixed flora on culture suggests improper urine collection.

C. Culture: Culture of the urine, to be meaningful, must be performed quantitatively. Properly collected urine is cultured in measured amounts on solid media, and the colonies that appear after incubation are counted to indicate the number of bacteria per milliliter. The usual procedure is to spread 0.1 mL of undiluted urine on blood agar plates and other solid media for quantitative culture. All media are incubated overnight at 37 °C; growth density is then compared to photographs of different densities of growth for similar bacteria, yielding semiquantitative data. Several simplified methods are available to estimate the number of bacteria in urine (eg, Dip-Slide, spoon with agar, agar-coated pipette, calibrated loop for streaking).

In active pyelonephritis, the number of bacteria in urine collected by ureteral catheter is relatively low.

While accumulating in the bladder, bacteria multiply rapidly and soon reach numbers in excess of 10^5/mL —far more than could occur as a result of contamination by urethral or skin flora or from the air. Therefore, it is generally agreed that if more than 10^5 colonies/mL are cultivated from a properly collected and properly cultured urine specimen, this constitutes strong evidence of active urinary tract infection. The presence of more than 10^5 bacteria of the same type per milliliter in 2 consecutive specimens establishes a diagnosis of active infection of the urinary tract with 95% certainty. If fewer bacteria are cultivated, repeated examination of urine is indicated to establish the presence of infection.

If fewer than 10^4/mL are present (especially if there are several types), this suggests that the organisms come from normal flora or are contaminants. Intermediate counts (10^4–10^5/mL) do not permit definitive interpretation from a single specimen, and cultures must be repeated with a fresh specimen. Obtaining such counts repeatedly suggests persistent, chronic, or suppressed infection, but if they are found only in a single specimen, they suggest contamination. If cultures are negative but clinical signs of urinary tract infection are present, "urethral syndrome," ureteral obstruction, tuberculosis, or other disease must be considered.

Bacteria most commonly found in urinary tract infections are enteric and other gram-negative rods.

Cerebrospinal Fluid

Meningitis ranks high among medical emergencies, and early, rapid, and precise diagnosis is essential. Diagnosis of meningitis depends upon maintaining a high index of suspicion, securing adequate specimens properly, and examining the specimens promptly. Because the risk of death or irreversible damage is great unless treatment is started immediately, there is rarely a second chance to obtain pretreatment specimens, which are essential for specific etiologic diagnosis and optimal management.

The most urgent diagnostic issue is the differentiation of acute purulent bacterial meningitis from "aseptic" and granulomatous meningitis. The immediate decision is usually based on the cell count and the glucose and protein content of cerebrospinal fluid (Table 32–6) and the results of microscopic search for microorganisms. The initial impression is modified by the results of culture, serologic tests, and other laboratory procedures. Table 32–6 illustrates some typical findings. In evaluating the results of cerebrospinal fluid glucose determinations, the simultaneous blood glucose level must be considered. In some central nervous system neoplasms, the cerebrospinal fluid glucose level is low. In bacterial and fungal meningitis, the cerebrospinal fluid lactic acid level is often above 35 mg/dL.

A. Specimens: As soon as infection of the central nervous system is suspected, blood samples are taken for culture, and cerebrospinal fluid is obtained. To obtain cerebrospinal fluid, perform lumbar puncture with strict aseptic technique, taking care not to risk compression of the medulla by too rapid withdrawal of fluid when the intracranial pressure is markedly elevated. Cerebrospinal fluid is usually collected in 3–4 portions of 2–5 mL each, in sterile tubes. This permits the most convenient and reliable performance of tests to determine the several different values needed to plan a course of action.

B. Microscopic Examination: Smears are made from fresh uncentrifuged cerebrospinal fluid that appears cloudy or from the sediment of centrifuged cerebrospinal fluid. Smears are stained with Gram's stain and occasionally with Ziehl-Neelsen stain. Study of stained smears under the oil immersion objective may reveal intracellular gram-negative diplococci (meningococci), intra- and extracellular lancet-shaped gram-positive diplococci (pneumococci), or small gram-negative rods (H influenzae or enteric gram-negative rods). Cryptococci are best seen in India ink preparations.

Table 32–6. Typical cerebrospinal fluid findings in various central nervous system diseases.

Diagnosis	Cells (per μL)	Glucose (mg/dL)	Protein (mg/dL)	Opening Pressure	Remark Below
Normal	0–5 lymphocytes	45–85	15–45	70–180 mm H$_2$O	1
Purulent meningitis (bacterial)	200–20,000 PMNs	Low (<45)	High (>50)	++++	2
Granulomatous meningitis (mycobacterial, fungal)	100–1000, mostly lymphocytes	Low (<45)	High (>50)	+++	2, 3
Aseptic meningitis, viral or meningoencephalitis	100–1000, mostly lymphocytes	Normal	Moderately high (>50)	Normal to +	3, 4
Spirochetal meningitis (syphilis, leptospirosis)	25–2000, mostly lymphocytes	Normal or low	High (>50)	+	3
"Neighborhood" reaction	Variably increased	Normal	Normal or high	Variable	5

1. CSF glucose level must be considered in relation to blood glucose level. Normally, CSF glucose level is 20–30 mg/dL lower than blood glucose level, or 50–70% of blood glucose normal value.
2. Organisms in smear or culture of CSF; antigen detection tests may be diagnostic.
3. PMNs may predominate early.
4. Virus isolation from CSF early; antibody titer rise in paired specimens of serum.
5. May occur in mastoiditis, brain abscess, epidural abscess, sinusitis, septic thrombus, brain tumor. CSF culture usually negative.

C. Antigen Detection and Counterimmunoelectrophoresis: If stained smears fail to reveal the presence of a microorganism, specific antisera against important central nervous system pathogens can be used in latex particle agglutination or coagglutination tests. Agglutination suggests the causative organism and can help in the selection of early specific treatment. Cryptococcal antigen in cerebrospinal fluid may be detected by a latex agglutination test.

D. Culture: The culture methods used must favor the growth of microorganisms most commonly encountered in meningitis. Virus isolation can be attempted in aseptic meningitis or meningoencephalitis. The virus can be successfully isolated from the cerebrospinal fluid in infections caused by mumps virus, echo- or coxsackieviruses, and herpes simplex virus.

E. Follow-Up Examination of Cerebrospinal Fluid: The return of the cerebrospinal fluid glucose level and cell count toward normal is good evidence of adequate therapy. The clinical response is of paramount importance.

Respiratory Secretions

Symptoms or signs often point to involvement of a particular part of the respiratory tract, and specimens are chosen accordingly. In interpreting laboratory results, it is necessary to consider the normal microbial flora of the area from which the specimen was collected.

A. Specimens:

1. Throat–Most "sore throats" are due to viral infection. Only 5–10% of "sore throats" in adults and 15–20% in children are associated with bacterial infections. The finding of a follicular yellowish exudate or a grayish membrane must arouse the suspicion that Lancefield group A β-hemolytic streptococcal, diphtherial, fusospirochetal (Vincent's), or candidal infection exists; such signs may also be present in infectious mononucleosis and herpesvirus, adenovirus, and other virus infections.

Throat swabs must be taken from each tonsillar area before a swab is taken from the posterior pharyngeal wall. The normal throat flora includes an abundance of viridans streptococci, neisseriae, diphtheroids, staphylococci, small gram-negative rods, and many other organisms. Microscopic examination of smears from throat swabs is of little value in streptococcal infections, because all throats harbor a predominance of streptococci, but it can help identify fusospirochetal disease.

Cultures of throat swabs are most reliable if inoculated promptly after collection. Media selective for streptococci can be used to culture for group A organisms. In streaking selective media or blood agar culture plates, it is essential to spread a small inoculum thoroughly and avoid overgrowth by normal flora. This can be done readily by touching the throat swab to one small area of the plate and using a second, sterile applicator (or sterile bacteriologic loop) to streak the plate from that area. Detection of β-hemolytic colonies is facilitated by slashing the agar (to provide reduced oxygen tension) and incubating the plate for 2 days at 37 °C.

Laboratory reports on throat cultures should state the types of prevalent organisms. If potential pathogens (eg, β-hemolytic streptococci) are found on cultures, their approximate number is important. In "strep throat," group A streptococci prevail. A few colonies of β-hemolytic streptococci may well represent only "transients" in the throat and have no pathogenic meaning. Group A β-hemolytic streptococci often are present in cultures when patients have diseases such as diphtheria or infectious mononucleosis.

2. Nasopharynx–Specimens from the nasopharynx are studied infrequently because special techniques must be used to obtain them. (See Viral Diagnosis, below.) Whooping cough is diagnosed by culture of B pertussis from a nasopharyngeal swab specimen or nasal washings.

3. Middle ear–Specimens are rarely obtained from the middle ear because puncture of the drum is necessary. In acute otitis media, 30–50% of aspirated fluids are bacteriologically sterile. The most frequently isolated bacteria are pneumococci, H influenzae, and hemolytic streptococci.

4. Lower respiratory tract–Bronchial and pulmonary secretions or exudates are often studied by examining sputum. The most misleading aspect of sputum examination is the almost inevitable contamination with saliva and mouth flora. Thus, finding Candida, S aureus, or even S pneumoniae in the sputum of a patient with pneumonitis has no etiologic significance unless supported by the clinical picture. Meaningful sputum specimens should be expectorated from the lower respiratory tract and should be grossly distinct from saliva. The presence of many squamous epithelial cells suggests heavy contamination with saliva; a large number of polymorphonuclear leukocytes (PMNs) suggests a purulent exudate. Sputum may be induced by the inhalation of heated hypertonic saline aerosol for several minutes. In pneumonia accompanied by pleural fluid, the pleural fluid may yield the causative organisms more reliably than does sputum. Most community-acquired bacterial pneumonias are caused by pneumococci. In suspected tuberculosis or fungal infection, gastric washings (swallowed sputum) may yield organisms when expectorated material fails to do so.

5. Transtracheal aspiration, bronchoscopy, lung biopsy, bronchoalveolar lavage–The flora in such specimens often reflects accurately the events in the lower respiratory tract. Specimens obtained by bronchoscopy or open lung biopsy may be necessary in the diagnosis of Pneumocystis pneumonia or infection due to Legionella or other organisms.

B. Microscopic Examination: Smears of purulent flecks or granules from sputum stained by Gram's stain or acid-fast methods may reveal causative organisms and PMNs. Some organisms (eg, Actinomyces) are best seen in unstained wet preparations. A direct "quellung" test for pneumococci can be performed with polyvalent serum on fresh sputum.

C. Culture: The media used for sputum cultures must be suitable for the growth of bacteria (eg, pneumococci, *Klebsiella*), fungi (eg, *Coccidioides immitis*), mycobacteria (eg, *M tuberculosis*), and other organisms. Specimens obtained by bronchoscopy and lung biopsy should also be cultured on other media (eg, for anaerobes, *Legionella*, and others). The relative prevalence of different organisms in the specimen must be estimated. Only a finding of one predominant organism or the simultaneous isolation of an organism from both sputum and blood can clearly establish its role in a pneumonic or suppurative process.

D. Viral Diagnosis: Most upper respiratory tract infections are caused by viruses. Throat swabs, throat washings, and sputum are fertile sources of virus if specialized laboratory facilities for virus isolation are available. Throat swabs immersed in broth, specimens obtained by gargling with broth, or sputum samples must be brought to the virus laboratory promptly or kept refrigerated or frozen until they are inoculated into cell cultures.

To support the possible causative role of viral agents, a rise in specific antibody titer must be demonstrated. Serum specimens are obtained aseptically as early as possible in the disease and again 2–3 weeks later. The first serum specimen is refrigerated until the second specimen has been secured, and both serum samples are then submitted to the virus laboratory at the same time, with an adequate clinical description, for specific serologic diagnosis.

Gastrointestinal Tract Specimens

Acute symptoms referable to the gastrointestinal tract, particularly nausea, vomiting, and diarrhea, are commonly attributed to infection. In reality, most such attacks are caused by intolerance to food or drink, enterotoxins (Table 18–4), drugs, or systemic illnesses.

Many cases of acute infectious diarrhea are due to viruses. On the other hand, many viruses (eg, adenoviruses, enteroviruses) can multiply in the gut without causing gastrointestinal symptoms. Similarly, some enteric bacterial pathogens may persist in the gut following an acute infection. Thus, it may be difficult to assign significance to a bacterial or viral agent cultured from the stool, especially in subacute or chronic illness.

These considerations should not discourage the physician from attempting laboratory isolation of enteric organisms but should constitute a warning of some common difficulties in interpreting the results.

The lower bowel has an exceedingly large normal bacterial flora. The most prevalent organisms are anaerobes (*Bacteroides*, gram-positive rods, and streptococci), gram-negative enteric organisms, and *S faecalis*. Any attempt to recover pathogenic bacteria from feces involves separation of pathogens from the normal flora, usually through the use of differential selective media and enrichment cultures. Important causes of acute gastrointestinal upsets include viruses, toxins (of staphylococci, clostridia, vibrios, toxigenic

E coli), invasive enteric gram-negative rods, slow lactose fermenters, shigellae and salmonellae, and campylobacteria. The relative importance of these groups of organisms differs greatly in various parts of the world.

A. Specimens: Feces and rectal swabs are the most readily available specimens. Bile obtained by duodenal drainage may reveal infection of the biliary tract. The presence of blood, mucus, or helminths must be noted on gross inspection of the specimen. Leukocytes seen in suspensions of stool examined microscopically are a useful means of differentiating invasive from noninvasive infectious diarrheas. Special techniques must be used to search for parasitic protozoa and helminths and their ova. Stained smears may reveal a prevalence of leukocytes and certain abnormal organisms, eg, *Candida* or staphylococci, but they cannot be used to differentiate enteric bacterial pathogens from normal flora.

B. Culture: Specimens are suspended in broth and cultured on ordinary as well as differential media (eg, MacConkey agar, EMB agar) to permit separation of non-lactose-fermenting gram-negative rods from other enteric bacteria. If *Salmonella* infection (typhoid fever or paratyphoid fever) is suspected, the specimen is also placed in an enrichment medium (eg, selenite F broth) for 18 hours before being plated on differential media (eg, Hektoen enteric or *Shigella-Salmonella* agar). *Yersinia enterocolitica* is more likely to be isolated after storage of fecal suspensions for 2 weeks at 4 °C, but it can be isolated on *Yersinia* or *Shigella-Salmonella* agar incubated at 25 °C. Vibrios grow best on thiosulfate citrate bile salts sucrose agar. Campylobacteria are isolated on Campy-BAP or Skirrow's selective medium incubated at 40–42 °C in 5% CO_2 with greatly reduced O_2 tension. Bacterial colonies are identified by standard bacteriologic methods, and blood is drawn from the patient for serologic diagnosis. Agglutination of bacteria from suspect colonies by pooled specific antiserum is often the fastest way to establish the presence of salmonellae or shigellae in the intestinal tract. A rise in the titer of specific serum antibody often supports the diagnosis of *Salmonella* infection.

Gastric washings represent swallowed sputum and may be cultured for tubercle bacilli and other mycobacteria on special media (see Chapter 26). For virus isolation, fecal specimens are submitted; paired serum specimens can be submitted later.

Intestinal parasites and their ova are discovered by repeated microscopic study of fresh fecal specimens. The specimens require special handling in the laboratory (see Chapter 48).

Wounds, Tissues, Bones, Abscesses, Fluids

Microscopic study of smears and culture of specimens from wounds or abscesses may often give early and important indications of the nature of the infecting organism and thus help in the choice of antimicrobial drugs. Specimens from tissue biopsies obtained for diagnostic purposes should be submitted for bacteriologic as well as histologic examination. Such specimens for bacteriologic examination are kept away from fixatives and disinfectants, minced and finely ground, and cultured by a variety of methods.

The pus in closed, undrained soft tissue abscesses frequently contains only one organism as the causative agent—most commonly staphylococci, streptococci, or enteric gram-negative rods. The same is true in acute osteomyelitis, where the organisms can often be cultured from blood before the local lesion has become chronic. Because a multitude of microorganisms are frequently encountered in abdominal abscesses and abscesses contiguous with mucosal surfaces as well as in open wounds, it is difficult to decide which organisms are significant in such cases. When deep suppurating lesions drain onto exterior surfaces through a sinus or fistula, the flora of the surface through which the lesion drains must not be mistaken for that of the deep lesion.

Bacteriologic examination of pus from closed or deep lesions must include culture by anaerobic methods. Anaerobic bacteria (*Bacteroides*, streptococci) sometimes play an essential causative role, and mixtures of anaerobes are often present, whereas aerobes may represent surface contaminants. The typical wound infections due to clostridia are readily suspected in gas gangrene.

The methods used must be suitable for the semiquantitative recovery of common bacteria and also for recovery of specialized microorganisms including mycobacteria and fungi. Eroded skin and mucous membranes are frequently the sites of yeast or fungus infections. *Candida, Aspergillus*, and other yeasts or fungi can be seen microscopically in smears or scrapings from suspicious areas and can be grown in cultures.

Exudates that have collected in the pleural, peritoneal, or synovial spaces must be aspirated with meticulous aseptic technique to avoid superinfection. If the material is frankly purulent, smears and cultures are made directly. If the fluid is clear, it can be centrifuged at high speed for 10 minutes and the sediment used for stained smears and cultures. The culture method used must be suitable for the growth of organisms suspected on clinical grounds—eg, mycobacteria, anaerobic organisms, neisseriae—as well as the commonly encountered pyogenic bacteria. Although direct tests for causative microorganisms yield the most important information, tests on oxalated fluids are also helpful. The following results are suggestive of infection: specific gravity > 1.018; protein content > 3 g/dL, often resulting in clotting; and cell counts > 500–1000/μL. Polymorphonuclear leukocytes predominate in acute untreated pyogenic infections; lymphocytes or monocytes predominate in chronic infections. Transudates resulting from neoplastic growth may grossly resemble infectious exudates by appearing bloody or purulent and by clotting on standing. Cytologic study of smears or of sections of centrifuged cells may prove the neoplastic nature of the process.

Genital Lesions

Gonorrhea, nongonococcal urethritis (chlamydial or mycoplasmal), and herpes simplex are prominent among the infections associated with local lesions of the external genitalia, discharge, and regional adenopathy. Syphilis, chancroid, lymphogranuloma venereum, and granuloma inguinale are less common but important diseases. Each has a characteristic natural history and evolution of lesions, but one can mimic another. The laboratory diagnosis of most of these infections is covered elsewhere in this book. A few diagnostic tests are listed below and outlined in Table 32–2.

A. Gonorrhea: A stained smear of urethral or cervical exudate shows intracellular gram-negative diplococci. Exudate, rectal swab, or throat swab must be plated promptly on special media to yield *N gonorrhoeae*. Serologic tests are not helpful.

B. Chlamydial Genital Infections: The genital tract is the usual source of many types of *Chlamydia trachomatis*, which can produce either asymptomatic or symptomatic infection. Symptomatic infections include nongonococcal urethritis (NGU), epididymitis, cervicitis, salpingitis, pelvic inflammatory disease, and lymphogranuloma venereum. These infections are sexually transmitted and may spread readily to the eye to produce inclusion conjunctivitis, which resembles trachoma.

Culture of exudates or secretions in specially treated cells may permit isolation of chlamydiae. When stained with Giemsa's stain or immunofluorescence stain and examined microscopically, smears of exudate or scrapings from the eye may reveal typical crescent-shaped inclusions in epithelial cells (see Chapter 29). Direct fluorescent antibody stains of urethral and endocervical exudates are more widely available than culture for diagnosis of chlamydial infection, but they are slightly less sensitive than culture.

Serologic tests (CF or microimmunofluorescence with group-reactive or immunotype-specific antigens) can be performed to show rising antibody titers in sera obtained at intervals of several weeks. Although skin tests can indicate past infection with *C trachomatis*, they have been abandoned because of inadequate specificity of the antigens.

C. Herpes Progenitalis: Primary or recurrent herpetic vesicles, evolving to ulcers and crusts and resembling the common "cold sores" on lips or skin, may occur on the genitalia. A positive diagnosis depends upon finding typical multinucleated giant cells or immunofluorescence in scrapings from the ulcer base or upon isolating and identifying herpes simplex virus from the aspirated contents of the vesicle. Monoclonal antibodies can be used for direct fluorescent antibody tests and to differentiate herpes simplex type I from type II. Culture is the best test for diagnosis; positive cultures are detected after 24–48 hours of incubation. A significant rise in antibody titer occurs during the primary infection.

D. Syphilis: Darkfield or immunofluorescence examination of tissue fluid expressed from the base of the chancre may reveal typical *T pallidum*. Serologic tests for syphilis become positive 3–6 weeks after infection. A positive flocculation test (eg, VDRL) requires confirmation. A positive immunofluorescent treponemal antibody test (eg, FTA-ABS) (see Chapter 27) proves syphilitic infection.

E. Chancroid: Smears from a suppurating lesion usually show a mixed bacterial flora. Swabs from lesions can be cultured on chocolate agar containing 1% Isovitalex and vancomycin, 3 μg/mL, to grow *Haemophilus ducreyi*. Serologic tests are rarely done.

F. Granuloma Inguinale: *Calymmatobacterium (Donovania) granulomatis*, the causative agent of this hard, granulomatous, proliferating lesion, can be grown in complex bacteriologic media, but this is rarely attempted in practice. Histologic demonstration of intracellular "Donovan bodies" in biopsy material most frequently supports the clinical impression. Serologic tests are not helpful.

G. Vaginitis: Vaginitis (bacterial vaginosis) associated with *G vaginalis* or *Mobiluncus* (see Chapter 24) is diagnosed in the examining room by inspection of the vaginal discharge; the discharge (1) is grayish and sometimes frothy, (2) has a pH above 4.6, (3) has an amine ("fishy") odor when alkalinized with potassium hydroxide, and (4) contains "clue cells," large epithelial cells covered with gram-negative or gram-variable rods. Similar observations are used to diagnose *Trichomonas vaginalis* (see Chapter 48) infection; the motile organisms can be seen in wet-mount preparations or cultured from genital discharge. *Candida albicans* vaginitis is diagnosed by finding pseudohyphae in a potassium hydroxide preparation of the vaginal discharge.

ANAEROBIC INFECTIONS

A large majority of the bacteria that make up the normal human flora are anaerobes (Table 32–5). When displaced from their normal sites into tissues or body spaces, anaerobes may produce disease. Certain characteristics are suggestive of anaerobic infections: (1) They are often contiguous with a mucosal surface. (2) They tend to involve mixtures of organisms. (3) They tend to form closed-space infections, either as discrete abscesses (lung, brain, pleura, peritoneum, pelvis) or by burrowing through tissue layers. (4) Pus from anaerobic infections often has a foul odor. (5) Most of the pathogenetically important anaerobes except *Bacteroides* are highly susceptible to penicillin G. (6) Anaerobic infections are favored by reduced blood supply, necrotic tissue, and a low oxidation-reduction potential—all of which also interfere with delivery of antimicrobial drugs. (7) It is essential to use special collection methods, transport media, and sensitive anaerobic techniques and media to isolate the organisms. Otherwise, bacteriologic examination may be negative or yield only incidental aerobes.

The following are sites of important anaerobic infections.

Respiratory Tract

Periodontal infections, perioral abscesses, sinusitis, and mastoiditis may involve predominantly *Bacteroides melaninogenicus, Fusobacterium,* and peptostreptococci. Aspiration of saliva (containing up to 10⁸ of these organisms) may result in necrotizing pneumonia, lung abscess, and empyema. Antimicrobial drugs and postural or surgical drainage are essential for treatment.

Central Nervous System

Anaerobes rarely produce meningitis but are common causes of brain abscess, subdural empyema, and septic thrombophlebitis. The organisms usually originate in the respiratory tract via extension or hematogenous spread.

Intra-Abdominal & Pelvic Infections

The flora of the colon consists predominantly of anaerobes, 10¹¹ per gram of feces. *Bacteroides fragilis*, clostridia, and peptostreptococci play a main role in abscess formation originating in perforation of the bowel. *Bacteroides bivius* and *Bacteroides disiens* are important in abscesses of the pelvis originating in the female genital organs. Like *B fragilis*, these *Bacteroides* species are often relatively resistant to penicillin; therefore, clindamycin, cefoxitin, or another effective agent should be used.

Bacteremia & Endocarditis

About 5% of these infections are now caused by anaerobes originating in the gut or the female genital tract. Specific bacteriologic diagnosis is essential for optimal treatment. Otherwise, the rate of treatment failure may be high.

Skin & Soft Tissue Infections

Anaerobes and aerobic bacteria often join to form synergistic infections (gangrene, necrotizing fasciitis, cellulitis). Surgical drainage, excision, and improved circulation are the most important forms of treatment, while antimicrobial drugs act as adjuncts. It is usually difficult to pinpoint one specific organism as being responsible for the progressive lesion, since mixtures of organisms are usually involved.

LABORATORY AIDS IN THE SELECTION OF ANTIMICROBIAL THERAPY

The first antimicrobial drug used in the treatment of an infection is chosen on the basis of clinical impression after the physician is convinced that an infection exists and has made a tentative etiologic diagnosis on clinical grounds. On the basis of this "best guess," a probable drug of choice can be selected (see Chapter 10). Before the probable drug of choice is administered, specimens are obtained for laboratory isolation of the causative agent. The results of these examinations may necessitate selection of a different drug. The identification of certain microorganisms that are uniformly drug-susceptible eliminates the necessity for further testing and permits the selection of optimally effective drugs solely on the basis of experience. Under other circumstances, tests for drug susceptibility of isolated microorganisms may be helpful (see Chapter 10).

The commonly performed disk diffusion susceptibility test must be used judiciously and interpreted with restraint. In general, only one member of each major class of drugs is represented. For staphylococci, penicillin G, nafcillin, cephalothin, erythromycin, gentamicin, and vancomycin are used. For gram-negative rods, ampicillin, cephalothin and second- and third-generation cephalosporins, ticarcillin and newer "antipseudomonal penicillins," chloramphenicol, trimethoprim-sulfamethoxazole, and the aminoglycosides (amikacin, tobramycin, gentamicin) are included. For urinary tract infections with gram-negative rods, nitrofurantoin, nalidixic acid and other quinolones, and trimethoprim may be added. The choice of drugs to be included in a routine susceptibility test battery should be based on the susceptibility patterns of isolates in the laboratory, the type of infection (community-acquired or nosocomial), and cost-efficacy analysis for the patient population.

Isolates of *H influenzae, N gonorrhoeae*, and *Bacteroides* species (except *B fragilis*) should be tested for β-lactamase production. Isolates of *B fragilis* might be tested for susceptibility to clindamycin and cefoxitin.

Methenamine salts (eg, methenamine mandelate) should never be used in a disk test. If sulfonamides (or their combinations) are to be tested by disk, the media must be free of PABA.

The sizes of zones of growth inhibition vary with the molecular characteristics of different drugs. Thus, the zone size of one drug cannot be compared to the zone size of another drug acting on the same organism. However, for any one drug the zone size can be compared to a standard, provided that media, inoculum size, and other conditions are carefully regulated. This makes it possible to define for each drug a minimum diameter of inhibition zone that denotes "susceptibility" of an isolate by the Kirby-Bauer technique.

The disk test measures the ability of drugs to *inhibit* the growth of microorganisms. Its results correlate reasonably well with therapeutic response in those disease processes where body defenses can frequently eliminate infectious microorganisms.

In a few types of human infections, the results of disk tests are of little assistance (and may be misleading) because a *bactericidal* drug effect is required for cure. Outstanding examples are infective endocarditis, acute osteomyelitis, and severe infections in a host whose antibacterial defenses are inadequate, eg, persons with neoplastic diseases that have been treated with radiation and antineoplastic chemotherapy, or persons who are being given corticosteroids in high dosage and are immunosuppressed.

Instead of the disk test, a semiquantitative test procedure can be used. It measures more exactly the concentration of an antibiotic necessary to inhibit growth of a standardized inoculum under defined conditions. In the past, this procedure employed individual tubes of broth. At present, a semiautomated microtiter method is used in which defined amounts of drug are dissolved in a measured small volume of broth and inoculated with a standardized number of microorganisms. The end point, or minimum inhibitory concentration (MIC), is considered the last broth cup remaining clear, ie, free from microbial growth. The minimum inhibitory concentration provides a better estimate of the probable amount of drug necessary to inhibit growth in vivo and thus helps in gauging the dosage regimen necessary for the patient.

In addition, bactericidal effects can be estimated by subculturing the clear broth onto antibiotic-free solid media. The result, eg, a reduction of colony-forming units by 99.9% below that of the control, is called the minimal bactericidal concentration (MBC).

The selection of a bactericidal drug or drug combination for each patient can be guided by specialized laboratory tests. Such tests measure either the rate of killing or the proportion of the microbial population that is killed in a fixed time.

Evaluation of the chemotherapeutic regimen in vivo can be performed by **serum assay** (see Chapter 10). This procedure consists of the following steps:

(1) An etiologic microorganism is isolated.

(2) Antimicrobial therapy is started.

(3) Blood is drawn from the patient receiving treatment at the time a peak or a trough (ie, maximum or minimum concentration of drug) is expected.

(4) Dilutions of the separated serum are tested for their ability to kill in vitro the microorganisms isolated from the patient.

This test can sometimes help decide whether the patient is receiving the proper drug in adequate amounts or whether the regimen should be altered.

In urinary tract infections, the antibacterial activity of urine is far more important than that of serum. The disappearance of infecting organisms from the urine during treatment can serve as a partial drug level assay.

In persons with renal impairment who must receive nephrotoxic drugs and in other special clinical cases, the concentration of drug in serum can be estimated by an assay of serum against special test microorganisms or, even better, by chemical or radioimmunoassay methods.

SEROLOGIC TESTS & THE DEMONSTRATION OF SPECIFIC ANTIBODY

In the course of many infections, serum antibodies are acquired relatively early, as microorganisms multiply, and these antibodies may persist for months or years. Thus, the serologic demonstration of antibody indicates effective exposure (by infection or vaccination) at some time in the past but may have no bearing on the current illness. For the diagnosis of a current infection, it is often necessary to demonstrate an increase in antibody concentration, ie, a rise of antibody level in the second of 2 blood specimens obtained at an interval of 10–20 days. The 2 specimens of sera must be examined simultaneously in the same test for meaningful results. Blood specimens must be taken aseptically and the serum separated with sterile precautions.

Diagnostic antibody titers are sometimes obtained in the following infections.

Amebiasis

Latex particles or red blood cells coated with *Entamoeba histolytica* antigens are agglutinated by serum in invasive amebiasis. Gel diffusion or counterimmunoelectrophoresis may reveal antibodies.

Brucellosis

During the acute infection, agglutinating antibodies appear; later, blocking (prozone, see p 266) IgA and IgG antibodies can be observed. Agglutinating IgM antibodies persist for years without manifest activity of the disease. The diagnosis of active brucellosis is suggested by the presence of IgG (over 1:80) agglutinating antibodies. Cross-reaction with tularemia is common.

Chlamydial Infections (Psittacosis [Ornithosis], Lymphogranuloma Venereum, Trachoma, Inclusion Conjunctivitis)

Antibodies to the group antigen often become demonstrable by CF tests within 2–4 weeks after symptoms appear. These antibodies cannot differentiate one infection of the group from another. Some group-reactive and species-specific antibodies can be found by the microimmunofluorescence test (see Chapter 29).

Coccidioidomycosis

Soon after the initial infection, precipitating and CF antibodies to *C immitis* appear. In the absence of complications, these tend to subside to very low levels within months. Dissemination of the infection is accompanied by a rising titer of CF antibodies ($> 1:32$), which carries a grave prognosis. Immunodiffusion (counterimmunoelectrophoresis) can be used as a screening test.

Mycoplasmal Pneumonia

In pneumonitis caused by *Mycoplasma pneumoniae*, cold agglutinins develop in the serum during the illness. These are substances that are capable of agglutinating human group O cells at 4 °C but not at 20 or 37 °C. Specific antibodies to *M pneumoniae* can be detected by CF, growth inhibition, or hemagglutination inhibition tests. CF is the most useful test and is more readily available than culture.

Histoplasmosis

Precipitating and CF antibodies to antigens of *H capsulatum* usually appear within 3–4 weeks of acute infection and, in the absence of complications, revert to low levels. If the infection disseminates and progresses, the CF titer rises in successive serum samples. Immunodiffusion tests for H and M precipitins (see p 328) can be useful. The histoplasmin skin test can cause elevation of serologic titers. Isolation of the fungus is the test of choice.

Infectious Mononucleosis

This disease is caused by the Epstein-Barr (EB) virus. Diagnosis of the clinically suggestive case usually rests on the identification of representative "atypical" lymphocytes in blood smears and on results of the "heterophil agglutination" test or commercial mononucleosis spot tests. The heterophil agglutination test is a nonspecific reaction: persons suffering from infectious mononucleosis develop a high titer (usually $> 1:40$) of antibodies that agglutinate fresh washed sheep red blood cells or horse red cells. Similar agglutinating antibodies appear in a variety of hypersensitivity reactions but can be differentiated by absorption tests. The mononucleosis agglutinins cannot be absorbed by boiled guinea pig kidney, whereas agglutinins following other reactions are removed by this absorption. Commercial mononucleosis spot tests combine these reactions and yield sensitive and specific results.

In special laboratories, antibodies to EB virus can be demonstrated in sera of mononucleosis patients by immunofluorescence. (See Chapter 44.)

Leptospirosis

Agglutination tests give very high titers (often over 1:1000) following infection. Serologic testing for diagnosis of leptospirosis is often more useful than culture.

Parasitic Diseases

In cysticercosis, trichinosis, echinococcosis, and other parasitic infections, CF, precipitation, or hemagglutination inhibition tests are occasionally employed for diagnosis.

Plague, Tularemia

Agglutination titers of 1:20 or higher, particularly with rising titers, can support the clinical diagnosis of acute infection. Low titers suggest cross-reactions (eg, with *Brucella* or *Shigella* organisms) or long-past infection.

Rickettsioses

CF, microagglutination, and immunofluorescence tests permit the demonstration of type-specific antibody rise if specific antigens are available. The Weil-Felix test (see p 302), which is based on the fact that various strains of *Proteus* organisms share certain antigens with the rickettsiae, is outmoded.

Salmonellosis
(Typhoid Fever, Enteric Fever)

A rising agglutination titer to O antigens is suggestive of active infection. Antibodies to H antigens occur commonly with vaccination and may persist for years. In previously vaccinated individuals with residual O or H titers, there may be no further titer rise with active infection. Serology is not very useful in the diagnosis of typhoid fever or other *Salmonella* infections. Cultures are preferred.

Streptococcal Infections
& Poststreptococcal Disease

Persons infected with β-hemolytic streptococci develop antibodies to a variety of streptococcal antigens and extracellular products. Most conveniently, antibodies to streptolysin O can be detected. If antistreptolysin O (ASO) is repeatedly found to be present in titers exceeding 166 units, this suggests recent infection with β-hemolytic streptococci or rheumatic disease. Antistreptolysin formation is readily suppressed by early and adequate penicillin therapy.

Syphilis

Serologic tests for syphilis employ either treponemal or nontreponemal antigens. Nontreponemal tests are based on the accidental relationship between lipid extracts of mammalian tissue and reagin, a substance that develops in the serum of persons after treponemal infection. Flocculation tests (VDRL, RPR) are standardized and can be automated. All of these tests estimate the presence of reagin and are therefore subject to false-positive results. The latter are particularly frequent in various infectious and febrile disorders, in collagen diseases, and after vaccinations. Nontreponemal tests can be performed in a quantitative manner if desired. Most biologic false-positive results are of low titer. Nontreponemal positive tests tend to revert to negative in adequately treated syphilis.

Treponemal tests are based on the reaction between treponemal suspensions and specific antitreponemal antibodies. The fluorescent treponemal antibody (FTA-ABS) test, which has high specificity and good sensitivity, is most commonly employed. It becomes positive early in syphilitic infection and tends to remain positive for years after adequate treatment. A treponemal hemagglutination (TPHA) test has similar sensitivity and specificity.

Toxoplasmosis

Toxoplasma gondii, a crescent-shaped protozoon, can be isolated with difficulty by inoculating mice with lymph node material taken from patients with acute infection. Several serologic tests can be applied. The dye test depends upon the ability of antibodies to prevent the uptake of methylene blue by living *Toxoplasma* organisms. The test results become positive (frequently > 1:1000) in 2–4 weeks after toxoplasmosis is acquired and may remain positive for years. In congenital toxoplasmosis, the dye test is often positive. The CF test becomes positive (up to 1:100) in 4–8 weeks and declines to very low levels in a few months. Immunofluorescent antibody tests in low titer indicate only past infection, but high titers (1:10,000 or more) suggest recent infection. Immunofluorescence tests for IgM antibody reveal congenital infection in newborns. Interpretation of positive high-titer tests in single samples of serum of adults must take into account the high frequency of asymptomatic infection.

Trichinosis

For the diagnosis of acute trichinosis, a bentonite flocculation test is useful. Bentonite particles coated with *Trichinella spiralis* antigen may be agglutinated to high titer by the serum of persons infected for 2 weeks or more.

Viral Infections

The diagnosis of viral infections is discussed in detail in Chapters 34 and 35.

SKIN TESTS

Under the antigenic stimulus of an infectious agent, the host may develop hypersensitivity, manifested by delayed type skin reactivity, to one or more antigens of that agent. The controlled application of known antigens can therefore give evidence of infection and serve as a valuable diagnostic aid. A positive skin reaction indicates only that the individual has, at some time in the past, been infected with the specific agent. It provides information about the relationship of a specific agent to a *current* illness only if conversion from a negative to a positive skin test occurs during or just preceding the current illness. The general skin reactivity declines markedly (anergy) during far-advanced stages of many infections and is a regular feature of sarcoidosis, Hodgkin's disease, and some childhood exanthematous diseases (eg, measles). Similarly, skin reactivity may be suppressed by the administration of corticosteroids or immunosuppressant drugs.

Most skin test reagents are not pure antigens but a complex mixture of potentially reactive substances. For proper interpretation, it is essential to include suitable control materials in the test. Both immediate and delayed skin reactions may occur with some skin test preparations. In general, the delayed reaction is the only meaningful one for the diagnosis of specific infection.

In a properly performed test, the entire test volume (usually 0.1 mL) of the standardized preparation must be injected intracutaneously. Unless the injection raises a well-circumscribed bleb, it is likely that part of the test volume has escaped into the subcutaneous tissue or onto the surface. This will diminish the reliability of the test. (Patch tests occasionally used in small children are not very reliable.) In most instances, the test should be read at 48 hours; additional readings at 24 and 72 hours are sometimes helpful.

The size of induration is the only important criterion of positive readings; erythema alone is not meaningful. When several strengths of test preparation are available, the smallest concentration of antigen must be injected initially, followed by increasingly higher concentrations if the previous test result was negative.

Diagnostic skin tests are sometimes applied in the following clinical conditions.

Candida

Candida antigens are used in skin tests to ascertain the individual's ability to respond with a delayed type hypersensitivity reaction as an indicator of active cell-mediated reactivity. Virtually all normal adults react positively.

Cat-Scratch Disease

Pus from active cases, diluted 1:5 and heated at 60 °C for 10 hours, can be used as a skin test antigen. It gives a positive reaction in some individuals with a typical clinical picture. The nature of the causative agent and the significance of the test are not known.

Coccidioidomycosis

Coccidioidin is a filtered, concentrated broth in which mycelium of *C immitis* has been grown for long periods. The usual test dilution is 1:100, and a positive reaction (more than 5 mm of induration) occurs in 24–48 hours. In 1:10 dilution, the material often gives cross-reactions with other fungal antigens. Positive skin tests commonly denote past subclinical infection and significant specific resistance to reinfection. A skin test with spherulin (derived from culture-grown spherules rather than from mycelium) is more sensitive but less specific.

Echinococcosis

The injection of inactivated hydatid fluid (Casoni reaction) obtained from human or animal cases may give both immediate and delayed reactions in individuals with *Echinococcus* infection. The test is less reliable than demonstration of antibody by immunoelectrophoresis.

Histoplasmosis

Histoplasmin is a concentrated filtrate prepared from broth in which *H capsulatum* has been grown for long periods. The usual test dilution is 1:100, and a positive reaction (more than 5 mm of induration) occurs in 24–48 hours. Cross-reactions with other fungal products occur relatively frequently. Positive skin tests commonly denote past subclinical infection and significant specific resistance to reinfection. The skin test may raise the antibody titer.

Leishmaniasis

Leishmanin is an inactivated suspension of cultured flagellate *Leishmania*. A positive delayed skin test to this preparation develops within 6–12 weeks after many *Leishmania* infections and remains positive for life. The test is often negative in active kala-azar but becomes positive after effective chemotherapy.

Leprosy

Lepromin, a standardized homogenate of lepromatous skin nodules, has no diagnostic value. Normal persons may react. However, in a person with known leprosy, a positive lepromin test is diagnostic of tuberculoid leprosy and a negative test indicates lepromatous (anergic) leprosy.

Mumps

Intradermal injection of inactivated mumps vaccine gives a delayed positive skin test reaction in 18–36 hours provided the individual has had a past infection. A negative mumps skin test is less reliable in identification of susceptible persons than is the absence of neutralizing serum antibodies. A positive mumps skin test does permit demonstration of the ability to respond with a delayed type hypersensitivity reaction.

Paracoccidioidomycosis

Skin tests with paracoccidioidin, a filtrate of an old broth culture of *Paracoccidioides brasiliensis*, are often positive in infected persons, but cross-reactions with blastomycin and histoplasmin are common.

Tuberculosis

The tuberculin skin test is performed with a purified protein derivative (PPD-S) standardized biologically in humans in terms of tuberculin units (TU) (see Chapter 26).

The initial test dose is usually 5 TU (intermediate strength PPD). Larger doses are injected when smaller doses have given negative results. The test is considered positive if induration 10 mm in diameter or more occurs in 48–72 hours following injection of 5 TU. In hypersensitive persons, not more than 1 TU should be injected to avoid serious reactions.

Years after a person has exhibited a positive tuberculin test, a repeat test may appear to be negative. However, the repeat test may exert a "booster" effect so that another tuberculin test 1–2 weeks later will give a positive (> 10 mm induration) result.

NONSPECIFIC CLINICAL LABORATORY TESTS

The usual laboratory procedures performed on most patients who undergo detailed medical examination frequently yield clues concerning possible infectious processes. Anemia and leukocytosis are suitable examples. Such abnormalities are compatible with a large variety of diagnoses and are helpful only if integrated with other findings into a meaningful pattern. No attempt is made here to list the many different laboratory findings that can thus aid in the diagnosis of infection. A few specific items will be discussed briefly for the sake of illustration.

Red Cell Count & Packed Cell Volume

Anemia is a feature of many protracted infections, eg, infective endocarditis and malaria. Conversely, in acute diarrheal diseases, there may be dehydration with elevated packed cell volume.

White Cell Count

In most suppurative infections, the white count is elevated and the proportion of young polymorphonuclear cells is increased. A low white count in pneumococcal or staphylococcal pneumonia, especially in elderly patients, is an unfavorable prognostic sign.

In some infections caused by gram-negative rods, there is a fall in the total white count. Similar findings occur in some viral infections (eg, myxoviruses). However, arbovirus infections with encephalitis commonly give rise to high white counts. In whooping cough, the white count is frequently high, with absolute lymphocytosis. Sudden widespread dissemination of any bacterial or fungal pathogen may be accompanied by a very rapid rise in the white count, at times to leukemoid levels. On the other hand, persons with depressed marrow activity do not develop white count elevations with infections.

These examples illustrate the complexity of interpreting white cell counts.

Erythrocyte Sedimentation Rate

In many acute infections, the sedimentation rate is normal; in prolonged infections, it becomes accelerated. Exceedingly high sedimentation rates tend to occur in only a few types of diseases: miliary tuberculosis, carcinomatosis, collagen-vascular diseases, and, occasionally, osteomyelitis. However, a rapid sedimentation rate can be associated with so many different processes which produce cell injury or derangements of blood proteins that it is rarely helpful in establishing the diagnosis of infection. It may be of use in evaluating therapeutic response, particularly in osteomyelitis.

C-Reactive Protein

C-reactive protein is a substance in the serum of certain patients that reacts with the somatic C polysaccharide of pneumococci in vitro but is commonly measured by precipitation with a specific antiserum prepared in rabbits. It is a β globulin that is found only in minute amounts in normal sera but occurs frequently in markedly increased amounts in sera of patients with inflammatory, neoplastic, or necrotizing processes. The laboratory test for the presence of C-reactive protein thus constitutes a nonspecific test for the presence of inflammation or tissue injury.

Tests for several mucoproteins in serum are likewise entirely nonspecific and so are of little help in specific diagnosis.

Transaminase & Similar Enzyme Tests

Aspartate transaminase (AST; formerly glutamic-oxaloacetic transaminase, GOT), alanine aminotransferase (ALT; formerly glutamic-pyruvic transaminase, GPT), lactate dehydrogenase (LDH), and others are intracellular enzymes involved in amino acid or carbohydrate metabolism. In the course of many disease processes involving cellular injury, the enzyme concentration in blood serum increases markedly. Consequently, elevated enzyme levels are found in acute infections, neoplasms, infarctions, and many degenerative processes and are not necessarily due to hepatic insult or myocardial infarction, with which they are commonly associated.

Serum Bilirubin

The serum bilirubin may be elevated, indicating jaundice, particularly in infections of the newborn and those caused by gram-negative enteric organisms.

Nonspecific Organ System Response to Infections

Whenever an infectious process involves primarily one organ system, nonspecific laboratory tests may show abnormal values. For example, in renal infections, proteinuria and abnormal urinary sediment may be present even without bacteriuria. In central nervous system infections, abnormal values of cerebrospinal fluid composition are of great help in diagnosis. In infections of the external eye, the cell picture of the conjunctival exudate assists in etiologic diagnosis. The x-ray appearance of bone or lung may not only support a diagnosis of infection but may even point to the causative agent.

Scanning Methods

Infective processes may alter blood supply to an area, produce necrotic foci, and change tissue cell behavior. Consequently, localized infections in some organs (eg, liver, spleen, brain) may be found by concentration or exclusion of isotopes such as gallium, technetium, and others. The technology of scanning methods and the interpretation of results tend to change very rapidly. Computerized tomography (CT scan), sonography, and nuclear magnetic resonance (NMR) are also very useful scanning procedures for diagnosis of localized infections.

REFERENCES

Balows A, Hausler WJ Jr (editors): *Diagnostic Procedures for Bacterial, Mycotic, and Parasitic Infections*, 6th ed. American Public Health Association, 1981.

Barry AL: *The Antimicrobic Susceptibility Test: Principles and Practices*. Lea & Febiger, 1976.

Campbell MC, Stewart JL: *The Medical Mycology Handbook*. Wiley, 1980.

Finegold SM: *Anaerobic Bacteria in Human Disease*. Academic Press, 1977.

Gorbach SL, Bartlett JG: Anaerobic infections. (3 parts.) *N Engl J Med* 1974;**290**:1177, 1237, 1289.

Haley LD, Callaway CS: *Laboratory Methods in Medical Mycology*, 4th ed. Center for Disease Control, US Department of Health, Education, and Welfare Publication No. (CDC)78-8361, 1978.

Hsiung GD: *Diagnostic Virology: Illustrated by Light and Electron Microscopy*, 3rd ed. Yale Univ Press, 1982.

Koneman EW et al: *Color Atlas and Textbook of Diagnostic Microbiology*, 2nd ed. Lippincott, 1983.

Kunin CM: *Detection, Prevention and Management of Urinary Tract Infections*, 3rd ed. Lea & Febiger, 1979.

Lennette EH, Schmidt NJ (editors): *Diagnostic Procedures for Viral, Rickettsial and Chlamydial Infections*, 5th ed. American Public Health Association, 1979.

Lennette EH et al (editors): *Manual of Clinical Microbiology*, 4th ed. American Society for Microbiology, 1985.

Lorian V (editor): *Antibiotics in Laboratory Medicine*, 2nd ed. Williams & Wilkins, 1986.

MacFaddin J: *Biochemical Tests for Identification of Medical Bacteria*, 2nd ed. Williams & Wilkins, 1980.

Morello JA et al: *Microbiology in Patient Care*, 4th ed. Macmillan, 1984.

Rippon JW: *Medical Mycology*, 2nd ed. Saunders, 1982.

Washington JA II (editor): *The Detection of Septicemia*. CRC Press, 1978.

Washington JA II, Henry JB (editors): *Medical Microbiology*. Part 5 of: *Clinical Diagnosis and Management by Laboratory Methods*, 16th ed. Henry JB (editor). Saunders, 1979.

General Properties of Viruses

DEFINITIONS

Viruses are the smallest infectious agents (20–300 nm in diameter), containing only one kind of nucleic acid (RNA or DNA) as their genome. The nucleic acid is encased in a protein shell, which may be surrounded by a lipid-containing membrane. The entire infectious unit is termed a virion. Viruses replicate only in living cells. They are inert in the extracellular environment. They are parasites at the genetic level. The viral nucleic acid contains information necessary for programming the infected host cell to synthesize a number of virus-specific macromolecules required for the production of virus progeny. During the replicative cycle, numerous copies of viral nucleic acid and coat proteins are produced. The coat proteins assemble together to form the capsid, which encases and stabilizes the viral nucleic acid against the extracellular environment and facilitates the attachment and perhaps penetration of the virus upon contact with new susceptible cells.

The nucleic acid, once isolated from the virion, can be hydrolyzed by either ribo- or deoxyribonuclease, whereas the nucleic acid within the intact virus is not affected by such treatment. In contrast, viral antiserum will neutralize the virion because it reacts with the antigens of the protein coat. However, the same antiserum has no effect on the free infectious nucleic acid isolated from the virion.

The host range for a given virus may be broad or extremely limited. Viruses are known to infect unicellular organisms such as mycoplasmas, bacteria, and algae and all higher plants and animals.

Much information on virus-host relationships has been obtained from studies on bacteriophages, the viruses that attack bacteria. This subject is discussed in Chapter 9. Properties of individual viruses are discussed in Chapters 36–47.

Some Useful Definitions in Virology (Fig 33–1)

Capsid: The protein shell, or coat, that encloses the nucleic acid genome. Empty capsids may be by-products of the replicative cycle of viruses with icosahedral symmetry.

Nucleocapsid: The capsid together with the enclosed nucleic acid.

Structural units: The basic protein building blocks of the coat. They are usually a collection of more than one nonidentical polypeptide.

Capsomeres: Morphologic units seen in the electron microscope on the surface of icosahedral virus particles. Capsomeres represent clusters of polypeptides, but the morphologic units do not necessarily correspond to the chemically defined structural units.

Envelope: A lipid-containing membrane that surrounds some virus particles. It is acquired during virus maturation by a budding process through a cellular membrane. Virus-encoded glycoproteins are exposed on the surface of the envelope.

Virion: The complete virus particle, which in some instances (adenoviruses, papovaviruses, picornaviruses) may be identical with the nucleocapsid. In more complex virions (herpesviruses, orthomyxoviruses), this includes the nucleocapsid plus a surrounding envelope. This structure, the virion, serves to transfer the viral nucleic acid from one cell to another.

Defective virus: A virus particle that is functionally deficient in some aspect of replication. De-

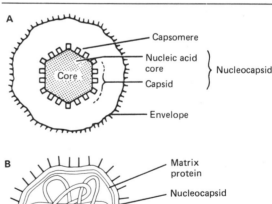

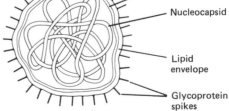

Figure 33–1. Schematic diagram illustrating the components of the complete virus particle (the virion). *A:* Enveloped virus with icosahedral symmetry. *B:* Virus with helical symmetry.

fective virus may interfere with the replication of normal virus.

Primary, secondary, and tertiary nucleic acid structure: Primary structure refers to the sequence of bases in the nucleic acid chain. Secondary structure refers to the spatial arrangement of the complete nucleic acid chain, ie, whether it is single- or double-stranded, circular or linear in conformation. Tertiary structure refers to other elements of fine spatial detail in the helix, eg, presence of supercoiling, breakage points, regions of strand separation.

Transcription: The mechanism by which specific information encoded in a nucleic acid chain is transferred to messenger RNA (mRNA).

Translation: The mechanism by which a particular base sequence in mRNA results in production of a specific amino acid sequence in a protein.

EVOLUTIONARY ORIGIN OF VIRUSES

The origin of viruses is not known. Two likely hypotheses are as follows:

(1) Viruses evolved from free-living cells. There is no evidence that viruses evolved from bacteria, although the possibility exists that other obligatory intracellular organisms, eg, chlamydiae, did so. However, poxviruses are so large and complex that they might represent evolutionary products of some cellular ancestor.

(2) Viruses may be components of host cells that became autonomous. They resemble genes that have acquired the capacity to exist independent of the cell. Sequences related to retroviruses are present in host cells (see Chapter 46). The likelihood is great that most viruses, including retroviruses, evolved in this fashion. On the other hand, large viruses of the pox and herpes groups show very limited resemblance to host cell DNA.

CLASSIFICATION OF VIRUSES

Basis of Classification

The following properties, listed in the order of preference or importance, have been used as a basis for the classification of viruses. The amount of information available in each category is not uniform for all viruses. For some agents, knowledge is available for only a few of the properties listed.

(1) Nucleic acid type: RNA or DNA; single-stranded or double-stranded; strategy of replication.

(2) Size and morphology, including type of symmetry, number of capsomeres, and presence or absence of membranes.

(3) Presence of specific enzymes, particularly RNA and DNA polymerases concerned with genome replication, and neuraminidase necessary for release of certain virus particles (influenza) from the cells in which they were formed.

(4) Susceptibility to physical and chemical agents, especially ether.

(5) Immunologic properties.

(6) Natural methods of transmission.

(7) Host, tissue, and cell tropisms.

(8) Pathology; inclusion body formation.

(9) Symptomatology.

Classification by Symptomatology

The oldest classification of viruses is based on the diseases they produce, and this system offers certain conveniences for the clinician. However, it is not satisfactory for the biologist because the same virus may appear in several groups if it causes more than one disease, depending upon the organ attacked.

A. Generalized Diseases: Diseases in which virus is spread throughout the body via the bloodstream and in which multiple organs are affected. Skin rashes may occur. These include smallpox, vaccinia, measles, rubella, chickenpox, yellow fever, dengue, enteroviruses, and many others.

B. Diseases Primarily Affecting Specific Organs: The virus may reach the organ via the bloodstream, along peripheral nerves, or by other routes.

1. Diseases of the nervous system–Poliomyelitis, aseptic meningitis (polio-, coxsackie-, and echoviruses), rabies, arthropod-borne encephalitides, lymphocytic choriomeningitis, herpes simplex, meningoencephalitis of mumps, measles, vaccinia, and "slow" virus infections.

2. Diseases of the respiratory tract–Influenza, parainfluenza, respiratory syncytial virus pneumonia and bronchiolitis, adenovirus pharyngitis, common cold (caused by many viruses).

3. Localized diseases of the skin or mucous membranes–Herpes simplex type 1 (usually oral) and type 2 (usually genital), molluscum contagiosum, warts, herpangina, herpes zoster, and others.

4. Diseases of the eye–Adenovirus conjunctivitis, herpes keratoconjunctivitis, and epidemic hemorrhagic conjunctivitis (enterovirus 70).

5. Diseases of the liver–Hepatitis type A (infectious hepatitis) and type B (serum hepatitis), yellow fever, and, in newborns, enteroviruses, herpesviruses, and rubella virus.

6. Diseases of the salivary glands–Mumps and cytomegalovirus.

7. Diseases of the gastrointestinal tract–Rotavirus, Norwalk virus.

8. Sexually transmitted diseases–Until recently, only bacteria (*Neisseria gonorrhoeae, Treponema pallidum,* and *Chlamydia trachomatis*) were included in this category of disease. It is now recognized that herpes simplex virus, hepatitis B virus, papilloma virus, molluscum contagiosum virus, the retroviruses associated with acquired immune deficiency syndrome (AIDS), and probably cytomegalovirus are all sexually transmitted pathogens.

Classification by Biologic, Chemical, & Physical Properties

Viruses can be clearly separated into major groupings, called families, on the basis of the type of nucleic acid genome and the size, shape, substructure, and mode of replication of the virus particle. Table 33–1 shows one scheme used for classification. However, there is not complete agreement among virologists on the relative importance of the criteria used to classify viruses.

Within each family, subdivisions, called genera, are usually based on physicochemical or serologic differences. Properties of the major families of animal viruses are summarized in Table 33–1, are discussed briefly below, and are considered in greater detail in the chapters that follow.

Survey of DNA-Containing Viruses

A. Parvoviruses: Very small viruses with a particle size of about 20 nm. They contain single-stranded DNA and have cubic symmetry, with 32 capsomeres 2–4 nm in diameter. They have no envelope. Replication and capsid assembly take place in the nucleus of the infected cell. Parvoviruses of rodents and swine replicate autonomously. The adenoassociated satellite viruses are defective, ie, they require the presence of an adenovirus or herpesvirus as "helper." Some satellite viruses occur in humans. (See Chapters 43 and 45.)

B. Papovaviruses: Small (45–55 nm), ether-resistant viruses containing double-stranded circular DNA and exhibiting cubic symmetry, with 72 capsomeres. Known human papovaviruses are the papilloma (wart) viruses (see Chapter 45) and agents isolated from brain tissue of patients with progressive multifocal leukoencephalopathy (JC virus) or from the urine of immunosuppressed renal transplant recipients (BK virus) (see Chapter 39). In animals, there are papilloma, polyoma, and vacuolating viruses. These agents have a slow growth cycle and replicate within the nucleus. Papovaviruses produce latent and chronic infections in their natural hosts, and all can induce tumors in some animal species. (See Chapter 46.)

C. Adenoviruses: Medium-sized (70–90 nm) viruses containing double-stranded DNA and exhibiting cubic symmetry, with 252 capsomeres. They have no envelope. At least 37 types infect humans, especially in mucous membranes, and they can persist in lymphoid tissue. Some adenoviruses cause acute respiratory diseases, pharyngitis, and conjunctivitis. Some human adenoviruses can induce tumors in newborn hamsters. There are many serotypes that infect animals. (See Chapters 43 and 46.)

D. Herpesviruses: Medium-sized viruses containing double-stranded DNA. The nucleocapsid is 100 nm in diameter, with cubic symmetry and 162 capsomeres. It is surrounded by a lipid-containing envelope (150–200 nm in diameter). Latent infections may last for the life span of the host.

Human herpesviruses include herpes simplex types

Table 33–1. Classification of viruses into families based on chemical and physical properties.

Nucleic Acid Core	Capsid Symmetry	Virion: Enveloped or Naked	Ether Sensitivity	No. of Capsomeres	Virus Particle Size (nm)*	Molecular Weight of Nucleic Acid in Virion (× 10⁶)	Physical Type of Nucleic Acid	No. of Genes (Approx.)	Virus Family
DNA	Icosahedral	Naked	Resistant	32	18–26	1.5–2.2	SS	3–4	Parvoviridae
				72	45–55	3–5	DS circular	5–8	Papovaviridae
				252	70–90	20–30	DS	30	Adenoviridae
		Enveloped	Sensitive	162	100†	90–130	DS	160	Herpesviridae
	Complex	Complex coats	Resistant‡		230 × 400	130–200	DS	300	Poxviridae
					42	1.6	DS circular§	4	Hepadnaviridae
RNA	Icosahedral	Naked	Resistant	32	20–30	2–2.8	SS	4–6	Picornaviridae
				**	60–80	12–15	DS segmented	10–12	Reoviridae
		Enveloped	Sensitive	32?	50–70	4	SS	10	Togaviridae
	Unknown or complex	Enveloped	Sensitive		45–50	4	SS	10	Flaviviridae
					50–300	3–5	SS segmented	10	Arenaviridae
					80–130	7	SS	30	Coronaviridae
					~100	7–10	SS segmented	4	Retroviridae
	Helical	Enveloped	Sensitive		90–100	6–15	SS segmented	>3	Bunyaviridae
					80–120	5	SS segmented	10	Orthomyxoviridae
					150–300	5–8	SS	>10	Paramyxoviridae
					70 × 175	3–4	SS	5	Rhabdoviridae

*Diameter, or diameter × length.

†The naked virus, ie, the nucleocapsid, is 100 nm in diameter; however, the enveloped virion varies up to 200 nm.

‡The genus *Orthopoxvirus*, which includes the better studied poxviruses (eg, vaccinia, variola, cowpox, ectromelia, rabbitpox, monkeypox), is ether-resistant. Some of the poxviruses belonging to other genera are ether-sensitive.

§One strand has a constant length of 3182 bases, and the other varies between 1700 and 2800 bases.

**Reoviruses possess a double protein capsid shell in which the exact number and spatial arrangement of capsomeres is difficult to determine.

1 and 2 (oral and genital lesions), varicella-zoster virus (shingles and chickenpox), cytomegalovirus, and EB virus (infectious mononucleosis and association with human neoplasms). Other herpesviruses occur in many animals. (See Chapters 44 and 46.)

E. Poxviruses: Large brick-shaped or ovoid (230 × 400 nm) viruses containing double-stranded DNA, with a lipid-containing envelope. All poxviruses share a common nucleoprotein antigen and contain several enzymes within the virion, including a DNA-dependent RNA polymerase. Poxviruses replicate entirely within the cell cytoplasm. All poxviruses tend to produce skin lesions. Some are pathogenic for humans (smallpox, vaccinia, molluscum contagiosum), others for animals. Some that are pathogenic for animals can infect humans, eg, cowpox, monkeypox. (See Chapter 42.)

F. Hepadnaviruses: Small (42-nm) viruses containing circular DNA molecules that are partially double-stranded. The virion also contains DNA polymerase that repairs the single-stranded region to make fully double-stranded molecules of 3200 base-pairs. The virus contains a nucleocapsid core and a lipid-containing envelope. The surface component is characteristically overproduced during replication of the virus, which takes place in the liver. Three virus types that infect mammals (humans, woodchucks, and ground squirrels) and one type that infects ducks are known. (See Chapter 38.)

Survey of RNA-Containing Viruses

A. Picornaviruses: Small (20–30 nm), ether-resistant viruses containing single-stranded RNA and exhibiting cubic symmetry. The RNA genome is positive-sense, ie, it can serve as an mRNA. The groups infecting humans are rhinoviruses (more than 100 serotypes causing common colds) and enteroviruses (polio-, coxsackie-, and echoviruses). Rhinoviruses are acid-labile and have a high density; enteroviruses are acid-stable and have a lower density. Picornaviruses infecting animals include foot-and-mouth disease of cattle and encephalomyocarditis of rodents. (See Chapter 37.)

B. Reoviruses: Medium-sized (60–80 nm), ether-resistant viruses containing a segmented double-stranded RNA and having cubic symmetry. Reoviruses of humans include rotaviruses, which cause infantile gastroenteritis, and have a distinctive wheel-shaped appearance. Antigenically similar reoviruses infect many animals. Orbiviruses constitute a distinct subgroup that includes Colorado tick fever virus of humans and other agents that infect plants, insects, and animals (bluetongue of cattle and sheep). (See Chapter 45.)

C. Arboviruses: An ecologic grouping of viruses with diverse physical and chemical properties. All of these viruses (more than 350) have a complex cycle involving arthropods as vectors that transmit the viruses to vertebrate hosts by their bite. Virus replication does not seem to harm the infected arthropod. Arboviruses infect humans, mammals, birds, and snakes and use mosquitoes and ticks as vectors. Human pathogens include dengue, yellow fever, encephalitis viruses, and others. Arboviruses belong to several virus families, including toga-, flavi-, bunya-, rhabdo-, arena-, and reoviruses. (See Chapter 36.)

D. Togaviruses: Many arboviruses, as well as rubella virus, belong here. They have a lipid-containing envelope and are ether-sensitive, and their genome is single-stranded, positive-sense RNA. The enveloped virion measures 50–70 nm. The virus particles mature by budding from the host cell plasma membrane. Some togaviruses, eg, Sindbis virus, possess a 35-nm nucleocapsid and within it a spherical core 12–16 nm in diameter. (See Chapters 36 and 41.)

E. Flaviviruses: Enveloped viruses, 45–50 nm in diameter, containing single-stranded, positive-sense RNA. Mature virions accumulate within cisternae of the endoplasmic reticulum. This group of arboviruses includes yellow fever virus. Most members are transmitted by blood-sucking arthropods.

F. Arenaviruses: RNA-containing, enveloped viruses ranging in size from 50 to 300 nm. The virions incorporate host cell ribosomes during maturation, which gives the particles a "sandy" appearance. Most members of this family are unique to tropical America (ie, the Tacaribe complex). All arenaviruses pathogenic for humans cause chronic infections in rodents. Lassa fever virus of Africa belongs here.

G. Coronaviruses: Enveloped, 80- to 130-nm particles containing an unsegmented genome of single-stranded RNA, the nucleocapsid is probably helical, 7–9 nm in diameter. They resemble orthomyxoviruses, but coronaviruses have petal-shaped surface projections arranged in a fringe like a solar corona. Coronavirus nucleocapsids develop in the cytoplasm and mature by budding into cytoplasmic vesicles. Human coronaviruses have been isolated from acute upper respiratory tract illnesses—"colds." Coronaviruses of animals include avian infectious bronchitis virus among many others. (See Chapter 40.)

H. Retroviruses: Enveloped viruses (90–120 nm in diameter) whose genome contains duplicate copies of high-molecular-weight, single-stranded RNA of the same polarity as viral mRNA. The virion contains a reverse transcriptase (RNA → DNA). The virus is replicated from an integrated "provirus" DNA copy in infected cells. Leukemia and sarcoma viruses of animals and humans (see Chapter 46), foamy viruses of primates, and some "slow" viruses (visna, maedi of sheep) (see Chapter 39) are included in this group. Retroviruses have allowed the identification of cellular "oncogenes" (see Chapter 46). Viruses associated with acquired immune deficiency syndrome (AIDS) are retroviruses (see Chapter 47).

I. Bunyaviruses: Spherical, 90- to 100-nm particles that replicate in the cytoplasm and acquire an envelope by budding into the Golgi apparatus. The genome is made up of a triple-segmented, single-stranded RNA that is negative-sense, ie, complementary to mRNA. The majority of these viruses are transmitted to vertebrates by arthropods. About 70 are antigenically related to Bunyamwera virus; 50 others are not but are morphologically similar. (See Chapter 36.)

J. Orthomyxoviruses: Medium-sized, 80- to 120-nm enveloped viruses containing a segmented, single-stranded, negative-sense RNA genome and exhibiting helical symmetry. Particles are either round or filamentous. Orthomyxoviruses have, as part of their surface, projections that contain hemagglutinin or neuraminidase activity. The internal nucleoprotein helix measures 6–9 nm, and the RNA is made up of 8 segments. During replication, the nucleocapsid is assembled in the nucleus, whereas the hemagglutinin and neuraminidase accumulate in the cytoplasm. The virus matures by budding at the cell membrane. All orthomyxoviruses are influenza viruses that infect humans or animals. The segmented nature of the viral genome permits ready genetic reassortment when 2 influenza viruses infect the same cell; this explains the high rate of natural variation among influenza viruses. (See Chapter 40.)

K. Paramyxoviruses: Similar to but larger (150–300 nm) than orthomyxoviruses. The internal nucleocapsid measures 18 nm, and the molecular weight of the single-stranded, nonsegmented, negative-sense RNA is greater than the sum of the RNA segments of the orthomyxoviruses. Both the nucleocapsid and the hemagglutinin are formed in the cytoplasm. Paramyxoviruses are resistant to dactinomycin. Those infecting humans include mumps, measles, parainfluenza virus, and respiratory syncytial virus. Others infect animals. (See Chapter 41.)

L. Rhabdoviruses: Enveloped virions resembling a bullet, flat at one end and round at the other (Fig 33–37), measuring about 70×175 nm. The envelope has 10-nm spikes. The genome is single-stranded, negative-sense RNA. Particles are formed by budding from the cell membrane. Rabies virus is a member of this group, along with many other viruses of animals and plants. (See Chapter 39.)

M. Other Viruses: Insufficient information to permit classification. This applies to non-A, non-B hepatitis viruses (see Chapter 38), to agents responsible for some immune complex diseases and for some "slow" virus diseases, including degenerative neurologic disorders such as kuru or Creutzfeldt-Jakob disease, or scrapie of sheep (see Chapter 39), and to some viruses of gastroenteritis (see Chapter 45).

N. Viroids: Small infectious agents causing diseases of plants. Viroids are agents that do not fit the definition of classical viruses. They are nucleic acid molecules (MW 70,000–120,000) without a protein coat. Plant viroids are single-stranded, covalently closed circular RNA molecules consisting of about 360 nucleotides and comprising a highly base-paired rodlike structure with unique properties. Each is arranged into 26 double-stranded regions separated by 25 regions of unpaired bases embodied in single-stranded internal loops; there is a loop at each end of the rodlike molecule. These features provide the viroid RNA molecule with structural, thermodynamic,

and kinetic properties very similar to those of a double-stranded DNA molecule of the same molecular weight and guanine-plus-cytosine (G + C) content. Viroids replicate by an entirely novel mechanism in which infecting viroid RNA molecules are copied by the host enzyme normally responsible for synthesis of nuclear precursors to mRNA. Viroid RNA has not been shown to encode any protein products; the devastating plant diseases induced by viroids occur by an unknown mechanism. To date, viroids have been detected only in plants; none have been demonstrated to exist in animals or humans.

PRINCIPLES OF VIRUS STRUCTURE

Types of Symmetry of Virus Particles

Electron microscopy and x-ray diffraction techniques have made it possible to resolve fine differences in the basic morphology of viruses. The study of virus symmetry in the electron microscope requires the use of heavy metal stains (eg, potassium phosphotungstate) to emphasize surface structure. The heavy metal permeates the virus particle as a cloud and brings out the surface structure of viruses by virtue of "negative staining."

Virus architecture can be grouped into 3 types based on the arrangement of morphologic subunits: (1) those with cubic symmetry, eg, adenoviruses; (2) those with helical symmetry, eg, orthomyxoviruses; and (3) those with complex structures, eg, poxviruses. Genetic economy requires that a virus structure be made from many identical molecules of one or a few proteins.

A. Cubic Symmetry: All cubic symmetry observed with animal viruses to date is of the icosahedral pattern, the most efficient arrangement for subunits in a closed shell. Knowledge of rules guiding icosahedral symmetry makes it possible to determine the number of capsomeres in a particle, an important characteristic in virus classification. The icosahedron has 20 faces (each an equilateral triangle), 12 vertices, and 5-fold, 3-fold, and 2-fold axes of rotational symmetry. Capsomeres can be arranged to comply with icosahedral symmetry in a limited number of ways, expressed by the formula $N = 10(n-1)^2 + 2$, where N is the total number of capsomeres and n the number of capsomeres on one side of each equilateral triangle. Table 33–2 shows the number of capsomeres where n varies from 2 to 6, in several virus groups.

Icosahedral structures can be built from one simple, asymmetric building unit, arranged as 12 pentamer (vertex) units and x number of hexamer units. The polypeptides that comprise the pentamers and hexamers of the capsid may be the same or different, depending on the particular virus. The smallest and most basic capsid is that of the phage ϕX-174, which simply consists of 12 pentamer units.

Viruses exhibiting icosahedral symmetry can also be grouped according to their triangulation number, T, which is the number of small triangles formed on the

Table 33–2. Number of capsomeres in several virus groups.

Virus Family	n	T	Capsomeres
Phage (ϕX-174)	2	1	12
Picorna*	2	3	32
Papova†	3	7	72
Reo	4	9	92(?)
Herpes	5	16	162
Adeno	6	25	252

*Picornaviruses are a special case and, for $n = 2$, fit the formula $N = 30(n - 1)^2 + 2$.

†Capsomeres in a skew arrangement.

single face of the icosahedron when all its adjacent morphologic subunits are connected by lines. The number of morphologic units (capsomeres) is expressed by the formula $M = 10T + 2$. Table 33–2 shows the triangulation number for several virus groups. It can be seen that the total number of capsomeres in a virus particle can be calculated if either the number of capsomeres on one edge or the triangulation number of the particle can be determined from electron micrographs.

An example of icosahedral symmetry is seen in Fig 33–2. The adenovirus ($n = 6$) model illustrated shows the 6 capsomeres along one edge (Fig 33–2[a]). Degradation of this virus with sodium lauryl sulfate releases the capsomeres in groups of 9 (Fig 33–2[b], [c]) and possibly groups of 6. The groups of 9 lie on the faces and include one capsomere from each of the 3 edges of the face, and the groups of 6 would be from the vertices. The groups of 9 form the faces of the 20 triangular facets, which account for 180 subunits, and the groups of 6 that form the 12 vertices account for 72 capsomeres; thus the total is 252 capsomeres in the particle.

The viral nucleic acid is condensed within the isometric particles; virus-encoded "core" proteins or, in the case of papovaviruses, cellular histones are involved in condensation of the nucleic acid into a form

suitable for packaging. The rules governing incorporation of nucleic acid into isometric particles are unknown; presumably there is a "packaging sequence" that is involved in assembly, although in general, primary, secondary, and tertiary structures of the nucleic acid are not crucial. There are size constraints on the nucleic acid molecules that can be packaged into a given icosahedral capsid. Icosahedral capsids are formed independent of nucleic acid. Most preparations of isometric viruses will contain some "empty" particles devoid of viral nucleic acid. Both DNA and RNA virus groups exhibit examples of cubic symmetry.

B. Helical Symmetry: In cases of helical symmetry, protein subunits are bound in a periodic way to the viral nucleic acid, winding it into a helix. The filamentous viral nucleic acid–protein complex (nucleocapsid) is then coiled inside a lipid-containing envelope. Thus, unlike the case with icosahedral structures, there is a regular, periodic interaction between capsid protein and nucleic acid in viruses with helical symmetry. It is not possible for "empty" helical particles to form.

An example of helical symmetry is shown in Fig 33–3. Tobacco mosaic virus, a plant virus, is most well-characterized with respect to the interaction between the viral RNA and capsid protein. However, it

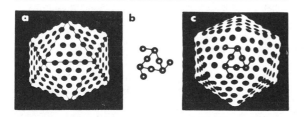

Figure 33–2. (a) Representation of the capsomere arrangement of an adenovirus particle, as viewed through the 2-fold axis of symmetry. (b) Arrangement of capsomere group of 9, obtained by treatment of an adenovirus with sodium lauryl sulfate. (c) Orientation of the capsomere group of 9 on the adenovirus particle. If the model were marked to show the maximum number of small triangles formed on one face of the icosahedron by drawing a line between each adjacent morphologic subunit, it would yield the triangulation number for the adenovirus particle, which turns out to be 25.

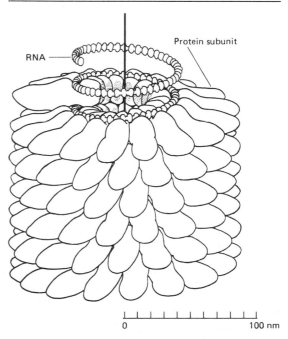

Figure 33–3. Schematic representation of tobacco mosaic virus. As can be seen in the cutaway section, the RNA helix is associated with protein molecules in the ratio of 3 nucleotides per protein molecule. (Reproduced, with permission, from Mattern CFT: Structure. Pages 707–715 in: *Medical Microbiology.* Baron S [editor]. Addison-Wesley, 1986. Modified from Caspar DLD: *Adv Prot Chem* 1963;**18**:37.)

is a rigid rod. All known examples of animal viruses with helical symmetry contain RNA genomes and, with the exception of rhabdoviruses, have flexible nucleocapsids that are wound into a ball inside envelopes (Figs 33–1B and 33–4).

C. Complex Structures: Some virus particles do not exhibit simple cubic or helical symmetry but are more complicated in structure. For example, poxviruses are brick-shaped with ridges on the external surface and a core and lateral bodies inside (Figs 33–4 and 42–1).

Measuring the Sizes of Viruses

Small size and ability to pass through filters that hold back bacteria are classic attributes of viruses. However, because some bacteria may be smaller than the largest viruses, filtrability is no longer regarded as a unique feature of viruses.

The following methods are used for determining the sizes of viruses and their components.

A. Filtration Through Collodion Membranes of Graded Porosity: These membranes are available with pores of different sizes. If the virus preparation is passed through a series of membranes of known pore size, the approximate size of any virus can be measured by determining which membranes allow the infective unit to pass and which hold it back. The size of the limiting APD (average pore diameter) multiplied by 0.64 yields the diameter of the virus particle. The passage of a virus through a filter will also depend on the physical structure of the virus; thus, only a very approximate estimate of size is obtained.

B. Sedimentation in the Ultracentrifuge: If particles are suspended in a liquid, they will settle to the bottom at a rate that is proportionate to their size. In an ultracentrifuge, forces of more than 100,000 times gravity may be used to drive the particles to the bottom of the tube. The relationship between the size and shape of a particle and its rate of sedimentation permits determination of particle size. Once again, the physical structure of the virus will affect the size estimate obtained.

C. Direct Observation in the Electron Microscope: As compared with the light microscope, the electron microscope uses electrons rather than light waves and electromagnetic lenses rather than glass lenses. The electron beam obtained has a much shorter wavelength than that of light, so that objects much smaller than the wavelength of visible or ultraviolet light can be visualized. Viruses can be visualized in preparations from tissue extracts and in ultrathin sections of infected cells. Electron microscopy is the most widely used method for estimating particle size.

D. Ionizing Radiation: When a beam of charged particles such as high-energy electrons, alpha particles, or deuterons passes through a virus, it causes an energy loss in the form of primary ionization. The release of ionization within the virus particle proportionately inactivates certain biologic properties of the virus particle such as infectivity, antigenicity, and hemagglutination. Thus, the size of the biologic unit responsible for a given function in a virus particle can be estimated.

E. Comparative Measurements: (Table 33–1.) For purposes of reference, the following data should be recalled: (1) *Staphylococcus* has a diameter of about 1000 nm. (2) Bacterial viruses (bacteriophages) vary in size (10–100 nm). Some are spherical or hexagonal and have short or long tails. (3) Representative protein molecules range in diameter from serum albumin (5 nm) and globulin (7 nm) to certain hemocyanins (23 nm).

The relative sizes and morphology of various virus families are shown in Fig 33–4. Particles with a 2-fold difference in diameter have an 8-fold difference in volume. Thus, the mass of a poxvirus is about 1000 times greater than that of the poliovirus particle, and the mass of a small bacterium is 50,000 times greater.

CHEMICAL COMPOSITION OF VIRUSES

Viral Protein

The structural proteins of viruses have several important functions. Their major purpose is to facilitate transfer of the viral nucleic acid from one host cell to another. They serve to protect the viral genome against inactivation by nucleases, participate in the attachment of the virus particle to a susceptible cell, and provide the structural symmetry of the virus particle.

The proteins determine the antigenic characteristics of the virus. The host's protective immune response is directed against antigenic determinants of proteins or glycoproteins exposed on the surface of the virus particle. Some surface proteins may also exhibit specific activities, eg, influenza virus hemagglutinin agglutinates red blood cells.

Some viruses carry enzymes (which are proteins) inside the virions. The enzymes are present in very small amounts and are probably not important in the structure of the virus particles; however, they are essential for the initiation of the viral replicative cycle when the virion enters a host cell. Examples include an RNA polymerase carried by viruses with negative-sense RNA genomes (eg, orthomyxoviruses, rhabdoviruses) that is needed to copy the first mRNAs, and reverse transcriptase, an enzyme in retroviruses that makes a DNA copy of the viral RNA, an essential step in replication and transformation. At the extreme in this respect are the poxviruses, the cores of which contain a transcriptional system; at least 15 different enzymes are packaged in poxvirus particles.

Viral Nucleic Acid

Viruses contain a single kind of nucleic acid, either DNA or RNA, that encodes the genetic information necessary for replication of the virus. The genome may be single-stranded or double-stranded, circular or linear, and segmented or nonsegmented. The type of nucleic acid, the strandedness, and the molecular weight are major characteristics used for classifying viruses into families (Table 33–1).

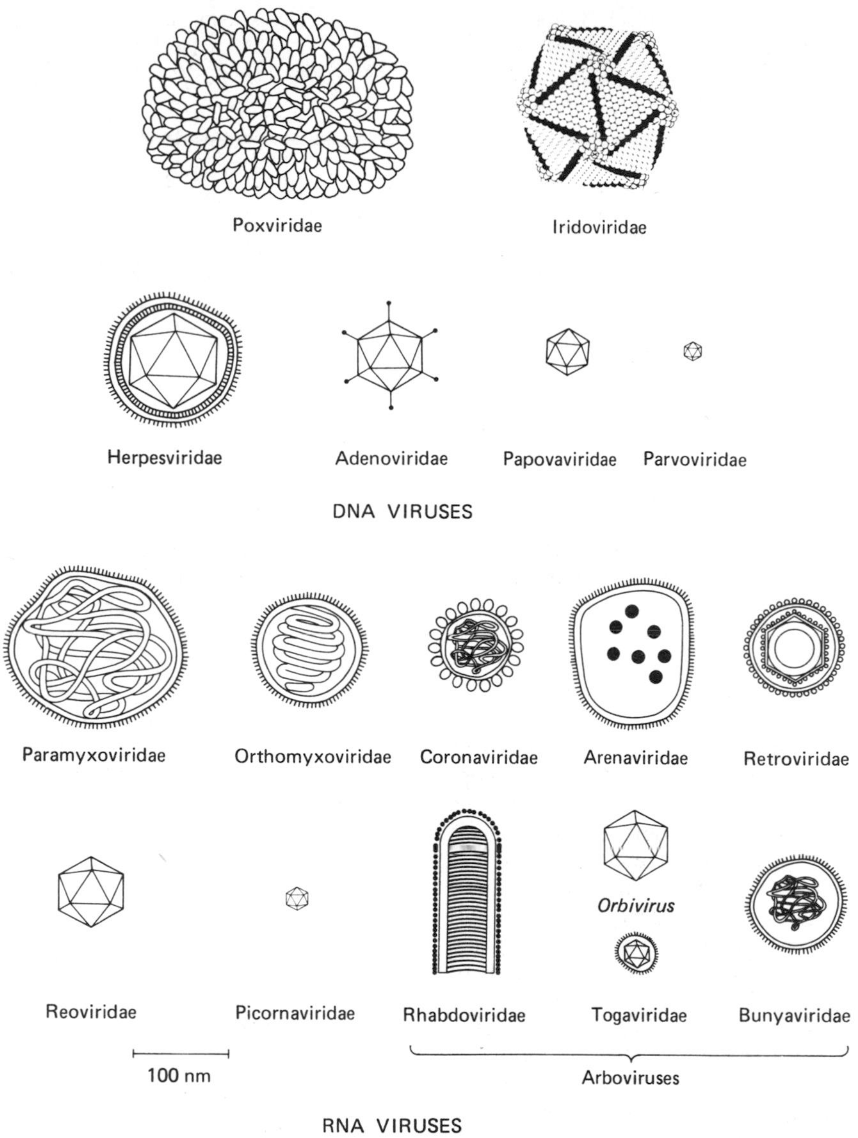

Figure 33–4. Shapes and relative sizes of animal viruses of the major families. (Reproduced, with permission, from Fenner F, White DO: *Medical Virology*, 2nd ed. Academic Press, 1976.)

The molecular weight of the viral DNA genome ranges from 1.5×10^6 (parvoviruses) to 200×10^6 (poxviruses). The molecular weight of the viral RNA genome ranges from 1×10^6 (for bromegrass mosaic virus) to 15×10^6 (for reoviruses).

Most viral genomes are quite fragile once they are removed from their protective protein capsid, but some nucleic acid molecules have been examined in the electron microscope without disruption, and their lengths have been measured. If linear densities of approximately 2×10^6 per μm for double-stranded nucleic acid and 1×10^6 per μm for single-stranded forms are used, molecular weights of viral genomes can be calculated from direct measurements (Table 33–1).

All major DNA virus groups in Table 33–1 have genomes that are single molecules of DNA and have a linear or circular configuration. This circle is often supercoiled (Fig 33–5) in the virion.

Viral RNAs exist in several forms. The RNA may be a single linear molecule (eg, picornavirus). For other viruses (eg, orthomyxovirus), the genome consists of several segments of RNA that may be loosely associated within the virion. The isolated RNA of picornaviruses and togaviruses, so-called positive-sense viruses, is infectious, and the entire molecule functions as an mRNA within the infected cell. The isolated RNA of the negative-sense RNA viruses, such as rhabdoviruses and orthomyxoviruses, is not infectious. For these virus families, the virions carry an RNA polymerase that in the cell transcribes the genome RNA molecules into several complementary

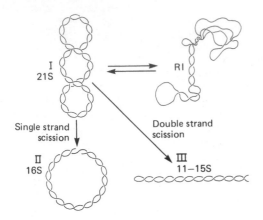

Figure 33–5. Forms of DNA of papovavirus SV40 and sedimentation coefficients in neutral sucrose gradients: supercoiled (I), nicked (II), linear (III), and replicative intermediate (RI). Linear DNA is formed by restriction endonucleases, which cleave both strands of the DNA at a single site. The RI shows 2 forks, 3 branches, and no ends, as seen in electron microscopy. (See Fig 33–26.)

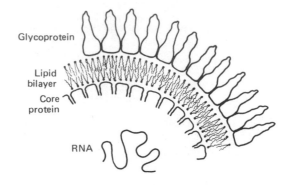

Figure 33–6. Proposed structure of Sindbis virus, an enveloped virus. (After Harrison et al.)

RNA molecules, each of which may serve as an mRNA.

The sequence and composition of nucleotides of each viral nucleic acid are distinctive. One of the properties useful for characterizing a viral nucleic acid is its G + C content. DNA virus genomes can be analyzed and compared using restriction endonucleases, enzymes that cleave DNA at specific nucleotide sequences. Each genome will yield a characteristic pattern of DNA fragments after cleavage with a particular enzyme. Using molecularly cloned DNA copies of RNA, restriction maps also can be derived for RNA virus genomes. Molecular hybridization techniques (DNA to DNA, DNA to RNA, or RNA to RNA) permit the study of transcription of the viral genome within the infected cell as well as comparison of the relatedness of different viruses.

The number of genes in a virus can be approximated if one makes certain assumptions about (1) triplet code, (2) the molecular weight of the genome, and (3) the average size of a protein (Table 33–1). It must also be assumed in such calculations that there are no overlapping genes in the viral genome; this assumption has been proved incorrect for some viruses (papovaviruses, orthomyxoviruses). Although such estimates are not precise, the values serve to illustrate the varying complexities and relative coding capacities of different virus groups.

Viral Lipids

A number of different viruses contain lipid envelopes as part of their structure (eg, Sindbis virus [Fig 33–6]). The lipid is acquired when the virus nucleocapsid buds through a cellular membrane in the course of maturation. Budding occurs only at sites where virus-specific proteins have been inserted into the host cell membrane. The different ways in which various

animal viruses acquire an envelope are suggested in Fig 33–7. The diagram serves to emphasize the diverse strategies that viruses have evolved in order to accomplish virus production by host cells.

The specific phospholipid composition of a virion envelope is determined by the specific type of cell membrane involved in the budding process. For example, herpesviruses bud through the nuclear membrane of the host cell, and the phospholipid composition of the purified virus reflects the lipids of the nuclear membrane. The acquisition of a lipid-containing membrane is an integral step in virion morphogenesis in some virus groups (see Replication of Viruses, below).

Lipid-containing viruses are sensitive to treatment with ether and other organic solvents (Table 33–1), indicating that disruption or loss of lipid results in loss of infectivity. Non-lipid-containing viruses are generally resistant to ether.

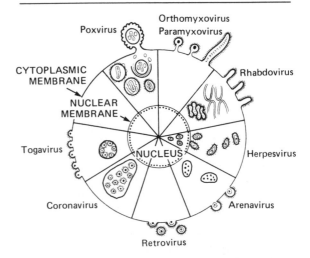

Figure 33–7. Diagram of relationships between several lipid-containing viruses and host cell membranes. (From Blough and Tiffany.)

Viral Carbohydrates

Virus envelopes contain glycoproteins. In contrast to the lipids in viral membranes which are derived from the host cell, the envelope glycoproteins are virus-coded. However, the sugars added to virus glycoproteins often reflect the host cell in which the virus is grown.

It is the surface glycoproteins of an enveloped virus that attach the virus particle to a target cell by interacting with a cellular receptor. The glycoproteins are also important virus antigens. As a result of their position at the outer surface of the virion, they are frequently involved in the interaction of the virus particle with Nt antibody. The 3-dimensional structures of the externally exposed regions of both of the influenza virus membrane glycoproteins (hemagglutinin, neuraminidase) have been determined by x-ray crystallography. Such studies are providing insights into the antigenic structure and functional activities of viral glycoproteins.

CULTIVATION & ASSAY OF VIRUSES

Cultivation of Viruses

Many viruses can be grown in cell cultures or in fertile eggs under strictly controlled conditions. Growth of virus in animals is still used for the primary isolation of certain viruses and for studies of the pathogenesis of virus diseases and of viral oncogenesis. Diagnostic laboratories attempt to recover viruses from clinical samples to establish disease etiologies (see Chapter 34). Research laboratories cultivate viruses as the basis for detailed analyses of virus expression and replication.

The availability of cells grown in vitro has facilitated the identification and cultivation of newly isolated viruses and the characterization of previously known ones. There are 3 basic types of cell culture. Primary cultures are made by dispersing cells (usually with trypsin) from freshly removed host tissues. In general, they are unable to grow for more than a few passages in culture, as secondary cultures. Diploid cell lines are secondary cultures which have undergone a change that allows their limited culture (up to 50 passages) but which retain their normal chromosome pattern. Continuous cell lines are cultures capable of more prolonged, perhaps indefinite growth that have been derived from diploid cell lines or from malignant tissues. They invariably have altered and irregular numbers of chromosomes. The type of cell culture used for virus cultivation depends on the sensitivity of the cells to that particular virus.

A. Detection of Virus-Infected Cells: Multiplication of a virus can be monitored in a variety of ways:

1. Development of cytopathic effects (CPE), ie, morphologic changes in the cells. Types of virus-induced cytopathic effects include cell lysis or necrosis, inclusion formation, giant cell formation, and cytoplasmic vacuolization. Most viruses produce some obvious cytopathic effect in infected cells that is generally characteristic of the virus group.

2. Appearance of a virus-coded protein, such as the hemagglutinin of influenza virus. Specific antisera can be used to detect the synthesis of viral proteins in infected cells.

3. Adsorption of erythrocytes to infected cells, called hemadsorption, due to the presence of viral-coded hemagglutinin (parainfluenza, influenza) in cellular membranes. This reaction becomes positive before cytopathic changes are visible and in some cases occurs in the absence of cytopathic effects.

4. Interference by a noncytopathogenic virus (eg, rubella) with the replication and induction of cytopathic effects by a second, challenge virus (eg, echovirus) added as an indicator.

5. Morphologic transformation by an oncogenic virus (eg, Rous sarcoma virus), usually accompanied by the loss of contact inhibition and the piling up of cells into discrete foci (see Chapter 46).

Virus growth in an embryonated chick egg may result in death of the embryo (eg, encephalitis virus), production of pocks or plaques on the chorioallantoic membrane (eg, herpes, smallpox, vaccinia), development of hemagglutinins in the embryonic fluids or tissues (eg, influenza), or development of infective virus (eg, poliovirus type 2).

B. Inclusion Body Formation: In the course of virus multiplication within cells, virus-specific structures called inclusion bodies may be produced (Fig 33–31). They become far larger than the individual virus particle and often have an affinity for acid dyes (eg, eosin). They may be situated in the nucleus (herpesvirus), in the cytoplasm (poxvirus), or in both (measles virus). In many viral infections, the inclusion bodies are the site of development of the virions (the virus factories). In some infections (poxviruses, reoviruses), the inclusion body consists of masses of virus particles in the process of replication. In others (as in the intranuclear inclusion body of herpes), the virus appears to have multiplied within the nucleus early in the infection, and the inclusion body appears to be a remnant of virus multiplication. Variations in the appearance of inclusion material depend largely upon the tissue fixative used.

The presence of inclusion bodies may be of considerable diagnostic aid. The intracytoplasmic inclusion in nerve cells, the Negri body, is pathognomonic for rabies.

C. Chromosome Damage: One of the consequences of infection of cells by certain viruses is derangement of the karyotype. The changes observed are random. Breakage, fragmentation, rearrangement of the chromosomes, abnormal chromosomes, and changes in chromosome number may occur. To date, no pathognomonic chromosome alterations have been identified in virus-infected cells in humans.

Cells transformed by viruses also exhibit random chromosomal abnormalities. Particular chromosomal alterations, including translocations, inversions, and deletions, are frequently observed in human cancer cells, especially specific types of leukemia. Over a dozen cellular oncogenes have been localized to specific human chromosomes; at least half are located at bands that are involved in translocations or deletions. The role of cellular oncogenes in human malignancy, however, remains unknown (see Chapter 46).

Quantitation of Viruses

A. Physical Methods: Virus particles can be counted directly in the electron microscope by comparison with a standard suspension of latex particles of similar small size. However, a relatively concentrated preparation of virus is necessary for this procedure, and infectious virus particles cannot be distinguished from noninfectious ones.

Certain viruses contain a protein (hemagglutinin) that has the ability to agglutinate red blood cells of humans or some animal. Hemagglutination assays are an easy and rapid method of quantitating these types of viruses (see Chapter 35). Both infective and noninfective particles give this reaction; thus, hemagglutination measures the total quantity of virus present.

A variety of serologic tests, such as radioimmunoassays (RIA) and enzyme-linked immunosorbent assays (ELISA; see Chapters 34 and 35), can be standardized to quantitate the amount of virus in a sample. Such tests do not distinguish infectious from noninfectious particles and sometimes detect viral proteins not assembled into particles.

B. Biologic Methods: End point biologic assays depend on the measurement of animal death, animal infection, or cytopathic effects in tissue culture at a series of dilutions of the virus being tested. The titer is expressed as the 50% infectious dose (ID_{50}), which is the reciprocal of the dilution of virus that produces the effect in 50% of the cells or animals inoculated. Precise assays require the use of a large number of test subjects.

The most widely used assay for infectious virus is the plaque assay. Monolayers of host cells are inoculated with suitable dilutions of virus and after adsorption are overlaid with medium containing agar or carboxymethylcellulose to prevent virus spreading throughout the culture. After several days, the cells initially infected have produced virus that spreads only to surrounding cells, producing a small area of infection, or plaque. Under controlled conditions, a single plaque can arise from a single infectious virus particle, termed a plaque-forming unit (PFU). The cytopathic effect of infected cells within the plaque can be distinguished from uninfected cells of the monolayer, with or without suitable staining, and plaques can usually be counted macroscopically (Fig 33–28). The ratio of the number of infectious particles to the total number of particles varies widely, from near unity to less than 1 per 1000.

Certain viruses, eg, herpes and vaccinia, form pocks when inoculated onto the chorioallantoic membrane of an embryonated egg. Such viruses can be quantitated by relating the number of pocks counted to the virus dilution inoculated.

PURIFICATION & IDENTIFICATION OF VIRUSES

Purification of Virus Particles

Pure virus must be available in order for meaningful studies on the properties and molecular biology of the agent to be carried out. For purification studies, the starting material is usually large volumes of tissue culture medium, body fluids, or infected cells. The first step frequently involves concentration of the virus particles by precipitation with ammonium sulfate, ethanol, or polyethylene glycol or by ultrafiltration. Hemagglutination and elution can be used to concentrate orthomyxoviruses (see Chapter 40). Once concentrated, virus can then be separated from host materials by differential centrifugation, density gradient centrifugation, column chromatography, and electrophoresis.

More than one step is usually necessary to achieve adequate purification. A preliminary purification will remove most nonviral material. This first step may include centrifugation; the final purification step almost always involves density gradient centrifugation. In rate-zonal centrifugation, a sample of concentrated virus is layered onto a preformed linear density gradient of sucrose or glycerol, and during centrifugation, the virus sediments as a band at a rate determined primarily by the size and weight of the virus particle. Samples are collected by piercing a hole in the bottom of the centrifuge tube. The band of purified virus may be detected by optical methods, by following radioactivity if the virus is radiolabeled, or by assaying for infectivity.

Viruses can also be purified by high-speed centrifugation in density gradients of cesium chloride (CsCl), potassium tartrate, potassium citrate, or sucrose. The gradient material of choice is the one that is least toxic to the virus. Virus particles migrate to an equilibrium position where the density of the solution is equal to their buoyant density and form a visible band. Virus bands are harvested by puncture through the bottom of the plastic centrifuge tube and assayed for infectivity.

Additional methods for purification are based on the chemical properties of the virus surface. In column chromatography, virus is bound to a substance such as DEAE or phosphocellulose and then eluted by changes in pH or salt concentration. Zone electrophoresis permits the separation of virus particles from contaminants on the basis of charge. Specific antisera also can be used to remove virus particles from host materials.

Icosahedral viruses are easier to purify than enveloped viruses. Because the latter usually contain variable amounts of envelope per particle, the virus population is heterogeneous in both size and density.

It is very difficult to achieve complete purity of viruses. Small amounts of cellular material tend to adsorb to particles and co-purify. The minimal criteria for purity are a homogeneous appearance in electron micrographs and the failure of additional purification procedures to remove "contaminants" without reducing infectivity.

Identification of a Particle as a Virus

When a characteristic physical particle has been obtained, it should fulfill the following criteria before it is identified as a virus particle:

(1) The particle can be obtained only from infected cells or tissues.

(2) Particles obtained from various sources are identical, regardless of the cellular species in which the virus is grown.

(3) The degree of infective activity of the preparation varies directly with the number of particles present.

(4) The degree of destruction of the physical particle by chemical or physical means is associated with a corresponding loss of virus activity.

(5) Certain properties of the particles and infectivity must be shown to be identical, such as their sedimentation behavior in the ultracentrifuge and their pH stability curves.

(6) The absorption spectrum of the purified physical particle in the ultraviolet range should coincide with the ultraviolet inactivation spectrum of the virus.

(7) Antisera prepared against the infective virus should react with the characteristic particle, and vice versa. Direct observation of an unknown virus can be accomplished by electron microscopic examination of aggregate formation in a mixture of antisera and crude virus suspension.

(8) The particles should be able to induce the characteristic disease in vivo (if such experiments are feasible).

(9) Passage of the particles in tissue culture should result in the production of progeny with biologic and serologic properties of the virus.

REACTION TO PHYSICAL & CHEMICAL AGENTS

Heat & Cold

There is great variability in the heat stability of different viruses. Icosahedral viruses tend to be stable, losing little infectivity after several hours at 37 °C. Enveloped viruses are much more heat-labile, rapidly dropping in titer at 37 °C. Virus infectivity is generally destroyed by heating at 50–60 °C for 30 minutes, although there are some notable exceptions (eg, hepatitis virus, adenoassociated satellite virus, scrapie agent).

Viruses can be preserved by storage at subfreezing temperatures, and some may withstand lyophilization and can thus be preserved in the dry state at 4 °C or even at room temperature. Viruses that withstand lyophilization are more heat-resistant when heated in the dry state. Enveloped viruses tend to lose infectivity after prolonged storage even at −90 °C and are particularly sensitive to repeated freezing and thawing.

Stabilization of Viruses by Salts

Many viruses can be stabilized by salts in concentrations of 1 mol/L, ie, the viruses are not inactivated even by heating at 50 °C for 1 hour. The mechanism by which the salts stabilize virus preparations is not known. Viruses are preferentially stabilized by certain salts. $MgCl_2$, 1 mol/L, stabilizes picorna- and reoviruses; $MgSO_4$, 1 mol/L, stabilizes orthomyxo- and paramyxoviruses; and Na_2SO_4, 1 mol/L, stabilizes herpesviruses.

The stability of viruses is important in the preparation of vaccines. The ordinary nonstabilized poliovaccine must be stored at freezing temperatures to preserve its potency. However, with the addition of salts for stabilization of the virus, potency can be maintained for weeks at ambient temperatures, even in the high temperatures of the tropics.

pH

Viruses are usually stable between pH values of 5.0 and 9.0. Some viruses (eg, enteroviruses) are resistant to acidic conditions. All viruses are destroyed by alkaline conditions. In hemagglutination reactions, variations of less than one pH unit may influence the result.

Radiation

Ultraviolet, x-ray, and high-energy particles inactivate viruses. The dose varies for different viruses. Infectivity is the most radiosensitive property, because replication requires expression of the entire genetic contents. Irradiated particles that are unable to replicate may still be able to express some specific functions in host cells.

Photodynamic Inactivation

Viruses are penetrable to a varying degree by vital dyes such as toluidine blue, neutral red, and proflavine. These dyes bind to the viral nucleic acid, and the virus then becomes susceptible to inactivation by visible light. Impenetrable viruses like poliovirus, when grown in the dark in the presence of vital dyes, incorporate the dye into their nucleic acid and are then susceptible to photodynamic inactivation. The coat antigen is unaffected by the process.

Neutral red is commonly used to stain plaque assays so that plaques are more readily seen. The assay plates must be protected from bright light once the neutral red has been added; otherwise, there is the risk that progeny virus will be inactivated and plaque development will cease.

Ether Susceptibility

Ether susceptibility can distinguish viruses that possess an envelope from those that do not. The following viruses are inactivated by ether: herpes-, orthomyxo-, paramyxo-, rhabdo-, corona-, retro-, arena-, toga-, flavi-, and bunyaviruses. The following viruses are resistant to ether: parvo-, papova-, adeno-, picorna-, and reoviruses. Poxviruses vary in sensitivity to ether.

Detergents

Nonionic detergents, eg, Nonidet P40 and Triton X-100, solubilize lipid constituents of viral membranes. The viral proteins in the envelope are released (undenatured). Anionic detergents, eg, sodium dodecyl sulfate, also solubilize viral envelopes; in addition, they disrupt capsids into separated polypeptides.

Formaldehyde

Formaldehyde destroys viral infectivity by reacting with nucleic acid. Viruses with single-stranded genomes are inactivated much more readily than those with double-stranded genomes. Formaldehyde has minimal adverse effects on the antigenicity of proteins and therefore has been used frequently in the production of inactivated viral vaccines.

Antibiotics & Other Antibacterial Agents

Antibacterial antibiotics and sulfonamides have no effect on viruses. Some antiviral drugs are available, however (see p 387).

Quaternary ammonium compounds, in general, are not effective against viruses. Organic iodine compounds are also ineffective. Larger concentrations of chlorine are required to destroy viruses than to kill bacteria, especially in the presence of extraneous proteins. For example, the chlorine treatment of stools adequate to inactivate typhoid bacilli is inadequate to destroy poliomyelitis virus present in feces. Formalin destroys resistant poliomyelitis and coxsackieviruses. Alcohols, such as isopropanol and ethanol, are relatively ineffective against certain viruses, especially picornaviruses.

REPLICATION OF VIRUSES

Overview

Viruses multiply only in living cells. The host cell must provide the energy and synthetic machinery and the low-molecular-weight precursors for the synthesis of viral proteins and nucleic acids. The viral nucleic acid carries the genetic specificity to code for all the virus-specific macromolecules in a highly organized fashion.

The unique feature of virus multiplication is that, soon after interaction with a host cell, the infecting virion is disrupted and its measurable infectivity lost. This phase of the growth cycle is called the **eclipse period;** its duration varies depending on both the particular virus and the host cell, and it ends with the formation of the first infectious progeny virus particles. The eclipse period is actually one of intense synthetic activity as the cell is redirected toward fulfilling the needs of the viral "pirate." In some cases, as soon as the viral nucleic acid enters the host cell, the cellular metabolism is redirected exclusively toward the synthesis of new virus particles. In other cases, the metabolic processes of the host cell are not altered significantly, although the cell synthesizes viral proteins and nucleic acids.

Virus multiplication was first studied successfully with bacteriophages. The mechanism of phage replication is presented in Chapter 9. For animal viruses,

the steps in the interaction between viruses and susceptible cells have now been elucidated in many systems. Details of virus replication come mainly from studies of one-step growth cycles. If populations of homogeneous cultured cells are infected with many virus particles per cell (high multiplicity of infection), the infection will progress in a carefully regulated pattern in all the cells in unison (ie, its progression is synchronized). This permits studies of the biochemistry and molecular biology of the infection. Details of a one-step growth cycle are illustrated in Fig 33–8 with adenovirus, a DNA-containing virus.

General Steps in Virus Replication Cycles

Viruses have evolved a variety of different strategies for accomplishing multiplication in parasitized host cells. Although the details vary from group to group, the general outline of the replication cycles is similar.

A. Attachment, Penetration, and Uncoating: The first step in virus infection is interaction of a virion with a specific receptor site on the surface of a cell. Receptor molecules differ for different viruses, being proteins in some cases (eg, picornaviruses) and oligosaccharides in others (eg, ortho- and paramyxoviruses). The presence or absence of receptors plays an important determining role in cell tropism and viral pathogenesis; for example, poliovirus is able to attach only to cells in the central nervous system and intesti-

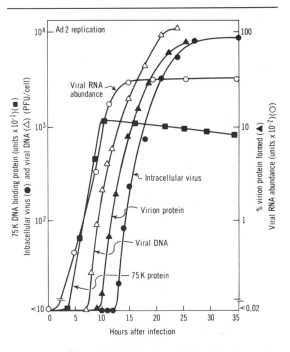

Figure 33–8. Time course of adenovirus replication cycle. The time between infection and the first appearance of progeny virus is the eclipse period. Note the sequential regulation of specific events in the virus replication cycle. (From Green.)

nal tract of primates. Receptor binding is believed to reflect fortuitous configurational homologies between a virion surface structure and a cell surface component. It has been suggested, for example, that rabies virus interacts with acetylcholine receptors and that Epstein-Barr virus recognizes the receptor for the third component of complement on B cells. It has been estimated that each susceptible cell contains at least 100,000 receptor sites for a given virus.

After binding, the virus particle is taken up inside the cell. This step is referred to as penetration, viropexis, or engulfment. In some systems, this is accomplished by receptor-mediated endocytosis, with delivery of the ingested virus particles to the lysosomes. In other systems, the details of penetration are less clear. Uncoating occurs concomitant with or shortly after penetration. Uncoating is the physical separation of the viral nucleic acid (or, in some cases, internal nucleocapsids) from the outer structural components of the virion. The infectivity of the parental virus is lost at this point. Viruses are the only infectious agents for which dissolution of the infecting agent is an obligatory step in the replicative pathway.

B. Synthesis of Virus Components: The synthetic phase of the viral replicative cycle ensues after uncoating of the viral genome. The essential theme in virus replication is that specific mRNAs must be transcribed from the viral nucleic acid for successful expression and duplication of genetic information. Once this is accomplished, viruses use cell components to translate the mRNA. Various classes of viruses use different pathways to synthesize the mRNAs depending upon the structure of the viral nucleic acid. Some viruses (eg, rhabdo-, orthomyxo-, and paramyxoviruses) carry RNA polymerases to synthesize mRNAs. RNA viruses of this type are called negative-strand (negative-sense) viruses, since their single-strand RNA genome is complementary to mRNA, which is conventionally designated positive-strand (positive-sense). Table 33–3 summarizes the various pathways of transcription (but not necessarily those of replication) of the nucleic acids of different classes of viruses.

In the course of virus replication, all the virus-specified macromolecules are synthesized in a highly organized sequence, although virus components are usually made in excess. In some virus infections, notably those involving double-stranded, DNA-containing viruses, early viral proteins are synthesized soon after infection and late proteins are made only late in infection, after viral DNA synthesis. Early genes may or may not be shut off when late products are made. In contrast, most if not all of the genetic information of RNA-containing viruses is expressed at the same time. In addition to these temporal controls, quantitative controls also exist, since not all virus proteins are made in the same amounts. Virus-specific proteins may regulate the extent of transcription of genome or the translation of viral mRNA.

Small animal viruses and bacteriophages are good models for studies of gene expression. Their small size has enabled the total nucleotide sequence of a few viruses to be elucidated. This has led to the discovery of overlapping genes in which some sequences in DNA are utilized in the synthesis of 2 different polypeptides, either by the use of 2 different reading frames or by 2 mRNA molecules using the same reading frames but different starting points. A virus system (adenovirus) first revealed the mRNA processing phenomenon called "splicing," whereby the mRNA sequences that code for a given protein are generated from separated sequences in the template, with noncoding intervening sequences spliced out of the transcript.

The widest variation in strategies of gene expression is found among the RNA-containing viruses.

Table 33–3. Pathways of nucleic acid transcription for various virus classes.

Type of Viral Nucleic Acid	Intermediates	Type of mRNA	Example	Comments
± DS DNA	None	+ mRNA	Most DNA viruses (eg, herpesvirus, T4 bacteriophage)	
+ SS DNA	± DS DNA	+ mRNA	φX bacteriophage	See Chapter 9.
± DS RNA	None	+ mRNA	Reovirus	Virion contains RNA polymerase that transcribes each segment to mRNA.
+ SS RNA	± DS RNA	+ mRNA	Picornaviruses, togaviruses, flaviviruses	Viral nucleic acid is infectious and serves as mRNA. For togaviruses, smaller + mRNA is also formed for certain proteins.
− SS RNA	None	+ mRNA	Rhabdoviruses, paramyxoviruses, orthomyxoviruses	Viral nucleic acid is not infectious; virion contains RNA polymerase which forms + mRNAs smaller than the genome. For orthomyxoviruses, + mRNAs are transcribed from each segment.
+ SS RNA	− DNA, ± DNA	+ mRNA	Retroviruses	Virion contains reverse transcriptase; viral RNA is not infectious but complementary DNA from transformed cell is.

DS = double-stranded
SS = single-stranded

− indicates negative strand
+ indicates positive strand

± indicates a helix containing a positive and a negative strand

Table 33–4. Comparison of replication strategies of several important RNA virus families.

| Characteristic | Grouping Based on Genomic RNA* | | | | | |
| | Positive-Strand Viruses | | | Negative-Strand Viruses | | Double-Stranded Viruses |
	Picornaviridae	Togaviridae	Retroviridae	Orthomyxoviridae	Paramyxoviridae	Reoviridae
Structure of genomic RNA	ss	ss	ss	ss	ss	ds
Sense of genomic RNA	Positive	Positive	Positive	Negative	Negative	
Segmented genome	0	0	0†	+	0	+
Genomic RNA infectious	+	+	0	0	0	0
Genomic RNA acts as messenger	+	+	+	0	0	0
Virion-associated polymerase	0	0	+‡	+	+	+
Subgenomic messages	0	+	+	+	+	+
Polyprotein precursors	+	+	+	0	0	0

*Abbreviations used: ss = single-stranded, ds = double-stranded, positive = same sense as mRNA, negative = complementary to mRNA, + = indicated property applies to that virus family, 0 = indicated property does not apply to that virus family.
†Retroviruses contain a diploid genome (2 copies of nonsegmented genomic RNA).
‡Retroviruses contain a reverse transcriptase (RNA-dependent DNA polymerase).

Some examples are shown in Table 33–4. Some virions carry polymerases (orthomyxoviruses, reoviruses); some systems utilize subgenomic messages, sometimes generated by splicing (orthomyxoviruses, retroviruses); and some viruses synthesize large polyprotein precursors that are processed and cleaved to generate the final gene products (picornaviruses, retroviruses).

The extent to which virus-specific enzymes are involved in these processes varies from group to group. In general, the larger viruses (herpesviruses, poxviruses) are more independent of cellular functions than are the smaller viruses. This is one reason the larger viruses are more susceptible to antiviral chemotherapy (see below), because more virus-specific processes are available as targets for drug action.

The intracellular sites where the different events in virus replication take place vary from group to group (Table 33–5). A few generalizations are possible. Viral protein is synthesized in the cytoplasm on polyribosomes composed of virus-specific mRNA and host cell ribosomes. Viral DNA is usually replicated in the nucleus. Viral genomic RNA is generally duplicated in the cell cytoplasm, although there are exceptions.

C. Morphogenesis and Release: Newly synthesized viral genomes and capsid polypeptides assemble together to form progeny viruses. As described above (Principles of Virus Structure), icosahedral capsids can condense in the absence of nucleic acid, whereas nucleocapsids of viruses with helical symmetry cannot form without viral RNA. There are no special mechanisms for the release of nonenveloped

Table 33–5. Summary of replication cycles of major virus families.

| Virus Family | Type of Nucleic Acid Genome | Presence of Virion Envelope | Intracellular Location* | | | | Duration of Multiplication Cycle (Hours)† |
			Synthesis of Viral Proteins	Replication of Genome	Formation of Nucleocapsid	Virion Maturation	
Papova	DNA	0	C	N	N	N	48
Adeno	DNA	0	C	N	N	N	25
Herpes	DNA	+	C	N	N	M	15–72
Pox	DNA	0	C	C	C	C	20
Picorna	RNA	0	C	C	C	C	6–8
Reo	RNA	0	C	C	C	C	15
Orthomyxo	RNA	+	C	N	N	M	15–30
Retro	RNA	+	C	N	C	M	
Toga	RNA	+	C	C	C	M	10–24
Paramyxo	RNA	+	C	C	C	M	10–48
Rhabdo	RNA	+	C	C	C	M	6–10
Bunya	RNA	+	C	C	C	M	24

*Abbreviations used: C = cytoplasm, N = nucleus, M = membranes.
†The values shown for duration of the multiplication cycle are approximate; ranges indicate that various members within a given family replicate with different kinetics. Different host cell types also influence the kinetics of virus replication.

viruses; the infected cells eventually lyse and release the virus particles.

Enveloped viruses mature by a budding process. Virus-specific envelope glycoproteins are inserted into cellular membranes; viral nucleocapsids then bud through the membrane at these modified sites and, in so doing, acquire an envelope. As noted above (Fig 33–7), budding frequently occurs at the plasma membrane but may involve other membranes in the cell. Enveloped viruses are not infectious until they have acquired their envelopes. Therefore, infectious progeny virions typically do not accumulate within the infected cell.

Virus maturation is sometimes an inefficient process. Excess amounts of viral components may accumulate and be involved in the formation of inclusion bodies in the cell (see above). As a result of the profound deleterious effects of virus replication, cellular cytopathic effects eventually develop and the cell dies. However, there are instances in which the cell is not damaged by the virus and long-term, persistent infections evolve (see Persistent, Latent, & Slow Virus Infections, below).

Summary of Virus Replication

The molecular events discussed above are summarized in Fig 33–9. Viruses with genomes containing double-stranded (ds) nucleic acid proceed along most of the steps shown in the figure. Viruses with single-stranded (ss) nucleic acid genomes utilize only some of the steps. With RNA-containing viruses, the replicative cycle is not divided cleanly into early and late phases, as it is with most DNA-containing viruses. Also, as noted above, not all viruses are enveloped in membranes.

The replicative cycle of a herpesvirus is summarized in Fig 33–10. Herpesviruses contain a DNA genome in an icosahedral capsid that obtains an envelope by budding through the nuclear membrane. The replication of picornaviruses is shown in Fig 33–11. Picornaviruses have an RNA genome in an icosahedral, nonenveloped capsid. The diagrams illustrate that steps in viral replication may involve different cellular compartments. Each virus effectively utilizes whichever cellular processes are necessary to achieve its multiplication and morphogenesis.

GENETICS OF ANIMAL VIRUSES

Genetic analysis is a powerful approach toward understanding the structure and function of the viral

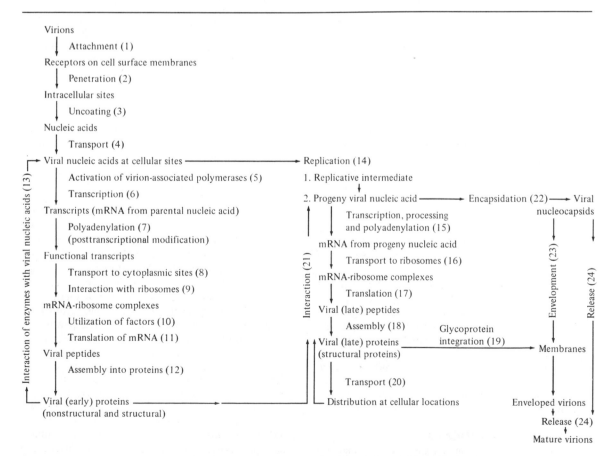

Figure 33–9. Molecular events in the replication of viruses. (From Becker.)

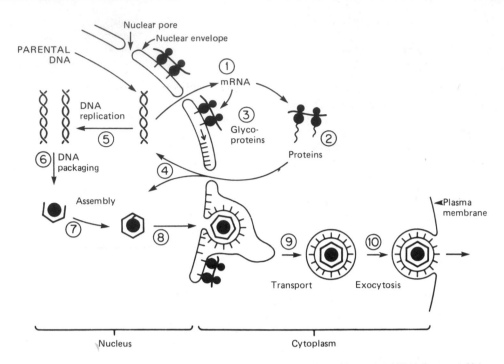

Figure 33–10. Herpesvirus replication and morphogenesis. Diagram begins with parental DNA (upper left) in nucleus of host cell. *(1)* Viral mRNAs are synthesized by host cell RNA polymerase on the viral DNA template. Messengers are exported from the nucleus and initiate the synthesis of viral proteins (free polyribosomes) *(2)* and glycoproteins (membrane-bound polyribosomes) *(3)*. Viral proteins enter the nucleus *(4)*, where they promote synthesis of additional classes of viral mRNAs. Viral DNA polymerase enters the nucleus and initiates viral DNA replication *(5)*. DNA is cut into unit lengths, packaged into nucleoids *(6)*, and encapsidated *(7)* within an icosahedral shell. The icosahedral shell buds through the nuclear membrane, acquiring a lipoprotein envelope containing viral glycoproteins *(8)*. The mature virus is transported in vesicles to the plasma membrane *(9)*. Fusion of the vesicle with the plasma membrane results in the release of the virus into the extracellular space *(10)*. (Reproduced, with permission, from Silverstein SC: Viral replication. Pages 94–100 in: *International Textbook of Medicine*. Vol 2: *Medical Microbiology and Infectious Diseases*. Braude AI [editor]. Saunders, 1981.)

genome, its gene products, and their roles in infection and disease. Meaningful genetic studies with animal viruses depend on 2 factors. The first is a plaque assay for virus infectivity, a sensitive and accurate quantitative assay method. The second is stable genetic markers, which ideally should result from single mutations. "Stable markers" refers to the use of mutants of various viral genes that are recognizable by some change in an observable property of the parental virus. Some markers commonly used include plaque size, specific virus-induced antigens, drug resistance, host range, and inability to grow at high temperatures. Mutants with such markers are obtained either after spontaneous mutation or after treatment with a mutagen.

The following terms are basic to a discussion of genetics: **Genotype** refers to the genetic constitution of an organism. **Phenotype** refers to the observable properties of an organism, which are produced by the genotype in cooperation with the environment. A **mutation** is a heritable change in the genotype. The **genome** is the sum of the genes of an organism.

Conditional-Lethal Mutants

Conditional-lethal mutants are mutants that are lethal (in that no infectious virus is produced) under one set of conditions—termed nonpermissive conditions—but that yield normal infectious progeny under other conditions—termed permissive conditions. Conditional-lethal mutants include temperature-sensitive (ts) and host range (hr) mutants. Ts mutants have been isolated from nearly all animal viruses; they grow at low (permissive) temperatures but not at high (nonpermissive) temperatures. Host range mutants are able to grow and form plaques in one kind of cell (permissive cell), whereas abortive infection occurs in another type (nonpermissive cell). Hr bacterial virus mutants may possess altered nucleic acid base sequences that are read as nonsense mutations by the nonpermissive host cell, resulting in polypeptide chain termination and consequently abortive infection. The permissive host cell, on the other hand, carries a transfer RNA that recognizes the altered sequence as a codon and inserts an amino acid, resulting in the formation of a functional polypeptide. It has not been established whether such a mechanism is also operative in host range mutants of animal viruses. Following the induction and isolation of a set of conditional-lethal mutants, mixed infection studies with pairs of mutants under permissive and nonpermissive conditions can yield information concerning gene function, gene se-

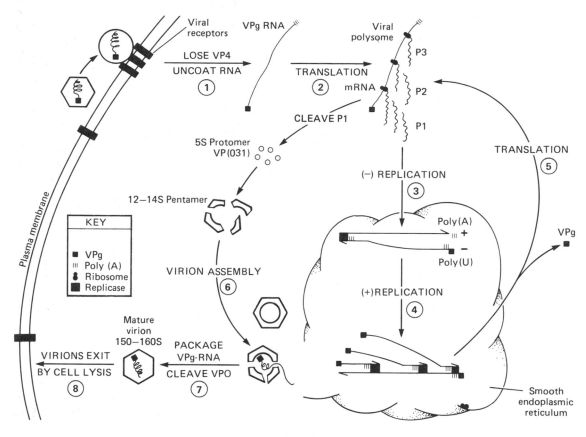

Figure 33–11. Overview of the picornavirus infection cycle. (Reproduced, with permission, from Rueckert RR: Picor naviruses and their replication. Pages 705–738 in: *Virology*. Fields BN et al [editors]. Raven Press, 1985.)

quence (genetic mapping), and mechanisms of virus replication at the molecular level.

Mutagens widely used for the induction of mutants fall into 3 classes: (1) base analogs that can replace the normal bases of DNA during replication; (2) substances that chemically alter the bases of nonreplicating DNA; and (3) those whose action is to remove DNA bases. An example of the first class of mutagens is 5-bromouracil, which replaces thymine quantitatively and which also base-pairs with guanine. This substance can thus induce mutations by causing 2 types of base-pair transitions depending upon whether the pairing error occurs during incorporation or during replication following incorporation. Nitrous acid is an example of the second class of mutagens. It can oxidatively deaminate either adenine or cytosine. Representative of the third class of mutagens is ethylene ethanesulfonate, which may remove guanine bases.

Defective Viruses

A defective virus is one that lacks one or more functional genes required for virus replication. Defective viruses require helper activity from another virus for some step in replication or maturation. Helper-dependent defective viruses frequently lack a portion of their genome (ie, deletion mutants). The extent of loss by deletion may vary from a short base sequence

to a large amount of the genome. Deletion mutants may arise spontaneously or may be constructed in the laboratory using biochemical techniques.

Spontaneous deletion mutants frequently arise when virus stocks are passaged repeatedly at high multiplicity. Such defective viruses may interfere with the replication of homologous virus and are called defective interfering (DI) virus particles. DI particles have lost essential segments of genome but contain normal capsid proteins; they require infectious homologous virus as helper for replication, and they interfere with the multiplication of that homologous virus. This interference with standard helper virus probably results from successful competition by DI particles for factors involved in genome replication.

DI particles were first recognized in the influenza virus system. When influenza virus is serially passed at high multiplicity, the yield of infectious virus decreases dramatically but the number of particles remains high (von Magnus phenomenon). Defective particles do not accumulate if the virus is passaged at low multiplicity. The most complete studies of DI particles have been made with vesicular stomatitis virus; the DI particles in that system are truncated (short rods) and are readily separable from the bullet-shaped, standard infectious virus.

DI particles may be biologically important. It has

been proposed that they may play a role in the establishment and maintenance of persistent infections.

Pseudovirions are a different type of defective particle. They contain host cell DNA rather than the viral genome. During viral replication, the capsid sometimes encloses random pieces of host nucleic acid rather than viral nucleic acid. Such particles look like ordinary virus particles when observed by electron microscopy, but they do not replicate. Pseudovirions theoretically might be able to transduce cellular nucleic acid from one cell to another.

Interactions Among Viruses

When 2 or more virus particles infect the same host cell, they may interact in a variety of ways. They must be sufficiently closely related, usually within the same virus family, for most types of interactions to occur. Genetic interaction results in some progeny that are heritably (genetically) different from either parent. Progeny produced as a consequence of nongenetic interaction are similar to the parental viruses. In genetic interactions the actual nucleic acid molecules interact, whereas the products of the genes are involved in nongenetic interactions.

A. Recombination: Recombination results in the production of progeny virus (recombinant) that carries traits not found together in either parent. The classical mechanism is that the nucleic acid strands break, and part of the genome of one parent is joined to part of the genome of the second parent. The recombinant virus is genetically stable, yielding progeny like itself upon replication. (See Chapter 40.) Viruses vary widely in the frequency with which they undergo recombination. Those with double-stranded DNA genomes recombine efficiently; most viruses with nonsegmented, single-stranded RNA genomes do not recombine. In the case of viruses with segmented genomes, eg, influenza virus, the formation of recombinants is due to reassortment of individual genome fragments rather than to an actual crossover event, and it occurs with ease.

B. Genetic Reactivation: This phenomenon represents a special case of recombination.

Marker rescue occurs between the genome of an active virion and the genome of a virus particle that has been inactivated in some way. A portion of the genome of the inactivated virus recombines with that of the active parent, so that certain markers of the inactivated parent are rescued and appear in the viable progeny. None of the progeny produced are identical to the inactivated parent. The progeny carrying the rescued markers of the inactivated parent are genetically stable (see examples in Chapter 40).

Multiplicity reactivation occurs when an inactive virus particle is rendered active by interaction with other inactive virus particles in the same cell. This may occur when a heavily damaged virus preparation is used to infect cells at high multiplicity of infection. Recombination occurs between the damaged nucleic acids of the parents, producing a viable genome that can replicate. The greater the damage to the parental

genomes, the larger the number of inactive particles required per cell to ensure the formation of a viable genome.

C. Complementation: This refers to the interaction of viral gene products in cells infected with 2 viruses, one or both of which may be defective. It results in the replication of one or both under conditions in which replication would not ordinarily occur. The basis for complementation is that one virus provides a gene product in which the second is defective, allowing the second virus to grow. The genotypes of the 2 viruses remain unchanged.

If both mutants are defective in the same gene product, they will not be able to complement the growth of one another. Therefore, this test is routinely used to group conditional-lethal mutants of a virus as a prelude to detailed biochemical analyses of the gene functions represented by the mutants.

D. Phenotypic Mixing: A special case of complementation is phenotypic mixing, or the association of a genotype with a heterologous phenotype. This occurs when the genome of one virus becomes randomly incorporated within capsid proteins specified by a different virus or a capsid consisting of components of both viruses (Fig 33–12). If the genome is encased in a completely heterologous protein coat (third and fourth progeny from left), this extreme example of phenotypic mixing may be called "phenotypic masking" or "transcapsidation." Such mixing is not a stable genetic change because, upon replication, the phenotypically mixed parent will yield progeny encased in capsids homologous to the genotype.

Phenotypic mixing usually occurs between different members of the same virus family; the intermixed capsid proteins must be able to interact correctly to form a structurally intact capsid. However, phenotypic mixing also can occur between enveloped viruses, and in this case, the viruses do not have to be closely related. The nucleocapsid of one virus becomes encased within an envelope specified by another, a phenomenon designated "pseudotype formation." There are many examples of pseudotype formation among the RNA tumor viruses (see Chapter 46). The nucleocapsid of vesicular stomatitis virus, a rhabdovirus, has an unusual propensity to be involved in pseudotype formation with unrelated envelope material.

E. Interference: Infection of either cell cultures or whole animals with 2 viruses often leads to an inhibition of multiplication of one of the viruses, an effect called interference. Interference in animals is distinct from specific immunity. Furthermore, interference does not occur with all virus combinations; 2 viruses may infect and multiply within the same cell as efficiently as in single infections.

Several mechanisms have been elucidated as causes of interference: (1) One virus may inhibit the ability of the second to adsorb to the cell, either by blocking its receptors (retroviruses, enteroviruses) or by destroying its receptors (orthomyxoviruses). (2) One virus may compete with the second for compo-

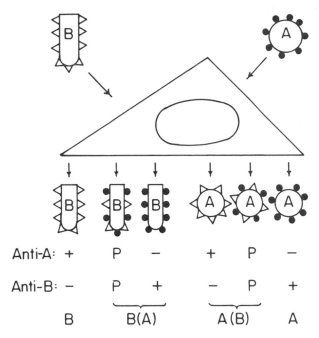

Figure 33–12. Schematic diagram of phenotypic mixing and neutralization of pseudotypes. + = Virus lesions present: no neutralization. P = Partial neutralization: resistant fraction present or slower neutralization kinetics. − = No virus lesions: virus completely neutralized. A and B are the pure virus types; A(B) is A genome with B envelope pseudotype; B(A) is B genome with A envelope pseudotype. (Reproduced, with permission, from Boettiger: *Prog Med Virol* 1979;**25**:37.)

nents of the replication apparatus (eg, polymerase, translation initiation factor). (3) The first virus may cause the infected cell to produce an inhibitor (interferon, see below) that prevents replication of the second virus.

When this phenomenon occurs between unrelated viruses, it is called **heterologous** interference. When it occurs between related viruses, it is called **homologous** interference. Most viruses have the capacity to interfere with their own replication (autointerference). In this case, DI particles are produced at the expense of complete virus when high multiplicities of infection are used (see above). Autointerference may have a role in the establishment of persistent virus infections.

Interference has been used as a basis for controlling outbreaks of infection with virulent strains of poliovirus by introducing into the population an attenuated poliovirus that interferes with the spread of the virulent virus. Interference between a preexisting virus infection and a superinfecting attenuated virus vaccine has sometimes been a problem in poliovirus vaccination programs.

Mapping of Viral Genomes

Efforts are under way to characterize and understand viral functions involved in replication and in disease production and to identify the regions of the viral genome encoding those specific functions.

Recent advances in animal virus genetics using restriction enzymes and other biochemical techniques have facilitated the identification of virus gene products and the mapping of these on the viral genome. Biochemical and physical mapping can usually be done much more rapidly than genetic mapping using classical genetic techniques.

The technique of reassortment mapping has been used with influenza A viruses, which have a genome of 8 segments of RNA, each coding for one virus protein. Under suitable conditions, the RNA genome segments and the polypeptides of different influenza A viruses migrate at different rates in polyacrylamide gels, so that strains can be distinguished. By analyzing the recombinants (reassortants) formed between different influenza viruses, the RNA segment coding for each protein has been determined. Similar experiments with temperature-sensitive mutants have shown the biologic function of various polypeptides. Recombinants are being analyzed to determine which virus proteins are responsible for virulence in humans.

The use of restriction endonucleases for identification of specific virus strains or isolates is illustrated in Fig 33–13. Viral DNA is isolated and incubated with a specific endonuclease until DNA sequences susceptible to the nuclease are cleaved. The fragments are then resolved on the basis of size by gel electrophoresis. The large fragments are most retarded by the sieving effect of the gel, so that an inverse relationship between size and migration is observed. The position of the DNA fragments can be determined by radioautography on x-ray film if the viral DNA is labeled. Such physical mapping techniques have been

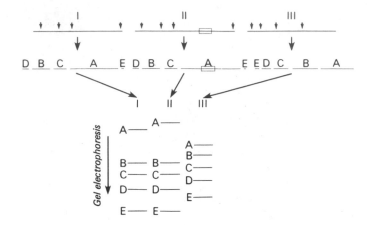

Figure 33–13. Illustration of principles of restriction endonuclease cleavage site analysis. The linear DNA (double-stranded) genomes of 3 hypothetical viruses to be compared are indicated as I, II, III. Suppose a specific nucleotide sequence, eg, GAATTC, the cleavage site for nuclease EcoRI, occurs at 4 sites in each genome as indicated by small arrows. Genomes I and II are identical except for a substantial DNA insertion mutation in genome II. Genome III has none of the sequences in question located in positions analogous to genomes I or II. Cleavage of these DNAs at the sites marked by arrows results in 5 fragments (A–E) in each case. If these DNA fragments are separated according to size in adjacent tracks in a gel electrophoresis experiment, the result will be as diagrammed: fragments B, C, D, and E of samples I and II will co-migrate and fragment A from each virus will differ. The fragments from genome III will co-migrate with none of those from genomes I and II. It should be noted that knowledge of the cleavage site maps at the top is not essential to be able to deduce the fact that genomes I and II are related to each other but not to genome III. (Reproduced, with permission, from Summers WC: *Yale J Biol Med* 1980;**53**:55.)

extremely useful in distinguishing virus types in systems in which the viruses cannot be cultured (eg, papillomaviruses).

Detailed physical maps can be prepared for DNA viruses by using a variety of restriction endonucleases. The position in the genome of given DNA sequences can be determined quite precisely.

Physical maps can be correlated with genetic maps if the latter are available. This allows virus gene products to be mapped to individual regions of the genome defined by the restriction enzyme fragments. Transcription of mRNAs throughout the replication cycle can be assigned to specific DNA fragments. Using mutagens, it is also possible to alter isolated fragments of viral DNA in order to introduce mutations into defined regions of the genome.

Viral Genomes as Vectors

A. Recombinant DNA: The insertion of DNA fragments into plasmids of bacteria has given rise to a new technology that holds great promise for the production of biologic materials, hormones, vaccines, interferon, and other gene products. Viral genomes have been engineered to serve as replication and expression vectors for both viral and cellular genes. The SV40 system has been used most extensively, but papillomavirus, adenovirus, and retrovirus vectors are also useful. Correct transcriptional signals must be included in order for the cloned genes to be expressed. The principles of recombinant DNA technology were described and illustrated in Chapter 4. Fig 33–14 shows the derivation of a recombinant. Fragments of hepatitis B virus DNA have been cloned and the im-

munizing antigen has been produced in bacteria as well as in eukaryotic cells. This approach offers the possibility of producing large amounts of such antigen for vaccine purposes.

B. Virus-Mediated Gene Transfer in Mammalian Cells: If external genetic information could be stably introduced into eukaryotic cells, this might permit repair of genetic defects. For instance, congenital galactosemia could be corrected by introducing the galactosidase gene into the patient's cells. No such repair has been accomplished in humans, but there are encouraging results in some experimental systems.

Gene transfer in bacteria can be accomplished by transformation, phage transduction, and conjugation (see Chapter 4). In eukaryotic cells, gene transfer has been accomplished by transformation, microinjection, and transfection of DNA fragments or recombinant genomes. The most promising approach for gene therapy of human genetic defects is by the use of defective retrovirus vectors carrying cloned replacement genes. Retrovirus vectors will efficiently integrate a replacement gene into chromosomal DNA. Technical difficulties face the delivery of the vector to appropriate target cells. After that problem is surmounted, there will still exist the problems of possible immunologic incompatibility of new gene products, possible transfer of undesirable genes together with desired ones, deleterious side effects due to the site of integration of the vector, and altered regulation of gene expression that may turn out to be damaging. Routine gene therapy of this type remains many years in the future.

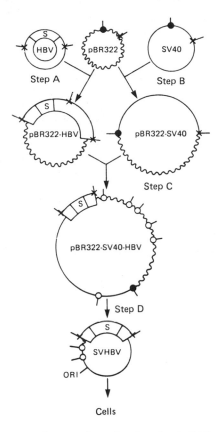

Figure 33–14. Construction of a functional SV40 papovavirus recombinant carrying about 40% of the hepatitis B virus (HBV) genome that includes the sequences coding for the immunizing surface antigen (HBsAg). The HBV DNA fragment is inserted into the late gene region of the papovavirus. x— = BamHI site; ●— = EcoRI site; ○— = HaeII site. *Steps A and B:* HBV DNA and SV40 DNA were each cleaved with restriction enzymes, ligated to cleaved plasmid pBR322 DNA, and then cloned and amplified in *E coli. Step C:* The new plasmids containing the viral DNAs were cleaved, ligated, and recloned in *E coli* to yield the double recombinant plasmid. *Step D:* HaeII digestion removed almost all of the plasmid DNA and a small part of SV40. The resultant recombinant DNA retained the SV40 origin of DNA replication (ORI) and the complete SV40 early gene region. For propagation in monkey kidney cells, an SV40 temperature-sensitive early gene mutant had to be used as helper, as it contained the required late genes. The mixed infection at the nonpermissive temperature (39 °C) yielded progeny virions only from cells doubly infected with the SV40-HBV recombinant (functional SV40 early genes) and the helper (functional late genes). The infected monkey kidney cells also synthesized HBsAg but no other HBV antigens. The antigen was excreted into the culture medium as 22-nm particles with the same properties as those found in the blood of patients with type B hepatitis. (Not shown at the top of the diagram are the HaeII sites in pBR322 and SV40 DNA.) (Reproduced, with permission, from Moriarty AM et al: *Proc Natl Acad Sci USA* 1981;**78**:2606.)

NATURAL HISTORY (ECOLOGY) & MODES OF TRANSMISSION OF VIRUSES

Ecology is the study of interactions between living organisms and their environment. Different viruses have evolved ingenious and often complicated mechanisms for survival in nature and transmission from one host to the next. The mode of transmission utilized by a given virus depends on the nature of the interaction between the virus and the host.

Viruses may be transmitted in the following ways: (1) Direct transmission from person to person by contact. The major means of transmission may be by droplet or aerosol infection (eg, influenza, measles, smallpox); by the fecal-oral route (eg, enteroviruses, rotaviruses, infectious hepatitis); by sexual contact (eg, hepatitis B, herpes simplex type 2, AIDS); by hand-mouth, hand-eye, or mouth-mouth contact (eg, herpes simplex, rhinovirus, Epstein-Barr virus); or by exchange of contaminated blood (eg, hepatitis B, AIDS). (2) Transmission from animal to animal, with humans an accidental host. Spread may be by bite (rabies) or by droplet or aerosol infection from rodent-contaminated quarters (eg, arenaviruses). (3) Transmission by means of an arthropod vector (eg, arboviruses, now classified primarily as togaviruses, flaviviruses, and bunyaviruses).

At least 3 different transmission patterns have been recognized among the arthropod-borne viruses:

1. Human-arthropod cycle—*Examples:* Urban yellow fever, dengue.

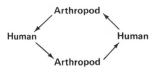

2. Lower vertebrate-arthropod cycle with tangential infection of humans—*Examples:* Jungle yellow fever, St. Louis encephalitis. The infected human is a "dead-end" host. This is a more common transmission mechanism.

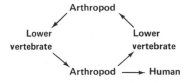

3. Arthropod-arthropod cycle with occasional infection of humans and lower vertebrates—*Examples:* Colorado tick fever, LaCrosse encephalitis.

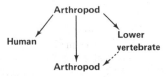

In this cycle, the virus may be transmitted from the adult arthropod to its offspring through the egg (transovarian passage); thus, the cycle may continue with or without intervention of a viremic vertebrate host.

In vertebrates, the invasion of most viruses evokes a violent reaction, usually of short duration. The result is decisive. Either the host succumbs or it lives through the production of antibodies that neutralize the virus. Regardless of the outcome, the sojourn of the active virus is usually short, although persistent or latent infections that last for months to years may occur (hepatitis B, herpes simplex, cytomegalovirus) (see p 386). In arthropod vectors of the virus, the relationship is usually quite different. The viruses produce little or no ill effect and remain active in the arthropod throughout the latter's natural life. Thus arthropods, in contrast to vertebrates, act as permanent hosts and reservoirs.

PATHOGENESIS OF VIRUS DISEASES

To produce disease, viruses must enter a host, come in contact with susceptible cells, replicate, and produce cell injury. Much is still not known about this process in many viral infections, but genetic and biochemical studies will eventually lead to an understanding of viral pathogenesis at the molecular level. Such understanding is necessary to design truly effective and specific antiviral strategies. Most of our knowledge of viral pathogenesis is based on animal models, because such systems can be more readily manipulated and studied.

Steps in Viral Pathogenesis
A. Entry and Primary Replication: Most viruses enter their hosts through the mucosa of the respiratory or gastrointestinal tracts. Major exceptions are those viruses that are introduced directly into the bloodstream by needles (hepatitis B, AIDS) or by insect vectors (arboviruses).

Many viruses replicate at the primary site of entry. Some, such as influenza viruses (respiratory infections) and rotaviruses (gastrointestinal infections), produce disease at the portal of entry and have no necessity for further systemic spread.

B. Virus Spread and Cell Tropism: Many viruses produce disease at sites distant from their point of entry (eg, enteroviruses, which enter through the gastrointestinal tract but produce central nervous system disease). After primary replication at the site of entry, these viruses then spread within the host. Mechanisms of viral spread vary, but the most common route is via the bloodstream or lymphatics. The viremic phase is short in many virus infections. In a few instances, neuronal spread is involved; this is apparently how rabies virus reaches the brain to cause disease and how herpes simplex virus moves to the ganglia to initiate latent infections.

Viral spread may be determined in part by specific viral genes. Studies with reovirus have demonstrated that the extent of spread from the gastrointestinal tract is determined by one of the outer capsid proteins. Cell and tissue tropism of a given virus usually reflects the presence of specific cell surface receptors for that virus. The chemical nature of virus receptors is not known in most cases. Receptors are components of the cell surface with which a region of the viral surface (capsid or envelope) can specifically interact and initiate infection. Presumably, the receptors are cell constituents that function in normal cellular metabolism but also happen to have an affinity for a particular virus. For example, it may be that rabies virus binds to acetylcholine receptors on neurons.

A second mechanism dictating tissue tropism involves proteolytic enzymes. Certain paramyxoviruses are not infectious until an envelope glycoprotein undergoes proteolytic cleavage. Multiple rounds of viral replication will not occur in tissues that do not express the appropriate activating enzymes.

C. Cell Injury and Clinical Illness: Destruction of virus-infected cells in the target tissues and the physiologic alterations produced in the host by the tissue injury are partly responsible for the development of disease. However, clinical illness from virus infection is the result of a complex series of events, and many of the factors that determine the degree of illness are unknown. Clinical illness is an insensitive indicator of virus infection; inapparent infections by viruses are very common.

D. Specific Examples: The pathogenesis of mousepox, a disease of the skin, and of human poliomyelitis, a disease of the central nervous system, are outlined in Fig 33–15. Both viruses multiply at the primary site of entry prior to systemic spread to target organs.

In mousepox, the virus enters the body through minute abrasions of the skin and multiplies in the epidermal cells. At the same time, it is carried by the lymphatics to the regional lymph nodes, where multiplication also occurs. The few virus particles entering the blood by way of the efferent lymphatics are taken up by the macrophages of the liver and spleen. The virus multiplies rapidly in both organs. Following release of virus from the liver and spleen, it moves by way of the bloodstream and localizes in the basal epidermal layers of the skin, in the conjunctival cells, and near the lymph follicles in the intestine. The virus may occasionally also localize in the epithelial cells of the kidney, lung, submaxillary gland, and pancreas. A primary lesion occurs at the site of entry of the virus. It appears as a localized swelling that rapidly increases in size, becomes edematous, ulcerates, and goes on to scar formation. A generalized rash follows that is responsible for the release of large quantities of virus into the environment.

In poliomyelitis, virus enters by way of the alimentary tract, multiplies locally at the initial sites of viral implantation (tonsils, Peyer's patches) or the lymph nodes that drain these tissues, and begins to appear in the throat and in the feces. Secondary virus spread oc-

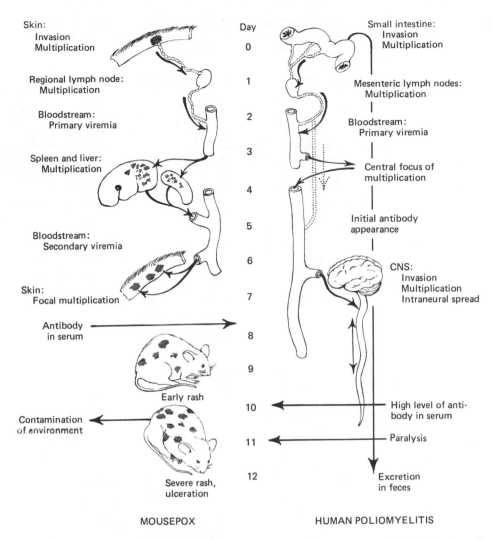

Figure 33–15. Schematic illustrations of the pathogenesis of mousepox and poliomyelitis. (Modified from Fenner.)

curs by way of the bloodstream to other susceptible tissues, namely, other lymph nodes, brown fat, and the central nervous system. Within the central nervous system, the virus spreads along nerve fibers. If a high level of multiplication occurs as the virus spreads through the central nervous system, motor neurons are destroyed and paralysis occurs. The shedding of virus into the environment does not depend upon secondary virus spread to the central nervous system. Secondary spread to the central nervous system is readily interrupted by the presence of antibodies induced by prior infection or vaccination.

Host Immune Response

Both humoral and cellular components of the immune response are involved in control of viral infections, but the precise roles of antibody and immune cells are still unknown. Viruses elicit a tissue response different from the response to pathogenic bacteria, not only in the parenchymatous cells but also in cellular infiltration. Whereas polymorphonuclear leukocytes

form the principal cellular response to the acute inflammation caused by pyogenic bacteria, infiltration with mononuclear cells and lymphocytes characterizes the inflammatory reaction of uncomplicated viral lesions.

Virus-encoded proteins, usually capsid proteins, serve as targets for the immune response. Virus-infected cells may be lysed by cytotoxic T lymphocytes as a result of their recognition of viral polypeptides on the cell surface. Humoral immunity protects the host against reinfection by the same virus. This is the basis for viral vaccine programs. Nt antibody blocks the initiation of viral infection, probably at the stage of attachment or uncoating. Secretory IgA antibody is important in protecting against infection by viruses through the respiratory or gastrointestinal tracts.

In addition to specific immunity, some nonspecific host defense mechanisms may be elicited by virus infection. The most prominent among the "nonimmune" responses is the induction of interferons (see below).

Special characteristics of certain viruses may have

profound effects on the host's immune response. Some viruses infect and damage cells of the immune system. The most dramatic example is the human retrovirus associated with acquired immune deficiency syndrome (AIDS) that infects T lymphocytes and destroys their ability to function (see Chapter 47).

Adverse effects of the immune response to virus infection are also known. Certain viruses do not invariably kill the cells they infect. The immunologic response of the host in these situations may be involved in the observed pathologic changes and clinical illness. This phenomenon is exemplified in lymphocytic choriomeningitis virus infection of mice. Infection of newborn mice before they develop immunologic competence results in a lifelong viral infection that is not associated with acute illness; however, later in life, many of the chronically infected mice develop a fatal debilitating disease involving the central nervous system. These animals also exhibit chronic glomerulonephritis, which is thought to be caused by deposition of virus antigen-antibody complexes (see Chapter 39).

Another type of immunopathologic disorder has been observed in humans previously immunized with vaccines containing killed measles or respiratory syncytial virus. Such persons may develop unusual immune responses that give rise to serious consequences when they later are exposed to the naturally occurring infective virus. Dengue hemorrhagic fever with shock syndrome, which develops in persons who already have had at least one prior infection with another dengue serotype, may be a naturally occurring manifestation of the same type of immunopathology (see p 427).

Another potential adverse effect of the immune response is the development of autoantibodies. If a viral antigen were to elicit antibodies that fortuitously recognized an antigenic determinant on a cellular protein in normal tissues, cellular injury or loss of function un-related to viral infection might result. The magnitude of this potential problem in human disease is currently unknown.

Effect of Host Age

Host age is a factor in virus pathogenicity. More severe disease is often produced in newborn animals. In addition to maturation of the immune response with age, there seem to be age-related changes in the susceptibility of certain cell types to virus infection. Virus infections usually can occur in all age groups but may have their major impact at different times of life, from rubella, which is most serious during gestation, to St. Louis encephalitis, which is most serious in the elderly (Table 33–6).

Viruses as Causes of Congenital Defects

Viral infection during pregnancy may be a significant cause of fetal damage and loss. Three principles involved in the production of congenital defects are (1) the ability of the virus to infect the pregnant woman and be transmitted to the fetus; (2) the stage of gestation at which infection occurs; and (3) the ability of the virus to cause damage to the fetus directly, by infection of the fetus, or indirectly, by infection of the mother resulting in an altered fetal environment (eg, fever). The sequence of events that may occur prior to and following viral invasion of the fetus is shown in Fig 33–16.

Rubella and cytomegalovirus are presently the primary agents responsible for congenital defects in humans (see Chapters 41 and 44). Congenital infection with herpes simplex, varicella-zoster, and coxsackie B viruses may also be of significance in inducing teratogenic effects in the fetus.

Persistent, Latent, & Slow Virus Infections

Virus infections are usually self-limiting. Some-

Table 33–6. Peak ages of incidence of serious viral diseases.*

Before Birth	At Birth	Infants	Children	Adolescents and Young Adults	Older Adults
			Herpes type 1		
	Herpes type 2	Respiratory syncytial disease	Rhinovirus colds	Herpes type 2	
Cytomegalovirus disease		Parainfluenza	Coronavirus disease	Hepatitis B	
Rubella	Hepatitis B	Adenovirus disease	Measles		
			Rubella		
			Mumps		
			Influenza		
			Polio and other enteroviral diseases		
		Rotavirus diarrhea	Hepatitis A	Infectious mononucleosis (EB virus)	St. Louis encephalitis
			Epidemic gastroenteritis (Norwalk virus)		
			Varicella (chickenpox)		Herpes zoster (shingles)

*Adapted from Wilson EB, NIH Publication No. 80–433.

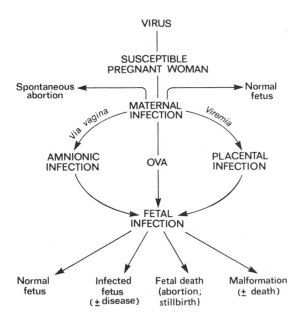

Figure 33–16. Viral infection of the fetus. (After Catalano and Sever.)

times, however, the virus persists for long periods of time in the host. The long-term virus-host interaction may take several forms. **Persistent infections** are those in which virus can be continuously detected; mild or no clinical symptoms may be evident. **Latent infections** are those in which the virus persists in an occult, or cryptic, form most of the time. There will be intermittent flare-ups of clinical disease; infectious virus can be recovered during flare-ups. **Slow virus infections** have a prolonged incubation period, lasting months or years, during which virus continues to multiply. Clinical symptoms are usually not evident during the long incubation period. **Inapparent** or subclinical infection covers, at the host-parasite level, the whole field of infections that give no overt sign of their presence.

Persistent infections occur with a number of animal viruses, and the persistence in certain instances depends upon the age of the host when infected. In human beings, for example, rubella virus and cytomegalovirus infections acquired in utero characteristically result in viral persistence that is of limited duration, probably because of development of the immunologic capacity to react to the infection as the infant matures. Infants infected with hepatitis B virus frequently become persistently infected (chronic carriers); most carriers are asymptomatic (see Chapter 38). Animal studies have shown that in persistent infections the virus population often undergoes many genetic and antigenic changes.

Persistent ("slow") viral infections may play a far-reaching role in human disease. Persistent virus infections are associated with leukemias and sarcomas of chickens and mice (see Chapter 46) as well as with progressive degenerative diseases of the central nervous system of humans and animals (see Chapter 39). The latter may represent a distorted immunopathologic reaction to chronic presence of the virus, leading to "immune complex disease" or chronic central nervous system disease.

Persistently infected cell cultures have been studied in the laboratory. Resistant healthy cells may emerge in infected cultures. The growth of the apparently healthy cells in culture for many generations is accompanied by a concomitant multiplication of virus. The number of cells supporting viral infection in such cultures is usually only a small portion of the entire population.

Herpesviruses typically produce latent infections. Herpes simplex viruses enter the sensory ganglia and persist in a noninfectious state that is not understood at the molecular level. There may be periodic reactivations during which lesions containing infectious virus appear at peripheral sites (eg, fever blisters). Chickenpox virus (varicella-zoster) also becomes latent in sensory ganglia. Recurrences are rare and occur years later, usually following the distribution of a peripheral nerve (shingles). Other members of the herpesvirus family also establish latent infections, including cytomegalovirus and Epstein-Barr virus. All may be reactivated by immunosuppression. Consequently, reactivated herpesvirus infections may be a serious complication for persons receiving immunosuppressant therapy.

Slow virus diseases are a group of chronic, progressive, fatal infections of the central nervous system caused by unconventional, transmissible, proteinaceous agents that have not yet been shown to contain nucleic acid. The best example of a slow virus infection is scrapie in sheep. Kuru and Creutzfeldt-Jakob disease occur in humans. The diseases have long incubation periods (months to years). When they do develop, the pathology is restricted to the central nervous system. The agents elicit no immune response and no inflammatory reaction from the host. The mechanism by which this baffling group of agents induce disease is unknown.

In Fig 33–17, examples of apparent, inapparent, persistent, latent, occult, and slow virus infections are presented.

PREVENTION & TREATMENT OF VIRAL INFECTIONS

Antiviral Chemotherapy

Unlike viruses, bacteria and protozoans do not rely on host cellular machinery for replication, so processes specific to these organisms provide ready targets for the development of antibacterial and antiprotozoal drugs. Because viruses are obligate intracellular parasites, antiviral agents must be capable of selectively inhibiting viral functions without damaging the host. Molecular virology studies have now succeeded in identifying virus-specific functions that can serve as realistic targets for inhibition. Theoretically,

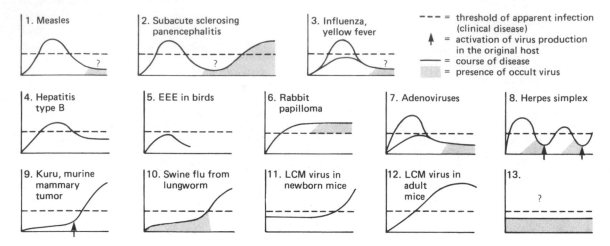

Figure 33–17. Apparent, inapparent, persistent, latent, occult, and slow virus infections. *(1)* Measles runs an acute, almost always clinically apparent course resulting in long-lasting immunity. *(2)* Measles may also be associated with persistence of latent infection in subacute sclerosing panencephalitis (see Chapter 41). *(3)* Yellow fever and influenza follow a pattern similar to measles except that infection may be more often subclinical than clinical. *(4)* In viral hepatitis type B, recovery from clinical disease may be associated with persistent infection in which fully active virus persists in the blood. *(5)* Some infections are, in a particular species, always subclinical, such as equine encephalomyelitis in some species of birds that then act as reservoirs of the virus. *(6)* In rabbit papilloma, the course of infection is chronic, and chronicity is associated with the virus becoming occult. *(7)* Infection of humans with certain adenoviruses may be clinical or subclinical. There may be a long latent infection during which virus is present in small quantity; virus may also persist after the illness. *(8)* The periodic activation of latent herpes simplex virus, which may recur throughout life in humans, often follows an initial acute episode of stomatitis in childhood. *(9)* In many instances, infection is wholly latent for long periods of time before it is activated. Examples of such "slow" virus infections characterized by long incubation periods are mammary tumor virus in mice, scrapie in sheep, and kuru in humans. *(10)* In pigs that have eaten virus-bearing lungworms, swine "flu" is occult until the appropriate stimulus induces virus production and, in turn, clinical disease. *(11)* Lymphocytic choriomeningitis (LCM) virus may be established in mice by in utero infection. A form of modified immunologic tolerance develops in which virus-specific T cells are not activated. Antibody is produced against viral proteins; this antibody and circulating LCM virus form antigen-antibody complexes that ultimately produce immune complex disease in the partially tolerant host. The presence of LCM virus in this persistent infection (circulating virus with little or no apparent disease) may be readily revealed by transmission to an indicator host, eg, adult mice from a virus-free stock. All adult mice develop classic acute symptoms of LCM and frequently die *(12)*. *(13)* The possibility is shown of latent infection with an occult virus that is not readily activated. Proof of the presence of such a virus remains a difficult task which, however, is attracting the attention of cancer investigators (see Chapter 46).

any stage in the viral replicative cycle (described above) could be a target for antiviral therapy. Recently, compounds have been found that are of value in treatment of virus diseases; other compounds appear promising (Fig 33–18).

Five antiviral drugs are currently licensed for use: acyclovir, amantadine, idoxuridine, trifluridine, and vidarabine. All are of use in only a limited number of situations and may be toxic to the host. Ideal antiviral agents remain to be developed.

A. Nucleoside Analogs: The majority of the available antiviral agents are nucleoside analogs. Most are limited in inhibitory activity to use against herpesviruses.

Analogs inhibit nucleic acid replication by inhibition of enzymes of the metabolic pathways for purines or pyrimidines or by inhibition of polymerases for nucleic acid replication. In addition, some of the analogs can be incorporated into the nucleic acid and block further synthesis or alter its function.

Analogs can inhibit cellular enzymes as well as virus-coded enzymes. The clinical use of such compounds depends on a high therapeutic ratio, so that the benefit of virus inhibition outweighs the inherent toxicity. The new generation of analogs are those able to specifically inhibit virus-coded enzymes, with minimal inhibition of analogous host cell enzymes.

Acyclovir (9-[2-hydroxyethoxymethyl]-guanine, acycloguanosine) is an analog of guanosine or deoxyguanosine that strongly inhibits herpes simplex virus but has little effect on other DNA viruses or on host cells. The drug is phosphorylated by the virus-coded thymidine kinase and causes a much greater inhibition of the virus-coded DNA polymerase than of the corresponding host cell enzymes. Herpesviruses that encode for their own thymidine kinase (herpes simplex, varicella-zoster) are much more susceptible than those that do not (cytomegalovirus, EB virus). Mutants of herpesvirus that lack thymidine kinase fail to phosphorylate the drug and are resistant to it.

Acyclovir has activity in vivo in mice with herpes encephalitis and topically for treatment of herpetic lesions in the eyes of rabbits or skin lesions of guinea pigs. It has been effective in topical application in the

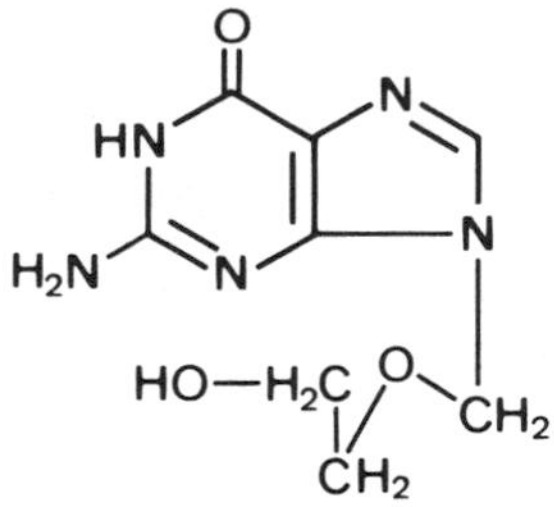

Acyclovir
(acycloguanosine)

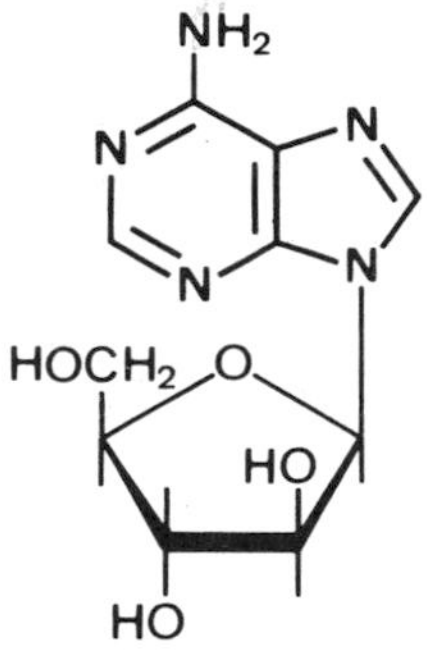

Vidarabine

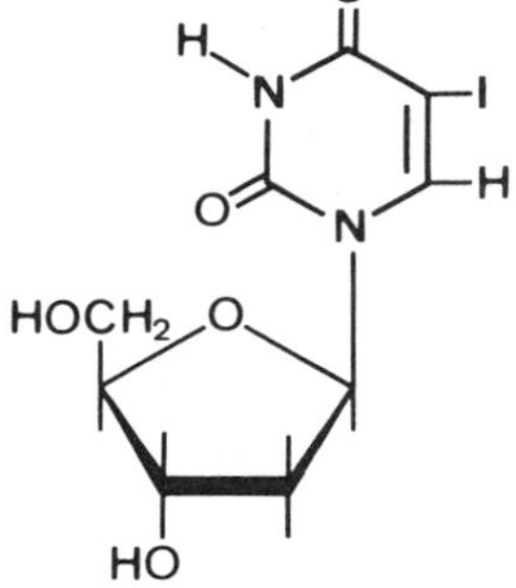

Idoxuridine

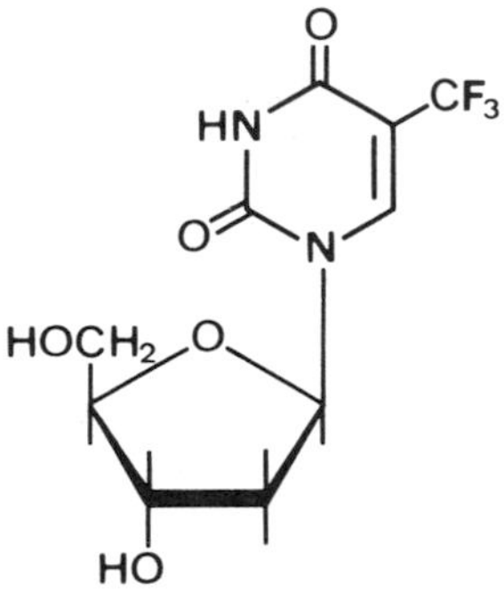

Trifluridine
(trifluorothymidine)

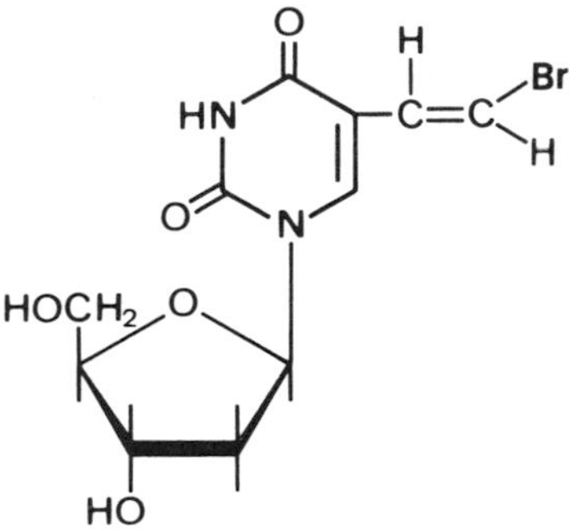

Bromovinyldeoxyuridine

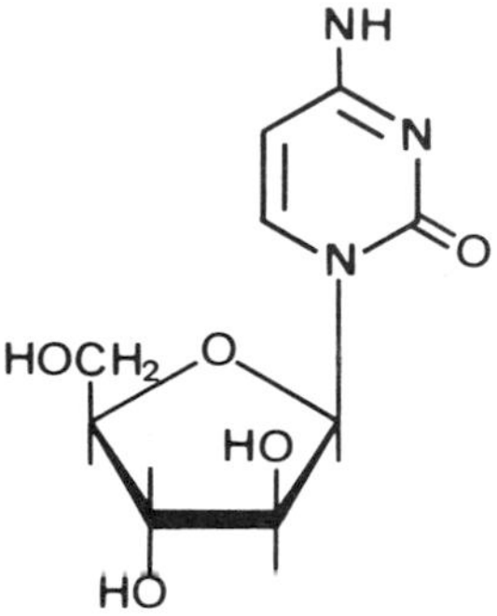

Cytarabine

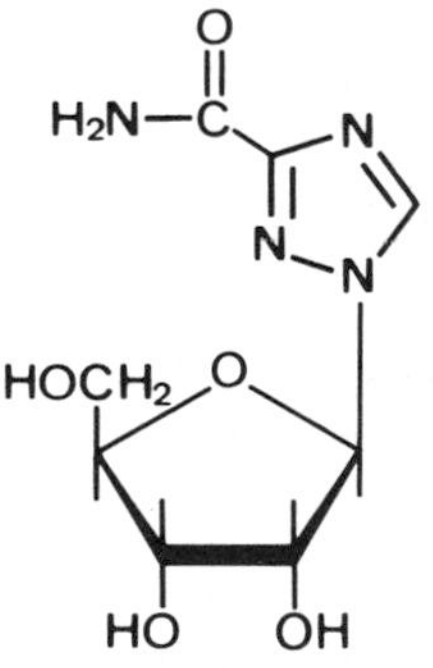

Ribavirin

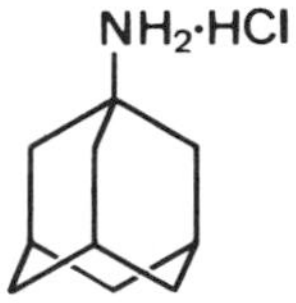

Amantadine

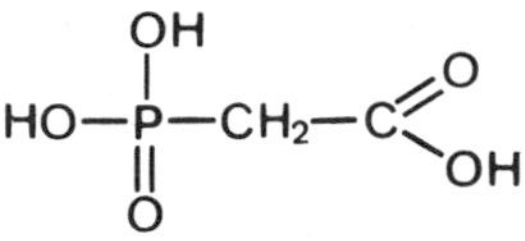

Phosphonoacetic acid

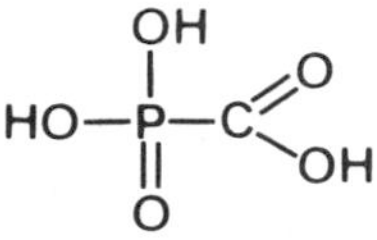

Phosphonoformic acid

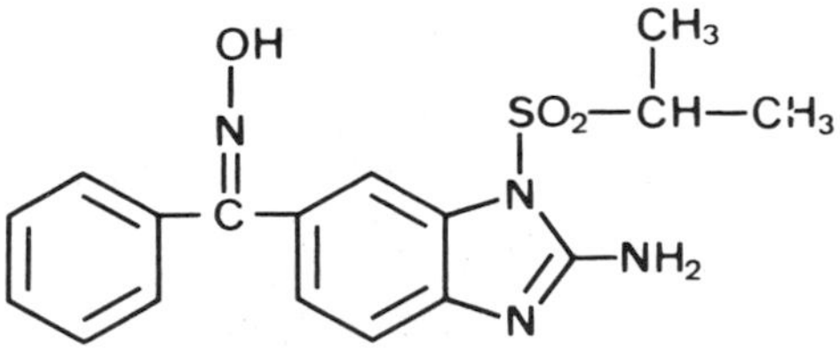

Enviroxime

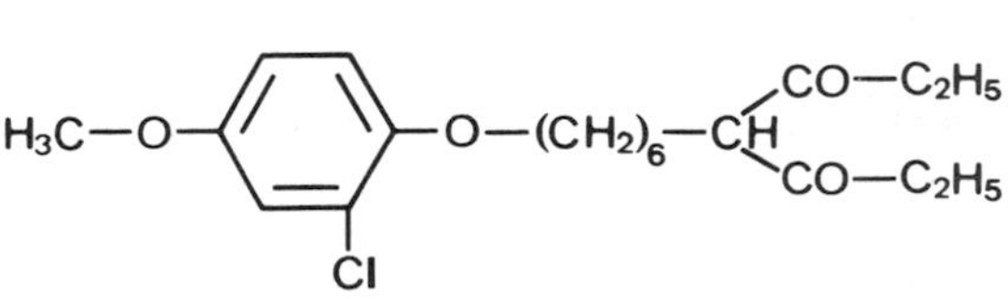

Arildone

Figure 33–18. Structural formulas for antiviral compounds.

control of herpetic eye lesions in humans and in the healing of primary but not recurrent herpetic skin lesions. Latent infections in the ganglia are not cured. Parenteral administration of acyclovir prevented the reactivation of latent herpesvirus infections and also was effective in the treatment of active herpetic lesions in patients undergoing immunosuppressive therapy.

Vidarabine (9-β-D-arabinofuranosyladenine, ara-A, adenine arabinoside) is a purine analog. Its precise mechanism of action is not clear, but it probably blocks viral DNA synthesis by inhibiting virus-specified enzymes such as DNA polymerase. Vidarabine has been used topically to treat corneal lesions due to herpes simplex virus. The clinical effectiveness of parenteral vidarabine against herpes simplex and varicella-zoster infection in humans has been significant. Vidarabine is the current drug of choice in serious systemic infections with these viruses. It must be given early before onset of coma in herpesvirus encephalitis. Unfortunately, no method exists for the early and reliable diagnosis of herpesvirus encephalitis. Vidarabine is relatively nontoxic but may cause nausea and phlebitis. It is not immunosuppressive. It is metabolized slowly in humans by deamination to arahypoxanthine.

Idoxuridine (5-iodo-2′-deoxyuridine [IDU]), a halogenated pyrimidine, inhibits thymidine kinase and is incorporated into DNA. Drug-resistant mutants of viruses regularly emerge in the presence of IDU. Topical administration of IDU is used in humans in the treatment of corneal lesions due to herpes simplex virus. Because of its toxicity due to inhibition of cellular DNA synthesis and its lack of efficacy, it is not used in systemic herpes infections. Idoxuridine was the first antiviral agent to be licensed for human use. It has been largely superseded by newer, less toxic analogs.

Trifluridine (trifluorothymidine, 5-trifluoro-methyl-2′-deoxyuridine) has also been used successfully in the topical treatment of herpes keratitis. Trifluridine is effective against strains of herpesvirus that are resistant to IDU.

Bromovinyldeoxyuridine ([E]-5-[2-bromovinyl]-2′-deoxyuridine, BVDU) offers many advantages over IDU. It is nontoxic, more active, and requires a virus-induced thymidine kinase for phosphorylation. It is even more active against varicella-zoster virus than against herpes simplex virus.

Cytarabine (1-β-D-arabinofuranosylcytosine monohydrochloride, Ara-C, cytosine arabinoside), another pyrimidine analog, inhibits cellular DNA synthesis and viral DNA synthesis about equally and, therefore, exhibits little viral specificity. Cytarabine is not effective as a systemic drug in virus infections and is immunosuppressive and cytotoxic.

Other halogenated pyrimidines, **5-fluoro-2′-deoxyuridine** and **5-bromo-2′-deoxyuridine**, inhibit virus DNA replication and have been useful for the study of virus replication but are not practical as chemotherapeutic agents.

Ribavirin (Virazole, 1-β-D-ribofuranosyl-1,2,4-triazole-3-carboxamide) is a synthetic nucleoside structurally related to guanosine that is effective to varying degrees against many DNA- and RNA-containing viruses in vitro. Its mechanism of action has not been defined, but it seems to interfere with an intracellular event, perhaps synthesis (capping) of viral mRNA. A small-particle aerosol delivery system has been devised to treat influenza and respiratory syncytial virus infections. Intravenous ribavirin has also proved effective in the treatment of Lassa fever.

B. Other Types of Antiviral Agents: A number of other types of compounds have been shown to possess some antiviral activity under certain conditions.

Amantadine (Symmetrel, 1-aminoadamantane hydrochloride), a synthetic amine, specifically inhibits all influenza A viruses by blocking viral penetration into the host cell or by blocking virus uncoating. When administered prophylactically, amantadine has a significant protective effect in experimental animals and humans against influenza A strains but not against influenza B or other viruses. **Rimantadine,** a derivative of amantadine, has the same spectrum of antiviral activity but is less toxic and has fewer side effects.

Phosphonoacetic acid (PAA) and **phosphonoformic acid (PFA, trisodium phosphonoformate, foscarnet)** inhibit herpes simplex virus replication. They are potent inhibitors of herpes simplex virus-induced DNA polymerase and have little effect on known cellular DNA polymerases. Herpesvirus mutants resistant to the drugs arise easily. PFA also inhibits to a lesser extent the polymerases of hepatitis B virus and retroviruses. PAA is very irritating when applied topically, whereas PFA is not. Both compounds accumulate in bone when given systemically.

Enviroxime (2,amino-1-[isopropyl sulphonyl]-6-benzimidazole phenyl ketone oxime) inhibits rhinoviruses in cell culture and markedly reduced the common cold symptoms in treated volunteers. Another benzimidazole derivative, **2-(α-hydroxybenzyl)-benzimidazole (HBB),** inhibits the replication of many picornaviruses in vitro.

Methisazone (Marboran), or N-methylisatin-β-thiosemicarbazone, is of historical interest as an inhibitor of poxviruses. The drug is highly virus-specific and does not affect normal cell metabolism; it inhibits poxvirus replication if given soon after exposure. It blocks a late stage in viral replication, resulting in the formation of immature, noninfectious virus particles. Methisazone was the first antiviral agent to be described. However, since smallpox has been eradicated, the drug is not used.

Arildone (4-[6-(2-chloro-4-methoxy) phenoxyl] hexyl-3,5-heptanedione), a phenoxyl diketone, is active in cultured cells against a number of DNA and RNA viruses. It appears to inhibit uncoating of viruses. Arildone is being tested for topical treatment of herpesvirus infections.

Interferons

Interferons are host-coded proteins that inhibit virus replication and are produced by intact animals or cultured cells in response to virus infection or other inducers. They are believed to be the body's first line of defense against virus infection.

A. Properties of Interferons: There are multiple species of interferons that fall into 3 general groups, designated IFN-α, IFN-β, and IFN-γ (Table 33–7). The IFN-α family is large, being coded by at least 14 genes in the human genome; the IFN-β and IFN-γ families are coded by one or a few genes each. Only the IFN-γ gene has been found to possess introns. The 3 multi-gene families have diverged so that the coding sequences now are not closely related.

The different interferons are similar in size, but the 3 classes are antigenically distinct. IFN-α and IFN-β are resistant to low pH. IFN-β and IFN-γ are glycosylated, but the sugars are not necessary for biologic activity, so cloned interferons produced in bacteria are biologically active.

B. Synthesis of Interferons: Interferons are produced by all vertebrate species. Normal cells do not generally synthesize interferon until they are induced to do so. Infection with viruses is a potent insult leading to induction; RNA viruses are stronger inducers of interferon than DNA viruses. Interferons also can be induced by double-stranded RNA, bacterial endotoxin, and small molecules such as tilorone. IFN-γ is not produced in response to most viruses but is induced by mitogen stimulation.

The different classes of interferon are produced by different cell types. IFN-α is synthesized predominantly by leukocytes, IFN-β mainly by fibroblasts, and IFN-γ only by lymphocytes.

Because the amounts of interferon synthesized by induced cells are quite small, it has been difficult to purify and characterize the proteins. With recombinant DNA techniques, cloned interferon genes are being expressed in large amounts in bacteria and in yeast, and the availability of genetically engineered interferons makes clinical studies feasible (see below).

C. Antiviral Activity and Other Biologic Effects: Interferons were first recognized by their ability to interfere with virus infection in cultured cells. Interferons are produced soon (less than 48 hours) after virus infection in intact animals, and virus production then decreases (Fig 33–19). Antibody does not

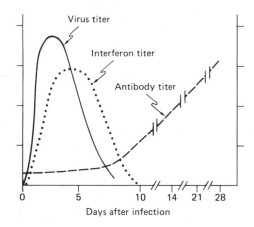

Figure 33–19. Illustration of kinetics of interferon and antibody synthesis after respiratory virus infection. The temporal relationships suggest that interferons are involved in the recovery process.

appear in the blood of the animal until several days after virus production has abated. This temporal relationship suggests that interferon plays a primary role in the defense of the host against virus infections. This conclusion is also supported by observations that agammaglobulinemic individuals usually recover from primary virus infections about as well as normal people.

The different types of interferon are roughly equivalent in antiviral activity. However, it is now known that interferons also exhibit a wide variety of cell regulatory activities. They are probably a family of hormones involved in regulation of cell growth and differentiation. Observed anticellular activities of interferons include inhibition of cell growth, effects on differentiation, and modulation of the immune response (ie, increased expression of histocompatibility antigens, enhancement of natural killer cell activity). The cell regulatory activity of IFN-γ is much greater than that of IFN-α or IFN-β. The multiplicity of effects of interferon upon host processes is summarized in Fig 33–20.

Interferons are almost always host species-specific in function. By contrast, interferon activity is not specific for a given virus; the replication of a wide variety of viruses can be inhibited. When interferon is added to cells prior to infection, there is marked inhibition of virus replication but nearly normal cell function. Interferons are extremely potent, so that very small amounts are required for function. It has been estimated that less than 50 molecules of interferon per cell are sufficient to induce the antiviral state.

The mechanism of interferon action is still poorly understood. However, it is clear that interferon is not the antiviral agent; rather, interferon induces an antiviral state by prompting the synthesis of other proteins that actually inhibit virus replication.

Interferon molecules bind to cell surface receptors, with IFN-α and IFN-β sharing a common receptor and

Table 33–7. Properties of human interferons.

Property	Type		
	Alpha	**Beta**	**Gamma**
Current nomenclature	IFN-α	IFN-β	IFN-γ
Former designation	Leukocyte	Fibroblast	Immune
Number of genes that code for family	14	≥ 2	1
Principal cell source	Leukocytes	Fibroblasts	Lymphocytes
Inducing agent	Viruses	Viruses	Mitogens
Size of protein (MW)	17,000	17,000	17,000
Stability at pH 2.0	Stable	Stable	Labile
Glycosylated	No	Yes	Yes
Introns in genes	No	No	Yes
Homology with IFN-α	80–95%	30–50%	<10%

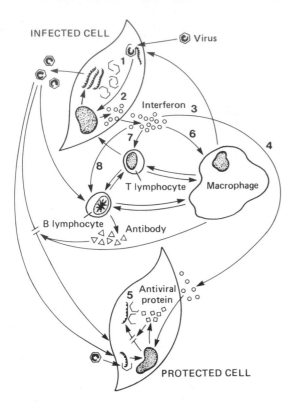

INFECTED CELL

T lymphocyte

Macrophage

B lymphocyte   Antibody

Antiviral
protein

PROTECTED CELL

Figure 33–20. Overview of different sites of action of interferons. Note that the original cell infected by virus produces interferon but is not protected by it. (Reprinted from Stringfellow DA [editor]. *Modern Pharmacology–Toxicology.* Vol 17: *Interferon and Interferon Inducers: Clinical Applications.* 1980. Courtesy of Marcel Dekker.)

IFN-γ recognizing a distinct receptor. This binding triggers the synthesis of several enzymes believed to be instrumental in the development of the antiviral state. These cellular enzymes subsequently block viral reproduction by inhibiting the translation of viral mRNA into viral protein (Fig 33–21). At least 2 enzymatic pathways appear to be involved: (1) a protein kinase phosphorylates and inactivates a cellular initiation factor and thus prevents formation of the initiation complex needed for viral protein synthesis, and (2) an oligonucleotide synthetase, 2,5-oligoA, that is needed for oligoadenylic acid formation activates a cellular endonuclease, RNase L, which degrades viral mRNA. Interferons also may affect viral assembly, perhaps as a result of changes at the plasma membrane. These explanations, however, may not represent the key mechanisms of interferon action; they also fail to reveal why the antiviral state acts selectively against viral mRNAs and not cellular mRNAs.

D. Clinical Studies: The antiviral effects of interferons were first tested clinically, but the results were not encouraging. It was originally hoped that interferons might be the answer to prevention of respiratory infections in which many different viruses may be involved. However, because high doses of interferons must be given frequently intranasally for several days

prior to virus exposure to be effective, their use turns out to be impractical. Interferon treatment may be helpful in certain severe virus infections (rabies, hemorrhagic fever, herpes encephalitis) and in some persistent virus infections (hepatitis B, laryngeal papillomas, herpes zoster). Topical interferon in the eye may suppress herpetic keratitis and accelerate healing.

Preliminary clinical trials testing interferons as anticancer agents (on the basis of their cell regulatory and immunomodulation properties) show limited but promising results. All interferons are being tested, but IFN-γ would be expected to be most effective due to its higher anticellular activity.

Large amounts of interferon are required for clinical trials, because million-unit injections are usually given daily. Such volumes of interferon could not be prepared from leukocytes or fibroblasts, so trials with partially purified preparations from these sources were not complete. The availability of cloned interferon will now permit large-scale testing of pure materials.

Interferons exhibit toxic side effects, even when purified material is tested. Gastrointestinal and nervous system side effects proportionate to the dose given are common. Bone marrow suppression also may occur.

Virus Vaccines

A. General Principles: Immunity to virus infection is based on the development of an immune response to specific antigens located on the surface of virus particles or virus-infected cells. For enveloped viruses, the important antigens are the surface glycoproteins. Although infected animals may develop antibodies against virion core proteins or nonstructural proteins involved in virus replication, that immune response is believed to play little or no role in the development of resistance to infection.

Vaccines are available for the prevention of several significant human diseases. Currently licensed vaccines, described in detail in the chapters dealing with specific virus families and diseases, are summarized in Table 33–8. Certain general principles apply to most virus vaccines for use in the prevention of human disease.

The pathogenesis of a particular viral infection influences the objectives of immunoprophylaxis. Mucosal immunity (local IgA) is important in resistance to infection by viruses that replicate exclusively in mucosal membranes (rhinoviruses, influenza viruses, rotaviruses). Viruses that have a viremic mode of spread (polio, hepatitis, measles) are controlled by serum antibodies. Cell-mediated immunity also is involved in protection against systemic infections (measles, herpes).

Neither vaccination nor recovery from natural infection always results in total protection against a later infection with the same virus. This situation holds for diseases for which successful control measures are available, including polio, smallpox, influenza, rubella, measles, mumps, and adenovirus infections. Control can be achieved by limiting the multiplication

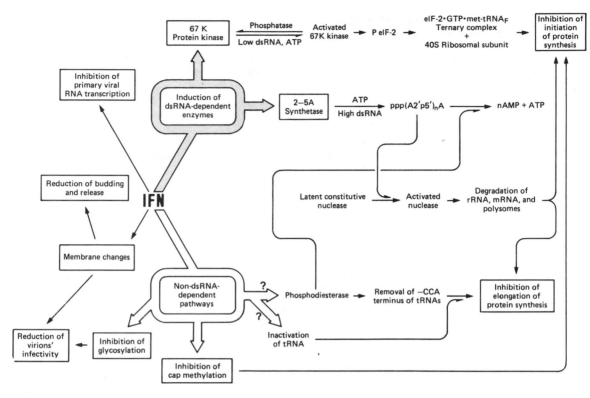

Figure 33–21. Suggested mechanisms for the antiviral action of interferon. (Reproduced, with permission, from Lebleu B, Content J. Mechanisms of interferon action: Biochemical and genetic approaches. Pages 47–94 in: *Interferon 1982.* Gresser I [editor]. Academic Press, 1982.)

of virulent virus upon subsequent exposure and preventing its spread to target organs where the pathologic damage is done (eg, polio and measles viruses kept from the brain and spinal cord; rubella virus kept from the embryo). Recently, Marek's disease, a widespread lymphoproliferative tumor caused by a herpesvirus of domestic chickens, has been brought under control by an attenuated virus vaccine. The vaccine results in a lifelong active infection of the chicken and does not prevent superinfection of the vaccinated animal with the virulent virus, but it does prevent the appearance of the tumor. This is the first practical cancer vaccine that has been developed. A second cancer vaccine—hepatitis B vaccine to prevent primary hepatocellular carcinoma— is now in field trial.

B. Killed Virus Vaccines: Killed virus vaccines are made by purifying virus harvests to a certain extent and then inactivating viral infectivity in a way that does minimal damage to the viral structural proteins; mild formalin treatment is frequently used.

Killed virus vaccines prepared from whole virions generally stimulate the development of circulating antibody against the coat proteins of the virus, conferring some degree of resistance. For some diseases, killed virus vaccines are currently the only ones available.

The following disadvantages apply to killed vaccines:

(1) Extreme care is required in their manufacture to

make certain that no residual live virulent virus is present in the vaccine.

(2) The immunity conferred is often brief and must be boosted, which not only involves the logistic problem of repeatedly reaching the persons in need of immunization but also has caused concern about the possible effects (hypersensitivity reactions) of repeated administration of foreign proteins.

(3) Parenteral administration of killed virus vaccine, even when it stimulates circulating antibody (IgM, IgG) to satisfactory levels, has sometimes given limited protection because local resistance (IgA) is not induced adequately at the natural portal of entry or primary site of multiplication of the wild virus infection—eg, nasopharynx for respiratory viruses, alimentary tract for poliovirus (see Fig 33–22 and Chapters 37 and 40).

(4) The cell-mediated response to inactivated vaccines is generally poor.

(5) Some killed virus vaccines have induced hypersensitivity to subsequent infection, perhaps owing to an unbalanced immune response to viral surface antigens that fails to mimic infection with natural virus.

C. Live Attenuated Virus Vaccines: Live virus vaccines utilize virus mutants that antigenically overlap with wild type virus but are restricted in some step in the pathogenesis of disease.

The development of virus strains suitable for live

Table 33–8. Principal vaccines used in prevention of virus diseases of humans.

Disease	Source of Vaccine	Condition of Virus	Route of Administration
Immunization Recommended for General Public			
Poliomyelitis	Tissue culture (human diploid cell line, monkey kidney)	Live attenuated	Oral
		Killed	Subcutaneous
Measles[1]	Tissue culture (chick embryo)	Live attenuated[2]	Subcutaneous[3]
Mumps[1]	Tissue culture (chick embryo)	Live attenuated	Subcutaneous
Rubella[1, 4]	Tissue culture (duck embryo, rabbit, or human diploid)	Live attenuated	Subcutaneous
Immunization Recommended Only Under Certain Conditions (Epidemics, Exposure, Travel, Military)			
Smallpox[5]	Lymph from calf or sheep (glycerolated, lyophilized) Chorioallantois, tissue cultures (lyophilized)	Live vaccinia	Intradermal: multiple pressure, multiple puncture
Yellow fever	Tissue cultures and eggs (17D strain)	Live attenuated	Subcutaneous or intradermal
Hepatitis type B	Purified HBsAg from "healthy" carriers	Killed	Subcutaneous
Influenza	Highly purified or subunit forms of chick embryo allantoic fluid (formalinized or UV-irradiated)	Killed	Subcutaneous or intradermal
Rabies	Duck embryo or human diploid cells	Killed	Subcutaneous
Adenovirus[6]	Human diploid cell cultures	Live attenuated	Oral, by enteric-coated capsule
Japanese B encephalitis[7]	Mouse brain (formalinized), tissue culture	Killed	Subcutaneous
Venezuelan equine encephalomyelitis[8]	Guinea pig heart cell culture	Live attenuated	Subcutaneous
Eastern equine encephalomyelitis[7]	Chick embryo cell culture	Killed	Subcutaneous
Western equine encephalomyelitis[7]	Chick embryo cell culture	Killed	Subcutaneous
Russian spring-summer encephalitis[7]	Mouse brain (formalinized)	Killed	Subcutaneous

[1]Available also as combined vaccines.

[2]Killed measles vaccine was available for a short period. However, a serious delayed hypersensitivity reaction often occurs when children who have received primary immunization with killed measles vaccine are later exposed to live measles virus. Because of this complication, killed measles vaccine is no longer recommended.

[3]With less attenuated strains, immune globulin USP is given in another limb at the time of vaccination.

[4]Neither monovalent rubella vaccine nor combination vaccines incorporating rubella should be administered to a postpubertal susceptible woman unless she is not pregnant and understands that it is imperative not to become pregnant for at least 3 months after vaccination. (The time immediately postpartum has been suggested as a safe period for vaccination.)

[5]Since smallpox virus seems to have been totally eradicated from the world, vaccination is no longer recommended. However, stocks of vaccine are held in depots if cases should reappear.

[6]Recently licensed but recommended only for military populations in which epidemic respiratory disease caused by adenovirus is a frequent occurrence. Types 4 and 7 are available as vaccines.

[7]Not available in the USA except for the Armed Forces or for investigative purposes.

[8]Available for use in domestic animals (from the US Department of Agriculture) and for investigative purposes.

virus vaccines previously was done chiefly by selecting naturally attenuated strains or by cultivating the virus serially in various hosts and cultures in the hope of deriving an attenuated strain fortuitously. The search for such strains is now being approached by laboratory manipulations aimed at specific, planned, genetic alterations in the virus (eg, rabies, influenza, respiratory syncytial viruses).

Attenuated vaccines have the advantage of acting like the natural infection with regard to their effect on immunity. They multiply in the host and tend to stimulate longer-lasting antibody production, to induce a good cell-mediated response, and to induce antibody production and resistance at the portal of entry (Fig 33–22).

The disadvantages of live attenuated vaccines include the following:

(1) The risk of reversion to greater virulence during multiplication within the vaccinee. Although reversion has not proved to be a problem in practice, its potential exists. Monitoring should be continued.

(2) Unrecognized adventitious agents latently infecting the culture substrate (eggs, primary cell cultures) may enter the vaccine stocks. Viruses found in vaccines have included avian leukosis virus, simian papovirus SV40, and simian cytomegalovirus. The

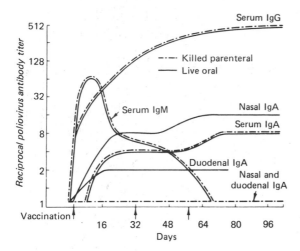

Figure 33–22. Serum and secretory antibody response to orally administered, live attenuated poliovaccine and to intramuscular inoculation of killed poliovaccine. (Reproduced, with permission, from Ogra et al: *Rev Infect Dis* 1980;2:352.)

problem of adventitious contaminants may be circumvented through the use of normal cells serially propagated in culture (eg, human diploid cell lines) as substrates for cultivation of vaccine viruses. Vaccines prepared in such cultures have been in use for years and have been administered to many millions.

(3) There is the potential problem that the live vaccine virus may produce persistent infections in the vaccinee. The actual risk of this is unknown, but it appears to be very low.

(4) The storage and limited shelf life of attenuated vaccines present problems, but this can be overcome in some cases by the use of viral stabilizers (eg, $MgCl_2$ for poliovaccine).

(5) Interference by co-infection with a naturally occurring, wild type virus may inhibit the replication of the vaccine virus and decrease its effectiveness. This has been noted with the vaccine strains of poliovirus, which can be inhibited by concurrent infections by various enteroviruses.

D. Proper Use of Present Vaccines: One fact cannot be overemphasized: An effective vaccine does not protect against disease until it is administered in the proper dosage to susceptible individuals. The failure to reach all sectors of the population with complete courses of immunization is reflected in the continued occurrence of paralytic poliomyelitis and measles in unvaccinated persons. Preschool children in poverty areas are the least adequately vaccinated group in the USA.

There was a theoretic possibility that antibody response might be diminished or that interference might occur if 2 or more live vaccines were given at the same time. In practice, however, simultaneous administration of live vaccines can be safe and effective. Trivalent live oral poliovaccine (when given in 3 doses) or a

combined live measles, mumps, and rubella vaccine, given by injection, is effective. Antibody response to each component of these combination vaccines is comparable with antibody response to the individual vaccines given separately.

As indicated in Table 33–8, certain virus vaccines are recommended for use by the general public. Other vaccines are recommended only for use by persons at special risk due to occupation, travel, or lifestyle.

E. Future Prospects: Molecular biology and modern technologies are combining to make possible novel approaches to vaccine development. The ultimate success of these new approaches remains to be determined.

1. Attenuation of viruses by genetic manipulation–This is being utilized to produce recombinants or mutants that can then serve as live virus vaccines.

The introduction of deletion mutations that damage the virus but do not completely inactivate it should yield a vaccine candidate unlikely to revert to virulence.

2. Use of avirulent virus vectors–The concept is to use recombinant DNA techniques to insert the gene coding for the protein of interest into the genome of an avirulent virus that can be administered as the vaccine. The prototype vector under study is vaccinia virus. The gene for hepatitis B surface antigen (HBsAg) has been introduced into a nonessential vaccinia gene. The resulting recombinant virus has elicited an immune response to HBsAg in test animals. Other virus vectors possessing large genomes (eg, herpesvirus) are also under study.

3. Purified proteins produced using cloned genes–Viral genes can now be easily cloned into plasmids. That cloned DNA can then be expressed in prokaryotic or eukaryotic cells if appropriately engineered constructions are used. The immunizing antigens of hepatitis B virus, rabies virus, herpes simplex virus, foot-and-mouth disease virus, and influenza virus have been successfully synthesized in bacteria or yeast cells. If the bacteria can be made to produce the antigen in sufficient quantity and immunogenicity, this will facilitate the production of a purified vaccine containing only the immunizing antigen. Interestingly, it is already apparent that the glycosylation of viral surface glycoproteins is not always essential for antigenicity. Unglycosylated herpesvirus proteins synthesized in bacteria have been able to induce Nt antibodies in test animals.

4. Synthetic peptides–Viral nucleic acids can be readily sequenced and the amino acid sequence of the gene products predicted. It is now technically possible to synthesize short peptides that correspond to antigenic determinants on a viral protein.

Antigenically active polypeptides synthesized for hepatitis B, influenza, and polioviruses have produced Nt antibodies in animals. The possibility of producing synthetic immunizing antigens for human vaccination is now being explored. Chemical synthesis would preclude exposure of vaccinees to viral nucleic acid, thereby avoiding any possibility of reversion to viru-

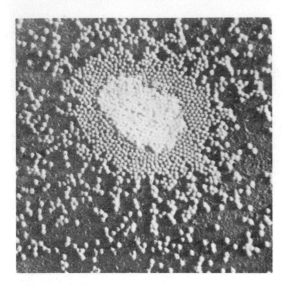

Figure 33–23. Electron micrograph typical of purified preparations of a spherical virus (20,000 ×). Shown are human wart virus particles (papovavirus family) having a diameter of 45 nm. (Melnick and Bunting.)

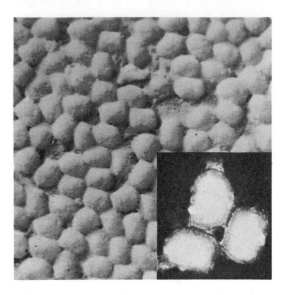

Figure 33–25. Electron micrograph of a purified sample of a brick-shaped poxvirus, molluscum contagiosum (20,000 ×). The virus particles, purified from human skin lesions by differential centrifugation, measure about 330 × 230 nm. (Melnick, Bunting, and Strauss.) *Inset:* Uranyl acetate stain of DNA-containing core of the virus (47,000 ×).

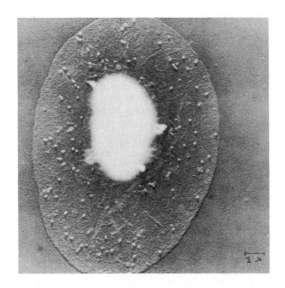

Figure 33–24. Influenza virus particles, PR8 stain, adsorbed on the membranes of a chicken erythrocyte. The particles are about 100 nm in diameter. (Werner and Schlesinger.)

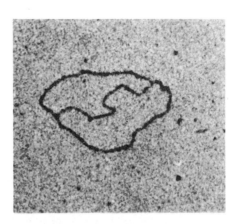

Figure 33–26. Replicating molecule of papovavirus SV40 DNA (see Fig 33–5). The electron micrograph shown above represents about 10% of the population of replicating DNA molecules. Most of the replicating molecules also contain a superhelical branch so tightly twisted that in electron micrographic preparations it is usually not possible to distinguish individual DNA duplexes. (Salzman et al.)

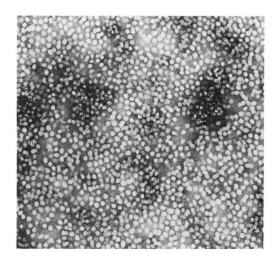

Figure 33–27. Purified hepatitis B surface antigen (HBsAg) (55,000 ×). (McCombs and Brunschwig.)

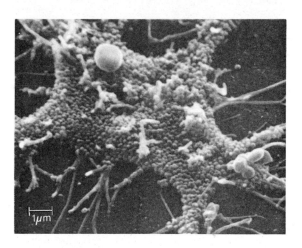

Figure 33–29. Scanning electron micrograph of a human epithelioid cell infected with herpes simplex virus type 1. Hundreds of virus particles may be seen on the surface of the cell. Bar = 1 μm. (Schlehofer and Hampl.)

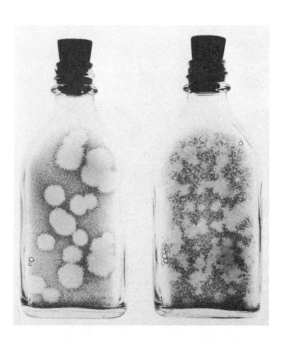

Figure 33–28. Plaques produced by poliovirus *(left)* and by an echovirus *(right)*. Both viruses are cultivated in bottle cultures of monkey kidney cells. After the viruses are seeded, the epithelial sheet is covered with an agar overlay containing a vital dye (neutral red). As the cytopathic effect of the virus becomes manifest, the cells lose their vital stain, and clear areas appear in the culture. The progeny of a single virus particle are located in each clear area. The plaque morphology of each of the viruses shown is sufficiently clear so that the 2 virus groups can readily be distinguished from each other by this method. (Hsiung and Melnick.)

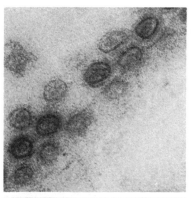
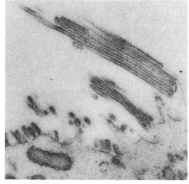

Figure 33–30. *Top:* Spherical forms of influenza virus (116,000 ×). The cell wall passes diagonally across the field, with host cell cytoplasm to the right. Several particles just beneath the cell membrane seem to be undergoing maturation toward the extracellular form. *Bottom:* Influenza virus at the cell surface (31,000 ×). Two bundles of filaments (one cut longitudinally, the other obliquely) extend into the extracellular space. At left, short filaments seem to be budding from the cell. (Morgan, Rose, and Moore.)

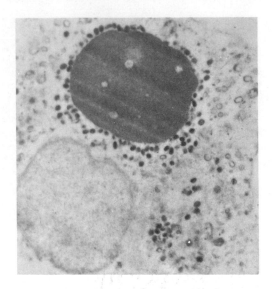

Figure 33–31. Mousepox virus within the infected cell (7400 ×). Nucleus at lower left; above it can be seen a dark cytoplasmic inclusion body surrounded by virus particles. A group of virus particles in the process of development is located to the right of the nucleus. (Gaylord and Melnick.)

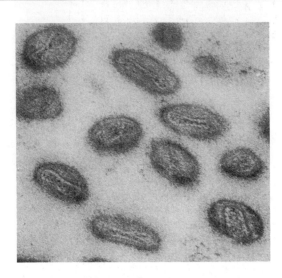

Figure 33–33. Ultrathin section of vaccinia virus particles within the cytoplasm of an infected cell (74,000 ×). The internal structure of the mature virus is evident. (Morgan, Rose, and Moore.)

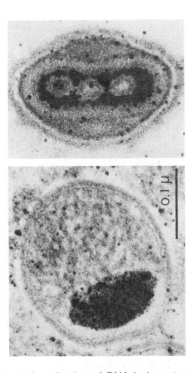

Figure 33–34. Localization of DNA in immature *(bottom)* and mature *(top)* vaccinia particles. After hydrolysis with HCl, a silver methenamine solution has been applied to Epon sections of the virus. Silver granules are specifically deposited at the sites of DNA. Other structures are made visible by counterstaining with uranyl acetate (170,000 ×). (Peters.)

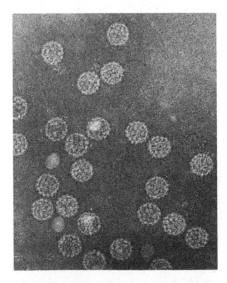

Figure 33–32. Papovavirus SV40. Purified preparation negatively stained with phosphotungstate (150,000 ×). (McGregor and Mayor.)

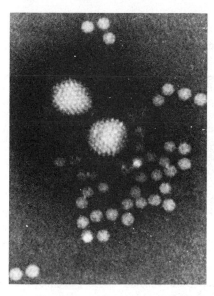

Figure 33–35. A group of adenoassociated satellite viruses surrounding 2 adenovirions that function as helpers for the defective parvoviruses (250,000 ×). (Mayor, Jordan, and Melnick.)

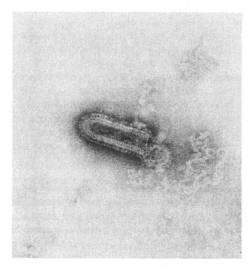

Figure 33–37. Electron micrograph of bullet-shaped particle typical of the rhabdovirus family (100,000 ×). Shown here is vesicular stomatitis virus negatively stained with potassium phosphotungstate. (McCombs, Benyesh-Melnick, and Brunschwig.)

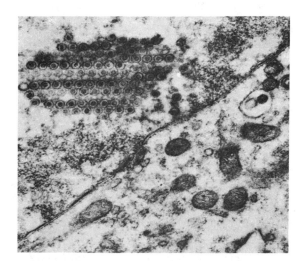

Figure 33–36. Herpesvirus in human amnion cell. The nuclear membrane runs from lower left to upper right. A regular array of virus particles, each possessing a dense central body and a single peripheral membrane, is present within the nucleus (27,000 ×). (Morgan.)

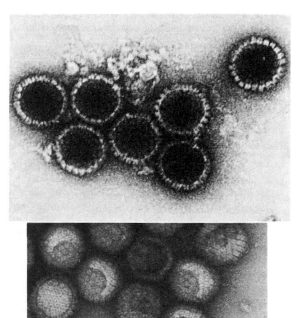

Figure 33–38. *Top:* Herpesvirus particles from human vesicle fluid, stained with uranyl acetate to show DNA core (140,000 ×). *Bottom:* Virions stained to show protein capsomeres of the virus coat (140,000 ×). (Smith and Melnick.)

lence. The problem of contaminating cellular proteins also would be avoided.

Although this approach holds promise, there are several obstacles to be overcome. The immune response induced by synthetic peptides is considerably weaker than that induced by intact protein or inactivated virus. It is not easy to identify peptide sequences able to induce a protective immune response. A single peptide representing a single epitope may not be able to induce resistance against a viral protein containing multiple antigenic determinants. Finally, not all antigenic determinants are sequential; it may be very difficult to simulate conformational determinants (ie, those determined by the tertiary configuration of the protein, which juxtaposes amino acids that may be widely separated in the primary sequence).

5. Subunit vaccines–Subviral components are being obtained by breaking apart the virion to include in the vaccine only those viral components needed to stimulate protective antibody.

This approach is coupled with better purification procedures. This can eliminate nonviral proteins and reduce the possibility of adverse reactions to the vaccine. Purified material can be administered in more concentrated form, containing greatly increased amounts of the specifically desired antigen.

6. Local administration of vaccine–Intranasally administered aerosol vaccines are being developed, particularly for respiratory disease viruses and also for measles virus. It is hoped this will stimulate local antibody at the portal of entry.

7. Conventional vaccines–While these new approaches are being pursued, efforts also continue to develop more conventional vaccines in certain systems.

Considerable success has been claimed for a varicella-zoster vaccine developed in Japan and currently under test in the USA. There is some concern about the possibility of vaccinated subjects contracting zoster in later life. Vaccines are also under development for cytomegalovirus and Epstein-Barr virus, but, as with the varicella-zoster vaccine, there is concern about the long-term effects. A vaccine is also being tested for respiratory syncytial virus.

REFERENCES

Burns WH et al: Isolation and characterisation of resistant herpes simplex virus after acyclovir therapy. *Lancet* 1982;**1**:421.

Cheville NF: *Cytopathology in Viral Diseases*. Vol 10 of: *Monographs in Virology*. Melnick JL (editor). Karger, 1975.

Choppin PW, Scheid A: The role of viral glycoproteins in adsorption, penetration, and pathogenicity of viruses. *Rev Infect Dis* 1980;**2**:40.

Diener TO: Viroids and their interactions with host cells. *Annu Rev Microbiol* 1982;**36**:239.

Fields BN, Greene MI: Genetic and molecular mechanisms of viral pathogenesis: Implications for prevention and treatment. *Nature* 1982;**300**:19.

Fields BN et al (editors): *Virology*. Raven Press, 1985.

Hirsch MS et al: Effects of interferon-alpha on cytomegalovirus reactivation syndromes in renal-transplant recipients. *N Engl J Med* 1983;**308**:1489.

Hsiung GD et al: The use of electron microscopy for diagnosis of virus infections: An overview. *Prog Med Virol* 1979;**25**:133.

Matthews REF: Classification and nomenclature of viruses: Fourth Report of the International Committee on Taxonomy of Viruses. *Intervirology* 1982;**17**:1.

McClung HW et al: Ribavirin aerosol treatment of influenza B virus infection. *JAMA* 1983;**249**:2671.

Merigan TC: Interferon: The first quarter century. *JAMA* 1982; **248**:2513.

Mims CA: Vertical transmission of viruses. *Microbiol Rev* 1981;**45**:267.

Oldstone MBA, Fujinami RS, Lampert PW: Membrane and cytoplasmic changes in virus-infected cells induced by interactions of antiviral antibody with surface viral antigen. *Prog Med Virol* 1980;**26**:45.

Reanney DC: The evolution of RNA viruses. *Annu Rev Microbiol* 1982;**36**:47.

Shinnick TM et al: Synthetic peptide immunogens as vaccines. *Annu Rev Microbiol* 1983;**37**:425.

Simons K, Garoff H, Helenius A: How an animal virus gets into and out of its host cell. *Sci Am* (Feb) 1982;**246**:58.

Smith GL, Mackett M, Moss B: Infectious vaccinia virus recombinants that express hepatitis B virus surface antigen. *Nature* 1983;**302**:490.

White DO: *Antiviral Chemotherapy, Interferons and Vaccines*. Vol 16 of: *Monographs in Virology*. Melnick JL (editor). Karger, 1984.

Whitley RJ et al: Herpes simplex encephalitis: Vidarabine therapy and diagnostic problems. *N Engl J Med* 1981;**304**:313.

Detection of Viruses & Antigens In Clinical Specimens

34

Viruses can be isolated and identified during the course of many diseases, thus establishing the etiologic diagnosis. Often, however, a specific diagnosis cannot be made in the first few days of the infection; the results of many diagnostic tests for viral diseases do not become available until the patient has recovered or died.

The time and cost entailed in isolating and identifying viruses necessitate careful selection of patients and proper collection and handling of specimens. As a general rule, the indications for attempting to isolate a virus from patients include the following: (1) Instances where the established diagnosis will directly affect the management of the patient, eg, laboratory-proved rubella in the first trimester of pregnancy would favor a decision to terminate pregnancy. (2) Instances where antiviral drugs are available for treatment, eg, herpes simplex infections. (3) Instances where the diagnosis is vital to the health of the community, eg, laboratory confirmation of smallpox, poliomyelitis, influenza, or arbovirus encephalitis will provide the information necessary for instituting immunization programs or insect control measures. (4) Instances where the etiologic agent of a disease is being sought. Studies of patients for etiologic association require prior planning and cooperation between the physician, the public health worker, and the virologist and must include the study of samples from control patients.

The laboratory procedures used in the diagnosis of viral diseases in human beings include the following:

(1) Isolation and identification of the agent.

(2) Measurement of antibodies developing during the course of the infection.

(3) Histologic examination of infected tissues. This should be performed on all fatal cases of virus infections and on animals suspected of infection with rabies virus.

(4) Detection of viral antigens in lesions by the use of fluorescein-labeled (or peroxidase-labeled) antibody. This method can be used on nasopharyngeal secretions (exfoliated cells), sputum, skin and conjunctival scrapings, brain biopsy specimens (for herpes encephalitis that can be treated), and autopsy tissues.

(5) Dot hybridization of viral nucleic acid by radiolabeled nucleic acid probes. This method is used for rapid detection of virus in common body secretions (urine, nasopharyngeal aspirates).

(6) Electron microscopic examination of vesicular fluids or tissue extracts treated with negative and positive stains to identify and count DNA and RNA virus particles (see Chapter 33). This procedure in the hands of trained personnel can provide diagnoses within hours when the specimens contain a sufficiently large number of virus particles, eg, 10^6 or more particles per milliliter. An important application in diagnostic virology is the detection of rotavirus in the feces of children suffering from acute gastroenteritis (Fig 34–1). Since the virus does not grow in conventional cell cultures, electron microscopy can serve to identify the causative agent directly.

CONSIDERATIONS IN THE DIAGNOSIS OF VIRAL DISEASES

The choice of methods for laboratory confirmation of a virus infection depends upon the illness. Antibody tests are more readily and cheaply performed than virus isolations, but they require adequately spaced serum samples, and the diagnosis often is not confirmed until convalescence. In addition, antibody tests can be carried out only for those illnesses for which the causative viruses have been grown in the

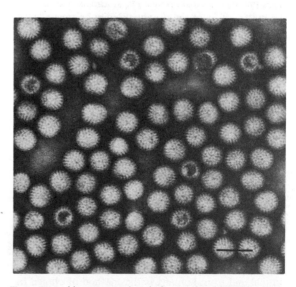

Figure 34–1. Human rotavirus in feces of a child with acute gastroenteritis (125,000 ×). Bar = 100 nm. (Barrera-Oro and Lombardi.)

laboratory. Virus isolation is required (1) when new epidemics occur, as with A2 (Hong Kong) influenza in 1968; (2) when serologic tests overlap and do not allow one to distinguish between 2 viruses, as with smallpox and vaccinia; (3) when it is necessary to confirm a presumptive diagnosis made by direct microscopic observation, eg, detecting a herpesvirus in vesicle fluid; and (4) when the same clinical illness may be caused by many different agents.

In the diagnostic evaluation of a patient with a suspected viral disease, one must bear in mind that the same clinical syndromes may be produced by a variety of agents. For example, aseptic (nonbacterial) meningitis may be caused by many different viruses as well as by spirochetes; similarly, respiratory disease syndromes may be caused by many viruses as well as mycoplasmas and other agents.

The isolation of a virus is not necessarily equivalent to establishing the cause of a given disease. A number of other factors must be taken into consideration. Some viruses persist in human hosts for long periods of time, and therefore the isolation of herpesviruses, poliomyelitis virus, echoviruses, or coxsackieviruses from a patient with an undiagnosed illness does not prove that the virus is the cause of the disease. A consistent clinical and epidemiologic pattern must be established by repeated studies before one can be sure that a particular agent is responsible for a specific clinical picture.

Dual infections present still another problem. Different viruses may have the same seasonal and geographic occurrence. Enteroviruses and arboviruses sometimes frequent the same area at the same time. Thus, in one summer a patient may have inapparent infection with one virus and clinical infection with the other. If the clinical infection should be mild, the syndrome (eg, aseptic meningitis) may have been produced by either virus. Antibody studies must be made for both viruses or the diagnosis may be missed altogether. Isolation of 2 viral agents similarly confuses the etiologic significance of each agent unless their roles in causing illness have been established by prior experience.

It must be emphasized that good diagnostic virology depends on rapid communication between the physician and the laboratory and on the quality of specimens and information supplied to the laboratory.

DIRECT EXAMINATION OF CLINICAL MATERIAL

The viral diseases for which direct microscopic examination of imprints or smears has been proved useful include rabies, herpes, and varicella-zoster. The staining of viral antigens by immunofluorescence in a brain smear and corneal impressions from the rabid animal and from humans is the method of choice for routine diagnosis of rabies. The procedure is carried out as follows:

Two impression smears on a glass slide are made with the suspect brain. The slide is fixed in acetone at −20 °C. One smear (control) is flooded with fluorescein-labeled antirabies globulin mixed with mouse brain containing rabies virus. The other smear (test) is flooded with the same fluorescein-labeled antirabies globulin mixed with norml mouse brain. The slide is incubated at 37 °C for 30 minutes in a moist chamber, then washed for 10 minutes in buffered saline, air dried, mounted, and examined in the fluorescence microscope by ultraviolet light. The positive test smear gives bright fluorescence, whereas the control smear gives no fluorescence because the specifically labeled antibodies have been bound by the rabies antigen added in mouse brain.

The same principle of identifying viral antigens using immunofluorescence is useful in rapid diagnosis of (1) certain respiratory virus diseases (eg, respiratory syncytial disease, where the virus is labile under ordinary laboratory conditions and cannot withstand freezing and thawing, and also influenza and parainfluenza) by examining smeared epithelial cells from the nasopharynx, and (2) herpetic lesions by examining cells scraped from the base of the lesion. Now that herpes encephalitis can be successfully managed if treatment is begun early, immunofluorescence microscopy of brain biopsy material may be indicated. Immunofluorescence microscopy is also used for detection of adenovirus, mumps, measles, varicella-zoster, and cytomegalovirus in appropriate clinical specimens. Buffy coat leukocytes or leukocytes of the cerebrospinal fluid obtained during the acute illness contain viral antigens (eg, enteroviruses), and this also offers a rapid method for obtaining a diagnosis.

SOLID-PHASE IMMUNOASSAYS

The recognition of hepatitis A virus and rotavirus by direct examination of fecal specimens led to the development of sensitive solid-phase immunoassays for their detection—inasmuch as these important pathogens are not readily grown in cell culture. Both radioimmunoassay (RIA) and enzyme-linked immunosorbent assay (ELISA) are available.

The principles of RIA and ELISA tests have been presented in Chapter 12. RIA applied to viral diagnosis is again discussed in Chapter 35.

ELISA for viral diagnosis consists of the following essential steps: (1) A specific antibody is adsorbed onto the wells in a plastic microtiter plate. (2) The material to be tested is added. If the viral antigen is present, it will combine with the antibody. The excess is washed off. (3) A conjugate is added that consists of antiviral antibody linked to an enzyme. If virus has been fixed to the plate, the antibody portion of the conjugate will attach. Unbound conjugate is washed off. (4) A substrate for the enzyme is added, and the colored product of hydrolyzed substrate is measured in a spectrophotometer. The resulting reading is proportionate to the amount of enzyme bound to the plate, which in turn is related to the quantity of virus antigen in the sample.

A more sensitive technique of antigen detection involves the use of a second specific antibody derived from a different animal species than the one used for preparing the coating antibody. The second antibody is reacted with virus antigen that has been bound to the original coating antibody. A third antibody conjugated with enzyme is added; this antibody is directed against the immunoglobulin of the animal species used to prepare the second specific antibody. Again, the amount of antibody bound, determined by the enzyme activity, is a function of antigen concentration.

NUCLEIC ACID HYBRIDIZATION

In clinical virology, rapid diagnostic methods usually involve the detection of virus proteins. Nucleic acid hybridization has recently proved to be highly sensitive and specific. For agents such as adenovirus (in nasopharyngeal aspirates) or cytomegalovirus (in urine), viral DNA in the specimen is spotted on a nitrocellulose membrane, where it is bound and denatured with alkali in situ; then the dot is hybridized with a radioactive-labeled viral DNA fragment. Recombinant DNA methods have been used to make available cloned viral DNA fragments from which the DNA probes are prepared. The dot is autoradiographed the next day. For rotavirus, which contains double-stranded RNA, the dot hybridization method is even more sensitive than ELISA. RNA in heat-denatured fecal samples containing rotavirus is immobilized as above, and in situ hybridization is carried out with radiolabeled single-stranded probes obtained by in vitro transcription of rotavirus. Complementary DNA probes to rotavirus and to enteroviruses may also be labeled and used in the dot hybridization method.

Dot hybridization is increasingly being used to detect viral DNA sequences in tissue samples not only from patients with acute infection but also from those with chronic diseases from which virus is not readily isolated. The latter include chronic hepatitis and primary hepatocellular carcinoma (hepatitis B virus DNA probe), latent varicella-zoster in sensory ganglia (varicella-zoster virus DNA probe), acquired immune deficiency syndrome (HTLV-III cDNA probe), cervical neoplasms (cloned papillomavirus DNA probe), and nasopharyngeal carcinoma and Burkitt's lymphoma (cloned EB virus DNA probe).

VIRUS ISOLATION TECHNIQUE

All specimens must be safely contained for transport to the laboratory. Each specimen must be clearly labeled and should be accompanied by relevant information.

The isolation of active virus requires the proper collection of appropriate specimens, their preservation both en route to and in the laboratory, and the inoculation of suitable cell cultures, susceptible animals, or embryonated eggs. Prior to the inoculation of the specimen, it may be necessary to eliminate bacteria from the specimen (see below). The presence of a virus is demonstrated by the appearance of characteristic histologic lesions, inclusion bodies, or viral antigens in the inoculated test system. Isolated viruses are specifically identified by using known antibodies that inhibit or neutralize the biologic effects of the virus or react with viral antigens (inhibit hemagglutination, fix complement, or induce specific fluorescence).

SPECIMENS FOR STUDY

Many viruses are most readily isolated in the first few days of the illness (Table 34–1). The specimens to be used in virus isolation attempts are listed in Table 34–2. Tissues obtained at autopsy may also serve this purpose. Each specimen must be handled in such a way that a virus will be kept infectious and will have a chance to grow (Table 35–8).

Material should, in general, be frozen (preferably at temperatures well below −20 °C) if there is a delay in bringing it to the laboratory. The principal exceptions are (1) whole blood drawn for antibody determination, which must have the serum separated before freezing; and (2) tissue for organ or cell culture (or urine for cytomegalovirus isolation), which should be kept at 4 °C and taken to the laboratory promptly.

In general, virus is present in respiratory illnesses in pharyngeal or nasal secretions. Virus can be demonstrated in the fluid and scrapings from the base of vesicular rashes. In eye infections, virus is detectable in conjunctival swabs or scrapings and in tears. Encephalitides are usually diagnosed more readily by serologic means. Arboviruses and herpesviruses are not usually recovered from spinal fluid, but brain tissue from patients with viral encephalitis may yield the causative virus. In illnesses associated with enteroviruses, such as central nervous system disease, acute pericarditis, and myocarditis, the viruses can be isolated from feces, throat swabs, or cerebrospinal fluid.

Table 34–1. Relation of stage of illness to presence of virus in test materials and to appearance of specific antibody.

Stage or Period of Illness	Virus Detectable in Test Materials	Specific Antibody Demonstrable*
Incubation	Rarely	No
Prodrome	Occasionally	No
Onset	Frequently	Occasionally
Acute phase	Frequently	Frequently
Recovery	Rarely	Usually
Convalescence	Very rarely	Usually

*Antibody may be detected very early in previously vaccinated persons.

Table 34–2. Specimens for isolation of viruses.

Clinical Manifestations and Common Causative Agents	Source of Specimen for Virus Isolation	
	Clinical	Postmortem or Biopsy
Upper respiratory tract infections		
Rhinovirus	Throat swab or nasal secretions	. . .
Parainfluenza		
Respiratory syncytial		
Adenovirus	Throat swab and feces	. . .
Enterovirus		
Reovirus		
Lower respiratory tract infections		
Influenza	Throat swab and sputum	Lung
Adenovirus		
Parainfluenza		
Rhinovirus		
Respiratory syncytial		
Pleurodynia		
Coxsackievirus	Throat swab and feces	. . .
Cutaneous and mucous membrane diseases		
Vesicular		
Smallpox and vaccinia	Vesicle fluid	Liver, spleen, and lung
Herpes simplex		
Varicella-zoster		
Enterovirus	Vesicle fluid, feces, and throat swab	. . .
Exanthematous		
Measles	Throat swab and blood	. . .
Rubella		
Enterovirus	Throat swab and feces	. . .
Diarrhea of infants		
Rotavirus	Feces	Intestinal wall and contents
Central nervous system infections		
Enterovirus	Feces, throat swab, and CSF	Brain tissue and intestinal contents
Herpes simplex	Throat swab and CSF	Brain tissue
Mumps	Throat swab, CSF, urine	Brain tissue
Lymphocytic choriomeningitis	Blood and CSF	Brain tissue
Arboviruses		
Western equine encephalitis	Blood and CSF	Brain tissue
Eastern equine encephalitis		
Venezuelan equine encephalitis		
California encephalitis	Usually not possible to isolate virus from clinical specimens	Brain tissue
St. Louis encephalitis		
Japanese B encephalitis		
Rabies	Saliva	Brain tissue
Chronic central nervous system infections		
Measles (subacute sclerosing panencephalitis)	. . .	Brain tissue
Human papovavirus (progressive multifocal leukoencephalopathy)	. . .	Brain tissue
Parotitis		
Mumps	Throat swab (Stensen's duct) and urine	. . .
Cytomegalovirus		
Severe undifferentiated febrile illnesses		
Colorado tick fever	Blood	. . .
Yellow fever		
Dengue		

Table 34–2 (cont'd). Specimens for isolation of viruses.

Clinical Manifestations and Common Causative Agents	Source of Specimen for Virus Isolation	
	Clinical	Postmortem or Biopsy
Congenital anomalies		
Cytomegalovirus	Urine and throat swab	Kidney, lung, and other tissues
Rubella	Throat swab and CSF	Lymph nodes, lung, spleen
Conjunctivitis		
Herpes simplex	Conjunctival swabs and tears	Conjunctival and corneal scrapings
Herpes zoster		
Adenovirus		
Enterovirus		
Vaccinia		
AIDS (acquired immune deficiency syndrome)		
Retrovirus LAV/HTLV-III	Blood	Lymph nodes

PRESERVATION OF VIRUSES

Freezing

A large wide-mouthed thermos jar or insulated carton, half-filled with pieces of solid CO_2 (dry ice), serves for transport and storage of material containing viruses. If dry ice is unavailable, the specimens should be kept cold and transported on ordinary ice. The temperature in a dry ice storage cabinet is close to $-76\,°C$. Electric deep-freeze cabinets can maintain temperatures of -50 to $-105\,°C$.

Lyophilization

This procedure consists of rapid freezing at low temperature (in a bath containing alcohol and dry ice) and dehydration from the frozen state at high vacuum.

Ten percent to 50% of normal plasma or serum in the fluid menstruum protects the virus to be frozen and dried. The plasma or serum must not contain neutralizing (Nt) antibodies. Skimmed milk is another "protective" menstruum in which virus-containing material may be suspended.

PREPARATION OF INOCULA

Bacteria-free fluid materials such as cerebrospinal fluid, whole blood, plasma, or serum may be inoculated into cell cultures, animals, or eggs, directly or after dilution with buffered phosphate solution (pH 7.6).

Preparation of Tissues

Tissue is washed in media or sterile water, minced into small pieces with scissors, and ground to make a homogeneous paste. Diluent is added in amounts sufficient to make a concentration of 10–20%. This suspension can be centrifuged at low speed (not more than 2000 rpm) for 10 minutes to sediment insoluble cellular debris. The supernatant fluid may be inoculated; if bacteria are present, they are eliminated as discussed below.

Tissues may also be trypsinized, and the resulting cell suspension may be (1) inoculated on an existing tissue culture cell monolayer, or (2) co-cultivated with another cell suspension of cells known to be virus-free.

Removal of Bacteria

If the material to be tested contains bacteria (throat washings, stools, urine, infected tissue, or insects), they must be inactivated or removed before inoculation.

A. Bactericidal Agents:

1. Antibiotics–Antibiotics are commonly employed in combination with differential centrifugation (see below).

2. Ether–If it is not harmful to the virus in question (eg, enteroviruses, vaccinia), ether may be added in concentrations of 10–15%.

B. Mechanical Methods:

1. Filters–Earthenware, porcelain, and asbestos filters reduce the virus concentration by adsorption and are therefore used infrequently. Millipore type membrane filters of cellulose acetate or similar inert material are preferred.

2. Differential centrifugation–This is a convenient method of removing many bacteria from heavily contaminated preparations of the small viruses. Bacteria are sedimented at low speeds that do not sediment the virus. High-speed centrifugation then sediments the virus. The virus-containing sediment is then resuspended in a small volume.

CULTIVATION IN CELL CULTURE

Cell culture techniques are the most widely used for isolating viruses from clinical specimens. When viruses multiply in cell culture, they produce biologic effects (cytopathic changes, viral interference, or the production of a hemagglutinin) that permit identification of the agent.

Test tube cultures are prepared by adding cells suspended in 1–2 mL of nutrient fluid that contains balanced salt solutions and various growth factors (usually serum, glucose, amino acids, and vitamins). Cells of fibroblastic or epithelial nature attach and grow on the wall of the test tube, where they may be examined with the aid of a low power microscope.

With many viruses, growth of the agent is paralleled by a degeneration of these cells (Fig 34–2). Some viruses produce characteristic cytopathic effects in cell culture, making a rapid presumptive diagnosis possible when the clinical syndrome is known. As examples, measles, mumps, parainfluenza, and respiratory syncytial viruses characteristically produce multinucleated giant cells, whereas adenoviruses produce grapelike clusters of large round cells, rhinoviruses produce focal areas of rounding and dendritic forms, and herpes simplex virus produces diffuse uniform rounding of cells.

Some viruses (eg, rubella virus) produce no direct cytopathic changes but can be detected by their interference with the cytopathic effect of a second challenge virus (viral interference).

Influenza virus and other orthomyxoviruses may be detected within 24–48 hours if erythrocytes are added to infected cultures. Viruses maturing at the cell membrane produce a hemagglutinin enabling the erythrocytes to adsorb at the cell surface (hemadsorption).

Organ cultures of ferret and human tracheal epithelium may support the growth of many viruses that cause upper respiratory tract disease, including some viruses that do not grow in conventional cell cultures (eg, coronaviruses). Viruses may cause general or focal necrosis of the ciliated epithelial cells or may be detected by a decline in ciliary movement.

The identity of a virus isolate is established with type-specific antiserum, which inhibits virus growth or which reacts with the viral antigens in the tests described in Chapter 35 (eg, complement fixation [CF], hemagglutination inhibition [HI], counterimmunoelectrophoresis, etc).

ANIMAL INOCULATION

In past decades, animal inoculation was often employed for virus isolation. Today, however, only relatively few specialized laboratories perform animal work. The laboratory animals employed include mice, hamsters, cotton rats, guinea pigs, rabbits, and mon-

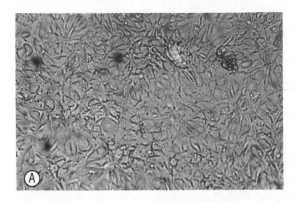
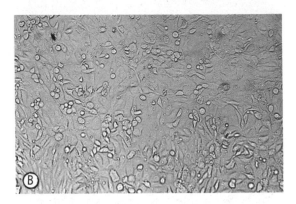
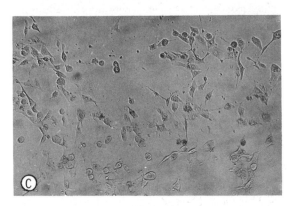

Figure 34–2. A: Monolayer of normal unstained monkey kidney cells in culture (120 x). **B:** Unstained monkey kidney cell culture showing early stage of cytopathic effects typical of enterovirus infection (120 x). Approximately 25% of the cells in the culture show cytopathic effects indicative of virus multiplication (1+ cytopathic effects). **C:** Unstained monkey kidney cell culture illustrating more advanced enteroviral cytopathic effect (3+ to 4+ cytopathic effects) (120 x). Almost 100% of the cells are affected, and most of the cell sheet has come loose from the wall of the culture tube.

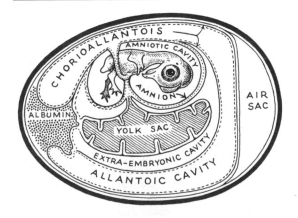

Figure 34–3. Schematic diagram showing developing chick embryo and indicating cavities and other structures used for various routes of inoculation.

keys. In some cases, infant mice (less than 48 hours old) are used. The animals of choice and the route of inoculation are listed in Table 35–8. Intracerebral and intranasal inoculation are employed particularly in mice; these routes require the special experience, skill, and methods available in public health or research laboratories that work with animals. The inoculated animals are observed for signs of illness, then are sacrificed, and their tissues are examined.

EMBRYONATED EGGS

Embryonated eggs in various stages of development (Fig 34–3) can be inoculated by one of several routes. After inoculation, the eggs are reincubated and examined daily for viability. Standardized methods permit inoculation of the chorioallantoic membrane, the amniotic sac, the allantoic sac, the yolk sac, or the embryo. After suitable incubation, fluid or tissue is removed and examined for viral growth or lesions (Table 35–8).

REFERENCES

Almeida JD et al: *Manual for Rapid Laboratory Viral Diagnosis*. WHO Publication No. 47. World Health Organization, 1979.

Chou S, Merigan TC: Rapid detection and quantitation of human cytomegalovirus in urine through DNA hybridization. *N Engl J Med* 1983;**308**:921.

Daisy JA, Lief FS, Friedman HM: Rapid diagnosis of influenza A infection by direct immunofluorescence of nasopharyngeal aspirates in adults. *J Clin Microbiol* 1979;**9**:688.

Dennis J, Oshiro LS, Bunter JW: Molluscum contagiosum, another sexually transmitted disease: Its impact on the clinical virology laboratory. *J Infect Dis* 1985;**151**:376.

Engleberg NC, Eisenstein BI: The impact of new cloning techniques on the diagnosis and treatment of infectious diseases. *N Engl J Med* 1984;**311**:892.

Gleaves CA et al: Comparison of standard tube and shell vial cell culture techniques for the detection of cytomegalovirus in clinical specimens. *J Clin Microbiol* 1985;**21**:217.

Lennette EH, Schmidt NJ (editors): Chapters 1 and 3 in: *Diagnostic Procedures for Viral, Rickettsial and Chlamydial Infections*, 5th ed. American Public Health Association, 1979.

Pothier P et al: Monoclonal antibodies against respiratory syncytial virus and their use for rapid detection of virus in nasopharyngeal secretions. *J Clin Microbiol* 1985;**21**:286.

Richman D et al: Summary of a workshop on new and useful methods in rapid viral diagnosis. *J Infect Dis* 1984;**150**:941.

Schmidt NJ et al: Direct immunofluorescence staining for detection of herpes simplex and varicella-zoster virus antigens in vesicular lesions and certain tissue specimens. *J Clin Microbiol* 1980;**12**:651.

Stålhandske P et al: Detection of adenoviruses in stool specimens by nucleic acid spot hybridization. *J Med Virol* 1985;**16**:213.

Serologic Diagnosis & Immunologic Detection of Virus Infections

Procedures Available

Typically, a virus infection elicits immune responses directed against one or more viral antigens. Both cellular and humoral immune responses usually develop, and measurement of either may be used to diagnose a virus infection. Cellular immunity may be assessed by dermal hypersensitivity, lymphocyte transformation, and cytotoxicity tests (see p 196). Humoral immune responses are of major diagnostic importance. Antibodies of the IgM class appear initially and are followed by IgG antibodies. The IgM antibodies disappear in several weeks, whereas the IgG antibodies persist for many years. Establishing the diagnosis of a virus infection is accomplished serologically by demonstrating a rise in antibody titer to the virus or by demonstrating antiviral antibodies of the IgM class.

Procedures for quantifying antibodies in virus diseases are based on classic antigen-antibody reactions (see Chapter 12), with some modifications for certain viruses. The commonly used methods include the neutralization (Nt) test, the complement fixation (CF) test, the hemagglutination inhibition (HI) test, and the immunofluorescence test. Less commonly used methods include passive hemagglutination, immunodiffusion, counterimmunoelectrophoresis, and radioimmunoassay. A summary of the tests available for viruses is listed in Table 35–8.

Measurement of antibodies by different methods does not necessarily give parallel results. This is illustrated in Table 35–1. Antibodies detected by CF are present during an enterovirus infection and in the convalescent period, but they do not persist. Antibodies detected by neutralization appear during infection and persist for many years. Assessment of antibodies by several methods in individuals or groups of individuals provides diagnostic information as well as information about epidemiologic features of the disease.

Collection of Blood Specimens

Serial samples of serum are essential for diagnostic purposes if antibodies are to be adequately tested and evaluated. In general, the first sample should be collected as soon as possible after the onset of the illness; the second, 2–3 weeks after onset. A third sample may be required later for special study. Antibodies appear earlier in some viral infections than in others, and so the times of collecting specimens must be varied according to circumstances.

Blood specimens should be drawn with aseptic precautions and without anticoagulants and the serum separated and stored at 4 °C or –20 °C. Before performing serologic tests it may be necessary to heat the serum (56 °C for 30 minutes) to remove nonspecific interfering or inhibiting substances and complement. This is essential for CF tests and also, with certain viruses, for Nt tests.

IgM Antibodies

If paired sera are not available, a presumptive diagnosis can sometimes be made by demonstrating IgM antibodies to the virus, even in the first serum sample taken. IgM antibodies may be detected by sensitivity to 2-mercaptoethanol or by immunofluorescence. (See Chapter 12.)

Table 35–1. Interpretation of laboratory data in enterovirus infection.

Virus Isolation	Complement-fixing (CF) Antibody	Neutralizing (Nt) Antibody	Antibody of IgM Class	Interpretation of Infection
−	−	−	−	None
+	−	−	−	Early
+	+	+	+	Current
−	+	+	+	Recent
−	−	+	−	Old

IgM antibodies develop simultaneously with or even before IgG antibodies but then disappear more quickly. However, IgM antibodies remain longer in persistent infections. In congenital infections, IgM antibody detection is of singular value, because IgM does not cross the placenta as does IgG. Thus, finding IgM antibodies to viruses in the serum of a newborn indicates that the child was infected in utero.

NEUTRALIZATION (Nt) TESTS

Virus-neutralizing antibodies are measured by adding serum containing these antibodies to a suspension of virus and then inoculating the mixture into susceptible cell cultures. The presence of Nt antibodies is demonstrated if the cell cultures fail to develop cytopathic effects (CPE) while control cell cultures, which have received virus plus a serum free of antibody, develop cytopathic effects. In some instances, the virus-antiserum mixture may be inoculated into susceptible experimental animals (as with type A coxsackieviruses) or embryonated eggs (as with mumps virus). The protection of the host from viral effects demonstrates Nt antibody.

The virus in a neutralized mixture is not destroyed. When some virus-antibody mixtures are treated with acid (pH 2.0), the acid denatures the antibody and liberates the virus in its original, fully infectious state.

The level of such antibodies can be determined by using a constant amount of virus and falling concentrations of serum, or undiluted serum and falling concentrations of virus. To establish a diagnosis, one looks for a significant rise in antibody titer—4-fold or greater is desirable—during the course of the infection. In recurrent infections, eg, herpes simplex, high antibody titers are commonly detected in serial serum samples; the diagnostic rise between acute and convalescent sera is not registered.

A positive test in a single sample of serum is not of diagnostic value in acute infections unless it can be demonstrated that the antibody belongs to the IgM class. Nt antibodies can persist for years, and their presence may indicate a past infection in a given individual. Thus, Nt tests are useful in serologic epidemiology, where one is interested in knowing which viral agents have infected a given population in the past.

Although simple in principle, Nt tests are expensive in time and in materials and must be standardized for each viral agent. Among the variables that must be considered are (1) the selection of the cell culture, experimental animal, or embryonated egg; (2) the route of inoculation of the virus-serum mixture; (3) the age of the test animals; (4) the stability of the test virus; (5) the reproducibility of the end point; (6) the relative heat-stability of the specific antibody and of possible interfering substances in serum; (7) the addition of an accessory factor found in fresh normal serum of the homologous species; (8) the use of one concentration of virus and varying dilutions of serum, or vice versa (and the relationship between varying concentrations of each); (9) the temperature of the neutralizing mixture; and (10) the time of incubation of the mixture.

Nt Test in Cell Culture

The details of this test vary in different laboratories, but the same principle underlies all of them: the viral antibody specifically neutralizes the cytopathogenic effects of the virus.

With each series of Nt tests, control titrations of virus are made. The highest concentration of each serum used is tested for possible nonspecific cell toxicity. A few tubes are left uninoculated to serve as cell controls. The typical results of sera obtained from a patient infected with type 1 poliovirus are shown in Table 35–2. The cultures were incubated at 36 °C for 3 days and then examined microscopically. At the end of that time, the virus titration showed that 100 TCID$_{50}$ doses had been added to each serum.

For viruses such as herpes, polio, or vaccinia, which produce plaques on cell sheets (Fig 33–28), neutralization may be measured by comparing the

Table 35–2. Cell culture neutralization (Nt) test with paired sera of patient infected with type 1 poliovirus.

Virus*	Serum (Day After Onset)	Cellular Degeneration (Cytopathic Effect) Final Serum Dilution					50% Serum Titer	
		1:2	1:10	1:50	1:250	1:1250	Logarithm	Antilog
Type 1	1	000	+++	+++	+++	+++	0.7	5
	20	000	000	000	00+	+++	2.5	320
Type 2	1	000	+++	+++	+++	+++	0.7	5
	20	000	000	0++	+++	+++	1.5	32
Type 3	1	+++	+++	+++	+++	+++	0	0
	20	+++	+++	+++	+++	+++	0	0
None	1	000						
	20	000						

*100 TCID$_{50}$ doses of each virus used in test. Three cultures were inoculated with each virus-serum mixture. + indicates cytopathic change in a culture because of virus growth. 0 indicates no growth of virus. (TCID$_{50}$ = 50% tissue culture infectious dose.)

number of plaques produced by the virus alone with the number produced in the presence of the serum. Such plaque reduction techniques are available for many viruses grown in cell culture and are commonly used where greater accuracy of quantitation is required.

Suspensions of monkey kidney cells or cells from a continuous cell line may be used directly in Nt tests. The same basic principle that underlies any virus Nt test, ie, antibody specifically neutralizes the infectivity of the virus, also applies to the color (or metabolic inhibition) test. The color test employs known quantities of cell suspensions that are added to test tubes or plastic panel cups 1 hour after the virus-serum mixture. This eliminates the need for cultures in which cells have already grown out on glass. The color test utilizes the fact that with continued cellular growth in control tubes or in the presence of an immune serum-virus mixture, acidic products of metabolism lower the pH of the medium. This effect is readily observed by incorporating the indicator dye phenol red into the medium. This dye is red at pH 7.4–7.8. It becomes salmon pink and finally yellow as the pH drops below 7.0. Conversely, cell necrosis induced by the virus leaves the medium red, because the dying cultures fail to reach the degree of acidity exhibited by the control cultures. The test can thus be read by color change alone rather than by the presence or absence of cellular degeneration as determined microscopically. Nt antibodies are measured by determining the serum dilution that in the presence of added virus will allow the cells to metabolize normally and the pH to fall as in the controls.

The test described in the above paragraph is used with the enteroviruses. Because adenoviruses cause a stimulation of cellular metabolism and more rapid lowering of the pH than that in the control cultures, the color reaction is the opposite of that described above.

Nt Tests in Eggs

The embryonated egg may also be used as an indicator system in virus Nt tests. With influenza and mumps viruses, after the inoculation of the virus-serum mixtures, the end point is measured by determining whether viral hemagglutinins have developed in the allantoic fluid (Fig 35–1).

With herpes simplex virus and the poxviruses, Nt antibody prevents the production of characteristic pocks in the chorioallantoic membrane (pock-reduction test).

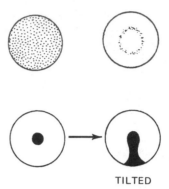

Figure 35–1. Patterns of positive (top) and negative (bottom) hemagglutination. When the tube is tilted, only nonagglutinated cells (bottom row) slide down the tube.

Nt Test in Mice

Mice of known uniform susceptibility and standard age are inoculated by a standard route with the virus-serum mixture. They are observed daily for signs of illness, such as weakness or paralysis, to establish specificity of the deaths. Illness and deaths are recorded daily for 21 days. Deaths within 24 hours after inoculation are attributed to traumatic or nonviral causes.

The virus suspension used is titrated by the adopted route of inoculation. The 50% lethal dose (LD_{50}) is calculated by an accepted method (eg, Reed-Muench, Kaerber), and a fixed number of LD_{50} is employed for each virus-serum mixture. Alternatively, the serum is kept constant and the virus dilutions are varied.

Interpretation of Nt Tests

Since Nt antibodies for viruses persist for years, it is customary to demonstrate a rise in titer in sequential sera in order to establish current or recent infection by the virus. A fall in titer in the third (late) serum sample and unusually high titers can be significant.

COMPLEMENT FIXATION (CF) TESTS

The principles underlying complement fixation (CF) tests have been described in Chapter 12. Because antiviral sera fix complement in the presence of the homologous antigens, such CF tests are employed in the diagnosis of many viral infections (Table 35–3). As in

Table 35–3. An example of a complement fixation (CF) test response.

Time of Taking Serum	Serum Dilution						Titer
	1:5	1:10	1:20	1:40	1:80	1:160	
Acute phase	0	0	0	0	0	0	0
Recovery phase	4+	3+	0	0	0	0	1:10
Convalescent	4+	4+	4+	3+	2+	0	1:80

4+ indicates complement fixation (no hemolysis); 0 indicates complete hemolysis.

all CF tests, strictly standardized procedures must be employed. The main problem in viral CF tests is the preparation of specific antigens that are stable and not anticomplementary. Most antigens at present are derived from viral cell cultures (fluids or disrupted cells), from embryonated eggs (fluids or tissues), or from extracted tissues of infected animals (eg, mouse brains extracted with acetone for diagnosis of arbovirus infections).

In some instances, viruses may have 2 types of antigens: one associated with the virus particle (V) and the other a separate small, "soluble" entity (S). Antibodies against different antigens may appear at different times during viral infection, as illustrated in mumps (see p 478). The interpretation of CF results depends on the antigen employed in the test and on the antibody titer rise observed.

HEMAGGLUTINATION INHIBITION (HI) TEST

Many viruses agglutinate erythrocytes, and this reaction may be specifically inhibited by immune or convalescent sera. As shown in Table 35–8, this reaction forms the basis of many diagnostic tests for viral infections.

Diseases in Which an Antibody Response May Be Demonstrated by the HI Test

Influenza
Rubella
Mumps
Measles
Newcastle disease
Variola
Vaccinia
California virus encephalitis
St. Louis encephalitis
Western equine encephalitis
Japanese B encephalitis
West Nile fever
Dengue
Adenovirus infections
Some enterovirus infections
Reovirus infections

General Principles

The same general principles apply for the HI tests used with different viral agents. However, a distinct species of erythrocytes may be necessary to agglutinate certain viruses, eg, some adenovirus types agglutinate only rat erythrocytes.

To be useful for diagnostic purposes, the erythrocyte suspension must be standardized and the viral antigen standardized and titrated. Positive and negative controls should be included in each test. The results are read (Fig 35–1) as follows:

(1) Positive agglutination is indicated by a red, granular, diffused lining on the bottom of the tube.

Table 35–4. An example of a hemagglutination inhibition (HI) test response.

Time of Taking Serum	Serum Dilution						Titer
	1:8	1:16	1:32	1:64	1:128	1:256	
Acute phase	0	+	+	+	+	+	1:8
Recovery phase	0	0	0	+	+	+	1:32
Convalescent	0	0	0	0	0	+	1:128

+ = Agglutination.
0 = No agglutination.

(2) Absence of agglutination is indicated by the formation of a compact red button at the bottom of the tube that slides when the tube is tilted.

(3) Partial agglutination is indicated by something in between a diffused lining on the bottom of the tube and a red button. This takes the form of a ring with a hollow center.

Specific antiviral antibody inhibits the agglutination of red cells by virus suspensions. This principle is used to quantify levels of antibody, to demonstrate rises in titer, and to establish the type-specific nature of the antibody rise in viral infections. Two serum specimens are needed from the patient, taken at an interval of 2–3 weeks. The first specimen should be obtained as promptly as possible after the onset of illness. Serial dilutions of the sera are made in diluent, a standard amount (usually 4 hemagglutinating units) of virus suspension is added, and after thorough mixing the red cell suspension is added. Incubation is often at room temperature for 60 minutes. Care must be taken not to disturb the mixtures. The test is then read by the criteria outlined above. The highest dilution of serum that inhibits hemagglutination under standard conditions is considered the HI titer (Table 35–4). A 4-fold or greater titer increase during a 2- to 3-week period is considered proof of active virus infection. For most viruses, HI micromethod tests are now employed.

IMMUNOFLUORESCENCE TEST

The principles of immunofluorescence tests are described in Chapter 12. The indirect immunofluorescence (fluorescent antibody, FA) tests use known specific labeled antiviral sera to identify viruses grown in cell culture (as an isolation procedure) or found in exfoliated cells of the respiratory tract (eg, influenza).

The indirect immunofluorescence test may be more sensitive. The unlabeled antiviral serum is used as an unknown reagent, eg, human serum tested against cells grown on coverslips and infected with a virus. Then fluorescein isothiocyanate-labeled antihuman globulin (prepared in an animal) is used as a "stain" for examination in ultraviolet light. Thus, immunofluorescence methods can be used either to identify a virus or to establish the presence of a specific antibody in a series of serum dilutions by employing known virus antigen.

IMMUNODIFFUSION TEST

In immunodiffusion tests, the antigen and antibody are allowed to diffuse toward each other in a semisolid medium such as agar. A line of precipitate is formed at the zone of optimal proportions. The number of precipitin lines formed will depend upon the number of distinct antigen-antibody reactions taking place; each line represents one antigen-antibody system. The technique is well suited for the analysis of soluble antigens associated with viruses (see Chapter 12). The test is more sensitive and rapid if combined with electrophoresis (see below).

In single radial diffusion tests, the viral antigen is included in the gel and antibody is then added in a well cut into the gel. A precipitate forms in a circular zone around the well. The area of the precipitate indicates the concentration of antibody.

The single radial diffusion hemolysis test is a modification that is particularly useful for detecting rubella antibodies. In this procedure, erythrocytes treated with viral hemagglutinin are mixed into the gel. After incubation to allow antibodies to diffuse into the gel, complement is added to destroy the erythrocytes with the attached antigen-antibody complex. The area of the clear zone is proportionate to the antibody titer.

COUNTERIMMUNOELECTROPHORESIS TEST

Counterimmunoelectrophoresis methods can be applied to virologic diagnosis. The principles of the method are presented in Chapter 12. Counterimmunoelectrophoresis applies when a viral antigen is negatively charged and moves toward the anode when the

electric current is applied. Antibody globulin tends to move toward the cathode. When antigen and antibody meet, a precipitin line forms in the gel. An example of hepatitis B surface antigen (HBsAg) interacting with human sera is shown in Fig 35–2.

RADIOIMMUNOASSAY

Radioimmunoassay (RIA) techniques measure immunologic rather than biologic activity (see Chapter 12). They are being widely adapted to the detection and measurement of viral antigens and antibodies in picogram concentrations. Two basic assay procedures have been utilized depending on whether the specific compound to be labeled is antigen or antibody. Conventional RIA systems are based on the principle of saturation analysis in which the protein or polypeptide to be measured competes with a labeled antigen for a limited amount of antibody. The final ratio of labeled antigen for the specific antibody depends on the proportion of unlabeled antigen present in the system. To quantify the amount of unlabeled antigen in the system, a means of separating the residual free radioactivity from that complexed with the antibodies is necessary. This can be achieved by immunologic precipitation of the bound fraction with a second antibody (double antibody) directed against the antigenic determinants of IgG in the first antibody.

Table 35–5 illustrates the general procedure for the double antibody RIA method as applied to the detection of hepatitis B surface antigen (HBsAg) or its antibody (anti-HBs). Antigen detection is based on determining whether a significant reduction occurs in the percentage of counts bound by the test sample when compared with the negative control samples. The amount of reduction is a function of the concentration

CATHODE (−)

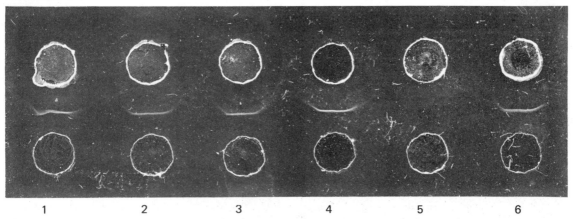

ANODE (+)

Figure 35–2. Counterimmunoelectrophoresis showing formation of precipitin lines between test samples and antibody to HBsAg (anti-HBs). Human serum samples were placed in the top row of wells, and anti-HBs was placed in all wells of the bottom row. In the top row, wells 1–4 contain 4 serum samples from patients with viral hepatitis type B. Well 5 contains a negative normal human serum control; well 6 contains a known positive for HBsAg.

Table 35-5. Double antibody radioimmunoassay.

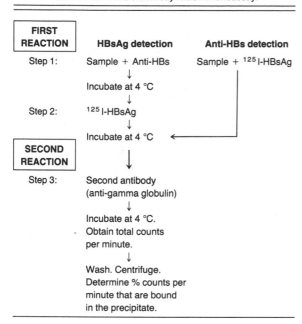

FIRST REACTION	HBsAg detection	Anti-HBs detection
Step 1:	Sample + Anti-HBs	Sample + ^{125}I-HBsAg
	↓	
	Incubate at 4 °C	
	↓	
Step 2:	^{125}I-HBsAg	
	↓	
	Incubate at 4 °C ←	
SECOND REACTION	↓	
Step 3:	Second antibody (anti-gamma globulin)	
	↓	
	Incubate at 4 °C. Obtain total counts per minute.	
	↓	
	Wash. Centrifuge. Determine % counts per minute that are bound in the precipitate.	

ENZYME-LINKED IMMUNOSORBENT ASSAY (ELISA)

The principles of this test are described in Chapter 12, and its application to the detection of viral antigen in clinical material is explained in Chapter 34. For serum antibody, the following procedure is used: Viral antigen is first applied to the solid phase. The test serum is added, and any specific antibody is bound to the antigen. Enzyme-linked antiglobulin is added; it attaches to the bound antibody in the test serum. Enzyme substrate is added and the color change measured. It is proportionate to the amount of enzyme bound, and that in turn is related to the amount of antibody in the test serum.

IMMUNE ELECTRON MICROSCOPY

Viruses not detectable by conventional techniques may be observed by immune electron microscopy (IEM). Antigen-antibody complexes or aggregates formed between virus particles in suspension and added homologous antiserum are detected more readily and with greater assurance than individual virus particles. Fig 35–3 shows the IEM examination of human stool filtrates in which hepatitis A virus is demonstrated.

With the IEM technique, the sample is first

of unlabeled antigen present. Conversely, antibody detection depends on finding an increased number of counts in the precipitate of the test specimens when compared with the counts observed in the control samples that do not contain antibody.

The second method of immunoassay, which has become a powerful analytic tool for the diagnostic laboratory, is illustrated in Table 35–6. This 2-site, solid-phase immunoradiometric assay involves adsorption of unlabeled antibody to an insoluble matrix, eg, polystyrene beads or polyvinyl microtiter wells. The test sample containing antigen is allowed to complex with the antibody-coated surface. Antigen is literally extracted immunologically from the test specimen by specific binding to its surface; it is measured following a second reaction, now with radioactive labeled antibody. The amount of radioactivity measured is proportionate to the concentration of antigen bound by the initial reaction. The test offers increased sensitivity and specificity and can be completed in a relatively short time.

The RIA technique is 100–200 times more sensitive than the CF test.

Table 35-6. Two-site immunoradiometric assay.

Step 1:	Specific unlabeled antibody adsorbed to insoluble matrix (polystyrene beads or polyvinyl microtiter wells).
	↓
Step 2:	Test sample added and antigen extracted immunologically.
	↓
Step 3:	Labeled antibody added as detector system for antigen bound in step 2.
	↓
	Wash. Measure radioactivity remaining on insoluble matrix.

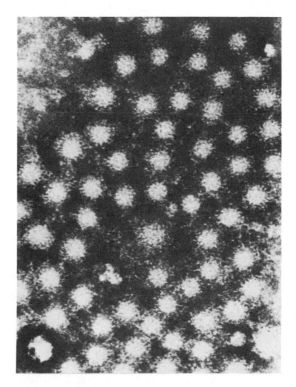

Figure 35-3. Electron micrograph of 27-nm hepatitis A virus aggregated with antibody (222,000 ×). Note the presence of an antibody "halo" around each particle. (Bradley, Hornbeck, and Maynard.)

clarified by centrifugation and then mixed with specific or convalescent serum. Following incubation, the complexes formed are sedimented by centrifugation; the supernatant is discarded and the pellet is resuspended in distilled water, mixed with 3% phosphotungstic acid, and examined by electron microscopy.

The IEM technique may permit the use of convalescent sera from patients with fever of undetermined origin to construct antigen-antibody complexes with serum obtained during the acute phase and to determine if infective agents were associated with the illness. This technique offers a sensitive method of identifying new agents and subsequently determining their role in infectious disease.

HETEROPHIL AGGLUTINATION TEST FOR INFECTIOUS MONONUCLEOSIS

Antibodies against the causative agent of infectious mononucleosis, the EB herpesvirus, can be demonstrated by immunofluorescence and a cell line that carries EB virus (see p 510). Far more commonly, the less specific heterophil agglutination test is used. In the course of infectious mononucleosis, substances appear in the serum that agglutinate sheep cells. If an early serum specimen is compared to a late one, the rise in titer occurs during mononucleosis. The agglutinins can be removed by absorbing serum with the materials shown in Table 35–7. If the sheep agglutinins are not removed by absorption with guinea pig kidney but are absorbed by beef erythrocytes, the diagnosis of infectious mononucleosis is confirmed. The accidental antigenic relationships that provide for the specificity of this result are not well understood.

A reliable, simple, and specific slide test (Mono-Diff, Monospot, Monostico, Monotest) has replaced the traditional sheep cell agglutination test as the most

Table 35–7. Absorption reactions of agglutinins in human serum.

Type of Serum	Agglutinins Absorbed by	
	Guinea Pig Kidney	Bovine Erythrocytes
Normal	Yes	No
Infectious mononucleosis	No	Yes
Serum sickness	Yes	Yes

frequently used serologic test in diagnosing infectious mononucleosis.

In this test, the absorbing materials are incorporated in the test circles on the slide. A single drop of serum is placed on each circle, and horse erythrocytes are added. Agglutination of these cells indicates the presence of agglutinins diagnostic for infectious mononucleosis.

TESTS FOR DERMAL HYPERSENSITIVITY (Skin Tests)

When available, tests for dermal hypersensitivity offer certain advantages in determining, easily and quickly, prior exposure to infectious agents. Tests have been described for mumps, herpes simplex, cat-scratch disease, western equine encephalitis, and vaccinia. The skin test may lead to increase in antibodies, eg, in the CF test.

The skin test antigen (0.1 mL) is injected intradermally into the flexor surface of one arm and the control material into the other arm. The sites of injection are examined after 12–48 hours. The mean diameter of erythematous reaction and induration is measured and compared to the control. A positive reaction is taken to indicate resistance to infection with some viruses.

Table 35–8. Laboratory diagnosis of viral diseases.

(CC, cell culture. Nt neutralization. CF, complement fixation. HI, hemagglutination inhibition. CAM, chorioallantoic membrane. ID, immunodiffusion. IF, immunofluorescence. CIE, counterimmunoelectrophoresis. RIA, radioimmunoassay. CPE, cytopathic effect. ELISA, enzyme-linked immunosorbent assay.)

Disease	Human Specimens to Be Tested	CC or Animals to Be Inoculated	Primary Isolation of Virus			Diagnostic Serologic Tests	
			Route	Tissue to Be Harvested for Passage	Positive Result in Test System: Signs and Pathology	Type of Test	Source of Virus or Antigen
ARTHROPOD-BORNE							
Encephalitides California St. Louis						Nt in mice or CC	Mouse brain or CC
Japanese B						CF	Mouse brain or CC
Western equine	Brain, blood	Mice	Intracerebral	Brain	Encephalitis	HI	Infant mouse brain
Eastern equine Venezuelan equine Russian spring-summer West Nile fever, etc.							

Table 35–8 (cont'd). Laboratory diagnosis of viral diseases.

(CC, cell culture. Nt neutralization. CF, complement fixation. HI, hemagglutination inhibition. CAM, chorioallantoic membrane. ID, immunodiffusion. IF, immunofluorescence. CIE, counterimmunoelectrophoresis. RIA, radioimmunoassay. CPE, cytopathic effect. ELISA, enzyme-linked immunosorbent assay.)

Disease	Human Specimens to Be Tested	CC or Animals to Be Inoculated	Primary Isolation of Virus			Diagnostic Serologic Tests	
			Route	Tissue to Be Harvested for Passage	Positive Result in Test System: Signs and Pathology	Type of Test	Source of Virus or Antigen
ARTHROPOD-BORNE (CONT'D)							
Yellow fever	Blood, viscera	Monkeys	Intraperitoneal	Viscera	Hepatic necrosis	Nt	Mouse brain
		Mice	Intracerebral	Brain	Encephalitis		
Rift Valley fever	Blood	Mice	Intraperitoneal	Liver	Hepatitis	Nt, CF	Mouse liver
Dengue	Blood	Mice	Intracerebral	Brain	Encephalomyelitis	Nt, CF	Mouse brain
Sandfly fever	Blood	Infant mice	Intracerebral	Brain	Encephalomyelitis	Nt, CF	Mouse brain
Colorado tick fever	Blood	Hamsters	Intraperitoneal	Brain	Encephalitis	Nt	Mouse brain
		Mice	Intracerebral	Brain	Encephalitis	CF	Mouse brain
NEUROTROPIC, NON-ARTHROPOD-BORNE							
Poliomyelitis	Spinal cord, feces, throat swabs	CC		CC fluid	CPE	Nt, CF	CC
Rabies	Brain	Mice	Intracerebral	Brain	Encephalitis, Negri inclusion bodies	IF	
Lymphocytic choriomeningitis	Brain, blood, spinal fluid	Mice	Intracerebral	Brain	Encephalitis and choroiditis	Nt	Mouse brain
		Guinea pig	Intraperitoneal	Spleen	Death with pneumonia, focal infiltration in liver	CF	Guinea pig spleen
B virus infection (Herpes B)	Brain, spleen	Rabbit	Intracutaneous	Spinal cord	Necrosis of skin, myelitis, intranuclear inclusion bodies	CF, Nt	Rabbit kidney CC
Herpes simplex		Rabbit kidney CC		CC fluid	CPE	CF, Nt, ELISA	Rabbit kidney CC
Human papovavirus	Brain	CC			CPE	HI	CC
Measles (SSPE)	Brain	Direct exam (or co-cultivation in CC)				IF	
DERMOTROPIC							
Variola (smallpox)	Skin lesions, vesicle fluid, blood	Embryonated egg	CAM	CAM	Pocks on membrane, cytoplasmic inclusion bodies	CF, HI, ID	Vesicle fluid of crusts
Vaccinia	Skin lesions, vesicle fluid	Embryonated egg	CAM	CAM	Pocks on membrane	CF	CAM, rabbit skin or testicle, mouse brain, CC
		Rabbit	Intracutaneous	Skin	Skin lesion, cytoplasmic inclusion bodies	Nt in eggs, rabbits, mice, CC; HI	
		CC		CC fluid	CPE		
Varicella (chickenpox)	Vesicle fluid	CC		CC cells	Intranuclear inclusions	CF, Nt, ELISA	CC
Zoster	Vesicle fluid	CC		CC cells	Intranuclear inclusions	CF, ELISA	CC
Measles	Nasopharyngeal secretions, blood	CC		CC fluid	Multinucleate giant cells and intranuclear inclusions	CF, Nt, ELISA	CC
Rubella (German measles)	Nasopharyngeal secretions, blood, amniotic fluid	CC		CC fluid	Interference or CPE	Nt, CF, HI, IF, ID, ELISA	CC

Table 35–8 (cont'd). Laboratory diagnosis of viral diseases.

(CC, cell culture. Nt, neutralization. CF, complement fixation. HI, hemagglutination inhibition. CAM, chorioallantoic membrane. ID, immunodiffusion. IF, immunofluorescence. CIE, counterimmunoelectrophoresis. RIA, radioimmunoassay. CPE, cytopathic effect. ELISA, enzyme-linked immunosorbent assay.)

Disease	Human Specimens to Be Tested	CC or Animals to Be Inoculated	Primary Isolation of Virus			Diagnostic Serologic Tests	
			Route	Tissue to Be Harvested for Passage	Positive Result in Test System: Signs and Pathology	Type of Test	Source of Virus or Antigen
DERMOTROPIC (CONT'D)							
Herpes simplex	Skin lesions, conjunctival swabs, tears	CC		CC fluid	CPE, inclusion bodies	Nt, CF, IF, ELISA	CC
Molluscum contagiosum	Skin lesions	(No satisfactory experimental animal. Characteristic cytoplasmic inclusion bodies. Virus can easily be seen in the electron microscope.)					
Verrucae (warts)	Skin lesions	(No satisfactory experimental animal. Electron microscopic examination of warts detects virus particles.)					
RESPIRATORY AND PAROTID							
Influenza A Influenza B Influenza C	Throat swabs, nasal washings, lung	Eggs	Amniotic and allantoic sacs	Embryonic fluids	Hemagglutinin produced	HI	Allantoic fluid
		Ferrets, mice	Intranasal	Lung	Pneumonitis	CF	Allantoic fluid
		CC		CC fluid	CPE, hemadsorption	Nt in eggs, mice, or CC	Allantoic fluid, mouse lung, CC
Parainfluenza		CC			Hemadsorption	Nt, CF	CC
Respiratory syncytial (RS) infection		CC		CC fluid	Multinucleate giant cells with cytoplasmic inclusions	Nt, CF	CC
Common cold (rhinovirus group)	Nasopharyngeal washings, swabs	CC		CC fluid	CPE	Nt	CC
Mumps	Saliva, spinal fluid, urine	Monkeys	Parotid gland	Parotid gland	Parotitis	CF	Amniotic fluid
		Eggs	Amniotic and yolk sacs	Amniotic fluid, yolk sac	Hemagglutinin produced	HI	Monkey parotid gland
		CC		CC fluid	CPE, hemadsorption	Nt in CC	CC
Adenovirus group	Throat swabs, pharyngeal washings, stool	CC		CC cells and fluid	CPE	CF, Nt, HI	CC
HEPATIC							
Infectious hepatitis (type A)	Blood, feces	(No satisfactory experimental system.)				RIA, ELISA	Serum, feces, liver, bile
Serum hepatitis (type B)	Blood, feces, urine					CIE, CF, ID, RIA, ELISA	Serum
MISCELLANEOUS							
Coxsackie infection	Feces, throat swabs, spinal fluid, vesicle fluid	Infant mice	Subcutaneous	Muscle	Paralysis with myositis and, with certain types, encephalitis, steatitis; pancreatitis	Nt in infant mice or CC	Mouse muscle
		CC		CC fluid	CPE	Nt, CF, HI	CC
Echovirus infection	Feces, throat swabs, spinal fluid	CC		CC fluid	CPE	Nt, CF, HI	CC

Table 35–8 (cont'd). Laboratory diagnosis of viral diseases.

(CC, cell culture. Nt, neutralization. CF, complement fixation. HI, hemagglutination inhibition. CAM, chorioallantoic membrane. ID, immunodiffusion. IF, immunofluorescence. CIE, counterimmunoelectrophoresis. RIA, radioimmunoassay. CPE, cytopathic effect. ELISA, enzyme-linked immunosorbent assay.)

Disease	Human Specimens to Be Tested	CC or Animals to Be Inoculated	Primary Isolation of Virus			Diagnostic Serologic Tests	
			Route	Tissue to Be Harvested for Passage	Positive Result in Test System: Signs and Pathology	Type of Test	Source of Virus or Antigen
MISCELLANEOUS (CONT'D)							
Rotavirus infection	Feces	(Electron microscopy to visualize virus.)				CF, IF, ELISA	(See p 514.)
Reovirus infection	Feces, throat swabs	CC		CC fluid	CPE	Nt, CF, HI	CC
Epidemic keratoconjunctivitis	Conjunctivas	CC		CC cells and fluid	CPE	Nt test for adenovirus 8	CC
Foot-and-mouth disease	Skin lesions	Guinea pigs	Intracutaneous, foot pads	Foot pads	Hyperkeratosis with vesicle formation, paralysis with myositis	CF	Guinea pig foot pad
		Newborn mice		Muscle			Mouse muscle
Cytomegalovirus disease	Oral swabs, urine, various organs	CC		CC cells and fluid	CPE, inclusion bodies	Nt, CF	CC

REFERENCES

Bonfanti C, Meurman O, Halonen P: Detection of specific immunoglobulin M antibody to rubella virus by use of an enzyme-labeled antigen. *J Clin Microbiol* 1985;**21**:963.

Budzko DB et al: Rapid test for detection of rabies antibodies in human serum. *J Clin Microbiol* 1983;**17**:481.

Burke DS, Nisalak A, Ussery MA: Antibody capture immunoassay detection of Japanese encephalitis virus immunoglobulin M and G antibodies in cerebrospinal fluid. *J Clin Microbiol* 1982;**16**:1034.

Burlington DB et al: Development of subtype-specific and heterosubtypic antibodies to the influenza A virus hemagglutinin after primary infection in children. *J Clin Microbiol* 1985;**21**:847.

Chan D, Hammond GW: Comparison of serodiagnosis of group B coxsackie virus infections by an immunoglobulin M capture enzyme immunoassay versus microneutralization. *J Clin Microbiol* 1985;**21**:830.

Cremer NE et al: Enzyme immunoassay versus plaque neutralization and other methods for determination of immune status to measles and varicella-zoster viruses and versus complement fixation for serodiagnosis of infections with those viruses. *J Clin Microbiol* 1985;**21**:869.

Hampar B et al: Enzyme-linked immunosorbent assay for determination of antibodies against herpes simplex virus types 1 and 2 in human sera. *J Clin Microbiol* 1985;**21**:496.

Hollinger FB, Dienstag JL: Hepatitis viruses. Pages 813–835 in: *Manual of Clinical Microbiology*, 4th ed. Lennette EH (editor). American Society for Microbiology, 1985.

Kapikian AZ et al: Visualization by immune electron microscopy of a 27-nm particle associated with acute infectious nonbacterial gastroenteritis. *J Virol* 1972;**10**:1075.

Lennette EH, Schmidt NJ (editors): Chapters 4, 5, 6, and 7 in: *Diagnostic Procedures for Viral, Rickettsial and Chlamydial Infections*, 5th ed. American Public Health Association, 1979.

Lennette EH et al: Standardization of viral reagents. *Medical Virology* 1983;**2**:347.

Vaananen P et al: Comparison of a simple latex agglutination test with hemolysis-in-gel, hemagglutination inhibition, and radioimmunoassay for detection of rubella virus antibodies. *J Clin Microbiol* 1985;**21**:793.

36   Arthropod-Borne & Rodent-Borne Viral Diseases

The **arthropod-borne viruses**, or **arboviruses**, are a group of infectious agents that are transmitted by blood-sucking arthropods from one vertebrate host to another. They multiply in the tissues of the arthropod without evidence of disease or damage. The vector acquires a lifelong infection through the ingestion of blood from a viremic vertebrate. Some arboviruses are maintained in nature by transovarian and possibly sexual transmission in arthropods.

Because of the importance of ecologic factors governing their transmission, **rodent-borne (robo) viral diseases** also are considered in this chapter. They are maintained in nature by direct intraspecies or interspecies transmission (or both) from rodent to rodent without participation of arthropod vectors. Virus infection is usually persistent. Transmission occurs through many routes by contact with body fluids or excretions.

Individual viruses were sometimes named after a disease (dengue, yellow fever) or after the geographic area where the virus was first isolated (St. Louis encephalitis, West Nile fever). Although arboviruses are found in all temperate and tropical zones, they are most prevalent in the tropical rain forest with its abundance of animals and arthropods.

There are more than 450 arboviruses and roboviruses; of these, 97 are pathogenic for humans. They are classified according to their chemical and physical properties and their antigenic relationships. As shown in Table 36–1, the arboviruses and roboviruses are placed among toga-, flavi-, bunya-, reo-, arena-, filo-, and rhabdovirus groups.

Togaviruses: The alphavirus subgroup consists of 28 viruses that are 70 nm in diameter and possess an enveloped, positive-sense RNA genome. The envelope contains 2 glycoproteins and lipid.

Flaviviruses: The genus consists of 65 viruses that are 40–50 nm in diameter and have an enveloped, positive-sense RNA. The envelope contains a single glycoprotein and lipid.

Both alphaviruses and flaviviruses replicate in the cytoplasm; alphaviruses mature by budding nucleocapsids through the plasma membrane, whereas flaviviruses mature through intracytoplasmic membranes (particularly the endoplasmic reticulum). Unlike alphaviruses, some flaviviruses may cause persistent infections, and many are transmitted between vertebrate hosts without intermediate arthropod vectors.

Bunyaviruses: Spherical particles contain a sin-

Table 36–1. Taxonomic status of some arboviruses and roboviruses.

Taxonomic Classification	Important Arbovirus and Robovirus Members
Togaviridae Genus *Alphavirus*	Chikungunya, eastern equine encephalitis, Mayaro, O'Nyong-nyong, Ross River, Semliki Forest, Sindbis, and Venezuelan and western equine encephalitis viruses
Flaviviridae Genus *Flavivirus*	Brazilian encephalitis (Rocio virus), dengue, Ilheus, Japanese B encephalitis, Kyasanur Forest disease, louping ill, Murray Valley encephalitis, Omsk hemorrhagic fever, Powassan, St. Louis encephalitis, tick-borne encephalitis, US bat salivary gland, West Nile fever, yellow fever, and Zika viruses
Bunyaviridae Genus *Bunyavirus*	Anopheles A and B, California, Guama, Simbu (Oropouche), and Turlock viruses
Genus *Phlebovirus*	Sandfly *(Phlebotomus)* fever viruses and Rift Valley fever viruses
Genus *Nairovirus*	Crimean-Congo hemorrhagic fever, Nairobi sheep disease, and Sakhalin viruses
Genus *Hantavirus*	Hantaan virus (Korean hemorrhagic fever, hemorrhagic fever with renal syndrome)
Reoviridae Genus *Orbivirus*	African horse sickness, bluetongue, and Colorado tick fever viruses
Rhabdoviridae Genus *Vesiculovirus*	Hart Park, Kern Canyon, and vesicular stomatitis viruses
Arenaviridae Genus *Arenavirus*	Junin, Lassa, Machupo, and Pichinde viruses
Filoviridae	Marburg and Ebola viruses

gle negative-sense RNA genome that is segmented. They have a lipid-containing envelope and measure 90–100 nm. The nucleocapsids have helical symmetry and contain a major viral protein. The envelope has 2 glycoproteins in the lipid bilayer and surface projections (10 nm) of glycopeptides clustered to form hollow cylinders. Several produce mosquito-borne encephalitides of humans and animals, others hemorrhagic fevers. Some are transmitted by sandflies *(Phlebotomus)*.

Reoviruses: (See Chapter 45.) A few arboviruses are members of the subgroup Orbivirus, including African horse sickness and Colorado tick fever (see below). Some infect birds, small mammals, and ticks.

Arenaviruses: (See Chapter 33.) Pleomorphic particles contain a segmented single negative-sense RNA genome, are surrounded by an envelope, and measure 50–300 nm. They contain granules believed to be ribosomes. Several hemorrhagic fever viruses that are antigenically related fall into this group. Most have a rodent host in their natural cycle (see below).

Rhabdoviruses: (See p 366.) Several bullet-shaped arboviruses fall into this group (Fig 33–37).

HUMAN ARBOVIRAL INFECTIONS

Almost 100 arboviruses can infect humans, but not all cause overt disease. Those infecting humans are all believed to be zoonotic, with humans the accidental hosts who play no important role in the maintenance or transmission cycle of the virus. Exceptions are urban yellow fever and dengue. Some of the natural cycles are simple and involve a nonhuman vertebrate host (mammal or bird) with a species of mosquito or tick (cg, jungle yellow fever, Colorado tick fever). Others, however, are quite complex. For example, many cases of Central European diphasic meningoencephalitis occur following ingestion of raw milk from goats and cows infected by grazing in tick-infested pastures where a tick-rodent cycle is occurring.

Diseases produced by the arboviruses may be divided into 3 clinical syndromes: (1) fevers of an undifferentiated type with or without a maculopapular rash and usually benign; (2) encephalitis, often with a high case fatality rate; and (3) hemorrhagic fevers, also frequently severe and fatal. These categories are somewhat arbitrary, and some arboviruses may be associated with more than one syndrome, eg, dengue.

The intensity of viral multiplication and its predominant site of localization in tissues determine the clinical syndrome. Thus, individual arboviruses can produce a minor febrile illness in some patients and encephalitis or a hemorrhagic diathesis in others. However, in an epidemic situation, one of the syndromes usually predominates, permitting a tentative diagnosis. A final diagnosis is based on further epidemiologic and serologic data.

After infection with an arbovirus, there is an incubation period during which viral multiplication takes place. This is followed by the abrupt onset of clinical manifestations that are closely related to viral dissemination. Malaise, headache, nausea, vomiting, and myalgia accompany fever, which is an invariable symptom and sometimes the only one. The illness may terminate at this stage, recur with or without a rash, or reveal hemorrhagic manifestations secondary to vascular abnormalities. Frequently, the period of viremia is asymptomatic, with the acute onset of encephalitis following localization of the virus in the central nervous system.

The above clinical categories are utilized in the following sections in discussing some of the most important diseases caused by the arboviruses.

Encephalitis can be produced by many different viruses. Arbovirus encephalitis occurs in distinct geographic distributions and vector patterns (Table 36–2). Each continent tends to have its own arbovirus pattern, and names are usually suggestive, eg, Venezuelan equine encephalitis (VEE), Japanese B encephalitis (JBE), Murray Valley (Australia) encephalitis (MVE). All of the preceding are alpha- and flavivirus infections spread by mosquitoes with a distinct ecologic distribution. California encephalitis is caused by bunyaviruses, as discussed below. However, on a given continent there may be a shifting distribution depending on virus hosts and vectors in a given year.

Encephalitis or meningoencephalitis can also occur with viruses that involve tissues other than the central nervous system—measles, mumps, hepatitis, chickenpox, zoster, herpes simplex, and others. Some of these viruses replicate actively in the central nervous system, producing inflammation. At other times, the viral infection sets off an immunologic reaction that results in "postinfectious" encephalomyelitis, with a prominent demyelinating component.

In some parts of the world, epidemics of arbovirus infection have involved thousands of individuals with symptomatic infection; many more were asymptomatically infected. In 1975 in the USA, 4308 cases of encephalitis were reported, with 340 deaths. Cases occurred in almost every state. Of the entire number, 42% were due to St. Louis encephalitis, 7% to other arboviruses, 4% to mumps, 3% to enteroviruses, 2% to herpesviruses, and 40% could not be identified by laboratory means. In 1984 in the USA, arboviral infections of the central nervous system occurred in over 100 persons. Thirty-three cases were caused by St. Louis encephalitis virus, 26 of them in California. Seventy-six cases were caused by California (La Crosse) encephalitis virus, 5 by eastern equine encephalitis virus, and 2 by western equine encephalitis virus.

TOGAVIRUS & FLAVIVIRUS ENCEPHALITIS (WEE, EEE, SLE)

Characteristics of the Viruses

A. Properties: The viruses are unstable at room

Table 36–2. Summary of 6 major human arbovirus infections that occur in the USA.

Diseases	Exposure	Distribution	Vectors	Infection: Case Ratio (Age Incidence)	Sequelae	Mortality Rate (%)
WEE	Rural	Pacific, Mountain, West Central, Southwest	*Culex tarsalis*	50:1 (under 5) 1000:1 (over 15)	+	3–7
EEE	Rural	Atlantic, southern coastal	*Aedes sollicitans* *Aedes vexans*	10:1 (infants) 50:1 (middle aged) 20:1 (elderly)	+	50–70
SLE	Urban-rural	Widespread	*Culex pipiens* *Culex quinquefasciatus* *Culex tarsalis* *Culex nigrapalpus*	800:1 (under 9) 400:1 (9–59) 85:1 (over 60)	±	5–10 (under 65) 30 (over 65)
VEE	Rural	South and Central America, southern USA	*Aedes* *Psorophora* *Culex*	25:1 (under 15) 1000:1 (over 15)	±	20–30 (children) < 10 (adults)
California encephalitis (La Crosse)	Rural	North Central, Atlantic, South	(*Aedes* sp?)	Unknown ratio (most cases under 20)	Rare	Fatalities rare
Colorado tick fever	Rural	Pacific, Mountain	*Dermacentor andersoni*	Unknown ratio (all ages affected)	Rare	Fatalities rare

temperature but stable at −70 °C. The viral envelope contains lipid, and thus the infectivity is rapidly inactivated by ether or by 1:1000 sodium deoxycholate. This property separates them easily from enteroviruses, which may have a similar seasonal occurrence.

The viruses infect many cell lines, embryonated eggs, mice, birds, bats, mules, horses, and other animals. In susceptible vertebrate hosts, primary virus multiplication occurs either in myeloid and lymphoid cells or in vascular endothelium. Multiplication in the central nervous system depends on the ability of the virus to pass the blood-brain barrier and to infect nerve cells. In natural infection of birds and mammals (and in experimental parenteral injection of the virus into animals), an inapparent infection develops in a majority. However, for several days there is viremia, and arthropod vectors acquire the virus by sucking blood during this period—the first step in its dissemination to other hosts. The above characteristics apply to the main flavi- and alphavirus infections in the western hemisphere, particularly St. Louis encephalitis (SLE), western equine encephalitis (WEE), eastern equine encephalitis (EEE), and Venezuelan equine encephalitis (VEE) (Table 36–2). They also apply to Japanese B encephalitis (JBE), which occurs in the Far East.

B. Replication: The togaviruses, alphavirus subgroup, have an RNA-associated nonglycosylated capsid protein and at least 2 envelope glycoproteins. The viruses replicate in the cytoplasm and mature by the budding of nucleocapsids through the plasma membrane. The genome serves as a positive-sense mRNA, producing 42–50S and 26S mRNAs during transcription. The 42–50S mRNA translates precursor polyproteins, including nonstructural proteins, whereas the 26S mRNA translates structural proteins. The proteins are elaborated by posttranslational cleavage.

The flaviviruses have an RNA-associated, nonglycosylated capsid protein, a small polypeptide, and one envelope glycoprotein. The viruses replicate in the cytoplasm and mature through intracytoplasmic membranes, mostly the endoplasmic reticulum. The genome RNA also is positive-sense and produces a 40–45S mRNA during transcription. A precursor protein has not been identified, and it has been proposed that multiple initiation sites account for the multiple proteins.

C. Measurement of Virus Concentration: Viral multiplication can be measured by cytopathic changes, virus-specific immunofluorescence, or the production of viral hemagglutinin as seen directly in the cell culture by the hemadsorption test. Plaque counts can be done in most cultures. Arboviruses exhibit homotypic and heterotypic interference, as well as susceptibility to interferon.

D. Antigenic Properties: CF antigens and viral hemagglutinins may be prepared from infected brains of newborn mice (because of their low fat content). The hemagglutinins of these viruses are part of the infectious virus particle and can agglutinate goose or newly hatched chick red blood cells. The union between hemagglutinin and red cell is irreversible. The erythrocyte-virus complex is still infective, but it can be neutralized by the addition of antibody, which results in large lattice formations.

Some of these viruses have an overlapping antigenicity, most readily demonstrated by cross-reactions in HI tests. The overlapping is due to the presence of one or more cross-reactive antigens in addition to the strain-specific antigen. Thus, immune sera prepared for one strain will contain strain-specific as well as group-specific antibodies.

An immune serum can be made more specific by adsorption with a heterologous virus of the same group. The adsorbed serum tested for HI activity reacts only with the homologous and not with the heterologous strain, facilitating the identification of newly isolated strains.

Pathogenesis & Pathology

The pathogenesis of the disease in humans has not been well studied, but the disease in experimental animals may afford a model for the human disease. The equine encephalitides in horses are diphasic. In the first phase (minor illness), the virus multiplies in nonneural tissue and is present in the blood 3 days before the first signs of involvement of the central nervous system. In the second phase (major illness), the virus multiplies in the brain, cells are injured and destroyed, and encephalitis becomes clinically apparent. The 2 phases may overlap. It is not known whether in humans there is a period of primary viral multiplication in the viscera with a secondary liberation of virus into the blood before its entry into the central nervous system. The viruses multiply in nonneural tissues of experimentally infected monkeys.

High concentrations of virus in brain tissue are necessary before the clinical disease becomes manifest. In mice, the level to which the virus multiplies in the brain is partly influenced by a genetic factor that behaves as a mendelian trait.

The primary encephalitides are characterized by lesions in all parts of the central nervous system, including the basal structures of the brain, the cerebral cortex, and the spinal cord. Small hemorrhages with perivascular cuffing and meningeal infiltration—chiefly with mononuclear cells—are common. Nerve cell degeneration associated with neuronophagia occurs. Purkinje's cells of the cerebellum may be destroyed. There are also patches of encephalomalacia; acellular plaques of spongy appearance in which medullary fibers, dendrites, and axons are destroyed; and focal microglial proliferation. Thus, not only the neurons but also the cells of the supporting structure of the central nervous system are attacked.

Widespread neuronal degeneration occurs with all arboviruses producing encephalitis, but some localization occurs.

Clinical Findings

Incubation periods of the encephalitides are between 4 and 21 days. There is a sudden onset with severe headache, chills and fever, nausea and vomiting, generalized pains, and malaise. Within 24–48 hours, marked drowsiness develops and the patient may become stuporous. Nuchal rigidity is common. Mental confusion, dysarthria, tremors, convulsions, and coma develop in severe cases. Fever lasts 4–10 days. The mortality rate in encephalitides varies (Table 36–2). With JBE, the mortality rate in older age groups may be as high as 80%. Sequelae may include mental deterioration, personality changes, paralysis, aphasia, and cerebellar signs.

Abortive infections simulate aseptic meningitis or nonparalytic poliomyelitis. Inapparent infections are common.

In California, where both WEE and SLE are prevalent, WEE has a predilection for children and infants. In the same area, SLE rarely occurs in infants, even though both viruses are transmitted by the same arthropod vector (*Culex tarsalis*).

Laboratory Diagnosis

A. Recovery of Virus: The virus occurs in the blood only early in the infection, usually before the onset of symptoms. The virus is most often recovered from the brains of fatal cases by intracerebral inoculation of newborn mice, and then it should be identified by serologic tests with known antisera.

B. Serology: Nt and HI antibodies are detectable within a few days after the onset of illness. CF antibodies appear later. The Nt and the HI antibodies endure for many years. The CF antibody may be lost within 2–5 years.

The HI test with newly hatched chick erythrocytes is the simplest diagnostic test, but it primarily identifies the group rather than the specific causative virus.

It is necessary to establish a rise in specific antibodies during infection in order to make the diagnosis. The first sample of serum should be taken as soon after the onset as possible and the second sample 2–3 weeks later. The paired specimens must be run in the same serologic test.

The cross-reactivity that takes place within the alphavirus or flavivirus group must be considered in making the diagnosis. Thus, following a single infection by one member of the group, antibodies to other members may also appear. These group-specific antibodies are usually of lower titer than the type-specific antibody. Serologic diagnosis becomes difficult when an epidemic caused by one member of the serologic group occurs in an area where another group member is endemic, or when an infected individual has been infected previously by a closely related virus. Under these circumstances, a definite etiologic diagnosis may not be possible. Nt, CF, and HI antibodies have a decreasing degree of specificity for the causative viral type (in the order listed).

Immunity

Immunity is believed to be permanent after a single infection. In endemic areas, the population may build up immunity as a result of inapparent infections; the proportion of persons with antibodies to the local arthropod-borne virus increases with age.

Effective killed vaccines have been developed to protect horses against EEE and WEE. No effective vaccines for these diseases are at present available for humans.

An excellent attenuated vaccine for VEE is available for curtailing epidemics among horses and has been used experimentally in humans. A vaccine for JBE is under study.

Because of antigens common to several members within a group, the response to immunization or to infection with one of the viruses of a group may be modified by prior exposure to another member of the same group. In general, the homologous response is greater than a cross-reacting one. This mechanism may be important in conferring protection on a community against an epidemic of another related agent (eg, no Japanese B encephalitis in areas endemic for West Nile fever).

Treatment

There is no specific treatment. In experimental animals, hyperimmune serum is ineffective if given after the onset of disease. However, if given 1–2 days after the introduction of the virus but before the signs of encephalitis are obvious, specific hyperimmune serum can prevent a fatal outcome of the infection.

Epidemiology

In severe epidemics caused by the encephalitis viruses, the case rate is about 1:1000. St. Louis encephalitis is the most important arthropod-borne viral disease of humans in the USA, having caused about 10,000 cases and 1000 deaths since it was first recognized in 1933. In the large urban epidemic of St. Louis encephalitis that occurred in 1966 in Dallas (population 1 million), there were 545 reported cases and 145 (27%) laboratory-confirmed cases, with a case-fatality rate of 10%. All deaths were in persons age 45 years or older. SLE continues to appear each year in the USA, the largest epidemic (1815 cases) being recorded in 1975.

The epidemiology of the arthropod-borne encephalitides must account for the maintenance and dissemination of the viruses in nature in the absence of humans. Most infections with the arboviruses occur in mammals or birds, with humans serving as accidental hosts. The virus is transmitted from animal to animal through the bite of an arthropod vector. Viruses have been isolated from mosquitoes and ticks, which serve as reservoirs of infection. In ticks, the viruses may pass from generation to generation by the transovarian route, and in such instances the tick acts as a true reservoir of the virus as well as its vector. In tropical climates, where mosquito populations are present throughout the year, arboviruses cycle continuously between mosquitoes and reservoir animals.

It is not known whether in temperate climates the virus is reintroduced each year from the outside (eg, by birds migrating from tropical areas) or whether it somehow survives the winter in the local area. The overwintering mechanism is not known. Three possible mechanisms are (1) that hibernating mosquitoes at the time of their emergence could reinfect birds and thus reestablish a simple bird-mosquito-bird cycle; (2) that the virus could remain latent in winter within birds, mammals, or arthropods; and (3) that cold-blooded vertebrates (snakes, turtles, lizards, alliga-

tors, frogs) may also act as winter reservoirs—eg, garter snakes experimentally infected with WEE virus can hibernate over the winter and circulate virus in high titers and for long periods the following spring. Normal mosquitoes can be infected by feeding on the emerged snakes and then can transmit the virus. Virus has been found in the blood of wild snakes.

A. Serologic Epidemiology: In highly endemic areas, almost the entire human population may become infected, and most infections are asymptomatic. This is true for Japanese B encephalitis infection in Japan. High infection-to-case ratios exist among specified age groups for many arbovirus infections (Table 36–2).

In the 1964 Houston SLE epidemic (712 reported cases), there was an inapparent infection rate of 8% in a random city survey, but in the epidemic area of the city the inapparent infection rate was 34%. The infection-to-case ratio remained about the same, however. It is obvious that the presence of infected mosquitoes is required before human infections can occur, although socioeconomic and cultural factors (air conditioning, screens, mosquito control) affect the degree of exposure of the population to these virus-carrying vectors.

In endemic areas of California, 11% of infants are born with maternal antibody to WEE and 27% have SLE maternal antibody. A direct relationship exists between the length of residence of the mother in the endemic area and the acquisition of antibody.

B. Mosquito-Borne Encephalitis: Infection of humans occurs when a mosquito like *Culex tarsalis, Culex quinquefasciatus, Culex pipiens,* or *Culex tritaeniorhynchus* (Japan) or another arthropod bites first an infected animal and later a human being.

The equine encephalitides, EEE, WEE, and VEE, are transmitted by culicine mosquitoes to horses or humans from a mosquito-bird-mosquito cycle. Equines, like humans, are unessential hosts for the maintenance of the virus. An epizootic of encephalitis in horses should alert physicians to the possibility that an arbovirus epidemic in humans may be developing. EEE and VEE in horses are severe, with up to 90% of the affected animals dying. Epizootic WEE is less frequently fatal for horses. In addition, EEE produces severe epizootics in certain domestic game birds. A mosquito-bird-mosquito cycle also occurs in SLE and JBE. Swine are an important host of JBE. Mosquitoes remain infected for life (several weeks to months). Only the female feeds on blood and can feed and transmit the virus more than once. The cells of the mosquito's mid gut are the site of primary virus multiplication. This is followed by viremia and invasion of organs—chiefly salivary glands and nerve tissue, where secondary virus multiplication occurs. The arthropod remains healthy.

Infection of insectivorous bats with arboviruses produces a viremia lasting 6–12 days without any illness or pathologic changes in the bat. While the virus concentration is high, the infected bat may infect mosquitoes that are then able to transmit the infection to wild birds and domestic fowl as well as to other bats.

In nature, mosquitoes are closely associated with bats, both in summer and during the winter (in hibernation sites). Experimentally, mosquitoes have been shown to transmit virus to bats. Bats thus infected could maintain a latent virus infection, with no detectable viremia, for over 3 months at 10 °C. When bats were returned to room temperature, viremia appeared after 3 days. The mosquito-bat-mosquito cycle may be a possible overwintering mechanism for some arboviruses.

C. Tick-Borne Encephalitis Complex:

1. Russian spring-summer encephalitis–This disease occurs chiefly in the early summer, particularly in humans exposed to the ticks *Ixodes persulcatus* and *Ixodes ricinus* in the uncleared forest. Ticks can become infected at any stage in their metamorphosis, and virus can be transmitted transovarially. The virus persists through the winter in hibernating ticks or in vertebrates such as hedgehogs or bats. Virus is secreted in the milk of infected goats for long periods, and infection may be transmitted to those who drink unpasteurized milk. Characteristics of the disease are involvement of the bulbar area or the cervical cord and the development of ascending paralysis or hemiparesis. The mortality rate is about 30%.

2. Louping ill–This disease of sheep in Scotland and northern England is spread by the tick *Ixodes ricinus*. Humans are occasionally infected.

3. Tick-borne encephalitis (Central European or diphasic meningoencephalitis)–This virus is antigenically related to Russian spring-summer encephalitis virus and louping ill virus. Typical cases have a diphasic course, the first phase being influenzalike and the second a meningoencephalitis with or without paralysis.

4. Kyasanur Forest disease–This is an Indian hemorrhagic disease caused by a virus of the Russian spring-summer encephalitis complex. In addition to humans, langur *(Presbytis entellus)* and bonnet *(Macaca radiata)* monkeys are naturally infected in southern India.

5. Powassan encephalitis–This tick-borne virus is the first member of the Russian spring-summer complex isolated in North America. Human infection is rare. Since 1959, when the original fatal case was reported from Canada, several additional cases have been confirmed in the northeastern portion of the USA.

Control

Biologic control of the natural vertebrate host is generally impractical, especially when the hosts are wild birds. The most effective method is arthropod control. Since the period of viremia in the vertebrate is of short duration (3–6 days for SLE infections of birds), any suppression of the vector for this period should break the transmission cycle. During the 1966 SLE epidemic in Dallas, low-volume, high-concentration malathion mist was sprayed aerially over most of Dallas County. A striking decrease in the number and infectivity rate of the mosquito vectors occurred, demonstrating the effectiveness of the treatment.

Killed virus vaccines have not met with success. Live attenuated encephalitis vaccines continue to be investigated. A live vaccine was successfully used to halt the severe epidemic of VEE in horses in Texas in 1971.

VENEZUELAN EQUINE ENCEPHALITIS

Venezuelan equine encephalitis (VEE) is a mosquito-borne viral disease that primarily produces an undifferentiated febrile illness in humans and encephalitis in equine animals. It is caused by a togavirus, subgroup alphavirus. There is a partial cross-immunity between VEE and EEE.

Clinical Findings

Over 50% of equines infected develop central nervous system symptoms after an incubation period of 24–72 hours, while the remainder have an undifferentiated febrile illness. Symptoms include high fever, depression, diarrhea, anorexia, and weight loss. In nonfatal cases, the fever subsides and convalescence is protracted. In fatal cases, fever persists, weakness ensues, and the horse loses balance and dies within 2–4 days.

The disease in humans is influenzalike in about 97% of patients who develop symptoms and consists of high fever, headache, and severe myalgia. Convalescence is often prolonged. Encephalitis occurs in about 3%. A mortality rate of 0.5% has been reported, usually in younger patients who develop neurologic signs. Leukopenia is common in both equines and humans.

Laboratory Diagnosis

The virus may be isolated from whole blood, serum, nasopharyngeal washings, many organs, and occasionally the cerebrospinal fluid during the acute phase of the illness. Isolations are made by intracerebral inoculation of suckling mice or in cell cultures. The antibody response is similar to that found in other arbovirus diseases. Nt and HI antibodies appear 2–3 weeks after onset but fall within 2–5 years. Serologic tests, listed in order of specificity, include Nt, CF, and HI. Cross-reactions with other alphaviruses are extensive using the HI test, although homologous titers are higher than the heterologous antibodies.

Epidemiology

The natural cycle for VEE involves mammals and mosquitoes. Birds and bats are susceptible. Humans are tangentially involved.

First reported in Venezuela in 1936, the disease gradually appeared in Panama and Mexico. In 1971, a severe epidemic occurred along the Texas-Mexico border, with the death of several thousand horses and the occurrence of several hundred human cases. Two human cases of VEE were reported in California in 1972. In Florida, VEE is enzootic in rodents. Serologic evidence indicates that much subclinical human infection with this agent occurs in Florida, but clinical central nervous system disease is rare.

Control

Because of the presence of virulent VEE in Mexican border states, immunization of all equines (including revaccination of previously vaccinated equines) with a live attenuated vaccine and local and aerial spraying of mosquitoes were begun on a routine basis in 1972. So far, these measures have proved effective in limiting the spread of the disease. Strict quarantine to prevent movement of equines into areas free of the disease is also necessary. The attenuated VEE vaccine has been used experimentally in humans but is not available for general use.

BUNYAVIRUS ENCEPHALITIS (California Encephalitis, La Crosse Encephalitis)

The California encephalitis virus complex comprises 14 antigenically related bunyaviruses, including La Crosse virus.

Clinical Findings & Diagnosis

The onset of California encephalitis virus infection is abrupt, typically with a severe bifrontal headache, a fever of 38–40 °C, sometimes vomiting, lethargy, and convulsions. Less frequently, there is only aseptic meningitis.

Histopathologic changes include neuronal degeneration and patchy inflammation, with perivascular cuffing and edema in the cerebral cortex and meninges.

The prognosis is excellent, although convalescence may be prolonged. Fatalities and neurologic sequelae are rare.

Serologic confirmation by HI, CF, or Nt tests is done on acute and convalescent specimens.

Epidemiology

These viruses were originally found in California, but they occur mainly in the Mississippi and Ohio river valleys, with scattered cases elsewhere. From 30 to 160 cases occur annually between July and September in the USA, particularly in the young (ages 4–14 years).

These viruses are probably transmitted between various woodland mosquitoes and small mammals such as squirrels and rabbits. Human infection is tangential. The mechanism by which the virus is maintained during the winter months is not known. However, overwintering in diapause eggs of the mosquito vector has been demonstrated. The virus is transmitted transovarially, and adults that develop from infected eggs can transmit the virus by bite.

OROPOUCHE FEVER

Oropouche (Oro) virus is a member of the Simbu serologic group of the bunyaviruses. It is a major cause of human febrile illness in Brazil. Outbreaks are frequent in urban centers in the eastern Amazon region. At least 220,000 persons were involved in 1978–1981, when the greatest wave yet recorded affected 19 localities. Outside of the Amazon region, human infection caused by Oro virus has been documented as yet only in Trinidad.

Three types of clinical syndromes have been associated with Oro virus infection: febrile illness, febrile illness with rash, and meningitis or meningismus. Many patients become severely ill, some to the point of prostration. The disease may be confused with malaria or other febrile conditions. The incubation period varies from 4 to 8 days. Fever, chills, severe headache, myalgias, arthralgia, dizziness, and photophobia are the most common clinical manifestations. Virtually all patients are viremic during the first 2 days of illness, but only 23% are still viremic on the fifth day.

Most of those infected develop clinical disease. In outbreaks in large cities, the distribution of virus is markedly uneven, whereas in small villages the agent is spread throughout. This pattern correlates with the distribution of the insect *Culicoides paraensis,* which is the main vector of Oro virus.

All outbreaks have occurred during the rainy season, and in several localities their decline has coincided with the end of this period. In some places, virus activity has been detected for a period of 6 months.

Oro virus probably occurs in nature in 2 distinct cycles: a jungle cycle (with the vector still unknown), which is responsible for maintaining the virus in nature, where primates, sloths, and possibly certain species of wild birds are implicated as vertebrate hosts; and an urban cycle, during which humans may be infected and, once infected, probably serve as an amplifying host of the virus among hematophagous insects.

Two insect species have been implicated as virus vectors in urban settings: the ceratopogonid midge *C paraensis* and the mosquito *Culex quinquefasciatus.* Transmission studies using hamsters have demonstrated that *C paraensis* is the more efficient of the 2 vectors. Furthermore, *C paraensis* can transmit the virus from humans to hamsters, which emphasizes the insect's role as a vector.

Methods for control of *C paraensis* are needed to prevent or interrupt epidemics, particularly in view of the increasing activity of the virus in urban centers of the eastern Amazon region and the report of an epidemic in 1981 in the western part of the Amazon region, where the large city of Manaus was extensively affected. It is also possible that Oropouche fever may spread to other areas, since *C paraensis* is widely distributed throughout South America, Central America, Mexico, and the eastern USA.

WEST NILE FEVER

West Nile fever is an acute, mild, febrile disease with lymphadenopathy and rash that occurs in the Middle East, tropical or subtropical Africa, and southwest Asia. It is caused by a flavivirus.

Clinical Findings

The virus is introduced through the bite of a *Culex* mosquito and produces viremia and a generalized systemic infection characterized by lymphadenopathy, sometimes with an accompanying maculopapular rash. Transitory meningeal involvement may occur during the acute stage. The virus may produce fatal encephalitis in older people, who have a delayed (and low) antibody response.

Laboratory Diagnosis

Virus can be recovered from blood taken in the acute stage of the infection. On paired serum specimens, CF, HI, and Nt titer rises may be diagnostic. Nt antibodies persist longer than CF antibodies. During convalescence, heterologous CF and Nt antibodies develop to JBE and SLE. The heterologous response is shorter and of lower titer than the homologous response.

Immunity

Only one antigenic type exists, and immunity is presumably permanent. Maternal antibodies are transferred from mother to offspring and disappear during the first 6 months of life.

Epidemiology & Control

Although West Nile fever appeared to be limited to the Middle East, antibodies to the virus have also been found in Africa, India, and Korea. In nonimmune populations, subclinical or clinical infections are common. In Cairo, 70% of persons over age 4 years have antibodies. In 1984, the virus was reported to have been isolated from the brains of 3 children who died of viral encephalitis.

The disease is more common in summer and more prevalent in rural than urban areas. The virus has been isolated from *Culex* mosquitoes during epidemics, and experimentally infected mosquitoes can transmit the virus. Mosquito abatement appears to be a logical, if unproved, control measure.

YELLOW FEVER

Yellow fever (YF) is an acute, febrile, mosquitoborne illness. Severe cases are characterized by jaundice, proteinuria, and hemorrhage. YF is a flavivirus. It multiplies in many different types of animals and in mosquitoes. It grows in embryonated chicks and in cell cultures made from chick embryos.

Strains freshly isolated from humans, monkeys, or mosquitoes are pantropic, ie, the virus invades all 3 embryonal layers. Fresh strains usually produce a severe (often fatal) infection with marked damage to the livers of monkeys after parenteral inoculation. After serial passage in the brains of monkeys or mice, such strains lose much of their viscerotropism; they cause encephalitis after intracerebral injection but only asymptomatic infection after subcutaneous injection. Cross-immunity exists between the pantropic and neurotropic strains of the virus.

During the serial passage of a pantropic strain of YF through tissue cultures, the relatively avirulent 17D strain was recovered. This strain lost its capacity to induce a viscerotropic or neurotropic disease in monkeys and in humans and is now used as a vaccine.

Hemagglutinins and CF antigens of YF virus may be prepared from infected tissues. Each antigen has 2 separable components: one is associated with the infectious particle, and the other is probably a product of the action of YF virus on tissues it infects.

Pathogenesis & Pathology

Our understanding of the pathogenesis of YF is based on work with the experimental infection in monkeys. The virus enters through the skin and then spreads to the local lymph nodes, where it multiplies. From the lymph nodes, it enters the circulating blood and becomes localized in the liver, spleen, kidney, bone marrow, and lymph glands, where it may persist for days.

The lesions of YF are due to the localization and propagation of the virus in a particular organ. Death may result from the necrotic lesions in the liver and kidney. The most frequent site of hemorrhage is the mucosa at the pyloric end of the stomach.

The distribution of necrosis in the liver may be spotty but is most evident in the mid zones of the lobules. The hyaline necrosis may be restricted to the cytoplasm; the hyaline masses are eosinophilic (Councilman bodies). Intranuclear eosinophilic inclusion bodies are also present and are of diagnostic value. During recovery, the parenchymatous cells are replaced, and the liver may be completely restored.

In the kidney, there is fatty degeneration of the tubular epithelium. Degenerative changes also occur in the spleen, lymph nodes, and heart. Intranuclear, acidophilic inclusion bodies may be present in the nerve and glial cells of the brain. Perivascular infiltrations with mononuclear cells also occur in the brain.

Clinical Findings

The incubation period is 3–6 days. At the onset, the patient has fever, chills, headache, and backache, followed by nausea and vomiting. A short period of remission often follows the prodrome. On about the fourth day, the period of intoxication begins with a slow pulse (90–100) relative to a high fever and moderate jaundice. In severe cases, marked proteinuria and hemorrhagic manifestations appear. The vomitus may be black with altered blood. Lymphopenia is present. When the disease progresses to the severe stage (black vomitus and jaundice), the mortality rate is high. On the other hand, the infection may be so mild as to go unrecognized. Regardless of severity, there are no sequelae; patients either die or recover completely.

Laboratory Diagnosis

A. Recovery of Virus: The virus may be recovered from the blood up to the fifth day of the disease by intracerebral inoculation of mice. The isolated virus is identified by neutralization with specific antiserum.

B. Serology: Nt antibodies develop early (by the fifth day) even in severe and fatal cases. In patients who survive the infection, circulating antibodies endure for life.

CF antibodies are rarely found after mild infection or vaccination with the attenuated, live 17D strain. In severe infections, they appear later than the Nt antibodies and disappear more rapidly.

The serologic response in YF may be of 2 types. In **primary infections** of YF, specific HI antibodies appear first, followed rapidly by antibodies to other flaviviruses. The titers of homologous HI antibodies are usually higher than those of heterologous antibodies. CF and Nt antibodies rise slowly and are usually specific.

In **secondary infections** where YF occurs in a patient previously infected with another flavivirus, HI and CF antibodies appear rapidly and to high titers. There is no suggestion of specificity. The highest HI and CF antibodies are usually heterologous. Accurate diagnosis even by Nt test may be impossible.

Histopathologic examination of the liver in fatal cases is useful in those regions where the disease is endemic.

Immunity

Subtle antigenic differences exist between YF strains isolated in different locations and between pantropic and vaccine (17D) strains.

An infant born of an immune mother has antibodies at birth that are gradually lost during the first 6 months of life. Reacquisition of similar antibodies is dependent upon the individual's exposure to the virus under natural conditions or by vaccination.

Epidemiology

Two major epidemiologic cycles of YF are recognized: (1) classic (or urban) epidemic YF and (2) sylvan (or jungle) YF. Urban YF involves person-to-person transmission by domestic *Aedes* mosquitoes. In the western hemisphere and West Africa, this species is primarily *Aedes aegypti,* which breeds in the accumulations of water that accompany human settlement. Mosquitoes remain close to houses and become infected by biting a viremic individual. Urban YF is perpetuated in areas where there is a constant influx of susceptible persons, cases of YF, and *A aegypti.* With the use of intensive measures for mosquito abatement, the incidence of urban YF has been markedly reduced in South America, even though 200–400 cases are recognized annually, mainly in persons occupationally

exposed in forested areas. The disease is probably underreported. In Africa, epidemics involving forest mosquito vectors affect tens of thousands of humans at intervals of a few years, but only a small number of cases are officially reported.

Jungle YF is primarily a disease of monkeys. In South America and Africa, it is transmitted from monkey to monkey by arboreal mosquitoes (ie, *Haemagogus, Aedes*) that inhabit the moist forest canopy. The infection in animals may be severe or inapparent. Persons such as woodcutters, nut-pickers, or road-builders come in contact with these mosquitoes in the forest and become infected. Jungle YF may also occur when an infected monkey visits a human habitation and is bitten by *A aegypti,* which then transmits the virus to a human being.

The virus multiplies in mosquitoes, which remain infectious for life. After the mosquito ingests a virus-containing blood meal, an interval of 12–14 days is required for it to become infectious. This interval is called the **extrinsic incubation period.**

All age groups are susceptible, but the disease in infants is milder than that in older groups. Large numbers of inapparent infections occur. The disease usually is milder in blacks. YF has never been reported in India or the Orient, even though the vector, *A aegypti,* is widely distributed there.

New outbreaks continue to occur. In Bolivia, 145 cases of jungle YF, with a mortality rate over 50%, were reported in 1975. The disease occurred in nonimmune persons coming from distant places for the rice harvests. The rice fields, with the jungle adjacent to them, are located near towns. Most cases were in male agricultural workers. The virus had established itself in this area in reservoirs close to the towns. Jungle YF rarely affects the local population, which has developed immunity by having been in contact with the virus through previous minor infections and also by frequent vaccinations. The real number of cases and deaths from jungle YF in such areas is much higher than the reports indicate, as many patients do not go to the hospital but recover or die without any report being made.

Control

Vigorous mosquito abatement programs have virtually eliminated urban YF. The last reported outbreak of YF in the USA occurred in 1905. However, with the speed of modern air travel, the threat of a YF outbreak exists wherever *A aegypti* is present. Most countries insist upon proper mosquito control on airplanes and vaccination of all persons at least 10 days before arrival in or from an endemic zone. The YF vaccination requirement for travelers entering the USA was eliminated in 1972.

In 1978, a YF outbreak occurred in Trinidad. Eight human cases and a number of infected forest monkeys were detected. The outbreak was quickly stopped by a mass immunization campaign and *A aegypti* control measures.

An excellent attenuated, live vaccine is available in

the 17D strain. Vaccine is prepared in eggs and dispensed as a dried powder. It is a live virus and must be kept cold. It is rehydrated just before use and injected subcutaneously by skin scarification or by jet injector. A single dose produces a good antibody response in more than 95% of vaccinated persons that persists for at least 10 years. After vaccination, the virus multiplies and may be isolated from the blood before antibodies develop.

DENGUE
(Breakbone Fever)

Dengue is a mosquito-borne infection characterized by fever, muscle and joint pain, lymphadenopathy, and rash and is caused by a flavivirus. Dengue and YF are antigenically related, but this does not result in significant cross-immunity.

Pathogenesis & Pathology
Viremia is present at the onset of fever and may persist for 3 days. The histopathologic lesion is in small blood vessels, with endothelial swelling, perivascular edema, and infiltration with mononuclear cells.

Clinical Findings
The onset of fever may be sudden or there may be prodromal symptoms of malaise, chills, and headache. Pains soon develop, especially in the back, joints, muscles, and eyeballs. The temperature returns to normal after 5–6 days or may subside on about the third day and rise again about 5–8 days after onset ("saddle-back" form). A rash (maculopapular or scarlatiniform) may appear on the third or fourth day and last for 24–72 hours, fading with desquamation. Lymph nodes are frequently enlarged. Leukopenia with a relative lymphocytosis is a regular occurrence. Convalescence may take weeks, although complications and death are rare. Especially in young children, dengue may be a mild febrile illness lasting 1–3 days.

A more severe syndrome—dengue hemorrhagic fever—may occur in individuals with passively acquired (as maternal antibody) or endogenously produced heterologous dengue antibody. Although initial symptoms simulate normal dengue, the patient's condition abruptly worsens and is associated with hypoproteinemia, thrombocytopenia, prolonged bleeding time, and elevated prothrombin time. Dengue shock syndrome, characterized by shock and hemoconcentration, may supervene. These altered manifestations of dengue have been observed, often in epidemic form, in the Philippines, Southeast Asia, and India—regions in which several dengue serotypes are regularly present; the mortality rate is 5–10%. In studies of the dengue diseases in Southeast Asia, dengue hemorrhagic fever, with or without shock, has been found to occur more frequently when dengue type 2 is the secondary infecting virus and the patient is a female age 3 years or older. In 1981, over 40 deaths from type 2

dengue occurred in Cuba as a result of hemorrhage and shock. Shock is probably a form of hypersensitivity reaction. It is postulated that virus-antibody complexes are formed within a few days of the second dengue infection which activate the complement system and lead to the disseminated intravascular coagulation seen in the hemorrhagic fever syndrome.

Laboratory Diagnosis
Isolation of the virus is difficult. Injection of early fresh serum into mice rarely produces disease, but the animals may subsequently be immune to challenge. Dengue viruses often grow in cell cultures.

Nt and HI antibodies appear within 7 days of onset of dengue fever and CF antibodies somewhat later. Homotypic antibodies tend to reach higher titers than heterotypic ones.

Immunity
At least 4 antigenic types of the virus exist.

Reinfection with a virus of a different serotype 2–3 months after the primary attack may give rise to a short, mild illness without a rash. Mosquitoes feeding on these reinfected patients can transmit the disease.

Epidemiology
The known geographic distribution of the dengue viruses today is India, the Far East, and the Hawaiian and Caribbean Islands. Dengue has occurred in the southern USA (1934) and in Australia. Most subtropical and tropical regions around the world where *Aedes* vectors exist are endemic or potentially endemic areas. For example, over 500,000 cases of dengue occurred in Colombia in 1972 following reinfestation of the Atlantic coastal areas by *A aegypti*. Over 100,000 cases occurred in 1981 in Cuba.

The infectious cycle is as follows:

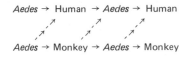

A aegypti is a domestic mosquito; *Aedes albopictus* exists in the bush or jungle and may be responsible for maintaining the infection among monkeys.

In urban communities, dengue epidemics are explosive and involve appreciable portions of the population. They often start during the rainy season, when the vector mosquito, *A aegypti,* is abundant. The mosquito has a short flight range, and urban spread of dengue is frequently house-to-house. The mosquito breeds in tropical or semitropical climates in artificial water-holding receptacles around human habitation or in tree holes or plants close to human dwellings. It apparently prefers the blood of humans to that of other animals. Since *A aegypti* is also the vector of yellow fever, the outbreak of dengue in the Caribbean serves as a warning of even more serious epidemics. Epidemics can be brought under control by aerial spraying with malathion to kill adult mosquitoes and by treatment of breeding sites to kill larvae.

A aegypti is the only known vector mosquito for dengue in the western hemisphere. The female acquires the virus by feeding upon a viremic human. Mosquitoes are infective after a period of 8–14 days (extrinsic incubation time). In humans, clinical disease begins 2–15 days after an infective mosquito bite. Once infective, a mosquito probably remains so for the remainder of her life (1–3 months or more). Dengue virus is not passed from one generation of mosquitoes to the next. In the tropics, mosquito breeding throughout the year maintains the disease.

Epidemics of dengue are usually observed when the virus is newly introduced into an area or if susceptible persons move into an endemic area. The endemic dengue in the Caribbean is a constant threat to the USA, where *A aegypti* mosquitoes are prevalent in the summer months.

In 1977, a dengue type 1 virus was isolated from mosquitoes and from patients in Jamaica, from where it spread to the Bahamas, Trinidad, Cuba, and the USA. This was the first time type 1 virus had been isolated in the western hemisphere.

In 1979, an epidemic of dengue type 4 broke out in Tahiti, the first known appearance of type 4 outside of Southeast Asia. There were 6800 reported cases on the island (population 97,000).

In 1981, dengue type 4 was first recognized in the western hemisphere, with the first cases in the French Antilles (contacts from French Polynesia) and then a spread to other islands, including Puerto Rico, Jamaica, Haiti, Trinidad, and St. Thomas. Dengue type 4 was the dominant virus isolated in Puerto Rico in 1981 and 1982, with over 100 strains being recovered. The virus has also been found on the mainland of Central America (Belize) and South America (Surinam and northern Brazil). As yet, these infections have been self-limited and relatively mild with no evidence of hemorrhagic fever.

Concurrent with the increased epidemic activity of dengue in the tropics, there has been an increase in the number of cases imported into the USA. Many of these cases continue to be imported into states where competent mosquito vectors are found, underscoring the need for effective surveillance, especially during periods of increased dengue activity in the tropics.

Control

Control depends upon antimosquito measures, eg, elimination of breeding places and the use of insecticides. An experimental attenuated virus vaccine has been produced but not tested.

SANDFLY FEVER
(Pappataci Fever, *Phlebotomus* Fever)

Sandfly fever is a mild, insect-borne disease that occurs commonly in countries bordering the Mediterranean Sea and in Russia, Iran, Pakistan, India,

Panama, Brazil, and Trinidad. The sandfly *Phlebotomus papatasii* is present in endemic areas between 20 and 45 degrees of latitude. Sandfly fever is caused by a bunyavirus (see p 418).

Clinical Findings

In humans, the bite of the sandfly results in small itching papules on the skin that persist for up to 5 days. The disease begins abruptly after an incubation period of 3–6 days. For 24 hours before and 24 hours after the onset of fever, the virus is found in the blood. The clinical features consist of headache, malaise, nausea, fever, conjunctival injection, photophobia, stiffness of the neck and back, abdominal pain, and leukopenia. All patients recover. There is no specific treatment. The pathology in humans is not known.

Laboratory Diagnosis

The diagnosis is made usually on clinical grounds. It may be confirmed by demonstrating a rise in antibody titer in paired serum specimens by Nt or HI tests.

Immunity

There are at least 20 separate antigenic types, but only 5 appear to cause human illness. Immunity is specific for each type and persists for at least 2 years.

Epidemiology

The disease is transmitted by the female sandfly, a midge only a few millimeters in size. In the tropics, the sandfly is prevalent all year; in cooler climates, only during the warm seasons. Transovarial transmission may occur.

The extrinsic incubation period in the sandfly is about 1 week. The insect feeds at night; during the day, it may be found in dark places (cracks in walls, caves, houses, and tree trunks). Eggs are laid a few days after a blood meal. About 5 weeks are required for the eggs to develop into winged insects. The adult lives only a few weeks in hot weather.

In endemic areas, infection is common in childhood. When nonimmune adults (eg, troops) arrive, large outbreaks can occur among the new arrivals and are occasionally mistaken for malaria.

Control

Sandflies are commonest just above the ground. Because of their small size, they can pass through ordinary screens and mosquito nets. Their flight range is up to 200 yards. Prevention of disease in endemic areas rests on application of insect repellents during the night and the use of residual insecticides in and around living quarters.

RIFT VALLEY FEVER
(Enzootic Hepatitis)

The agent of this disease, a bunyavirus of the phlebovirus subgroup, is primarily pathogenic for sheep and other domestic animals. Humans are secondarily infected during the course of epizootics in domesticated animals in Africa and the Middle East. Infection among laboratory workers is common.

The clinical features are similar to those of dengue: acute onset, fever, prostration, pain in the extremities and joints, and gastrointestinal distress. The temperature curve is like that of dengue and yellow fever (saddle-back type). There is a marked leukopenia. The disease is short-lived, and recovery almost always is complete.

The virus can be isolated from human blood early in the disease. CF, Nt, and HI antibodies develop and persist for years.

Rift Valley fever was believed to be relatively benign for humans until 1977, when it spread to Egypt. There it caused enormous losses of sheep and cattle, and thousands of human cases occurred, with 600 deaths. Although mosquitoes are known to transmit the virus in epizootics and epidemics, the reservoir of the virus in nature and the means of interepizootic maintenance are not known. Vaccination of livestock with available killed or live attenuated vaccines should prevent transmission to both humans and animals. Movement of animals should be restricted when an epizootic is in progress. Rift Valley fever can be expected to spread from Africa to countries of the Mediterranean basin and southwest Asia.

COLORADO TICK FEVER
(Mountain Fever, Tick Fever)

Colorado tick fever is a mild febrile disease, without rash, that is transmitted by a tick. It is caused by an orbivirus (Table 36–1). During the acute stage, the virus is present in the blood and can be isolated in cell culture or suckling mice. It appears to be antigenically distinct. The pathologic features of the disease in humans are not known, since the disease is self-limited.

Clinical Findings
The incubation period is 4–6 days. The disease has a sudden onset with chilly sensations and myalgia. Symptoms include headache, deep ocular pain, muscle and joint pains, lumbar backache, and nausea and vomiting. The temperature is usually diphasic. After the first bout of 2 days, the patient may feel well. Symptoms and fever then reappear and last 3–4 more days.

Laboratory Diagnosis
The virus may be isolated from whole blood by inoculation of suckling mice. Viremia may persist for 2 weeks. Specific Nt and CF antibodies appear in the second week of illness and persist for years.

Immunity
Only one antigenic type is known. A single infection is believed to produce lasting immunity.

Epidemiology
Colorado tick fever is limited to areas where the

wood tick *Dermacentor andersoni* is distributed, primarily Colorado, Oregon, Utah, Idaho, Montana, and Wyoming. Patients have been in a tick-infested area 4–5 days before onset of symptoms, and in many cases ticks are found attached, as their bite is painless. Cases occur chiefly in adult males, the group with greatest exposure to ticks.

D andersoni collected in nature can carry the virus. This tick is a true reservoir, and the virus is transmitted transovarially by the adult female. Natural infection occurs in rodents, which act as hosts for immature stages of the tick.

Control
The disease can be prevented by avoiding tick-infested areas, and by using protective clothing or repellent chemicals. An experimental live vaccine has been made.

RODENT-BORNE HEMORRHAGIC FEVERS

Rodent- and arthropod-borne hemorrhagic fevers have been reported from Africa, Siberia, Central and Southeast Asia, Europe, and South America. The arboviral hemorrhagic fevers borne by ticks (Russian spring-summer encephalitis complex, Crimean-Congo hemorrhagic fever group) and by mosquitoes (dengue, Chikungunya, yellow fever viruses) are described above. The zoonotic rodent-borne hemorrhagic fevers—Korean (Hantaan virus), South American (Junin and Machupo viruses), and Lassa fevers—are considered in this section. Although the natural reservoir and mode of transmission of Marburg and Ebola viruses (African hemorrhagic fever) are not known, it is strongly suspected that they are harbored by rodents.

Common clinical features of the epidemic hemorrhagic fevers include fever; petechiae or purpura; gastrointestinal, nasal, and uterine bleeding; leukopenia; hypotension; shock; proteinuria; thrombocytopenia; and central nervous system signs, often ending in death.

HEMORRHAGIC FEVER WITH RENAL SYNDROME (HFRS) (Hantaan Virus)

HFRS is an acute viral infection that causes an interstitial nephritis which can lead to acute renal insufficiency and renal failure in the clinically severe forms of the disease that occur in Asia, particularly in Korea. Generalized hemorrhage and shock may occur, with a case-fatality rate of 10%. In a milder clinical form—nephropathia epidemica, which is prevalent in Scandinavia—the interstitial nephritis generally resolves without hemorrhagic complications, and fatalities are rare.

Hantaan virus is classified as a bunyavirus. Virion particles are spherical, with a diameter of about 95 nm, and have an envelope. They contain single-stranded, 3-segmented, negative-sense RNA genomes with a total molecular weight of about 4.5×10^6. Three viral nucleocapsids, each composed of a nucleocapsid protein and a single RNA species, and 2 virus-specified glycoproteins associated with virion membrane components have been identified. Virus replication occurs in the cytoplasm of infected cells, and morphogenesis involves budding, primarily into the Golgi cisternae. The hantavirus subgroup has a specific antigenic reaction and a characteristic RNA oligonucleotide pattern.

Over 2000 cases of HFRS occurred among United Nations troops during the Korean war, but Hantaan virus was isolated only in 1976. The agent was recovered in Korea from *Apodemus agrarius,* a rodent previously shown by epidemiologic investigations to be associated with the transmission of epidemic hemorrhagic fever. In the 1980s, HFRS caused by Hantaan virus has been recognized in different areas of France.

HFRS is not restricted to rural areas where infected field and sylvatic rodents constitute the animal-host reservoir. Urban rats are now known to be persistently infected with Hantaan virus, and infected laboratory rats were proved to be sources of Hantaan outbreaks in scientific institutes in Europe and Asia. Serosurveys indicated that rats in the USA also were infected with a Hantaan-related virus, and this virus has recently been isolated from a domestic rat, *Rattus norvegicus*. Hantaan-related infections have not been detected in laboratory rats raised in the USA, perhaps because large-scale suppliers of laboratory animals employ the cesarean-originated, barrier-sustained system, which reduces the opportunity for vertical and horizontal transmission of rodent pathogens. Laboratories that obtain rodents from sources with unknown standards of animal care and breeding may be subject to the risk of laboratory-acquired HFRS.

Human illness caused by Hantaan virus has not been reported in the USA. However, Hantaan virus-related infections have occurred in persons whose occupations place them in contact with seropositive rats. For example, 6% of longshoremen in Baltimore had neutralizing antibody to Hantaan virus.

AFRICAN HEMORRHAGIC FEVERS
(Marburg & Ebola Viruses)

Marburg and Ebola viruses are members of the filovirus family. They cause acute diseases characterized by high fever, with bleeding into skin (petechiae, purpura) and from the nose, gastrointestinal tract, and genitourinary tract; thrombocytopenia; and marked toxicity, often leading to shock and death. Marburg virus disease was recognized in 1967 among laboratory workers exposed to tissues of African green monkeys *(Cercopithecus aethiops)* imported into Germany and Yugoslavia. Transmission from patients to medical personnel occurred, with high mortality rates.

There have been no cases since then in Europe or America, but antibody surveys have indicated that the virus is present in East Africa and causes infection in monkeys and humans.

Marburg virus has been isolated in guinea pigs and various cell culture systems. The virus particle contains RNA and has a cylindric or filamentous shape by electron microscopy. It superficially resembles a rhabdovirus but has no antigenic relationship with any known virus. Experimentally inoculated monkeys developed a uniformly fatal disease resembling hemorrhagic fever in humans.

Treatment is directed at maintaining renal function and electrolyte balance and combating hemorrhage and shock. Transfusion of convalescent plasma may have some benefit. Extreme care is needed to prevent exposure of medical personnel to blood, saliva, and urine of patients.

In 1976, two severe epidemics of hemorrhagic fever occurred in Sudan and Zaire. The virus responsible, provisionally named Ebola virus after a river in Zaire, resembles Marburg virus morphologically but is antigenically distinct. The outbreaks involved over 500 cases and at least 400 deaths due to clinical hemorrhagic fever. The illness was marked by a sudden onset of severe headache, fever, muscle pains, and prostration, quickly followed by profuse diarrhea and vomiting. In each outbreak, hospital staff became infected through close and prolonged contact with patients, their blood, or their excreta. In one hospital, 41 of 76 infected staff members died.

It is probable that Marburg and Ebola viruses have a reservoir host, perhaps a rodent, and become transmitted to humans only accidentally. Human infection, however, is highly communicable to human contacts. By means of rapid travel, such diseases may spread to distant nonendemic areas and present a risk.

Because the natural reservoirs of Marburg and Ebola viruses are still unknown, no control activities can be organized. Hospital spread has been a marked feature of both diseases, and management of patients therefore requires special attention. Patients should be nursed in medical units in the locality where the cases occur. A team trained in the techniques of barrier nursing and management of infectious patients should be available.

LASSA FEVER

The first recognized cases of this disease occurred in 1969 among Americans stationed in the Nigerian village of Lassa. Lassa virus is extremely virulent: the mortality rate was 36–67% in 4 epidemics in West Africa involving about 100 cases. Transmission can occur by human-to-human contact, presenting a hazard to hospital personnel. Nine of 20 medical workers have died from infections. Lassa fever can involve almost all the organ systems, although symptoms may vary in the individual patient. The disease is characterized by very high fever, mouth ulcers, severe muscle aches, skin rash with hemorrhages, pneumonia, and heart and kidney damage. Benign, febrile cases occur. The virus can be isolated from the patient's blood in Vero monkey cell cultures.

Lassa virus is an arenavirus (see pp 365 and 419). Four arenaviruses cause human disease—Lassa, lymphocytic choriomeningitis, Junin, and Machupo. They can be distinguished by immunofluorescent antibody tests.

Lassa virus seems to be transmitted by human contact and also to have a nonhuman cycle. A house rat *(Mastomys natalensis)* is the principal rodent reservoir of Lassa virus. When the virus spreads within a hospital, human contact is the mode of transmission.

Lassa virus is active in all western African countries situated between Senegal and Zaire. In Sierra Leone, Lassa fever accounts for 10% of all febrile patients admitted to hospitals and for almost 2% of the general mortality rate.

The only available therapy for Lassa fever has employed hyperimmune serum from recovered patients. Interferon is being considered now. Rodent control may limit the natural cycle of the virus.

SOUTH AMERICAN HEMORRHAGIC FEVERS (Junin & Machupo Viruses)

Junin hemorrhagic fever (JHF) is a major public health problem in certain agricultural areas of Argentina; over 18,000 cases were reported between 1958 and 1980, with a mortality rate of 10–15% in untreated patients. A gradual increase in the endemic area of JHF has been observed since 1958. The disease has a marked seasonal variation, and the infection occurs almost exclusively among workers in maize and wheat fields who are exposed to the reservoir rodent, *Calomys musculinus*.

Junin virus produces both humoral and cell-mediated immunodepression; deaths due to JHF may be related to an inability to initiate a cell-mediated immune response. The administration of convalescent human plasma to patients during the first week of illness reduced the mortality rate from 15% to 1%. Were it not for the humoral immunodepression regularly induced by Junin virus and the related Machupo virus (see below), the infection in humans would be no more than a brief, nonspecific illness.

The first outbreak of Machupo hemorrhagic fever (MHF) was identified in Bolivia in 1962, and several others subsequently were detected. It is estimated that 2000–3000 persons were affected by the disease, with a case-fatality rate of 20%. A small nosocomial outbreak involving 6 persons, 5 of whom died, was reported in 1971.

An effective rodent control program directed against infected *Calomys callosus*, the host of Machupo virus, was undertaken in Bolivia, and as a result no human cases of MHF have been recorded since 1974.

REFERENCES

Calisher CH et al: Arbovirus subtyping: Applications to epidemiologic studies, availability of reagents, and testing services. *Am J Epidemiol* 1981;**114**:619.

Edelman R et al: Evaluation in humans of a new, inactivated vaccine for Venezuelan equine encephalitis virus (C-84). *J Infect Dis* 1979;**140**:708.

George S et al: Isolation of West Nile virus from the brains of children who had died of encephalitis. *Bull WHO* 1984; **62**:879.

Grimstad PR et al: Serologic evidence for widespread infection with La Crosse and St. Louis encephalitis viruses in the Indiana human population. *Am J Epidemiol* 1984;**119**:913.

Halstead SB: Viral hemorrhagic fevers. *J Infect Dis* 1981; **143**:127.

Huang CH, Liang HC, Jia FL: Beneficial role of a nonpathogenic orbi-like virus: Studies on the interfering effect of M14 virus in mice and mosquitoes infected with Japanese encephalitis virus. *Intervirology* 1985;**24**:147.

Johnson KM, Elliott LH, Heymann DL: Preparation of polyvalent viral immunofluorescent intracellular antigens and use in human serosurveys. *J Clin Microbiol* 1981;**14**:527.

Luby JP: St. Louis encephalitis. *Epidemiol Rev* 1979;**1**:55.

McCormick JB et al: Lassa fever: Effective therapy with ribavirin. *N Engl J Med* 1986;**314**:20.

Monath TP et al: Immunoglobulin M antibody capture enzyme-linked immunosorbent assay for diagnosis of St. Louis encephalitis. *J Clin Microbiol* 1984;**20**:784.

Reeves WC: Overwintering of arboviruses. *Prog Med Virol* 1974;**17**:193.

Rice CM et al: Nucleotide sequence of yellow fever virus: Implications for flavivirus gene expression and evolution. *Science* 1985;**229**:726.

Sangkawibha N et al: Risk factors in dengue shock syndrome: A prospective epidemiologic study in Rayong, Thailand. 1. The 1980 outbreak. *Am J Epidemiol* 1984;**120**:653.

Schmaljohn CS et al: Antigenic and genetic properties of viruses linked to hemorrhagic fever with renal syndrome. *Science* 1985;**227**:1041.

Shope RE, Peters CJ, Davies FG: The spread of Rift Valley fever and approaches to its control. *Bull WHO* 1982;**60**:299.

Theiler M, Downs WG: *The Arthropod-Borne Viruses of Vertebrates: An Account of the Rockefeller Foundation Virus Program, 1951–1970.* Yale Univ Press, 1973.

Tsai TF et al: Serological and virological evidence of a Hantaan virus-related enzootic in the United States. *J Infect Dis* 1985; **152**:126.

WHO Scientific Group: Arthropod-borne and rodent-borne viral diseases. *WHO Tech Rep Ser* 1985;**No. 719.**

Work TH: Arbovirus diseases of North America. Pages 1065–1082 in: *Textbook of Pediatric Infectious Diseases.* Feigin RD, Cherry JD (editors). Saunders, 1981.

Picornavirus Family (Enterovirus & Rhinovirus Groups)

Picornaviruses are small (20–30 nm) and nonenveloped and contain a single-stranded RNA genome (MW 2–3×10^6). The structural features of the virions of each genus are similar. The virion is composed of 4 structural proteins (VP1–VP4) plus one or 2 copies of VP0, the uncleaved precursor of VP2 and VP4. VP1 is the predominantly exposed surface protein. VP4 is located internally within the virion, in close association with the viral RNA. The genome of the picornaviruses is a single-stranded messenger molecule that is covalently linked to a small protein. Upon infection of a susceptible cell, the RNA is translated to yield a large polyprotein that is posttranslationally cleaved into the viral specific proteins.

Enterovirus

Enteroviruses exist in many animals, including humans, cattle, pigs, and mice.

Enteroviruses of human origin include the following:

(1) Polioviruses, types 1–3.

(2) Coxsackieviruses of group A, types 1–24.

(3) Coxsackieviruses of group B, types 1–6.

(4) Echoviruses, types 1–34

(5) Enteroviruses, types 68–72. Since 1969, new enterovirus types have been assigned enterovirus type numbers rather than being subclassified as coxsackieviruses or echoviruses. The vernacular names of the previously identified enteroviruses have been retained.

Enteroviruses are transient inhabitants of the human alimentary tract and may be isolated from the throat or lower intestine. Rhinoviruses, on the other hand, are isolated chiefly from the nose and throat. Among the enteroviruses that are cytopathogenic (polioviruses, echoviruses, and some coxsackieviruses), growth can be readily obtained at 36–37°C in primary cultures of human and monkey kidney cells and certain cell lines (such as HeLa); in contrast, most rhinovirus strains can only be recovered in cells of human origin (embryonic human kidney or lung, human diploid cell strains) at 33 °C.

The enterovirus capsid is thought to be composed of 32 morphologic subunits, possibly in the form of a rhombic triacontahedron rather than a regular icosahedron. Rhinovirus capsid architecture appears to be similar. Infective nucleic acid has been extracted from several enteroviruses and rhinoviruses.

Enteroviruses are stable at acid pH (3.0–5.0) for 1–3 hours, whereas rhinoviruses are acid-labile. Enteroviruses and some rhinoviruses are stabilized by magnesium chloride against thermal inactivation.

Enteroviruses and rhinoviruses differ in buoyant density. Enteroviruses have a buoyant density in cesium chloride of about 1.34 g/mL; human rhinoviruses, about 1.40 g/mL.

Rhinovirus

Human rhinoviruses include more than 100 antigenic types. Rhinoviruses of other host species include those of horses and cattle.

Other Genera

Other picornaviruses are foot-and-mouth disease of cattle *(Aphthovirus)* and encephalomyocarditis of rodents *(Cardiovirus)*.

The host range of the picornaviruses varies greatly from one type to the next and even among strains of the same type. They may readily be induced, by laboratory manipulation, to yield variants that have host ranges and tissue tropisms different from those of certain wild strains; this has led to the development of attenuated poliovirus strains now used as vaccines.

Many picornaviruses cause diseases in humans ranging from severe paralysis to aseptic meningitis, pleurodynia, myocarditis, hepatitis, vesicular and exanthematous skin lesions, mucocutaneous lesions, respiratory and intestinal illnesses, undifferentiated febrile illness, and conjunctivitis. However, subclinical infection is far more common than clinically manifest disease. Different viruses may produce the same syndrome; on the other hand, the same picornavirus may cause more than a single syndrome. Furthermore, some clinical symptoms produced by enteroviruses cannot be distinguished from those caused by some non-enteroviruses. Hence, laboratory tests are required to establish etiology.

ENTEROVIRUS GROUP

POLIOMYELITIS

Poliomyelitis is an acute infectious disease that in its serious form affects the central nervous system.

The destruction of motor neurons in the spinal cord results in flaccid paralysis. However, most poliovirus infections are subclinical.

Properties of the Virus

A. General Properties: Poliovirus particles are typical enteroviruses, 28 nm in diameter. They are inactivated when heated at 55 °C for 30 minutes, but Mg^{2+}, 1 mol/L, prevents this inactivation. Milk or ice cream is also protective, but proper pasteurization inactivates the virus. While purified poliovirus is inactivated by a chlorine concentration of 0.1 ppm, much higher concentrations of chlorine are required to disinfect sewage containing virus in fecal suspensions and in the presence of other organic matter. In contrast to arboviruses, which may be prevalent at the same time of year, polioviruses are not affected by ether or sodium deoxycholate.

B. Animal Susceptibility and Growth of Virus: Polioviruses have a very restricted host range. Most strains will infect monkeys when inoculated directly into the brain or spinal cord. Chimpanzees and cynomolgus monkeys can also be infected by the oral route; in chimpanzees, the infection thus produced is usually asymptomatic. The animals become intestinal carriers of the virus; they also develop a viremia that is quenched by the appearance of antibodies in the circulating blood. Unusual strains have been transmitted to mice or chick embryos.

Most strains can be grown in primary or continuous cell line cultures derived from a variety of human tissues or from monkey kidney, testis, or muscle, but not in cells of lower animals.

Poliovirus requires a primate-specific membrane receptor for infection, and the absence of this receptor on the surface of nonprimate cells makes them virus-resistant. This restriction can be overcome by introducing poliovirus into resistant cells by means of synthetic lipid vesicles called liposomes. Once inside the cell, poliovirus replicates normally.

C. Virus Replication: After attaching to virus receptors (which seem to be controlled in humans by genes on chromosome 19), poliovirus undergoes replication as diagrammed in Fig 33–11. Poliovirus RNA serves both as its own messenger RNA and as the source of the genetic information. Viral protein is synthesized on polysomes held together by viral RNA.

Guanidine in concentrations greater than 1 mmol/L and 2-(α-hydroxybenzyl)-benzimidazole inhibit poliovirus multiplication in tissue culture. Guanidine acts by inhibiting the release of newly made viral RNA from the replicative complex.

D. Antigenic Properties: There are 3 antigenic types. CF antigens for each type may be prepared from tissue culture or infected central nervous system specimens. Inactivation of the virus by formalin, heat, or ultraviolet light liberates a soluble CF antigen. This antigen is cross-reactive and fixes complement with heterotypic poliomyelitis antibodies. A type-specific precipitin reaction occurs when concentrated virus is used with immune animal or convalescent human sera. Two type-specific antigens are contained in poliovirus preparations and can be detected by precipitin and CF tests. They are the N (native) and H (heated) antigens. The N form can be converted to the H form by heating. The N form represents full particles containing RNA; the H form, empty particles.

Pathogenesis & Pathology

The mouth is the portal of entry of the virus, and primary multiplication takes place in the oropharynx or intestine. The virus is regularly present in the throat and in the stools before the onset of illness. One week after onset there is little virus in the throat, but virus continues to be excreted in the stools for several weeks, even though high antibody levels are present in the blood.

The virus may be found in the blood of patients with abortive and nonparalytic poliomyelitis and in orally infected monkeys and chimpanzees in the preparalytic phase of the disease. Antibodies to the virus appear early in the disease, usually before paralysis occurs.

Viremia is also associated with immunization with type 2 oral vaccine. Free virus is usually present in the blood between days 2 and 5 after vaccination, and virus is bound to antibody for an additional few days. Bound virus is detected by acid treatment, which inactivates the antibody and liberates active virus.

These findings have led to the view that the virus first multiplies in the tonsils, the lymph nodes of the neck, Peyer's patches, and the small intestine. The central nervous system may then be invaded by way of the circulating blood. In monkeys infected by the oral route, small amounts of antibody prevent the paralytic disease, whereas large amounts are necessary to prevent passage of the virus along nerve fibers. In humans also, antibody in the form of pooled human gamma globulin (immune globulin USP) may prevent paralysis if given before exposure to the virus.

Poliovirus can spread along axons of peripheral nerves to the central nervous system, and there it continues to progress along the fibers of the lower motor neurons to increasingly involve the spinal cord or the brain. Operations on the oropharynx and tonsillectomy enhance the likelihood of central nervous system involvement during prevalence of polioviruses in the community. This may be attributable to the access of cut nerve fibers to virus in the pharynx or to the removal of immunologically active lymphoid tissue.

Poliovirus invades certain types of nerve cells, and in the process of its intracellular multiplication it may damage or completely destroy these cells. The anterior horn cells of the spinal cord are most prominently involved, but in severe cases the intermediate gray ganglia and even the posterior horn and dorsal root ganglia are often involved. In the brain, the reticular formation, vestibular nuclei, and deep cerebellar nuclei are most often affected. The cortex is virtually spared, with the exception of the motor cortex along the precentral gyrus.

Poliovirus does not multiply in muscle in vivo. The

changes that occur in peripheral nerves and voluntary muscles are secondary to the destruction of nerve cells. Changes occur rapidly in nerve cells, from mild chromatolysis to neuronophagia and complete destruction. Cells that lose their function may recover completely. Inflammation occurs secondary to the attack on the nerve cells; the focal and perivascular infiltrations are chiefly lymphocytes, with some polymorphonuclear cells, and microglia.

In addition to pathologic changes in the nervous system, there may be myocarditis, lymphatic hyperplasia, ulceration of Peyer's patches, prominence of follicles, and enlargement of lymph nodes.

Clinical Findings

When an individual susceptible to infection is exposed to the virus, one of the following responses may occur: (1) inapparent infection without symptoms, (2) mild illness, (3) aseptic meningitis, (4) paralytic poliomyelitis. As the disease progresses, one response may merge with a more severe form, often resulting in a biphasic course: a minor illness, followed first by a few days free of symptoms and then by the major, severe illness. Only about 1% of infections are recognized clinically.

The incubation period is usually 7–14 days, but it may range from 3 to 35 days.

A. Abortive Poliomyelitis: This is the commonest form of the disease. The patient has only the minor illness, characterized by fever, malaise, drowsiness, headache, nausea, vomiting, constipation, and sore throat in various combinations. The patient recovers in a few days. The diagnosis of abortive poliomyelitis can be made only when the virus is isolated or antibody development is measured.

B. Nonparalytic Poliomyelitis (Aseptic Meningitis): In addition to the above symptoms and signs, the patient with the nonparalytic form has stiffness and pain in the back and neck. The disease lasts 2–10 days, and recovery is rapid and complete. In a small percentage of cases, the disease advances to paralysis. Poliovirus is only one of many viruses that produce aseptic meningitis.

C. Paralytic Poliomyelitis: The major illness usually follows the minor illness described above, but it may occur without the antecedent first phase. The predominating complaint is flaccid paralysis resulting from lower motor neuron damage. However, incoordination secondary to brain stem invasion and painful spasms of nonparalyzed muscles may also occur. The amount of damage varies greatly. Muscle involvement is usually maximal within a few days after the paralytic phase begins. The maximal recovery usually occurs within 6 months, with residual paralysis lasting much longer.

Laboratory Diagnosis

A. Cerebrospinal Fluid: The cerebrospinal fluid contains an increased number of leukocytes—usually 10–200/μL, seldom more than 500/μL. In the early stage of the disease, the ratio of polymorphonuclear cells to lymphocytes is high, but within a few days the ratio is reversed. The total cell count slowly subsides to normal levels. The protein content of the cerebrospinal fluid is elevated (average, about 40–50 mg/dL), but high levels may occur and persist for weeks. The glucose content is normal.

B. Recovery of Virus: Cultures of human or monkey cells may be used. The virus may be recovered from throat swabs taken soon after onset of illness and from rectal swabs or feces collected for longer periods. The virus has been found in about 80% of patients during the first 2 weeks of illness but in only 25% during the third 2-week period. No permanent carriers are known. Poliovirus is uncommonly recovered from the cerebrospinal fluid, unlike some coxsackieviruses and echoviruses.

In fatal cases, the virus should be sought in the cervical and lumbar enlargements of the spinal cord, in the medulla, and in the colon contents. Histologic examination of the spinal cord and parts of the brain should be made. If paralysis has lasted 4–5 days, it is difficult to recover the virus from the cord.

Specimens should be kept frozen during transit to the laboratory. After treatment with antibiotics, cell cultures are inoculated, incubated, and observed. Cytopathogenic effects appear in 3–6 days. An isolated virus is identified and typed by neutralization with specific antiserum.

C. Serology: Paired serum specimens are required to show a rise in antibody titer (Table 35–2).

During poliomyelitis infection, complement-fixing H antibodies form before N antibodies (see Antigenic Properties, above). The level of H antibodies declines first. Early acute stage sera thus contain H antibodies only; 1–2 weeks later, both N and H antibodies are present; in late convalescent sera, only N antibodies are present. Only first infection with poliovirus produces strictly type-specific CF responses. Subsequent infections with heterotypic polioviruses recall or induce antibodies, mostly against the heat-stable group antigen shared by all 3 types of poliovirus.

Nt antibodies appear early and are usually already detectable at the time of hospitalization. If the first specimen is taken sufficiently early, a rise in titer can be demonstrated during the course of the disease.

Immunity

Immunity is permanent to the type causing the infection. There may be a low degree of heterotypic resistance induced by infection, especially between type 1 and type 2 polioviruses.

Passive immunity is transferred from mother to offspring. The maternal antibodies gradually disappear during the first 6 months of life. Passively administered antibody lasts only 3–5 weeks.

Virus neutralizing antibody forms soon after exposure to the virus, often before the onset of illness, and apparently persists for life. Its formation early in the disease implies that viral multiplication occurs in the body before the invasion of the nervous system. As the virus in the brain and spinal cord is not influenced by high titers of antibodies in the blood (which are found in the preparalytic stage of the disease), immunization is of value only if it precedes the onset of symptoms referable to the nervous system.

The VP1 surface protein of poliovirus contains several virus neutralizing epitopes, each of which may contain less than 10 amino acids. Each epitope is capable of inducing virus neutralizing antibodies, and the epitopes may serve as the basis for future vaccines.

Treatment

Treatment involves reduction of pain and muscle spasm and maintenance of respiration and hydration. When the fever subsides, early mobilization and active exercise are begun. There is no role for antiserum.

Epidemiology

Poliomyelitis occurs worldwide—year-round in the tropics and during summer and fall in the temperate zones. Winter outbreaks are rare.

The disease occurs in all age groups, but children are usually more susceptible than adults because of the acquired immunity of the adult population. In isolated populations (Arctic Eskimos), poliomyelitis attacks all ages equally. In underdeveloped areas, where conditions favor the wide dissemination of virus, poliomyelitis continues to be a disease of infancy. In developed countries, before the onset of vaccination, the age distribution shifted so that most patients were over age 5 and 25% were over age 15 years. With rising levels of hygiene and sanitation, a similar trend is now occurring in developing countries. Since poliomyelitis in older persons is more likely to be a clinically manifest infection than a subclinical one, the reported incidence of clinical disease is actually rising in areas where vaccination is not widespread, and outbreaks of poliomyelitis are being recorded in some such areas.

The case-fatality rate is variable. It is highest in the oldest patients and may reach 5–10%.

Humans are the only known reservoir of infection. Under conditions of poor hygiene and sanitation in warm areas, where almost all children become immune early in life, polioviruses maintain themselves by continuously infecting a small part of the population. In temperate zones with high levels of hygiene, epidemics have been followed by periods of little spread of virus, until sufficient numbers of susceptible children have grown up to provide a pool for transmission in the area. Warm weather favors the spread of virus by increasing human contacts, the susceptibility of the host, or the dissemination of virus by extrahuman sources. Virus can be recovered from the pharynx and intestine of patients and healthy carriers. The prevalence of infection is highest among household contacts. When the first case is recognized in a family, all susceptibles in the family are already infected, the result of rapid dissemination of virus.

During periods of wide prevalence of poliovirus in an area, flies become contaminated and may distribute virus to food. The role of flies in disease transmission is unsettled. Virus is present in sewage during such periods and can serve as a source of contamination of flies or water used for drinking, bathing, or irrigation.

In temperate climates, infection with enteroviruses, including polio, occurs mainly during the summer. There is a direct correlation between poor hygiene, sanitation, and crowding and the acquisition of infection and antibodies at an early age.

Prevention & Control

Both live and killed virus vaccines are available. Formalinized vaccine (Salk) is prepared from virus grown in monkey kidney cultures. At least 4 inoculations over a period of 1–2 years have been recommended in the primary series. Periodic booster immunizations have been necessary to maintain immunity. Killed vaccine induces humoral antibodies, but, upon exposure, virus is still able to multiply in the gut (Fig 33–22).

Oral vaccines contain live attenuated virus grown in primary monkey or human diploid cell cultures. The vaccine is stabilized by magnesium chloride, 1 mol/L, so that it can be kept without losing potency for a year at 4 °C and for a month at moderate room temperature (about 25 °C). Nonstabilized vaccine must be kept frozen until used.

The live poliovaccine multiplies, infects, and thus immunizes. In the process, infectious progeny of the vaccine virus are disseminated in the community. Although the viruses, particularly type 3 and type 2, mutate in the course of their multiplication in vaccinated children, only extremely rare cases of paralytic poliomyelitis have occurred in recipients of oral poliovaccine or their close contacts. Repeat vaccinations seem to be important to establish permanent immunity. The vaccine produces not only IgM and IgG antibodies in the blood but also secretory IgA antibodies in the intestine, which then becomes resistant to reinfection (Fig 33–22).

A potential limiting factor for oral vaccine is interference. If the alimentary tract of a child is infected with another enterovirus at the time the vaccine is given, the establishment of polio infection and immunity may be blocked. This may be an important problem in areas (particularly in tropical regions) where enterovirus infections are common.

Trivalent oral poliovaccine is used in the USA (see Table 12–6). The American Academy of Pediatrics recommends that primary immunization of infants begin at 2 months of age simultaneously with the first DTP inoculation. The second and third doses should be given at 2-month intervals thereafter, and a fourth dose at $1\frac{1}{2}$ years of age. The multiple doses are recommended to maximize immunity for all 3 serotypes. A trivalent vaccine booster is recommended for all children entering elementary school. No further boosters are presently recommended.

Adults residing in the continental USA have only a small risk of exposure. However, adults who are at increased risk because of contact with a patient or who are anticipating travel to an endemic or epidemic area should be immunized. Pregnancy is neither an indication for nor a contraindication to required immunization.

Before the beginning of vaccination campaigns in the USA, there were about 21,000 cases of paralytic poliomyelitis per year. In 1977, only 18 such cases occurred. Twelve cases of type 1 poliomyelitis occurred in the USA in 1979—all among unvaccinated Amish groups. The disease failed to spread to surrounding vaccinated communities. In 1984, only 4 cases were reported in the USA. There is no longer any endogenous reservoir of wild viruses within the USA. However, there is a continuing need for adequate vaccination programs in all population groups in order to limit the spread of wild viruses when they are introduced from other countries, particularly from Mexico.

Both killed and live virus vaccines induce antibodies and protect the central nervous system from subsequent invasion by wild virus. Low levels of antibody resulting from killed vaccine have little effect on intestinal carriage of virus. The gut develops a far greater degree of resistance after live virus vaccine, which seems to be dependent on the extent of initial vaccine virus multiplication in the alimentary tract rather than on serum antibody level.

Live vaccine should not be administered to immunodeficient or immunosuppressed individuals. Only killed (Salk) vaccine is to be used.

On very rare occasions, a live vaccine strain can induce neurologic or paralytic disease in persons who are not evidently immunodeficient. Such cases are carefully studied by public health agencies, and it is estimated that there has been one vaccine-associated case for every 10 million persons vaccinated.

Immune globulin USP (gamma globulin), 0.3 mL/kg, can provide protection for a few weeks against the paralytic disease but does not prevent subclinical infection. Gamma globulin is effective only if given shortly before infection; it is of no value after clinical symptoms develop.

The prevention of poliomyelitis depends on vaccination. Quarantine of patients or intimate contacts is ineffective in controlling the spread of the disease. This is understandable in view of the large number of inapparent infections that occur.

During epidemic periods (defined now as 2 or more local cases caused by the same type in any 4-week period), children with fever should be placed at bed rest. Undue exercise or fatigue, elective nose and throat operations, and dental extractions should be avoided. Food and human excrement should be protected from flies. Once the poliovirus type responsible for the epidemic is determined, oral poliovaccine should be administered to susceptible persons in the population.

Patients with poliomyelitis can be admitted to general hospitals provided appropriate isolation precautions are employed. All pharyngeal and bowel discharges are considered infectious and should be disposed of quickly and safely.

COXSACKIEVIRUSES

The coxsackieviruses, a large subgroup of the enteroviruses, are divided into 2 groups, A and B, having different pathogenic potentials for mice. They produce a variety of illnesses in human beings. Herpangina; hand, foot, and mouth disease; and acute hemorrhagic conjunctivitis are caused by certain coxsackievirus group A serotypes; and pleurodynia (devil's grip), myocarditis, pericarditis, and meningoencephalitis are caused by some group B coxsackieviruses. In addition to these, a number of group A and B serotypes can give rise to aseptic meningitis, respiratory and undifferentiated febrile illnesses, hepatitis, and paralysis. Generally, paralysis produced by nonpolio enteroviruses is incomplete and reversible. Coxsackie B viruses are the most commonly identified causative agents of viral heart disease in humans.

Properties of the Viruses

A. General Properties: Coxsackieviruses are typical enteroviruses, with a diameter of 28 nm.

B. Animal Susceptibility and Growth of Virus: Coxsackieviruses are highly infective for newborn mice. Certain strains (B1–6, A7, 9, 16, and 24) also grow in monkey kidney cell culture. Some group A strains grow in human amnion and human embryonic lung fibroblast cells. Chimpanzees and cynomolgus monkeys can be infected subclinically; virus appears in the blood and throat for short periods and is excreted in the feces for 2–5 weeks. Type A14 produces poliomyelitislike lesions in adult mice and in monkeys, but in suckling mice this type produces only myositis. Type A7 strains produce paralysis and severe central nervous system lesions in monkeys.

Group A viruses produce widespread myositis in the skeletal muscles of newborn mice, resulting in flaccid paralysis without other observable lesions. Group B viruses may produce focal myositis, encephalitis, and, most typically, necrotizing steatitis involving mainly fetal fat lobules. The genetic makeup of inbred strains determines their susceptibility to coxsackie B viruses. Some B strains also produce pancreatitis, myocarditis, endocarditis, and hepatitis in both suckling and adult mice. Corticosteroids may enhance the susceptibility of older mice to infection of the pancreas. Normal adult mice tolerate infections with group B coxsackieviruses. However, severely malnourished or immunodeficient mice have greatly enhanced susceptibility.

C. Antigenic Properties: At least 29 different immunologic types of coxsackieviruses are now recognized; 23 are listed as group A and 6 as group B types.

Pathogenesis & Pathology

Virus has been recovered from the blood in the early stages of natural infection in humans and of experimental infection in chimpanzees. Virus is also found in the throat for a few days early in the infection and in the stools for up to 5–6 weeks. The distribution of virus is similar to that found with the other enteroviruses.

Group B coxsackieviruses may cause acute fatal encephalomyocarditis in infants. This appears to be a generalized systemic disease with virus replication and lesions in the central nervous system, heart muscle, and other organs.

Clinical Findings

The incubation period of coxsackievirus infection ranges from 2 to 9 days. The clinical manifestations of infection with various coxsackieviruses are diverse and may present as distinct disease entities.

A. Herpangina: This disease is caused by certain group A viruses (2, 4, 5, 6, 8, 10). There is an abrupt onset of fever, sore throat, anorexia, dysphagia, vomiting, or abdominal pain. The pharynx is usually hyperemic, and characteristic discrete vesicles occur on the anterior pillars of the fauces, the palate, uvula, tonsils, or tongue. The illness is self-limited and most frequent in small children.

B. Summer Minor Illnesses: Coxsackieviruses are often isolated from patients with acute febrile illnesses of short duration that occur during the summer or fall and are without distinctive features.

C. Pleurodynia (Epidemic Myalgia, Bornholm Disease): This disease is caused by group B viruses. Fever and chest pain are usually abrupt in onset but are sometimes preceded by malaise, headache, and anorexia. The chest pain may be located on either side or substernally, is intensified by movement, and may last from 2 days to 2 weeks. Abdominal pain occurs in approximately half of cases, and in children this may be the chief complaint. The illness is self-limited, and recovery is complete, although relapses are common.

D. Aseptic Meningitis and Mild Paresis: This syndrome is caused by all types of group B coxsackieviruses and by coxsackieviruses A7, A9, and A24. Fever, malaise, headache, nausea, and abdominal pain are common early symptoms. Signs of meningeal irritation, stiff neck or back, and vomiting may appear 1–2 days later. The disease sometimes progresses to mild muscle weakness suggestive of paralytic poliomyelitis. Patients almost always recover completely from nonpoliovirus paresis. Early in aseptic meningitis, the cerebrospinal fluid shows pleocytosis (up to 500 cells/μL) with up to 50% polymorphonuclear neutrophils.

E. Neonatal Disease: Neonatal disease may be caused by group B coxsackieviruses, with lethargy, feeding difficulty, and vomiting, with or without fever. In severe cases, myocarditis or pericarditis can occur within the first 8 days of life; it may be preceded by a brief episode of diarrhea and anorexia. Cardiac and respiratory embarrassment are indicated by tachycardia, dyspnea, cyanosis, and changes in the ECG. The clinical course may be rapidly fatal, or the patient may recover completely. The disease may sometimes be acquired transplacentally. Myocarditis has also been caused by some group A coxsackieviruses.

F. Colds: A number of the enteroviruses have been associated with common colds; among these are coxsackieviruses A10, A21, A24, and B3.

G. Hand, Foot, and Mouth Disease: This disease has been associated particularly with coxsackievirus A16, but A4, A5, A7, A9, and A10 have also been implicated. Virus may be recovered not only from the stool and pharyngeal secretions but also from vesicular fluid.

The syndrome is characterized by oral and pharyngeal ulcerations and a vesicular rash of the palms and soles that may spread to the arms and legs. Vesicles heal without crusting, which clinically differentiates them from the vesicles of herpes- and poxviruses. The rare deaths are caused by pneumonia.

H. Myocardiopathy: Coxsackievirus B infections are increasingly recognized as a cause of primary myocardial disease in adults as well as children. Coxsackieviruses of group A and echoviruses have been implicated to a lesser degree.

At autopsy, virus has been demonstrated in the myocardium, endocardium, and pericardial fluid by immunofluorescence, peroxidase-labeled antibody, or ferritin-labeled antibody. About 5% of all symptomatic coxsackievirus infections induce heart disease. The virus may affect the endocardium, pericardium, myocardium, or all three. Acute myocardiopathies have been shown to be caused by coxsackieviruses A4, A14, B1–5, and others and also by echovirus types 9 and 22 and others.

Monkeys infected with coxsackievirus B4 develop pancarditis, with a pathologic picture strikingly similar to that of rheumatic heart disease.

In experimental animals, the severity of acute viral myocardiopathy is greatly increased by vigorous exercise, hydrocortisone, alcohol consumption, pregnancy, and undernutrition and is greater in males than in females. In human illnesses, these factors may similarly increase the severity of the disease.

I. Acute Hemorrhagic Conjunctivitis: Coxsackievirus A24 is one of the agents that can cause this disease (see below).

J. Diabetes Mellitus: Serologic studies suggest an association of type 1 diabetes with past infection by coxsackievirus B4 and perhaps other members of the B group. Experimental studies support the findings in humans. In mice, another picornavirus, encephalomyocarditis virus, induces lesions in the pancreatic islets of Langerhans as well as an accompanying diabetes.

K. Swine Vesicular Disease: The agent of this disease is an enterovirus antigenically related to coxsackievirus B5. Furthermore, the swine virus can also infect humans.

Laboratory Diagnosis

A. Recovery of Virus: The virus is isolated readily from throat washings during the first few days of illness and in the stools during the first few weeks. In coxsackievirus A21 infections, the largest amount of virus is found in nasal secretions. In cases of aseptic meningitis, strains have been recovered from the cerebrospinal fluid as well as from the alimentary tract. In hemorrhagic conjunctivitis cases, A24 virus is isolated from conjunctival swabs, throat swabs, and feces.

Specimens are inoculated into tissue cultures and also into suckling mice. In tissue culture, a cytopathic effect appears within 5–14 days. In suckling mice, signs of illness appear usually within 3-8 days with group A strains and 5–14 days with group B strains. The virus is identified by the pathologic lesions it produces and by immunologic means.

B. Serology: Nt antibodies, which are detected as shown in Fig 37–1, appear early during the course of infection. Nt antibodies tend to be specific for the infecting virus and persist for years. CF antibodies exhibit cross-reactions and disappear in 6 months. Serologic tests are difficult to evaluate (because of the multiplicity of types) unless the antigen used in the test has been isolated from a specific patient or during an epidemic outbreak.

Serum antibodies can also be detected and titrated by the immunofluorescence technique, using infected cell cultures on coverslips as antigens. These can be preserved frozen for years.

Immunity

In humans, Nt and CF antibodies are transferred passively from mother to fetus. Adults have antibodies against more types of coxsackieviruses than do children, which indicates that multiple experience with these viruses is common and increases with age.

Epidemiology

Viruses of the coxsackie group have been encountered around the globe. Isolations have been made mainly from human feces, pharyngeal swabbings, sewage, and flies. Antibodies to various coxsackieviruses are found in serum collected from persons all over the world and in pooled gamma globulin.

Coxsackieviruses are recovered much more frequently in summer and early fall. Also, children develop Nt and CF antibodies in summer, indicating infection by coxsackieviruses during this period. Such children have much higher incidence rates for acute, febrile minor illnesses during the summer than children who fail to develop coxsackievirus antibodies.

Familial exposure is important in the acquisition of infections with coxsackieviruses. Once the virus is introduced into a household, all susceptible persons usually become infected, although all do not develop clinically apparent disease.

In herpangina, only about 30% of infected persons within households develop faucial lesions. Others may present a mild febrile illness without throat lesions. Virus has been found in 85% of patients with herpangina, in 65% of their neighbors, in 40% of family contacts, and in 4% of all persons in the community.

The coxsackieviruses share many properties with the echo- and polioviruses. Because of their epidemiologic similarities, enteroviruses may occur together in nature, even in the same human host or the same specimens of sewage or flies.

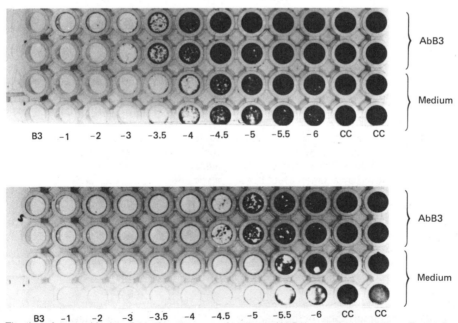

Figure 37–1. Titration of coxsackievirus B3 in the presence of antibody (AbB3) and control medium. From left to right, as the virus dilution increases, complete cytopathic effect, incomplete cytopathic effect, and then individual plaques are seen. The last 2 rows on the right side are cell controls (CC). B3 line shows 0.5 log$_{10}$ dilutions of virus. *Top:* Assayed 48 hours postinfection. *Bottom:* Assayed 72 hours postinfection; further progression of cytopathic effect is evident. (From Randhawa AS et al: *J Clin Microbiol* 1977;5:535.)

ECHOVIRUSES

The echoviruses (*e*nteric *c*ytopathogenic *h*uman *o*rphan viruses) are grouped together because they infect the human enteric tract and because they can be recovered from humans only by inoculation of certain tissue cultures. Over 30 serotypes are known, but not all cause human illness. Aseptic meningitis, febrile illnesses with or without rash, common colds, and acute hemorrhagic conjunctivitis are among the diseases caused by echoviruses.

Properties of the Viruses

A. General Properties: Echoviruses are typical enteroviruses measuring 24–30 nm.

B. Growth of Virus: Monkey kidney cell culture is the method of choice for the isolation of these agents. Some also multiply in human amnion cells and cell lines such as HeLa.

Certain echoviruses agglutinate human group O erythrocytes. The hemagglutinins are associated with the infectious virus particle but are not affected by neuraminidase.

Initially, echoviruses were distinguished from coxsackieviruses by their failure to produce pathologic changes in newborn mice, but echovirus 9 can produce paralysis in newborn mice. Conversely, strains of some coxsackievirus types (especially A9) lack mouse pathogenicity and thus resemble echoviruses. This variability in biologic properties is the chief reason why new enteroviruses are no longer being subclassified as echo- or coxsackieviruses.

C. Antigenic Properties: Over 30 different antigenic types have been identified. The different types may be separated on the basis of cross-Nt or cross-CF tests. Variants exist that do not behave exactly like the prototypes. After human infections, Nt antibodies persist longer than CF antibodies.

D. Animal Susceptibility: To be included in the echo group, prototype strains must not produce disease in suckling mice, rabbits, or monkeys. In the chimpanzee, no apparent illness is produced, but infection can be demonstrated by the presence and persistence of virus in the throat and in the feces and by the type-specific antibody responses.

Pathogenesis & Pathology

The pathogenesis of the alimentary infection is similar to that of the other enteroviruses. Virus may be recovered from the throat and stools; in certain types (4, 5, 6, 9, 14, and 18) associated with aseptic meningitis, the virus has been recovered from the cerebrospinal fluid.

Clinical Findings

To establish etiologic association of echovirus with disease, the following criteria are used: (1) There is a much higher rate of recovery of virus from patients with the disease than from healthy individuals of the same age and socioeconomic level living in the same area at the same time. (2) Antibodies against the virus develop during the course of the disease. If the clinical syndrome can be caused by other known agents, then virologic or serologic evidence must be negative for concurrent infection with such agents. (3) The virus is isolated from body fluids or tissues manifesting lesions, eg, from the cerebrospinal fluid in cases of aseptic meningitis.

Echoviruses 4, 6, 9, 11, 14, 16, 18, and others have been associated with aseptic meningitis. Rashes are common in types 4, 9, 16 ("Boston exanthem disease"), and 18. Rashes are commonest in young children. Occasionally, there is conjunctivitis, muscle weakness, and spasm (types 6, 9, and others). Infantile diarrhea may be associated with some types (eg, 18, 20). Echovirus type 28 isolated from upper respiratory illness causes "colds" in volunteers and has been reclassified as rhinovirus type 1. For many echoviruses (and some coxsackieviruses), no disease entities have been defined.

With the virtual elimination of poliomyelitis in developed countries, the central nervous system syndromes associated with echo- and coxsackieviruses have assumed greater prominence. The latter in children under age 1 year may lead to neurologic sequelae and mental impairment. This does not appear to happen in older children.

Laboratory Diagnosis

It is impossible in an individual case to diagnose an echovirus infection on clinical grounds. However, in the following epidemic situations, echoviruses must be considered: (1) summer outbreaks of aseptic meningitis; (2) summer epidemics, especially in young children, of a febrile illness with rash; and (3) outbreaks of diarrheal disease in young infants from whom no pathogenic enterobacteria can be recovered.

The diagnosis is dependent upon laboratory tests. The procedure of choice is isolation of virus from throat swabs, stools, rectal swabs, and, in aseptic meningitis, cerebrospinal fluid. Serologic tests are impractical—because of the many different virus types—except when a virus has been isolated from a patient or during an outbreak of typical clinical illness. Nt and HI antibodies are type-specific and may persist for years. CF antibodies give many heterotypic responses.

If an agent is isolated in tissue culture, it is tested against different pools of antisera against enteroviruses. Determination of the type of virus present depends upon neutralization by a single serum. Infection with 2 or more enteroviruses may occur simultaneously.

Epidemiology

The epidemiology of echoviruses is similar to that of other enteroviruses. They occur in all parts of the globe. Unlike the enterobacteria, which are constantly present in the intestinal tract, the enteroviruses produce only transitory infections. They are more apt to be found in the young than in the old. In the temperate zone, infections occur chiefly in summer and autumn and are about 5 times more prevalent in children of lower-income families than in those living in more favorable circumstances.

Studies of families into which enteroviruses were introduced demonstrate the ease with which these agents spread and the high frequency of infection in persons who had formed no antibodies from earlier exposures. This is true for all enteroviruses.

Wide dissemination is the rule. In a period when 149 inhabitants of a city of 740,000 were hospitalized with echo 9 disease, approximately 6% of the population, or 45,000 persons, had a compatible illness.

Control

Avoidance of contact with patients exhibiting acute febrile illness, especially those with a rash, is advisable for very young children. Members of institutional staffs responsible for caring for infants should be tested to determine whether they are carriers of enteroviruses. This is particularly important during outbreaks of diarrheal disease among infants.

OTHER ENTEROVIRUS TYPES

Four enteroviruses (types 68–71) grow in monkey kidney cultures, and 3 of them cause human disease.

Enterovirus 68 was isolated from the respiratory tracts of children with bronchiolitis or pneumonia.

Enterovirus 70 is the chief cause of acute hemorrhagic conjunctivitis. It was isolated from the conjunctiva of patients with this striking eye disease, which occurred in pandemic form in 1969–1971 in Africa and Southeast Asia. It was not diagnosed in the USA until its importation into Florida in 1981. Acute hemorrhagic conjunctivitis has a sudden onset of subconjunctival hemorrhage ranging from small petechiae to large blotches covering the bulbar conjunctiva. There may also be epithelial keratitis and occasionally lumbar radiculomyelopathy. The disease is commonest in adults, with an incubation period of 1 day and a duration of 8–10 days. Complete recovery is the rule. The virus is highly communicable and spreads rapidly under crowded or unhygienic conditions. There is no effective treatment.

Enterovirus 71 was isolated from patients with meningitis, encephalitis, and paralysis resembling poliomyelitis. It continues to be one of the main causes of central nervous system disease, sometimes fatal, around the world. In some areas, particularly in Japan and Sweden, the virus has caused outbreaks of hand, foot, and mouth disease.

RHINOVIRUS GROUP

Rhinoviruses are isolated commonly from the nose and throat but very rarely from feces. These viruses, as well as coronaviruses and some reo-, adeno-, entero-, parainfluenza, and influenza viruses, cause upper respiratory tract infections, including the "common cold."

Properties of the Virus

A. General Properties: Rhinoviruses are picornaviruses similar to enteroviruses but differing from them in having a buoyant density in cesium chloride of 1.40 g/mL and in being acid-labile.

B. Animal Susceptibility and Growth of Virus: These viruses are infectious only for humans and chimpanzees. They have been grown in cultures of human embryonic lung fibroblasts (WI-38) and in organ cultures of ferret and human tracheal epithelium. They are grown best at 33 °C in rolled cultures.

C. Antigenic Properties: Over 100 serotypes are known. Some cross-react (eg, types 9 and 32).

Pathogenesis & Pathology

The virus enters via the upper respiratory tract. High titers of virus in nasal secretions—which can be found as early as 2–4 days after exposure—are associated with maximal illness. Thereafter, viral titers fall, although illness persists.

Histopathologic changes are limited to the submucosa and surface epithelium. These include engorgement of blood vessels, edema, mild cellular infiltration, and desquamation of surface epithelium, which is complete by the third day. Nasal secretion increases in quantity and in protein concentration.

Experiments under controlled conditions have shown that chilling, including the wearing of wet clothes, does not produce a cold or increase susceptibility to the virus. Chilliness is an early symptom of the common cold.

Clinical Findings

The incubation period is brief, from 2 to 4 days, and the acute illness usually lasts for 7 days although a nonproductive cough may persist for 2–3 weeks. The average adult has 1–2 attacks each year. Usual symptoms in adults include irritation in the upper respiratory tract, nasal discharge, headache, mild cough, malaise, and a chilly sensation. There is little or no fever. The nasal and nasopharyngeal mucosa become red and swollen, and the sense of smell becomes less keen. Mild hoarseness may be present. Prominent cervical adenopathy does not occur. Secondary bacterial infection may produce acute otitis media, sinusitis, bronchitis, or pneumonitis, especially in children. Type-specific antibodies appear or rise with each infection.

Immunity

Natural immunity may exist but may be brief. Only 30–50% of volunteers can be infected with infectious material; yet the "resistant" volunteers may catch colds of the same serotype at other times. Furthermore, people in isolated areas have more severe colds and a higher incidence of infection when a cold is introduced than people in areas regularly exposed to the virus. It has also been observed that older adults experience fewer colds than young adults and children. One 3-year study of acute respiratory tract illness in college and medical students showed that the same serotype was never isolated from separate illnesses in any student who had 2 or more illnesses.

Recent work with human volunteers has shown that resistance to the common cold is independent of measurable serum antibody but perhaps is related to specific antibody in the nasal secretions. These secretory antibodies are primarily 11S IgA immunoglobulins, produced locally in the mucosa and not a transudate from the serum. These 11S IgA antibodies do not persist as long as those in serum, and this could explain the paradox of reinfection in a person with adequate serum antibodies.

Volunteers infected with one rhinovirus serotype resist challenge with both homologous and heterologous virus for 2–16 weeks after the initial infection. Resistance to homologous challenge is complete during this period, while resistance to heterologous challenge is incomplete. This nonspecific resistance may be a factor in the control of naturally occurring colds.

Epidemiology

The disease occurs throughout the world. In the temperate zones, the attack rates are highest in early fall and winter, declining in the late spring. Members of isolated communities form highly susceptible groups.

The virus is believed to be transmitted through close contact, by large droplets. The fingers of a person with a cold are usually contaminated because of frequent contact with the virus-shedding nose. Transmission to susceptible persons then occurs by hand to hand or hand to object (eg, doorknob) to hand contamination. Self-inoculation after hand contamination may be a more important mode of spread than that by airborne particles.

Colds in children spread more easily to others than do colds in adults. Adults in households with a child in school have twice as many colds as adults in households without school children.

In a single community, many rhinovirus serotypes cause outbreaks of disease in a single season, and different serotypes predominate during different respiratory disease seasons.

Treatment & Control

No specific treatment is available. The development of a potent rhinovirus vaccine is unlikely because of the difficulty in growing rhinoviruses to high titer in culture, the fleeting immunity, and the many serotypes causing colds. In addition, many rhinovirus serotypes are present during single respiratory disease outbreaks and may recur only rarely in the same area. Injection of purified vaccines has shown that the high levels of serum antibody are frequently not associated with similar elevation of local secretory antibody, which may be the most significant factor in disease prevention.

In field studies, the use of virucidal paper tissues (containing 3.5 mg of citric acid, 1.7 mg of malic acid, and 0.7 mg of sodium lauryl sulfate per square inch) markedly reduced hand contamination by rhinoviruses during nose blowing and also lessened the infectiousness of the virus shedder. Daily intranasal spraying with interferon has been reported to prevent the natural transmission of rhinoviruses to susceptible persons.

FOOT-AND-MOUTH DISEASE (Aphthovirus of Cattle)

This highly infectious disease of cattle, sheep, pigs, and goats is rare in the USA but endemic in Mexico and Canada. It may be transmitted to humans by contact or ingestion. In humans, the disease is characterized by fever, salivation, and vesiculation of the mucous membranes of the oropharynx and of the skin of the palms, soles, fingers, and toes.

The disease in animals is highly contagious in the early stages of infection when viremia is present and when vesicles in the mouth and on the feet rupture and liberate large amounts of virus. Excreted material remains infectious for long periods. The mortality rate in animals is usually low but may reach 70%. Infected animals become poor producers of milk and meat. Many cattle serve as foci for infection for up to 8 months.

The virus is a typical picornavirus, measuring 24 nm in diameter, and is acid-labile, with a buoyant density in cesium chloride of 1.43 g/mL. There are at least 7 types with over 50 subtypes.

Immunity after infection is adequate but of short duration.

A variety of animals are susceptible to infection. The typical disease can be reproduced by inoculating the virus into the pads of the foot. The reaction in infant mice inoculated with the virus of foot-and-mouth disease is similar to their reaction to inoculation with coxsackieviruses: paralysis results as a consequence of myositis. The virus grows readily in tissue culture of cattle tongue or hamster BHK-21 cells. Formalin-treated vaccines have been prepared from virus grown in such tissue cultures. However, such vaccines do not produce a long-lasting immunity, and frequent booster inoculations are necessary. New vaccines are being developed by 2 techniques: recombinant DNA in bacteria (*Escherichia coli*), and synthesis of the immunogenic epitope.

The methods of control of the disease are dictated by its high degree of contagiousness and the resistance of the virus to inactivation. When foci of infection occur in the USA, all exposed animals are slaughtered and their carcasses destroyed. Strict quarantine is established, and the area is not presumed to be safe until susceptible animals fail to develop symptoms within 30 days. Another method is to quarantine the herd and vaccinate all unaffected animals. Other countries have successfully employed systematic vaccination schedules. Some nations (eg, the USA and Australia) forbid the importation of potentially infective materials such as fresh meat, and the disease has been eliminated in these areas. Even so, migrating birds may play a role in carrying the virus from one country to another, as from France and Holland to England.

REFERENCES

Banatvala JE et al: Coxsackie B, mumps, rubella, and cytomegalovirus specific IgM responses in patients with juvenile-onset insulin-dependent diabetes mellitus in Britain, Austria, and Australia. *Lancet* 1985;**1:**1409.

Chow M et al: Synthetic peptides from four separate regions of the poliovirus type 1 capsid protein VP1 induce neutralizing antibodies. *Proc Natl Acad Sci USA* 1985;**82:**910.

Couch RB: The common cold: Control? *J Infect Dis* 1984; **150:**167.

Dorries R, ter Meulen V: Specificity of IgM antibodies in acute human coxsackievirus B infections, analysed by indirect solid phase enzyme immunoassay and immunoblot technique. *J Gen Virol* 1983;**64:**159.

Emini EA et al: Antigenic conservation and divergence between the viral-specific proteins of poliovirus type 1 and various picornaviruses. *Virology* 1985;**140:**13.

Evans AS: Criteria for control of infectious diseases with poliomyelitis as an example. *Prog Med Virol* 1984;**29:**141.

Hayden GF, Hendley JO, Gwaltney JM Jr: The effect of placebo and virucidal paper handkerchiefs on viral contamination of the hand and transmission of experimental rhinoviral infection. *J Infect Dis* 1985;**152:**403.

Kandolf R, Hofschneider PH: Molecular cloning of the genome of a cardiotropic coxsackie B3 virus: Full-length reverse-transcribed recombinant cDNA generates infectious virus in mammalian cells. *Proc Natl Acad Sci USA* 1985;**82:**4818.

Kew OM et al: Multiple genetic changes can occur in the oral poliovaccine upon replication in humans. *J Gen Virol* 1981;**56:**337.

Khatib R et al: Alterations in coxsackievirus B4 heart muscle disease in ICR Swiss mice by anti-thymocyte serum. *J Gen Virol* 1983;**64:**231.

Kitamura N et al: Primary structure, gene organization and polypeptide expression of poliovirus RNA. *Nature* 1981;**291:**547.

Melnick JL: Enterovirus type 71 infections: A varied clinical pattern sometimes mimicking paralytic poliomyelitis. *Rev Infect Dis* 1984;**6:**S387.

Melnick JL: Enteroviruses: Polioviruses, coxsackieviruses, echoviruses, and newer enteroviruses. Pages 739–794 in: *Virology.* Fields BN et al (editors). Raven Press, 1985.

Melnick JL, Wenner HA, Phillips CA: Enteroviruses. Pages 471–534 in: *Diagnostic Procedures for Viral, Rickettsial, and Chlamydial Infections,* 5th ed. Lennette EH, Schmidt NJ (editors). American Public Health Association, 1979.

Nathanson N, Martin JR: The epidemiology of poliomyelitis: Enigmas surrounding its appearance, epidemicity, and disappearance. *Am J Epidemiol* 1979;**110:**672.

Yin-Murphy M: Acute hemorrhagic conjunctivitis. *Prog Med Virol* 1984;**29:**23.

Hepatitis Viruses

Viral hepatitis is a systemic disease primarily involving the liver. Most cases of acute viral hepatitis in children and adults are caused by one of the following agents: hepatitis A virus (HAV), the etiologic agent of viral hepatitis type A (infectious hepatitis or short incubation hepatitis); hepatitis B virus (HBV), which is associated with viral hepatitis B (serum hepatitis or long incubation hepatitis); and the more recently recognized hepatitis C, D, etc, viruses. Because these viruses are associated with hepatitis that cannot be ascribed to either HAV or HBV, the disease is designated non-A, non-B hepatitis. They account for most of the transfusion-associated hepatitis cases seen in the USA since 1976 and a sizable portion of sporadic hepatitis. Additional well-characterized viruses that can cause sporadic hepatitis, such as yellow fever virus, cytomegalovirus, Epstein-Barr virus (infectious mononucleosis), herpes simplex virus, rubella virus, and the enteroviruses, are discussed in other chapters. Hepatitis viruses produce acute inflammation of the liver, resulting in a clinical illness characterized by fever, gastrointestinal symptoms such as nausea and vomiting, and jaundice. Regardless of the virus type, identical histopathologic lesions are observed in the liver during acute disease.

HAV, transmitted primarily by the fecal-oral route, may be transmitted rarely by the parenteral route. HBV produces sporadic infections principally after parenteral inoculation of virus-infected blood or blood products, although transmission by close, intimate contact is also common.

Appreciation of the existence of these lesser known modes of transmission is important when attempting to correlate presently established clinical classifications of viral hepatitis with the presence or absence of hepatitis B surface antigen (HBsAg). This antigen was originally detected in 1963 in the serum of an apparently healthy Australian aborigine by reacting the serum in immunodiffusion tests with serum from a multiply transfused hemophiliac, but the association of the Australia (Au) antigen (HBsAg) with viral hepatitis was not recognized until 1967.

The incidence of this unique antigen in acute hepatitis associated with transfusions was 50–75% prior to the introduction of sensitive screening methods to ban the use of blood donors circulating HBsAg. In chronic active hepatitis, the prevalence rate has varied but is around 30% in most series. A high prevalence of HBsAg has been observed in cases of primary liver cancer in most areas of the world. The antigen is not present in sera from well-documented cases of common-source epidemics of viral hepatitis A.

Nomenclature of the hepatitis viruses, antigens, and antibodies is as follows:

Hepatitis A

HAV	Hepatitis A virus. Etiologic agent of infectious hepatitis. Enterovirus 72, single serotype.
Anti-HAV	Antibody to HAV. Detectable at onset of symptoms; lifetime persistence.
IgM anti-HAV	IgM class antibody to HAV. Indicates recent infection with hepatitis A; positive up to 4–6 months after infection.

Hepatitis B

HBV	Hepatitis B virus. Etiologic agent of serum hepatitis (long-incubation hepatitis).
HBsAg	Hepatitis B surface antigen. Surface antigen(s) of HBV detectable in large quantity in serum; several subtypes identified.
HBeAg	Hepatitis B e antigen. Soluble antigen; associated with HBV replication, with high titers of HBV in serum, and with infectivity of serum.
HBcAg	Hepatitis B core antigen. No test available for routine use.
Anti-HBs	Antibody to HBsAg. Indicates past infection with and immunity to HBV, presence of passive antibody from HBIG, or immune response from HBV vaccine.
Anti-HBe	Antibody to HBeAg. Presence in serum of HBsAg carrier suggests lower titer of HBV.
Anti-HBc	Antibody to HBcAg. Indicates infection with HBV at some undefined time in the past.
IgM anti-HBc	IgM class antibody to HBcAg. Indicates recent infection with HBV; positive for 4–6 months after infection.

Delta hepatitis

δ virus	Delta virus. Etiologic agent of delta hepatitis; may only cause infection in presence of HBV.
δ-Ag	Delta antigen. Detectable in early acute δ virus infection.
Anti-δ	Antibody to δ-Ag. Indicates past or present infection with δ virus.

Non-A, non-B hepatitis

NANB — Non-A, non-B hepatitis virus. Diagnosis by exclusion. At least 2 viruses in group. Epidemiology parallels that of hepatitis B.

Epidemic non-A, non-B hepatitis

Epidemic NANB — Epidemic non-A, non-B hepatitis virus. Causes large epidemics in Asia and North Africa; fecal-oral or waterborne transmission.

Immune globulins

IG — Immune globulin USP (previously called ISG, immune serum globulin, or gamma globulin). Contains antibodies to HAV, low titers of antibodies to HBV.

HBIG — Hepatitis B immune globulin. Contains high titers of antibodies to HBV.

General Properties of the Viruses

A. Hepatitis Type A: Recent studies indicate that HAV should be classified with the enteroviruses as enterovirus 72. It is a 27- to 32-nm spherical particle with cubic symmetry, containing a linear single-stranded RNA genome with a molecular weight of about 2.25×10^6. Lipid is not an integral component of HAV, which is stable to treatment with ether, acid, and heat (60 °C for 1 hour), and its infectivity can be preserved for at least 1 month after being dried and stored at 25 °C and 42% relative humidity or for years at −20 °C. The virus is destroyed by autoclaving (121 °C for 20 minutes), by boiling in water for 5 minutes, by dry heat (180 °C for 1 hour), by ultraviolet irradiation (1 minute at 1.1 watts), by treatment with formalin (1:4000 for 3 days at 37 °C), or by treatment with chlorine (10–15 ppm for 30 minutes). The relative resistance of HAV to disinfection procedures emphasizes the need for extra precautions in dealing with hepatitis patients and their products.

Electron microscopic examination of infected liver reveals intracytoplasmic localization of virus particles. Only one serotype is known. There is no antigenic cross-reactivity with HBV.

HAV initially was identified in stool and liver preparations by employing immune electron microscopy as the detection system (Fig 35–3). The addition of specific hepatitis A antisera from convalescent patients to fecal specimens obtained from patients early in the incubation period of their illness prior to the onset of jaundice permitted concentration and visibility of virus particles by the formation of antigen-antibody aggregates. More sensitive serologic assays such as the microtiter solid-phase immunoradiometric assay and immune adherence have made it possible to detect HAV in stools, liver homogenates, and bile and to measure specific antibody in serum.

Chimpanzees and 2 South American monkeys, the white-moustached (*Saguinus mystax*) and rufiventer marmosets, are susceptible to HAV and have provided laboratories with a source of virus for experimentation and for preparation of diagnostic reagents. HAV from marmoset-adapted material and from extracts of patients' feces has recently been cultivated serially in primary explant cultures of adult *Saguinus labiatus* marmoset livers and in cell culture. A noncytopathic infection occurs, which is identified by immunofluorescence and by radioimmunoassay.

B. Hepatitis Type B: HBsAg is closely associated with hepatitis B infections. Electron microscopy of HBsAg-reactive serum has revealed 3 morphologic forms (Fig 38–1). The most numerous are spherical particles measuring 22 nm in diameter (Fig 33–27). These small particles appear to be made up exclusively of HBsAg—as do tubular or filamentous forms, which have the same diameter but may be over 200 nm long. Larger, 42-nm spherical particles (HBV, originally referred to as Dane particles) are less frequently observed. These particles are more complex. The outer surface, or envelope, contains HBsAg and surrounds a 27-nm inner core that contains HBcAg (Figs 38–2 and 38–3). Overproduction of the surface component apparently results in the 22-nm particles. DNA polymerase activity and endogenous DNA template are associated with the inner core of HBV. The DNA template consists of double-stranded DNA with a molecular weight of approximately 2×10^6.

It is the variable length of a single-stranded region of the circular DNA molecules that results in genetically heterogeneous particles with a wide range of buoyant densities.

Two major polypeptides with molecular weights of 25,000 and 30,000 constitute approximately 55% by weight of the HBsAg-containing 22-nm particle. A third major polypeptide has a molecular weight of 68,000, has HBsAg reactivity, and cross-reacts with human serum albumin. The viral envelope may be assembled from the 2 smaller polypeptides, one of which (MW 30,000) is glycosylated.

HBeAg is believed to be a hidden antigenic component of the HBV core particle. Nucleotide sequences found in the HBcAg region of the HBV genome may

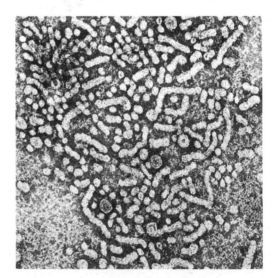

Figure 38–1. Unfractionated HBsAg-positive human plasma. Filaments, 22-nm spherical particles, and a few 42-nm virions are shown (77,000 x).

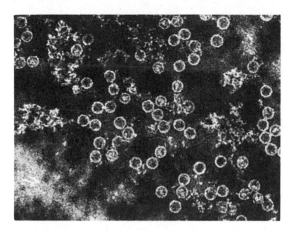

Figure 38–2. HBcAg purified from infected liver nuclei (122,400 x). The diameter of the core particles is 27 nm. (Fields, Dreesman, and Cabral.)

code for this polypeptide, which has a molecular weight of 15,000–20,000.

The stability of HBsAg does not always coincide with that of the infectious agent. However, both are stable at −20 °C for more than 20 years and stable to repeated freezing and thawing. The virus also is stable at 37 °C for 60 minutes and remains viable after being dried and stored at 25 °C for at least 1 week. HBV (but not HBsAg) is sensitive to higher temperatures (100 °C for 1 minute) or to longer incubation periods (60 °C for 10 hours) depending on the amount of virus present in the sample. HBsAg is stable at pH 2.4 for up to 6 hours, but HBV infectivity is lost. Sodium hypochlorite, 0.5% (eg, 1:10 Clorox), destroys antigenicity within 3 minutes at low protein concentrations, but undiluted serum specimens require higher concentrations (5%). HBsAg is not destroyed by ultraviolet irradiation of plasma or other blood products, and viral infectivity may also resist such treatment. HBV is unevenly distributed during Cohn ethanol fractionation of plasma. Most of the virus is retained in fraction I (fibrinogen, factor VIII) or III (prothrombin complex), whereas HBsAg is relegated to fractions II (gamma globulin) and IV (plasma protein).

C. Non-A, Non-B Hepatitis: Clinical and epidemiologic studies and cross-challenge experiments in chimpanzees have suggested that at least 2 non-A, non-B hepatitis agents exist. Distinct ultrastructural changes are observed in the liver of infected animals. These consist of cytoplasmic inclusions, thickening of the membranes of the smooth endoplasmic reticulum through apposition of cisternae, and the appearance of a unique cytoplasmic protein matrix of densely packed microtubules. Viruslike particles have been identified by immune electron microscopy in serum and liver tissue. The best defined particles are approximately 27 nm in diameter. The agents of non-A, non-B hepatitis are apparently susceptible to inactivation by heat and by formalin. Because of a lack of sufficient and specific antigen and a suitable antibody reagent, no confirmed serologic test has been developed for identifying infected persons.

D. Delta (δ) Agent: A new antigen-antibody system, termed the delta (δ) antigen and antibody (anti-δ), is detected in some HBV infections. The antigen is found within certain HBsAg particles. The δ antigen is distinct from the known antigenic determinants of HBV. It is localized to hepatocyte nuclei that do not contain HBcAg and has a buoyant density in cesium chloride of 1.28 g/mL and a molecular weight of 68,000. In blood, the δ agent is surrounded by an HBsAg envelope and has a particle size of 35–37 nm and a buoyant density of 1.24–1.25 g/mL. It is precipitated by anti-HBs. The genome of the δ agent consists of RNA with a molecular weight of 5.5×10^5. No homology with the HBV genome has been found using hybridization techniques. The δ agent is believed to be a defective virus that replicates only in HBV-infected cells.

The δ antigen has been subjected to chemical and enzymatic treatment. No loss of activity occurred following treatment with EDTA, detergents, ether, nucleases, glycosidases, or acid; but partial or complete loss of activity was detected after treatment with alkali, thiocyanate, guanidine hydrochloride, trichloracetic acid, and proteolytic enzymes.

Pathology

Microscopically, there is spotty parenchymal cell degeneration, with necrosis of hepatocytes, a diffuse lobular inflammatory reaction, and disruption of liver cell cords. These parenchymal changes are accompanied by reticuloendothelial (Kupffer) cell hyperplasia, periportal infiltration by mononuclear cells, and cell degeneration. Localized areas of necrosis with ballooning or acidophilic bodies are frequently observed. Later in the course of the disease, there is an accumulation of macrophages containing lipofuscin near degenerating hepatocytes. Disruption of bile canaliculi or blockage of biliary excretion may occur following liver cell enlargement or necrosis. Preservation of the reticulum framework allows hepatocyte regeneration so that the highly ordered architecture of the liver lobule can be ultimately regained. The damaged hepatic tissue is usually restored in 8–12 weeks.

In 5–15% of patients, the initial lesion consists of confluent (bridging) hepatic necrosis with impaired regeneration, resulting in collapsed stroma. The occurrence of this lesion in patients over age 40 frequently presages a precarious clinical course leading to fibrosis, cirrhosis, and death.

Chronic carriers of HBsAg may or may not have demonstrable evidence of liver disease. Persistent (unresolved) viral hepatitis, a mild benign disease that may follow acute hepatitis B in 8–10% of adult patients, is characterized by sporadically abnormal transaminase values and hepatomegaly. Histologically, the lobular architecture is preserved, with portal inflammation, swollen and pale hepatocytes (cobblestone arrangement), and slight to absent fibrosis. This lesion is frequently observed in asymptomatic carri-

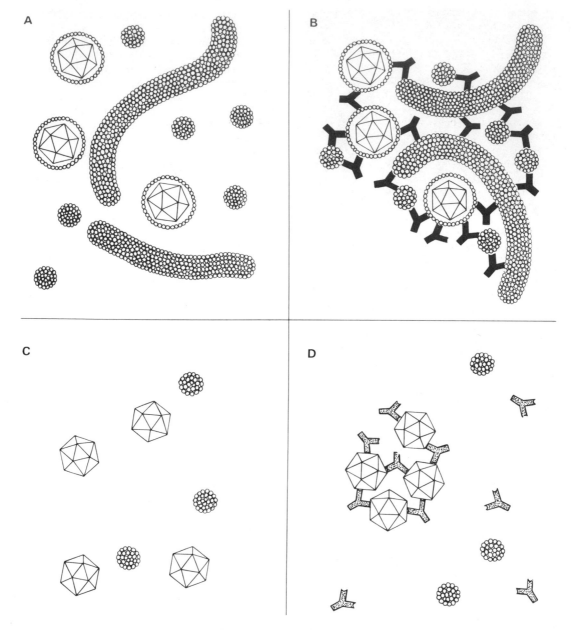

Figure 38–3. Various hepatitis B particles are related and differentiated by their antigenicity. The forms seen in patients' blood are the 22-nm spheres, the filaments 22 nm wide, and the 42-nm virus itself (HBV), which consists of an outer shell and a 27-nm inner core *(A)*. All 3 forms are characterized by the presence of HBsAg, as indicated by the fact that the antibody (black) to that antigen combines with and agglutinates them all *(B)*. Adding detergent to virus particles strips the surface antigen outer shell off them, yielding free cores *(C)*. These are agglutinated by a different antibody (stippled), the antibody to core antigen, distinguishing them from the surface particles *(D)*. (From: Melnick JL, Dreesman GR, Hollinger FB: Viral hepatitis. *Sci Am* [July] 1977;**237**:44. Copyright © 1977 by Scientific American, Inc. All rights reserved.)

ers, usually does not progress toward cirrhosis, and has a favorable prognosis.

Chronic active (aggressive) hepatitis features a spectrum of histologic changes from inflammation and necrosis to collapse of the normal reticulum framework with bridging between the portal triads or terminal hepatic veins. HBsAg is observed in 10–50% of

these patients. The prognosis is guarded, with progression to macronodular cirrhosis frequently occurring.

Occasionally during acute viral hepatitis, more extensive damage may occur that prevents orderly liver cell regeneration. Such fulminant or massive hepatocellular necrosis is seen in 1–2% of jaundiced patients with hepatitis B but is less common in hepatitis A.

In hepatitis B patients, electron microscopic studies have revealed in liver cell nuclei 27-nm particles that are morphologically similar to the inner core of the virus. Correspondingly, immunofluorescence studies indicate that during HBV infection HBcAg is found primarily in the nucleus, whereas HBsAg is localized in the cytoplasm. HBsAg and HBcAg are rarely found in the same cell, and there appears to be an inverse relationship between the severity of the lesion and the abundance of HBsAg. Hepatocytes with a ground-glass appearance are laden with cytoplasmic HBsAg and are often found in biopsy specimens from patients with persistent viral hepatitis. Nuclear HBcAg predominates in patients whose immune system is compromised.

HBV DNA sequences have been detected in bone marrow cells and in peripheral blood lymphocytes of patients who may or may not be positive for HBs antigenemia. Patients with acquired immune deficiency syndrome (AIDS) may have HBV DNA sequences in bone marrow, semen, and lymph nodes as well as in mononuclear blood cells, even in the absence of serologic markers of HBV. Thus, HBV may play a role in the pathogenesis of AIDS as well as in hepatitis and primary hepatocellular carcinoma.

Clinical Findings
(Table 38–1)

In individual cases, it is not possible to make a reliable clinical distinction between hepatitis A, hepatitis B, and non-A, non-B hepatitis. Other viral diseases that may present as hepatitis are infectious mononucleosis, yellow fever, cytomegalovirus infection, herpes simplex, rubella, and some enterovirus infections. Hepatitis may occasionally occur as a complication of leptospirosis, syphilis, tuberculosis, toxoplasmosis, and amebiasis, all of which are susceptible to specific drug therapy. Noninfectious causes include biliary ob-

Table 38–1. Epidemiologic and clinical features of viral hepatitis A, B, and non-A, non-B.

	Viral Hepatitis Type A	Viral Hepatitis Type B	Non-A, Non-B Viral Hepatitis
Incubation period	15–45 days (avg, 25–30).	50–180 days (avg, 60–90).	14–120 days (avg, 35–70).*
Principal age distribution	Children,† young adults.	15–29 years.‡	?
Seasonal incidence	Throughout the year but tends to peak in autumn.	Throughout the year.	Throughout the year.
Route of infection	Predominantly fecal-oral.	Predominantly parenteral.	Predominantly parenteral.
Occurrence of virus			
Blood	2 weeks before to ≤ 1 week after jaundice.	Months to years.	Months to years.
Stool	2 weeks before to 2 weeks after jaundice.	Absent.	Probably absent.
Urine	Rare.	Absent.	Probably absent.
Saliva, semen	Rare (saliva).	Frequently present.	Unknown.
Clinical and labratory features			
Onset	Abrupt.	Insidious.	Insidious.
Fever > 38 °C (100.4 °F)	Common.	Less common.	Less common.
Duration of transaminase elevation	1–3 weeks.	1–6+ months.	1–6+ months.
Immunoglobulins (IgM levels)	Elevated.	Normal to slightly elevated.	Normal to slightly elevated.
Complications	Uncommon, no chronicity.	Chronicity in 5–10%	Chronicity in 30–50%.
Mortality rate (icteric cases)	< 0.5%.	< 1–2%.	0.5–1%
HBsAg	Absent.	Present.	Absent.
Immunity			
Homologous	Yes.	Yes.	?
Heterologous	No.	No.	No.
Duration	Probably lifetime.	Probably lifetime.	?
Gamma globulin (immune globulin USP) prophylaxis	Regularly prevents jaundice.	Prevents jaundice only if gamma globulin is of sufficient potency against HBV.	?

*Shorter (14 days) and much longer (120 days) incubation periods have been observed.
†Nonicteric hepatitis A is common in children.
‡Among the 15–29 year age group, hepatitis B is often associated with drug abuse or promiscuous sexual behavior. Patients with transfusion-associated hepatitis B are generally over age 29.

struction, primary biliary cirrhosis, Wilson's disease, drug toxicity, and drug hypersensitivity reactions.

In viral hepatitis, the onset of jaundice is often preceded by gastrointestinal symptoms such as nausea, vomiting, severe anorexia, and fever that may mimic influenza. Jaundice may appear within a few days of the prodromal period, but anicteric hepatitis is more common.

Extrahepatic manifestations of viral hepatitis (primarily type B) include (1) a transient serum sickness-like prodrome consisting of urticaria, rash, and nonmigratory polyarthralgia or arthritis occurring 1–6 weeks prior to the onset of hepatitis in 15–20% of patients; (2) polyarteritis nodosa; and (3) glomerulonephritis. Circulating immune complexes have been suggested as the cause of these syndromes. Mixed cryoglobulinemia is a syndrome characterized by purpura, arthralgia, and weakness, often with renal involvement. Vasculitis and immune complex deposition are common. In most cases, the cryoprecipitates contain either HBsAg or anti-HBs.

Complete recovery occurs in most hepatitis A cases and in over 85% of type B hepatitis cases. Hepatitis A is more severe in adults than in children, in whom it often goes unnoticed. Approximately 3% of patients with acute icteric type B hepatitis ultimately develop chronic active hepatitis. Case-fatality rates appear to vary with age and may reflect underlying conditions rather than any increased virulence of the specific causative agent. For the epidemiologic years 1973–1974, the case-fatality rate for hepatitis B among persons age 29 years or younger was 0.5–0.6%; for the age group 30 years and over, it was 2%. The rates are highest for transfusion-associated cases (2.7%). Fulminant hepatitis is lethal in 60–90% of cases and is highly correlated with age. In most patients who survive, complete restoration of the hepatic parenchyma and normal liver function is the rule. Patients who develop confluent (bridging) hepatic necrosis (submassive hepatic necrosis) also have a poor prognosis, and 15–30% of those who survive develop chronic active hepatitis.

The potential courses of acute viral hepatitis have been discussed in the section on pathology. Uncomplicated viral hepatitis rarely continues for more than 10 weeks without improvement. Relapses occur in 5–20% of cases and are manifested by abnormalities in liver function with or without the recurrence of clinical symptoms. A posthepatitis syndrome may occur, especially in postmenopausal women. It is characterized by repeated episodes of anorexia, irritability, lethargy, weakness, headaches, and right upper quadrant pain. This syndrome is due to interference with normal estrogen metabolism in the liver and can be successfully treated with estrogens and progesterone in women.

Non-A, non-B hepatitis is usually clinically mild, with only minimal to moderate elevation of liver enzymes. Hospitalization is unusual, and jaundice occurs in less than 25% of patients. Despite the mild nature of the disease, a relatively large number of cases (30–50%) progress to chronic liver disease. Most patients are asymptomatic, but histologic evaluation often reveals evidence of chronic active hepatitis, especially in those whose disease is acquired following transfusion.

Laboratory Features

Liver biopsy permits a tissue diagnosis of hepatitis. Tests for abnormal liver function, such as serum alanine aminotransferase (ALT; formerly SGPT) and bilirubin, supplement the clinical, pathologic, and epidemiologic findings. Transaminase values in acute hepatitis range between 500 and 2000 units and are almost never below 100 units. ALT values are usually higher than serum aspartate transaminase (AST; formerly SGOT) values. A sharp rise in ALT with a short duration (3–19 days) is more indicative of viral hepatitis A, whereas a gradual rise with prolongation (35–200 days) appears to characterize viral hepatitis B and non-A, non-B infections.

Leukopenia is typical in the preicteric phase and may be followed by a relative lymphocytosis. Large atypical lymphocytes such as are found in infectious mononucleosis may occasionally be seen but do not exceed 10% of the total lymphocyte population.

Further evidence of liver dysfunction and host response is reflected in decreased serum albumin and increased serum globulin levels. Elevation of gamma globulin and serum transaminase is frequently used to gauge chronicity and activity of liver disease. In many patients with hepatitis A, an abnormally high level of IgM is found that appears 3–4 days after the ALT begins to rise. Hepatitis B patients have normal to slightly elevated IgM levels.

The clinical, virologic, and serologic events following exposure to HAV are shown in Fig 38–4. Virus particles have been detected by immune electron microscopy in fecal extracts of hepatitis A patients (Fig 35–3). Virus appears early in the disease and disappears within 3 weeks following the onset of jaundice.

By means of radioimmunoassay, the HAV antigen has been detected in liver, stool, bile, and blood of naturally infected humans and experimentally infected chimpanzees and marmosets. The detection of HAV in the blood of infected chimpanzees and humans supports previous epidemiologic evidence of viremia during the acute stage of the disease. Peak titers of HAV are detected in the stool about 1–2 weeks prior to the first detectable liver enzyme abnormalities.

Anti-HAV appears in the IgM fraction during the acute phase, peaking about 3 weeks after elevation of liver enzymes. During convalescence, anti-HAV is in the IgG fraction, where it persists for decades. Thus, detection of IgM-specific anti-HAV in the blood of an acutely infected patient confirms the diagnosis of hepatitis A. The methods of choice for measuring HAV antibodies are radioimmunoassay, ELISA, and immune adherence hemagglutination (see Chapter 35).

The most sensitive and specific methods for detecting HBsAg or anti-HBs are radioimmunoassay and ELISA (see Chapters 34 and 35). These assays and the red cell agglutination (RCA) technique, which em-

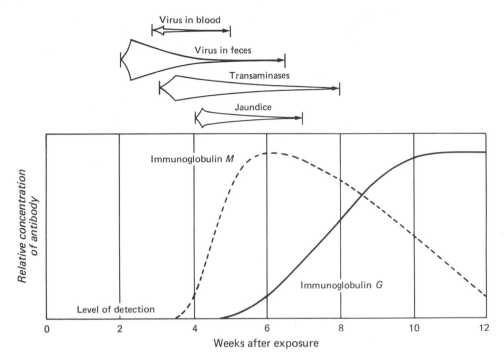

Figure 38–4. Immunologic and biologic events associated with viral hepatitis type A. (From Hollinger FB, Dienstag JL: *Manual of Clinical Microbiology*, 4th ed. American Society for Microbiology, 1985.)

ploys anti-HBs-coated cells in a microtiter system, have replaced counterelectrophoresis as the methods of choice for detecting HBsAg.

The particles containing HBsAg are antigenically complex. Each contains a group-specific antigen, *a*, in addition to 2 pairs of mutually exclusive subdeterminants, *d/y* and *w/r*. Thus, 4 phenotypes of HBsAg have been observed: *adw, ayw, adr,* and *ayr*. In the USA, *adw* is the predominant subtype, although *ayw* is also commonly seen, especially among parenteral drug abusers. These virus-specific markers are useful in epidemiologic investigations, since secondary cases have the same subtype as the index case. The evidence indicates that these antigenic determinants are the phenotypic expression of HBV genotypes and are not determined by host factors.

The clinical and serologic events following exposure to HBV are depicted in Fig 38–5 and Table 38–2. DNA polymerase activity, which is representative of the viremic stage of hepatitis B, occurs early in the incubation period, shortly after the first appearance of HBsAg. The latter is usually detectable 2–6 weeks in advance of clinical and biochemical evidence of hepatitis and persists throughout the clinical course of the disease but typically disappears by the sixth month after exposure. A diagnosis of chronic hepatitis is entertained in those patients in whom HBsAg persists for more than 6 months. In patients destined to become carriers, the initial illness may be mild or inapparent, manifested only by an elevated transaminase level.

Anti-HBc is frequently detected at the onset of clinical illness approximately 2–4 weeks after HBsAg re-

activity appears. Because this antibody is directed against the internal core component of HBV, its appearance in the serum is indicative of viral replication. In the typical case of acute type B hepatitis, high titers of IgM-specific anti-HBc are detected. In contrast, low titers of IgM anti-HBc are found in the sera of most chronic HBsAg carriers. Antibody to HBsAg is first detected at a variable period after the disappearance of HBsAg. It is present in low concentrations usually detectable only by the most sensitive methods.

The anti-HBc test is of limited clinical value when the HBsAg test is positive. However, in perhaps 5% of the acute cases of hepatitis B, and more frequently during early convalescence, HBsAg may be undetectable in the serum. Examination of these sera for high titers of IgM-specific anti-HBc may help establish the correct diagnosis. In the absence of anti-HBc and HBsAg, active hepatitis B can be excluded. In contrast, the presence of anti-HBc alone is presumptive evidence for an active HBV infection. However, this relationship is not infallible, and some patients who have recovered from hepatitis B with the development of anti-HBs and anti-HBc eventually lose one or the other antibody.

Another antigen-antibody system of importance involves HBeAg and its antibody. If the specimen contains HBsAg, certain situations may warrant further testing of the serum for HBeAg or anti-HBe. These include assessing the risk of transmission of HBV following exposure to contaminated blood and advising health care professionals who are chronically infected. Specimens positive for HBeAg (or positive for HBsAg

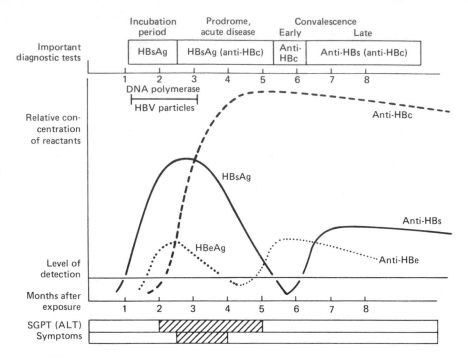

Figure 38–5. Clinical and serologic events occurring in a patient with hepatitis B. The common diagnostic tests and their interpretation are presented in Table 38–2. (From Hollinger FB, Dienstag JL: *Manual of Clinical Microbiology*, 4th ed. American Society for Microbiology, 1985.)

at a dilution of 1:10,000) are considered to be very infectious, ie, they contain high concentrations of HBV. Infectivity is reduced, but probably not eliminated, in specimens containing anti-HBe (or low titers of HBsAg).

Attempts to isolate HBV in a cell or organ culture system have generally not been successful. However, successful transmission of HBV to chimpanzees has been achieved. The infection results in serologic, biochemical, and histologic evidence of type B hepatitis. Immunofluorescence and electron microscopy reveal HBsAg in the cytoplasm and viruslike particles with HBcAg in the nuclei of hepatocytes. Serial passage has been successful. No evidence for hepatitis B transmission from chimpanzees to humans has been reported.

Virus-Host Immune Reactions

Currently there is evidence for at least 3 hepatitis viruses—type A, type B, and the agent or agents of non-A, non-B hepatitis. A single infection with any confers homologous but not heterologous protection against reinfection. Infection with HBV of a specific subtype, eg, HBsAg/*adw*, appears to confer immunity to other HBsAg subtypes, probably because of their common group *a* specificity.

Most cases of hepatitis type A presumably occur without jaundice during childhood, and by late adulthood there is a widespread resistance to reinfection. However, serologic studies in the USA indicate that the incidence of infection among certain populations may be declining as a result of improvements in sanitation commensurate with a rise in the standard of liv-

Table 38–2. Common serologic tests for HBV and their interpretation.

Positive Tests	Interpretation
HBsAg (surface antigen)	Active hepatitis B infection, either acute or chronic.
Anti-HBs (in absence of HBsAg)	Protection against reinfection (immunity). Remains for years.
Anti-HBc (in absence of anti-HBs)	Active HBV infection cannot be excluded. A recent HBV infection can be confirmed by examining the sample for high titers of IgM anti-HBc.
HBeAg*	Active hepatitis infection, acute or chronic. Found in presence of HBsAg. Indicates specimens that exhibit potential for enhanced infectivity.
Anti-HBe	When present in HBsAg carrier, blood is potentially less infectious.

*Other HBV serologic markers that may be present at the same time include HBV (Dane particles), observable by electron microscopy. Core antigen and viral DNA polymerase can be measured by disrupting HBV.

ing. It has been estimated that as many as 60–90% of young middle- to upper-income adults in the USA may be susceptible to type A hepatitis. Younger people who live in poorer circumstances or crowded institutions (eg, military forces) are at increased risk.

The immunopathogenetic mechanisms that result in viral persistence and hepatocellular injury in type B hepatitis remain to be elucidated. Since the virus is not believed to be cytopathic, it is postulated that hepatocellular injury during acute disease represents T cell lysis of HBV-infected hepatocytes, whereas piecemeal necrosis may be a reflection of an autoimmune response to native liver membrane antigens induced by the virus. It is not known which of the various HBV-specified antigens are being recognized by the immunocompetent T cells. The degree of cell-mediated immunologic activity attained and the effects of immunoregulatory lipoprotein molecules generated by the infection may be responsible for continuation of the disease and for focal distribution of the hepatic necrosis. The role of antibody-dependent, complement-mediated cytolysis; defective suppressor cell function; and humoral immune mechanisms in the pathogenesis of this disease also is unclear at present.

Various host responses, immunologic and genetic, have been proposed to account for the frequency of HBsAg persistence, which has been observed to be higher in infants and children than in adults and higher in certain disease states, eg, Down's syndrome, leukemia (acute and chronic lymphocytic), leprosy, thalassemia, and chronic renal insufficiency. In comparison with other mentally retarded patients, patients with Down's syndrome are particularly prone to persistent antigenemia. This does not imply that patients with Down's syndrome have an increased susceptibility to HBV. On the contrary, among equally exposed patients who are residents within the same institution, the total serologic evidence of HBV infection is similar except that the antigen carrier rate is low and the antibody prevalence rate is high in patients who do not have Down's syndrome. An immunologic difference in the host response to the infectious virus is apparently responsible for this serologic dichotomy.

Persistent antigenemia and mild or subclinical infections are more frequently observed in individuals who have been infected with low doses of virus. Correspondingly, an inverse relationship between virus dose and time of appearance of HBsAg or an abnormal ALT value has been reported; ie, the incubation period becomes longer as the dose of virus diminishes.

The frequency of the chronic HBsAg carrier state following acute type B hepatitis is about 10%. More than half of these patients continue to exhibit biochemical and histologic evidence of chronic liver disease, ie, chronic persistent or chronic active hepatitis.

Treatment

Treatment of patients with hepatitis is directed at allowing hepatocellular damage to resolve and repair itself under optimal conditions. In previously healthy young military recruits, ad libitum ward privileges or strenuous exercise did not appear to alter the acute course of viral hepatitis. Therapeutic administration of corticosteroids with or without azathioprine has been successful in inducing remissions and prolonging survival in patients with progressive chronic active hepatitis, especially those with non-A, non-B hepatitis. These drugs are not recommended for use in cases of acute viral hepatitis, especially hepatitis B, since the development of a carrier state appears to be enhanced in this situation. Corticosteroids do not alter the clinical course of severe or fulminant hepatitis. Patients should be advised to avoid hepatotoxins such as alcohol during convalescence.

Interferon, vidarabine, and acyclovir have been remarkably successful in reducing the level of HBV markers and related antigens in the blood of chronic active hepatitis B patients and in improving the health of some patients so treated. However, the response has been temporary in most instances, with resumption of viral replication after discontinuation of the drug.

Epidemiology

The incidence of reported hepatitis in the USA had varied from 26 to 33 cases per 100,000 population, with about 70% categorized as hepatitis A, until 1983, when cases of hepatitis B exceeded those of hepatitis A for the first time. The actual incidence is undoubtedly much higher, because many persons contract so mild a form of hepatitis that they do not seek treatment, and physicians report only 10–20% of the cases they see. To permit more accurate hepatitis surveillance and to identify epidemiologic trends, all acute cases and confirmed carriers of type B hepatitis should be promptly reported to the local or state health department as required by law. The incidence of hepatitis A and B is highest in persons in the 20- to 29-year-old age group.

As shown in Table 38–1, there are marked differences in the epidemiologic features of hepatitis A, B, and non-A, non-B infections.

A. Viral Hepatitis Type A (Short Incubation Hepatitis): Outbreaks of type A hepatitis are common in families and institutions, summer camps, and especially among troops. The most likely mode of transmission under these conditions is by the fecal-oral route through close personal contact. Intestinal carriers probably do not exist. The clinical disease is most often manifest in children and young adults, with the highest rates in those between 15 and 30 years of age. The ratio of anicteric to icteric cases in adults is about 1:3; in children, it may be as high as 12:1.

Sudden, explosive epidemics of type A hepatitis usually result from fecal contamination of a single source (eg, drinking water, food, or milk). The consumption of raw oysters or improperly steamed clams obtained from water polluted with sewage has also resulted in several outbreaks of hepatitis.

Other recently identified sources of potential infection are nonhuman primates. There have been over 35 outbreaks in which primates, usually chimpanzees, have infected humans in close personal contact with them. These animals probably acquire the infection after arrival and transmit the virus to their caretakers. A persistent carrier state is unlikely, since the number of new cases diminishes with residence.

HAV seems to be hardly ever transmitted by the use of contaminated needles and syringes or through the administration of blood. Hemodialysis plays no role in the spread of hepatitis A infections to either patients or staff. The prevalence of anti-HAV is identical in persons with past histories of multiple blood transfusions or accidental inoculations with blood-contaminated instruments and in those from the same socioeconomic background without such exposures. About 30–60% of American adults possess antibodies, with a higher prevalence in those from lower socioeconomic groups.

B. Viral Hepatitis Type B (Long Incubation Hepatitis): HBV is also worldwide in distribution. There are about 200 million carriers, of whom close to 1 million live in the USA; 25% of carriers develop chronic active hepatitis. Each year in the USA, about 4000 persons die of HBV-associated cirrhosis and 800 die of HBV-related primary hepatocellular carcinoma.

There is no seasonal trend and no high predilection for any age group, although there are definite high-risk groups such as parenteral drug abusers, institutionalized persons, health care personnel, individuals who have recently received blood transfusions, hemodialysis patients and staff, highly promiscuous persons, and newborn infants born to mothers with hepatitis B. The incidence of hepatitis B among recipients of blood transfusions is about 1%. Since mandatory screening of blood donors for HBsAg was instituted and commercial donors are being replaced with all-volunteer donor sources, the number of icteric cases of transfusion-associated hepatitis has been substantially reduced. At present, non-A, non-B hepatitis accounts for the majority of transfusion-associated hepatitis cases in the USA.

Cases of hepatitis B appear sporadically and are often associated with the parenteral inoculation of infective human blood (or its products), usually obtained from an apparently healthy carrier. Thousands of cases have occurred following parenteral administration of human serum, plasma, whole blood or blood products, or vaccines that contained human serum. Many persons have been infected by improperly sterilized syringes, needles, or scalpels or even by tattooing or ear piercing. The estimated ratio of anicteric to icteric infections is reported to be as high as 4:1.

Other modes of transmission of hepatitis B exist. Volunteers who ingested infectious plasma developed infection. HBsAg can be detected in saliva, nasopharyngeal washings, semen, menstrual fluid, and vaginal secretions as well as in blood. Transmission from carriers to close contacts by the oral route or by sexual or other intimate exposure occurs. There is particularly strong evidence of transmission from persons with subclinical cases and carriers of HBsAg to homosexual and heterosexual long-term partners, although the precise mechanism of transmission is not clear. Transmission by the fecal-oral route has not been documented.

Health care personnel (surgeons, pathologists, and other physicians, dentists, nurses, laboratory technicians, and blood bank personnel) have a higher incidence of hepatitis and prevalence of detectable HBsAg or anti-HBs than those who have no occupational exposure to patients or blood products. The risk that these apparently healthy HBsAg carriers (especially medical and dental surgeons) represent to the patients under their care remains to be determined but is probably small.

Hepatitis B infections are common among patients and staff of hemodialysis units. Family contacts are also at increased risk. As many as 50% of the renal dialysis patients who contract hepatitis B may become chronic carriers of HBsAg compared with 2% of the staff group, emphasizing differences in the host immune response.

The presence of HBeAg, or a high concentration of HBsAg, in a person's serum is a useful marker for potentially high infectivity; in contrast, lower levels of infectivity appear to correlate best with the presence of anti-HBe.

Persons who have received a transfusion, especially from a paid donor, have a higher incidence of hepatitis and HBs antigenemia than nontransfused persons. This has led to the recommendation that anyone who has received a transfusion should not be allowed to serve as a blood donor. However, as commercial sources of blood donors are eliminated and newer, more sensitive methods for detecting HBsAg (radioimmunoassay, red cell agglutination) are employed, this recommendation is becoming less important.

Engorged mosquitoes and bedbugs, particularly if collected in homes of HBsAg carriers, may be positive for virus. Under suitable circumstances, they may play a role in viral dissemination.

The incubation period of hepatitis B is 50–180 days, with a mean between 60 and 90 days. It appears to vary with the dose of HBV administered and the route of administration, being prolonged in patients who receive a low dose of virus or who are infected by a nonpercutaneous route.

Gamma globulin and albumin are blood products that appear free from the risk of hepatitis B. Their method of preparation includes cold ethanol fractionation. In addition, albumin is heated to 60 °C for 10 hours.

C. Non-A, Non-B Hepatitis: In 1983, non-A, non-B hepatitis accounted for 6% of all reported cases of hepatitis in the USA but for 90% of the cases of transfusion-associated hepatitis. In addition, up to 25% of sporadic hepatitis cases may be caused by the agent or agents responsible for this disease entity. The incubation period ranges from 5 to 10 weeks, although both shorter (2 weeks) and longer (4 months) intervals have been observed. Serologic markers for active HAV, HBV, or other viral agents occasionally associated with hepatitis are absent. Thus, the diagnosis is one of exclusion in a patient with biochemical evidence of viral hepatitis. Specific methods for identifying this agent are not yet available. In the absence of such markers, attention has turned to other risk factors associated with this disease. The most meaningful predictor of the disease in a blood donor appears to be a high alanine aminotransferase (ALT, SGPT) value. Transfusion of a donor unit with an elevated ALT level of $\geq$ 45 IU/L significantly increases the recipient's risk of contracting non-A, non-B hepatitis.

D. Delta (δ) Agent: The δ agent is found throughout the world, but its highest prevalence is reported among Italians, persons who have received multiple transfusions (including intravenous drug abusers), and their close contacts. The primary routes of transmission are believed to be similar to those of HBV. Infection is dependent on HBV replication with synthesis of HBsAg. HBV provides a rescue function for the δ agent. Once infection is established, it interferes with the expression of HBV gene products and reduces the concentration of hepatitis B markers associated with infectivity. The incubation period varies from 2 to 12 weeks, being shorter in HBV carriers who are superinfected with the agent than in susceptible persons who are simultaneously infected with both HBV and the δ agent. Infection with the δ agent can be diagnosed by identifying an IgM anti-δ response during the acute or chronic stage of the disease. Persons who have recovered from δ infection are immune to rechallenge with that agent or with HBV.

Two epidemiologic patterns of δ infection have been identified. In Mediterranean countries (northern Africa, southern Europe, and the Middle East), δ infection is endemic among persons with hepatitis B, and most infections are thought to be transmitted by intimate contact. In nonendemic areas, such as the USA and northern Europe, δ infection is confined to persons exposed frequently to blood and blood products, primarily drug addicts and hemophiliacs. Whether in endemic or nonendemic countries, the only persons with any appreciable risk of transfusion-associated δ hepatitis are those who receive pooled blood derivatives obtained from thousands of donors. This group includes persons with inherited or acquired coagulation problems who are receiving commercial clotting factor concentrates. The same demographic factors that increase the likelihood of hepatitis B and non-A, non-B hepatitis in commercial blood donors also contribute to their enhanced risk of exposure to the δ agent.

Delta hepatitis was not found in Swedish drug addicts before 1973. In the ensuing decade, its incidence in that population increased to about 75% of all addicts who were hepatitis B carriers; the disease involved their intimate contacts as well. Delta hepatitis also may occur in explosive outbreaks and affect entire localized pockets of hepatitis B carriers. Outbreaks of severe, often fulminant and chronic δ hepatitis have occurred for decades in isolated populations in the Orinoco and Amazon basins of South America and have been given such exotic names as "Labrea fever" and "hepatitis of the Sierra Nevada de Santa Marta." Severe outbreaks of δ hepatitis are not confined to isolated, remote regions of developing countries. In Worcester, Massachusetts, more than 200 drug addicts and their sexual partners have been affected, and 9 have died since 1983. In the USA, δ virus has been found to participate in 20–30% of cases of chronic hepatitis B, acute exacerbations of chronic hepatitis B, and fulminant hepatitis B; and 3–12% of blood donors with serum HBsAg have antibodies to the δ virus. Delta hepatitis is not a new disease, because globulin lots prepared from plasma collected in the USA 40 years ago contain antibodies to the δ virus.

Prevention & Control

A vaccine for hepatitis B is available. Vaccine is prepared by purifying HBsAg associated with the 22-nm particles from healthy HBsAg-positive carriers and treating the particles with virus-inactivating agents (formalin, urea, heat). Protection is conferred by antibody to the *a* antigen, an antigen common to all subtypes. Preparations containing intact 22-nm particles have been highly effective in reducing HBV infection in hemodialysis patients and staff, among homosexuals, and in newborns born to HBV-infected mothers. Other sources of immunogen are being developed: (1) HBsAg produced by a recombinant DNA in yeast cells containing a plasmid into which the gene for HBsAg has been incorporated, (2) polypeptides derived from the 22-nm particles, and (3) a recombinant of live vaccinia virus and the HBsAg gene. All of these new sources have been used successfully in immunizing chimpanzees, and new vaccines should soon replace the plasma-derived vaccine.

The vaccine made from yeast will be a second-generation vaccine. The purified HBsAg used for this vaccine exists as particles 15–30 nm in diameter, with the morphologic characteristics of free surface antigen in plasma and of the purified antigen now used in plasma-derived hepatitis B vaccine. In contrast to HBsAg from human plasma, the antigen produced by recombinant yeast is not glycosylated. Under reducing conditions, sodium dodecyl sulfate electrophoresis of the antigen purified from yeast reveals a single band with a molecular weight of 23,000; this corresponds to the nonglycosylated polypeptide that is the major component of the HBV envelope. The vaccine formulated using this material has now been shown to be immunogenic for animals and for humans, with a potency similar to that of vaccine made from plasma-derived antigen. In addition, chimpanzees immunized with this yeast recombinant hepatitis B vaccine (HBsAg, subtype *adw*) were protected when challenged with virus of subtype *adr* or *ayw*, whereas nonimmunized animals were infected when challenged with live virus.

Since a source of large amounts of HAV has not been found, the development of a vaccine for hepatitis A depends on the future success of cell culture systems for growing the agent. An experimental (attenuated virus) vaccine is currently undergoing phase I clinical trials in humans.

Until all susceptible at-risk groups are immunized, prevention and control of hepatitis must be directed toward interrupting the chain of transmission and using passive immunization.

A. Viral Hepatitis Type A: The appearance of hepatitis in camps or institutions is often an indication of poor sanitation and poor personal hygiene. Control measures are directed toward the prevention of fecal contamination of food, water, or other sources by the individual. Reasonable hygiene—such as hand washing after bowel movements or before meals, the use of disposable plates and eating utensils, and the use of 0.5% sodium hypochlorite (eg, 1:10 dilution of Clorox) as a disinfectant—is essential in preventing the spread of HAV during the acute phase of the illness. Extraordinarily conservative measures, such as the use of gowns, masks, and gloves, are usually unnecessary unless there is exposure to feces or fecally contaminated items. Infectivity studies indicate that the risk of transmitting hepatitis A is greatest from 2 weeks before to 1 week after the onset of jaundice. Transmission by the aerosol route appears relatively unimportant. (See General Properties of the Viruses, p 444.)

Immune human globulin (IG) is prepared from large pools of normal adult plasma and confers passive protection in about 90% of those exposed when given within 1–2 weeks after exposure to hepatitis A. Its prophylactic value decreases with time, and its administration more than 4 weeks after exposure or after the onset of clinical symptoms is probably not indicated.

In the doses generally prescribed, IG does not prevent infection but rather makes the infection mild or subclinical and permits active immunity to develop. For ordinary exposure, the dose is 0.02 mL/kg given once intramuscularly during the incubation period. For persons with continuing exposure (Peace Corps workers, military personnel, chimpanzee handlers, travelers to endemic areas), 0.05–0.1 mL/kg can be given every 4–6 months. Simplified guidelines for IG prophylaxis against hepatitis A are shown in Table 38–3.

B. Viral Hepatitis Type B: Persons who have had hepatitis probably should not be used as blood donors. Even persons without a history of hepatitis and with normal liver function tests may be carriers of

the virus. In addition, HBV carriers (or those with non-A, non-B hepatitis) may develop acute hepatitis A and the underlying condition may go unrecognized. Sensitive methods for detecting HBsAg in blood donors are now being employed by all blood banks to avoid administering HBsAg-positive blood. Nevertheless, cases of posttransfusion hepatitis B continue to occur, although at a reduced frequency. Since the incidence of posttransfusion hepatitis (both B and non-B) is higher among recipients of commercial (paid donor) blood or blood from first-time donors, the establishment of an all-volunteer population who donate periodically is an important measure for eliminating transfusion-associated hepatitis. However, registries of minimal-risk donors who are known to be in good health should also provide satisfactory sources of blood, even if such persons are paid.

Proper donor selection and the development of a central registry for identification of carriers can lower the incidence of transfusion-associated hepatitis. In addition, blood or its products should be used only when necessary, since the risk of hepatitis appears to increase with the number of units administered. Hepatitis B virus may be transmitted to personnel in blood transfusion laboratories, but there is no evidence for the transmission of infection from members of the staff to blood or blood products.

Patients with acute type B hepatitis generally need not be isolated so long as blood and instrument precautions are stringently observed, both in the general patient care areas and in the laboratories. Staff members should wear gloves or other protective clothing when in contact with blood or blood-contaminated objects from these patients. Because spouses and intimate contacts of persons with acute type B hepatitis are at greater risk of acquiring clinical type B hepatitis than those exposed to healthy carriers, they need to be warned about practices that might increase the risk of infection or transmission.

There is no justification for removing HBsAg-positive carriers from patient contact in the absence of evidence of disease transmission. The use of gloves should reduce the potential for HBV transmission. There is no evidence that asymptomatic HBsAg-positive food handlers pose a health risk to the general public.

The resistance of HBV to physical and chemical agents makes it difficult to treat human blood and its products to render them safe for human inoculation. Autoclaving and the use of ethylene oxide gas are both acceptable methods for disinfecting metal objects, instruments, or heat-sensitive equipment. Another useful germicide is 2% activated glutaraldehyde.

Since as little as 0.0001 mL of plasma can transmit the disease, a single carrier of hepatitis B virus might "infect" a large batch of pooled plasma. It has been recommended, therefore, that pooled plasma not be used. If pools must be used, they should be made from blood from no more than 5 donors and each unit tested for HBsAg by one of the more sensitive methods (eg, radioimmunoassay) prior to pooling. Pooled plasma

Table 38–3. Guidelines for IG prophylaxis against hepatitis A.

Person's Weight (kg)	IG Dose (mL)	
	Routine	High Risk* (Prolonged Exposure)
< 22	0.5	1.0
22–45	1.0	2.5
> 45	2.0	5.0

*Within limits, larger doses of IG provide longer-lasting but not necessarily more protection. Therefore, more IG is prescribed in high-risk situations where continuous exposure is anticipated (institutional contacts, travelers to foreign countries).

should be used only in cases of emergency, because of the possibility of transmitting hepatitis B to a patient who is already ill.

Studies on passive immunization using specific hepatitis B immune globulin (HBIG) have been encouraging. A special immune globulin from plasma containing anti-HBs with a titer 50,000 times greater than standard commercial IG was prepared and administered to 10 susceptible children 4 hours after they had been exposed to infectious serum containing HBV. Six subjects failed to develop HBs antigenemia or biochemical evidence of hepatitis, for a 60% level of protection. In contrast, all 11 control children who received the same dose of virus but without IG became infected (HBsAg-positive).

Studies that have compared placebo with IG containing anti-HBs have indicated a protective effect if the latter is given soon after exposure. However, the concentration of antibody required for protection has not been adequately ascertained. In one study, the protective activity of 3 preparations of immune globulin containing varying levels of antibody to HBsAg was compared. Subjects included hospital personnel accidentally exposed to hepatitis B and newly admitted patients or recently hired employees of renal dialysis units. Since there was no placebo group and the results did not favor one anti-HBs preparation over another, any protective results are difficult to interpret. However, the incubation period of hepatitis B was prolonged significantly in those volunteers receiving the high-titer preparation.

Evidence of passive-active immunity was more frequently observed among newly admitted institutionalized patients who received standard IG containing a low concentration of anti-HBs than among those treated with an anti-HBs-rich preparation of IG. It is noteworthy that both preparations successfully prevented the development of a chronic carrier state. Similarly, administration of specific HBIG (or conventional IG with titers of anti-HBs greater than 1:256) to spouses of patients with acute type B hepatitis has been shown to be effective in preventing not only symptomatic type B hepatitis but the infection itself. However, passive-active immunity appeared to occur more frequently in susceptible individuals receiving conventional IG.

Prevention of transfusion-associated hepatitis by the administration of standard IG has not been consistently demonstrated in carefully conducted trials. Therefore, although HBIG has been officially released for clinical use in exposure to small amounts of HBV, such as might occur with an accidental prick with a contaminated needle or direct mucous membrane contact arising from a splash or pipetting accident, its routine administration to recipients of blood transfusions is not recommended.

Women who are HBV carriers or who acquire type B hepatitis while pregnant can transmit the disease to their infants. The risk of transmission is increased during the third trimester and the postpartum period. Infants who become HBsAg-positive generally do so within 1–2 months, but testing should continue at monthly intervals for at least 6 months. Most develop persistent antigenemia, especially if the mother is also HBeAg-positive. The effectiveness of HBIG in preventing hepatitis B in infants born to these HBV-positive mothers has been substantiated in several studies. Infants are given 0.5 mL of HBIG plus 10 μg of vaccine concurrently but at a different site within a few hours of birth. If vaccine is not immediately available, it should be given within the next 7 days. A second dose of vaccine should be given at 1 month and a third dose at 6 months of age.

Preexposure prophylaxis with a commercially available hepatitis B vaccine currently is recommended by the World Health Organization, the Centers for Disease Control, and the Advisory Committee on Immunization Practices for all susceptible, at-risk groups. The human-plasma-derived vaccine (Heptavax-B) has been administered in many countries, with extensive follow-up of vaccinees. Except for mild discomfort at the injection site, the product has been shown to be safe, immunogenic, and effective in preventing hepatitis B.

The plasma-derived hepatitis B vaccine became available in the USA in mid 1982, and about 800,000 persons had been vaccinated by mid 1985. However, at this writing, there has not been any significant decrease in incidence of acute hepatitis B. About 23,000 cases have been reported annually in the period 1982–1985, but the estimated number of cases is 200,000 per year. Apparently the high-risk groups—with the exception of health-care workers—are not taking the vaccine; these include homosexual males, heterosexuals with multiple sexual partners, intravenous drug abusers, prisoners, residents and staff members of mental institutions, and immigrants from Vietnam, Haiti, and other areas of high endemicity.

HBV vaccination in hemodialysis patients has not always been successful. Seroconversion rates vary with the intensity of their cell-mediated immune response as determined by the skin reaction to dinitrochlorobenzene. Patients with a strong skin reaction react as well as healthy persons to the vaccine, but those with a weak skin reaction need higher doses of vaccine.

Guidelines for postexposure prophylaxis have been established by the Center for Infectious Diseases, Centers for Disease Control (Tables 38–4 and 38–5). Persons exposed to HBV percutaneously or by contamination of the mucosal surfaces should immediately receive both HBIG and HBsAg vaccine administered simultaneously at different sites to provide immediate protection with passively acquired antibody followed by active immunity generated by the vaccine. IG or HBsAg vaccine is of no demonstrable benefit in the treatment of HBsAg carriers.

Delta hepatitis can be prevented by vaccinating HBV-susceptible persons with hepatitis B vaccine. However, vaccination does not protect hepatitis B carriers from superinfection by δ virus.

Table 38–4. Hepatitis B virus postexposure recommendations.

| Exposure | HBIG | | Vaccine | |
	Dose	Recommended Timing	Dose	Recommended Timing
Perinatal	0.5 mL IM	Within 12 hours of birth.	0.5 mL (10 μg) IM	Within 12 hours of birth;* repeat at 1 and 6 months.
Sexual	0.06 mL/kg IM	Single dose within 14 days of sexual contact.	†	—

*The first dose can be given the same time as the HBIG dose but at a different site.
†Vaccine is recommended for homosexual men and for regular sexual contacts of HBV carriers and is optional in initial treatment of heterosexual contacts of persons with acute HBV.

Table 38–5. Recommendations for hepatitis B prophylaxis following percutaneous exposure.

| Source | Exposed Person | |
	Unvaccinated	Vaccinated
HBsAg-positive	1. HBIG once immediately.* 2. Initiate HB vaccine† series.	1. Test exposed person for anti-HBs. 2. If inadequate antibody,‡ HBIG once immediately plus HB vaccine booster dose.
Known source High-risk HBsAg-positive	1. Initiate HB vaccine series. 2. Test source for HBsAg. If positive, HBIG once.	1. Test source for HBsAg only if exposed person is vaccine nonresponder; if source is HBsAg-positive, give HBIG once immediately plus HB vaccine booster dose.
Low-risk HBsAg-positive	Initiate HB vaccine series.	Nothing required.
Unknown source	Initiate HB vaccine series.	Nothing required.

*HBIG dose 0.06 mL/kg IM.
*HB vaccine dose 20 μg IM for adults; 10 μg IM for infants or children under 10 years of age. First dose within 1 week; second and third doses, 1 and 6 months later.
‡Less than 10 sample ratio units by RIA, negative by enzyme immunoassay.

REFERENCES

Blumberg BS: Australia antigen and the biology of hepatitis B. *Science* 1977;**197**:17.

Bramwell SP et al: Dinitrochlorobenzene skin testing predicts response to hepatitis B vaccine in dialysis patients. *Lancet* 1985;**1**:1412.

Deinhardt F, Gust ID: Viral hepatitis. *Bull WHO* 1982;**60**:661.

Gerin JL et al: Chemically synthesized peptides of hepatitis B surface antigen duplicate the *d/y* specificities and induce subtype-specific antibodies in chimpanzees. *Proc Natl Acad Sci USA* 1983;**80**:2365.

Harmon FR, Melnick JL: Synthetic vaccines for viral hepatitis. In: *Synthetic Vaccines*. Arnon R (editor). CRC Press, 1986.

Hollinger FB, Dienstag JL: Hepatitis viruses. Pages 813–835 in: *Manual of Clinical Microbiology*, 4th ed. Lennette EH (editor). American Society for Microbiology, 1985.

Hollinger FB, Melnick JL, Robinson WS: *Viral Hepatitis: Biological and Clinical Features, Specific Diagnosis, and Prophylaxis*. Raven Press, 1985.

Immunization Practices Advisory Committee: Recommendations for protection against viral hepatitis. *MMWR* 1985; **34**:313.

Krugman S, Giles JP: Viral hepatitis, type B (MS-2 strain): Further observations on natural history and prevention. *N Engl J Med* 1973;**288**:755.

Laure F et al: Hepatitis B virus DNA sequences in lymphoid cells from patients with AIDS and AIDS-related complex. *Science* 1985;**229**:561.

Maupas P, Melnick JL (editors): Hepatitis B virus and primary hepatocellular carcinoma. *Prog Med Virol* 1981;No. 27.

Melnick JL, Dreesman GR, Hollinger FB: Approaching the control of viral hepatitis type B. *J Infect Dis* 1976;**133**:210.

Milich DR et al: Enhanced immunogenicity of the pre-S region of hepatitis B surface antigen. *Science* 1985;**228**:1195.

Nishioka NS, Dienstag JL: Delta hepatitis: A new scourge? *N Engl J Med* 1985;**312**:1515.

Rosina F, Saracco G, Rizzetto M: Risk of post-transfusion infection with the hepatitis delta virus: A multicenter study. *N Engl J Med* 985;**312**:1488.

Smith GL, Mackett M, Moss B: Infectious vaccinia virus recombinants that express hepatitis B virus surface antigen. *Nature* 1983;**302**:490.

Szmuness W et al: Hepatitis B vaccine: Demonstration of efficacy in a controlled clinical trial in a high-risk population in the United States. *N Engl J Med* 1980;**303**:833.

Tabor E: The three viruses of non-A, non-B hepatitis. *Lancet* 1985;**1**:743.

Ticehurst JR et al: Molecular cloning and characterization of hepatitis A virus cDNA. *Proc Natl Acad Sci USA* 1983; **80**:5885.

Vyas GN, Dienstag JL, Hoofnagle JH (editors): *Viral Hepatitis and Liver Disease*. Grune & Stratton, 1984.

Rabies & Other Viral Diseases of the Nervous System; Slow Viruses

39

RABIES

Rabies is an acute infection of the central nervous system that is almost always fatal. The virus is usually transmitted to humans from the bite of a rabid animal.

Properties of the Virus

A. Structure: Rabies virus is a rhabdovirus with morphologic and biochemical properties in common with vesicular stomatitis virus of cattle and several animal, plant, and insect viruses. The rhabdoviruses are rod- or bullet-shaped particles measuring 60–400 nm × 60–85 nm (Fig 33–37). The particles are surrounded by a membranous envelope with protruding spikes 10 nm long. Inside the envelope is a ribonucleocapsid. The genome is single-stranded RNA (MW $3–5 \times 10^6$) that is not infectious and does not serve as a messenger. Virions contain an RNA-dependent RNA polymerase.

B. Reactions to Physical and Chemical Agents: Rabies virus survives storage at 4 °C for weeks but is inactivated by CO_2. On dry ice, therefore, it must be stored in glass-sealed vials. Rabies virus is killed rapidly by exposure to ultraviolet radiation or sunlight, by heat (1 hour at 50 °C), by lipid solvents (ether, 0.1% sodium deoxycholate), and by trypsin.

C. Animal Susceptibility and Growth of Virus: Rabies virus has a wide host range. All warm-blooded animals, including humans, are susceptible. The virus is widely distributed in infected animals, especially in the nervous system, saliva, urine, lymph, milk, and blood. Recovery from infection is rare except in certain bats, where the virus has become peculiarly adapted to the salivary glands. Vampire bats may transmit the virus for months without themselves ever showing any signs of disease.

When freshly isolated in the laboratory, the strains are referred to as street virus. Such strains show long and variable incubation periods (usually 21–60 days in dogs) and regularly produce intracytoplasmic inclusion bodies. Inoculated animals may exhibit long periods of excitement and viciousness. The virus may invade the salivary glands as well as the central nervous system.

Serial brain-to-brain passage in rabbits yields a "fixed" virus that no longer multiplies in extraneural tissues. This fixed virus multiplies rapidly, and the incubation period is shortened to 4–6 days. At this stage, inclusion bodies are found only with difficulty.

The virus may be propagated in chick embryos, baby hamster kidney cells, and human diploid cell cultures. One strain (Flury), after serial passage in chick embryos, has been modified so that it fails to produce disease in animals injected extraneurally. This attenuated virus is used for vaccination of animals.

The replication of rabies virus is similar to that of the most studied rhabdovirus, vesicular stomatitis virus. The single-stranded RNA genome of molecular weight 4.6×10^6 is transcribed by the virion-associated RNA polymerase to 5 mRNA species that are complementary to parts of the genome. These mRNAs code for the 5 virion proteins. The genome is a template for a replicative intermediate responsible for the generation of progeny RNA. After encapsidation, the bullet-shaped particles acquire the envelope by budding through the cytoplasmic membrane.

D. Antigenic Properties: The purified spikes elicit Nt antibody in animals. Antiserum prepared against the purified nucleocapsid is used in diagnostic immunofluorescence.

Pathogenesis & Pathology

Rabies virus multiplies in muscle or connective tissue and is propagated through the endoneurium of the Schwann cells or associated tissue spaces of the sensory nerves to the central nervous system. It multiplies there and may then spread through peripheral nerves to the salivary glands and other tissues. Rabies virus has not been isolated from the blood of infected persons.

The incubation period may depend on the amount of inoculum, severity of lacerations, and distance the virus has to travel from its point of entry to the brain. There is a higher attack rate and shorter incubation period in persons bitten on the face or head.

There are hyperemia and nerve cell destruction in the cortex, midbrain, basal ganglia, pons, and especially the medulla. Demyelinization occurs in the white matter, and degeneration of axons and myelin sheaths is common. In the spinal cord, the posterior horns are most severely involved, with neuronophagia and cellular infiltrates (mononuclear, perivascular, and perineural).

Rabies virus produces a specific cytoplasmic inclusion, the Negri body, in infected nerve cells. The presence of such inclusions is pathognomonic of rabies but may not be observed in all cases. The inclusions are eosinophilic, sharply demarcated, and more or less spherical, with diameters of 2–10 μm. Several may be found in the cytoplasm of large neurons. They occur throughout the brain and spinal cord but are most frequent in Ammon's horn. Negri bodies contain rabies virus antigens and can be demonstrated by immunofluorescence.

Rabies virus multiplies outside the central nervous system and may produce cellular infiltrates and necrosis in salivary and other glands, in the cornea, and elsewhere.

The post-rabies vaccine reaction is an allergic encephalomyelitis (see p 201).

Clinical Findings

The usual incubation period in dogs ranges from 3 to 8 weeks, but it may be as short as 10 days. Clinically, the disease in dogs is divided into 3 phases: prodromal, excitative, and paralytic. The prodromal phase is characterized by fever and a sudden change in the temperament of the animal; docile animals may become snappy and irritable, whereas aggressive animals may become more affectionate. The excitative phase lasts 3–7 days, during which the dog shows symptoms of irritability, restlessness, nervousness, and exaggerated response to sudden light and sound stimuli. At this stage the animal is most dangerous because of its tendency to bite. The animal has difficulty in swallowing, suffers from convulsive seizures, and enters into a paralytic stage with paralysis of the whole body, coma, and death. Sometimes the animal goes into the paralytic stage without passing through the excitative stage.

The incubation period in humans varies from 2 to 16 weeks or more, but in many cases it is only 2–3 weeks. It is usually shorter in children than in adults. The clinical spectrum can be divided into 4 phases: a short prodromal phase, a sensory phase, a period of excitement, and a paralytic or depressive phase. The prodrome, lasting 2–4 days, may show any of the following: malaise, anorexia, headache, nausea and vomiting, sore throat, and fever. Usually there is an abnormal sensation around the site of infection. The patient may show increasing nervousness and apprehension. General sympathetic overactivity is observed, including lacrimation, pupillary dilatation, and increased salivation and perspiration. The act of swallowing precipitates a spasm of the throat muscles; a patient may allow saliva to drool from the mouth simply to avoid swallowing and the associated painful spasms. (Because of the patient's apparent fear of water, the disease has been known as hydrophobia since ancient days.) This phase is followed by convulsive seizures or coma and death, usually 3–5 days following onset. Progressive paralytic symptoms may develop before death.

Hysteria may simulate certain features of rabies, particularly in persons who have been near a rabid animal or have been bitten by a nonrabid one.

Laboratory Diagnosis

A. Microscopy: Tissues infected with rabies virus are currently identified most rapidly and accurately by means of direct immunofluorescence using antirabies hamster serum. (See Chapter 34.) Impression preparations of brain or cornea tissue are often used.

A definitive pathologic diagnosis of rabies is based on the finding of Negri bodies in the brain (especially Ammon's horn) or the spinal cord. Negri bodies are found in impression preparations or histologic sections. They are sharply demarcated, more or less spherical, and 2–10 μm in diameter, and they have a distinctive internal structure with basophilic granules in an eosinophilic matrix. Negri bodies (and rabies antigen) can usually be found in animals or humans suffering from rabies or dead from the infection, but they are rarely found in bats.

B. Virus Isolation: Available tissue (or saliva) is inoculated intracerebrally into mice. Infection in mice results in flaccid paralysis of legs, encephalitis, and death. The central nervous system of the inoculated animal is examined for Negri bodies and rabies antigen. In specialized laboratories, hamster and mouse cell lines can be inoculated for rapid (2–4 day) growth of rabies virus; this is much faster than growth in mice. An isolated virus is identified by Nt tests with specific antiserum.

C. Serology: Antibodies to rabies can be detected by immunofluorescence, CF, or Nt tests. Such antibodies may develop in infected persons or animals during progression of the disease.

All animals considered "rabid or suspected rabid" (Table 39–1) should be sacrificed immediately for laboratory examination of tissues. Other animals, if available, should be held for observation for 10 days. If they show any signs of encephalitis, rabies, or unusual behavior, they should be killed humanely and the tissues examined in the laboratory. On the other hand, if they appear normal after 10 days, decisions must be made on an individual basis in consultation with public health officials.

Immunity & Prevention

Only one antigenic type of rabies virus is known. More than 99% of infections in humans and mammals who develop symptoms end fatally. Survival after proved rabies infection is extremely rare. It is therefore essential that individuals at high risk receive preventive immunization, that the nature and risk of any exposure be evaluated (Table 39–1), and that individuals be given postexposure prophylaxis if their exposure is believed to have been dangerous.

A. Pathophysiology of Rabies Prevention by Vaccine: It is likely that rabies virus remains latent in tissues for some time after virus is introduced from a bite. If immunogenic vaccine or antibody can be administered promptly, the virus can be prevented from invading the central nervous system. The action of passively administered antibody is to provide additional time for a vaccine to stimulate active **antibody**

Table 39–1. Rabies postexposure prophylaxis guide, 1980.*

The following recommendations are only a guide. In applying them, take into account the animal species involved, the circumstances of the bite or other exposure, the vaccination status of the animal, and presence of rabies in the region. *Local or state public health officials should be consulted if questions arise about the need for rabies prophylaxis.*

Animal Species	Condition of Animal at Time of Attack	Treatment of Exposed Person†
Domestic Dog and cat	Healthy and available for 10 days of observation	None, unless animal develops rabies‡
	Rabid or suspected rabid	RIG§ and HDCV**
	Unknown (escaped)	Consult public health officials. If treatment is indicated, give RIG§ and HDCV**
Wild Skunk, bat, fox, coyote, raccoon, bobcat, and other carnivores	Regard as rabid unless proved negative by laboratory tests††	RIG§ and HDCV**
Other Livestock, rodents, and lagomorphs (rabbits and hares)	Consider individually. Local and state public health officials should be consulted on questions about the need for rabies prophylaxis. Bites of squirrels, hamsters, guinea pigs, gerbils, chipmunks, rats, mice, other rodents, rabbits, and hares almost never call for antirabies prophylaxis.	

*Reproduced, with permission, from *MMWR* (June) 1980;**29**:279.
†*All bites and wounds should immediately be thoroughly cleansed with soap and water.* If antirabies treatment is indicated, both rabies immune globulin (RIG) and human diploid cell rabies vaccine (HDCV) should be given as soon as possible, *regardless* of the interval from exposure.
‡During the usual holding period of 10 days, begin treatment with RIG and vaccine (preferably HDCV) at first sign of rabies in a dog or cat that has bitten someone. The symptomatic animal should be killed immediately and tested.
§If RIG is not available, use antirabies serum, equine (ARS). Do not use more than the recommended dosage.
**If HDCV is not available, use duck embryo vaccine (DEV). Local reactions to vaccines are common and do not contraindicate continuing treatment. Discontinue vaccine if fluorescent antibody (FA) tests of the animal are negative.
††The animal should be killed and tested as soon as possible. Holding for observation is not recommended.

production before the central nervous system is invaded.

B. Types of Vaccines: All vaccines for human use contain only inactivated rabies virus.

1. Nerve tissue vaccine–This is made from infected sheep, goat, or mouse brains and used in many parts of the world including Asia, Africa, and South America. It causes sensitization to nerve tissue and results in postvaccinal encephalitis (an allergic disease) with substantial frequency (0.05%). It has not been used in the USA for several decades. Estimates of its efficacy in persons bitten by rabid animals vary from 5% to 50%.

2. Duck embryo vaccine–This was developed to minimize the problem of postvaccinal encephalitis. The rabies virus is grown in embryonated duck eggs, but the head is removed before the vaccine is prepared so as to remove nervous tissue and avoid allergic encephalitis. It produces local reactions regularly and systemic reactions (fever, malaise, myalgia) in one-third of recipients. Neuroparalytic (< 0.001%) and anaphylactic (< 1%) reactions are infrequent, but the antigenicity of the vaccine is low. Consequently, many (16–25) doses have to be given to obtain a satisfactory postexposure antibody response. This was the vaccine used in the USA in the recent past.

3. Human diploid cell vaccine (HDCV)–To obtain a rabies virus suspension free from nervous system and foreign proteins, rabies virus was adapted to growth in the WI-38 human normal fibroblast cell line.

The rabies virus harvest is concentrated by ultrafiltration and inactivated with beta propiolactone or tri-N-butyl phosphate. This material is sufficiently antigenic that only 4–6 doses of virus (Table 39–2) need to be given to obtain a substantial antibody response in most recipients. Local reactions (erythema, itching, swelling at the injection site) occur in 25% of recipients, and mild systemic reactions (headache, nausea, myalgia, dizziness) occur in about one-fifth of recipients. No serious anaphylactic, neuroparalytic, or encephalitic reactions have been reported. This vaccine has been used in the USA since 1979. A vaccine made in a diploid cell line derived from the lung of a fetal rhesus monkey also became available in 1985.

4. Live attenuated viruses–Live attenuated viruses adapted to growth in chick embryos (eg, Flury strain) are used for animals but *not* for humans. Occasionally, such vaccines can cause death from rabies in injected cats or dogs. Rabies viruses grown in various animal cell cultures have also been used as vaccines for domestic animals.

C. Types of Available Rabies Antibody:

1. Rabies immune globulin, human (RIG)–This is a gamma globulin prepared by cold ethanol fractionation from the plasma of hyperimmunized humans. The neutralizing antibody content is standardized to 150 IU/mL. The dose is 20 IU/kg, half given around the bite wound and the other half intramuscularly.

2. Antirabies serum, equine (ARS)–This is

Table 39–2. Rabies immunization regimens, 1980.*

Preexposure: Preexposure rabies prophylaxis for persons with special risks of exposure to rabies, such as animal-care and control personnel and selected laboratory workers, consists of immunization with either human diploid cell rabies vaccine (HDCV) or duck embryo vaccine (DEV), according to the following schedule.

Rabies Vaccine	Number of 1-mL Doses	Route of Administration	Intervals Between Doses	If No Antibody Response to Primary Series, Give–†
HDCV	3	Intramuscular	One week between 1st and 2nd; 2–3 weeks between 2nd and 3rd‡	One booster dose‡
DEV	3 or 4	Subcutaneous	One month between 1st and 2nd; 6–7 months between 2nd and 3rd‡ *or* One week between 1st, 2nd, and 3rd; 3 months between 3rd and 4th‡	Two booster doses,‡ 1 week apart

Postexposure: Postexposure rabies prophylaxis for persons exposed to rabies consists of the immediate, thorough cleansing of all wounds with soap and water, administration of rabies immune globulin (RIG) or, if RIG is not available, antirabies serum, equine (ARS), and the initiation of either HDCV or DEV, according to the following schedule.§

HDCV	5**	Intramuscular	Doses to be given on days 0, 3, 7, 14, and 28‡	An additional booster dose‡
DEV	23	Subcutaneous	Twenty-one daily doses followed by a booster on day 31 and another on day 41‡ *or* Two daily doses in the first 7 days, followed by 7 daily doses. Then one booster on day 24 and another on day 34‡	Three doses of HDCV at weekly intervals‡

*Reproduced, with permission, from *MMWR* (June) 1980;**29**:280.
†If no antibody response is documented after the recommended additional booster dose(s), consult the state health department or CDC.
‡Serum for rabies antibody testing should be collected 2–3 weeks after the last dose.
§The postexposure regimen is greatly modified for someone with previously demonstrated rabies antibody.
**The World Health Organization recommends a sixth dose 90 days after the first dose.

concentrated serum from horses hyperimmunized with rabies virus. The neutralizing antibody content is standardized to contain 1000 IU per vial (approximately 5 mL). The dose is 40 IU/kg.

D. Choice of Rabies Immunizing Products: This is an application of the risk/benefit ratio, as far as known for each product. HDCV has the greatest efficacy among known vaccines in stimulating antibody production, and few adverse effects are associated with it. There are fewer reactions to RIG (especially rare serum sickness, anaphylaxis) than to ARS, and RIG has a much longer half-life, since it is protein homologous for the human recipient.

E. Preexposure Prophylaxis: This is indicated for persons at high risk of contact with rabid animals. The goal is to attain an antibody level presumed to be protective by means of vaccine administration prior to any exposure. Current suggested schedules are shown in Table 39–2.

F. Postexposure Prophylaxis: Since 1960, 1–5 cases of human rabies have occurred in the USA per year, but every year 20–30 thousand persons receive some treatment for possible bite-wound exposure. *All* bites should be thoroughly cleaned with soap and water immediately, and tetanus prophylaxis should be considered. The decision to administer rabies antibody, rabies vaccine, or both, depends on (1) the nature of the biting animal (Table 39–1) and its vaccination status; *all* bites by wild animals and bats require RIG and HDCV; (2) the existence of rabies in the area; (3) the manner of attack (provoked or unpro-

voked) and the severity of bite and contamination by saliva of the animal; and (4) advice from local public health officials. Schedules for postexposure prophylaxis involving the administration of RIG (or ARS) and HDCV (or DEV) are shown in the 1980 recommendations for the USA (Table 39–2). Different materials and schedules may be proposed in other parts of the world depending on availability of products and local experience.

Epidemiology

About 1000 cases of human rabies are reported each year to the World Health Organization, most of them in developing countries, eg, India, Southeast Asia, the Philippines, North Africa, and South America. In these countries, most human cases develop from the bite of rabid dogs, and perhaps 1 million persons are given postexposure prophylaxis yearly.

In the USA, Canada, and western Europe, cases of human rabies develop from bites of wild animals (especially skunks, foxes, and bats) or are imported by travelers bitten elsewhere in the world. In South America, near Trinidad, rabies is transmitted especially by vampire bats that normally suck the blood of cattle (and may cause outbreaks among them) but may also bite humans. The increase in wildlife rabies in the USA and some other developed countries presents a far greater risk to humans than dogs or cats do. Wild animals trapped and sold as pets can be the source of human exposure.

In 1981, over 7000 laboratory-confirmed cases of

animal rabies were reported in the USA and its territories. Seven kinds of animals accounted for 97% of these cases: skunks (62%), bats (12%), raccoons (7%), cattle (6%), cats (4%), dogs (3%), and foxes (3%). Of these, 85% of cases occurred in wild animals and 15% in domestic animals. Approximately 95,000 animals were tested, giving a positive detection rate of 8%.

Bats present a special problem because they may carry rabies virus while they appear to be healthy, excrete it in saliva, and transmit it to other animals, including other bats, and to humans. South American vampire bats may transmit rabies to insectivorous bats living in caves. The latter, in turn, may transmit rabies to fruit-eating bats that visit such caves and migrate elsewhere. Bat caves may contain aerosols of rabies virus and present a risk to spelunkers. Migrating fruit-eating bats exist in all 48 contiguous states of the USA, in Canada, and in Latin America. They are a source of infection for many animals and humans. They may exhibit unusual behavior (because of encephalitis) that attracts the attention of people and leads to bites. *All persons bitten by bats must receive postexposure prophylaxis.*

Human-to-human rabies infection is very rare. It can originate from the saliva of a patient who has rabies and exposes attending personnel. Recently, rabies has been transmitted from corneal transplants—the corneas came from donors who died with undiagnosed central nervous system diseases; the recipients died from rabies 50–80 days later.

Ten of the 23 human rabies cases reported to the Centers for Disease Control from 1975 through 1984 were acquired outside the USA; these included 6 cases acquired by United States citizens living outside the USA and 4 cases acquired by noncitizens outside the USA but diagnosed in the USA. In 8 of the 10 cases, there were histories of probable exposure to rabies from a dog bite; in those 8 cases, the development of rabies was attributable to failure to seek treatment (3 cases), postexposure therapy not recommended (2 cases), and delay in seeking treatment, failure to receive rabies immune globulin as part of postexposure therapy, and misdiagnosis of the exposing animal (1 case each). Rabies in humans is much more frequent in other countries: in Latin America, an annual average of 280 cases—all fatal—was reported during the decade 1970–1979.

Control

Isolated countries, eg, Britain, that have no indigenous rabies in wild animals can establish quarantine procedures. Dogs and other pets to be imported are quarantined for 6–12 months. In countries where dog rabies exists, stray animals should be destroyed and vaccination of pet dogs and cats should be mandatory. In countries where wildlife rabies exists and where contact between domestic animals, pets, and wildlife is inevitable, all domestic animals and pets should be vaccinated and the incidence of rabies in wild animals should be continually ascertained.

Preexposure vaccination is desirable for all persons who are at high risk of contact with rabid animals (Table 39–2). This applies particularly to veterinarians, animal care personnel, certain laboratory workers, and spelunkers. Persons traveling to developing countries where rabies control programs for domestic animals are not optimal should be offered preexposure prophylaxis if they plan to stay for more than 30 days. Persons on long-term international assignments in rabies-endemic areas who are at risk of inapparent exposure to rabies or a delay in postexposure prophylaxis should be advised to have a booster every 2 years or to have their serum tested for rabies-neutralizing antibody every 2 years and, if their titer is inadequate, have a booster. It should be emphasized that preexposure prophylaxis does not eliminate the need for prompt postexposure prophylaxis if an exposure to rabies occurs.

Rabies should be considered in any case of encephalitis or myelitis of unknown etiology, even in the absence of an exposure history, particularly in a person who has lived or traveled outside the USA.

Dogs and cats that appear healthy but have made an unprovoked attack upon and bitten a person should be quarantined for at least 10 days (see Laboratory Diagnosis, above).

ASEPTIC MENINGITIS

This syndrome is characterized by acute onset, fever, headache, and stiff neck. There is pleocytosis of the spinal fluid, consisting largely of mononuclear cells. The fluid is bacteria-free, with a normal glucose content and often a slightly elevated protein content.

Etiology

Aseptic meningitis may be caused by a variety of agents: (1) primarily neurotropic viruses (poliomyelitis, lymphocytic choriomeningitis, and arthropod-borne encephalitis viruses); (2) viruses not primarily neurotropic (enteroviruses, mumps, herpes simplex, herpes zoster, infectious mononucleosis, infectious hepatitis, varicella, and measles); (3) spirochetes (*Treponema pallidum* and leptospirae); (4) bacteria, as in silent brain abscess and inadequately treated bacterial meningitis; and (5) mycoplasmas or chlamydiae.

Diagnosis

The diagnosis of aseptic viral meningitis is made by exclusion of bacterial causes of the symptom complex. Specific etiologic causes of aseptic meningitis can usually be determined only by isolation of the agent or the demonstration of a rise in specific antibodies. However, epidemiologic features have diagnostic value. (See discussions of specific agents.)

Laboratory Findings

The peripheral white count is usually normal, but in lymphocytic choriomeningitis, eosinophilia may appear a few days after onset. There is pleocytosis of the cerebrospinal fluid; polymorphonuclear cells often predominate during the first 24 hours, but a shift to lymphocytes usually occurs thereafter. The range is 100–800 cells or more. In lymphocytic choriomeningitis there may be 500–3000 cells or more. Protein levels of the spinal fluid are often elevated, but the glucose level is within normal limits.

LYMPHOCYTIC CHORIOMENINGITIS

Lymphocytic choriomeningitis (LCM) is an acute disease with aseptic meningitis or a mild systemic influenzalike illness. Occasionally there is a severe encephalomyelitis or a fatal systemic disease. The incubation period is usually 18–21 days but may be as short as 1–3 days. The mild systemic form is rarely recognized clinically. There may be fever, malaise, generalized muscle aches and pains, weakness, sore throat, and cough. The fever lasts for 3–14 days.

LCM is an RNA-containing arenavirus (see Chapter 36) 50–150 nm in diameter.

Diagnosis

Specific diagnosis can be made by the isolation of virus from spinal fluid or blood during the acute phase and by tests demonstrating a rise in antibody titer between acute and convalescent serum specimens. CF antibodies rise to diagnostic levels in 3–4 weeks, then fall gradually and reach normal levels after several months. Nt antibodies appear later and reach diagnostic levels 7–8 weeks after onset; they may persist for 4–5 years.

Laboratory Findings

In the prodromal period (or mild systemic form), leukopenia with relative lymphocytosis is frequently present. In the meningitic form, there is pleocytosis in the spinal fluid (100–3000 cells/μL), with a predominance of lymphocytes. The glucose level is normal and the protein level slightly elevated.

Epidemiology & Control

The disease is endemic in mice and other animals (dogs, monkeys, guinea pigs) and is occasionally transmitted to humans. One large epidemic in the USA was caused by infected pet hamsters. There is no evidence of person-to-person spread.

Infected gray house mice, probably the most common source of human infection, excrete the virus in urine and feces. The virus may be harbored by mice throughout their lives, and females transmit it to their offspring, which in turn become healthy carriers. Mice inoculated as adults develop a rapidly fatal generalized infection. In contrast, congenitally or neonatally infected mice do not become acutely ill, but 10–12 months later many develop a fatal debilitating disease involving the central nervous system. The animals exhibit chronic glomerulonephritis and hypergammaglobulinemia; the glomerular lesions are due to deposition of antigen-antibody complexes, and the in-

fection in mice is considered an immune complex disease (see Slow Virus Diseases, below). The mode of transmission from mice to humans is uncertain. Mice and their droppings should be controlled.

EPIDEMIC NEUROMYASTHENIA (Benign Myalgic Encephalomyelitis)

A number of outbreaks of epidemic neuromyasthenia have been reported in Europe and the USA. No causative agent has been isolated, although viruses are believed to play a role. The main features of the disease are fatigue, headache, intense muscle pain, slight and transient paresis, mental disturbances, and objective evidence of diffuse involvement of the central nervous system. The illness is sometimes confused with poliomyelitis. Young and middle-aged adults are principally afflicted. Sporadic cases have also been reported.

ENCEPHALOMYOCARDITIS VIRUS INFECTION (Mengo Fever)

The virus has been recovered in several regions of the world, but only rare human infections have been reported. In one well studied case, the patient had fever, headache, nuchal rigidity, vomiting, and short periods of delirium. The virus was isolated from the blood on the first and second days of illness, and antibodies appeared during convalescence. In a few cases, sera from individuals suffering from central nervous system diseases neutralized the virus.

The virus is pathogenic for many animals, including mice, guinea pigs, monkeys, and chick embryos. It has been isolated in nature from the cotton rat, mongoose, rhesus monkey, baboon, chimpanzee, and *Taeniorhynchus* mosquitoes. The virus can cause lesions in the central nervous system and in skeletal and cardiac muscle. An outbreak of fatal myocarditis caused by this virus has been observed in pigs.

The agent belongs to the picornavirus family. It has a diameter of about 25 nm and contains 30% RNA. It is a satisfactory antigen in the CF test and also agglutinates sheep erythrocytes. Antibodies can be measured by Nt, CF, and HI methods.

SLOW & UNCONVENTIONAL VIRUS DISEASES

Some chronic degenerative diseases of the central nervous system of humans are caused by "slow" or chronic, persistent virus infections. Among these are subacute sclerosing panencephalitis and progressive multifocal leukoencephalopathy. Other diseases, such as kuru and Creutzfeldt-Jakob disease, appear to be caused by unconventional transmissible agents (Table 39–3).

Table 39–3. Slow and unconventional virus diseases.

Disease	Agent	Host(s)	Incubation Period	Nature of Disease
Diseases of humans				
Kuru	Prion	Humans (chimpanzees, monkeys)	Months to years	Spongiform encephalopathy
Creutzfeldt-Jakob (C-J) disease	Prion	Humans (chimpanzees, monkeys)	Months to years	Spongiform encephalopathy
Subacute sclerosing panencephalitis (SSPE)	Measles virus variant	Humans	2–20 years	Chronic sclerosing panencephalitis
Progressive multifocal leukoencephalopathy (PML)	Papovavirus (JC)	Humans	Years	CNS demyelination
Diseases of animals				
Scrapie	Prion	Sheep (goats, mice)	Months to years	Spongiform encephalopathy
Transmissible mink encephalopathy (TME)	Prion	Mink (other animals)	Months	Spongiform encephalopathy
Visna	Retrovirus	Sheep	Months to years	CNS demyelination

Several animal viruses produce chronic infections of the central nervous system that result in progressive degenerative changes. These animal infections serve as models for similar disorders of humans. These diseases include visna of sheep in Iceland, scrapie of sheep in Britain, and transmissible mink encephalopathy. The progressive neurologic diseases produced by these viruses may have incubation periods of up to 5 years before the clinical manifestations of the infections become evident (Table 39–3).

Slow Virus Infections

A. Visna: Visna and **progressive pneumonia (maedi) viruses** are closely related agents that cause slow infections in sheep. These viruses are classified as retroviruses (subfamily Lentivirinae) because of structural similarities (see Chapter 46), although they are not tumorigenic. The viruses that cause acquired immune deficiency syndrome (AIDS; see Chapter 47) are more closely related to visna virus than to the oncogenic retroviruses.

Visna virus infects all of the organs of the body of the infected sheep; however, pathologic changes are confined primarily to the brain, lungs, and reticuloendothelial system. Inflammatory lesions develop in the central nervous system soon after infection, but there is usually a long incubation period (months to years) before observable neurologic symptoms appear. Disease progression can be either rapid (weeks) or slow (years).

Virus can be recovered for the life of the animal, but virus expression is restricted in vivo so that only minimal amounts of infectious virus are present in the infected host. Once recovered in culture, the virus is cytolytic and kills infected cells.

Antigenic variation occurs during the long-term persistent infections. Many mutations occur in the structural gene that codes for viral envelope glycoproteins. However, the role antigenic drift might play in the pathogenesis of disease is unknown.

Infected animals develop antibodies to the virus;

these can be detected in the cerebrospinal fluid as well as the serum of sick animals. Some animals develop Nt antibodies, whereas in other animals the antibodies appear to be nonneutralizing.

B. Subacute Sclerosing Panencephalitis (SSPE): SSPE is a rare disease of teenagers and young adults, with slowly progressive demyelination in the central nervous system ending in death. In electron microscopic studies of involved brain cells, structures are visible that resemble the nucleocapsid of paramyxoviruses. By co-cultivation with HeLa cells, lymph node material or brain material from SSPE patients has yielded isolates of viruses that closely resemble measles virus. Some isolates differ from measles in the electrophoretic behavior of a single protein, the internal membrane or M viral protein, which plays a key role in viral assembly at the cell membrane. SSPE patients have high titers of antimeasles antibody (IgG) in both serum and cerebrospinal fluid. However, antibody to the M protein is lacking. The lack of M protein explains one characteristic of SSPE: persistence of infection but no production of mature infectious virus.

It is possible that SSPE represents a tolerant infection with defective cell-mediated responses in which latent measles virus persists for years. This may be the result of an immunologic dysfunction of the host, of a change in the virus so that some antigens are missing or are not expressed while the viral genetic information persists in host cells, or of both features. Experimentally, persistent infection with measles virus can be established in cell culture where some viral antigens are not expressed on the host cell surface, and such cells are not killed by lymphocytes (see Chapter 41).

A progressive panencephalitis has also been reported in patients with **congenital rubella.** The neurologic illness developed in the second decade and consisted of spasticity, ataxia, seizures, and progressive decline in intellectual ability.

C. Progressive Multifocal Leukoencephalop-

athy (PML): Papovaviruses (see Chapter 46) have been isolated from brain tissue of patients with progressive multifocal leukoencephalopathy, a rare central nervous system complication found in patients suffering from chronic leukemia, Hodgkin's disease, lymphosarcoma, or carcinomatosis or in others receiving immunosuppressants. Demyelination in the central nervous system of patients with PML (usually immunosuppressed individuals) results from oligodendrocyte infection by papovaviruses.

The virus isolated, designated JC virus, is antigenically and biologically distinct from known papovaviruses. A related papovavirus, BK virus, has been isolated from the urine of renal transplant patients receiving immunosuppressive therapy but is not known to induce disease. JC and BK viruses are antigenically related to each other and to SV40. The human papovaviruses BK and JC commonly infect humans; antibodies to them are found in 70–80% of human sera. Antibody specific to SV40 occurs in about 3% of human sera.

In hamsters, the JC isolate induces brain tumors that resemble glioblastomas and medulloblastomas but without demyelination. BK lacks this oncogenicity but can transform hamster cells in culture.

Spongiform Encephalopathies of Humans & Animals

Four degenerative central nervous system diseases—kuru and **Creutzfeldt-Jakob disease** of humans, **scrapie** of sheep, and **transmissible encephalopathy** of mink—have similar pathologic features. These diseases have been described as subacute spongiform virus encephalopathies. The causative agents do not appear to be conventional viruses; infectivity is associated with proteinaceous material devoid of detectable amounts of nucleic acid. The term prion has been proposed to designate this novel class of agents (see p 2).

These agents are unusually resistant to standard means of inactivation. They are resistant to treatment with formaldehyde, β-propiolactone, ethanol, proteases, deoxycholate, and ionizing radiation. However, they are sensitive to phenol (90%), household bleach, ether, acetone, urea (6 mol/L), strong detergents (10% sodium dodecyl sulfate), iodine disinfectants, and autoclaving.

A. Characteristics of Diseases: There are several distinguishing hallmarks of diseases caused by these unconventional agents. The diseases are confined to the nervous system and exhibit reactive astrocytosis. Neurons may be vacuolated, or amyloid plaques may be present, or both. Long incubation periods (months to decades) precede the onset of clinical illness and are followed by chronic progressive pathology (weeks to years). The diseases are always fatal, with no known cases of remissions or recoveries. The host shows no inflammatory response and no immune response (the agents do not appear to be antigenic), no production of interferon is elicited, and there is no effect on host B or T cell function. Finally, immunosup-

pression of the host has no effect on pathogenesis of the disease.

B. Scrapie: Scrapie, which behaves as a recessive genetic trait in sheep, shows marked differences in susceptibility of different breeds. Susceptibility to experimentally transmitted scrapie ranges from zero to over 80% in sheep, whereas goats are almost 100% susceptible. Scrapie has also been transmitted to laboratory monkeys. The transmission of scrapie to mice and hamsters, in which the incubation period is greatly reduced, has facilitated study of the disease.

Infectivity can be recovered from lymphoid tissues early in infection, but high titers of the agent are found only in the brain, spinal cord, and eye (which are also the only places where pathologic changes are observed). Maximal titers of infectivity are reached in the brain long before neurologic symptoms appear. A feature of the disease is the development of amyloid plaques in the central nervous system of infected animals. These areas represent extracellular accumulations of protein; they stain with Congo red.

A protein designated PrP (MW 27,000–30,000) has recently been purified from scrapie-infected brain. It co-purifies with scrapie infectivity, aggregates, and behaves like amyloid. Preparations containing only PrP and no detectable nucleic acid have been found to be infectious. PrP is encoded by a cellular gene. Transcripts from this gene are found in many normal tissues and in similar levels in normal and infected brains. The level of PrP, however, is elevated in infected brains. It has been possible to produce antibody against purified PrP. It is still uncertain whether this protein represents the essential structural element of the infectious agent or a pathologic product that accumulates as a result of the disease.

C. Transmissible Mink Encephalopathy (TME): This disease is caused by an agent that induces clinical disease and neurologic lesions in the gray matter of the brain similar to those of scrapie. It also has a long incubation period in mink that are naturally infected—presumably by the oral route. TME probably represents a strain of sheep scrapie acquired when mink on mink ranches were fed scrapie-infected sheep carcasses.

D. Kuru: Two human spongiform encephalopathies are caused by "slow viruses," producing lesions similar to those of scrapie and TME. These are kuru and Creutzfeldt-Jakob disease. Brain material from patients who died from either disease can produce similar diseases when injected into chimpanzees, and the serial passage of diseased chimpanzee brain into healthy chimpanzees or rodents transfers the illness.

Kuru occurs only in the eastern highlands of New Guinea. The disease consists of relentless progressive cerebellar ataxia, tremors, dysarthria, and emotional lability without significant dementia. It occurs more frequently in women than in men, which coincides with the customs surrounding cannibalism. The remains of dead relatives were handled and eaten primarily by women and children. Since cannibalism has been outlawed, the incidence of the disease has decreased, and it is now felt that this was the primary mode of transmission of the agent.

E. Creutzfeldt-Jakob Disease (CJD): C-J disease (subacute presenile dementia) develops gradually, with progressive dementia, myoclonic fasciculations, ataxia, and somnolence, and leads to death in 8–12 months. The histologic lesions resemble those of kuru and scrapie, including the presence of amyloid plaques. C-J disease occurs with a frequency of approximately 1 case per million population per year in the USA and Europe. Most cases occur sporadically and involve patients over 50 years of age. C-J disease has been transmitted accidentally by contaminated growth hormone preparations from human cadaver pituitary glands and by a corneal transplant, leading to the death of the recipient 18 months later. Both kuru and C-J disease fail to show cerebrospinal fluid pleocytosis or abnormalities in sedimentation rate, blood chemistry, or body temperature.

A protein very similar to the scrapie PrP has recently been purified from brain tissue infected with C-J disease. It has been speculated that the agent of C-J disease was derived originally from scrapie-infected sheep and transmitted to humans by ingestion of poorly cooked sheep brains or eyeballs.

Other Central Nervous System Degenerative Disorders

Chronic virus infections or infections with unconventional agents may be associated with other progressive degenerative diseases of the central nervous system of humans. Many chronic diseases might be considered to originate in this way. These include multiple sclerosis, Alzheimer's disease, and amyotrophic lateral sclerosis.

A. Multiple Sclerosis (MS): This is a degenerative disorder of the central nervous system, with diffuse involvement beginning in early adult life and a varied course for 10–20 years. The gamma globulin in the cerebrospinal fluid is elevated, but antibodies to no one virus are regularly elevated. The etiology is not understood, and there may be viral, immunologic, and genetic aspects. Possibly, MS represents an autoimmune reaction to central nervous system involvement by viruses that may remain latent for the life of the host.

In chronic diseases mentioned above (progressive multifocal leukoencephalopathy, subacute sclerosing panencephalitis) and multiple sclerosis, as well as in systemic lupus erythematosus and sarcoidosis, antibodies to different viruses are often present at levels higher than in matched controls. What is not yet known is whether the high levels (1) occur before the chronic disease, indicating a viral cause; (2) occur at the same time the chronic disease becomes manifest, as a result of a common defect in immunity; or (3) occur after the chronic disease is visible, as a result of a decrease in cell-mediated immunity brought on by the disease.

B. Alzheimer's Disease: There are some neuropathologic similarities between C-J disease and Alzheimer's disease, including the appearance of amyloid plaques. However, attempts to transmit disease to primates or rodents using brain samples from patients with Alzheimer's disease have been unsuccessful to date.

Immune Complex Diseases

In a number of the human progressive degenerative disorders of suspected viral cause, the immunologic response of the host to the virus may be responsible for the pathologic changes and for the clinical illness (see Chapter 33). Two diseases of animals that serve as models in exploring this type of pathogenesis are lymphocytic choriomeningitis (LCM) in mice and Aleutian disease of mink. In both diseases, the virus appears to persist in the chronically infected animal as a virus-antibody complex in which the antibody is unable to neutralize and eliminate the virus. Deposition of these antigen-antibody complexes throughout a relatively long period of infection may produce the basic lesions of the disease.

Aleutian disease of mink is a chronic immune complex disease initiated by a 25-nm virus. Aleutian mink die in 3–6 months after infection, but other genetic types of mink survive longer. Virus circulates from the acute stage of infection onward and can be found in many organs and in serum and urine. Antibody is produced in large quantity, so there is IgG hyperglobulinemia. The virus complexes with the antibody without being neutralized. Virus-antibody complexes circulate and then deposit in glomeruli, leading to renal failure and death. The failure of virus neutralization and elimination by the excess antibody is not entirely understood.

Postinfectious or postvaccinal demyelinating encephalomyelitis and neuritis may be due to immunologic cross-reactions evoked by specific viral antigenic epitopes that are homologous to regions in the target myelins of the central and peripheral nervous systems. Such homologies have been found by computer searches in which decapeptides in 2 human myelin proteins were compared with those in proteins of viruses known to infect humans. The viruses included measles, Epstein-Barr, influenza A and B, and adenoviruses.

REFERENCES

Anderson LJ et al: Rapid antibody response to human diploid rabies vaccine. *Am J Epidemiol* 1981;**113**:270.

Bockman JM et al: Creutzfeldt-Jakob disease prion proteins in human brains. *N Engl J Med* 1985;**312**:73.

Brahic M et al: Gene expression in visna virus infection in sheep. *Nature* 1981;**292**:240.

Brown P et al: Alzheimer's disease and transmissible virus dementia (Creutzfeldt-Jakob disease). *Ann NY Acad Sci* 1982; **396:**131.

Burgoyne GH et al: Rhesus diploid rabies vaccine (adsorbed): A new rabies vaccine using FRhL-2 cells. *J Infect Dis* 1985;**152:**204.

Chatigny MA, Prusiner SB: Biohazards of investigations on the transmissible spongiform encephalopathies. *Rev Infect Dis* 1980;**2:**713.

Dietzschold B et al: Characterization of an antigenic determinant of the glycoprotein that correlates with pathogenicity of rabies virus. *Proc Natl Acad Sci USA* 1983;**80:**70.

Gajdusek DC: Hypothesis: Interference with axonal transport of neurofilament as a common pathogenetic mechanism in certain diseases of the central nervous system. *N Engl J Med* 1985;**312:**714.

Haase AT et al: Natural history of restricted synthesis and expression of measles virus genes in subacute sclerosing panencephalitis. *Proc Natl Acad Sci USA* 1985;**82:**3020.

Hall WW, Choppin PW: Measles-virus proteins in the brain tissue of patients with subacute sclerosing panencephalitis: Absence of the M protein. *N Engl J Med* 1981;**304:**1152.

Jahnke U, Fischer EH, Alvord EC Jr: Sequence homology between certain viral proteins and proteins related to encephalomyelitis and neuritis. *Science* 1985;**229:**282.

Johnson KP et al: Experimental subacute sclerosing panencephalitis: Selective disappearance of measles virus matrix protein from the central nervous system. *J Infect Dis* 1981;**144:**161.

Johnson RT: The contribution of virologic research to clinical neurology. *N Engl J Med* 1982;**307:**660.

Katzman R: Alzheimer's disease. *N Engl J Med* 1986;**314:**964.

Manuelidis L, Valley S, Manuelidis EE: Specific proteins associated with Creutzfeldt-Jakob disease and scrapie share antigenic and carbohydrate determinants. *Proc Natl Acad Sci USA* 1985;**82:**4263.

Norkin LC: Papovaviral persistent infections. *Microbiol Rev* 1982;**46:**384.

Oldstone MBA: Virus neutralization and virus-induced immune complex disease: Virus-antibody union resulting in immunoprotection or immunologic injury—two sides of the same coin. *Prog Med Virol* 1975;**19:**84.

Prusiner SB: Prions: Novel infectious pathogens. *Adv Virus Res* 1984;**29:**1.

Stroop WG, Baringer JR: Persistent, slow and latent viral infections. *Prog Med Virol* 1982;**28:**1.

Warrell MJ et al: Economical multiple-site intradermal immunisation with human diploid-cell-strain vaccine is effective for post-exposure rabies prophylaxis. *Lancet* 1985;**1:**1059.

Wechsler SL, Meissner HC: Measles and SSPE viruses: Similarities and differences. *Prog Med Virol* 1982;**28:**65.

Wiktor TJ et al: Protection from rabies by a vaccinia virus recombinant containing the rabies virus glycoprotein gene. *Proc Natl Acad Sci USA* 1984;**81:**7194.

Orthomyxovirus (Influenza) & Coronavirus Families

40

ORTHOMYXOVIRUSES

The name myxovirus was originally applied to influenza viruses. It meant virus with an affinity for mucins. There are 2 main groups—the orthomyxoviruses and the paramyxoviruses. Their differences in simple terms are shown in Table 40–1. Paramyxoviruses are discussed in Chapter 41.

All orthomyxoviruses are influenza viruses. Isolated strains are named after the virus *type* (A, B, C), the host and location of initial isolation, the year of isolation, and the antigenic designation of the hemagglutinin and neuraminidase. At least 11 hemagglutinin antigenic subtypes and 8 neuraminidase antigenic subtypes are known. Both antigens are glycoproteins under separate genetic control, and they vary independently. Examples of influenza designations follow:

A/swine/New Jersey/8/76 (H1N1), previously (Hsw1N1)
A/Philippines/2/82 (H3N2)
A/Chile/1/83 (H1N1)
B/USSR/100/83

The last 3 strains were incorporated in the vaccine for use in the 1985–1986 season.

INFLUENZA

Influenza is an acute respiratory tract infection that usually occurs in epidemics. Three immunologic types of influenza virus are known: A, B, and C. Antigenic changes continually take place within the A group of influenza viruses and to a lesser degree in the B group, whereas influenza C appears to be antigenically stable. Influenza A strains are also known for pigs, horses, ducks, and chickens (fowl plague). Some animal iso-

lates are antigenically similar to the strains circulating in the human population.

Influenza virus type C differs from the type A and type B viruses; its receptor-destroying enzyme does not appear to be a neuraminidase, and its virion structure is not fully understood. The following descriptions are based on influenza virus type A.

Properties of the Virus

A. Structure: Influenza virus consists of pleomorphic, approximately spherical particles having an external diameter of about 110 nm and an inner electron-dense core of 70 nm.

The surface of the virus particles is covered with 2 types of projections, or spikes, approximately 10 nm long that possess either the hemagglutinin or the neuraminidase activity of the virus. A model of the influenza virion is shown in Fig 40–1.

The RNA genome consists of 8 distinct pieces with an aggregate molecular weight of $2-4 \times 10^6$.

Because of a divided genome, viruses of this group exhibit several biologic phenomena such as high recombination frequency, multiplicity reactivation, and ability to synthesize hemagglutinin and neuraminidase after chemical inactivation of viral infectivity.

Although viral RNA has not proved to be infectious, viral ribonucleoprotein appears to be so. This structure contains the virion-associated RNA-dependent RNA polymerase as well as the genome. Viral messenger RNA that is formed is complementary to the virion RNA.

The results of hybridization studies on RNA have supported the immunologic grouping of the hemagglutinins of the influenza A viruses. Results of similar studies of the neuraminidase genes have been in agreement with N antigen subtype designations based on the results of serologic tests.

B. Reactions to Physical and Chemical Agents: Influenza viruses are relatively stable and may be stored at 0–4 °C for weeks. The virus is less stable at −20 °C than at +4 °C. Ether and protein denaturants destroy infectivity. The hemagglutinin and CF antigens are more stable than the infective virus. Ultraviolet irradiation destroys infectivity, hemagglutinating activity, neuraminidase activity, and CF antigen, in that order. Infectivity and hemagglutination are more stable at alkaline pH than at acid pH.

C. Animal Susceptibility and Growth of Virus: Human strains of the virus can infect different

Table 40–1. Differences between orthomyxoviruses and paramyxoviruses.

	Orthomyxoviruses	Paramyxoviruses
Viruses and diseases	Influenza A, B, C	Mumps, measles, respiratory syncytial, parainfluenza
Genome	Single-stranded RNA in 8 pieces, MW $2-4 \times 10^6$	Single-stranded RNA in single piece, MW $5-8 \times 10^6$
Inner ribonucleoprotein helix	9-nm diameter	18-nm diameter

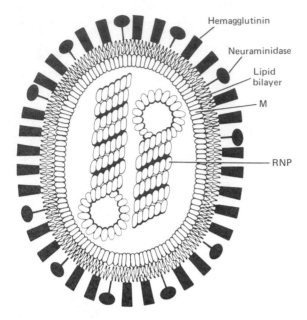

Hemagglutinin

Neuraminidase

Lipid bilayer

M

RNP

Figure 40–1. A model of the influenza virion. The innermost component is the helical ribonucleoprotein (RNP), which is 9 nm in diameter. It is as yet unknown whether the RNP is one long molecule or is divided into pieces like the virus RNA. The nucleocapsid is further organized by the coiling of the whole RNP strand into a double helix 50–60 nm in diameter. The protein component of this structure has a molecular weight of 60,000 and is associated with the group-specific CF antigen. A protein (M) shell surrounds the nucleoprotein and forms the inner part of the virus envelope. It is composed of a small protein (MW 26,000) and constitutes about 40% of the virus protein. About 20% of the virus particle is composed of lipid, apparently derived from the host cell. The lipid is formed into a bilayer structure. The hemagglutinin spike is responsible for the agglutination of erythrocytes by this virus. It is composed of 2 molecules of a glycoprotein (MW 75,000) that may or may not be cleaved to form 2 disulfide-linked glycopeptides of molecular weight 27,000 and 53,000. The smaller of these is present at the end of the molecule which is attached to the lipid. The neuraminidase spike is responsible for the receptor-destroying activity of the virus; this activity results in elution of the virus from host cells or erythrocytes. The role of its activity in virus replication is unknown. It is composed of 4 polypeptide molecules with a molecular weight of about 60,000. The arrangement of these molecules is still a matter of debate. Both the hemagglutinin and the neuraminidase spikes have been purified, and a study of the purified protein has helped to explain antigenic changes of the virus. (From Compans and Choppin.)

animals; ferrets are most susceptible. Serial passage in mice increases its virulence, producing extensive pulmonary consolidation and death. The developing chick embryo readily supports the growth of virus, but there are no gross lesions.

Wild influenza viruses do not grow well in tissue cultures. In most instances, only an abortive growth cycle occurs, ie, viral subunits are synthesized but little or no new infectious progeny is formed. From most influenza strains, mutants can be selected that will grow in cell culture. Because of the poor growth of many strains in cell culture, initial isolation attempts should employ inoculation both of the amniotic cavity of the embryonated egg and of monkey cell cultures.

The process of infection begins by adsorption of the virus onto its receptor sites (neuraminic acid-containing glycoproteins). The hemagglutinin protein is involved in this reaction. The other spike protein, neuraminidase, can destroy the site. The virus particle is taken into the cell, where it is disrupted, causing a decrease in detectable virus shortly after infection.

Intracellular synthesis of the viral RNA and protein then occurs. Viral RNA pieces are synthesized individually in the nucleus within 2–3 hours. All viral proteins are synthesized in the cytoplasm. Structural proteins bind to the cell membrane and are joined by the ribonucleoprotein. At 8 hours, new virus particles bud through the membrane. Neuraminidase may be important in release of the completed virion.

In most influenza systems, noninfectious virus capable of hemagglutination is produced (von Magnus phenomenon). These virions are "incomplete" and increase in number upon serial, high-multiplicity passage of the virus. The incomplete viruses are smaller and more pleomorphic than standard virus, and they interfere with replication of standard virus. They are known as *d*efective *i*nterfering, or DI, viruses. The largest virus RNA piece is missing from them.

D. Biologic Properties:

1. Hemagglutination–All strains of influenza virus agglutinate erythrocytes from chickens, guinea pigs, and humans and—unlike paramyxoviruses—agglutinate erythrocytes from many other species as well. Agglutination of red blood cells occurs when the hemagglutinin interacts with a specific receptor on the red blood cell membrane. This receptor is a glycoprotein (MW 3×10^4) that contains sialic acid. This glycoprotein serves both as the receptor site for the hemagglutinin and as the substrate for the viral neuraminidase. Cleavage of the glycoprotein by the enzyme dissociates the virion from the red cell, resulting in spontaneous elution. After elution, the cell receptors are destroyed and hence can no longer be agglutinated with fresh virus; however, the eluted virus can reattach to and agglutinate additional cells.

2. Group antigen–All influenza A virus strains share a common antigen, distinct from those of influenza B and C. This soluble (S) antigen is found in the medium from infected cell cultures and is a component of the ribonucleoprotein of the virus. It can be identified by CF. Antibody to this nucleoprotein antigen does not induce resistance to the virus in humans. The other internal proteins and the RNA polymerase also have group-specific antigenic activity.

3. Specific antigens–The infectious virus particles induce in animals the development of virus-neutralizing and other antibodies, and the inoculated animals become resistant to infection. Influenza virus administered in large amounts is toxic. The effect is apparently associated directly with the virus particles and can be prevented by specific antibody.

Virions contain 2 subtype- or strain-specific antigens—the hemagglutinin and the neuraminidase. The hemagglutinin is the principal specific envelope antigen, and differences in this antigen among strains of virus can be shown by HI tests. Antibody to the hemagglutinin neutralizes virus and is a protective mechanism.

Neuraminidase is antigenically distinct from the hemagglutinin and is governed by a separate gene (RNA fragment); hence, it can vary independently of the hemagglutinin. The antigens of the hemagglutinin and the neuraminidase of the virus are the basis for classifying new strains. Antibody against the neuraminidase does not neutralize the virus, but it modifies the infection, probably by its effect on the release of virus from the cells. The antibody against the neuraminidase occurs in sera of humans who experience infection. The presence of antineuraminidase antibody results in marked protection against disease.

4. Filamentous forms–In addition to the spherical particles, elongated forms possessing the same surface projections exist. The filamentous forms also agglutinate red cells and elute from them. In its early passages in chick embryos, the virus is usually in filamentous form, but with serial passage it takes on a spherical appearance.

5. Recombination–The multisegment nature of the influenza virus genome allows recombination to occur with high frequency by reassortment between orthomyxoviruses of the same group. The RNA fragments of different influenza A viruses migrate at different rates in polyacrylamide gels. Similarly, the polypeptides of different influenza A viruses can be differentiated. Thus, using 2 different parental viruses and obtaining recombinants between them, it is possible to tell which parent donated which RNA fragment to the recombinant. These techniques enable rapid and more complete analysis of recombinants that emerge in nature.

Pathogenesis & Pathology

The ability of enveloped viruses to fuse with cellular membranes is important for entry into host cells. For influenza virus, the hemagglutinin mediates this function. The mechanism involves binding of the virus to a cell surface receptor, followed by endocytosis and subsequent fusion of the endocytosed vesicle with a lysosome. Within the lysosome, fusion occurs between the viral envelope and lysosomal membrane, resulting in the release of the nucleocapsid into the cell cytoplasm.

The virus enters the respiratory tract in airborne droplets. Viremia is rare. Virus is present in the nasopharynx from 1–2 days before to 1–2 days after onset of symptoms. The neuraminidase lowers the viscosity of the mucous film in the respiratory tract, laying bare the cellular surface receptors and promoting the spread of virus-containing fluid to lower portions of the tract. Even when Nt antibodies are in the blood, they may not protect against infection. Antibodies must be present in sufficient concentration at the superficial cells of the respiratory tract. This can be achieved only if the antibody level in the blood is high or if antibody is secreted locally.

Inflammation of the upper respiratory tract causes necrosis of the ciliated and goblet cells of the tracheal and bronchial mucosa but does not affect the basal layer of epithelium. Interstitial pneumonia may occur with necrosis of bronchiolar epithelium and may be fatal. The pneumonia is often associated with secondary bacterial invaders: staphylococci, pneumococci, streptococci, and *Haemophilus influenzae*.

Clinical Findings

The incubation period is 1 or 2 days. Chills, malaise, fever, muscular aches, prostration, and respiratory symptoms may occur. The fever persists for about 3 days; complications are not common, but pneumonia, myocarditis, pericarditis, and central nervous system complications occur rarely. The latter include encephalomyelitis, polyneuritis, Guillian-Barré syndrome, and Reye's syndrome (see below).

When influenza appears in epidemic form, the clinical findings are consistent enough so that the disease can be diagnosed in most cases. Sporadic cases cannot be diagnosed on clinical grounds. Mild as well as asymptomatic infections occur. The severity of the pandemic of 1918–1919 has been attributed to the fact that bacterial pneumonia often developed.

The lethal impact of an influenza epidemic is reflected in the excess deaths due to pneumonia and cardiovascular and renal diseases. Pregnant women and elderly persons with chronic illnesses have a higher risk of complications and death.

Methods currently used in the USA for estimating excess mortality underestimate the serious morbidity associated with epidemic influenza. Community virologic surveillance has demonstrated that influenza viruses have produced epidemics of acute respiratory disease (ARD) every winter since 1974. The examination of recent hospitalizations for ARD has shown a strong correlation of ARD with influenza virus activity in the community. Analysis of the underlying condition of persons hospitalized with ARD during epidemic periods indicates that only 41% had an underlying condition for which vaccine is currently recommended. Deaths in the hospitalized group correlated with the trend of virus-proved community morbidity and followed that trend by 3 weeks. Of 514 deaths among 8003 hospitalizations for ARD during epidemic periods, 441 (86%) occurred among persons for whom immunization should have been recommended.

Reye's syndrome occurs mainly in children. It is characterized by encephalopathy and fatty degeneration of the liver, and the mortality rate is high. In 1979–1980, more than 400 cases were reported in the USA, with a mortality rate near 30%. Reye's syndrome is associated with influenza B, particularly in 10- to 14-year-old children, and sometimes with other viral diseases such as chickenpox in 5- to 9-year-old children. Salicylates may be a factor in the pathogenesis of Reye's syndrome.

Laboratory Diagnosis

Influenza is readily diagnosed by laboratory procedures. For antibody determinations, the first serum sample should be taken less than 5 days after onset and the second 10–14 days later.

For rapid detection of influenza virus in clinical specimens, positive smears from nasal swabs may be demonstrated by specific staining with fluorescein-labeled antibody.

A. Recovery of Virus: Throat washings or garglings are obtained within 3 days after onset and should be tested at once or stored frozen. Penicillin and streptomycin are added to limit bacterial contamination, and embryonated eggs are inoculated by the amniotic route. Amniotic and allantoic fluids are harvested 2–4 days later and tested for hemagglutinins. If results are negative, passage is made to fresh embryos. If hemagglutinins are not detected after 2 such passages, the result is negative.

If a strain of virus is isolated—as demonstrated by the presence of hemagglutinins—it is titrated in the presence of type-specific influenza sera to determine its type. The isolate belongs to the same type as the serum that inhibits its hemagglutinating power.

Primate cell cultures (human or monkey) are susceptible to certain human strains of influenza virus. Rapid diagnosis can be made by growing the virus from the clinical specimen in cell culture and then staining the cultured cells with fluorescent influenza antibody 24 hours later, when infected cells are rich in antigen even though they may appear normal.

The phenomenon of hemadsorption is utilized for the early detection of virus growth in cell cultures. Guinea pig red cells or human O cells are added to the cultures 24–48 hours after the clinical specimens have been inoculated and are viewed under the low power lens. Positive hemadsorption shows red blood cells firmly attached to the cell culture sheets as rosettes or chains. The cytopathogenic effects of the influenza viruses are often negligible. Hemadsorption provides a more sensitive testing procedure.

B. Typing of New Isolates: A double immunodiffusion (DID) test is used for typing influenza virus isolates. The allantoic fluid content of a single infected embryonated egg may be used for the DID test. Reference antisera are placed in the outer wells, and the virus harvest, after disruption by detergent, is added to the center well. The plates are incubated overnight in a moist atmosphere, and precipitin lines are read the following morning.

Membrane immunofluorescence has also been recommended as a simple, rapid, and accurate method for typing current influenza A isolates. Surface antigens of infected, unfixed monkey kidney cells are stained in suspension by indirect immunofluorescence using anti-H3N2 and anti-H1N1 antisera.

C. Serology: Paired sera are used to detect rises in HI, CF, or Nt antibodies. The HI antibody is used most often. Normal sera often contain nonspecific mucoprotein inhibitors that must first be destroyed by treatment with RDE (receptor-destroying enzyme of *Vibrio cholerae* cultures), trypsin, or periodate. Because normal persons usually have influenza antibodies, a 4-fold or greater increase in titer is necessary to indicate influenza infection. Peak levels of antibodies are present 2–4 weeks after onset, persist for about 4 weeks, and then gradually fall during the course of a year to preinfection levels.

Within one type of influenza virus, strains may differ markedly in antigenicity. It is best to use recently isolated strains.

CF antigens are of 2 types. One is soluble (S antigen) and type-specific but not strain-specific. The other is part of the virus particle (V antigen) and is highly strain-specific. It is useful for demonstrating antibody rise when the first serum specimen was not taken early in the disease, because the peak CF titer occurs in the fourth week.

Immunity

Three immunologically unrelated types of influenza virus are known and are referred to as influenza A, B, and C. In addition, the swine, equine, and avian influenza viruses are antigenically related to the human influenza A virus. Influenza C virus exists as a single and stable antigenic type.

At least 18 different antigenic components have been determined in type A strains of influenza virus by quantitative adsorption methods. More undoubtedly exist. Strains share their antigenic components, but in varying proportions. A strain generally shares its antigens with strains prevalent within a few years of its isolation.

Two possible mechanisms for the antigenic variation of influenza virus have been suggested:

(1) All possible configurations may be present in a pool of antigens that exist worldwide; from these, highly infectious strains arise and initiate epidemics. High antibody levels to recent strains in the human population will inhibit strains with major antigens that were dominant in recently prevalent strains and will select strains of different antigenic composition.

Serial passage of virus in mice vaccinated with the homologous strain yields a virus with an apparent rearrangement of antigens or the appearance of new antigens. The change in antigenic character evolves slowly on passage (antigenic drift).

(2) Antigenically different strains may be selected by genetic recombination induced by selection factors such as passage in a partially immune host. When 2 strains of influenza virus are simultaneously injected into mice or eggs, a new strain sharing the properties of each parent strain may be recovered; this has been attributed to genetic recombination (antigenic shift).

Antibodies are important in immunity against influenza, but they must be present at the site of virus invasion. Resistance to initiation of infection is related to antibody against the hemagglutinin. Decreased extent of viral invasion and decreased ability to transmit virus to contacts are related to antibody directed against the neuraminidase.

Virus neutralizing antibody occurs earlier in nasal secretions and rises to high titers sooner among those already possessing high concentrations of IgA in their nasal washings prior to the infection. Even though infected with influenza virus, such individuals remain well. In contrast, those with low IgA levels in nasal washings prior to infection are highly susceptible not only to infection but also to clinical illness.

Prevention & Treatment by Drugs

Amantadine hydrochloride and its analog rimantadine are antiviral drugs for systemic use in the prevention of influenza A. The drugs block penetration of or uncoat influenza A virus in the host cell and prevent virus replication. The established effect is prophylaxis, and amantadine (200 mg/d) must be given to high-risk persons during epidemics of influenza A if protection is to result. Amantadine is relatively nontoxic but may produce central nervous system stimulation with dizziness and insomnia, particularly in the elderly. It should be considered for persons with chronic obstructive respiratory disease, cardiac insufficiency, or renal disease, particularly if they have not been vaccinated yearly or if a new influenza A strain is epidemic. Amantadine may also modify the severity of influenza A if started within 24–48 hours after onset of illness.

Epidemiology

Influenza occurs in successive waves of infection, with peak incidences during the winter. Influenza A infections may vary from a few isolated cases to extensive outbreaks that within a few weeks involve 10% or more of the population, with rates of 50–75% in children of school age. The period between epidemic waves of influenza A is 2–3 years. All known pandemics were caused by influenza A strains. During the pandemic of 1918–1919, more than 20 million persons died, mainly from complicating bacterial pneumonias. Recent pandemics occurred in 1957–1958 owing to A influenza (H2N2) and in 1968 owing to A influenza (H3N2). In 1976 in New Jersey, a new type of influenza arose that resembled swine influenza (Hsw1N1), but it failed to spread in spite of a lack of immunity in most people under age 50 years. An enormous government-sponsored vaccination campaign was stopped because Guillain-Barré syndrome appeared in some vaccinated individuals. However, subsequent influenza vaccination programs have not been associated with Guillain-Barré syndrome. The predominant influenza A in the USA in 1978–1979 was an H1N1 variant of the strains prevalent in the 1950s. During the 1984–1985 season, influenza A (H3N2) viruses were isolated in every state in the USA; they were associated with 7.2% of all deaths due to pneumonia and influenza, the highest percentage since 1976, when it reached 7.7%. Type A (H3N2) viruses predominated, accounting for 97% of the reported 2100 isolates. Low levels of influenza B activity occurred late in the season, and influenza A (H1N1) virus was reported rarely.

Influenza B tends not to spread through communities as quickly as influenza A. Its interepidemic period is from 3 to 6 years. In the USA, type B accounted for 3% of influenza virus isolates in the 1984–1985 season.

The main reason for the periodic occurrence of epidemic influenza is the accumulation of a sufficient number of susceptible persons in a population that harbors the virus in a few subclinical or minor infections throughout the year. Epidemics may be started when the virus mutates to a new antigenic type that has survival advantages and when antibodies in the population are low to this new type. **Antigenic drift**, illustrated in Fig 40–2, involves point mutation in the gene that leads to amino acid sequence changes and altered antigenic sites, so that the virus is no longer recognized by the host immune system. A much more drastic change in the segmented RNA genome occurs when **antigenic shift** occurs. This involves the recombination or reassortment of the RNA segments of human and animal influenza viruses. Outbreaks may also be caused by the emergence of viruses that have previously caused epidemics and have remained unaltered for many years.

In early life, the range of the influenza antibody spectrum is narrow, but it becomes progressively broader in later years. The antibodies (and immunity) acquired from the initial infections of childhood are of limited range and reflect the dominant antigens of the prevailing strains. Later exposures to viruses of related but differing antigenic composition result in an antibody spectrum broadening toward a larger number of the common antigens of influenza viruses. Exposures later in life to antigenically related strains result in a progressive reinforcement of the primary antibody. The highest antibody levels in a particular age group therefore reflect the dominant antigens of the virus responsible for the childhood infections of the group. Thus, a serologic recapitulation of past infection with influenza viruses of different antigenic makeup can be obtained by studying the age distribution of influenza antibodies in normal populations.

Antibodies against swine influenza (perhaps related to the pandemic influenza strain of 1918) have not been found in persons born after 1923. Persons born during 1923–1933 had their first influenza experience with a type A virus closely related to the 1933 WS strain. Those born between 1934 and 1943 do not possess swine or WS antibodies but have antibodies against another type A virus, PR-8 (H0N1).

Another antigenic change occurred among the A viruses in 1946. Strains occurring between 1946 and 1957 have been called A1, or H1N1, strains. The influenza antibodies in persons born between 1946 and 1957 are chiefly against the H1N1 strains. With the widespread appearance of the type A2 Asian strain in 1957, the H1N1 subtypes were replaced by H2N2 viruses.

Type A2 virus seemed to be related to previous

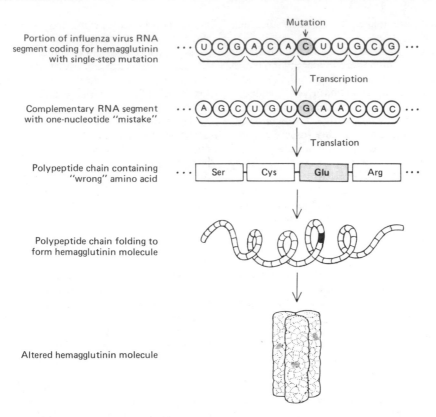

Portion of influenza virus RNA segment coding for hemagglutinin with single-step mutation

Mutation

Transcription

Complementary RNA segment with one-nucleotide "mistake"

Translation

Polypeptide chain containing "wrong" amino acid

Ser — Cys — Glu — Arg

Polypeptide chain folding to form hemagglutinin molecule

Altered hemagglutinin molecule

Figure 40–2. Antigenic drift consists of a series of minor genetic alterations within a group of similar strains. One such alteration is depicted here. The short portion of a viral RNA segment shown at the top contains the genetic information that codes for the hemagglutinin molecule; the segment contains a single-step mutation (shaded). The RNA, represented simply as a string of lettered beads, is actually a chain of nucleotides each of which is made up of a ribose sugar, a phosphate group, and one of 4 organic bases: adenine (A), uracil (U), guanine (G), and cytosine (C). The viral RNA is copied by the polymerase in the virion to yield a complementary RNA strand, A generally pairing with U and G with C. In this case, however, a "mistake" has been made: the mutant C pairs with a G. As a result, the 3-letter "triplet" coding for a specific amino acid inserts a "wrong" amino acid in the polypeptide chain of the H protein. The new amino acid may in turn interfere with the folding of the polypeptide chain, distorting the H molecule, or it may appear in the antigenic region of the molecule, producing a minor antigenic variant that cannot be neutralized by antibodies to the parent influenza virus. (Reproduced, with permission, from Kaplan and Webster: The epidemiology of influenza. *Sci Am* [Dec] 1977;**237**:88. Copyright © 1977 by Scientific American, Inc. All rights reserved.)

influenza viruses, in that sera in 1957 from people who were age 70 years or older often contained antibody against A2 isolates. Furthermore, anti-A2 antibody increases were found in sera from this age group after injections of type A vaccine that did not contain the A2 virus (anamnestic response). This suggests that viruses prevalent during the 1889 pandemic contained H2N2 antigens shared with the 1957 Asian strains.

Influenza B appears to be changing antigenically, since almost all strains isolated in 1965–1966 were closely related to B/Singapore/3/64, which differed significantly from the formerly prevalent variant represented by B/Maryland/1/59. In 1972, a new variant was isolated in Hong Kong (B/HK/5/72) and then became the predominant type B virus around the world. In 1979–1980, for the first time in 6 years, type B viruses caused most of the reported cases in the USA. Most of the type B strains were closely related to B/Singapore/79.

Surveillance for influenza outbreaks is more extensive than for any other disease in order to identify the early appearance of new strains, with the aim of preparing vaccines against them before an epidemic occurs.

Surveillance also extends into animal populations, especially birds, pigs, and horses. Some believe that pandemic strains arise from recombinants of human and animal strains.

Since the virus causing fowl plague was identified as human influenza A type in 1955, many influenza viruses have been isolated from a wide variety of domestic and wild bird species. Some of these include the major H and N antigens related to human strains.

Avian influenza ranges from highly lethal infections in chickens and turkeys to inapparent infections in these and other avian species that harbor the same strains. Domestic ducks and quail often manifest influenza infection by coughing, sneezing, and swelling around the beak, with variable mortality rates. Wildlife species and most domestic fowl show little or no signs of disease.

The possibility that influenza viruses are transmitted between birds and mammals, including humans, may seem unlikely, particularly if the transfer were to be only by the respiratory route. However, influenza viruses of ducks multiply in the cells lining the intestinal tract and are shed in high concentrations into water. These viruses remain viable for days or weeks in water. It is possible that influenza among birds is a waterborne infection, moving from wild to domestic birds and even to humans.

Control Through Immunization

In the 1940s, it appeared that killed influenza vaccine given by subcutaneous injection might provide protection against epidemic influenza. This hope was dashed when the H1N1 strain appeared in 1947, making existing vaccines useless because of major antigenic changes. Each subsequent major antigenic shift—they occur every 10–15 years—made existing vaccines useless.

It is possible that the number of antigens of influenza viruses might be finite but might vary in proportion from one strain to the next. If several strains of broad antigenic composition were combined, such a vaccine might yield an antigenic mass capable of protecting against present and future epidemics. On the other hand, the number of antigenic shifts and the possibility of antigenic drift among influenza viruses might be infinite, emphasizing the need for new research approaches (see below).

A. Who should be vaccinated? At present, it is recommended in the USA that vaccination be limited to those at high risk—the elderly and persons with chronic bronchopulmonary or cardiac disease, metabolic and renal disorders, chronic anemia, or conditions that compromise the immune mechanism, including certain cancers and immunosuppressive therapy. They should be vaccinated every year, according to dosage directions provided by the manufacturer. However, if a major antigenic shift becomes apparent, the entire population might be considered for vaccination—as was the case in the 1976 "swine flu" epidemic.

B. When should vaccination be done? At present, yearly vaccinations should be given before the influenza season begins, ie, in early fall.

C. How are antigens for killed influenza vaccines selected and prepared?

1. If only minor antigenic drift is expected for the next influenza season, the most recent strains of A and B viruses representative of the main antigens are included. They are grown in embryonated eggs, harvested, purified, inactivated, concentrated to a standard hemagglutinin content, and stored for administration in the fall.

2. If a strain representing a major antigenic shift has been isolated (usually in Southeast Asia, where influenza occurs 6 months before it becomes epidemic

in Europe or the USA), then ways must be found to grow the important new antigen in bulk. This is accomplished by the **recombination** method. Stable hybrids can be made of the low-yield new antigen strain and a high-yield egg-adapted influenza virus. By cocultivation of the new, different isolate with an established high-egg-yield virus, recombinant progeny are obtained. These hybrids are selected out, grown in bulk, and incorporated into the "vaccine for the next season." Whenever such recombinant vaccines have been tested, their potency was equal to that of wild-strain vaccines.

3. From either of these 2 methods, subviral antigens can be prepared. Such "split viruses" result from chemical treatment of virion suspensions, with subsequent purification and concentration, and they contain the most important antigenic proteins. The split-virus vaccines produce fewer side effects than whole-virus vaccines. They are preferred for that reason but may require several injections instead of a single one, because of lower antigenicity. They are recommended for children.

D. What are the major risks of and untoward reactions associated with influenza vaccines?

1. All killed vaccines can produce fever, local inflammation at the site of subcutaneous injection, and systemic toxicity with poorly defined nonspecific symptoms of illness for 1–2 days.

2. Since the vaccine strains are grown in eggs, some egg protein antigens are present in the vaccine. Persons allergic to eggs may develop symptoms and signs of hypersensitivity.

3. Whatever immunity results from an inactivated vaccine appears to be of short duration—probably 1–3 years against the homologous virus.

4. Guillain-Barré syndrome, an ascending paralysis, has been statistically associated with mass vaccination programs, eg, the "swine flu" vaccination of 1976. It occurred 5–7 times more frequently in vaccinated than in matched, unvaccinated persons. While most persons affected by this syndrome recover completely, 5–10% have residual muscle weakness and 3–5% a fatal outcome. However, no such increased risk of contracting Guillain-Barré syndrome has been associated with subsequent standard influenza vaccines.

E. Current research approaches to better influenza vaccines.

1. A neuraminidase-specific vaccine, which induces antibodies only to the neuraminidase antigen of the prevailing influenza virus. Antibody to neuraminidase reduces the amount of virus replicating in the respiratory tract and the ability to transmit virus to contacts. It reduces clinical symptoms in the infected person but permits subclinical infection that may give rise to more lasting immunity.

2. A live vaccine using temperature-sensitive (ts) mutants. Such ts mutants grow well at the cooler (33 °C) temperature of the upper respiratory tract but fail to grow at the higher (37 °C) temperature of the lung. Mutants selected for this ts property appear to be

attenuated or avirulent. Thus, they might be given as a live vaccine into the respiratory tract, stimulating local as well as systemic immunity. By recombination of the *ts* gene with the gene for the current major antigen, potent live vaccines could theoretically be produced and rapidly administered to cope with an influenza epidemic.

Attenuated live influenza virus vaccine has been used in the USSR with reported success. The attenuated virus was selected by serial transfer through embryonated eggs rather than by genetic manipulation.

3. Reassortant viruses containing the hemagglutinin and neuraminidase genes of a human influenza A virus and the other 6 RNA segments (ie, "internal genes") of an avian influenza virus are being developed as possible live virus vaccine strains. The safety of such an avian-human influenza reassortant virus has been demonstrated in susceptible volunteers. The reassortant was satisfactorily attenuated and was not transmissible, these factors being consistent with the low level of virus shed by the infected volunteers. The reassortant virus resembled human influenza A virus in that infection was confined to the respiratory tract. Evidence for systemic spread or enterotropism, both of which are characteristic of avian influenza A viruses in their natural hosts, was not found. The stability of the attenuation phenotype must now be addressed.

4. Combined yearly vaccination of persons at high risk, using the best mix of important antigens, and administration of amantadine or other anti-influenza drugs at times of particular stress, eg, surgery, hospitalization.

CORONAVIRUSES

The coronaviruses include human strains from the respiratory tract, avian *i*nfectious *b*ronchitis *v*irus (IBV), *m*ouse *h*epatitis *v*irus (MHV), an enteritis virus of swine, and others. The human coronaviruses cause common colds and have been implicated in gastroenteritis in infants. Coronaviruses of lower animals establish persistent infections in their natural hosts. Because the murine infection can result in a high incidence of subacute to chronic demyelinating disease, it is being studied as a model for multiple sclerosis in humans.

Properties of the Viruses

Coronaviruses are enveloped, 80- to 130-nm particles that contain an unsegmented genome of single-stranded RNA (MW 7×10^6). The helical nucleocapsid is 7–9 nm in diameter; it matures in the cytoplasm by budding into cytoplasmic vesicles. There are 20-nm-long club-shaped or petal-shaped projections that are widely spaced on the outer surface of the envelope, resembling a solar corona. The 3 chief virus proteins include a 60K phosphorylated nucleocapsid protein, a 90K glycoprotein making up the petal-shaped structures, and a 23K glycoprotein embedded in the envelope lipid bilayer. Viral antigens are found only in the cytoplasm of infected cells.

Growth of Virus

The human coronaviruses are difficult to grow in cell cultures. Some strains require human embryonic tracheal and nasal organ cultures; others will grow in human embryonic intestine or kidney cell cultures. The optimal temperature for growth is 33–35 °C.

Antigenic Properties

The human prototype strain is 229E. Some human isolates are closely related; others are not. Cross-reactions occur between some human and some animal strains, but avian IBV appears to be unrelated to human agents. All or most strains have CF antigens; some have hemagglutinins.

Clinical Features & Laboratory Diagnosis

The human coronaviruses produce "colds," usually afebrile, in adults. If virus is isolated, diagnosis can be confirmed by demonstrating a significant rise in CF or Nt antibody titer in paired serum specimens.

In the absence of virus isolation, serologic diagnosis can be made on the basis of significantly increased antibody titers. The CF test is a more sensitive index of human coronavirus infections than is virus isolation with cell and organ culture methods available at present. Serologic diagnosis of infections with strain 229E is now possible by means of the passive hemagglutination test. Red cells coated with coronavirus antigen are agglutinated by antibody-containing sera. The test is type-specific, as sensitive as the Nt test, rapid, and convenient.

Epidemiology

As indicated in the foregoing, the coronaviruses are a major cause of respiratory illness in adults during some winter months when the incidence of colds is high but the isolation of rhinoviruses or other respiratory viruses is low. These viruses are a common cause of virus-induced exacerbations in patients with chronic bronchitis.

The apparent infrequency of coronavirus infections in children may be a result of the type of test used: initial infections with strain 229E are accompanied by only a transient CF antibody response, whereas in reinfections in adults, the CF response is enhanced and the Nt antibody response is diminished. Therefore, the Nt test should be the procedure of choice for infants and children and the CF test more sensitive for adults.

Coronaviruses of lower animals can establish long-term infections in their natural hosts (pigs, chickens, mice). They may also set up inapparent persistent infections in humans.

REFERENCES

Bailowitz A, Kaslow RA: Use of amantadine in the United States, 1977–1982. *J Infect Dis* 1985;**151:**372.

Burnet FM: Portraits of viruses: Influenza virus A. *Intervirology* 1979;**11:**201.

Carson JL, Collier AM, Hu SS: Acquired ciliary defects in nasal epithelium of children with acute viral upper respiratory infections. *N Engl J Med* 1985;**312:**463.

Couch RB et al: Efficacy of purified influenza subunit vaccines and relation to the major antigenic determinants on the hemagglutinin molecule. *J Infect Dis* 1979;**140:**553.

Frank AL et al: Influenza B virus infections in the community and the family: The epidemics of 1976–1977 and 1979–1980 in Houston, Texas. *Am J Epidemiol* 1983;**118:**313.

Gerna G et al: Human enteric coronaviruses: Antigenic relatedness to human coronavirus OC43 and possible etiologic role in viral gastroenteritis. *J Infect Dis* 1985;**151:**796.

Gething MJ, Sambrook J: Cell-surface expression of influenza haemagglutinin from a cloned DNA copy of the RNA gene. *Nature* 1981;**293:**620.

Jackson DC, Nestorowicz A: Antigenic determinants of influenza virus hemagglutinin. 11. Conformational changes detected by monoclonal antibodies. *Virology* 1985;**145:**72.

Langmuir AD et al: An epidemiologic and clinical evaluation of Guillain-Barré syndrome reported in association with the administration of swine influenza vaccines. *Am J Epidemiol* 1984;**119:**841.

Murphy BR et al: Avian-human reassortant influenza A viruses derived by mating avian and human influenza A viruses. *J Infect Dis* 1984;**150:**841.

Palese P, Young JF: Variation of influenza A, B, and C viruses. *Science* 1982;**215:**1468.

Riddiough MA, Sisk JE, Bell JC: Influenza vaccination: Cost-effectiveness and public policy. *JAMA* 1983;**249:**3189.

Tyrrell DAJ: Approaches to the control of respiratory virus diseases. *Bull WHO* 1980;**58:**513.

Webster RG et al: Molecular mechanisms of variation in influenza viruses. *Nature* 1982;**296:**115.

41

Paramyxovirus Family & Rubella Virus

Paramyxoviruses include important human (mumps, measles, parainfluenza, respiratory syncytial) and animal viruses. Some features that distinguish them from orthomyxoviruses are shown in Table 40–1. Rubella virus resembles togaviruses (see Chapter 33) in chemical and physical properties but fits with paramyxoviruses on an epidemiologic basis.

Properties of the Paramyxoviruses

A. Structure: The particle has a lipid-containing envelope covered with spikes; a helical ribonucleoprotein nucleocapsid 18 nm in diameter is enclosed. The RNA is a single molecule (MW $5–8 \times 10^6$). Features of the particle are shown in Fig 41–1.

The envelope of paramyxoviruses contains 2 glycoproteins, HN and F, that form spikelike projections from the surface of the viral membrane. These glycoproteins are involved in the early interactions between virus and cell. The larger glycoprotein, HN, has neuraminidase and hemagglutinating activities and is responsible for virus adsorption. The other glycoprotein, F, is involved in virus-induced cell fusion and hemolysis and in virus penetration through fusion of viral and cell membranes. The membrane-fusing activity of the F protein is activated by proteolytic cleavage of a precursor (F_0) by a host enzyme to yield 2 disulfide-linked polypeptides (F_1 and F_2) (Fig 41–2). Only then can viral replication begin.

B. Biologic Properties:

1. Cell fusion–In the course of infection, paramyxoviruses cause cell fusion, long recognized as giant cell formation. This ability to fuse cells is now used for the creation of cell hybrids, an important tool in somatic cell genetics.

2. Persistent infection–Most paramyxoviruses can produce a persistent noncytocidal infection of cultured cells. The clinical importance of this property may explain subacute sclerosing panencephalitis (SSPE) (see pp 463 and 480).

3. Antigenic properties–Measles, canine distemper, and rinderpest viruses have related antigens. Another antigenically related group includes mumps, parainfluenza, and Newcastle disease viruses.

C. Replication: The RNA genome of viruses of this group is not infectious and does not function as mRNA. Instead, the viral genome is transcribed into shorter RNA molecules that serve as messenger and are complementary to the genome. The paramyxoviruses possess an RNA-dependent RNA polymerase that is a structural component of the virion and produces the initial mRNA.

MUMPS
(Epidemic Parotitis)

Mumps is an acute contagious disease characterized by a nonsuppurative enlargement of one or both of the parotid glands, although other organs may also be involved.

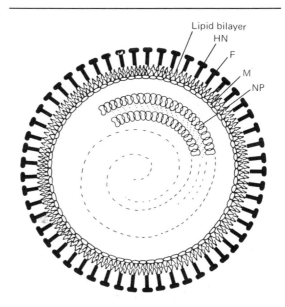

Figure 41–1. The components of paramyxoviruses. HN: Larger virus glycoprotein, responsible both for hemagglutination and receptor-destroying activities of the virus particle. F: Smaller virus glycoprotein, involved in cell fusion by these viruses and probably in the entry of the virus into the cell. F is composed of 2 disulfide bond–linked polypeptides cleaved from a high-molecular-weight precursor. Lipid bilayer: The lipid is cell-derived but probably altered in composition from that of the normal cell. M: Nonglycosylated membrane protein. The HN, F, M, and lipid bilayer can be disrupted, destroying hemolytic activity, and then reassembled without the nucleocapsid, whereupon hemolytic activity is restored. NP: Ribonucleoprotein, the major CF antigen. There is another small protein of about 47,000 molecular weight whose location and function in the virion are unknown. (From Choppin and Compans.)

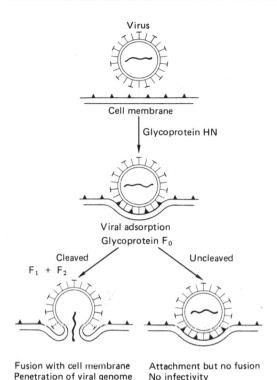

Figure 41–2. Initiation of infection. Adsorption of paramyxovirus to receptors on the cell membrane is mediated by the HN glycoprotein. Penetration of the virus into the cell by means of fusion of viral and cell membranes is mediated by the F_0 glycoprotein, which must be cleaved into 2 subunits, F_1 and F_2, to be active. If the F protein is not cleaved, the virus will attach but it will not fuse with the cell membrane and the viral genome cannot penetrate the cell. (After Choppin and Scheid.)

Properties of the Virus

Mumps virus is a typical paramyxovirus.

A. Morphology and Biochemical Properties: The mumps virus particle has the typical paramyxovirus morphology. Typical also are the biologic properties of hemagglutination, neuraminidase, and hemolysin. Hemagglutination can be inhibited by specific antisera to mumps virus, and this inhibition can be used to measure antibody responses. Similarly, the nucleocapsid of the virus particle forms the major component of the "S" (soluble) CF antigen.

B. Reactions to Physical and Chemical Agents: The hemagglutinin, the hemolysin, and the infectivity of the virus are destroyed by heating at 56 °C for 20 minutes. The CF antigen is more heat-stable.

C. Animal Susceptibility and Growth of Virus: In monkeys, mumps can produce a disease very much like that in human beings. Parotitis is produced by introducing the virus into Stensen's duct or directly into the gland by injection. By the use of fluorescent antibody, the virus has been located in the cytoplasm of acinar cells.

The virus grows readily in embryonated eggs and in cell culture. Passage in embryonated eggs reduces pathogenicity for humans, and this method was used to obtain a vaccine strain. Mumps virus growing in cell culture produces multinucleated giant cells (syncytia).

Pathogenesis & Pathology

Two theories exist regarding the pathogenesis of mumps. (1) The virus travels from the mouth by way of Stensen's duct to the parotid gland, where it undergoes primary multiplication. This is followed by a generalized viremia and localization in testes, ovaries, pancreas, thyroid, or brain. (2) Primary replication occurs in the superficial epithelium of the respiratory tract. This is followed by a generalized viremia and simultaneous localization in the salivary glands and other organs.

Little tissue damage is associated with uncomplicated mumps. The ducts of the parotid glands show desquamation of the epithelium, and polymorphonuclear cells are present in the lumens. There are interstitial edema and lymphocytic infiltration. With severe orchitis, the testis is congested, and punctate hemorrhage as well as degeneration of the epithelium of the seminiferous tubules is observed. Central nervous system pathology may vary from perivascular edema to inflammatory reaction, glial reaction, hemorrhage, or demyelination.

Clinical Features

The incubation period is commonly 18–21 days. A prodromal period of malaise and anorexia is followed by rapid enlargement of parotid glands as well as other salivary glands. Swelling may be confined to one parotid gland, or one gland may enlarge several days before the other. The gland enlargement is associated with pain, especially when tasting acid substances. The salivary adenitis is commonly accompanied by low-grade fever and lasts for approximately a week.

The testes and ovaries may be affected, especially after puberty. Twenty percent of males over 13 years of age who are infected with mumps virus develop orchitis, which is often unilateral and does not usually lead to sterility. Because of the lack of elasticity of the tunica albuginea, which does not allow the inflamed testis to swell, atrophy of the testis may follow secondary to pressure necrosis. Secondary sterility does not occur in women because the ovary, which has no such limiting membrane, can swell when inflamed.

Mumps accounts for 10–15% of cases of aseptic meningitis observed in the USA and is more common among males than females. Meningoencephalitis usually occurs 5–7 days after inflammation of the salivary glands, but it may occur simultaneously or in the absence of parotitis and is usually self-limiting. The cerebrospinal fluid shows pleocytosis (10–2000/μL, mostly lymphocytes) that may persist after clinical recovery.

Rare complications of mumps include (1) a self-limiting polyarthritis that resolves without residual deformity; (2) pancreatitis associated with transient hyperglycemia, glycosuria, and steatorrhea (it has been suggested that diabetes mellitus may occasionally follow); (3) nephritis; (4) thyroiditis; and (5) unilateral nerve deafness (hearing loss is complete and permanent). Mumps may be a possible causative agent in the production of aqueductal stenosis and hydrocephalus in children. Injection of mumps virus into suckling hamsters has produced similar lesions.

Laboratory Diagnosis

Laboratory studies are not usually required to establish the diagnosis of typical cases. However, mumps can sometimes be confused with enlargement of the parotids due to suppuration, foreign bodies in the salivary ducts, tumors, etc. In cases without parotitis, particularly in aseptic meningitis, the laboratory can be helpful in establishing the diagnosis.

A. Recovery of Virus: Virus can be isolated from saliva, cerebrospinal fluid, or urine collected within 4 days after onset of illness. After treatment with antibiotics, the specimens are inoculated into monkey kidney cell cultures. Virus growth can be detected in 5–6 days by adsorption of suitable erythrocytes by the infected cells. The isolate can be identified with specific antiserum that can inhibit the hemadsorption. Immunofluorescent serum can also identify a virus isolate in cell culture within 2–3 days.

B. Serology: Antibody rise can be detected in paired sera. The CF test is best for specificity and accuracy, although the HI test may be used. A 4-fold or greater rise in antibody titer is evidence of mumps infection.

A CF test on a single serum sample obtained soon after onset of illness may serve for a presumptive diagnosis. S (soluble) antibodies develop within a few days after onset and sometimes can reach a high titer before V (viral) antibodies can be detected. In early convalescence, both S and V antibodies are present at high levels. Subsequently, S antibodies disappear more rapidly, leaving V antibodies as a marker of previous infection for several years. The intradermal injection of inactivated virus results in reappearance of V antibodies in high titer. Nt antibodies also appear during convalescence and can be determined in cell culture.

Immunity

Immunity is permanent after a single infection. Only one antigenic type exists. Passive immunity is transferred from mother to offspring; thus it is rare to see mumps in infants under age 6 months.

Treatment

Immune globulin USP is of no value for decreasing the incidence of orchitis, even when given immediately after parotitis is first noted.

Epidemiology

Mumps occurs throughout the world endemically throughout the year. Outbreaks occur where crowding favors dissemination of the virus. The disease reaches its highest incidence in children age 5–15 years, but epidemics occur in army camps. Although morbidity rates are high, the mortality rate is negligible. However, in the USA until 1975, mumps was the leading cause of viral encephalitis of known etiology. The incidence has been greatly reduced since the introduction of the combined measles-mumps-rubella vaccine.

Humans are the only known reservoir of virus. The virus is transmitted by direct contact, airborne droplets, or fomites contaminated with saliva and, perhaps, urine. The period of communicability is from about 4 days before to about a week after the onset of symptoms. More intimate contact is necessary for the transmission of mumps than for measles or varicella.

About 30–40% of infections with mumps virus are inapparent. Individuals with subclinical mumps acquire immunity. During the course of inapparent infection, they can serve as sources of infection for others.

Antibodies to mumps virus are transferred across the placenta and are gradually lost during the first year of life. In urban areas, antibodies are then acquired gradually, so that the 15-year-old group has about the same prevalence of persons with antibodies as the adult group. Antibodies are acquired at the same rate by persons living under favorable and unfavorable socioeconomic conditions.

Control

Mumps is usually a mild childhood disease. A live attenuated vaccine made in chick embryo cell culture is available. It produces a subclinical noncommunicable infection.

The vaccine is recommended for children over age 1 year and for adolescents and adults who have not had mumps parotitis. A single dose of the vaccine given subcutaneously produces detectable antibodies in 95% of vaccinees, and antibody persists for at least 8 years.

Combination live virus vaccines (measles-mumps-rubella) produce antibodies to each of the viruses in about 95% of vaccinees.

In 1967, the year mumps vaccine was licensed, there were about 200,000 mumps cases (and 900 patients with encephalitis) in the USA. After 17 years of vaccine use, the number of mumps cases in 1984 was less than 3000, with fewer than 20 cases of encephalitis. Further declines in the incidence of mumps are expected as more children entering school are required to provide proof of mumps vaccination. The mumps incidence in states requiring such proof is 50% of that in states without such a law.

PARAINFLUENZA VIRUS INFECTIONS

The parainfluenza viruses are paramyxoviruses with morphologic and biologic properties typical of the genus. They grow well in primary monkey or human epithelial cell culture but poorly or not at all in the embryonated egg. They produce a minimal cytopathic effect in cell culture but are recognized by the hemadsorption method. Laboratory diagnosis may be made by the hemadsorption, CF, and Nt tests.

Parainfluenza 1

Included here are **Sendai virus,** also known as the **hemagglutinating virus of Japan (HVJ),** and **hemadsorption virus type 2 (HA-2).** Sendai virus may be a causative agent of pneumonia in pigs and newborn infants. Sendai virus is important in somatic cell genetics, where it is used to produce cell fusion. Clinically, the most important member of this group appears to be the widespread HA-2 virus. It is not cytopathogenic for monkey kidney cell cultures but is detected in such cultures by the hemadsorption test. It is one of the main agents producing croup in children, but it can also cause coryza, pharyngitis, bronchitis, bronchiolitis, or pneumonia. In adults, it produces respiratory symptoms like those of the common cold, with reinfection occurring in persons with antibodies from earlier infections.

Parainfluenza 2

This group includes the **croup-associated (CA) virus** of children. The virus grows in human cells (HeLa, lung, amnion) and monkey kidney. Syncytial masses are produced, with loss of cell boundaries. The virus agglutinates chick and human type O erythrocytes. Adsorption and hemagglutination occur at 4 °C, and elution of virus takes place rapidly at 37 °C. However, the cells reagglutinate when returned to 4 °C. Mumps patients develop type 2 antibodies.

Parainfluenza virus 2 occurs spontaneously in 30% of lots of monkey kidney cells grown in culture. The monkey virus SV5 is antigenically related.

Parainfluenza 3

The viruses in this group are also known as **hemadsorption virus type 1 (HA-1).** They are detected in monkey kidney cultures by the hemadsorption technique. Serial passage in culture may lead to cytopathic changes. Multinucleated giant cell plaques are produced under agar in certain human cell lines.

The virus has been isolated from children with mild respiratory illnesses, croup, bronchiolitis, or pneumonitis. Strains of type 3 virus have been isolated from nasal secretions of cattle ill with a respiratory syndrome known as "shipping fever." At least 70% of market cattle bled at slaughter have parainfluenza 3 antibodies.

Parainfluenza 4 & 5

These viruses are not known to cause any human illness, although antibodies are widespread. Their growth in cell culture can be recognized by the hemadsorption method.

Clinical Features & Control

Children in the first year of life with primary infections caused by parainfluenza virus type 1, 2, or 3 may have serious illness ranging from laryngotracheitis and croup (particularly type 2) to bronchitis, bronchiolitis, and pneumonitis (particularly type 3).

Virtually all infants have maternal antibodies to parainfluenza viruses in serum, yet such antibodies do not prevent infection or disease. Reinfection of older children and adults also occurs in the presence of antibodies arising from an earlier infection. Such reinfections usually present as nonfebrile upper respiratory infections ("colds").

The incubation for type 1 is 5–6 days; that for type 3 is 2–3 days. Most children have acquired antibodies to all 3 types before age 10.

Natural infection stimulates antibody appearance in nasal secretions and concomitant resistance to reinfection. An experimental killed vaccine induces serum antibodies but does not protect against infection. Live vaccines are being investigated.

NEWCASTLE DISEASE CONJUNCTIVITIS

Newcastle disease virus is a typical paramyxovirus that is primarily pathogenic for fowl. It produces pneumoencephalitis in young chickens and "influenza" in older birds. In humans, it may produce an inflammation of the conjunctiva. Recovery is complete in 10–14 days. The infection in humans is an occupational disease limited to laboratory workers and to poultry workers handling infected birds.

The virus grows readily in the embryonated egg, in chick embryo cell culture, or in HeLa cells and produces hemagglutination.

Human erythrocytes treated with the virus are agglutinated by specific serum against Newcastle virus.

Newcastle antibodies can be measured by the HI, CF, and Nt tests using chick embryos or tissue cultures. Cross-reacting HI antibodies can develop in mumps, hepatitis, and infectious mononucleosis. Normal human sera possess a heat-labile, nonspecific inhibitor that can be destroyed by heating at 56 °C for 30 minutes.

There are several other avian paramyxoviruses.

MEASLES (Rubeola)

Measles is an acute, highly infectious disease characterized by a maculopapular rash, fever, and respiratory symptoms.

Properties of the Virus

A. Morphology and Biologic Properties: Measles virus is a typical paramyxovirus, related to canine distemper and bovine rinderpest. All 3 lack neuraminidase activity. Measles agglutinates monkey erythrocytes at 37 °C but does not elute, and it interacts with a distinct cell receptor. Measles virus also causes hemolysis, and this activity can be separated from that of the hemagglutinin.

B. Animal Susceptibility and Growth of Virus: The experimental disease has been produced in monkeys. They develop fever, catarrh, Koplik's spots, and a discrete papular rash. The virus has been grown in chick embryos; in cell cultures of human, monkey, and dog kidney tissue; and in human continuous cell lines. In cell cultures, multinucleate syncytial giant cells form by fusion of mononucleated ones, and other cells become spindle-shaped in the course of their degeneration. Nuclear changes consist of margination of the chromatin and its replacement centrally with an acidophilic inclusion body. Measles virus is relatively unstable after it is released from cells. During the culture of the virus, the intracellular virus titer is 10 or more times the extracellular titer.

Pathogenesis & Pathology

The virus enters the respiratory tract, enters cells, and multiplies there. During the prodrome, the virus is present in the blood, throughout the respiratory tract, and in nasopharyngeal, tracheobronchial, and conjunctival secretions. It persists in the blood and nasopharyngeal secretions for 2 days after the appearance of the rash. Transplacental transmission of the virus can occur.

Koplik's spots are vesicles in the buccal mucosa formed by focal exudations of serum and endothelial cells, followed by focal necrosis. In the skin, the superficial capillaries of the corium are first involved, and it is here that the rash makes its appearance. Generalized lymphoid tissue hyperplasia occurs. Multinucleate giant cells are found in lymph nodes, tonsils, adenoids, spleen, appendix, and skin. In encephalomyelitis, there are petechial hemorrhages, lymphocytic infiltration, and, later, patchy demyelination in the brain and spinal cord.

Subacute sclerosing panencephalitis (SSPE) is a rare, persistent, and fatal disease resulting from measles virus infection of the brain. Measles nucleoprotein antigens have been identified by immunofluorescence within inclusion bodies of the infected nerve cells. The inability to complete viral reproduction may be due to a defect in the expression or accumulation of a single virus gene product, the matrix protein. The virus has been grown by co-cultivating HeLa cells with brain biopsy material or lymph node material from patients. The presence of latent intracellular measles virus in these specimens suggests a tolerant infection with defective cell-mediated immunity.

If measles antibody is added to cells infected with measles virus, the viral antigens on the cell surface are altered. By expressing fewer viral antigens on the surface, cells may avoid being killed by antibody- or cell-mediated cytotoxic reactions, yet may retain viral genetic information. This may lead to persistent infection as found in SSPE patients.

Clinical Findings

The incubation period is about 10 days to onset of fever and 14 days to appearance of rash. The prodromal period is characterized by fever, sneezing, coughing, running nose, redness of eyes, Koplik's spots (enanthems of the buccal mucosa), and lymphopenia. The fever and cough persist until the rash appears and then subside within 1–2 days. The rash spreads over the entire body within 2–4 days, becoming brownish in 5–10 days. Symptoms of the disease are most marked when the rash is at its peak but subside rapidly thereafter.

In measles, the respiratory tract becomes more susceptible to invasion by bacteria, especially hemolytic streptococci; bronchitis, pneumonia, and otitis may follow in 15% of cases.

Encephalomyelitis occurs in about 1:1000 cases. There appears to be no correlation between the severity of the measles and the appearance of neurologic complications. The cause of measles encephalitis is unknown. It has been suggested that early central nervous system involvement is caused by direct viral invasion of the brain. Later appearance of central nervous system symptoms is associated with demyelination and may be an immunopathologic reaction. Symptoms referable to the brain usually appear a few days after the appearance of the rash, often after it has faded. There is a second bout of fever, with drowsiness or convulsions and pleocytosis of the cerebrospinal fluid. Survivors may show permanent mental disorders (psychosis or personality change) or physical disabilities, particularly seizure disorders. The mortality rate in encephalitis associated with measles is about 10–30%, and many survivors (40%) show sequelae.

Measles virus appears to be responsible for subacute sclerosing panencephalitis (SSPE), a fatal degenerative brain disorder. The disease manifests itself in children and young adults by progressive mental deterioration, myoclonic jerks, and an abnormal electroencephalogram with periodic high-voltage complexes. The disease develops a number of years after the initial measles infection.

Atypical measles. After the introduction of killed measles virus vaccine in 1965, a new clinical syndrome was observed in children who had a history of receiving the vaccine. The syndrome, called atypical measles, was associated with measles virus infection and was characterized by high fever, pneumonia, and an unusual rash (raised papules, wheals, and tiny hemorrhages in the skin) without Koplik's spots. Killed measles virus vaccine is no longer used. Atypical measles is now seen occasionally in young adults who had received killed vaccine as children.

Laboratory Diagnosis

Measles is usually easily diagnosed on clinical grounds. About 5% of cases lack Koplik's spots and are difficult to differentiate clinically from infection with rubella virus, certain enteroviruses, and adenoviruses.

A. Recovery of Virus: Measles virus can be isolated from the blood and nasopharynx of a patient from 2–3 days before the onset of symptoms to 1 day after the appearance of rash. Human amnion or kidney cell cultures are best suited for isolation of virus.

B. Serology: Specific Nt, HI, and CF antibodies develop early, with maximal titers near the time of onset of rash. Serologic confirmation of measles depends upon a 4-fold rise in antibody titer or upon demonstration of measles-specific IgM antibody in a single serum specimen drawn between 1 and 2 weeks after onset of the rash. False negatives may occur if the serum is taken earlier than 1 week or later than 2 weeks after onset of the rash.

Measles and canine distemper share an antigen. Measles patients develop antibodies that cross-react with canine distemper virus. Similarly, dogs, after infection with distemper virus, develop antibodies that fix complement with measles antigen. Rinderpest virus is also related to measles.

Immunity

There appears to be only one antigenic type of measles virus, since one attack generally confers lifelong immunity. Most so-called second attacks represent errors in diagnosis of the initial or the second illness.

Epidemiology

Measles is endemic throughout the world. In general, epidemics recur regularly every 2–3 years. The state of immunity of the population is the determining factor. The disease flares up when there is an accumulation of susceptible children. By age 20 years, more than 80% of those who were susceptible have had an attack of the disease. The severity of an epidemic is a function of the number of susceptible individuals. Only about 1% of susceptible persons fail to contract measles on their first close contact with a patient.

When the disease is introduced into isolated communities where it has not been endemic, all age groups develop clinical measles. A classic example of this was the introduction of measles into the Faroe Islands in 1846; only people over age 60 years, who had been alive during the last epidemic, escaped the disease. In places where the disease strikes rarely, its consequences are often disastrous, and the mortality rate may be as high as 25%.

The highest incidence of measles is in the late winter and spring. Infection is contracted by inhalation of droplets expelled in sneezing or coughing. Measles is spread chiefly by children during the catarrhal prodromal period; they are infectious from 1–2 days prior to the onset of symptoms until a few days after the rash has appeared.

Control

Live attenuated measles virus vaccine effectively prevents measles. Prior to the introduction of the vaccine, over 500,000 cases of measles occurred annually in the USA, and over 300 developed encephalitis. Following mass immunization in 1966–1967, the number of cases decreased to 67,000 and 22,000 annually in the next 2 years, with a corresponding decrease in measles encephalitis. Nevertheless, measles continued to occur, and in 1976 and 1977, the reported numbers of cases increased to 40,000 and 56,000 respectively—90% among the nonvaccinated. About 95% of children properly inoculated with live virus vaccine develop antibodies that persist for at least 18 years.

As of 1979, an effective measles vaccine had been given to 70% of the children in the USA. The result has been the disappearance of the major epidemics of the 1950s that infected and immunized 98% of children by age 10. However, the 30% of children who had not been immunized in the 1960s became the susceptible adolescents of the 1970s. In 1980, more than 25% of measles cases in the USA occurred among those 10–14 years of age and more than 20% among those 15–19 years of age. To prevent adult measles from becoming a major problem, the vaccination program for children has been intensified, with the result that measles cases in 1983 decreased to about 1500, a record low. The prevaccination rate of measles deaths per year was 400, but measles deaths are now a rarity. In 1983, 20% of all measles cases reported occurred on college campuses; the largest outbreak included 128 cases with 3 deaths (due to respiratory complications) among a total student population of 712. As of this writing, about 15% of college students may be susceptible to measles, largely because they were children at the start of the national measles vaccination programs and may have been missed or may not have been properly immunized. They should be vaccinated to decrease their vulnerability.

Less attenuated vaccine virus may produce fever and a modified skin rash in a proportion of vaccinees; this reaction can be prevented by the simultaneous administration of immune globulin USP (0.02 mL/kg body weight) *at a separate site from the vaccine*. The more attenuated vaccine viruses do not produce symptoms and do not require the use of immune globulin. The different vaccine strains appear to be equally effective in producing immunity.

Measles antibodies cross the placenta and protect the infant during the first 6–10 months of life. Vaccination with the live virus fails to take during this period, and measles immunization should be deferred until 15 months of age. This applies both to monovalent measles vaccine and to combined measles-mumps-rubella vaccine.

When the live vaccine was first introduced in the USA, it was often given to infants in the first year of life. This did not produce long-lasting immunity, and such children must be revaccinated.

Because of the severe disease caused by measles virus in many developing countries, vaccine is often given in 2 doses, the first at age 8–9 months and the second a year later. During measles outbreaks, vaccine should be given at age 6 months and again a year later. The latter regimen should also be followed in developing countries in cases where the risk of exposure is high, eg, infants in hospitals. As nations achieve measles control, the age of immunization should be raised to 15 months.

Vaccination is not recommended in persons with febrile illnesses or allergies to eggs or other products used in the production of the vaccine, and in persons with immune defects.

Epidemiologic studies have shown that the risk, if any, of SSPE occurring in vaccinated persons is far less than the risk of its occurring in persons who have natural measles.

Killed measles vaccine should not be used, as certain vaccinees become sensitized and develop either local reactions when revaccinated with live attenuated virus or severe atypical measles when infected with wild virus or even with live vaccine virus (see Atypical measles, above).

Measles may be prevented or modified by administering antibody early in the incubation period. Human gamma globulin (immune globulin USP) contains antibody titers of 200–1000 against 100 $TCID_{50}$ of virus. With small doses, the disease can be made mild and immunity ensues. With a large dose of immune globulin, the disease can be prevented; however, the person remains susceptible to infection at a later date. Antibodies given later than 6 days after exposure are not likely to influence the course of the disease.

An aerosolized form of the measles vaccine has been introduced recently for vaccination in the first few months of life. It should be particularly useful for widespread early immunization of children in developing countries where measles before the age of 9 months is common and where mortality rates are high.

RESPIRATORY SYNCYTIAL (RS) VIRUS

This labile paramyxovirus produces a characteristic syncytial effect, the fusion of cells in human cell culture. It is the single most serious cause of bronchiolitis and pneumonitis in infants. RS virus occurs spontaneously in chimpanzees and has been associated with coryza in these primates.

Properties of the Virus

The particle is slightly smaller (80–120 nm) than other paramyxoviruses, and the nucleocapsid measures 11–15 nm. The envelope of RS virus contains 2 surface glycoproteins. Glycoprotein G (MW 84,000–90,000) mediates attachment to target cells, and glycoprotein F (MW 68,000–70,000) is the viral fusion glycoprotein. The F protein directs fusion of viral and cellular membranes (Fig 41–2), resulting in viral penetration, and can direct fusion of infected cells with adjoining cells, resulting in the formation of syncytia. Syncytia formation is both a prominent cytopathic effect and an additional mechanism of viral spread. Neutralization of fusion activity is important in host immunity.

The RS viral genome, a single negative strand of RNA, encodes 10 unique mRNAs. One of the products of mRNA translation in vitro was identified by peptide mapping as the nonglycosylated and uncleaved form of the F protein, which has now been sequenced.

Although RS is one of the most labile of viruses, it can be stabilized by $MgSO_4$, 1 mol/L (like measles and other paramyxoviruses). RS virus does not hemagglutinate. A soluble CF antigen can be separated from the virus particle.

RS virus produces a respiratory tract infection in cotton rats. The virus grows relatively slowly in cell cultures (4–8 days). For rapid diagnostic results, the direct immunofluorescence test with RS antiserum can be applied to nasopharyngeal smears containing exfoliated cells.

Monoclonal antibodies have been prepared that immunoprecipitate the nucleoprotein, glycoprotein G, or glycoprotein F. Through the use of immunofluorescence or ELISA tests, 3 subgroups of RS virus have been proposed. However, when tested by cross-neutralization, RS virus isolates from different outbreaks show minimal antigenic variation.

Clinical & Epidemiologic Features

Most RS virus infections are confined to the upper respiratory tract, but the disease can extend to the lower respiratory tract with a broad spectrum of severity. In its extreme form, it can be fatal. On autopsy, the lungs of infants who die of RS virus infection show extensive bronchopneumonia, accompanied by sloughing of bronchiolar epithelium and infiltration by monocytes and other immunologic cells.

RS virus can be isolated from about 40% of infants under age 6 months suffering from bronchiolitis and from about 25% with pneumonitis, but it is almost never isolated from healthy infants. RS virus infection in older infants and children results in milder respiratory tract infection than in those under 6 months of age. Adult volunteers can be reinfected with RS virus (in spite of the presence of specific antibodies), but the resulting symptoms are those of an upper respiratory infection, a "cold."

RS virus spreads extensively in children every year during the winter season. Reinfection commonly occurs in children, even with the homologous virus, but each subsequent infection is milder than the preceding ones. Nosocomial infections occur in nurseries and on pediatric hospital wards. Transmission occurs primarily via the hands of staff members. Hand washing after every patient contact, wearing gowns and gloves, and isolation of infected patients reduce nosocomial spread.

Very high levels (1:400) of Nt antibody that is maternally transmitted and present in the first 2 months of life are believed to be critical in protective immunity. Severe RS disease begins to occur in infants at 2–4 months of age, when maternal antibody levels are falling. The natural rate of decrease is about 50% each month; thus, the antibody level soon falls below the protective level. Healthy 1-month-old infants have antibody titers that are up to 4 times higher than those of age-matched infants with RS virus bronchiolitis or pneumonia.

Formalin-inactivated RS virus has been tried as a vaccine in infants. The results were poor, because the vaccinated infants who subsequently became naturally infected with RS virus developed more severe disease than did the nonvaccinated infants. Since this occurred despite the Nt antibodies induced by the vaccine, it led to the belief that RS antibody might be harmful. Thus, RS disease was felt to be the result of an immunopathologic process mediated by maternal antibodies. However, it now seems that the level of antibodies is the critical factor. In addition, an immediate hypersensitivity to virus-IgE interactions may be involved. The nasal secretions of children experiencing severe reactions to RS virus contain histamine and also anti-RS virus IgE.

Passive transfer of postinfection viral antibodies or monoclonal antibodies to either of the virus glycoproteins (see above) protected the respiratory tract of experimental rodents against RS virus infection. The possibility of passive immunization of human infants is being explored. Efforts also are in progress to develop an attenuated vaccine that infects subclinically and induces nasal antibody.

Ribavirin administered in a continuous aerosol for 3–6 days was clinically beneficial to hospitalized infants. In addition, viral shedding was decreased.

RUBELLA
(German Measles)

Rubella is an acute febrile illness characterized by a rash and posterior auricular and suboccipital lymphadenopathy that affects children and young adults. Infection in early pregnancy may result in serious abnormalities of the fetus.

Properties of the Virus

The virus is RNA-containing, ether-sensitive, and about 60 nm in diameter. It contains a 30-nm internal nucleocapsid with a double membrane and forms by budding from the endoplasmic reticulum into intracytoplasmic vesicles and at the marginal cell membrane. Projections of the virion, 6 nm long, possess hemagglutinin for some avian erythrocytes. Receptor-destroying enzyme has no effect, and there is no spontaneous elution after hemagglutination.

Rubella virus can be propagated in cell culture. In some cultures, eg, human amnion cells, rabbit kidney cells, and a line of monkey kidney (VERO) cells, the virus produces detectable cytopathologic changes. In other cell cultures, rubella virus replicates without causing a cytopathic effect; however, interference is induced that protects the cells against the cytopathic effect of other viruses. One method of isolating rubella virus consists of inoculating green monkey kidney cells with the specimen and, after 7–10 days of incubation, challenging the cultures with echovirus 11. If echovirus cytopathic effect develops, the specimen is considered negative for rubella virus; conversely, the absence of echovirus cytopathic effect implies the presence of rubella virus in the original specimen.

1. POSTNATAL RUBELLA

Pathogenesis

Infection occurs through the mucosa of the upper respiratory tract. The virus probably replicates primarily in the cervical lymph nodes. After a period of 7 days, viremia develops that lasts until the appearance of antibody on about day 12–14. The development of antibody coincides with the appearance of the rash, suggesting an immunologic basis for the rash. After the rash appears, the virus remains detectable only in the nasopharynx.

Clinical Features

Rubella usually begins with malaise, low-grade fever, and a morbilliform rash appearing on the same day. Less often, systemic symptoms may precede the rash by 1 or 2 days, or the rash and lymphadenopathy may occur without systemic symptoms. The rash starts on the face, extends over the trunk and extremities, and rarely lasts more than 3 days. Posterior auricular and suboccipital lymphadenopathy are present. Transient arthralgia and arthritis are commonly seen in adult females. Rare complications include thrombocytopenia and encephalitis.

Unless an epidemic occurs, the disease is difficult to diagnose clinically, since the rash caused by other viruses such as the enteroviruses is similar. However, rubella has a peak occurrence in the spring, whereas enterovirus infections occur mainly in the summer and fall.

Immunity

Rubella antibodies appear in the serum of patients as the rash fades, and the titer of antibody rises rapidly over the next 1–3 weeks. Much of the initial antibody consists of IgM. IgM rubella antibodies found in a single serum sample obtained 2 weeks after the rash give evidence of recent rubella infection.

One attack of the disease confers lifelong immunity, as only one antigenic type of the virus exists. A history of rubella is not a reliable index of immunity. The presence of antibody at a 1:8 dilution implies immunity. Immune mothers transfer antibodies to their offspring, who are then protected for 4–6 months.

Treatment

No specific treatment is given unless the patient is pregnant. Rubellalike illness in the first trimester of pregnancy should be substantiated by demonstrating a 4-fold rise in antibody titer to the virus by means of the HI, CF, Nt, or ELISA test. A high antibody level in a single serum specimen or a rise in antibody titer in 2 samples taken 1–2 weeks apart should be confirmed by a test for rubella-specific IgM. As seen in Fig 41–3, HI antibody appears earlier and persists longer than CF antibody; HI is the test of choice, since rapid diagnosis is essential for therapeutic management. Isolation of virus from the throat is possible, but this takes longer than conducting serologic tests.

Laboratory-proved rubella in the first 10 weeks of

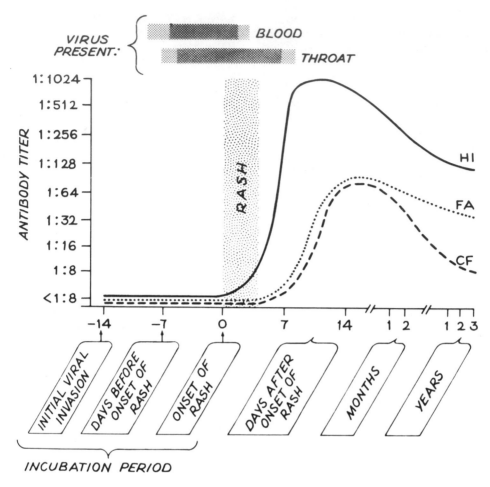

Figure 41–3. Virus and antibody dynamics in rubella. HI = hemagglutination-inhibiting antibody; FA = fluorescent antibody; CF = complement-fixing antibody.

pregnancy is almost uniformly associated with fetal infection. Therapeutic abortion is strongly recommended in laboratory-proved cases to avoid the risk of malformed infants.

Immune globulin USP injected into the mother does not protect the fetus against rubella infection.

2. CONGENITAL RUBELLA SYNDROME

Pathogenesis

Rubella infection during pregnancy may result in infection of the placenta and fetus. A limited number of cells of the fetus become infected. Although the virus does not destroy the cells, the growth rate of the infected cells is reduced, which results in fewer than normal numbers of cells in the organs at birth. The earlier in pregnancy infection occurs, the greater the chance of extensive involvement, with the birth of an infant afflicted with severe anomalies. Infection in the first month of pregnancy results in abnormalities in about 80% of cases, whereas detectable defects are found in about 15% of infants acquiring the disease

during the third month of gestation. The intrauterine infection is associated with chronic persistence of the virus in the newborn, which may last for 12–18 months after birth.

Clinical Findings

Infants with congenital rubella syndrome may have one or more abnormalities, which include defects of the heart and great vessels (patent ductus arteriosus, pulmonary artery stenosis, pulmonary valvular stenosis, ventricular septal defect, and atrial septal defect), eye defects (cataracts, glaucoma, and chorioretinitis), and neurosensory deafness. Infants may also display growth retardation, failure to thrive, hepatosplenomegaly, thrombocytopenia with purpura, anemia, osteitis, and an encephalitic syndrome leading to cerebral palsy.

The spectrum of neurologic and neurosensory involvement in surviving infants is wide. Among 100 patients with congenital rubella infection, neurologic manifestations were found in 81 at some time between birth and 18 months. Sequelae include hearing impairment, visual impairment, growth disturbance, microcephaly, mental retardation, and cerebral dysfunction. Problems with balance and motor skills develop in preschool children. Psychiatric disorders and behavioral manifestations occur in preschool and school-age children.

In one study, the neurologic course of congenital rubella syndrome was traced in nonretarded children. During the first 2 years, manifestations involved abnormal tone and reflexes (69%), motor delays (66%), feeding difficulties (48%), and abnormal clinical behavior (45%). Hearing loss was documented in 76%. At 3–7 years, poor balance, motor incoordination (69%), and behavioral disturbances (66%) predominated. Hearing losses increased to 86%. At 9–12 years, the following were noted: residua that included learning deficits (52%), behavioral disturbances (48%), poor balance (61%), muscle weakness (54%), and deficits in tactile perception (41%). Thus, the encephalitic manifestations of congenital rubella syndrome are persistent and diverse.

Infants with congenital rubella syndrome often have increased susceptibility to infection and abnormal immunoglobulins, most commonly elevated IgM with low levels of IgG and IgA. There is a 20% mortality rate among congenitally virus-infected infants symptomatic at birth. Some virus-infected infants who appear normal at birth may manifest abnormalities at a later date. Severely affected infants may require institutionalization.

Immunity

Normally, maternal rubella antibody in the form of IgG is transferred to infants and gradually lost over a period of 6 months. In infants infected in utero, persistence of rubella virus causes a rising titer of rubella-specific IgM as well as a rise in the specific IgG level that persists long after the fall in maternal IgG.

Epidemiology

The virus has been recovered from the nasopharynx, throat, blood, cerebrospinal fluid, and urine. The infection is spread by respiratory pathways (droplets).

Infants continue to be infectious, with virus found in the throat for up to 18 months after birth. Virus has been recovered from many tissues tested postmortem.

Congenitally infected infants who appear normal but who shed virus are capable of transmitting rubella to susceptible contacts such as nurses and physicians caring for the infants. This represents a serious hazard to women in the first trimester of pregnancy, who should avoid contact with these babies.

Rubella without rash is of importance because inapparent rubella infection (with viremia) acquired during pregnancy has the same deleterious effect on the fetus as rubella with the typical rash.

3. CONTROL OF RUBELLA

In the 20th century, epidemics of rubella have occurred every 6–9 years. After each epidemic, cases declined for the next 5 years, then increased to epidemic levels 6–9 years after the last major outbreak. In the 1964 epidemic, more than 20,000 infants were born with severe manifestations of congenital rubella.

In the USA, the control of rubella is being attempted by routine vaccination of children age 1–12 years and selected immunization of adolescents and women of childbearing age. Before vaccine became available in 1969, about 70,000 cases were being reported annually. In the next 15 years, about 123 million doses of vaccine were administered, which resulted in a decrease in rubella incidence to only 750 cases in 1984, a decrease of 99% in reported cases. However, the decrease occurred primarily in children. Persons 15 years of age and older experienced only a small decrease in incidence and now account for over 70% of cases. (Before 1969, they accounted for only 20%.) Since vaccine-induced antibodies persist for at least 10 years, the changing pattern may not be due to vaccine failure as much as to failure to adequately vaccinate susceptible adults.

Since the introduction of vaccine, scattered outbreaks have been reported, chiefly among nonvaccinated adolescents in high school and college who had not received vaccine in the routine immunization program. The changing age incidence of rubella since introduction of vaccine is similar to the changing epidemiologic pattern with measles (see above).

In postpubertal females, the vaccine produces self-limited arthralgia and arthritis in about one-third of the vaccinees. Since rubella vaccine virus may infect the placenta, the vaccine should not be given to a postpubertal female unless she is not pregnant, is susceptible (ie, serologically negative), understands that she should not become pregnant for at least 3 months after vaccination, and is adequately warned of the complications of arthralgia. Nevertheless, since rubella vaccination is an effective way of preventing birth defects, it should be vigorously encouraged in women of childbearing age.

In children, the vaccine may also produce mild febrile episodes with arthralgia, often several months after vaccination, but without any permanent residual effects. Vaccinated children are not infectious and do not transmit the vaccine or wild virus to contacts at home, even to mothers who are susceptible and pregnant. In contrast, nonimmunized children can bring home wild virus and spread it to susceptible family contacts.

Opinions have been expressed that vaccination of children cannot prevent future infection of pregnant women exposed to wild virus. Therefore, vaccination of prepubertal girls and women in the immediate postpartum period has also been proposed. It would seem wise for all pregnant women to undergo a serum antibody test for rubella and, if found to be susceptible, receive a vaccination immediately after delivery. Conception in the 6–8 weeks after delivery is rare, so the risk of harming a fetus would be minimal.

There is conflicting evidence on the nature and duration of postvaccination immunity with the first

(HPV77) rubella vaccine, the risk of superinfection with wild virus, and the subsequent spread of such virus to pregnant women.

In 1979, the second rubella vaccine, RA27/3, grown in human diploid cells, was licensed, and this is the vaccine of choice. It produces much higher antibody titers and a more enduring and more solid immunity than HPV77, and there is evidence that it largely prevents subclinical superinfection with wild virus. This vaccine is available as a single antigen or combined with measles and mumps vaccine. It may effectively produce IgA antibody in the respiratory tract and thus interfere with infection by wild virus.

Congenital rubella disease is being brought under control. In the USA, its incidence has declined from a high of about 30,000 cases in 1964 (in the prevaccine period) to 55 cases in 1979, 9 cases in 1982, and only 2 cases in 1984. To eliminate rubella and the congenital rubella syndrome, it is necessary to immunize women of childbearing age as well as all school-age children. In addition to the recommendations set forth above, it is advised that women be vaccinated as part of routine medical and gynecologic care, particularly during visits to family-planning clinics, and that proof of immunity (positive serologic tests or documented rubella vaccination) be required for female students entering college and for female hospital personnel who might come in contact with rubella patients or pregnant women.

REFERENCES

Amler RW et al: Imported measles in the United States. *JAMA* 1982;**248:**2129.

Anderson LJ et al: Antigenic characterization of respiratory syncytial virus strains with monoclonal antibodies. *J Infect Dis* 1985;**151:**626.

Black NA et al: Post-partum rubella immunisation: A controlled trial of two vaccines. *Lancet* 1983;**2:**990.

Brunell PA et al: Antibody response following measles-mumps-rubella vaccine under conditions of customary use. *JAMA* 1983;**250:**1409.

Choppin PW, Scheid A: The role of viral glycoproteins in adsorption, penetration, and pathogenicity of viruses. *Rev Infect Dis* 1980;**2:**40.

Fujinami RS, Oldstone MBA: Antiviral antibody reacting on the plasma membrane alters measles virus expression inside the cell. *Nature* 1979;**279:**529.

Hall CB et al: Aerosolized ribavirin treatment of infants with respiratory syncytial viral infection: A randomized double-blind study. *N Engl J Med* 1983;**308:**1443.

Krugman S et al: Measles: Current impact, vaccines and control. *Rev Infect Dis* 1983;**5:**389.

Orenstein WA et al: The opportunity and obligation to eliminate rubella from the United States. *JAMA* 1984;**251:**1988.

Prince GA et al: Quantitative aspects of passive immunity to respiratory syncytial virus infection in infant cotton rats. *J Virol* 1985;**55:**517.

Rawls WE: Congenital rubella: The significance of virus persistence. *Prog Med Virol* 1968;**10:**238.

Remington PL et al: Airborne transmission of measles in a physician's office. *JAMA* 1985;**253:**1574.

Sabin AB et al: Successful immunization of children with and without maternal antibody by aerosolized measles vaccine. (2 parts.) *JAMA* 1983;**249:**2651 and 1984;**251:**2673.

Serdula MK et al: Serological response to rubella revaccination. *JAMA* 1984;**251:**1974.

Sheppard RD et al: Measles virus matrix protein synthesized in a subacute sclerosing panencephalitis cell line. *Science* 1985;**228:**1219.

Whittle HC et al: Immunisation of 4–6 month old Gambian infants with Edmonston-Zagreb measles vaccine. *Lancet* 1984;**2:**834.

Wright PF et al: Administration of a highly attenuated, live respiratory syncytial virus vaccine to adults and children. *Infect Immun* 1982;**37:**397.

Poxvirus Family

42

Poxviruses are the largest and most complex of viruses. The family encompasses a large group of agents that are morphologically similar and share a common nucleoprotein antigen. Infections with most poxviruses are characterized by a rash, whereas lesions induced by some members of the family are markedly proliferative. The group includes variola virus, the etiologic agent of smallpox, the viral disease that has most affected humans throughout recorded history until 1977.

The so-called orthopoxviruses have a broad host range, affecting several vertebrates. They include ectromelia (mousepox), rabbitpox, cowpox, monkeypox, vaccinia, and variola (smallpox) viruses. The last 4 are infectious for humans. Some subgroups have a restricted host range and infect only arthropods, or only rodents (fibroma and myxoma), or only birds. Other subgroups infect mainly sheep (orf, sheeppox), goats (goatpox), and cattle (eg, milker's nodule).

Even though smallpox (variola) has been declared eradicated from the world after an intensive campaign coordinated by the World Health Organization (WHO), there is a continuing need to be familiar with vaccinia virus and its possible complications in hu-

mans. There is also a need to be aware of other poxvirus diseases that may resemble smallpox and thus must be differentiated from it by laboratory means. Lastly, vaccinia virus is under intensive study as a vector for introducing active immunizing genes as live vaccines for a variety of virus diseases of humans and domestic animals.

PROPERTIES OF POXVIRUSES

Classification

Most of the poxviruses that can cause disease in humans are contained in the orthopoxvirus and parapoxvirus subgroups; there are also several that are currently unclassified.

Vaccinia virus differs in only minor morphologic respects from variola and cowpox viruses. It is the prototype of poxviruses in terms of structure and replication. Monkeypox can infect both monkeys and humans and may resemble smallpox clinically. Parapoxviruses are morphologically distinctive, their surfaces exhibiting a crisscross pattern (Fig 42–1). Their genomes are smaller (MW 85×10^6) and have a

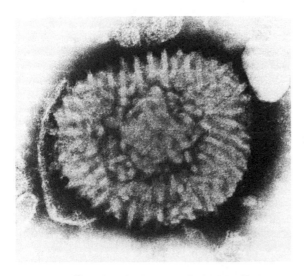 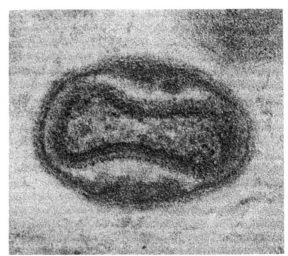

Figure 42–1. Electron micrographs of vaccinia (*Orthopoxvirus*) virions. **A:** Negatively stained particle showing ridges or tubular elements covering the surface (228,000 ×). (Reproduced, with permission, from Dales S: *J Cell Biol* 1963;**18**:51.) **B:** Thin section of vaccinia virion showing a central biconcave core, 2 lateral bodies, and an outer membrane (220,000 ×). (Reproduced, with permission, from Pogo BGT, Dales S: *Proc Natl Acad Sci USA* 1969;**63**:820.) Cross sections of immature and mature vaccinia virions are shown in Figs 33–33 and 33–34.

higher guanine-plus-cytosine (G + C) content (63%) than those of the orthopoxviruses (MW 120 × 10⁶; G + C 35%).

All poxviruses share a common nucleoprotein (NP) antigen in the inner core. There is serologic cross-reactivity among viruses within a given genus but very limited reactivity across genera. Consequently, immunization with vaccinia virus affords no protection against disease induced by parapoxviruses or the unclassified poxviruses.

Morphology & Composition

Poxviruses are large enough to be seen as featureless particles by light microscopy. By electron microscopy, they can be seen to be brick-shaped or ellipsoid particles measuring about 230 × 400 nm. There is an outer lipoprotein membrane, or envelope, that encloses a core and 2 structures of unknown function, called lateral bodies (Fig 42–1). The core contains the large viral genome, linear double-stranded DNA (MW 85–240 × 10⁶); the DNA strands are connected at the ends by terminal hairpin loops (Figs 33–33 and 33–34).

The virion contains a multiplicity of enzymes, including a transcriptional system that can synthesize, polyadenylate, cap, and methylate viral mRNA. More than 100 structural polypeptides have been detected. The chemical composition of a poxvirus resembles that of a bacterium.

Vaccinia virus is composed predominantly of protein (90%), lipid (5%), and DNA (3%). A number of the proteins are glycosylated or phosphorylated. The lipids are cholesterol and phospholipids. The DNA is rich in adenine and thymine bases. In addition to being covalently linked at the ends, poxvirus DNA contains inverted terminal repeats of variable length.

Multiplication

The replication cycle of vaccinia virus is summarized in Fig 42–2. Poxviruses are unique among DNA viruses in that the entire multiplication cycle takes place in the cytoplasm of infected cells. They are further distinguished from all other animal viruses by the fact that the uncoating step requires a newly synthesized, virus-coded protein.

A. Virus Attachment, Penetration, and Uncoating: Virus particles establish contact with the cell surface and are then engulfed in phagocytic vacuoles of the cell. First-stage uncoating takes place by means of hydrolytic enzymes in the vacuole. This releases the virus core into the cytoplasm. Among the several enzymes inside the poxvirus particle, there is a viral RNA polymerase that transcribes about half of the viral genome into early mRNA. These mRNAs are transcribed within the virus core and then released into the cytoplasm. Because the necessary enzymes are contained within the viral core, early transcription is not affected by inhibitors of protein synthesis. The "uncoating" protein that acts on the cores is among the more than 50 polypeptides made early after infection.

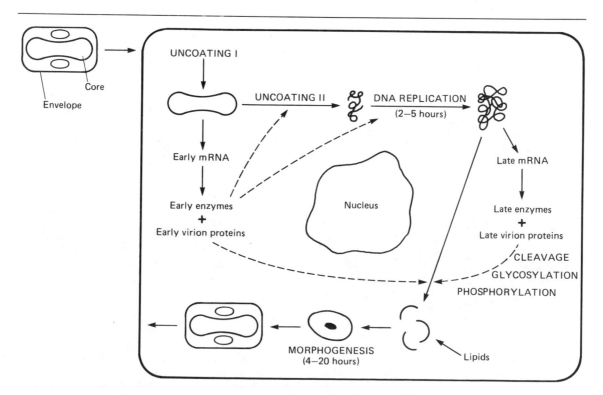

Figure 42–2. Outline of replication cycle of vaccinia virus. (Reproduced, with permission, from Moss B: Replication of poxviruses. Pages 685–703 in: *Virology*. Fields BN et al [editors]. Raven Press, 1985.)

The second-stage uncoating step liberates viral DNA from the cores; it requires both RNA and protein synthesis. The synthesis of host cell macromolecules is inhibited at this stage.

Poxviruses inactivated by heat can be reactivated either by viable poxviruses or by poxviruses inactivated by nitrogen mustards (which inactivate the DNA). This process is called nongenetic reactivation and is due to the stimulation of the uncoating protein. Heat-inactivated virus alone cannot cause second-stage uncoating, because of the heat lability of the RNA polymerase. Any poxvirus can reactivate any other poxvirus.

B. Replication of Viral DNA and Synthesis of Viral Proteins: Among the early proteins made after vaccinia virus infection are enzymes involved in DNA replication, including a DNA polymerase and thymidine kinase. Viral DNA replication starts soon after the release of viral DNA in the second stage of uncoating. It occurs from 2 to 6 hours after infection in discrete areas of the cytoplasm, which appear as "factories" or inclusion bodies (Fig 33–31) in electron micrographs. Inclusion bodies can form anywhere in the cytoplasm. The number observed per cell is proportionate to the multiplicity of infection, suggesting that each infectious particle can induce a "factory."

The pattern of viral gene expression changes markedly with the onset of replication of viral DNA. The synthesis of many of the early proteins is inhibited. Late viral mRNA is translated into large amounts of structural proteins and small amounts of other viral proteins and enzymes. DNA replication then ceases.

C. Maturation: The assembly of the virus particle from the manufactured components is a complex process. Many of the polypeptides that become part of the virus particle are modified by the addition of sugars (glycosylation) or phosphorus (phosphorylation) or by proteolytic cleavage. Poxviruses are unique in that de novo formation of virus membranes occurs (Figs 33–33 and 33–34).

Morphogenesis of poxvirus particles can be followed by electron micrographs of thin cell sections. Different structural phases can be correlated with the biochemical steps described above. Mature virions appear as a DNA-containing core encased in double membranes, surrounded by protein, and all enclosed within 2 outer membranes.

Some of the particles are released from the cell by budding and gain a cell-related envelope. The means by which these particles leave the inclusions and move to the cell periphery is unknown. However, the majority of poxvirus particles remain within the host cell. About 10,000 virus particles are produced per cell.

Two antiviral drugs affect the morphogenesis of poxvirus particles. Rifampin can block the formation and assembly of the vaccinia virus envelope. Methisazone interferes with the formation of late proteins and assembly of the particle. (See Chapter 33.)

D. Virus-Coded Growth Factor: A 140-residue polypeptide encoded by one of the early genes of vaccinia virus is closely related to epidermal growth factor (EGF) and to transforming growth factor. The presence of putative signal and transmembranous sequences further suggests that the viral protein might be an integral membrane protein but that, as in the case of EGF itself, the membrane-associated form may be the precursor of a soluble growth factor. Production of EGF-like growth factors by virus-infected cells could account for the proliferative diseases associated with members of the poxvirus family such as Shope fibroma, Yaba tumor, and molluscum contagiosum viruses.

VACCINIA & VARIOLA

Comparison of Vaccinia & Variola Viruses

Both vaccinia and variola viruses grow on the chorioallantoic membrane of the 10- to 12-day-old chick embryo, but the latter produces much smaller pocks. Both grow in several types of chick and primate cell lines. Variola infects only humans and monkeys, whereas vaccinia also infects rabbits.

Although poxviruses have a complex antigenic pattern, vaccinia and variola differ from each other by only one antigen.

In addition to structural antigens, poxviruses produce soluble antigens and hemagglutinins. Vaccinia virus contains a heat-labile (L) antigen that is destroyed at 60 °C and a heat-stable (S) antigen that withstands treatment at 100 °C. Both antigens may be present in soluble form in infected tissue (ie, not associated with virus particles). LS antigens from variola and from vaccinia virus are antigenically similar. The serologic tests for smallpox diagnosis depend upon the LS antigens. The hemagglutinin of vaccinia or variola virus is not an integral part of the virion. It is a lipoprotein complex associated with a 65-nm particle. The hemagglutination reaction with chicken red cells can be inhibited by vaccinia immune serum or by convalescent smallpox serum.

Vaccinia virus, the agent used for smallpox vaccination, is a distinct species of orthopoxvirus. Restriction endonuclease maps of the genome of vaccinia virus are distinctly different from those of cowpox virus, which had been believed to be its ancestor. Vaccinia virus may be the product of genetic recombination, a new species derived from cowpox virus or variola virus by serial passage, or the descendant of a now extinct virus genus.

Pathogenesis & Pathology of Smallpox

The portal of entry of variola virus is the mucous membranes of the upper respiratory tract. After the entry of the virus, the following are believed to take place: (1) primary multiplication in the lymphoid tissue draining the site of entry; (2) transient viremia and infection of reticuloendothelial cells throughout the body; (3) a secondary phase of multiplication in these cells, leading to (4) a secondary, more intense viremia; and (5) the clinical disease.

The skin lesion follows the localization of virus in the epidermis from the bloodstream. The virus can be isolated from the blood in the first few days of the disease. Clinical improvement follows the development of the skin eruption, perhaps owing to the appearance of antibodies. The pustulation of the skin lesions may give rise to a secondary fever; this may be due to absorption of the products of cell necrosis rather than to secondary bacterial infection.

Skin pustules may become contaminated, usually with staphylococci, sometimes leading to bacteremia and sepsis.

In the preeruptive phase, the disease is hardly infective. By the sixth to ninth days, lesions in the mouth tend to ulcerate and discharge virus. Thus, early in the disease, infectious virus originates in lesions in the mouth and upper respiratory tract. Later, pustules break down and discharge virus into the environment of the smallpox patient.

Histopathologic examination of the skin shows that proliferation of the prickle-cell layer occurs early. These proliferated cells contain many cytoplasmic inclusions. There is infiltration with mononuclear cells, particularly around the vessels in the corium. Epithelial cells of the malpighian layer become swollen through distention of cytoplasm and undergo "ballooning degeneration." The vacuoles in the cytoplasm enlarge. The cell membrane breaks down, and coalescence with neighboring, similarly affected cells results in the formation of vesicles. The vesicles enlarge and then become filled with white cells and tissue debris. In variola and vaccinia all the layers are involved, and there is actual necrosis of the corium. Thus, scarring is seen after variola and vaccinia.

Clinical Findings

The incubation period of variola (smallpox) is about 12 days. The onset may be gradual or sudden. One to 5 days of fever and malaise precede the appearance of the exanthems, which are papular for 1–4 days, vesicular for 1–4 days, and pustular for 2–6 days, forming crusts that fall off 2–4 weeks after the first sign of the lesion and leaving pink scars that fade slowly. In each area affected, the lesions are generally found in the same stage of development. The temperature falls within 24 hours after the rash appears.

The distribution of the rash is characteristic. Lesions are most abundant on the face and less so on the trunk. The nature and extent of the rash are functions of the severity of the disease. Vaccinated contacts may develop a febrile illness without rash that progresses no further. In severe cases, the rash is hemorrhagic. The case-fatality rate may vary from 5 to 40%. In mild variola or in vaccinated persons, the mortality rate is under 1%.

Mild variola (variola minor) gives rise to a mild disease in contacts, whereas modified variola major in immunized persons often gives rise to severe smallpox in contacts.

Laboratory Diagnosis

Several tests are available to confirm the diagnosis of smallpox. Now that the disease is presumably eradicated, it is important to diagnose any cases that resemble smallpox. The tests depend upon direct microscopic examination of material from skin lesions, recovery of virus from the patient, identification of viral antigen from the lesion, and demonstration of antibody in the blood.

A. Electron Microscopy: Direct examination of clinical material in the electron microscope can also be used for rapid identification of virus particles (about 1 hour) and can readily differentiate smallpox from chickenpox (the latter is caused by a herpesvirus).

B. Smears: Carefully prepared and properly stained smears from lesions of the papular and vesicular stages may give a positive result within 30 minutes. Smears from lesions are made on slides. The superficial epidermis is removed and the base of the lesion gently scraped with a blade. The dried smears are washed with distilled water and ether, fixed with alcohol, and stained with a mixture of equal parts of 1% gentian violet and 2% sodium bicarbonate for 5 minutes, with steaming. If elementary bodies are seen in large numbers, a presumptive diagnosis of smallpox can be made.

C. Virus Culture: The detection of virus on the chorioallantoic membrane of the 12- to 14-day-old chick embryo is the most reliable laboratory test. It is the easiest way of distinguishing cases of smallpox from generalized vaccinia, for the lesions produced by these viruses on the membrane differ markedly. In 2–3 days, vaccinia pocks are large with necrotic centers whereas variola pocks are much smaller. Cowpox and monkeypox produce hemorrhagic lesions. All of these can also be grown in various cell cultures and identified by hemadsorption or immunofluorescence.

D. Antigen Detection: Antigen can be detected readily by immunodiffusion or by CF test in material collected from the skin lesion.

E. Antibody Determination: After the first week, Nt, CF, and HI antibodies appear. However, these are of no practical importance in diagnosis, and their levels may decline within several months. A specific rise in antibody titer in paired sera can be used to confirm a diagnosis.

Differential Diagnosis

Smallpox may be confused with varicella, pustular acne, meningococcemia, blood dyscrasias, drug rashes, and other illnesses associated with a skin eruption, but none of these illnesses yield materials that give positive laboratory tests for variola virus.

The use of restriction enzyme cleavage of viral DNA and the analysis of polypeptides in poxvirus-infected cells can demonstrate distinct characteristics for variola, vaccinia, monkeypox, and cowpox. This is important because smallpoxlike illnesses must be identified to ascertain that variola has indeed been eradicated.

Immunity

Children of vaccinated, immune mothers receive maternal antibody transplacentally, which persists for several months. After that time, artificial immunity can be produced by vaccination (see Control & Eradication of Smallpox, below). Immunity is demonstrable 8–9 days following vaccination, reaches its maximum within 2–3 weeks, and is maintained at an appreciable level for a few years.

Antibodies alone are not sufficient for recovery from primary poxvirus infection. In the human host, Nt antibodies develop within a few days after onset of smallpox but do not prevent progression of lesions, and patients may die in the pustular stage with high antibody levels. Cell-mediated immunity may be as important as circulating antibody. Patients with hypogammaglobulinemia generally react normally to vaccination and develop immunity despite the apparent absence of antibody. Immunity is accompanied by delayed cutaneous hypersensitivity to vaccinia. Patients who have defects in both cellular immune response and antibody response develop a progressive, usually fatal disease upon vaccination.

Production of interferon (see Chapter 33) is another possible immune mechanism. Irradiated animals without detectable antibody or delayed hypersensitivity recovered from vaccinia infection as rapidly as untreated control animals.

Treatment

Vaccinia immune globulin (VIG) is prepared from blood provided by revaccinated military personnel. Indications for use of vaccinia immune globulin are accidental inoculation of vaccine in the eye or eczema vaccinatum.

Methisazone (Marboran) is effective as prophylaxis but is not useful in treatment of established disease (see Chapter 33).

Epidemiology

Transmission of smallpox could usually be traced to contact between cases. Rarely, the dried virus survived on clothes or other materials and resulted in infections.

Patients may be infectious during the incubation period. Virus has been isolated from throat swabs obtained from family contacts of patients with smallpox. Respiratory droplets are infectious earlier than skin lesions.

The following epidemiologic features made smallpox amenable to total eradication: There is no known nonhuman reservoir. Subclinical infectious cases do not occur. Chronic, asymptomatic carriage of the virus does not occur. Since virus in the environment of the patient derives from lesions in the mouth and throat (and later in the skin), patients with infection sufficiently severe to transmit the disease are likely to be so ill that they quickly reach the attention of medical authorities. The close contact requisite for effective spread of the disease generally makes for ready identification of a patient's contacts so that specific control measures can be instituted to interrupt the cycle of transmission.

Control & Eradication of Smallpox

Control of smallpox by deliberate infection with mild forms of the disease was practiced for centuries. This process, called variolation, was dangerous but decreased the disastrous effects of major epidemics, reducing the case-fatality rate from 25% to 1%. Jenner introduced vaccination with live vaccinia virus in 1798.

In 1967, WHO introduced a worldwide campaign to eradicate smallpox. Epidemiologic features of the disease (described above) made it feasible to attempt total eradication. At that time, there were 33 countries with endemic smallpox and 10–15 million cases per year. The last Asiatic case occurred in Bangladesh in 1975, and the last natural victim in Somalia in 1977. There were 3 main reasons for this outstanding success: The vaccine was easily prepared, stable, and safe; it could be given simply by personnel in the field; and mass vaccination of the world population was not necessary. Cases of smallpox were traced, and contacts of the patient and those in the immediate area were vaccinated.

Even though there is no evidence of smallpox transmission anywhere in the world, WHO has coordinated the investigation of 173 possible cases of smallpox between 1979 and 1984. All have been diseases other than smallpox, most commonly chickenpox or other illnesses that produce a rash. Even so, a suspected case of smallpox becomes a public health emergency and must be promptly investigated by means of clinical evaluation, collection of laboratory specimens, and preliminary laboratory diagnosis.

The presence of stocks of virulent smallpox virus in laboratories is of concern because of the danger of laboratory infection and subsequent spread into the community. Variola virus stocks have been destroyed in all laboratories except 2 WHO collaborating centers (one in Atlanta and one in Moscow) that pursue diagnostic and research work on variola-related poxviruses.

Vaccination With Vaccinia

Vaccinia virus for vaccination is prepared from vesicular lesions ("lymph") produced in the skin of calves or sheep or grown in chick embryos. The latter can be harvested under bacteriologically sterile conditions. The final product contains 40% glycerol to stabilize the virus and 0.4% phenol to destroy bacteria. WHO standards require that smallpox vaccines have a potency of not less than 10^8 pock-forming units per milliliter.

Calf-lymph vaccine is kept frozen until issued to physicians. It can then be stored for some weeks in a refrigerator without significant loss of potency, but when removed to room temperature it must be used promptly. Deterioration of vaccine is a problem in tropical countries. There, a stable lyophilized vaccine prepared from infected chorioallantoic membranes of embryonated eggs ("avianized vaccine") has been used.

The success of smallpox eradication has meant that routine vaccination is no longer recommended. The following summary of vaccination is given because vaccinia virus continues to be administered to millions of persons in military and other populations, and complications from such use continue to occur.

A. Time of Vaccination: Complications of vaccination (see below) occur most commonly under the age of 1 year. Therefore, when necessary, vaccinating between 1 and 2 years of age is preferable to vaccinating in the first year of life. Infants suffering from skin diseases or those with siblings who have skin diseases should not be vaccinated because the vaccinia virus may localize in the lesions of the vaccinated child or of the contact (eczema vaccinatum). Revaccination has been done at 3-year intervals.

B. Technique: The methods used are multiple pressure, multiple puncture, or jet injection. In all techniques, inoculation should be intradermal, never subcutaneous. The skin (arm or thigh) is cleaned with acetone, ether, or soap and water. After the area is dry, a drop of the vaccine is placed on the skin and the side of the needle is then pressed firmly through the drop of vaccine into the superficial layers of the skin. At least 5 pressures should be made. The point of the needle should not draw blood. After the vaccination has been completed, excess vaccine is removed from the skin with dry, sterile gauze. No dressing is applied.

C. Reactions and Interpretations:

1. Primary take–In the fully susceptible person, a papule surrounded by hyperemia appears on the third or fourth day. The papule increases in size until vesiculation appears (on the fifth or sixth day). The vesicle reaches its maximum size by the ninth day and then becomes pustular, usually with some tenderness of the axillary nodes. Desiccation follows and is complete in about 2 weeks, leaving a depressed pink scar that ultimately turns white. The reading of the result is usually made on the seventh day. If this reaction is not observed, vaccination should be repeated with vaccine from another lot until a successful result is obtained.

2. Revaccination–A **successful revaccination** shows in 1 week (6–8 days) a vesicular or pustular lesion or an area of palpable induration surrounding a central lesion, which may be a scab or an ulcer. Only this reaction indicates with certainty that virus multiplication has taken place. **Equivocal reactions** may represent immunity but may also represent merely allergic reactions to a vaccine that has become inactivated. When an equivocal reaction occurs, the revaccination should be repeated using a new lot of vaccine known to give "takes" in other persons. A second reading should be made after 6–8 days.

D. Complications of Vaccination:

1. Bacterial infection of the vaccination site– This virtually never occurs.

2. Generalized vaccinia–This is manifested by the occurrence of crops of vaccinial lesions over the surface of the body. Following vaccination, children suffering from eczema may develop vaccinial lesions on the eczematous areas (eczema vaccinatum). Children with a current or past history of eczema should not be vaccinated, since the mortality rate in untreated generalized vaccinia is 30–40%. Neither should children who have siblings with eczema be vaccinated, because of the danger of transmitting the virus and producing generalized vaccinia in the siblings. Generalized vaccinia can occur in the absence of eczema, but this is rare. The use of vaccinia immune globulin has reduced the mortality rate of eczema vaccinatum from 40% to 7%.

3. Contact vaccinia–Several episodes involving patients with vaccinal infections have been reported among contacts of recently vaccinated military personnel within the last few years. The WHO recommendations on posteradication policy urge that military personnel who have been vaccinated be confined to their bases and prevented from contacting unvaccinated persons for a period of 2 weeks following vaccination.

4. Postvaccinal encephalitis–The mortality rate of this serious complication may be as high as 40%. The incidence in the USA was about 3 per million among primary vaccinees of all ages. The onset is sudden and occurs about 12 days after vaccination. There is a pleocytosis of the cerebrospinal fluid, the lymphocyte count being 100–200/μL. Focal lesions are widely distributed throughout the gray and white matter of the brain and cord. Perivascular infiltrations of mononuclear cells and areas of demyelination are the chief histologic lesions.

The cause is not clear. Several possibilities exist: (1) Vaccinia virus may invade the central nervous system. (2) Vaccination may activate a latent virus of the nervous system. (3) The reaction may be due to an antigen-antibody reaction that is allergic in character. Similar demyelinating disease has been reported after infection with variola, measles, and varicella and after vaccination against rabies.

5. Vaccinia necrosum or progressive vaccinia–This results from inability to make antibody or to develop cellular resistance and may be fatal. Treatment with vaccinia immune globulin or methisazone (see below) may be of value.

6. Fetal vaccinia–Very rarely, a woman vaccinated late in pregnancy transmitted vaccinia virus to the fetus, and stillbirth resulted. Therefore, vaccination should be avoided in pregnancy.

Smallpox vaccination is associated with a definite measurable risk. In the USA the risk of death from all complications was 1 per million for primary vaccinees and 0.1 per million for revaccinees. For children under 1 year of age, the risk of death was 5 per million primary vaccinations. Among primary vaccinees, the combined incidence of postvaccinal encephalitis and vaccinia necrosum was 3.8 per million in persons of all ages. In revaccinees, these 2 complications occurred at a rate of 0.7 per million.

Even though routine smallpox vaccination of children in the USA was stopped in 1971, more than 4 million doses of smallpox vaccine were administered in 1978. Severe complications of vaccination occurred in conjunction with immunodeficiency, immunosuppression, hematologic or other malignancies, and pregnancy.

Prophylaxis

Methisazone (Marboran) can provide transitory protection to an individual who has been exposed to smallpox. The drug is no substitute for vaccination. It is of no value in the treatment of smallpox once the patient has become febrile. It may be beneficial in severe cases of eczema vaccinatum that do not quickly respond to vaccinia immune globulin. Rifampin inhibits the replication of vaccinia virus in cell culture, but it has not been proved to be effective against smallpox in field trials.

COWPOX

This disease of cattle is milder than the pox diseases of other animals, the lesions being confined to the teats and udders. Infection of humans occurs by direct contact during milking, and the lesion in milkers is usually confined to the hands. The disease is more severe in unvaccinated persons than in the vaccinated. The local lesion is associated with fever and lymphadenitis. Generalized eruption is rare.

Cowpox virus is similar to vaccinia virus immunologically and in host range. It is also closely related immunologically to variola virus. Jenner observed that those who have had cowpox are immune to smallpox. Cowpox virus can be distinguished from vaccinia virus by the deep red hemorrhagic lesions that cowpox virus produces on the chorioallantoic membrane of the chick embryo. The strains of vaccinia virus used for vaccination of humans are of uncertain origin. If originally derived from cowpox strains, their artificial passage in laboratory animals has resulted in new properties. The natural reservoir of cowpox seems to be a rodent, and both cattle and humans are only accidental hosts.

Domestic cats also are susceptible to cowpox virus. More than 50 cases in felines have been reported from the United Kingdom, but transmission from cats to humans is believed to be uncommon. Cowpox is no longer enzootic in cattle, although bovine and associated human cases occasionally occur. Feline cowpox is sporadic, and transmission is probably from a small wild rodent. Human cases (with hemorrhagic skin lesions, fever, and general malaise) may occur without any known animal contact and may not be diagnosed.

MONKEYPOX

This disease is known to occur in monkeys held in captivity. No simian outbreaks in nature have ever been recorded. In 1970, the first known human cases of infection with this virus occurred; these were suspected cases of smallpox occurring in villages in Africa where no smallpox cases had been observed for 2 years. Continued surveillance has led to the diagnosis of over 130 human cases from western and central Africa, all in tropical rain forest areas. Most patients experienced what appeared to be reasonably typical smallpox illnesses, but the isolates were found to have properties of typical monkeypox strains and to differ markedly from variola virus. Monkeys are frequently used by the villagers for food and skins. The smallpox surveillance system was able to detect the rare human infections due to monkeypox virus. There does not seem to be a simian reservoir of smallpox, and monkeypox when present does not seem to spread readily among humans. It is estimated that only about 15% of susceptible family contacts acquire monkeypox from patients. Thus, human monkeypox infection is not easily transmitted from person to person. In the 19 instances involving presumed transmission among humans during 1982–1983, transmission stopped at secondary infection in 12 episodes and may have proceeded to third- or fourth-generation transmission in only 7 episodes.

YABA MONKEY VIRUS & TANAPOX VIRUS

Yaba virus, a simian poxvirus, causes benign histiocytomas 5–20 days after subcutaneous or intramuscular administration to monkeys. The tumors regress after about 5 weeks; this is ascribed to the cytopathic effect of the virus itself. True neoplastic changes do not occur. Intravenous administration of the virus causes the appearance of multiple histiocytomas in the lungs, heart, and skeletal muscles. The virus is easily isolated from tumor tissue, and characteristic inclusions are found in the tumor cells.

Monkeys of various species and humans are susceptible to the cellular proliferative effects of the virus, but other laboratory animals are insusceptible. Under natural conditions, the virus is possibly transmitted by bloodsucking vectors (as is myxoma, a poxvirus of rabbits).

Yaba poxvirus is similar to Tanapox virus, which caused epidemics of an acute febrile illness associated with pocklike lesions in Kenya in 1957–1962 and is now active in Africa, particularly in Zaire. It is thought to be spread from infected animals to humans by contaminated arthropods.

In morphology, the Yaba virus particles are similar to vaccinia and molluscum contagiosum virions. No immunologic relationship has been found between Yaba virus and other poxviruses (except Tanapox virus). The virus multiplies only in cultures of monkey cells, with cytopathic and proliferative effects. Characteristic eosinophilic inclusions in the cytoplasm of the cell have been found.

The Yaba virus DNA has a G + C content of 32.5%, which is significantly different from the 36%

G + C content of vaccinia, rabbitpox, cowpox, and ectromelia viruses.

MOLLUSCUM CONTAGIOSUM

The lesions of this disease are small, pink, wartlike tumors on the face, arms, back, and buttocks. The disease occurs throughout the world, in both sporadic and epidemic forms, and is more frequent in children than in adults. It is spread by direct and indirect contact (eg, by barbers, common use of towels). Lesions may persist for up to 2 years, and second attacks are common. The virus is a poor immunogen: about one-third of patients never produce antibodies against the virus.

Histologically, inclusions form in basal layers of the epithelium, gradually enlarge, crowd the nucleus to one side, and eventually fill the cell.

The virus has not been transmitted to animals but has been studied in the human lesion by electron microscopy. The purified virus is oval or brick-shaped and measures 230 × 330 nm. Antibodies to the virus do not cross-react with other poxviruses.

In ultrathin sections of infected cells, the inclusion bodies are divided into compartments by extremely thin walls, with nests of mature virus particles filling the cavities between the septa. The matrix of the cytoplasm surrounding the cavities appears honeycombed and undergoes segmentation into spherical objects that are larger than the virus itself. The virus appears to form within this larger sphere.

The incidence of molluscum contagiosum as a sexually transmitted disease in young adults is increasing. Although the typical lesion is an umbilicated papule, lesions in moist genital areas may become inflamed or ulcerated and may be confused with those produced by herpes simplex virus (HSV). Specimens from such lesions are often submitted to viral diagnostic laboratories for isolation of HSV.

Although molluscum contagiosum virus has not been serially propagated in cell culture, it undergoes an abortive infection with a resulting characteristic cytopathic effect. The cellular changes can be mistaken for those produced by HSV; thus, isolates from specimens suspected to contain HSV should be specifically identified by immunologic methods. Because the cytopathic effect disappears with serial passage, it might be considered to be a toxic effect and the specimen may be reported as negative for a viral agent. In a 1985 study of 137 specimens cultured for HSV by using human fibroblast cells, 49 contained HSV; 6 others produced cytopathic effects but were negative for HSV by immunofluorescence staining. Electron microscopy of the original clinical specimen or the first-passage cell-culture material confirmed the presence of molluscum contagiosum virus. Thus, electron microscopic examination of lesion specimens which produce a cytopathic effect that is not specifically attributable to HSV and which cannot be serially passaged may reveal the presence of molluscum contagiosum virus.

REFERENCES

Baxby D: Identification and interrelationships of the variola/vaccinia subgroup of poxviruses. *Prog Med Virol* 1975;**19**:215.

Baxby D, Bennett M, Gaskell RM: Medical implications of feline cowpox. *Lancet* 1985;**2**:45.

Breman JG, Arita I: The confirmation and maintenance of smallpox eradication. *N Engl J Med* 1980;**303**:1263.

Brown JP et al: Vaccinia virus encodes a polypeptide homologous to epidermal growth factor and transforming growth factor. *Nature* 1985;**313**:491.

Committee on Orthopoxvirus Infections: Smallpox: Post-eradication vigilance continues. *WHO Chron* 1982;**36**:87.

Dennis J, Oshiro LS, Bunter JW: Molluscum contagiosum, another sexually transmitted disease: Its impact on the clinical virology laboratory. *J Infect Dis* 1985;**151**:376.

Dumbell KR, Archard LC: Comparison of white pock (h) mutants of monkeypox virus with parental monkeypox and with variola-like viruses isolated from animals. *Nature* 1980;**286**:29.

Essani K, Dales S: Biogenesis of vaccinia: Evidence for more than 100 polypeptides in the virion. *Virology* 1979;**95**:385.

Fenner F: Portraits of viruses: The poxviruses. *Intervirology* 1979;**11**:137.

Mutombo MW, Arita I, Jezek Z: Human monkeypox transmitted by a chimpanzee in a tropical rain-forest area of Zaire. *Lancet* 1983;**1**:735.

Pickup DJ et al: Spontaneous deletions and duplications of sequences in the genome of cowpox virus. *Proc Natl Acad Sci USA* 1984;**81**:6817.

Zuckerman AJ: Palaeontology of smallpox. *Lancet* 1984;**2**:1454.

Adenovirus Family

43

Adenoviruses can replicate and produce disease in the respiratory tract, eye, gastrointestinal tract, and urinary bladder. Occasionally, other organs, such as the central nervous system, may be affected. Many adenovirus infections are subclinical. About one-third of the 41 known human serotypes are responsible for most cases of human adenovirus disease. A few types serve as models for cancer induction in animals. Adenoviruses are especially valuable systems for molecular and biochemical studies of eukaryotic cell processes.

PROPERTIES OF ADENOVIRUSES

Classification

Adenoviruses have been recovered from a wide variety of species and grouped into 2 genera, one that infects birds and another that infects mammals. Human adenoviruses are divided into 7 groups (A–G) on the basis of their physical, chemical, and biologic properties. There are at least 41 antigenic types of human adenoviruses.

Morphology & Composition

Adenoviruses are 70–90 nm in diameter and display icosahedral symmetry, with capsids composed of 252 capsomeres. There is no envelope. They contain 13% DNA and 87% protein. Adenoviruses are unique among icosahedral viruses in that they have a structure called a "fiber" projecting from each of the 12 vertices, or penton bases (Fig 43–1 and Table 43–1). The rest of the capsid is composed of 240 hexon capsomeres. The hexons, pentons, and fibers constitute the major adenovirus antigens important in virus classification and disease diagnosis (see below).

The DNA (MW 20–30 × 10^6) is linear and double-stranded. The guanine plus cytosine (G + C) content of the DNA is lowest (48–49%) in group A (types 12, 18, and 31) adenoviruses, the most strongly oncogenic types, and ranges as high as 61% in other types. This is one criterion used in subgrouping human isolates. Viral DNA contains a virus-coded protein that is covalently linked to each 5′ end of the linear genome. The DNA can be isolated in an infectious form, and the relative infectivity of that DNA is reduced at least 100-fold if the terminal protein is removed by proteolysis.

Molecular characterization of viral DNA from 41 human adenovirus serotypes shows that they can be divided into 7 subgroups (A–G; see Table 43–2). The degree of homology between viral genomes belonging to the same subgroup is at least 90%, with the exception of subgroup A, which shows a larger heterogeneity. Viral genomes belonging to different subgroups show less than 25% DNA homology. It has been suggested that type 4, which cross-reacts with members of several subgroups, is most closely related to the archetypes of human adenoviruses.

The DNA is condensed in the core of the virion in an arrangement resembling 12 large spheres packed tightly together. A virus-coded protein, polypeptide VII (Table 43–1), is important in forming the core structure.

The major adenovirus antigens, their size, and their structural position in the virion are shown in Table 43–1. Three structural proteins, produced in large excess, constitute "soluble antigens" A, B, and C. Group-reactive CF antigens are hexons that form a majority of capsomeres. All human adenoviruses possess this common soluble hexon antigenicity. It persists in suspensions of virus treated with heat or formalin to inactivate infectivity. Pentons occur at the 12 vertices of the capsid and have fibers protruding from them. The fibers contain the type-specific antigens that are important in serotyping. At least 41 distinct antigenic types have been isolated from humans and many additional ones from various animals. They are typed by cross-neutralization or HI tests. The penton base carries a toxinlike activity that results in rapid appearance of cytopathic effects and detachment of cells from the surface on which they are growing. Pentons and fibers are associated with hemagglutinating activity. The hemagglutinin is type-specific.

Adenovirus Multiplication

Adenoviruses replicate well only in cells of epithelial origin. The replicative cycle is sharply divided into early and late events. The carefully regulated expression of sequential events in the adenovirus cycle is summarized in Fig 33–8.

A. Virus Attachment, Penetration, and Uncoating: The virus probably attaches to cells via the fiber structures. There are about 100,000 fiber receptors per cell. The virus particle is internalized, and uncoating commences in the cytoplasm and is completed in the nucleus.

B. Early Events: The steps that occur before the onset of viral DNA synthesis are defined as early events. Soon after infection, host macromolecular

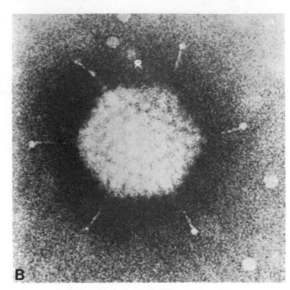

Figure 43–1. Electron micrographs of adenovirus. *A:* The virus particle displays cubic symmetry and is nonenveloped. A hexon capsomere (surrounded by 6 identical hexons) and a penton capsomere (surrounded by 5 hexons) are marked with dots. *B:* Note the fiber structures projecting from the vertex penton capsomeres (285,000 ×). (Reproduced, with permission, from Valentine RC, Pereira HG: Antigens and structure of the adenovirus. *J Mol Biol* 1965;**13**:13.)

Table 43–1. Comparative data on adenovirus type 2 morphologic and antigenic subunits and protein components.

Appearance	Name	Number Per Virion	Molecular Weight	Antigen	Specificity	Protein Components
Virion	DNA		23,000,000			
	Protein		150,000,000			
◯	Hexon	240	210,000 400,000 320,000 360,000	A	Group	II
⬡hexons	Hexons	20	3,600,000			II, VIII, IX
◯—◯	Penton	12	280,000 1,100,000			III, IV
◯	Penton base	12	210,000	B	Subgroup	III
══◯	Fiber	12	70,000	C	Type	IV
Core	DNA	1	23,000,000	P		
	Protein		29,000,000			V, VI, VII
	Protein		13,000			VII, IX
	Protein		7,500			X

Column headers: Morphologic Subunits (Appearance, Name, Number Per Virion, Molecular Weight); Antigenic Subunits (Antigen, Specificity); Protein Components

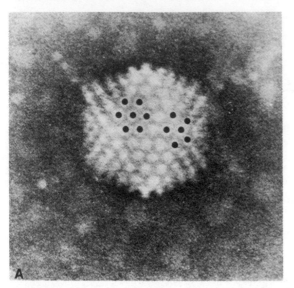

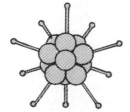

Dodecon: Hemagglutinin made up of 12 pentons with their fibers.

Table 43–2. Association of human adenoviruses with disease.

Subgroup	Type	Disease
A	12, 18, 31	Not defined in humans; induce tumors in newborn hamsters.
B	3, 7, 11, 14, 16, 21, 34, 35	Acute respiratory infections with fever, conjunctivitis, pharyngitis, pneumonia, gastroenteritis, hemorrhagic cystitis.
C	1, 2, 5, 6	Respiratory infection in small children, latent infection in lymphatic tissue.
D	8–10, 13, 15, 17, 19, 20, 22–30, 32, 33, 36, 37, 39	Types 8 and 19 cause epidemic keratoconjunctivitis; type 37, sporadic keratoconjunctivitis.
E	4	Acute respiratory infections with fever, epidemic keratoconjunctivitis.
F, G	38, 40, 41	Gastroenteritis.

synthesis is inhibited by an unknown mechanism. The cessation of host protein synthesis is particularly rapid and is undoubtedly part of the reason infected cells are killed.

The early transcripts come from 7 widely separated regions of the viral genome and from both viral DNA strands (Fig 43–2). The E1A gene is especially important; it must be expressed in order for the other early regions to be transcribed. The E1A/E1B regions contain the only adenovirus genes involved in cell transformation. More than 20 early proteins, many of which are nonstructural and are involved in viral DNA replication, are synthesized in adenovirus-infected cells. The E3 region is nonessential for virus growth in tissue culture but presumably performs some necessary function during virus infection of human hosts.

C. Replication of Viral DNA and Late Events: Viral DNA replication takes place in the nucleus. The virus-coded, covalently linked terminal protein functions as a primer for initiation of viral DNA synthesis.

Late events begin concomitant with the onset of viral DNA synthesis. Late genes coding for virus structural proteins (Fig 43–2) are transcribed, processed, and transported to the cytoplasm, where the viral proteins are synthesized. Although host genes continue to be transcribed in the nucleus late in infection, few host genetic sequences are transported to the cytoplasm. It was studies with adenovirus hexon mRNA that led to the profound discovery that eukaryotic mRNAs are usually not colinear with their genes but are spliced products of separated coding regions in the genomic DNA. Very large amounts of viral structural proteins are made.

D. Virus Maturation: Virion morphogenesis occurs in the nucleus, but the initial step in the assembly process begins in the cytoplasm. Newly synthesized polypeptides assemble into capsomeres in the cytoplasm. Each hexon capsomere is a trimer of identical polypeptides. The penton is composed of 5 penton base polypeptides and 3 fiber polypeptides. A virus-coded "scaffold protein" assists in the aggregation of hexon polypeptides but is not part of the final structure.

Capsomeres self-assemble into empty shell capsids in the nucleus. Naked DNA then enters the preformed capsid by an unknown mechanism, followed by precursor core proteins. Finally, precursor core proteins are cleaved, which allows the particle to tighten its configuration, and several or all of the pentons are added. The mature particle is then stable, infectious, and resistant to nucleases. The assembly process is inefficient, producing some empty particles devoid of DNA and leaving many structural proteins unused in the cell. Structural proteins associated with mature virus particles are catalogued in Fig 43–1.

E. Virus Effects on Cells in Culture: Adenoviruses are cytopathic for human cell cultures, particularly primary kidney and continuous epithelial cells. Growth of virus in tissue culture is associated with a stimulation of acid production (increased glycolysis) in the early stages of infection. The cytopathic effect usually consists of marked rounding and aggregation of affected cells into grapelike clusters. The infected cells do not lyse even though they round up and leave the glass surface on which they have been grown.

In cells infected with adenovirus types 3, 4, and 7, rounded intranuclear inclusions containing DNA are seen. The virus particles in the nucleus frequently exhibit crystalline arrangements. Cells infected with group B viruses also contain crystals composed of protein without nucleic acid. About 7000 virus particles are produced per infected cell, and most of them remain within the cell after the cycle is complete and the cell is dead. Crude infected cell lysates show huge quantities of capsomeres, sometimes partially assembled into viral components.

Human adenoviruses exhibit a narrow host range. When cells derived from species other than humans are infected, the human adenoviruses undergo an abortive replication cycle. Adenovirus early antigens, mRNA, and DNA are all synthesized, but not all capsid proteins and no infectious progeny are produced.

F. Adenovirus Interactions With Other Viruses:

1. Adenovirus-SV40 "hybrids"–Human adenovirus replication in monkey kidney cells can be achieved by coinfection with SV40. Certain adenovirus vaccine strains grown in monkey kidney cell cultures inadvertently became "contaminated" with SV40. Some SV40 sequences became covalently linked to the adenovirus DNA, so that stable "hybrids" were formed. Two types of hybrids have been identified. One is a defective adenovirus-SV40 genome encased in an adenovirus capsid; it requires a helper adenovirus for replication. The other consists of nondefective (ie, self-replicating) adenovirus type 2 that carries a portion of the SV40 genome. These hybrids have been very useful in genetic analyses but have no manifest medical relevance.

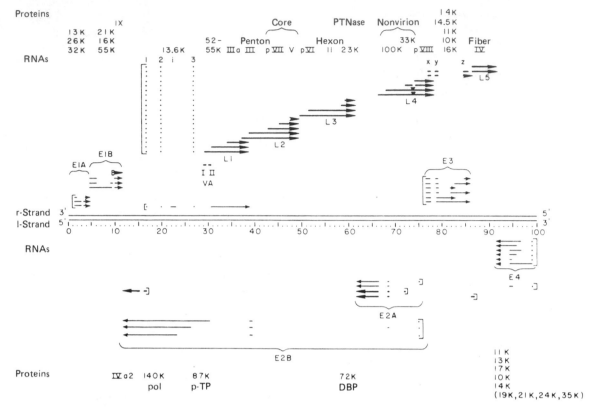

Figure 43–2. Transcription and translation map of adenovirus type 2. The early mRNAs are designated E, and the late mRNAs are labeled L. All late transcripts contain the tripartite leader, denoted 1, 2, and 3. Polypeptides designated by roman numerals are part of the virion; proteins identified in kilodaltons (K) are nonstructural translation products. (Reproduced, with permission, from Broker TR: Animal virus RNA processing. Pages 181–212 in: *Processing of RNA.* Apirion D [editor]. CRC Press, 1984.)

2. Adenoassociated virus (AAV)–In some adenovirus preparations, small 20-nm particles were found (Fig 33–35). These proved to be parvoviruses that could not replicate unless adenovirus (or sometimes herpesvirus) was present as a helper. AAV contains single-stranded DNA (MW 1.6×10^6) and is serologically unrelated to adenovirus. Although AAV can infect cells in the absence of an adenovirus helper and induce a latent infection, AAV is not involved in the production of any known adenovirus-induced human disease.

Animal Susceptibility & Transformation of Cells

Most laboratory animals are not readily infected with adenoviruses. Newborn hamsters sustain a fatal infection with type 5 and develop malignant tumors when inoculated with any of 8 or more types, including types 12, 18, and 31. Transformed cells produce tumors when inoculated into adult hamsters or rats but do not contain infectious virus. Only a small part ($< 10\%$) of the adenovirus genome is present in many transformed cells; this explains the inability to recover infectious virus from transformed cells.

The transforming region in human adenoviruses has been narrowed to the early region (E1A/E1B) at the left-hand end of the viral genome (Fig 43–2). Because these regions encode several polypeptides, the gene products most involved in transformation have not been identified with certainty.

The highly oncogenic nature of adenovirus type 12 may well be related to the observation that one effect of its E1A region is to turn off the synthesis of class I major histocompatibility antigens (H2 or HLA) in infected and transformed cells.

It is of interest that the adenovirus E1A gene has been found to share some structural features with the *myc* cellular oncogene (see Chapter 46).

Adenovirus DNA or mRNA has never been found in human tumors.

ADENOVIRUS INFECTIONS IN HUMANS

Pathogenesis

Adenoviruses infect epithelial cells of mucous membranes, the cornea, and other organ systems. They can be isolated from such structures during acute illness and may persist for long periods. Types 1, 2, 5, and 6 can be isolated from surgically removed adenoids or tonsils of most children by growing the epithelium in vitro. Gradual removal of antibody during long culture in vitro permits the viruses to grow, but they cannot be isolated directly from suspensions of such tissues.

Most human adenoviruses grow in intestinal epithelium after ingestion but usually do not produce symptoms or lesions.

Clinical Findings

The association of human adenoviruses with clinical diseases is listed in Table 43–2.

A. Respiratory Diseases: Respiratory diseases associated with adenoviruses include syndromes designated as undifferentiated acute respiratory disease, pharyngoconjunctival fever, nonstreptococcal exudative pharyngitis, and primary atypical pneumonia not associated with the development of cold agglutinins.

About 5% of acute respiratory disease in young children is due to adenoviruses. Respiratory symptoms of cough, nasal congestion, and coryza may be accompanied by systemic symptoms of fever, chills, malaise, headache, and myalgia. Adenovirus types 1, 2, 5, and 6 are most commonly involved. Acute respiratory disease of military recruits is similar except that it is caused predominantly by types 4 and 7 and occurs in young recruits under conditions of fatigue and crowding.

Pharyngoconjunctival fever may be caused by several adenovirus types. It is characterized by fever, conjunctivitis, pharyngitis, malaise, and cervical lymphadenopathy. Under natural conditions, only types 3 and 7 regularly cause outbreaks in which conjunctivitis is a predominant symptom. Types 1, 2, 5, 6, 37, and many others have produced sporadic cases that included conjunctivitis.

B. Eye Infections: Mild ocular involvement may be part of the respiratory-pharyngeal syndromes caused by adenoviruses. Complete recovery with no lasting sequelae is the common outcome. "Swimming pool conjunctivitis" may be caused by adenovirus types 3, 7, and many others.

The follicular conjunctivitis caused by many adenovirus types resembles chlamydial conjunctivitis (see Chapter 29) and is self-limited.

A more serious disease is epidemic keratoconjunctivitis (shipyard eye). The disease is characterized by an acute conjunctivitis, with enlarged, tender preauricular nodes, followed by keratitis that leaves round, subepithelial opacities in the cornea for up to 2 years. It is caused by types 8, 19, and 37. Type 8 infections have been characterized by their lack of associated systemic symptoms except in infants.

C. Gastrointestinal Disease: Many adenoviruses replicate in intestinal cells and are present in stools, but the presence of many common types is not associated with gastrointestinal disease. However, two newly discovered serotypes (types 40 and 41) have been etiologically associated with infantile gastroenteritis. These viruses are abundantly present in diarrheic stools. The enteric adenoviruses are very difficult to cultivate and are detected by electron microscopy or antigen-based assays.

Intussusception of infancy has been ascribed to adenoviruses 1, 2, 5, and 6.

D. Other Diseases: Types 11 and 21 may be a cause of acute hemorrhagic cystitis in children. Virus commonly occurs in the urine of such patients. Type 37 occurs in cervical lesions and in male urethritis and may be sexually transmitted.

Immunocompromised patients may suffer from adenovirus infections, although not as often as from herpesvirus infections. The most common problem caused by adenovirus infection in transplant patients is pneumonia, which may be fatal. Renal impairment and hepatitis may develop.

Laboratory Diagnosis

A. Recovery and Identification of Virus: Viruses are isolated by inoculation of tissue cultures of human cells in which characteristic cytopathic changes are produced. The viruses have been recovered from throat swabs, conjunctival swabs, rectal swabs, stools of patients with acute pharyngitis and conjunctivitis, and urine of patients with acute hemorrhagic cystitis. Virus isolations from the eye are obtained mainly from patients with conjunctivitis.

The fastidious enteric adenoviruses can be detected by direct examination of fecal extracts by electron microscopy or by ELISA. They can be isolated in a line of human embryonic kidney cells transformed with a fragment of adenovirus 5 DNA.

Isolates can be identified as adenoviruses by using fluorescent antibody or CF tests to detect group-specific antigens. HI and Nt tests measure type-specific antigens and can be used to identify specific serotypes.

Characterization of viral DNA by hybridization or by restriction endonuclease digestion patterns can identify an isolate as an adenovirus and subgroup it. These approaches are especially useful for types that are difficult to cultivate.

B. Serology: In most cases, the Nt antibody titer of infected persons shows a 4-fold or greater rise against the type recovered from the patient and a lesser response to other types. Nt antibodies are measured in human cell cultures using the cytopathic end point in tube cultures or the color test in panel cups. The latter test depends upon the phenomenon that adenovirus growing in cell cultures produces an excess of acid over that of uninfected control cultures. This viral lowering of pH can be prevented by immune serum. The pH is measured by incorporating phenol red into the medium and observing the color changes after 3 days of incubation.

Infection of humans with any adenovirus type stimulates a rise in CF antibodies to adenovirus antigens of all types. The CF test, using the common antigen, is an easily applied method for detecting infection by any member of the adenovirus group.

Immunity

Studies in volunteers revealed that type-specific Nt antibodies protect against the disease but not always against reinfection. Infections with the viruses were frequently induced without the production of overt illness.

Nt antibodies against one or more types may be present in over 50% of infants 6–11 months old. Normal healthy adults generally have antibodies to several types. Nt antibodies to types 1 and 2 occur in 55–70% of individuals age 6–15, but antibodies to types 3 and 4 are less prevalent. Nt antibodies probably persist for life.

Infants are usually born without CF antibodies but develop these by age 6 months. Older individuals with Nt antibodies to 4 or more strains frequently give completely negative CF reactions. For military recruits, the incidence of infection (especially due to types 3 and 4) was not influenced by the presence of group CF antibodies.

Epidemiology

Adenoviruses can readily spread from person to person. Type 1, 2, 5, and 6 infections occur chiefly during the first years of life and are associated with fever and pharyngitis or asymptomatic infection. These are the types most frequently obtained from the adenoids and tonsils.

In children and young adults, types 3 and 7 commonly cause upper respiratory illness, pharyngitis, and conjunctivitis. While the illness is usually mild, occasionally there is high fever, cervical lymphadenitis, and even pneumonitis. Sometimes enteric infection produces gastroenteritis, but more commonly it is asymptomatic.

In adolescents and young adults, eg, college populations, only 2–5% of respiratory illness is caused by adenoviruses. In sharp contrast, respiratory disease due to types 3, 4, 7, 14, and 21 is common among military recruits. Adenovirus disease causes great morbidity when large numbers of persons are being inducted into the Armed Forces; consequently, its greatest impact is during periods of mobilization. During a 1-year study, 10% of recruits in basic training were hospitalized for a respiratory illness caused by an adenovirus. During the winter, adenovirus accounted for 72% of all the respiratory illness. However, adenovirus disease is not a problem in seasoned troops.

Epidemic keratoconjunctivitis caused by type 8 spread in 1941 from Australia via the Hawaiian Islands to the Pacific Coast. There it spread rapidly through the shipyards and other industries, thence to the East Coast, and finally to the Midwest. A large outbreak caused by type 8 occurred in 1977 in Georgia among patients subjected to invasive eye procedures by one ophthalmologist. The initial case was a nurse who returned from a vacation in Korea with severe keratoconjunctivitis. In the USA, the incidence of Nt antibody to type 8 adenovirus in the general population has been about 1%, whereas in Japan it has been over 30%. In Japan, type 8 spreads via the respiratory route in children. Since 1973, adenovirus type 19—and since 1977, adenovirus type 37—have caused epidemics of typical epidemic keratoconjunctivitis.

In prospective family studies, adenovirus infections have been found to be predominantly enteric; they may be abortive or invasive and followed by persistent intermittent excretion of virus. Such excretion is most characteristic of types 1, 2, 3, and 5, which are usually endemic. Infection rates are highest among infants, but siblings who introduce the infection into a household are more effective in spreading the disease than are infants; similarly, duration of excretion is more important than the mode. In the families studied, Nt antibodies provided immunity (85% protective) against homotypic but not heterotypic infection. The contribution of adenoviruses to all infectious illness in the families, based on virus-positive infections only, was 5% in infants and 3% in the 2- to 4-year-old age group.

The observed incidence of adenovirus infection in patients undergoing marrow transplantation is about 5%, an underestimate of the true incidence of infection because of the lack of serologic studies and of sensitive methods for routine cultures of rectal specimens. However, the distribution of serotypes found in transplant patients is distinct from that found in community surveys. Types 11, 34, and 35 are found most often and have also been reported in renal transplant recipients and in the urine of patients with acquired immune deficiency syndrome (AIDS). Type 4 also has been found in immunocompromised patients. The most likely source of infection in transplant patients is endogenous viral reactivation, because the patients become more immunosuppressed after marrow transplantation. Because laminar airflow rooms do not protect patients from infection or even postpone the infection, infection from environmental sources and person-to-person transmission is unlikely in these cases.

Prevention & Control

A trivalent vaccine was prepared by growing type 3, 4, and 7 viruses in monkey kidney cultures and then inactivating the viruses with formalin. However, when it was found that the vaccine strains were contaminated genetically with SV40 tumor virus determinants, this vaccine was withdrawn from use. Subsequently, it was found that most adenovirus strains do not replicate in monkey cells unless SV40 is present as a helper virus. Thus, a vaccine had to be made from noncontaminated live virus that could be grown in human diploid cells. The vaccine is given orally in a coated capsule to liberate the virus into the intestine. By this route, the live vaccine produces a subclinical infection that confers a high degree of immunity against wild strains. It does not spread from a vaccinated person to contacts. Such live virus vaccines against type 4 and type 7 are licensed and recommended for immunization of military populations. When both are administered simultaneously, vaccinees respond with Nt antibodies against both virus types.

Rigid asepsis during eye examination is essential in the control of epidemic keratoconjunctivitis.

REFERENCES

D'Angelo LJ et al: Epidemic keratoconjunctivitis caused by adenovirus type 8: Epidemiologic and laboratory aspects of a large outbreak. *Am J Epidemiol* 1981;**113**:44.

De Jong JC et al: Candidate adenovirus 40 and 41: Fastidious adenoviruses from human infant stool. *J Med Virol* 1983; **11**:215.

Fife KH, Ashley R, Corey L: Isolation and characterization of six new genome types of human adenovirus types 1 and 2. *J Clin Microbiol* 1985;**21**:20.

Fox JP, Hall CE, Cooney MK: The Seattle virus watch. 7. Observations of adenovirus infections. *Am J Epidemiol* 1977; **105**:362.

Kemp MC et al: The changing etiology of epidemic keratoconjunctivitis: Antigenic and restriction enzyme analyses of adenovirus types 19 and 37 isolated over a 10-year period. *J Infect Dis* 1983;**148**:24.

Logan JS, Shenk T: Transcriptional and translational control of adenovirus gene expression. *Microbiol Rev* 1982;**46**:377.

McPherson RA, Ginsberg HS, Rose JA: Adeno-associated virus helper activity of adenovirus DNA binding protein. *J Virol* 1982;**44**:666.

Shields AF et al: Adenovirus infections in patients undergoing bone-marrow transplantation. *N Engl J Med* 1985;**312:529.**

Takafuji ET et al: Simultaneous administration of live, enteric-coated adenovirus types 4, 7, and 21 vaccines: Safety and immunogenicity. *J Infect Dis* 1979;**140**:48.

Wadell G, De Jong JC, Wolontis S: Molecular epidemiology of adenoviruses: Alternating appearance of two different genome types of adenovirus 7 during epidemic outbreaks in Europe from 1958 to 1980. *Infect Immun* 1981;**34**:368.

Wadell G et al: Molecular epidemiology of adenoviruses: Global distribution of adenovirus 7 genome types. *J Clin Microbiol* 1985;**21**:403.

All **herpesviruses** have a core of double-stranded DNA surrounded by a protein coat that exhibits icosahedral symmetry and has 162 capsomeres. The nucleocapsid is surrounded by an envelope. The enveloped form measures 120–200 nm; the "naked" virion, 100 nm. The double-stranded DNA (MW 85–150 × 10⁶) has a wide range of guanine + cytosine content in different herpesviruses. There is little DNA homology among different herpesviruses, except herpes simplex types 1 and 2.

Various classifications for herpesviruses have been proposed, but individual virus names are generally used. Common and important herpesviruses of humans include herpes simplex virus types 1 and 2, varicella-zoster virus, Epstein-Barr (EB) virus, and cytomegalovirus. They have a propensity for subclinical infection, latency following the primary infection, and reactivation thereafter.

Herpesviruses that infect lower animals are B virus of Old World monkeys; herpesviruses saimiri, aotus, and ateles; marmoset herpesvirus of New World monkeys; pseudorabies virus of pigs; virus III of rabbits; infectious bovine rhinotracheitis virus; and many others. Herpesviruses are also known for birds, fish, fungi, and oysters, although the only link between some of these viruses is their appearance in the electron microscope.

Herpesviruses have been linked with malignant diseases in humans and lower animals: herpes simplex virus type 2 with cervical and vulvar carcinoma; EB virus with Burkitt's lymphoma of African children and with nasopharyngeal carcinoma; Lucké virus with renal adenocarcinomas of the frog; Marek's disease virus with a lymphoma of chickens; Hinze virus with a lymphoma of rabbits; and a number of New World primate herpesviruses with reticulum cell sarcomas and lymphomas in these animals.

HERPES SIMPLEX
(Human Herpesvirus 1 & 2)
(Herpes Labialis, Herpes Genitalis, & Many Other Syndromes)

Infection with herpes simplex virus (herpesvirus hominis) may take several clinical forms. The infection is most often inapparent. The usual clinical manifestation is a vesicular eruption of the skin or mucous membranes. Infection is sometimes seen as severe keratitis, meningoencephalitis, and a disseminated illness of the newborn.

Properties of the Virus

A. The Virion: (Fig 44–1.) Morphologically and chemically, herpes simplex virus has been studied in great detail. The envelope is derived from the nuclear membrane of the infected cell (Fig 33–10). It contains lipids, carbohydrate, and protein and is removed by ether treatment. The double-stranded DNA genome (MW 85–106 × 10⁶) is linear. Types 1 and 2 show 50% sequence homology. Treatment with restriction endonucleases (see Chapters 4 and 33) yields characteristically different cleavage patterns for type 1 and 2 viruses and even for different strains of each type. This "fingerprinting" of strains allows epidemiologic tracing of a given strain (Fig 33–13), whereas in the past, the ubiquitousness of herpes simplex virus made such investigations impossible.

B. Animal Susceptibility and Growth of Virus: The virus has a wide host range and can infect rabbits, guinea pigs, mice, hamsters, rats, and the chorioallantois of the embryonated egg.

In rabbits, herpesvirus produces a vesicular eruption in the skin of the inoculated area, sometimes progressing to fatal encephalitis. Corneal inoculation results in dendritic keratitis, which may progress to encephalitis. The virus may remain latent in the brains of survivors, and anaphylactic shock can precipitate an acute relapse of encephalomyelitis. Herpetic keratitis heals, but infective herpesvirus may be recovered from the eye intermittently with or without clinical activity. The virus remains latent in the trigeminal ganglion.

In the chorioallantoic membrane of embryonated eggs the lesions are raised white plaques, each induced by one infectious virus particle. The plaques produced by herpesvirus type 2 are larger than the tiny plaques produced by type 1 virus. The virus grows readily and produces plaques in almost any cell culture. Infected cells develop inclusion bodies and then undergo necrosis (cytopathic effect).

In Chinese hamster cells, which contain 22 chromosomes, the virus causes breaks in region 7 of chromosome No. 1 and in region 3 of the X chromosome. The Y chromosome is unaffected.

C. Virus Replication: The virus enters the cell either by fusion with the cell membrane or by pinocytosis. It is then uncoated, and the DNA becomes associated with the nucleus. Normal cellular DNA and protein synthesis virtually stop as virus replication begins. The virus induces a number of enzymes, at least 2 of which—thymidine kinase and DNA poly-

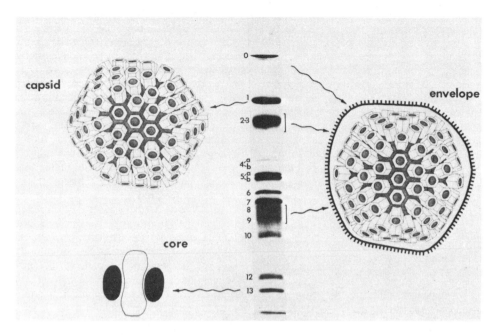

Figure 44–1. Herpesvirus. Several proteins have been identified in the virion. The protein in band 1 by gel electrophoresis is associated with the viral capsid; the glycoproteins present in bands 0, 2–3, 8, and 9 are associated with the envelope; and a DNA-binding protein (band 13) is associated with the internal core. (Powell and Purifoy.)

merase—are virus-coded. Thymidine kinases produced by different herpesviruses are serologically different from each other and different from the enzyme in uninfected cells.

Acyclovir, a purine nucleoside analog with an acyclic side chain (see Chapter 33), is a clinically useful inhibitor of herpesvirus replication. It enters both infected and uninfected cells, but it must be phosphorylated before it is active as an antiviral agent. Thymidine kinases (but not cellular kinases) of herpes simplex and varicella-zoster viruses form large quantities of acyclovir monophosphate; cellular kinases then continue the phosphorylation to produce acyclovir triphosphate, a selective inhibitor of viral DNA polymerase. (The DNA polymerase of cytomegalovirus is also sensitive to acyclovir triphosphate, but cytomegalovirus lacks thymidine kinase activity and thus cannot initiate the activation of acyclovir.)

Viral proteins are made in a controlled sequence that must proceed stepwise. They are made in the cytoplasm and most are transported to the nucleus, where they take part in virus DNA synthesis and the assembly of nucleocapsids. Maturation occurs by budding of nucleocapsids through the altered inner nuclear membrane. Enveloped virus particles are then released from the cell through tubular structures that are continuous with the outside of the cell or from vacuoles that release their contents at the surface of the cell (Fig 33–10).

D. Defective Interfering Herpesvirions: Serial passage of undiluted herpes simplex virus results in cyclic production of infectious and defective virions. The DNA in defective virions is made up of reiterated sequences of small fragments of the virus DNA. Defective virions interfere with the replication of standard virus and stimulate overproduction of a large polypeptide, which may have a regulatory function. The biologic role of the defective virions is not known.

E. Antigenic Properties: Herpesvirus-infected cells produce a large number of antigens that represent structural and nonstructural viral proteins. Some of these antigens are common to both types 1 and 2 and some are specific for one type. A number of tests, eg, fluorescent antibody, CF, virus neutralization, and radioimmunoassay, have been used to detect herpesvirus antigens.

F. Differentiation of Types 1 and 2: Herpes simplex virus types 1 and 2 cross-react serologically but may be distinguished by a number of tests: (1) The use of type-specific antiserum prepared by absorption of the viral antiserum with heterotypically infected cells or by inoculation of rabbits with individual type-specific proteins. (2) The greater temperature sensitivity of type 2 infectivity. (3) Preferential growth in different cell species. (4) Restriction enzyme patterns of virus DNA molecules. (5) Differences in the polypeptides produced by type 1 and type 2.

G. Oncogenic Properties: After inactivation of their lytic capabilities by ultraviolet irradiation or other means, herpesvirus types 1 and 2 can cause transformation of cultured hamster cells, which may induce tumors when inoculated into newborn hamsters. Viral genetic information can be demonstrated in the tumor cells. (See Chapter 46.)

Pathogenesis & Pathology

The lesion in the skin involves proliferation, ballooning degeneration, and intranuclear acidophilic inclusions. In fatal cases of herpes encephalitis, there are meningitis, perivascular infiltration, and nerve cell destruction, especially in the cortex. Neonatal generalized herpes infection causes areas of focal necrosis with a mononuclear reaction and formation of intranuclear inclusion bodies in all organs. Survivors may sustain permanent damage.

The fully formed early inclusion (Cowdry type A inclusion body is rich in DNA and virtually fills the nucleus, compressing the chromatic to the nuclear margin. Later, the inclusion loses its DNA and is separated by a halo from the chromatin at the nuclear margin.

Clinical Findings

Herpesvirus may cause many clinical entities, and the infections may be primary or recurrent. Primary infections occur in persons without antibodies and often result in the virus assuming a latent state in sensory ganglia of the host. Latent infections persist in persons with antibodies, and recurrent lesions are common (eg, recurrent herpes labialis). The primary infection in most individuals is clinically inapparent but is invariably accompanied by antibody production.

The recurrent attacks, in the presence of viral neutralizing antibody, follow nonspecific stimuli such as exposure to excess sunlight, fever, menstruation, or emotional stresses.

A. Herpesvirus Type 1: The clinical entities attributable to herpesvirus type 1 include the following:

1. Acute herpetic gingivostomatitis (aphthous stomatitis, Vincent's stomatitis)–This is the most common clinical entity caused by primary infections with type 1 herpesvirus. It occurs most frequently in small children (1–3 years of age) and includes extensive vesiculoulcerative lesions of the mucous membranes of the mouth, fever, irritability, and local lymphadenopathy. The incubation period is short (about 3–5 days), and lesions heal in 2–3 weeks.

2. Eczema herpeticum (Kaposi's varicelliform eruption)–This is a primary infection, usually with herpesvirus type 1, in a person with chronic eczema. In this illness, there may be extensive vesiculation of the skin over much of the body and high fever. In rare instances, the illness may be fatal.

3. Keratoconjunctivitis–The initial infection with herpesvirus may be in the eye, producing severe keratoconjunctivitis. Recurrent lelsions of the eye appear as dendritic keratitis or corneal ulcers or as vesicles on the eyelids. With recurrent keratitis, there may be progressive involvement of the corneal stroma, with permanent opacification and blindness.

4. Encephalitis–A severe form of encephalitis may be produced by herpesvirus. In adults, the neurologic manifestationsd suggest a lesion in the temporal lobe. Pleocytosis (chiefly of lymphocytes) is present in the cerebrospinal fluid; however, definite diagnosis during the illness can usually be made only by isolation of the virus (or by demonstrating viral antigens by immunofluorescence) from brain tissue obtained by biopsy or at postmortem. The disease carries a high mortality rate, and those who survive often have residual neurologic defects.

5. Herpes labialis (cold sores, herpes febrilis–This is the most common recurrent disease produced by type 1. Clusters of localized vesicles occur, usually at the mucocutaneous junction of the lips. The vesicle ruptures, leaving a painful ulcer that heals without scarring. The lesions may recur, repeatedly and at various intervals of time, in the same location. The permanent site of latent herpes simplex virus is the trigeminal ganglion.

B. Herpesvirus Type 2: The clinical entities associated with herpesvirus type 2 include the following:

1. Genital herpes (herpes progenitalis)–Genital herpes is characterized by vesiculoulcerative lesions of the penis of the male or the cervix, vulva, vagina, and perineum of the female. The lesions are more severe during primary infection and may be associated with fever, malaise, and inguinal lymphadenopathy. In women with herpesvirus antibodies, only the cervix or vagina may be involved, and the disease may therefore be asymptomatic. Recurrence of the lesions is common. Type 2 virus remains latent in lumbar and sacral ganglia. Changing patterns of sexual behavior are reflected by an increasing number of type 1 virus isolations from genital lesions and of type 2 from facial lesions, presumably as a result of oralgenital sexual activity.

2. Neonatal herpes–Herpesvirus type 2 may be transmitted to the newborn during birth by contact with herpetic lesions in the birth canal. The spectrum of illness produced in the newborn appears to vary from subclinical or local to severe generalized disease with a fatal outcome. Severely affected infants who survive may have permanent brain damage. To avoid infection, delivery by cesarean section has been used in pregnant women with genital herpes lesions. To be effective, cesarean section must be performed before rupture of the membranes.

Severe generalized disease of the newborn can be acquired postnatally by exposure to either type 1 or 2. Efforts should be made to prevent exposure to active lesions among family and especially among hospital personnel.

Transplacental infection of the fetus with types 1 and 2 herpes simplex virus may cause congenital malformations, but this phenomenon is rare.

C. Miscellaneous: Localized lesions of the skin caused by type 1 or 2 may occur in abrasions that become contaminated with the virus (traumatic herpes). These lesions are seen on the fingers of dentists, hospital personnel (herpetic whitlow), or persons with genital lesions and on the bodies of wrestlers.

Primary and recurrent herpes can occur in the nose (acute herpetic rhinitis).

Mild aseptic meningitis has been attributed to the virus, and recurrent episodes of meningeal irritation have been observed.

Epidemiologic evidence has shown that in most geographic areas, patients with cervical and vulvar cancer have a high frequency of type 2 antibodies. In addition, herpesvirus type 2 nonstructural antigens have been detected by immunofluorescence in biopsies of cervical and vulvar carcinomas. (See Chapter 46.)

Laboratory Diagnosis

A. Recovery of Virus: The virus may be isolated from herpetic lesions (skin, cornea, or brain). It may also be found in the throat, saliva, and stools, both during primary infection and during asymptomatic periods. Therefore, the isolation of herpesvirus is not in itself sufficient evidence to indicate that this virus is the causative agent of a disease under investigation.

Inoculation of tissue cultures is used for virus isolation. The appearance of typical cytopathic effects in cell culture suggests the presence of herpesvirus in 18–36 hours. The agent is then identified by Nt test or immunofluorescence staining with specific antiserum.

Scrapings or swabs from the base of early herpetic lesions contain multinucleated giant cells.

B. Serology: Antibodies may be measured quantitatively by Nt tests in cell cultures. In the early stage of the primary immune response, Nt antibody appears that is detectable only in the presence of fresh complement. This antibody soon is replaced by Nt antibody that can function without complement.

Since the only hope for treatment of herpes simplex virus encephalitis lies in early diagnosis, a rapid means of diagnosis is needed. The fluorescent antibody test using brain biopsy material is the method of choice.

Antibodies appear in 4–7 days; can be measured by Nt, CF, ELISA, radioimmunoassay, or immunofluorescence; and reach a peak in 2–4 weeks. They persist with minor fluctuations for the life of the host. Most adults have antibodies in their blood at all times.

After a primary type 1 infection, the IgM Nt antibody response is type-specific, but after a primary type 2 infection, the IgM that develops neutralizes both type 1 and type 2 virus. Subsequently, IgG antibodies react with both type 1 and type 2 antigens, albeit in varying ratios.

There is also some cross-stimulation between herpes simplex and varicella-zoster antigens in patients with preexisting antibody to the other virus.

Immunity

Many newborns have passively transferred maternal antibodies. This antibody is lost during the first 6 months of life, and the period of greatest susceptibility to primary herpes infection occurs between ages 6 months and 2 years. Type 1 antibodies begin to appear in the population in early childhood; by adolescence, they are present in most persons. Antibodies to type 2 (genital herpesvirus) rise during the age of adolescence and sexual activity.

After recovery from a primary infection (inapparent, mild, or severe), the virus is usually carried in a latent state, in the presence of antibodies.

Treatment

Topically applied idoxuridine (5-iodo-2'-deoxyuridine, IDU), trifluridine (trifluorothymidine), vidarabine (adenine arabinoside, ara-A), acyclovir (acycloguanosine), and other inhibitors of viral DNA synthesis have been used for herpetic keratitis (see Chapter 33). These drugs inhibit herpesvirus replication and may suppress clinical manifestations. However, the virus remains latent in the sensory ganglia, and the rate of relapse is similar in drug-treated and untreated individuals. Some drug-resistant virus strains have emerged.

Intravenous acyclovir is now the drug of choice for treating herpes encephalitis diagnosed by biopsy. Best results are obtained if treatment is begun early in the disease, before coma sets in.

Acyclovir has low toxicity and also has been administered systemically to suppress the activation of a latent herpes infection in immunosuppressed patients. Topically administered, it is of no value for treatment of recurrent type 1 or type 2 lesions but has decreased the duration of primary lesions. An oral dosage form of acyclovir recently has been approved for treatment of initial episodes and for management of recurrent episodes of genital herpes in certain patients. Although it provides symptomatic relief when taken for initial disease, the oral form of acyclovir does not prevent virus latency or recurrent disease. When taken to treat or suppress recurrent episodes, acyclovir does not eliminate latent virus. It may actually increase the severity and frequency of recurrences after therapy is discontinued.

Epidemiology

The epidemiology of type 1 and type 2 herpesvirus differs. Herpesvirus type 1 is probably more constantly present in humans than any other virus. Primary infection occurs early in life and is often asymptomatic or produces acute gingivostomatitis. Antibodies develop, but the virus is not eliminated from the body; a carrier state is established that lasts throughout life and is punctuated by transient attacks of herpes. If primary infection is avoided in childhood, it may not occur in later life, perhaps because the thicker adult epithelium is less susceptible or because the opportunity for contact with the virus is diminished (less contact with saliva of infected persons).

The highest incidence of type 1 virus carriage in the oropharynx of healthy persons occurs among children 6 months to 3 years of age. By adulthood, 70–90% of persons have type 1 antibodies.

Type 1 virus is transmitted more readily in families of lower socioeconomic groups; the most obvious explanation is their more crowded living conditions and lower hygienic standards. The virus is spread by direct contact (saliva) or through utensils contaminated with the saliva of a virus shedder. The source of infection for children is usually a parent with an active herpetic lesion.

Type 2 is usually acquired as a sexually transmitted

disease. A newborn may acquire type 2 infection from an active lesion in the mother's birth canal.

Control

Newborns and persons with eczema should be protected from evident active herpetic lesions.

Although certain drugs are effective in treatment of herpesvirus infections, once a latent infection is established there had been no known treatment that would prevent recurrences and reduce virus shedding until the recent successful results with oral or parenteral acyclovir. However, acyclovir must be taken daily to be effective, and once the drug is stopped, recurrences appear.

Experimental vaccines are being developed from glycoprotein antigens found in the viral envelope and from recombinant attenuated viruses cultivated in *Escherichia coli*. Another approach has been through the development of modified vaccinia virus into which herpesvirus DNA coding for an immunizing glycoprotein is inserted. Infection by the modified vaccinia virus allows the herpesvirus DNA to be expressed and has protected mice from lethal herpesvirus disease and from establishment of latent infection.

Herpes recurs in the presence of circulating antibody, so a vaccine would seem to be of little use in a person who already had a primary infection.

VARICELLA-ZOSTER VIRUS (Human Herpesvirus 3)

VARICELLA (Chickenpox) ZOSTER (Herpes Zoster, Shingles, Zona)

Varicella (chickenpox) is a mild, highly infectious disease, chiefly of children, characterized clinically by a vesicular eruption of the skin and mucous membranes. However, the disease may be severe in immunocompromised children. The causative agent is indistinguishable from the virus of zoster.

Zoster (shingles) is a sporadic, incapacitating disease of adults (rare in children) that is characterized by an inflammatory reaction of the posterior nerve roots and ganglia, accompanied by crops of vesicles (like those of varicella) over the skin supplied by the affected sensory nerves.

Both diseases are caused by the same virus. Varicella is the acute disease that follows primary contact with the virus, whereas zoster is the response of the partially immune host to a reactivation of varicella virus present in latent form in sensory ganglia.

Properties of the Virus

Varicella-zoster virus is morphologically identical with herpes simplex virus. The virus propagates in cultures of human embryonic tissue and produces typical intranuclear inclusion bodies. Supernatant fluids from such infected cultures contain a CF antigen but no infective virus. Infectious virus is easily transmitted by infected cells. The virus has not been propagated in laboratory animals. Virus can be isolated from the vesicles of chickenpox or zoster patients or from the cerebrospinal fluid in cases of zoster aseptic meningitis.

Inoculation of vesicle fluid of zoster into children produces vesicles at the site of inoculation in about 10 days. This may be followed by generalized skin lesions of varicella. Generalized varicella may occur in such inoculated children without local vesicle formation. Contacts of such children develop typical varicella after a 2-week incubation period. Children who have recovered from zoster virus-induced infection are resistant to varicella, and those who have had varicella are no longer susceptible to primary zoster virus.

Antibody to varicella-zoster virus can be measured by CF, gel precipitation, Nt, or indirect immunofluorescence to virus-induced membrane antigens.

The virus has a colchicinelike effect on human cells. Arrest in metaphase, overcontracted chromosomes, chromosome breaks, and formation of micronuclei are often seen.

Pathogenesis & Pathology

A. Varicella: The route of infection is probably the mucosa of the upper respiratory tract. The virus probably circulates in the blood and localizes in the skin. Swelling of epithelial cells, ballooning degeneration, and the accumulation of tissue fluids result in vesicle formation. In nuclei of infected cells, particularly in the early stages, eosinophilic inclusion bodies are found.

B. Zoster: In addition to skin lesions—histopathologically identical with those of varicella—there is an inflammatory reaction of the dorsal nerve roots and sensory ganglia. Often only a single ganglion may be involved. As a rule, the distribution of lesions in the skin corresponds closely to the areas of innervation from an individual dorsal root ganglion. There is cellular infiltration, necrosis of nerve cells, and inflammation of the ganglion sheath.

Varicella virus seems able to enter and remain within dorsal root ganglia for long periods. Years later, various insults (eg, pressure on a nerve) may cause a flare-up of the virus along posterior root fibers, whereupon zoster vesicles appear. Thus, varicella-zoster and herpes simplex viruses are similar in their ability to induce latent infections with clinical recurrence of disease in humans. However, zoster rarely occurs more than once.

Clinical Findings

A. Varicella: The incubation period is usually 14–21 days. Malaise and fever are the earliest symptoms, soon followed by the rash, first on the trunk and then on the face, the limbs, and the buccal and pharyngeal mucosa. Successive fresh vesicles appear in crops during the next 3–4 days, so that all stages of papules, vesicles, and crusts may be seen at one time. The eruption is found together with the fever and is proportionate to its severity. Complications are rare, although encephalitis does at times occur about 5–10 days after the rash. The mortality rate is much less than 1% in uncomplicated cases. In neonatal varicella (contracted from the mother just before or just after birth), the mortality rate may be 20%. In varicella encephalitis, the mortality rate is about 10%, and another 10% are left with permanent injury to the central nervous system. Primary varicella pneumonia is rare in children but may occur in about 20–30% of adult cases, may produce severe hypoxia, and may be fatal.

Children with immune deficiency disease or those receiving immunosuppressant or cytotoxic drugs are at high risk of developing very severe and sometimes fatal varicella or disseminated zoster.

B. Zoster: The incubation period is unknown. The disease starts with malaise and fever that are soon followed by severe pain in the area of skin or mucosa supplied by one or more groups of sensory nerves and ganglia. Within a few days after onset, a crop of vesicles appears over the skin supplied by the affected nerves. The eruption is usually unilateral; the trunk, head, and neck are most commonly involved. Lymphocytic pleocytosis in the cerebrospinal fluid may be present.

In patients with localized zoster and no underlying disease, vesicle interferon levels peak early during infection (by the sixth day), whereas those in patients with disseminated infection peak later. Peak interferon levels are followed by clinical improvement within 48 hours. Vesicles pustulate and crust, and dissemination is halted.

Zoster tends to disseminate when there is an underlying disease, especially if the patient is taking immunosuppressive drugs or has lymphoma treated by irradiation.

Laboratory Diagnosis

In stained smears of scrapings or swabs of the base of vesicles, multinucleated giant cells are seen. In similar smears, intracellular viral antigens can be demonstrated by immunofluorescence staining.

Virus can be isolated in cultures of human or other fibroblastic cells in 3–5 days. It does not grow in epithelial cells, in contrast to herpes simplex, and does not infect laboratory animals or eggs. An isolate in fibroblasts is identified by immunofluorescence or Nt tests with specific antisera.

Herpesviruses can be differentiated from poxviruses by (1) the morphologic appearance of particles in vesicular fluids examined by electron microscopy, and (2) the presence of antigen in vesicle fluid or in an extract of crusts as determined by gel diffusion tests with specific antisera to herpes, varicella, or vaccinia viruses, which give visible precipitation lines in 24–48 hours.

A rise in specific antibody titer can be detected in the patient's serum by CF, Nt (in cell culture), and indirect immunofluorescence tests or by enzyme immunoassay. Zoster can occur in the presence of relatively high levels of Nt antibody in the blood just prior to onset. The role of cell-mediated immunity is unknown.

Immunity

Varicella and zoster viruses are identical, the 2 diseases being the result of differing host responses. Previous infection with varicella leaves the patient with enduring immunity to varicella. However, zoster may occur in persons who have contracted varicella earlier. This is a reactivation of a varicella virus infection that has been latent for years.

Prophylaxis & Treatment

Gamma globulin of high specific antibody titer prepared from pooled plasma of patients convalescing from herpes zoster (varicella-zoster immune globulin, VZIG) can be used to prevent the development of the illness in immunocompromised children who have been exposed to varicella. Standard immune globulin USP is without value because of the low titer of varicella antibodies.

VZIG is available from the American Red Cross Blood Services (through 13 regional blood centers) for prophylaxis of varicella in exposed high-risk persons and is especially recommended for immunodeficient or immunosuppressed children. It has no therapeutic value once varicella has started.

Idoxuridine and cytarabine inhibit replication of the viruses in vitro but are not effective in treatment of patients.

Vidarabine has been beneficial in adults with severe varicella pneumonia, immunocompromised children with varicella, and adults with disseminated zoster. Intravenous acyclovir can halt the progression of zoster, especially if given within 3 days after the onset of rash, even in immunocompromised patients.

Epidemiology

Zoster occurs sporadically, chiefly in adults and without seasonal prevalence. In contrast, varicella is a common epidemic disease of childhood (peak incidence is in children age 2–6 years, although adult cases do occur). It is much more common in winter and spring than in summer. Almost 200,000 cases are reported annually in the USA.

Varicella readily spreads, presumably by droplets as well as by contact with skin. Contact infection is rare in zoster, perhaps because the virus is absent in the upper respiratory tract.

Zoster in children or adults can be the source of varicella in children and can initiate large outbreaks.

Control

None is available for the general population.

Varicella may spread rapidly among patients, especially among children with immunologic dysfunctions or leukemia or in those receiving corticosteroids or cytotoxic drugs. Varicella in such children poses the threat of pneumonia, encephalitis, or death. Efforts should be made to prevent their exposure to varicella. VZIG may be used to modify the disease in such children who have been exposed to varicella.

A live attenuated varicella vaccine has been developed and tested successfully in hospitalized immunosuppressed children who were exposed to varicella. The vaccine is particularly useful in preventing the spread of varicella in such children at high risk.

A number of problems are envisioned for the use of such a vaccine for the general population as opposed to high-risk patients. The vaccine would need to confer immunity comparable to that of natural infections. A short-lasting immunity might result in an increased number of susceptible adults, in whom the disease is more severe. Furthermore, any such vaccine would need to be evaluated for later morbidity due to zoster as compared to that following natural childhood infections with varicella virus.

CYTOMEGALOVIRUS
(Human Herpesvirus 5)
(Cytomegalic Inclusion Disease)

Cytomegalic inclusion disease is a generalized infection of infants caused by intrauterine or early postnatal infection with the cytomegaloviruses. The disease causes severe congenital anomalies in about 10,000 infants in the USA per year. Cytomegalovirus has been detected in the cervix of up to 10% of healthy women. Cytomegalic inclusion disease is characterized by large intranuclear inclusions that occur in the salivary glands, lungs, liver, pancreas, kidneys, endocrine glands, and, occasionally, the brain. Most fatalities occur in children under 2 years of age. Inapparent infection is common during childhood and adolescence. Severe cytomegalovirus infections are frequently found in adults receiving immunosuppressive therapy.

Properties of the Virus
A. General Properties: Morphologically, cytomegalovirus is indistinguishable from herpes simplex or varicella-zoster virus.

In infected human fibroblasts, virus particles are assembled in the nucleus. The envelope of the virus is derived from the inner nuclear membrane. The growth cycle of the virus is slower and infectious virus is more cell-associated than herpes simplex virus.

B. Animal Susceptibility: All attempts to infect animals with human cytomegalovirus have failed. A number of animal cytomegaloviruses exist, all of them species-specific in rats, hamsters, moles, rabbits, and monkeys. The virus isolated from monkeys propagates in cultures of monkey as well as human cells.

Human cytomegalovirus replicates in vitro only in human fibroblasts, although the virus is often isolated from epithelial cells of the host. The virus can transform human and hamster cells in culture, but whether it is oncogenic in vivo is unknown.

Pathogenesis & Pathology
In infants, cytomegalic inclusion disease is congenitally acquired, probably as a result of primary infection of the mother during pregnancy. The virus can be isolated from the urine of the mother at the time of birth of the infected baby, and typical cytomegalic cells, 25–40 μm in size, occur in the chorionic villi of the infected placenta.

Foci of cytomegalic cells are found in fatal cases in the epithelial tissues of the liver, lungs, kidneys, gastrointestinal tract, parotid gland, pancreas, thymus, thyroid, adrenals, and other regions. The cells can be found also in the urine or adenoid tissue of healthy children. The route of infection in older infants, children, and adults is not known.

The isolation of the virus from urine and from tissue cultures of adenoids of healthy children suggests subclinical infections at a young age. The virus may persist in various organs for long periods in a latent state or as a chronic infection. Virus is not recovered from the mouths of adults. Disseminated inclusions in adults occur in association with acquired immune deficiency syndrome (AIDS) and other conditions with immunosuppression (eg, patients undergoing organ transplantation).

Clinical Findings
Congenital infection may result in death of the fetus in utero or may produce the clinical syndrome of cytomegalic inclusion disease, with signs of prematurity, jaundice with hepatosplenomegaly, thrombocytopenic purpura, pneumonitis, and central nervous system damage (microcephaly, periventricular calcification, chorioretinitis, optic atrophy, and mental or motor retardation).

Infants born with congenital cytomegalic inclusion disease may appear well and live for many years. It has been estimated that one in every 1000 infants born in the USA is seriously retarded as a result of this congenital infection.

Inapparent intrauterine infection seems to occur frequently. Elevated IgM antibody to cytomegalovirus or isolation of the virus from the urine occurs in up to 2% of apparently normal newborns. This high rate occurs in spite of the fact that women may already have cytomegalovirus antibody before becoming pregnant. Such intrauterine infections have been implicated as possible causes of mental retardation and hearing loss.

Many women who have been infected naturally with cytomegalovirus at some time prior to pregnancy begin to excrete the virus from the cervix during the last trimester of pregnancy. At the time of delivery, infants pass through the infected birth canal and become infected, although they possess high titers of maternal antibody acquired transplacentally. These infants begin to excrete the virus in their urine at about 8–12 weeks of age. They continue to excrete the virus for several years but remain healthy.

Acquired infection with cytomegalovirus is common and usually inapparent. In children, acquired infection may result in hepatitis, interstitial pneumonitis, or acquired hemolytic anemia. The virus is shed in the saliva and urine of infected individuals for weeks or months.

Cytomegalovirus can cause an infectious mononucleosis-like disease without heterophil antibodies. "Cytomegalovirus mononucleosis" occurs either spontaneously or after transfusions of fresh blood during surgery ("postperfusion syndrome"). The incubation period is about 30–40 days. Cytomegaloviruria and a rise of cytomegalovirus antibody are present. Cytomegalovirus has been isolated from the peripheral blood leukocytes of such patients. Perhaps the postperfusion syndrome is caused by cytomegalovirus harbored in the leukocytes of the blood donors.

Patients with malignancies or immunologic defects or those undergoing immunosuppressive therapy for organ transplantation may develop cytomegalovirus pneumonitis or hepatitis and occasionally generalized disease. In such patients, a latent infection may be reactivated when host susceptibility to infection is increased by immunosuppression. In seronegative patients without evidence of previous cytomegalovirus infection, the virus may be transmitted exogenously. Eighty-three percent of seronegative patients who received kidneys from seropositive transplant donors developed infection. Thus, the kidneys seemed to be the source of virus.

Laboratory Diagnosis

A. Recovery of Virus: The virus can be recovered from mouth swabs, urine, liver, adenoids, kidneys, and peripheral blood leukocytes by inoculation of human fibroblastic cell cultures. In cultures, 1–2 weeks are usually needed for cytologic changes consisting of small foci of swollen, rounded, translucent cells with large intranuclear inclusions. Cell degeneration progresses slowly, and the virus concentration is much higher within the cell than in the fluid. Prolonged serial propagation is needed before the virus reaches high titers.

The cell culture methods of virus isolation are too slow to be useful in guiding therapy, particularly in immunosuppressed patients. Rapid diagnostic methods that have been developed include observation of inclusion bodies in tissue or in desquamated cells found in urine, direct detection of viral antigen, and visualization of virus by electron microscopy. The most promising is a quantitative method employing DNA hybridization; 10-mL samples of urine are used in this test. The virus in urine is concentrated by ultracentrifugation, after which its denatured DNA is retained on a filter and quantitatively identified within 24 hours by hybridization with radioactively labeled cytomegalovirus DNA.

B. Serology: Antibodies may be detected by Nt, CF, radioimmunoassay, or immunofluorescence tests.

Such tests may be useful in detecting congenitally infected infants with no clinical manifestations of disease.

Immunity

Antibodies occur in most human sera. Virus may occur in the urine of children for many months even though serum Nt antibody is present. This suggests that the virus propagates in the urinary tract rather than being filtered from the bloodstream. Virus is not found in young children who lack antibody.

Treatment

There is no specific treatment. Neither immune globulin USP nor DNA virus-inhibitory drugs have any effect.

Epidemiology

Epidemics in open populations are unknown, and new infections are almost always asymptomatic. After infection, virus is shed from multiple sites (urine, saliva, tears, semen, cervical secretions, breast milk). Shedding may continue for years, often intermittently, as latent virus becomes reactivated. Thus, exposures to and infections by cytomegalovirus are widespread, even though the precise mechanism of virus transmission in the population remains unknown except in congenital infections and those acquired by organ transplantation, blood transfusion, and reactivation of latent virus. The prolonged shedding of virus in urine and saliva suggests a urine-hand-mouth route of infection. Cytomegalovirus can also be transmitted by sexual contact.

Intrauterine infection may produce a serious disease in the newborn. Infants infected during fetal life may be born with antibody that continues to rise after birth in the presence of persistent virus excretion.

Most infants infected with cytomegalovirus in the perinatal period are asymptomatic, and infection continues in the presence of high antibody titers.

The prevalence of infection varies with socioeconomic status and hygienic practices. The antibody prevalence may be relatively low (40–50%) in adults in high socioeconomic groups in developed countries, in contrast to a prevalence of 90–100% in adults in developing nations and in low socioeconomic groups in developed countries.

Control

Specific control measures are not available. Isolation of newborns with generalized cytomegalic inclusion disease from other newborns is advisable.

Screening of transplant donors and recipients for cytomegalovirus antibody may prevent some transmissions of primary cytomegalovirus. The cytomegalovirus-seronegative transplant recipient population represents a high-risk group for cytomegalovirus infections as well as other lethal superinfections. Administration of human IgG or α interferon is effective in decreasing the number of viral infections in transplant recipients.

A live cytomegalovirus "vaccine" has been developed and has had some preliminary clinical trials. The vaccine virus was given to humans after its 129th passage in human diploid cells. In contrast to the wild virus, the vaccine virus did not induce latency; this is a very favorable factor in evaluation of vaccine safety. Another approach to immunization involves the use of cytomegalovirus polypeptides, which induce Nt antibodies.

EB HERPESVIRUS
(Human Herpesvirus 4)
(Infectious Mononucleosis, Burkitt's Lymphoma, Nasopharyngeal Carcinoma)

EB (Epstein-Barr) virus is the causative agent of infectious mononucleosis and has been associated with Burkitt's lymphoma and nasopharyngeal carcinoma. The virus is an antigenically distinct herpesvirus.

Properties of the Virus

A. Morphology: EB virus is indistinguishable in size and structure from other herpesviruses.

B. Antigenic Properties: EB virus is distinct from all other human herpesviruses. Many different EB virus antigens can be detected by CF, immunodiffusion, or immunofluorescence tests. A lymphocyte-detected membrane antigen (LYDMA) is the earliest-detected virus-determined antigen. EBNA is a complement-fixing nuclear antigen. Early antigen (EA) is formed in the presence of DNA inhibitors, and membrane antigen (MA), the Nt antigen, is a cell surface antigen. The virus capsid antigen (VCA) is a late antigen representing virions and structural antigen.

C. Virus Growth: Human blood B lymphocytes infected in vitro with EB virus have resulted in the establishment of continuous cell lines, suggesting that these cells have been transformed by the virus.

This transformation by EB virus enables B lymphocytes to multiply continuously, and all cells contain many EB virus genomes and express EBNA. Some EB virus cell lines express certain antigens but produce no virus particles or VCA; others produce virus particles. EB virus is carried in lymphoid cell lines derived from patients with African Burkitt's lymphoma, nasopharyngeal carcinoma, or infectious mononucleosis. Non-virus-producing B lymphocyte cell lines can be established in vitro from the blood of patients with infectious mononucleosis. Such lines represent a latent state of the virus; the cells contain EB virus genomes but express only the earliest antigen (LYDMA) and possibly EBNA.

Owl monkeys and marmosets inoculated with cell-free EB virus can develop fatal malignant lymphomas. Lymphoblastoid cells from such monkeys cultured as continuous cell lines give positive reactions with EB virus antisera by immunofluorescence.

Immunity

The most widely used and most sensitive serologic procedure for detection of EB virus infection is the indirect immunofluorescence test with acetone-fixed smears of cultured Burkitt's lymphoma cells. The cells containing the EB virus exhibit fluorescence after treatment with fluorescent antibody. Detectable levels of antibody persist for many years.

Early in acute disease, a transient rise in IgM antibodies to VCA occurs, replaced within 2 weeks by IgG antibodies to VCA, which persist for life. Slightly later, antibodies to MA and to EBNA arise and persist throughout life.

EB virus is often present in saliva of immunosuppressed patients. About 50% of transplant recipients yield virus-positive throat washings, in contrast to about 10% of healthy adults.

Epidemiology

Seroepidemiologic studies using the immunofluorescence technique and CF reaction indicate that infection with EB virus is common in different parts of the world and that it occurs early in life. In some areas, including urban parts of the USA, about 50% of children 1 year old, 80–90% of children over age 4, and 90% of adults have antibody to EB virus.

In groups at a low socioeconomic level, EB virus infection occurs in early childhood without any recognizable disease. These inapparent infections result in permanent seroconversion and total immunity to infectious mononucleosis. In groups living in comfortable social circumstances, infection is often postponed until adolescence and young adulthood. Again, the majority of these adult infections are asymptomatic, but in almost half of cases the infection is manifested by heterophil-positive infectious mononucleosis.

Antibody to EB virus is also present in nonhuman primates.

EB Virus & Human Disease

Most EB virus infections are clinically inapparent. The virus causes infectious mononucleosis and is strongly associated with Burkitt's lymphoma and nasopharyngeal carcinoma.

Infectious mononucleosis (glandular fever) is a disease of children and young adults characterized by fever and enlarged lymph nodes and spleen. The total white blood count may range from 10,000/μL to 80,000/μL, with a predominance of lymphocytes. Many of these are large "atypical" cells with vacuolated cytoplasm and nucleus. These atypical lymphocytes, probably T cells, are diagnostically important. During mononucleosis, there often are signs of hepatitis.

During the course of infection, the majority of patients develop heterophil antibodies, detected by sheep cell agglutination or the mononucleosis spot test (see Chapter 35).

Although the pathogenesis of infectious mononucleosis is still not understood, infectious EB virus can be recovered from throat washings and saliva of patients ("kissing disease"). Infectious virus is produced by B lymphocytes in the oropharynx and perhaps in special epithelial cells of this region. Virus cannot be recovered from blood, but EB virus genome-containing B lymphocytes are present in up to 0.05% of the circulating mononuclear leukocytes as demonstrated by the establishment of cell lines. These EB virus genome-containing cells express the earliest antigen, LYDMA, which is specifically recognized by killer T cells.

These T cells reach large numbers and can lyse EB virus genome-positive but not EB virus genome-negative target cells. Part of the infectious mononucleosis syndrome may reflect a rejection reaction against virally converted lymphocytes. Virus may be isolated intermittently from oropharyngeal washings and circulating leukocytes for over a year after clinical recovery from the disease.

Patients with infectious mononucleosis develop antibodies against EB virus, as measured by immunofluorescence with virus-bearing cells. Antibodies appear early in the acute disease, rise to peak levels within a few weeks, and remain high during convalescence. Unlike the short-lived heterophil antibodies, those against EB virus persist for years.

The role that EB virus may play in Burkitt's lymphoma (a tumor of the jaw in African children and young adults) and nasopharyngeal carcinoma (common in males of Chinese origin) is less well established. The association with EB virus is based primarily on the finding that the prevalence of antibody is greater and the antibody titers are higher among patients with Burkitt's lymphoma and nasopharyngeal carcinoma than in healthy matched controls or individuals with other types of malignancies. The significance of these associations is uncertain at present. All cells from Burkitt's lymphoma of African origin and from nasopharyngeal carcinoma carry multiple copies of the EB virus genome and express the antigen EBNA.

B VIRUS
(Herpesvirus of Old World Monkeys)

B virus infection of humans is an acute, usually fatal, ascending myelitis and encephalitis. Cases have followed (1) the bites of apparently normal carrier monkeys or (2) contact with tissue cultures derived from monkeys. Human cases were rare but have increased as the number of persons handling monkeys and preparing vaccines from monkey kidney cultures increased. Herpes B virus is most commonly found in rhesus, cynomolgus, and bonnet macaque monkeys.

Because B virus infection occurs naturally in macaque monkeys, it has been named herpesvirus simiae. It is related as measured by the Nt test to herpes simplex virus and by one immunoprecipitation line to pseudorabies virus. The virus is transmissible to monkeys, rabbits, guinea pigs, and newborn mice. The virus grows in the chick embryo, producing pocks on the chorioallantoic membrane, and in cultures of rabbit, monkey, or human cells. Experimentally infected animals exhibit intranuclear inclusions and multinucleated giant cells.

The virus enters through the skin and localizes at the site of the monkey bite, producing vesicles and then necrosis of the area. From the site of the skin lesion, the virus enters the central nervous system by way of the peripheral nerves. The picture is predominantly that of a meningoencephalomyelitis. About 3 days after exposure, the patient develops vesicular lesions at the site; regional lymphangitis and adenitis follow. About 7 days later, motor and sensory abnormalities occur; this is followed by acute ascending paralysis, involvement of the respiratory center, and death.

Virus can be recovered from the brain, spinal cord, and spleen of fatal cases. Suspensions of these tissues are inoculated into rabbit kidney cell cultures or intradermally into rabbits; a necrotic lesion of the skin occurs, and the rabbit develops myelitis. The agent is established as B virus by serologic identification. Herpes antiserum hardly neutralizes B virus, whereas B virus antiserum neutralizes both herpes simplex and B viruses equally well.

There is no specific treatment once the clinical disease is manifest. However, immune globulin containing B virus antibodies is recommended as a preventive measure immediately after a monkey bite.

An experimental killed B virus vaccine has induced antibody responses in human recipients, but its protective value has not yet been proved.

B virus infection occurs in monkeys as a latent infection much as herpes simplex occurs in humans. The virus has been recovered from monkey saliva, brain, and spinal cord and from many lots of monkey kidney culture (once the starting material for preparing poliomyelitis and other vaccines for human use).

In 24 cases of monkey B virus infection, half from the USA, 23 patients contracted encephalitis and 18 died after a bite wound, a puncture with a contaminated needle, or a cut by glass from monkey tissue cell culture.

MARMOSET HERPESVIRUS
(Herpesvirus of New World Monkeys)

Several herpesviruses have been isolated from New World monkeys, including herpesviruses T, saimiri, ateles, saguinus, and aotus. These viruses seem to have a natural monkey host in which they are present with little apparent effect, but they can produce serious disease when they infect monkeys of another genus. Thus, they resemble herpes simplex virus in humans. Some of these viruses are antigenically related to herpes simplex, and some are distinct.

Two of these viruses—herpesviruses saimiri and ateles—produce malignant disease in other primates. They thus form useful model systems for viral oncologists. Monkeys can be protected from the malignant effect of these viruses by vaccination with live attenuated or killed virus.

REFERENCES

Chou S, Merigan TC: Rapid detection and quantitation of human cytomegalovirus in urine through DNA hybridization. *N Engl J Med* 1983;**308:**921.

Corey L: The diagnosis and treatment of genital herpes. *JAMA* 1982;**248:**1041.

Cremer KJ et al: Vaccinia virus recombinant expressing herpes simplex virus type 1 glycoprotein D prevents latent herpes in mice. *Science* 1985;**228:**737.

Gershon AA et al: Live attenuated varicella vaccine. Efficacy for children with leukemia in remission. *JAMA* 1984;**252:**355.

Handsfield HH et al: Cytomegalovirus infection in sex partners: Evidence for sexual transmission. *J Infect Dis* 1985;**151:**344.

Kieff E et al: The biology and chemistry of Epstein-Barr virus. *J Infect Dis* 1982;**146:**506.

Lung ML et al: Evidence that respiratory tract is major reservoir for Epstein-Barr virus. *Lancet* 1985;**1:**889.

Onorato IM et al: Epidemiology of cytomegaloviral infections: Recommendations for prevention and control. *Rev Infect Dis* 1985;**7:**479.

Pellett PE et al: Anatomy of the herpes simplex virus 1 strain F glycoprotein B gene: Primary sequence and predicted protein structure of the wild type and of monoclonal antibody-resistant mutants. *J Virol* 1985;**53:**243.

Plotkin SA, Huang ES: Cytomegalovirus vaccine virus (Towne strain) does not induce latency. *J Infect Dis* 1985;**152:**395.

Sköldenberg B et al: Acyclovir versus vidarabine in herpes simplex encephalitis: Randomised multicentre study in consecutive Swedish patients. *Lancet* 1984;**2:**707.

Spector SA et al: Detection of human cytomegalovirus in clinical specimens by DNA-DNA hybridization. *J Infect Dis* 1984;**150:**121.

Weller TH: Varicella and herpes zoster. *N Engl J Med* 1983;**309:**1362.

Whitley R et al: DNA restriction-enzyme analysis of herpes simplex virus isolates obtained from patients with encephalitis. *N Engl J Med* 1982;**307:**1060.

World Health Organization: Prevention and control of herpesvirus diseases. (2 parts.) *Bull WHO* 1985;**63:**185, 427.

Reoviruses, Rotaviruses, & Other Human Viral Infections

45

REOVIRUSES

Reoviruses are medium-sized viruses with a double-stranded, segmented RNA genome. The family includes the original reovirus genus plus the orbiviruses, the rotaviruses, and insect and plant viruses.

Properties of the Reoviruses

A. Structure: The virions measure 60–80 nm in diameter and possess 2 distinct capsid shells. The outer shell can be digested by chymotrypsin to reveal the core, which has 12 short spikes at the vertices of the icosahedron. The genome consists of double-stranded RNA in 10 discrete segments (total MW 15×10^6).

B. Reactions to Physical and Chemical Agents: Reoviruses are unusually stable to heat, acid pH, and many chemicals, but they are inactivated by 70% ethanol. Limited treatment with proteolytic enzymes increases infectivity.

C. Antigenic Properties: Three distinct but related types of reovirus are demonstrable by Nt and HI tests. All 3 types share a common CF antigen. Reoviruses contain a hemagglutinin for human O or bovine erythrocytes. The human red cell receptors for the reovirus hemagglutinin are not affected by the receptor-destroying enzyme of *Vibrio cholerae* but are destroyed by 1:1000 potassium periodate. The cell surface receptor for reovirus type 3 has recently been isolated and characterized as a glycoprotein with a molecular weight of 67,000; it may also function as the β-adrenergic receptor.

D. Growth of Virus: After adsorption, reovirus reaches the cytoplasm of the host cell. There, the outer shell of the virus is removed and a core-associated RNA transcriptase transcribes mRNA molecules from one strand of the genome RNA still contained in the core. The 10 functional mRNA molecules correspond in size to the 10 genome segments. The reovirus cores contain as structural proteins all enzymes necessary for transcribing, capping, and extruding the mRNAs from the core, leaving the double-stranded RNA genome segments inside.

Once extruded from the core, the 10 mRNA pieces are translated into 11 polypeptides, the primary gene products of reoviruses. It has been shown that the number of primary gene products exceeds the number of genome segments because segment S1 encodes 2 polypeptide species in overlapping reading frames. Further cleavage of these peptides occurs in the infected cell. Reovirus protein synthesis occurs in the cytoplasm, associated with structures of the cytoskeleton.

A virus-induced RNA-dependent RNA polymerase is responsible for synthesizing negative-sense strands from mRNA-like molecules to form the double-stranded genome segments. Apparently, replication to form progeny RNA thus occurs in partially completed core structures.

Reoviruses produce a distinctive cytopathic effect in monkey kidney cells. The nucleus is intact, but the cytoplasm contains inclusion bodies in which the virus particles are found. Some reoviruses grow in newborn mice or in monkeys and may produce central nervous system disease. The virus also multiplies in chick embryos.

Pathogenesis

Reovirus has become an important model system for the study of the pathogenesis of viral infection at the molecular level. Defined recombinants from 2 reoviruses with differing pathogenic phenotypes are used to infect mice. Segregation analysis is then used to associate particular features of pathogenesis with specific viral genes and gene products. The pathogenic properties of reoviruses are primarily determined by the protein species ($\sigma 1$, $\mu 1C$, or $\sigma 3$) found on the outer capsid of the virion. The viral hemagglutinin ($\sigma 1$) is responsible for the receptor interactions that control cell and tissue tropisms; $\sigma 1$ is also the major determinant of the host humoral and cellular immune responses. The $\mu 1C$ protein determines the ability of the virus to replicate at the primary site of infection, the gastrointestinal tract, and subsequently undergo systemic spread; it also modulates the immune response to $\sigma 1$. The $\sigma 3$ protein is responsible for inhibiting the synthesis of host cell RNA and protein; thus, it controls the ability of reoviruses to kill and lyse cells. The picture which is emerging is that virion surface proteins play a critical role in pathogenesis. Studies also indicate that virulence is multigenically determined and represents the interactions of multiple viral and cellular genes and gene products.

Epidemiology

The reoviruses are found in humans, chimpanzees,

monkeys, mice, and cattle. Antibodies are also present in other species.

All 3 types have been recovered from healthy children, from young children during outbreaks of minor febrile illness, from children with diarrhea or enteritis, and from chimpanzees with epidemic rhinitis.

Human volunteer studies have failed to demonstrate a clear cause-and-effect relationship of reoviruses to human illness. In inoculated volunteers, reovirus is recovered far more readily from feces than from the nose or throat. An association of reovirus type 3 with biliary atresia has been suggested.

ORBIVIRUSES

Orbiviruses are a genus within the reovirus family. They commonly infect insects, and many are transmitted by insects to vertebrates. None of these viruses cause serious clinical disease in humans, but they may cause mild fevers (see Colorado Tick Fever in Chapter 36). Serious animal pathogens include bluetongue virus of sheep and African horse sickness virus. Antibodies to orbiviruses are found in many vertebrates, including humans.

Orbiviruses have a double protein shell in which a fuzzy, indistinct layer covers the main capsid, which has 32 ring-shaped capsomeres arranged in icosahedral symmetry. This feature gives the group its name (Latin *orbis* "ring").

The genome consists of 10 segments of double-stranded RNA, with a total molecular weight of 12×10^6. The replicative cycle is similar to that of reoviruses. Orbiviruses are sensitive to low pH.

ROTAVIRUSES
(Infantile Gastroenteritis)

The rotaviruses are closely related to reoviruses. They are a major cause of diarrheal illness in human infants and young animals, including calves, mice, piglets, chickens, turkeys, and others. Among rotaviruses are the agents of human infantile diarrhea, Nebraska calf diarrhea, epizootic diarrhea of infant mice, and SA11 virus of monkeys.

Properties of the Viruses

A. Structure: The name rotavirus (Latin *rota* "wheel") is based on the electron microscopic appearance of the outer capsid margin as the rim of a wheel surrounding radiating spokes from the inner hublike core. The particles have a double-shelled capsid and are about 60–75 nm in diameter. Single-shelled viral particles that lack the outer capsid exhibit rough outer edges and are 50–60 nm in diameter. The inner core of the particles is 33–40 nm in diameter (Fig 45–1).

The virus particle contains 11 segments of double-stranded RNA (total MW 10×10^6). Virions contain an RNA-dependent RNA polymerase that can be activated by chelating agents and a poly A polymerase. The double-shelled particle is the infectious form of the virus. Infectivity of the virions is enhanced by

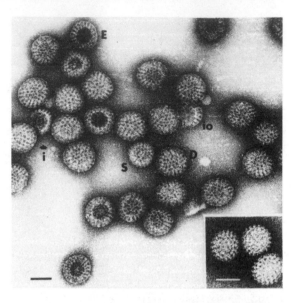

Figure 45–1. Electron micrograph of a negatively stained preparation of human rotavirus. D = double-shelled particles; S = single-shelled particles; E = empty capsids; i = fragment of inner shell; io = fragments of a combination of inner and outer shell. Inset: single-shelled particles obtained by treatment of the virus preparation with sodium dodecyl sulfate, 100 μg/mL, immediately prior to processing for electron microscopy. Bars = 50 nm. (Esparza and Gil.)

treatment with proteolytic enzymes, eg, trypsin, and this is used in virus isolation in cell culture.

B. Animal Susceptibility and Pathogenesis: Cross-species infections can occur in experimental inoculations, but it is not clear if they occur in nature. In experimental studies, human rotavirus can induce diarrheal illness in newborn colostrum-deprived animals (eg, piglets, calves). Homologous infections may have a wider age range. Swine rotavirus infects both newborn and weanling piglets. Newborns often exhibit subclinical infection due perhaps to the presence of maternal antibody, while overt disease is more common in weanling animals.

Rotaviruses infect cells in the villi of the small intestine. They multiply in the cytoplasm of these enterocytes and damage their transport mechanisms. Damaged cells may slough into the lumen of the intestine and release large quantities of virus, which appear in the stool. The diarrhea caused by rotaviruses may be due to impaired sodium and glucose absorption as the damaged cells on villi are replaced by nonabsorbing immature crypt cells.

C. Virus Replication: Optimal growth requires treatment with proteolytic enzymes (trypsin, pancreatin) and sometimes rolling of the infected cultures. Such cultivated viruses now serve as antigens for serologic testing.

In vitro, rotavirus growth is maximal at 18–20 hours. Viral antigens are detected within 4–8 hours in the cytoplasm of infected cells stained by the immunofluorescence technique, where they appear initially as distinct perinuclear granules. Later, antigen is present throughout the cytoplasm. Different types of cell culture manifest great differences in susceptibility to rotavirus infection.

D. Antigenic Properties: The rotaviruses possess common antigens located on the inner shell. These can be detected by immunofluorescence, immune electron microscopy, and many other methods. Type-specific antigens are located on the outer capsid layers. These type-specific antigens differentiate among rotaviruses from different species and are demonstrable by Nt tests. At least 4 serotypes have been identified among human rotaviruses, but more may exist. Some animal and human rotaviruses share serotype specificity. Rotaviruses lacking the common antigens described above have been detected in diarrheic stools of calves, chickens, humans, and piglets.

The viruses usually associated with human gastroenteritis are classified as group A rotaviruses, but antigenically and genomically distinct rotaviruses have also caused diarrheal outbreaks.

Molecular epidemiologic studies have analyzed the number of human strains based on differences in the migration of the 11 genome segments following electrophoresis of the RNA in polyacrylamide gels. Extensive genome heterogeneity has been demonstrated in numerous studies. These differences in electropherotypes reflect changes in serotypes. Although electropherotyping cannot predict serotype, it can be a useful epidemiologic tool to monitor virus transmission. The gene-coding assignments responsible for the antigenic specificities of rotavirus proteins are shown in Fig 45–2.

Clinical Findings & Laboratory Diagnosis

Rotaviruses cause the major portion of diarrheal illness in infants and children but not in adults. Typical symptoms include diarrhea, fever, abdominal pain, and vomiting, leading to dehydration.

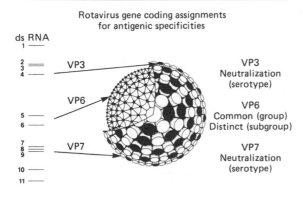

Figure 45–2. Gene-coding assignments for antigenic specificities of rotavirus proteins. (Reproduced, with permission, from Kapikian AZ et al: *J Infect Dis* 1986; 153:815.)

Adult contacts may be infected, as evidenced by seroconversion, but they rarely exhibit symptoms, and virus is infrequently detected in their stools. However, epidemics of severe disease have occurred in adults.

In infants and children, severe loss of electrolytes and fluids may be fatal unless treated. Patients with milder cases have symptoms for 3–5 days, then recover completely. Asymptomatic infections, with seroconversion, occur.

Laboratory diagnosis rests on demonstration of virus in stool collected early in the illness and on a rise in antibody titer. Virus in stool is demonstrated by immune electron microscopy, immunodiffusion, and other methods. Many serologic tests can be used to detect an antibody titer rise, particularly CF and ELISA.

Epidemiology & Immunity

Rotaviruses are the single most important worldwide cause of gastroenteritis in children. Typically, 50–60% of cases of acute gastroenteritis of hospitalized children throughout the world are caused by rotaviruses. Rotavirus infections usually predominate during the winter season, with an incubation period of 2–4 days. Symptomatic infections are most common in children between ages 6 months and 12 years, and transmission appears to be by the fecal-oral route. Nosocomial infections are frequent.

Rotaviruses are ubiquitous. By age 6, 60–90% of children have serum antibodies to one or more types. Both humans and animals can become infected even in the presence of antibodies. Local immune factors, such as secretory IgA or interferon, may be important in protection against rotavirus infection. Alternatively, reinfection in the presence of circulating antibody could reflect the presence of multiple serotypes of virus. Asymptomatic infections are common in infants before age 6 months, the time during which protective maternal antibody acquired passively by newborns should be present. Such neonatal infection does not prevent reinfection, but it may protect against the development of severe disease during reinfection. Rotavirus antibody has been detected in colostrum for up to 9 months postpartum.

Treatment & Control

Treatment of gastroenteritis is supportive, to correct the loss of water and electrolytes that may lead to dehydration, acidosis, shock, and death. Management consists of replacement of fluids and restoration of electrolyte balance either intravenously or orally, as feasible.

In view of the fecal-oral route of transmission, waste-water treatment and sanitation are significant control measures.

A live bovine rotavirus has been reported to function as a vaccine. Oral administration has protected children from developing gastroenteritis when naturally exposed to rotaviruses in the community. Other approaches toward a vaccine include the use of attenuated and cold-adapted human rotavirus mutants and of interspecies reassortant rotaviruses. Another approach is the feeding of bovine milk to young children. Raw and pasteurized milk (but not commercially available infant formulas) contains Nt antibodies against rotaviruses because of the widespread distribution of rotavirus among cows.

EPIDEMIC GASTROENTERITIS VIRUS
(Norwalk Virus)

Epidemic nonbacterial gastroenteritis is characterized by (1) the absence of bacterial pathogens; (2) gastroenteritis with rapid onset and recovery and relatively mild systemic signs; and (3) an epidemiologic pattern of a highly communicable disease that spreads rapidly with no particular predilection in terms of age or geography. Although various terms have been used in reports of different outbreaks (eg, epidemic viral gastroenteritis, viral diarrhea, winter vomiting disease, epidemic diarrhea and vomiting) in which a particular clinical feature predominated, studies of outbreaks and of the illness transmitted to volunteers suggest that distinct syndromes may be different manifestations of infection by the same agent.

Virus particles with a diameter of 27 nm have been demonstrated by immune electron microscopy (see Chapter 35) in stools from adults with acute gastroenteritis in a Norwalk, Ohio, outbreak and other outbreaks. There appear to be at least 3 serotypes.

The Norwalk agent has not been grown in tissue culture. However, volunteer experiments have clearly shown that the appearance of the virus coincides with the clinical illness. Antibody develops during the illness and is protective against reinfection with that agent. Experimental infection of chimpanzees results in infection and seroconversion of animals in the absence of clinical illness.

Viral gastroenteritis has an incubation period of 16–48 hours. Onset is rapid, and the clinical course lasts 24–48 hours; symptoms include diarrhea, nausea, vomiting, low-grade fever, abdominal cramps, headache, and malaise. Hospitalization is rarely required. No sequelae have been reported.

Immune electron microscopy was required initially for detection of virus and antibody. A radioimmunoassay blocking test and an immune adherence method can more readily detect antibody to Norwalk type viruses. Whereas rotavirus antibody develops early in childhood, Norwalk virus antibody is acquired later in life; by the fifth decade, 50% of adults have such antibody.

Treatment is symptomatic. Because of the infectious nature of the stools, care should be taken in their disposal.

WARTS
(Verrucae, Human Papovavirus)

Human wart virus (human papilloma virus) has been classified in the papovavirus group (*pa*pilloma, *polyoma*, *va*cuolating viruses). Papillomaviruses (diameter 55 nm) include viruses of rabbits, cattle, and humans; polyomaviruses (diameter 45 nm) include polyomaviruses of mice, vacuolating viruses of rabbits and monkeys (SV40), and a virus associated with progressive multifocal leukoencephalopathy (PML) of humans. Papovaviruses produce tumors in their natural host or in another species (see Chapter 46).

Common skin warts (verrucae) can be spread by autoinoculation through scratching, or by direct or indirect contact. A filtrable agent recovered from warts has produced warts in volunteers. Virus particles with a diameter of 55 nm can be obtained from those warts that have intranuclear inclusions in their rete cells. Thin sections of such papillomas have revealed crystalline masses within the nucleus. By electron microscopic counting procedures, warts are seen to contain their highest concentration of virus particles when they are about 6 months old; 6–12 months is also the period of peak antibody titers in the patient.

The nuclei of normal skin cells are uniform in size, and the DNA content shows little variation from cell to cell. In contrast, wart-infected skin exhibits large and variable nuclear sizes and also much higher and more variable DNA values that cannot be explained by increased polyploidy or by increased cell division.

Patients who carry warts possess specific antibodies against this human papovavirus. By immunodiffusion, IgM and IgG antibodies can be measured; by CF, IgG antibodies only. The outlook for healing and disappearance of warts is best if high-titer IgG antibodies can be measured by CF. Antibodies are detectable also in some persons with no history of warts.

Patients with transplanted kidneys who are receiving immunosuppressive drugs experience an increased incidence of warts and of active infections with herpesviruses (see Chapter 44).

Characteristics of papillomaviruses have been investigated by restriction enzyme mapping, nucleic acid hybridization, and polypeptide patterns. Serologic tests are limited, since virus has not been grown in cell culture.

Differences in their DNA distinguish more than 34 papillomavirus types. Types 16 and 18, in particular, are associated with cervical, vulvar, and penile cancer.

Hand warts and plantar warts appear to be antigenically identical. Genital and perianal warts (condylomata acuminata) are caused by a similar but not identical agent. Laryngeal papillomas are caused by a similar and perhaps identical virus, type 11, suggesting that infants may be infected by the genital wart virus of their mothers. While laryngeal papillomas are rare, the growths may obstruct the larynx and have to be removed repeatedly by surgical means. Viral DNA can be detected in normal tissues of the larynx of patients in remission. This latent infection may serve as a source of new lesions. Interferon has been used to treat laryngeal papillomas with some success.

Papovaviruses have also been associated with progressive multifocal leukoencephalopathy (PML).

Large numbers of virus particles can be seen under the electron microscope in infected brain cells, and a number of isolations of a human papovavirus resembling SV40 have been made in cell cultures (see Slow Virus Diseases in Chapter 39). The virus can be present in the urine of normal pregnant women and of renal allograft recipients.

EXANTHEM SUBITUM
(Roseola Infantum)

Exanthem subitum is a mild disease occurring mainly in infants between 6 months and 3 years of age. At times it is confused with rubella. The causative agent is found in the serum and throat washings during the febrile period. The febrile disease (but without rash) can be transmitted to monkeys with bacteria-free serum.

The incubation period is about 10–14 days. The onset is abrupt; the temperature may rise to 40–41 °C and last 5 days. There is usually lymphadenopathy. Seizures are frequent. The rubelliform rash characteristically follows the disappearance of fever by a few hours and affects most of the body but not the face. Leukopenia is present with a relative lymphocytosis. All patients recover promptly without any specific therapy.

The disease may occur in small outbreaks, but often only single cases occur in families.

PARVOVIRUS DISEASES
(Bone Marrow Aplasia, Erythema Infectiosum)

Human parvovirus (HPV), which is sometimes present in symptom-free blood donors, may cause febrile illness in blood recipients. In addition, it may cause aplastic crisis in patients with hemolytic anemias.

The virus is widespread. Antibody was found in 97% of children and young adults with hemophilia treated with clotting factor concentrates but in only 36% of those who had received multiple blood transfusions and in 20% of age-matched controls. HPV infection is common in childhood; in one study, antibody to HPV most often developed between the ages of 5 and 10 years, and 60% of an adult blood donor population was seropositive.

When HPV infection occurs in either a child or an adult with chronic hemolytic anemia, an aplastic crisis may result from the temporary arrest of erythropoiesis. In bone marrow culture, the virus infects and lyses erythroid progenitor cells. In the body, HPV lowers the production of erythrocytes, causing a reduction in the hemoglobin level of the peripheral blood. The temporary arrest of production of red blood cells becomes apparent only in patients with chronic hemolytic anemia, because of the short life span of their erythrocytes; a 7-day interruption in erythropoiesis would not be expected to cause a detectable anemia in a normal person.

HPV infection in normal persons causes erythema infectiosum, or fifth disease. This erythematous illness is most common in children of early school age and occasionally affects adults. Mild constitutional symptoms may accompany the rash, and joint involvement is often found in adult cases. Both sporadic cases and epidemics have been described.

Infection seems to be transmitted via the respiratory tract. Patients with an aplastic crisis often report a recent respiratory tract illness. Involvement of the respiratory tract is the most commonly reported symptom associated with epidemic erythema infectiosum.

After intranasal inoculation, systemic HPV infection developed in 4 of 5 seronegative volunteers, whereas 3 volunteers who had detectable IgG antibody to HPV at the time of inoculation did not become infected. Viremia occurred 1 week after inoculation, persisted for about 5 days, and reached high titers comparable to those observed in natural infections in both blood donors and persons with an aplastic crisis. During the period of viremia, virus was detected in nasal washes and gargle specimens from 3 of the 4 infected volunteers, identifying the upper respiratory tract—most probably the pharynx—as the site of viral shedding. The immune response of volunteers exhibiting such viremia was characteristic of primary systemic viral infection. In the volunteers who lacked demonstrable antibody to HPV at inoculation, specific antibody (in the form of IgM-HPV immune complexes) was first detected during the latter days of viremia. After the clearance of viremia, only IgM antibody to HPV was detectable for a period of about 1 week before IgG antibody to HPV developed in the third week after inoculation.

Infected volunteers became clinically ill at 2 quite distinct times after inoculation. The first phase of illness occurred at the end of the first week, and symptoms included fever, malaise, myalgia, chills, and itching. Fever and at least one of the other symptoms occurred in all infected volunteers. The first episode of illness coincided in time with viremia and, more particularly, with the detection of circulating IgM-HPV immune complexes. After an incubation period of 17 days, a second phase of illness began. A fine, pink, maculopapular rash appeared on the limbs or trunk, or both; and joint symptoms and signs began on the second day of the rash. The illness was short-lived, with the rash fading after 2 or 3 days, although the joint symptoms persisted for 1 or 2 days longer. The rash was typical of adult cases of epidemic erythema infectiosum, and the occurrence of joint symptoms was compatible with the high incidence of this complication in adult cases.

There was a period of at least 1 week during which reticulocytes were not detected; this demonstrates that erythropoiesis in normal individuals is susceptible to interruption by HPV infection. This interruption occurred at the end of the viremic phase and was associated with a slight but significant fall in hemoglobin levels.

GUILLAIN-BARRÉ SYNDROME
(Inflammatory Polyradiculopathy)

This is an inflammatory and demyelinating disorder of the nervous system. It is a rare sequela to acute viral infections, especially measles, rubella, varicella-zoster, or mumps. It can also follow vaccination, especially with vaccinia virus or some types of influenza vaccine. In 1976, swine influenza vaccine inoculation of humans was followed by the Guillain-Barré syndrome 5 times more often than occurred in matched individuals who had not been given this vaccine. Very rarely, this syndrome has followed infections by enteroviruses and cytomegalovirus.

The symptoms may range from minor neuropathy with paresthesias or weakness to rapidly progressive ascending paralysis and occasional death. Treatment is symptomatic.

DIABETES MELLITUS

Viruses have been suspected as one of the causes of diabetes mellitus in humans. There have been many reports showing a temporal relationship between onset of various virus infections and the onset of diabetes. Patients with insulin-dependent type 1 diabetes had significantly higher titers or greater prevalence of Nt antibodies against coxsackieviruses B1, B4, or B5 than did nondiabetic controls. Furthermore, encephalomyocarditis virus of mice, a member of the same family as the coxsackieviruses, can produce a disease resembling diabetes in mice; development of the disease depends also upon the genetic constitution of both virus and host. Coxsackie B4 virus has been isolated from a diabetic child. This virus produced diabetes when injected into mice and was recovered from the mice, further substantiating the hypothesis that a viral agent may cause diabetes. The severity of the murine disease is directly related to the number of B cells destroyed by the infection, and in some cases, several insults are required to produce sufficient B cell damage to result in clinically apparent diabetes. Variants of coxsackie B viruses and reoviruses have also been shown to damage B cells and produce diabetes.

There is a different mechanism by which viruses might cause non-insulin-dependent type 2 diabetes. Lymphocytic choriomeningitis (LCM) virus produces a persistent infection of B cells. The infected cells have normal morphology, their insulin content remains within the normal range, and there is no inflammation. Nonetheless, glucose levels are elevated and glucose tolerance tests show marked impairment. Thus, persistent viral infections might sometimes be involved in type 2 diabetes.

The likelihood of developing diabetes in the first several decades of life is 10–20% in patients with congenital rubella, compared to 0.1–0.2% in a control population.

VIRAL ARTHRITIS

A number of viruses, including the agents that cause some of the common childhood diseases, may cause arthritis. Virus-induced arthritis usually resolves within weeks and does not cause permanent joint damage. However, for proper therapy, it is important to differentiate viral arthritis from the debilitating rheumatologic disease. The following viruses have been associated with the arthritic syndrome: hepatitis B, rubella (including the vaccine virus), mumps, varicella, adenovirus, enterovirus, parvovirus, and some of the arboviruses and respiratory viruses.

REFERENCES

Anderson MJ et al: An outbreak of erythema infectiosum associated with human parvovirus infection. *J Hyg* 1984;**93**:85.

Anderson MJ et al: Experimental parvoviral infection in humans. *J Infect D* is 1985;**152**:257.

Baron RC et al: Serological responses among teenagers after natural exposure to Norwalk virus. *J Infect Dis* 1984;**150**:531.

Bishop RF et al: Clinical immunity after neonatal rotavirus infection: A prospective longitudinal study in young children. *N Engl J Med* 1983;**309**:72.

Cukor G, Blacklow NR: Human viral gastroenteritis. *Microbiol Rev* 1984;**48**:157.

Dimitrov DH, Graham DY, Estes MK: Detection of rotaviruses by nucleic acid hybridization with cloned DNA of simian rotavirus SA11 genes. *J Infect Dis* 1985;**152**:293.

Fields BN, Green MI: Genetic and molecular mechanisms of viral pathogenesis: Implications for prevention and treatment. *Nature* 1982;**300**:12.

Midthun K et al: Reassortant rotaviruses as potential live rotavirus vaccine candidates. *J Virol* 1985;**53**:949.

Nakata S et al: Humoral immunity in infants with gastroenteritis caused by human calicivirus. *J Infect Dis* 1985;**152**:274.

Plummer FA et al: An erythema infectiosum-like illness caused by human parvovirus infection. *N Engl J Med* 1985;**313**:74.

Rayfield EJ, Mento SJ: Viruses may be etiologic agents for non-insulin-dependent (type II) diabetes. *Rev Infect Dis* 1983;**5**:341.

Stals F, Walther FJ, Bruggeman CA: Faecal and pharyngeal shedding of rotavirus and rotavirus IgA in children with diarrhoea. *J Med Virol* 1984;**14**:333.

Steinberg BM et al: Laryngeal papillomavirus infection during clinical remission. *N Engl J Med* 1983;**308**:1261.

Yolken RH et al: Antibody to human rotavirus in cow's milk. *N Engl J Med* 1985;**312**:605.

Yoon J-W et al: Virus-induced diabetes mellitus: Isolation of a virus from the pancreas of a child with diabetic ketoacidosis. *N Engl J Med* 1979;**300**:1173.

Tumor Viruses & Oncogenes

46

The role that viruses play in causing human cancer remains ambiguous, but recent studies have greatly strengthened the likelihood of their involvement. The viruses that have been strongly associated epidemiologically with human cancers are listed in Table 46–1. Many viruses can cause tumors in animals, either as a consequence of natural infection or after experimental inoculation (discussed below), and it is assumed that similar virus-neoplasm relationships may occur in humans.

Animal viruses are being studied intensively to learn how a limited amount of genetic information (one or a few virus genes) can so profoundly alter the growth behavior of cells, ultimately converting a normal cell into a neoplastic one. Such studies will inevitably reveal insights into growth regulation in normal cells as well. By definition, tumor viruses are agents that can produce tumors when they infect appropriate animals. However, most studies on tumor viruses are now done on cultured animal cells rather than on intact animals. In vitro studies are preferred, because it is possible to analyze events at cellular and subcellular levels. In such cultured cells, tumor viruses can cause "transformation."

It was studies with RNA tumor viruses that uncovered the involvement of cellular oncogenes in neoplasia. Those discoveries revolutionized thinking in the 1980s about the molecular mechanisms of carcinogenesis.

GENERAL FEATURES OF CELL TRANSFORMATION BY TUMOR VIRUSES

What Is Transformation?

Transformation is a stable, heritable change in the growth control of cells in culture. No set of characteristics invariably distinguishes transformed cells from their normal counterparts. In practice, transformation is recognized by the cells' permanent acquisition of some growth property not exhibited by the parental cell type. The most prominent changes associated with transformed cells can be divided into 4 general categories:

A. Alterations in Cell Growth Patterns: Growth to higher cell density, increased rate of growth, decreased requirement for serum growth factors, decreased cell adhesion to a substrate, enhanced ability to grow in semisolid medium (anchorage independence), and loss of "contact inhibition." The latter property means that transformed cells are no longer inhibited by contact with other cells, as normal cells are, but tend to pile up to form a "focus." Induction of foci can provide the basis for a quantitative assay for certain tumor viruses.

B. Alterations in Cell Surface: Increased rate of transport of cell nutrients, increased secretion of proteases or protease activators, increased agglutinability by plant lectins, and changes in composition of glycoproteins and glycolipids, sometimes including the presence of virus-coded proteins.

C. Alterations in Intracellular Components and Biochemical Processes: Increased metabolic rate; increased glycolysis; altered levels of cyclic nucleotides; activation or repression of certain cellular genes; presence of viral DNA, mRNA, and viral coded proteins; and changes in cell cytoskeleton, often resulting in more rounded cell shape.

D. Tumorigenicity: Production of tumors when transformed cells are injected into appropriate test animals, especially immunologically deficient animals. Many transformed cells exhibit changes in growth behavior in vitro but are not transplantable in vivo. No in vitro growth characteristic can successfully predict tumorigenicity.

Types of Tumor Viruses

Like other viruses, tumor viruses are classified among different virus families according to the nucleic acid of their genome and the biophysical characteristics of their virions. DNA tumor viruses are classified

Table 46–1. Association of viruses with human cancers.

Virus Family	Virus Genus	Human Cancer
Herpesviridae	EB herpesvirus	Nasopharyngeal carcinoma African Burkitt's lymphoma B-cell lymphoma
	Herpes type 2 virus	Cervical carcinoma
Papovaviridae	Papillomavirus	Urogenital tumors (cervical, vulvar, penile cancers) Squamous cell carcinomas?
Hepadnaviridae	Hepatitis B virus	Primary hepatocellular carcinoma
Retroviridae	HTL virus	Adult T-cell leukemia

into the papova-, adeno-, herpes-, hepadna-, and pox-virus groups.

RNA tumor viruses were once called oncor-naviruses but now are designated as retroviruses. Retroviruses are unique in that they carry an RNA-directed polymerase (reverse transcriptase) that constructs a DNA copy of the RNA genome of the virus. The DNA copy becomes integrated into the DNA of the infected host cell, and it is from this integrated DNA copy (provirus) that all proteins of the virus are translated. Among widely studied RNA tumor viruses are those causing avian sarcomas, avian leukoses, mouse leukemias, mouse sarcomas, mouse mammary tumors, feline leukemias, and human T-cell leukemia.

Interactions of Tumor Viruses With Host Cells

Host cells are either permissive or nonpermissive for replication of a given virus. Permissive cells support virus growth, while nonpermissive cells do not. In general, permissive cells are not transformed by the virus, but nonpermissive cells may be transformed. Cells that are permissive for one virus may be nonpermissive for another.

DNA tumor viruses usually replicate in certain cells of their natural host (ie, homologous cells) but rarely, if ever, produce tumors in those hosts. Conversely, DNA tumor viruses are unable to replicate in heterologous host cells but can, on occasion, transform them. An example is simian virus SV40, a prototype DNA tumor virus that naturally infects rhesus monkeys. The virus replicates in monkey kidney cells but does not transform them. SV40 cannot replicate in cells of rodent origin (ie, heterologous cells) but is able to transform them at low efficiency. These 2 types of virus-host interaction are illustrated in Fig 46-1.

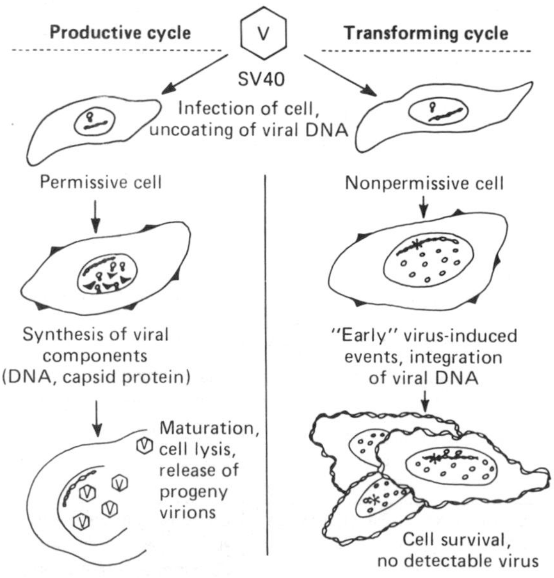

In contrast, RNA tumor viruses may cause cancers in their natural hosts. They can both replicate in and transform homologous cells. Certain viruses may be able to transform heterologous cells as well, usually in the absence of virus replication. Thus, RNA tumor viruses differ from DNA tumor viruses in that the former can transform both permissive and nonpermissive cells. A characteristic property of RNA tumor viruses is that they are not lethal for the cells in which they replicate (Fig 46-2). Cells infected with leukemia viruses exhibit no morphologic or cytopathic changes and continue to grow normally, while cells infected with sarcoma viruses undergo morphologic changes and grow like tumor cells.

Not all cells from the natural host species are susceptible to virus infection or transformation or both. Most tumor viruses exhibit marked tissue specificity, a property that probably reflects the variable presence of surface receptors for the virus or intracellular factors necessary for viral gene expression.

Integration of Tumor Virus Nucleic Acid Into a Host Cell

The stable genetic change from a normal to a neoplastic cell is attributed to the integration of certain viral genes into the host cell genome. This may be similar to the integration of a temperate bacteriophage into the bacterial genome in lysogeny (see Chapter 9). However, a repressor is required for the maintenance of lysogeny, and no analogous repressor has yet been found in transformed mammalian cells.

With DNA tumor viruses, a portion of the DNA of the viral genome becomes integrated into the host cell chromosome (Fig 46-3). With RNA tumor viruses, viral RNA serves as a template for the synthesis of viral DNA (through the agency of a virus-coded reverse transcriptase), and that DNA copy of the viral RNA is integrated into the host cell DNA (Fig 46-3). Gener-

Figure 46–1. Schematic comparison of 2 types of interaction between a DNA tumor virus and a host cell (productive and transforming cycles). (Courtesy of Benyesh-Melnick and Butel.)

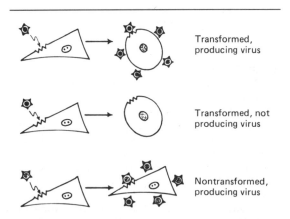

Figure 46–2. Schematic representation of the responses of fibroblasts to infection by retroviruses. (Courtesy of Weiss.)

DNA tumor virus

RNA tumor virus

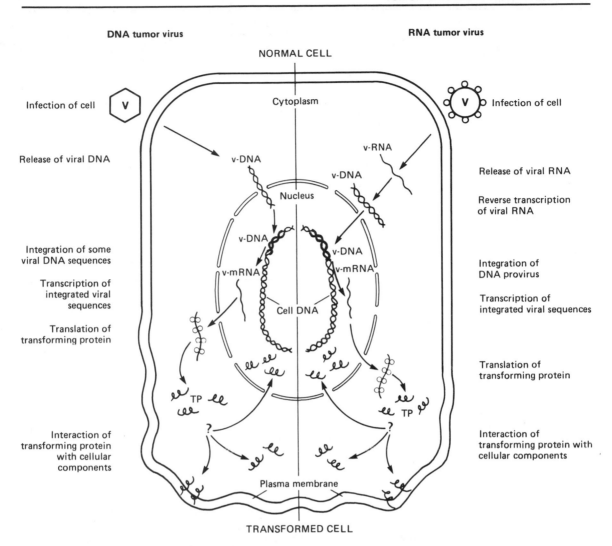

Figure 46–3. Molecular mechanism of cell transformation by tumor viruses carrying a transforming gene. Transformation by a DNA tumor virus is summarized on the left and transformation by an RNA tumor virus on the right. Viral nucleic acid (v-DNA, v-RNA) is released after infection of a normal cell by a virus (V) and, in the case of RNA tumor viruses, a DNA copy is reverse transcribed from the viral genomic RNA. Viral DNA is then integrated into a host cell chromosome. Messenger RNA (v-mRNA) is transcribed from the integrated viral sequences, transported to the cytoplasm, and translated on polyribosomes. The transforming protein (TP) product is then transported to appropriate locations within the cell to interact with cellular components, eg, the plasma membrane, the cytoplasm, the nucleus, or all of these. Some virus-specific transforming proteins appear to localize in only one cellular compartment, whereas others are found in more than one location. Cell regulatory processes are altered in some way by the transforming protein with the result that the cell is transformed. As described in the text, known viral transforming proteins differ structurally and functionally. The transforming genes carried by RNA tumor viruses are derived from cellular genes; no known cellular homologs exist for the DNA tumor virus transforming genes.

ally, very few copies (perhaps one) of the viral genome are integrated in a transformed cell.

Mechanisms of Cell Transformation by Viruses

Tumor viruses mediate changes in cell behavior by means of a limited amount of genetic information. There are 2 general patterns by which this is accomplished: (1) the tumor virus introduces a new "transforming gene" into the cell (Fig 46–3), and (2)

the virus induces the expression of a preexisting cellular gene. The result in either case is that the cell loses control of normal regulation of growth processes.

A. DNA Tumor Viruses: With DNA tumor viruses, eg, SV40, the viral genome contains "early" and "late" regions (Fig 46–4). The late region consists of genes that code for the synthesis of coat proteins; they are not expressed in transformed cells. The early region is expressed soon after infection of cells; it contains genes that code for early proteins, eg, the SV40

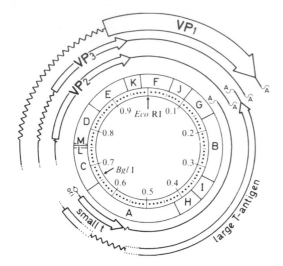

Figure 46–4. Physical map of SV40 DNA indicating localization of the main biologic functions. The single cleavage site of the restriction enzyme *Eco*RI is used as a reference point for the physical map (inner circle). The origin of DNA replication (ori) is at or close to 0.663; this site corresponds to a large palindromic sequence, part of which represents the recognition sequence of *Bgl*I. The 5 virus-coded proteins are indicated by blocked arrows; note that the T antigen is coded by 2 noncontiguous segments on the genome. Untranslated parts of the mRNA are shown as solid lines; dots indicate uncertainty as to the exact position of the 5′ end. Zigzag lines are used for the segments that are spliced out. A wavy line with an A illustrates the 3′ terminal poly(A) tail. (Courtesy of Fiers W et al: *Nature* 1978;**273**:113.)

tumor (T) antigen, which are necessary for the replication of viral DNA in permissive cells and for the transformation of nonpermissive cells. The transforming protein must be continuously synthesized for the cells to stay transformed. Even with the larger DNA viruses such as adenoviruses, only one or 2 genes are involved in cell transformation.

B. RNA Tumor Viruses: RNA tumor viruses encode very few genes, only one of which mediates transformation. The transforming gene is not required for replication of these viruses, in contrast to the situation with DNA tumor viruses. It is now established that the transforming genes carried by various RNA tumor viruses (known as *onc* genes) represent cellular genes that have been appropriated by those viruses at some time in the distant past and incorporated into their genomes (Fig 46–5). The avian sarcoma virus is one of the most intensively studied agents; its transforming gene is designated *src*. The *src* gene product is a phosphoprotein that localizes primarily in plasma membranes of transformed cells, functions as a protein kinase, and phosphorylates proteins at tyrosine residues. This and other cellular oncogenes, as well as their normal cell proto-oncogene predecessors, are described below.

The mechanism of transformation by the leukemia

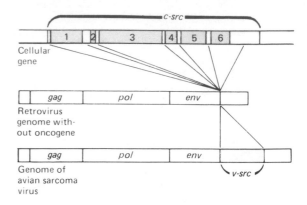

Figure 46–5. Split cellular gene c-*src* *(top)* consists of exons (light gray) and introns (dark gray). The cellular gene was somehow picked up by a preexisting retrovirus; the introns were eliminated and the exons, spliced together, were inserted into the viral genome *(middle)* to complete the avian sarcoma virus genome *(bottom)*. In addition to *src*, the genes are *gag* (which encodes the protein of the viral capsid), *pol* (which encodes reverse transcriptase), and *env* (which encodes glycoprotein spikes of the viral envelope). Other retrovirus oncogenes are thought to have similar origins but represent different cellular genes. (After Bishop JM: *Sci Am* [March] 1982;**246**:80.)

viruses is more indirect. They do not carry an *onc* gene in their genome. The promoter for viral transcription is contained in a sequence designated the long terminal repeat (LTR). Insertion of the viral promoter adjacent to a cellular oncogene (see p 523) may result in enhanced expression of that gene and, subsequently, neoplasia. Fig 46–6 shows a model of such "promoter-insertion oncogenesis." In other instances, expression of the cellular gene may be increased

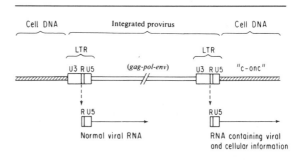

Figure 46–6. Structure and transcriptional products of an integrated leukemia virus provirus. The integrated provirus is flanked by sequences termed long terminal repeats (LTRs). Synthesis of normal viral RNA (genomic RNA and mRNAs) initiates within the left LTR. Initiation within the right LTR would generate a molecule containing viral 5′ sequences plus cellular information encoded in the adjacent cellular DNA. If, as shown, the provirus integrated upstream from a potentially oncogenic cellular gene (designated c-*onc*), initiation within the right LTR could cause elevated expression of the c-*onc* gene. (Courtesy of Hayward et al: *Nature* 1981;**290**:475.)

through the action of nearby viral "enhancer" sequences.

In summary, neoplastic transformation by retroviruses is the result of a cellular gene that is normally expressed at low, carefully regulated levels becoming activated and expressed constitutively. In the case of the acute transforming viruses, a cellular gene has been inserted by recombination into the viral genome and is expressed as a viral gene under the control of the viral promoter. In the case of the leukemia viruses, the viral promoter or enhancer element is inserted adjacent to or near the cellular gene in the cellular chromosome.

Recovery of Viral Genes & Transforming Genes From Transformed Cells That Do Not Produce Virus

A. Rescue of Infectious Virus: Transformed cells do not always produce virus. Cells transformed by DNA tumor viruses never do, and those transformed by RNA tumor viruses may not. It is sometimes desirable to recover the transforming virus from such nonproducer tumor cells. Three general approaches have been used to "rescue" infectious virus. The methods apply to both DNA and RNA tumor virus systems, and their effectiveness depends on the characteristics of the particular tumor cell line. Obviously, infectious virus can be recovered only if a complete viral genome has been integrated into the DNA of the tumor cell. Recombinant DNA techniques can be used to recover viral specific sequences regardless of whether a complete genome is present.

1. Addition of a helper virus—A permissive cell may be transformed by a virus that is defective in a necessary replicative function. When such a cell is superinfected with a "helper" virus that expresses normal replicative functions, the superinfecting virus "helps" the defective transforming virus by providing the missing function, and both types of viruses are produced by the cell (Fig 46–7).

2. Chemical induction—A variety of chemicals (eg, inhibitors of nucleic acid and protein synthesis) can affect a host cell genome carrying integrated viral genes. As a result of such chemical treatment, gene expression is activated and tumor virus may be produced. This can occur when chemical treatment is applied to nonpermissive cells that have been transformed by tumor viruses. Such treatment can also prompt virus expression from apparently normal cells that carry endogenous RNA tumor viruses in their genomes (see below).

3. Cell fusion—A transformed nonpermissive cell can be fused with an uninfected permissive cell to form a heterokaryon (ie, a cell with 2 different nuclei). An inactivated paramyxovirus or a chemical may be employed to fuse the cell membranes. The permissive cell components provide missing factors needed for virus replication, and the heterokaryon will produce infectious tumor virus.

B. Rescue of Transforming Activity: Cellular DNA can be extracted from tumor cells and inoculated

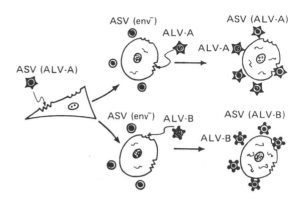

Figure 46–7. Diagram showing the rescue of the envelope-defective ASV(env⁻) strain by helper leukemia viruses (ALV) of different subgroups (A and B). (After Weiss.)

onto a normal recipient cell line in the presence of a chemical facilitator that promotes ingestion of the DNA. This technique is called transfection. The transfected cells are observed for morphologic changes, eg, focus formation, as evidence of transforming activity expressed by the applied tumor cell DNA. The cellular sequences carrying the transforming activity can then be recovered using molecular cloning techniques. This approach has identified additional cellular oncogenes not carried by any known RNA tumor viruses (Table 46–2).

CELLULAR ONCOGENES

Oncogene is the general term given to genes that cause cancer. "Friendly" versions of these transforming genes are present in normal cells and have been designated proto-oncogenes.

The discovery of cellular oncogenes came from studies with acutely transforming retroviruses. Surprisingly, it was found that normal cells contained nearly exact (but not identical) copies of various retrovirus transforming genes; cellular sequences had been picked up and incorporated into the retrovirus genomes. Transduction of the cellular genes was probably an accident, reflecting the way the retroviruses replicate. The presence of the cellular sequences is of no benefit to the virus, and each particular "hybrid" virus probably would have perished with the death of the host animal had not an industrious tumor virologist isolated it from the tumor. About 20 different cellular oncogenes have been identified by virtue of their presence in retrovirus isolates. There are probably other potential cellular oncogenes that have not been segregated into retrovirus vectors. Gene transfer techniques (see above) have been successful in recovering a few novel oncogenes from tumors of nonviral origin (Table 46–2).

Cellular proto-oncogenes represent highly conserved sequences found in cells of species ranging from fruit flies to humans. This suggests that their

Table 46–2. Representative cellular oncogenes.

General Class	Name of Oncogene	Origin		Protein Product*	
		Prototype Retrovirus	Host Species	Property	Subcellular Location
Tyrosine protein kinases	src	Rous sarcoma virus	Chicken	Tyrosine kinase	PM
	abl	Abelson murine leukemia virus	Mouse		PM, Cyt
	fes†	ST feline sarcoma virus	Cat		
	fps†	Fujinami sarcoma virus	Chicken		
	fms	McDonough feline sarcoma virus	Cat	Related to colony-stimulating factor (CSF-1) receptor	PM, ER
Potential protein kinases (related to above group)	mos	Moloney murine sarcoma virus	Mouse		Cyt
	erb-B	Avian erythroblastosis virus	Chicken	EGF receptor (truncated)	PM, ER
Growth factor	sis	Simian sarcoma virus	Woolly monkey	PDGF-like	Cyt, secreted
Binder of guanosine nucleotides	Ha-ras	Harvey murine sarcoma virus	Rat	GDP/GTP binding	PM
	Ki-ras	Kirsten murine sarcoma virus			
	N-ras	None	Human (neuroblastomas)		
Nuclear proteins	myb	Avian myeloblastosis virus	Chicken		Nuc
	myc	MC29 myelocytomatosis virus		DNA binding	
	fos	FBJ osteosarcoma virus	Mouse		
Unclassified	rel	Reticuloendotheliosis virus	Turkey		
	ets	E26 virus	Chicken		Nuc
	neu	None	Rat (neuroglioblastomas)	Related to EGF receptor	PM
	B-lym		Chicken (lymphomas)		

*Abbreviations used: PM = plasma membrane, Cyt = cytoplasm, ER = endoplasmic reticulum, EGF = epidermal growth factor, PDGF = platelet-derived growth factor, GDP/GTP = guanosine di- and triphosphate, Nuc = nucleus.
†fes and fps are equivalent.

functions are essential to normal activities of cells. Cellular oncogenes can be broadly grouped on the basis of presumed function and predominant properties (Table 46–2). They are structurally and functionally heterogeneous entities. Examples now exist of tyrosine-specific protein kinases (eg, src), a growth factor (sis is similar to human platelet-derived growth factor, a potent mitogen for cells of connective tissue origin), a growth factor receptor (erb-B is a truncated epidermal growth factor receptor), and GTP-binding proteins (eg, Ha-ras). The picture emerging is that recognized oncogenes probably represent individual components of complicated pathways responsible for regulating cell growth. Incorrect expression of any component might interrupt that regulation, resulting in uncontrolled growth of cells (cancer).

The molecular mechanisms believed to be responsible for activating a benign proto-oncogene and converting it into a cancer gene vary. Documented mechanisms of activation include the following: overexpression of a proto-oncogene as a result of a newly provided strong transcriptional promoter, "enhancer" sequences, or amplification of the gene; a chromosomal translocation that removes a proto-oncogene from its normal regulatory sequences and juxtaposes it near a strong promoter (such as used in immunoglobulin

production); and alterations in the structure of the protein product owing to a point mutation or deletion in the gene. These mechanisms might result in gene expression at the wrong time during the cell cycle or in inappropriate tissue types.

Carcinogenesis is believed to be a multistep process, ie, multiple genetic changes must occur to convert a normal cell into a malignant one. A long time is usually required for the appearance of tumors. The natural history of spontaneously occurring human and animal cancers suggests a multistep process of cellular evolution, probably involving repeated selection of rare cells with some selective growth advantage. The number of mutationlike changes underlying this process is not known. Studies with cultured primary cells have shown that different oncogenes (eg, myc and ras) can cooperate to cause morphologic cell transformation. Some viral genes, eg, myc and polyoma large T antigen, can immortalize primary cells so that they will grow continuously in culture but not exhibit properties of complete transformation. Such observations suggest that multiple cellular oncogenes may be involved in the evolution of tumors.

To date, the patterns of oncogene expression have not correlated well with different tumor types. Therefore, the actual roles that oncogenes may play in the development of human cancer remain unknown. Their possible involvement, however, remains a central focus of modern studies of carcinogenesis.

DNA TUMOR VIRUSES

Five families of DNA-containing viruses have been shown to contain members capable of tumor induction or cell transformation. Representative examples are included in Table 46–3, along with a summary of their general properties. A brief description of each of these families, with particular reference to oncogenesis, is given below.

Papovaviruses

These are small viruses (diameter 45–55 nm) that possess a circular genome of double-stranded DNA (MW $3–5 \times 10^6$) enclosed within a nonenveloped capsid exhibiting icosahedral symmetry. Virus particles mature in the nucleus of permissive host cells.

A. Polyomaviruses: SV40 and polyoma viruses are the best-characterized DNA-containing tumor viruses, since they contain a limited amount of genetic information (6–7 genes). Papovavirus-transformed cells exhibit new virus-determined tumor (T) antigens that are unrelated to viral capsid (structural) antigens. Most of the T antigens are found in the nucleus of transformed cells, but small amounts are localized in

Table 46–3. Some properties of DNA-containing tumor viruses.

Virus	Host of Origin	Natural Tumors (Host of Origin)	Experimental Host Range		Size (nm)	Structure	Site of Virus Maturation	Persistence of Infectious Virus in Tumor
			In Vivo Tumors	In Vitro Cell Transformation				
Papovaviruses								
Papilloma								
Human	Human	Yes	Human	Mouse	45–55	Icosahedral symmetry	Nuclear	Yes, but not always
Rabbit	Rabbit	Yes	Rabbit					
Bovine	Cow	Yes	Cow, horse	Bovine, mouse				
Canine	Dog	Yes	Dog					
Polyoma	Mouse	No	Mouse, hamster, other rodents	Mouse, hamster, rat				
SV40	Monkey	No	Hamster	Hamster, mouse, monkey, human				No
BK, JC	Human	No	Hamster	Hamster				
Adenoviruses								
Human types 3, 7, 11, 12, 14, 16, 18, 21, 31	Human	No	Hamster, rat, mouse	Hamster, rat, human	70–90	Icosahedral symmetry	Nucleus	No
Simian (some)	Monkey	No						
Bovine type 3	Cow	No						
Avian (CELO)	Chicken	No						
Herpesviruses								
Human								
Type 2	Human		Hamster	Hamster				
EB virus	Human	Yes	Monkey	Human, monkey				
Cytomegalovirus	Human			Hamster, mouse	100	Icosahedral symmetry	Nuclear membrane	No
Monkey (Melendez)	Monkey	No	Monkey					
Avian (Marek)	Chicken	Yes	Chicken					
Frog (Lucké)	Frog	Yes	Frog					
Rabbit (Hinze)	Rabbit	No	Rabbit					
Hepadnaviruses								
Human hepatitis B	Human	Yes			42	Complex	Nucleus	No
Woodchuck hepatitis	Woodchuck	Yes						
Poxviruses								
Molluscum contagiosum	Human	Yes	Human		230 × 300	Complex symmetry	Cytoplasm	Yes
Yaba	Monkey	Yes	Monkey					
Fibroma-myxoma	Rabbit, squirrel, deer	Yes	Rabbit, squirrel, deer					

the plasma membrane, where they may be involved in virus-specific transplantation antigen reactions. The T antigens are necessary for initiation of transformation and for maintenance of the transformed phenotype. One of the T antigens binds to viral DNA at the site of initiation of DNA synthesis and is essential for virus replication in permissive cells.

Polyoma virus causes many different types of tumors following injection into newborn mice. Tumors do not develop as a result of natural infection among young mice. Polyoma virus replicates in mouse cells and transforms certain heterologous (eg, hamster) nonpermissive cells.

SV40, vacuolating virus, causes characteristic vacuole formation during replication in cells of the natural host (monkey). SV40 causes tumors in experimentally inoculated newborn hamsters and transforms various nonpermissive rodent cells. Tumor induction in the natural host—the rhesus monkey—has not been observed. SV40 contaminated early lots of live poliomyelitis vaccines that had been grown in monkey cells. Although many persons, including newborns, accidentally received such SV40-contaminated vaccines, these individuals have been followed for over 25 years, and no SV40-related tumors have been reported.

The human papovaviruses (BK and JC) have been isolated from immunocompromised patients, and JC virus has been isolated from brains of patients with progressive multifocal leukoencephalopathy. These viruses are widely distributed in human populations, as evidenced by the presence of specific antibody in adult sera. Both viruses may persist in the kidneys of healthy individuals after primary infection and may reactivate when the host's immune response is impaired. These human viruses are similar to SV40 and can transform nonpermissive rodent cells and induce tumors in newborn hamsters. However, they have not been associated with any human tumors, just as SV40 has not been associated with tumors in its natural host.

B. Papillomaviruses: The papillomaviruses are slightly larger in diameter (55 nm) than the polyomaviruses (45 nm) and contain a larger genome (MW 5×10^6 versus 3×10^6). The organization of the papillomavirus genome appears to be more complex, although all the early gene products of the virus have not been identified. Papillomaviruses cause benign or malignant tumors in many types of mammals. They are one of the few types of DNA viruses known to cause natural tumors in their hosts of origin. Papillomaviruses are highly tropic for epithelial cells of the skin and mucous membranes. Molecular and biologic studies with these agents have progressed slowly, because they have not been propagated in vitro in cell culture. This difficulty in culturing is probably a reflection of the strong dependence of virus replication on the differentiated state of the host cell.

There is widespread diversity among papillomaviruses. Since neutralization tests cannot be done in the absence of infectivity assays, papillomavirus isolates have been classified using molecular criteria.

Virus "types" share less than 50% DNA homology. Over 40 distinct human papillomavirus (HPV) types have been recovered. Papillomaviruses cause several different kinds of warts in humans, including skin warts, plantar warts, flat warts, genital condylomas, and laryngeal papillomas. The multiple types of human isolates seem to be preferentially associated with certain clinical lesions, although distribution patterns are not absolute. HPV types 6, 11, and 16 have been especially associated with lesions that have a tendency to undergo malignant conversion. Recent studies strongly suggest an association of certain serotypes with genital and anal cancers and laryngeal carcinoma of humans. The majority of cervical, penile, and vulvar cancers carry HPV DNA. Most frequently, HPV16 is found, although some cancers contain DNA from HPV 11, 18, 31, 33, or 35. HeLa cells, a widely used tissue culture cell line derived many years ago from a cervical carcinoma, have been found to contain HPV 18 DNA. Both integrated and unintegrated copies of viral DNA may be present in cancer cells, although HPV DNA is generally not integrated (episomal) in noncancerous cells.

Papillomaviruses are biologically distinguished from the related polyomaviruses by the induction of tumors in natural hosts, the presence of virus particles in some tumor tissues, and the maintenance of viral DNA as episomal copies in some transformed cells.

Adenoviruses (See Chapter 43.)

The adenoviruses comprise a large group of agents widely distributed in nature (in humans and many animals). They are medium-sized viruses (diameter 70–90 nm) containing a linear genome of double-stranded DNA (MW $20–25 \times 10^6$) and naked capsids with icosahedral symmetry. Replication is species-specific, occurring in cells of the natural hosts. Adenoviruses can transform nonpermissive heterologous cells and induce the synthesis of virus-specific T antigens that localize in both the nucleus and the cytoplasm of transformed cells. Different serotypes of adenoviruses manifest varying degrees of oncogenicity in newborn hamsters, with the most oncogenic having the property of transforming cells that are able to escape from T cell immunity. Adenoviruses commonly infect humans, causing mild acute illnesses, mainly of the respiratory and intestinal tracts. No association of adenoviruses with human neoplasms has been found.

Herpesviruses
(See Chapter 44.)

These large viruses (diameter 100–200 nm) contain a linear genome of double-stranded DNA (MW 100×10^6) and have a capsid with icosahedral symmetry surrounded by an outer lipid-containing envelope. Herpesviruses typically cause acute infections followed by latency and eventual recurrence in each host, including humans. Herpesviruses replicate in cells of their natural hosts. Some herpesviruses (herpes simplex virus types 1 and 2 and cytomegalovirus) can transform certain cells in culture, but at a very low frequency. Transformed hamster cells produce tumors when injected into hamsters.

Some herpesviruses are associated with tumors in lower animals. Marek's disease is a highly contagious lymphoproliferative disease of chickens that can be prevented by vaccination with an attenuated strain of the Marek's disease virus. The prevention of cancer by vaccination in this case establishes the virus as the causative agent and suggests the possibility of a similar approach to prevention of some human tumors if a virus is identified as a causative agent. Other examples of herpesvirus-induced tumors in animals include lymphomas of certain types of monkeys and adenocarcinomas of frogs.

In humans, herpesviruses have been linked epidemiologically to a few specific types of tumors. Carcinoma of the cervix shows an association with herpes simplex virus type 2, although that association is not as strong as for HPV and cervical cancer (described above). No specific herpesvirus-transforming gene has yet been identified, however. It is possible that herpesvirus-induced oncogenesis may be fundamentally different from transformation mediated by viruses that encode transforming proteins.

Epstein-Barr herpesvirus (EBV) causes acute infectious mononucleosis when it infects B lymphocytes of susceptible humans. In a few immunodeficient children, such EBV infections have progressed to a B cell lymphoma. One tragic case of severe combined immunodeficiency recently demonstrated that EBV can cause B cell lymphoma. A 12-year-old child kept in a gnotobiotic environment since birth received a bone marrow transplant and died 124 days later of multiple B cell proliferations proved to be due to EBV. EBV also has been linked to Burkitt's lymphoma, a tumor most commonly found in children in central Africa, and to nasopharyngeal carcinoma, the incidence of which is higher in Chinese male populations in Southeast Asia than elsewhere. Cells from these 2 types of tumors contain Epstein-Barr viral DNA and antigens. Normal human lymphocytes have a limited life span in vitro, but EBV can transform such lymphocytes into lymphoblast cell lines that grow indefinitely in culture. All cells that carry EBV genomes express a virus-specific nuclear antigen (called EBNA) regardless of whether mature virus is released.

With the exception of the case of severe combined immunodeficiency, no definite proof yet exists that any herpesvirus is directly responsible for any human tumor. Because of their low efficiencies of transformation in vitro and the difficulties in defining a transforming gene, it is possible that herpesvirus effects represent only one step in a complex sequence leading to neoplasia (see p 524). For example, EBV appears to be one cofactor in the pathogenesis of Burkitt's lymphoma. A chromosomal translocation that activates the c-*myc* proto-oncogene also may play a role in transformation.

Poxviruses (See Chapter 42.)

Poxviruses are large, brick-shaped viruses (diameter 230×400 nm) with a linear genome of double-stranded DNA (MW $130–240 \times 10^6$), a capsid with complex symmetry, and a lipid-containing envelope. Yaba virus produces benign tumors (histiocytomas) in its natural host, monkeys. Shope fibroma virus produces fibromas in some rabbits and is able to alter cells in culture. Very little is known about the nature of the interaction of the virus with the host cells. Molluscum contagiosum virus produces small benign growths in humans.

Hepatitis B Virus (See Chapter 38.)

On the basis of its physical and chemical properties, hepatitis B virus (HBV) has recently been classified as the prototype of a new virus family, Hepadnaviridae, characterized by 42-nm spherical virions with a circular genome of double-stranded DNA (MW 1.6×10^6). One strand of the DNA is incomplete and variable in length; the virus contains a DNA polymerase that can complete the strand length. Studies of the virus are hampered because it has not been grown in cell culture.

Recent investigations have shown HBV to be a risk factor in the development of cancer in humans. Epidemiologic and laboratory studies have proved persistent infection with HBV to be an important cause of chronic liver disease and have strongly implicated the virus in the development of hepatocellular carcinoma. Several tumor samples and tumor cell lines have been found to contain hepatitis B viral DNA. However, the precise mechanism of the initiation of oncogenesis and maintenance of the carcinoma remains obscure. The advent of an effective hepatitis B vaccine for the prevention of primary infection raises the possibility of prevention of hepatocellular carcinoma, particularly in areas of the world where infection with HBV is hyperendemic (eg, Africa, China, Southeast Asia). Because of the long latent period before cancer development, however, the effects of vaccination will not be apparent for at least 20 years.

RNA TUMOR VIRUSES

RNA tumor viruses were formerly called **oncorna** *(onco*genic *RNA)* **viruses** but are now classified as **retroviruses** because they contain an RNA-directed DNA polymerase (reverse transcriptase). RNA tumor viruses mainly cause tumors of connective tissue (sarcomas) or of the reticuloendothelial and hematopoietic systems (leukemias, leukoses). The RNA tumor viruses most widely studied experimentally are the sarcoma viruses of birds and mice and the leukemia viruses of mice, cats, birds, and humans. Some representative examples are shown, with a summary of their properties, in Table 46–4.

General Features of RNA Tumor Viruses

(1) The genome consists of 2 identical subunits of single-stranded, positive-sense RNA, each of molecular weight $2–3 \times 10^6$.

Table 46–4. Some properties of RNA-containing tumor viruses (retroviruses).

Virus*	Abbreviations Used	Host of Origin	Natural Tumors (Host of Origin)	Experimental Host Range		Size (nm)	Morphology (Particle Type)	Site of Virus Maturation	Persistence of Infectious Virus in Tumor
				In Vivo Tumor	In Vitro Cell Transformation				
Avian complex Leukemia	ALV	Chicken	Yes	Chicken, turkey	Chicken†		C	Budding at cell membrane	Yes, but not always
Sarcoma (Rous)	ASV			Avian, rodent, monkey	Avian, rodent, bovine, monkey, human				
Murine complex Leukemia	MLV	Mouse	Yes	Mouse, rat, hamster	Mouse‡		C		
Sarcoma	MSV		No	Mouse, rat, hamster	Mouse, rat, hamster				
Murine mammary tumor (Bittner)	MMTV	Mouse	Yes	Mouse		70–100	B		
Feline complex Leukemia	FeLV	Cat	Yes	Cat			C		
Sarcoma	FeSV			Cat, dog, rabbit, monkey	Cat, dog, monkey, human				
Primate Woolly monkey, sarcoma	SSV-1	Monkey	Yes	Monkey	Monkey, mouse, rat		C		
Gibbon, leukemia	GALV	Ape	Yes				C		
Monkey, mammary carcinoma (Mason-Pfizer)	M-PMV	Monkey	?		Monkey		D		
Human T-cell lymphotropic	HTLV	Human	Yes		Human		C		
Other Viper		Viper	Yes				C		
Hamster, leukemia	HaLV	Hamster	?				C		
Rat, leukemia	RaLV	Rat	?				C		
Bovine, lymphoma		Cow	Yes				C		

*A series of endogenous C type viruses exist that are not oncogenic but replicate in tissue culture.
†With avian myeloblastosis virus and avian erythroblastosis virus only.
‡With the Abelson strain of MLV only.

(2) Virus particles contain an RNA-directed DNA polymerase (reverse transcriptase).

(3) Virus particles mature and emerge from infected host cells by budding from cytoplasmic membranes (Fig 46–8).

(4) Typically, virus particles have an electron-dense nucleoid surrounded by an outer membrane (envelope) containing glycoprotein and lipid. A model of a retrovirus particle is shown in Fig 46–9. The particles are divided into 4 classes, A, B, C, and D (see below), on the basis of morphology.

(5) Two types of antigens are found in retroviruses: type-specific or subgroup-specific antigens associated with the glycoproteins in the viral envelope, which are coded by the *env* gene (Fig 46–5); and group-specific antigens associated with the virion core, which are coded by the *gag* gene. Cross-reactions do not occur between the envelope antigens of retroviruses from different species.

Replication of RNA Tumor Viruses

After virus particles have adsorbed to and penetrated host cells, the viral RNA serves as the template for the synthesis of viral DNA through the action of the enzyme reverse transcriptase, which is encoded by the viral genome and carried within the core of the viral particle. The newly formed viral DNA becomes integrated into the host cell DNA as a provirus (Fig 46–3). Progeny viral genomes may then be transcribed from the provirus DNA into viral RNA. The structure of the provirus is constant, but its integration into the host cell genome can occur at different sites.

Some RNA tumor viruses (eg, nondefective sarcoma or leukemia viruses) can replicate without the aid of helper viruses, but other RNA tumor viruses (eg, defective sarcoma or acute leukemia viruses) cannot replicate alone because they lack essential replicative functions that must be supplied by a helper virus. The helper virus is typically a leukemia virus (Fig

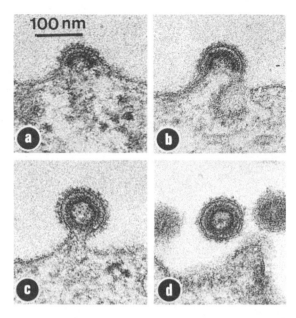

Figure 46–8. Sequential stages of the budding process of replicating retroviruses. Pictured is the Friend strain of murine leukemia virus. (Courtesy of H. Frank.)

C. C Type Viruses: The C type viruses comprise a large group of well-characterized agents. The particles are 90–110 nm in diameter, and the electron-dense nucleoids are centrally located. The C type viruses may exist as exogenous or endogenous entities (see below). It should be noted that there are some C type viruses, called lentiviruses (eg, visna virus), which cause chronic infections with slowly progressive neurologic impairment. The lentiviruses are not tumorigenic.

D. D Type Viruses: This group of retroviruses is poorly characterized. Both intracellular and extracellular forms exist. Immature intracellular particles are ring-shaped and usually slightly smaller than the intracytoplasmic A type particles. The mature particles are 100–120 nm in diameter, contain an eccentric nucleoid, and characteristically exhibit surface spikes shorter than those on B type particles. Some D type particles are transmitted horizontally in monkeys and may cause breast carcinoma; others are endogenous viruses in primates.

Exogenous C Type Tumor Viruses

These viruses are transmitted horizontally among host animal groups and initiate infection and transformation only after contact. In contrast to endogenous

46–7). As noted above (Fig 46–2), a salient feature of retroviruses is that they are not cytolytic, ie, they do not kill the cells in which they replicate.

Morphologic Groups of RNA Tumor Viruses

Three morphologic classes of extracellular retrovirus particles, as well as an intracellular form, are known. Examples of each are shown in Fig 46–10.

A. A Type Particles: These occur only intracellularly and consist of a ring-shaped nucleoid surrounded by a membrane. They often occur in mouse cells and appear to be noninfectious. Intracytoplasmic A type particles, 75 nm in diameter, are precursors of extracellular B type viruses. In contrast, intracisternal A type particles, 60–90 nm in diameter, are distinct entities that are not a stage in the life cycle of either B type or C type viruses.

B. B Type Viruses: These particles are 100–130 nm in diameter and contain an eccentric nucleoid. The prototype of this group is the mouse mammary tumor virus (MMTV), which occurs in "high mammary cancer" strains of inbred mice (eg, C3H) and is found in particularly large amounts in lactating mammary tissue and milk. Thus, it is readily transferred to suckling mice, in whom the incidence of subsequent development of adenocarcinoma of the breast is high. Endogenous MMTV provirus sequences (see below) are present in cells of mouse strains of both low and high mammary tumor incidence but are transcribed much more efficiently in the latter. Virus expression is regulated by both genetic and hormonal factors of the host animals.

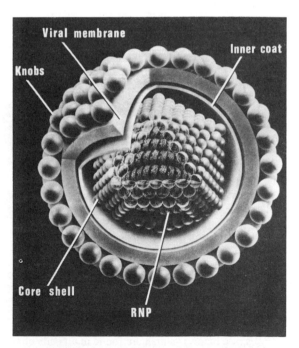

Figure 46–9. Three-dimensional model of Friend leukemia virus as prototype for mammalian C type retroviruses. Removal of the front triangle of the icosahedral core shell allows the ribonucleoprotein to be seen. RNP = ribonucleoprotein. Knobs (KN) + viral membrane (VM) + inner coat (IC) = viral envelope. Core shell (CS) + RNP = core. (Reproduced, with permission, from Frank H et al: *Z Naturforsch* 1978;**33**:124.)

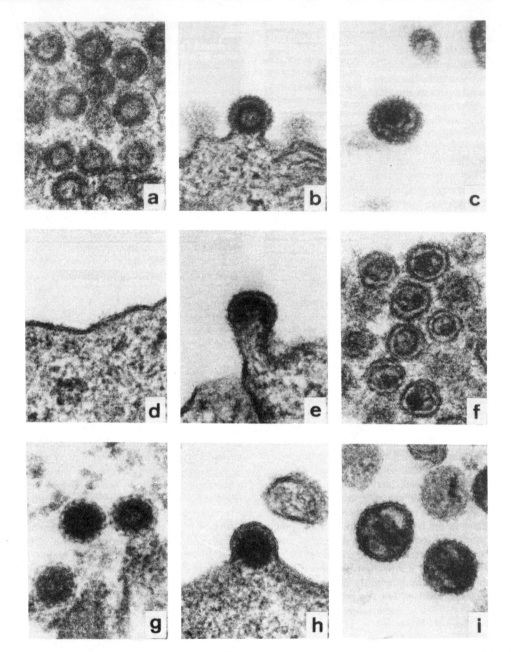

Figure 46–10. Comparative morphology of type A, B, C, and D retroviruses. *(a)* Intracytoplasmic A type particles (representing immature precursor of budding B type virus). *(b)* Budding B type virus. *(c)* Mature, extracellular B type virus. *(d)* Lack of morphologically recognizable intracytoplasmic form for C type virus. *(e)* Budding C type virus. *(f)* Mature, extracellular C type virus. *(g)* Intracytoplasmic A type particle (representing immature precursor form of D type virus). *(h)* Budding D type virus. *(i)* Mature, extracellular D type virus. All micrographs are approximately × 87,000. Thin sections were double-stained with uranyl acetate and lead citrate. (Courtesy of Fine and Gonda.).

viruses (see below), which are found in all cells of all individuals of a given species, gene sequences of exogenous viruses are found only in infected cells. Several general types of exogenous retroviruses have been identified.

A. Avian Sarcoma Viruses (eg, Rous Sarcoma Virus of Chickens): These agents possess and express 4 genes, including a transforming gene ac-

tive in focus assays in vitro. The transforming genes are derived from cellular genes (Fig 46–5; see Cellular Oncogenes, above). These competent viruses do not require helper viruses for replication.

B. Leukemia Viruses of Birds, Rodents, Cats, and Monkeys; This group contains the majority of C type retroviruses. These viruses possess only 3 genes: they lack an *onc* gene and cannot transform cells in vitro. However, they retain the ability to transform precursor cells in blood-forming tissues in vivo, perhaps by a promoter-insertion mechanism. The leukemia viruses replicate without the aid of helper viruses. Many representatives of this group are present in the blood of their host animals for short or long periods before a neoplastic process becomes manifest. Some of the infected animals eventually develop leukemias or solid lymphoid tumors.

C. Defective Acute Avian Leukemia Viruses and Mammalian Sarcoma Viruses: These viruses are highly oncogenic in appropriate host animals. They carry characteristic *onc* genes but lack replication genes. Consequently, progeny virus is produced only in the presence of helper viruses. The helper viruses are generally other RNA tumor viruses (leukemia viruses), which may recombine in various ways with the defective viruses. These defective transforming retroviruses have been the source of most of the recognized cellular oncogenes (see p 523).

D. Human Retroviruses: In numerous cases, a human retrovirus has been isolated from patients with adult T-cell leukemias and lymphomas. The human T-cell lymphotropic viruses (HTLV) have a marked affinity for mature T cells. HTLV is expressed at very low levels in infected individuals, and its initial discovery hinged on the use of T-cell growth factor (interleukin-2) to amplify populations of malignant T cells in vitro, coupled with the use of sensitive molecular techniques to assay for virus markers. The virus is distributed worldwide, with clusters of HTLV-associated disease in certain geographic areas (southern Japan, the Caribbean basin, and the southern USA). The fact that proviral sequences are found in the DNA of neoplastic T cells but not in normal human cells establishes that the virus is an exogenous agent. It is possible to transmit HTLV from donor cells to recipient cord blood or bone marrow cells by co-cultivation experiments; transformed immortalized recipient cell lines of T-cell origin will emerge.

A related human retrovirus has been established as the causative agent of acquired immune deficiency syndrome (AIDS; see Chapter 47). It is a cytolytic virus more similar to the lentiviruses than to the noncytolytic leukemia viruses.

Endogenous C Type Viruses

Viral genetic information that is a constant part of the genetic constitution of an organism is designated as "endogenous." An integrated retroviral provirus behaves like a cluster of cellular genes and is subject to regulatory control by the cell. This cellular control usually results in partial or complete repression of viral gene expression. In fact, it is not uncommon for normal cells to maintain the endogenous viral infection in a quiescent form for extended periods of time. The same endogenous viral genome may be actively expressed in one cell and completely repressed in another.

Many vertebrates possess endogenous RNA virus sequences. In most instances, the endogenous viruses are not pathogenic for their host animals. Endogenous retrovirus genes are present in the germ cells of animals and are transmitted through an indefinite number of generations with no detriment to the animal. The endogenous virus sequences are of no apparent benefit to the animal. The reasons for the retention and conservation of these sequences are not known. The proto-oncogene sequences present in all normal cells are not located in the cellular chromosome adjacent to any endogenous virus sequences.

The growth of endogenous viruses is usually restricted in cells derived from the original host. Cells from a different, susceptible species must be found for the virus to replicate. Such viruses are said to be "xenotropic."

One method to detect the presence of heritable viral genes in normal cells is to "activate" virus expression in tissue culture. Exposure of virus-free chick or mouse embryo cells to ionizing radiation, chemical carcinogens, or metabolic inhibitors resulted in the production of an RNA virus with all the characteristics of a leukemia virus. Such experiments prompted the conclusion that normal murine and avian cells have the genetic potential for specifying a complete nontransforming retrovirus. More commonly, endogenous virus sequences are now detected and characterized at the molecular level by using nucleic acid hybridization techniques.

Important features of endogenous viruses can be summarized briefly as follows: (1) DNA copies of RNA tumor virus genome are covalently linked to cellular DNA and are present in all somatic and germ cells in the host; (2) endogenous viral genomes are transmitted genetically from parent to offspring; (3) the integrated state subjects the endogenous viral genomes to host genetic control; and (4) the endogenous virus may be induced to replicate either spontaneously or by treatment with extrinsic (chemical) factors.

REFERENCES

Bernards R, van der Eb AJ: Adenovirus: Transformation and oncogenicity. *Biochim Biophys Acta* 1984;**783**:187.

Bishop JM: Exploring carcinogenesis with retroviral and cellular oncogenes. *Prog Med Virol* 1985;**32**:5.

Bishop JM: Oncogenes. *Sci Am* (March) 1982;**246**:80.

Bishop JM: Viral oncogenes. *Cell* 1985;**42**:23.

de The G, Henle W, Rapp F (editors): *Oncogenesis and Her-pesviruses III*. International Agency for Research on Cancer, 1978.

Francis DP, Essex M: Leukemia and lymphoma: Infrequent manifestations of common viral infections? A review. *J Infect Dis* 1978;**138**:916.

Gallo RC, Blattner WA: Human T-cell leukemia/lymphoma viruses: ATL and AIDS. Pages 104–138 in: *Important Ad-*

vances in Oncology. De Vita VT Jr, Hellman S, Rosenberg SA (editors). Lippincott, 1985.

Gissmann L: Papillomaviruses and their association with cancer in animals and in man. *Cancer Surveys* 1984;**3**:161.

Heldin C-H, Westermark B: Growth factors: Mechanism of action and relation to oncogenes. *Cell* 1984;**37**:9.

Melnick JL: Hepatitis B virus and liver cancer. Pages 337–367 in: *Viruses Associated With Human Cancer*. Phillips LA (editor). Marcel Dekker, 1983.

Melnick JL et al: The role of herpes simplex virus in cervical and vulvar cancer. *Devel Biol Stand* 1982;**52**:87.

Moore DH et al: Mammary tumor viruses. *Adv Cancer Res* 1979;**29**:347.

Rapp F: The challenge of herpesviruses. *Cancer Res* 1984;**44**:1309.

Rigby PWJ, Lane DP: Structure and function of simian virus 40 large T-antigen. *Adv Viral Oncol* 1983;**3**:31.

Shearer WT et al: Epstein-Barr virus-associated B-cell proliferations of diverse clonal origins after bone marrow transplantation in a 12-year-old patient with severe combined immunodeficiency. *N Engl J Med* 1985;**312**:1151.

Takemoto KK: Human papovaviruses. *Int Rev Exp Pathol* 1978;**18**:281.

Tooze J (editor): *The Molecular Biology of Tumor Viruses*, 2nd ed. *DNA Tumor Viruses*, 1981; *RNA Tumor Viruses*, 1982. Cold Spring Harbor Laboratory.

Varmus HE: Form and function of retroviral proviruses. *Science* 1982;**216**:812.

Acquired Immune Deficiency Syndrome (AIDS)   47

AIDS is a profound immunoregulatory disorder that is often fatal, because it predisposes the host to severe opportunistic infections or neoplasms. Susceptibility to opportunists or neoplasms occurs as a result of the depletion of helper T cells owing to infection by a retrovirus, HTLV-III (human T-lymphotropic virus type III).* The disease was first recognized in 1981, when a dramatically increased incidence of Kaposi's sarcoma and *Pneumocystis carinii* pneumonia was reported in male homosexuals as a result of their immune defects. HTLV-III also is known as lymphadenopathy virus (LAV) and AIDS-related virus (ARV).

PROPERTIES OF THE VIRUS

Classification

It is a tribute to modern molecular virology that, only 4 years from the time an unusual disease syndrome was first recognized, the causative agent was isolated and identified and the genomes of multiple isolates sequenced.

HTLV-III is a retrovirus and exhibits many of the physicochemical features typical of the family (see Chapter 46). The unique morphologic characteristic of HTLV-III is a cylindric nucleoid in the mature virion (Fig 47–1). The diagnostic bar-shaped nucleoid is visible in electron micrographs in those extracellular particles that happen to be sectioned at the appropriate angle.

HTLV-III displays only limited genetic similarity to the human retroviruses associated with certain human T cell leukemias (HTLV-I and HTLV-II; see Chapter 46). On the basis of several properties (nucleic acid homology, genome and protein sizes, virion morphology, and biologic characteristics of infections), HTLV-III more closely resembles members of the retrovirus subfamily designated Lentivirinae. The prototype lentivirus is visna virus, a slowly replicating, pathogenic but nononcogenic retrovirus of sheep (see Chapter 39). The significant differences in fundamental biologic properties between HTLV-III and the

previously known transforming retroviruses probably account for the unique disease features of AIDS.

Biologic Properties

HTLV-III is T-lymphotropic, especially for helper T cells identified by monoclonal antibody OKT4 (Leu-3). Virus infection causes a pronounced cytopathic effect, including the formation of multinucleated giant cells, followed by cell death. This explains the quantitative and functional depletion of the T4 lymphocyte subset that is a hallmark of AIDS. A burst of virus production accompanies loss of cell viability. Cells are not transformed (Fig 47–2). This is in marked contrast to the effect on T cells of the transforming human retrovirus HTLV-I, which is associated with certain types of human leukemia (see Chapter 46). It is possible that not all HTLV-III-infected cells are killed immediately; virus-producing cells that survive for a long time might serve as reservoirs of infection in the affected host.

HTLV-III can infect other cell types at low levels as well. These include B lymphocytes and monocytes in vivo and a variety of human cell lines in vitro. The virus is able to spread throughout the body and has been detected in lymphoid cells, brain, thymus, spleen, and testes. There is a marked difference in the ability of natural isolates to infect cells and grow in vitro, which probably reflects the fact that variants exist in nature.

The cytopathology produced by HTLV-III and other lentiviruses is associated with the presence of unintegrated replicating forms of the viral genome in the cytoplasm of cells. This phenomenon provides a possible focus for chemotherapeutic strategies.

No animal model has been developed for AIDS. Chimpanzees can be infected by HTLV-III, as evidenced by the development of antibodies and transient changes in T cell ratios, but they do not develop clinical signs of AIDS.

Genetic Characteristics

HTLV-III is a completely exogenous virus; in contrast to the transforming retroviruses, the viral genome does not contain any conserved cellular genes (see Chapter 46). Individuals become infected by the introduction of virus from outside sources and not by the activation of silent sequences contained in cellular

*As this book goes to press, a decision has been reached to change the name of the virus associated with AIDS to human immunodeficiency virus (HIV).

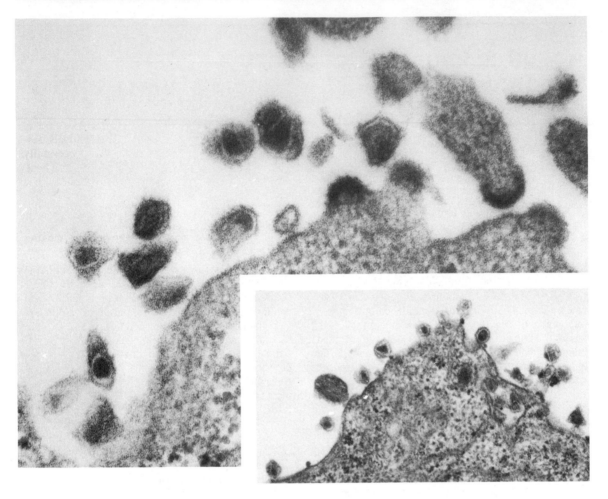

Figure 47–1. Characteristic budding of virus particles from peripheral blood lymphocytes of 2 patients with AIDS. Magnification of larger figure 142,000 ×, that of inset 47,500 ×.

DNA. After an individual is exposed to HTLV-III, proviral DNA is integrated into the cellular DNA of infected cells.

The virus contains the 3 genes required for a replicating retrovirus—*gag, pol,* and *env* (see Chapter 46). However, 2 additional open reading frames found by sequence analysis of the HTLV-III genome may play a role in the unusual pathogenicity of the virus. These extra coding sequences distinguish the HTLV group from other retroviruses. One unique product is involved in "transactivation," whereby a viral gene product is involved in transcriptional activation of other viral genes. Transactivation in HTLV-III is highly efficient and may account, in part, for the virulent nature of HTLV-III infections. It is speculated that the same viral protein might alter the transcriptional regulation of specific host cell genes, eg, those involved in control of lymphocyte cell growth, and be responsible for the observed cellular phenotypic changes.

The many different isolates of HTLV-III are not identical but appear to comprise a spectrum of related viruses. The regions of greatest divergence among different isolates are localized to the *env* gene, which codes for the viral envelope proteins. Another lentivirus, visna virus, typically undergoes progressive antigenic variation in reaction to the host's immune response during persistent infection. Whether the divergence in the envelope of HTLV-III will complicate efforts to develop an effective vaccine for AIDS remains to be determined.

Disinfection & Inactivation

HTLV-III is completely inactivated ($\geq 10^5$ units of infectivity) by treatment for 10 minutes at room temperature (37 °C) with any of the following: 10% household bleach, 50% ethanol, 35% isopropanol, 1% NP40, 0.5% Lysol, 0.5% paraformaldehyde, or 0.3% hydrogen peroxide. The virus is also inactivated by extremes in pH (pH 1.0 and 13.0).

The virus is not inactivated by 2.5% Tween-20. Although paraformaldehyde inactivates virus free in solution, it is not yet known if it penetrates tissues sufficiently to inactivate all virus that might be present in cultured cells or tissue specimens.

HTLV-III is readily inactivated in liquids or 10%

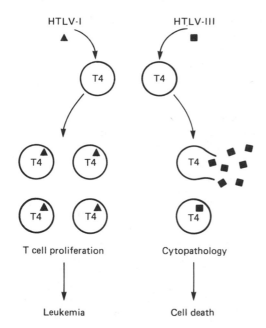

Figure 47–2. Comparison of response of human T lymphocytes to infection with HTLV-I, a transforming retrovirus, and HTLV-III, a cytopathogenic retrovirus that is the causative agent of AIDS. Not all HTLV-III-infected cells are killed immediately; surviving virus-infected cells serve as reservoirs of infection in the host.

serum by heating at 56 °C for 10 minutes, but dried proteinaceous material affords marked protection. Lyophilized blood products would need to be heated at 68 °C for 72 hours to ensure inactivation of contaminating virus.

AIDS INFECTIONS IN HUMANS

Pathogenesis

AIDS patients have an absolute reduction in the level of the helper (OKT4-reactive) T lymphocyte subset, and this results in an inversion of the normal helper T cell:suppressor (OKT8-reactive) T cell ratio in peripheral blood. In addition, leukopenia, lymphopenia, and suppressed T cell functions both in vivo (skin test anergy) and in vitro (mitogen-induced T cell blastogenesis) are observed. Humoral immune responses also may be diminished.

HTLV-III virus is the initiator of the disorder. T lymphocytes are the target cells for the virus. In vitro, the virus grows in T lymphocytes and destroys them in the process (cytolytic infection).

HTLV-III also can infect B cells and macrophages in vivo, although the infection is milder than that of T lymphocytes. Virus has been detected in various organs including testes and spleen but most notably in the brain and cerebrospinal fluid of AIDS patients with neurologic findings. It appears that HTLV-III plays a role in the pathogenesis of encephalopathy or demen-

tia—or both—associated with AIDS in addition to its role in causing the immune deficiency characteristic of the disease.

Whether HTLV-III is the sole etiologic agent of AIDS is still not known. Other infectious agents may be important as cofactors in the development of AIDS, perhaps by affecting the immune status of the individual. For example, the vast majority of AIDS patients have evidence of infection with hepatitis B virus. It is not known what distinguishes those individuals destined to develop AIDS from those who successfully suppress the virus infection. It is possible that a host partially immunocompromised from other causes may be most susceptible to HTLV-III infection.

Clinical Findings

The incubation period appears to be long, ranging from 6 months to more than 2 years. The highest percentage of cases (75%) has occurred in male homosexuals, but other populations known to be at risk include bisexual males, heterosexual intravenous drug users, and hemophiliacs treated with blood products or factor VIII concentrates.

AIDS is characterized by a pronounced suppression of the immune system and the development of unusual neoplasms (especially Kaposi's sarcoma) or a wide variety of severe opportunistic infections. The more serious symptoms are often preceded by a prodrome that can include fatigue, malaise, unexplained weight loss, fever, shortness of breath, chronic diarrhea, white patches on the tongue (hairy leukoplakia, oral candidiasis), and lymphadenopathy. It has been estimated that 5–10% of homosexual males with prolonged unexplained lymphadenopathy and impaired immune function may develop AIDS.

The most common infectious complications of AIDS include the following:

(1) Protozoa — *Pneumocystis carinii, Toxoplasma gondii, Isospora belli, Cryptosporidium.*

(2) Fungi — *Candida albicans, Cryptococcus neoformans, Coccidioides immitis, Histoplasma capsulatum.*

(3) Bacteria — *Mycobacterium avium, Mycobacterium tuberculosis, Listeria monocytogenes, Nocardia asteroides, Salmonella.*

(4) Viruses — Cytomegalovirus, herpes simplex virus, adenovirus, JC human papovavirus, hepatitis B virus.

The incidence of cancer in homosexuals with AIDS is about 40%; 90% of these cases are Kaposi's sarcoma and 10% are malignant lymphomas. Kaposi's sarcoma is a vascular tumor thought to be of endothelial origin that appears in skin, mucous membranes, lymph nodes, and visceral organs. Before this type of malignancy was observed in AIDS patients, it was considered to be a very rare cancer that occurred infrequently in older men and with a higher frequency in children and young adults in equatorial Africa. In addition to the primary infection with HTLV-III virus that allows Kaposi's sarcoma to develop, cytomegalovirus also may play a role. Cytomegalovirus particles have been seen in several Kaposi's sarcoma tumors by electron microscopy, and all the patients with Kaposi's sarcoma who were studied showed serologic evidence of past cytomegalovirus infection. Cytomegalovirus-specific DNA, RNA, and antigens have been reported in Kaposi's sarcoma tumors and cell lines. Finally, all the groups with an unusually high incidence of Kaposi's sarcoma (ie, elderly men, young Africans, organ transplant recipients, immunocompromised individuals, and homosexual men) show a high degree of prior exposure to cytomegalovirus. The exact role, if any, of cytomegalovirus in the induction of Kaposi's sarcoma or AIDS remains to be established, but it is well to remember that cytomegalovirus can establish both persistent and latent infections in humans. Cytomegalovirus also can be sexually transmitted, and studies with homosexuals also implicate oral-genital contact as a mode of transmission. Cytomegalovirus-induced mononucleosis manifests many of the symptoms that occur during the prodromal phase of AIDS (eg, fever, lymphadenopathy, atypical lymphocytes, transient polyclonal increases in immunoglobulins, suppression of both specific and nonspecific cell-mediated immunity, and a reversal in the helper T cell:suppressor T cell ratio, which may persist for more than a year).

Diagnosis

In patients with AIDS or pre-AIDS, the HTLV-III retrovirus can be isolated from lymphocytes in peripheral blood or bone marrow as well as from cell-free plasma. It can be grown in lymphocyte cultures containing abundant OKT4-reactive target cells. Primary cells must be stimulated with a mitogen, eg, phytohemagglutinin, and supplemented with T cell growth factor (interleukin-2). A continuous T cell line has recently been developed that is susceptible to HTLV-III. Viral growth is detected by the appearance of a magnesium-dependent, high-molecular-weight reverse transcriptase about 7–14 days after infection together with a pronounced cytopathic effect. Virus-specific antigens also develop and are measured by indirect immunofluorescence or radioimmunoprecipitation methods using serum from antibody-positive persons or hyperimmune serum prepared by using purified virus. For reasons that are not clear, T cells from infected persons must be cultured in vitro before they will yield positive assays for viral antigen.

Test kits are commercially available for measuring antibodies by enzyme-linked immunosorbent assay (ELISA). In about 90% of persons with positive antibody tests, HTLV-III retrovirus can be recovered from cultured lymphocytes. Viremia may persist for years in both symptomatic and asymptomatic persons. When ELISA-based antibody tests are used for screening populations with a low prevalence of HTLV-III infections, a positive test in a serum sample must be confirmed by a repeat test before the serum donor is notified. If the repeat ELISA test is negative, the specimen should be tested by another method. Alternative tests have included immunofluorescence and radioimmunoprecipitation assays, but the most extensive experience has been with the Western blot technique, in which antibodies to HTLV-III proteins of specific molecular weights can be detected. Antibodies to viral core protein p24 or envelope glycoprotein gp41 are most commonly detected.

Epidemiology

AIDS was first recognized in the USA in 1981. By October 1985, more than 14,000 cases had occurred, with over 7000 deaths, and the number of infected asymptomatic carriers was estimated to be over 1 million. By September 1985, the World Health Organization also had reported about 1300 cases in Europe, 725 cases in Latin America, and 100 cases in Australia. About 5–10% of carriers may show early signs of AIDS-related complex: swollen lymph glands, malaise, fever, night sweats, diarrhea, and loss of weight. However, most carriers seem to have normal immune function. It is not known how many of the virus-infected individuals will eventually develop clinical symptoms or progress to full-blown AIDS, but at this writing it appears to be about 1%.

The disease is believed to have originated in central Africa, where monkeys may originally have harbored the virus. In contrast to the situation in the USA and Europe, where over 90% of patients are male, cases in Africa are distributed equally between males and females. Although AIDS in the USA was originally confined to homosexuals, by 1985 a significant number of AIDS patients were being reported among heterosexuals, particularly illicit drug users and their infants. About 1% of the cases resulted solely from heterosexual contacts. The rate of increase of AIDS cases in heterosexuals is much lower than the rate of increase among homosexuals when AIDS first appeared.

Antibodies to HTLV-III are found in almost all patients with clinical AIDS. In addition, patients with persistent generalized lymphadenopathy, fever, and wasting—conditions described as lymphadenopathy syndrome, pre-AIDS, or AIDS-related complex (ARC)—have a very high prevalence of antibodies. Promiscuous homosexual men and intravenous drug users also have a high prevalence of antibodies. In contrast, antibodies are rare in normal individuals, persons with a variety of other viral infections (eg, cytomegalovirus mononucleosis), and immunosuppressed individuals (eg, renal transplant recipients, patients with various unrelated immunodeficiency disorders). Among individuals with no traditional risk factors for AIDS, antibodies have developed among recipients of contaminated blood transfusions or blood products, notably hemophiliacs, and among female sexual partners of men with HTLV-III infection.

AIDS is a disease most often transmitted by sexual contact. Since the first description of AIDS as a new disease entity in previously healthy homosexual men, promiscuous homosexual activity has been recognized as a major risk factor for acquisition of the disease. The risk increases in proportion to the number of sexual encounters with different partners. Particular sexual practices appear to be higher risk factors than others; there is a higher prevalence of AIDS among homosexual men who practice passive anal intercourse than among those who practice insertive anal intercourse. Transmission of virus or virus-infected cells in semen may be the critical factor. Other body fluids, eg, saliva and tears, also may contain virus, but there is little if any evidence that the virus is transmitted by body fluids other than blood or semen. It has been convincingly documented that asymptomatic, virus-positive individuals can transmit the virus, and the recipient may develop AIDS while the donor remains free of disease.

Women may acquire the disease from bisexual men, and children of virus-infected mothers are increasingly being diagnosed. Pediatric AIDS cases, acquired from mothers in high-risk groups, usually present with clinical symptoms by 2 years of age. Clinical findings may include interstitial pneumonitis, severe oral candidiasis, generalized lymphadenopathy, bacterial sepsis, hepatomegaly or splenomegaly (or both), diarrhea, and failure to thrive.

Transfusion of infectious blood or blood products is an effective route for virus transmission. Thus, hemophiliacs who receive contaminated clotting factor concentrates have been placed at high risk. Over 90% of recipients of factor VIII concentrates in the USA were reported to have developed antibodies to HTLV-III by 1985. Users of illicit drugs are commonly infected through the use of contaminated needles.

Control

There is currently no effective method for the prevention or cure of this devastating disease. Without intervention by drugs or vaccines, the only way to avoid epidemic spread of HTLV-III is to have a lifestyle that minimizes or eliminates the high-risk factors discussed above. It is striking that the disease has not occurred among medical and health-care workers who care for AIDS patients but do not have lifestyles which place them in the high-risk groups. No cases have been documented to result from such common exposures as sneezing, coughing, sharing meals, or other casual contacts.

The cytopathic nature of HTLV-III infection suggests that the infected cells involved in immune function are destroyed and that fresh cells must be infected continuously to maintain the infected state. Unlike cellular oncogenes, HTLV-III genes are not present in normal uninfected cells. Thus, if viral replication could be inhibited by the use of some of the drugs now under study, infection of new cells and maintenance of the disease should theoretically be prevented. Other approaches under investigation include inducing antibodies to the viral envelope glycoprotein or the cell surface receptor for the virus. New sources of immunizing antigens may come from cloning of the viral genes.

Because HTLV-III may be transmitted in blood, all donor blood should be tested for antibody and, when such tests become commercially available, for virus. Properly conducted antibody tests appear to detect almost all HTLV-III carriers. Since the introduction of widespread screening of blood donors for virus exposure and the rejection of contaminated blood, transmission by blood transfusion has virtually disappeared.

In 1986, the US Public Health Service and other public health agencies recommend that persons reported to have an HTLV-III infection should be provided the following information and advice:

1. The prognosis over the long term for an individual infected with HTLV-III is not known. However, available data indicate that most persons will remain infected and about 1% will develop the disease.

2. Although asymptomatic, these individuals may transmit HTLV-III to others. Regular medical evaluation and follow-up is advised, especially for those who develop signs or symptoms suggestive of AIDS.

3. Infected persons should refrain from donating blood, plasma, body organs, other tissue, or sperm.

4. There is a risk of infecting others by sexual intercourse, by sharing of needles, and possibly by saliva through oral-genital contact or intimate kissing. The efficacy of condoms in preventing infection with HTLV-III is unproved, but consistent use of condoms may reduce transmission of the virus.

5. Toothbrushes, razors, or other implements that could become contaminated with blood should not be shared.

6. Seropositive women or women with seropositive sexual partners are themselves at increased risk of acquiring AIDS. If they become pregnant, their offspring also are at increased risk of acquiring AIDS.

7. After accidents that result in bleeding, contaminated surfaces should be cleaned with household bleach freshly diluted 1:10 in water.

8. Devices that have punctured the skin, eg, hypodermic and acupuncture needles, should be steam sterilized by autoclaving before reuse or should be safely discarded. Whenever possible, disposable needles and equipment should be used.

9. When seeking medical or dental care for intercurrent illness, infected persons should inform those responsible for their care that they are seropositive, so that appropriate evaluation can be undertaken and precautions taken to prevent transmission to others.

10. Testing for HTLV-III antibody should be offered to persons who may have been infected as a result of their contact with seropositive individuals (eg, sexual partners, persons with whom needles have been shared, infants born to seropositive mothers).

11. Most persons with a positive test for HTLV-III do not need to consider a change in employment unless their work involves significant potential for exposing others to their blood or other body fluids. There is no evidence of virus transmission by food handling.

12. Seropositive persons in the health care professions who perform invasive procedures or have skin lesions should take precautions similar to those recom-

mended for hepatitis B carriers to protect patients from the risk of infection.

13. Children with positive tests should be allowed to attend school, since casual person-to-person contact of school children poses no risk. However, a more restricted environment is advisable for preschool children or children who lack control of their body secretions, display biting behavior, or have oozing lesions.

REFERENCES

Broder S (editor): Symposium on HTLV. *Cancer Res* 1985;**45 (Suppl):**4519s.

Brun-Vezinet F et al: The possible role of a new lymphotropic retrovirus (LAV) in the pathogeny of AIDS and AIDS-related diseases. *Prog Med Virol* 1985;**32:**189.

Cooper DA et al: Acute AIDS retrovirus infection: Definition of a clinical illness associated with seroconversion. *Lancet* 1985;**1:**537.

Feorino PM et al: Transfusion-associated acquired immunodeficiency syndrome: Evidence for persistent infection in blood donors. *N Engl J Med* 1985;**312:**1293.

Fisher AG et al: A molecular clone of HTLV-III with biological activity. *Nature* 1985;**316:**262.

Gallo RC et al: Frequent detection and isolation of cytopathic retroviruses (HTLV-III) from patients with AIDS and at risk for AIDS. *Science* 1984;**224:**500.

Hirsch MS et al: Risk of nosocomial infection with human T-cell lymphotropic virus III (HTLV-III). *N Engl J Med* 1985;**312:**1.

Jaffe HW et al: Infection with HTLV-III/LAV and transfusion-associated acquired immunodeficiency syndrome: Serologic evidence of an association. *JAMA* 1985;**254:**770.

Johnson RE et al: Acquired immunodeficiency syndrome among patients attending hemophilia treatment centers and mortality experience of hemophiliacs in the United States. *Am J Epidemiol* 1985;**121:**797.

Kaminsky LS et al: High prevalence of antibodies to acquired immune deficiency syndrome (AIDS)-associated retrovirus (ARV) in AIDS and related conditions but not in other disease states. *Proc Natl Acad Sci USA* 1985;**82:**5535.

Landesman SH, Ginzburg HM, Weiss SH: The AIDS epidemic. *N Engl J Med* 1985;**312:**521.

Laurence J et al: Lymphadenopathy-associated viral antibody in AIDS. *N Engl J Med* 1984;**311:**1269.

Melnick JL, Ochoa S, Oró J (editors): Viruses, oncogenes and cancer. *Prog Med Virol* 1985;**32:**1.

Moss AR et al: Incidence of the acquired immunodeficiency syndrome in San Francisco, 1980–1983. *J Infect Dis* 1985;**152:**152.

Rabson AB, Martin MA: Molecular organization of the AIDS retrovirus. *Cell* 1985;**40:**477.

Salahuddin SZ et al: Isolation of infectious human T-cell leukemia/lymphotropic virus type III (HTLV-III) from patients with acquired immunodeficiency syndrome (AIDS) or AIDS-related complex (ARC) and from healthy carriers: A study of risk groups and tissue sources. *Proc Natl Acad Sci USA* 1985;**82:**5530.

Weiss RA et al: Neutralization of human T-lymphotropic virus type III by sera of AIDS and AIDS-risk patients. *Nature* 1985;**316:**69.

Weiss SH et al: Screening test for HTLV-III antibodies: Specificity, sensitivity, and applications. *JAMA* 1985;**253:**221.

Wong-Staal F et al: Genomic diversity of human T-lymphotropic virus type III (HTLV-III). *Science* 1985;**229:**759.

Medical Parasitology

48

Donald Heyneman, PhD*

Although all of the medically significant microorganisms considered in this *Review* are parasitic in their human hosts, the biomedical discipline of **parasitology** has traditionally been concerned only with the parasitic protozoa, helminths, and arthropods. This chapter offers a brief survey of the protozoan and helminthic parasites of medical importance. The text is supplemented by tabular materials and illustrations.[†] The following books and articles are recommended for reference:

Ash LR, Orihel TC: *Atlas of Human Parasitology,* 2nd ed. American Society of Clinical Pathologists, 1984.

Barrett J: *Biochemistry of Parasitic Helminths.* University Park Press, 1981.

Beaver PC, Jung RC, Cupp EW: *Clinical Parasitology,* 9th ed. Lea & Febiger, 1984.

Brown HW, Neva FA: *Basic Clinical Parasitology,* 5th ed. Appleton-Century-Crofts, 1982.

Bruce-Chwatt LJ: *Essential Malariology.* Heinemann, 1980.

Cohen S, Warren KS (editors): *Immunology of Parasitic Infections,* 2nd ed. Blackwell, 1982.

Desowitz RS: *Ova and Parasites: Medical Parasitology for the Laboratory Technologist.* Harper & Row, 1980.

Drugs for parasitic infections. *Med Lett Drugs Ther* 1984;**26:**27.

Garcia LS, Ash LR: *Diagnostic Parasitology: Clinical Laboratory Manual,* 2nd ed. Mosby, 1979.

Goldsmith RS: Infectious diseases: Protozoal (Chapter 25) and Infectious diseases: Helminthic (Chapter 26) in: *Current Medical Diagnosis & Treatment 1986.* Krupp MA, Chatton MJ, Tierney LM Jr (editors). Lange, 1986.

Harwood RF, James MT: *Entomology in Human and Animal Health,* 7th ed. Macmillan, 1979.

Hunter GW III, Swartzwelder JC, Clyde DF: *Tropical Medicine,* 6th ed. Saunders, 1984.

Maegraith B: *Adams & Maegraith Clinical Tropical Diseases,* 8th ed. Blackwell, 1984.

Manson-Bahr PEC, Apted FIC: *Manson's Tropical Diseases,* 18th ed. Ballière Tindall, 1982.

Markell EK, Voge M: *Medical Parasitology,* 5th ed. Saunders, 1981.

Melvin DM, Brooke MM: *Laboratory Procedures for the Diagnosis of Intestinal Parasites,* revised 1974. Centers for Disease Control, US Department of Health & Human Services Publication No. (CDC) 79-8282, 1979.

Reeder MM, Palmer PES: *The Radiology of Tropical Disease With Epidemiological, Pathological and Clinical Correlation.* Williams & Wilkins, 1980.

*Professor of Parasitology, Department of Epidemiology and International Health, University of California, San Francisco.
[†]The illustrations on pp 561–571 are by P.H. Vercammen-Grandjean, DSc.

Schmidt GD, Roberts LS: *Foundations of Parasitology,* 3rd ed. Mosby, 1985.

Strickland GT: *Hunter's Tropical Medicine,* 6th ed. Saunders, 1984.

VonBrand T: *Biochemistry and Physiology of Endoparasites.* Elsevier/North Holland, 1979.

Wakelin D: *Immunity to Parasites: How Animals Control Parasite Infections.* Arnold, 1984.

Warren KS, Mahmoud AAF (editors): *Geographic Medicine for the Practitioner: Algorithms in the Diagnosis and Management of Exotic Diseases.* Univ of Chicago Press, 1978.

Warren KS, Mahmoud AAF (editors): *Tropical and Geographical Medicine.* McGraw-Hill, 1984.

Yamaguchi T (editor): *Color Atlas of Clinical Parasitology.* Lea & Febiger, 1981.

CLASSIFICATION

The parasites of humans in the kingdom *Protozoa* are now classified under 3 phyla. *Sarcomastigophora* (containing the flagellates and amebas); *Apicomplexa* (containing the sporozoans); and *Ciliophora* (containing the ciliates). Within these great assemblages are found the important human parasites. Illustrations of parasitic protozoa can be found on pp 561–564.

(1) *Mastigophora,* the flagellates, have one or more whiplike flagella and, in some cases, an undulating membrane (eg, trypanosomes). These include intestinal and genitourinary flagellates *(Giardia, Trichomonas, Retortamonas, Dientamoeba, Enteromonas, Chilomastix)* and blood and tissue flagellates *(Trypanosoma, Leishmania).*

(2) *Sarcodina* are typically ameboid and are represented in humans by species of *Entamoeba, Endolimax, Iodamoeba, Naegleria,* and *Acanthamoeba.*

(3) *Sporozoasida* undergo a complex life cycle with alternating sexual and asexual reproductive phases, usually involving 2 different hosts (eg, arthropod and vertebrate, as in the blood forms). The subclass *Coccidia* contains the human parasites *Isospora, Toxoplasma,* and others. Among the *Haemospororina* (blood sporozoans) are the malarial parasites (*Plasmodium* species) and the subclass *Piroplasmasina,* which includes *Babesia* species.

(4) *Ciliophora* are complex protozoa bearing cilia distributed in rows or patches, with 2 kinds of nuclei in each individual. *Balantidium coli,* a giant intestinal ciliate of humans and pigs, is the only human parasite representative of this group.

The parasitic worms, or helminths, of human beings belong to 2 phyla:

(1) **Platyhelminthes** (flatworms) lack a true body cavity (celom) and are characteristically flat in dorsoventral section. All medically important species belong to the classes **Cestoda** (tapeworms) and **Trematoda** (flukes). The tapeworms are bandlike and segmented; the flukes are typically leaf-shaped; and the schistosomes are elongate. The important tissue and intestinal cestodes of humans belong to the genera *Diphyllobothrium, Spirometra, Taenia, Echinococcus, Hymenolepis,* and *Dipylidium*. Medically important trematode genera include *Schistosoma, Paragonimus, Clonorchis, Opisthorchis, Heterophyes, Metagonimus, Fasciolopsis,* and *Fasciola*.

(2) **Nemathelminthes** (wormlike, unsegmented roundworms) include many parasitic species that infect humans.

These are listed in Table 48–4 together with the other parasitic helminths. An essential procedure in diagnosis of many helminthic infections is microscopic recognition of ova or larvae in feces, urine, blood, or tissues. Illustrations of diagnostically important stages can be found on pp 565–571; important characteristics are listed in Table 48–5.

GIARDIA LAMBLIA

Giardia lamblia, a flagellate, is the only common protozoan found in the duodenum and jejunum of humans. It is the cause of giardiasis.

Morphology & Identification

A. Typical Organisms: The trophozoite of *G lamblia* is a heart-shaped, symmetric organism 10–18 μm in length. There are 4 pairs of flagella, 2 nuclei with prominent central karyosomes, and 2 axostyles. A large concave sucking disk in the anterior portion occupies much of the ventral surface. The swaying or dancing motion of *Giardia* trophozoites in fresh preparations is unmistakable. As the parasites pass into the colon, they typically encyst. Cysts are found in the stool—often in enormous numbers. These cysts, 8–14 μm in length, are ellipsoid and thick-walled and contain 2–4 nuclei.

B. Culture: This organism has not been cultivated for prolonged periods on artificial media.

Pathogenesis & Clinical Findings

G lamblia is usually only weakly pathogenic for humans. Cysts may be found in large numbers in the stools of entirely asymptomatic persons. In some persons, however, large numbers of parasites attached to the bowel wall may cause irritation and low-grade inflammation of the duodenal or jejunal mucosa, with consequent acute or chronic diarrhea. The stools may be watery, semisolid, greasy, bulky, and foul-smelling at various times during the course of the infection. Malaise, weakness, weight loss, abdominal cramps, distention, and flatulence can occur. Children are more liable to clinical giardiasis than adults. Immunosuppressed individuals are especially liable to massive infection with severe clinical manifestations. Symptoms may continue for long periods.

Diagnostic Laboratory Tests

Diagnosis depends upon finding the distinctive cysts in formed stools, or cysts and trophozoites in liquid stools. Examination of the duodenal contents may be necessary to establish the diagnosis. Duodenal aspiration or use of the duodenal capsule technique (Entero-Test) is often superior to fecal examination for diagnosis.

Treatment

Oral quinacrine hydrochloride (Atabrine) will cure about 90% of *G lamblia* infections. Metronidazole (Flagyl) and furazolidone (Furoxone) are alternatives. Tinidazole (Fasigyn), used for 1-day treatment, is widely used but is not available in the USA. Treatment may be repeated if necessary. Only symptomatic patients require treatment.

Epidemiology

G lamblia occurs worldwide. Humans are infected by ingestion of fecally contaminated water or food containing *Giardia* cysts or by direct fecal contamination, as may occur in day-care centers for children, refugee camps, or jails. Epidemic outbreaks have been reported at ski resorts in the USA where overloading of sewage facilities or contamination of the water supply has resulted in sudden outbreaks of giardiasis. Outbreaks among campers in wilderness areas suggest that humans may be infected with various animal *Giardia* species harbored by rodents, deer, cattle, sheep, horses, or household pets. This suggests that human infection can also be a zoonosis.

TRICHOMONAS

The trichomonads are flagellate protozoa with 3–5 anterior flagella, other organelles, and an undulating membrane. *Trichomonas vaginalis* causes trichomoniasis in humans.

Morphology & Identification

A. Typical Organisms: *T vaginalis* is pear-shaped, with a short undulating membrane lined with a flagellum, and has 4 anterior flagella. It measures 15–30 μm in length. The organism moves with a characteristic wobbling and rotating motion. The nonpathogenic trichomonads, *Trichomonas hominis* and *Trichomonas tenax,* cannot readily be distinguished from *T vaginalis* when alive. When fixed and stained, *T tenax* measures 6–10 μm in length. *T hominis* measures 8–12 μm and bears 5 anterior flagella and a long undulating membrane. For all practical purposes, trichomonads found in the mouth are *T tenax;* in the intestine, *T hominis;* and in the genitourinary tract (both sexes), *T vaginalis*.

B. Culture: *T vaginalis* may be cultivated in many solid and fluid cell-free media, in tissue cultures, and in the chick embryo, but it requires more complex media, eg, CPLM (cysteine-peptone-liver-maltose) medium, for optimal growth. Simplified trypticase serum is usually used for semen cultures.

C. Growth Requirements: *T vaginalis* grows best at 35–37 °C under anaerobic conditions, less well aerobically. The optimal pH for growth in vitro (5.5–6.0) suggests why vaginal trichomoniasis is more severe in women with abnormally low vaginal acidity.

Pathogenesis, Pathology, & Clinical Findings

T hominis and *T tenax* are generally considered to be harmless commensals. *T vaginalis* is capable of causing low-grade inflammation. The intensity of infection, the pH and physiologic status of the vaginal and other genitourinary tract surfaces, and the accompanying bacterial flora are among the factors affecting pathogenicity. The organisms do not survive at normal vaginal acidity of pH 3.8–4.4.

In females, the infection is normally limited to vulva, vagina, and cervix; it does not usually extend to the uterus. The mucosal surfaces may be tender, inflamed, eroded, and covered with a frothy yellow or cream-colored discharge. In males, the prostate, seminal vesicles, and urethra may be infected. Signs and symptoms in females, in addition to profuse vaginal discharge, include local tenderness, vulval pruritus, and burning. About 10% of infected males have a thin, white urethral discharge.

Diagnostic Laboratory Tests

A. Specimens and Microscopic Examination: Vaginal or urethral secretions or discharge should be examined microscopically in a drop of saline for characteristic motile trichomonads. Dried smears may be stained with hematoxylin or other stains for later study.

B. Culture: Culture of vaginal or urethral discharge, of prostatic secretion, or of a semen specimen may reveal organisms when direct examination is negative.

Immunity

Infection confers no apparent immunity. Little is known about the immune responses to trichomonads.

Treatment

Successful treatment of vaginal infection requires destruction of the trichomonads, for which topical and systemic metronidazole (Flagyl) is best. The patient's sexual partner should be examined and treated simultaneously if necessary. Postmenopausal patients may require treatment with estrogens to improve the condition of the vaginal epithelium. Prostatic infection can be cured with certainty only by systemic treatment with metronidazole.

Epidemiology & Control

T vaginalis is a common parasite of both males and females. Infection rates vary greatly but may be quite high (40% or higher). Transmission is by sexual intercourse, but contaminated towels, douche equipment, examination instruments, and other objects may be responsible for some new infections. Infants may be infected during birth. Most infections, in both sexes, are asymptomatic or mild. Control of *T vaginalis* infections always requires simultaneous treatment of both sexual partners. Mechanical protection (condom) should be used during intercourse until the infection is eradicated in both partners.

OTHER INTESTINAL FLAGELLATES

Retortamonas intestinalis, Chilomastix mesnili, and *Enteromonas hominis* are nonpathogenic intestinal parasites of humans that must be distinguished in the laboratory from the pathogenic amebas and flagellates (see p 562).

Chilomastix mesnili

This parasite can be confused with *Trichomonas* in the laboratory. It is found throughout the world. The trophozoite is pear-shaped and resembles *Trichomonas,* but the spiral motion of the trophozoite is unlike that of *Trichomonas.* The cyst is lemon-shaped, uninucleate, and 7–10 μm long.

THE HEMOFLAGELLATES

The hemoflagellates of humans include the genera *Trypanosoma* and *Leishmania.* There are 2 distinct types of human trypanosomes: (1) African, which causes sleeping sickness and is transmitted by tsetse flies *(Glossina): Trypanosoma brucei rhodesiense* and *Trypanosoma brucei gambiense;* and (2) American, which causes Chagas' disease and is transmitted by cone-nosed bugs *(Triatoma,* etc): *Trypanosoma (Schizotrypanum) cruzi.* The genus *Leishmania,* divided into several species infecting humans, causes cutaneous (Oriental sore), mucocutaneous (espundia), and visceral (kala-azar) leishmaniasis. All of these infections are transmitted by sandflies *(Phlebotomus, Lutzomyia,* and *Psychodopygus).*

The genus *Trypanosoma* appears in the blood as trypomastigotes, with elongated bodies supporting a lateral undulating membrane and a flagellum that borders the free edge of the membrane and emerges at the anterior end as a whiplike extension (see p 564). The kinetoplast is a darkly staining body lying immediately adjacent to the tiny node (blepharoplast) from which the flagellum arises. Other developmental forms among the hemoflagellates include (1) a leishmanial rounded intracellular stage, the amastigote; (2) a flagellated extracellular stage, the promastigote, a lanceolate form without an undulating membrane, with a kinetoplast at the anterior end; and (3) an epimastigote, a more elongated extracellular stage with a short undulating membrane and a kinetoplast placed more posteriorly.

In *Leishmania* life cycles, only the amastigote and promastigote are found, the latter being restricted to the insect vector. In *T cruzi,* all 3 may occur in humans, and trypomastigote and epimastigote in the vector. In African trypanosomes, the latter 2 flagellated stages also occur in the tsetse fly vector, but only the trypomastigote in humans.

1. LEISHMANIA

The genus *Leishmania,* widely distributed in nature, has a number of species that are nearly identical morphologically. Differentiation is based on the electrophoretic mobility profile of a battery of isoenzymes (zymodeme pattern); excretory factor serotyping; kinetoplast DNA restriction analysis (schizodemes); lectin conjugation patterns on the parasite surface; use of monoclonal probes to detect specific antigens; promastigote growth patterns in vitro in the presence of antisera; developmental characteristics of promastigotes in the specific sandfly vector; vectors, reservoir hosts, and other epidemiologic factors; and the clinical characteristics of the disease produced. Visceral leishmaniasis results from infection with members of the *Leishmania donovani* complex, which includes many different species and subspecies that are often found in limited geographic areas. The New World forms are all carried by sandflies of the genera *Lutzomyia* and *Psychodopygus;* Old World leishmanias are transmitted by sandflies of the genus *Phlebotomus.* The different leishmanias present a range of clinical and epidemiologic characteristics that, for convenience only, are combined under 3 clinical groupings: (1) visceral leishmaniasis (kala-azar), (2) cutaneous leishmaniasis (Oriental sore, Baghdad boil, wet cutaneous sore, dry cutaneous sore, chiclero ulcer, uta, and other names), and (3) mucocutaneous or naso-oral leishmaniasis (espundia). However, some species can induce several disease syndromes, and the same clinical condition can be caused by different agents.

Morphology & Identification

A. Typical Organism: Only the nonflagellated amastigote (Leishman-Donovan or LD body; see p 563) occurs in mammals. The sandfly transmits the infective promastigotes by bite. The promastigotes rapidly change to amastigotes after phagocytosis by macrophages, then multiply, filling the cytoplasm of the macrophages. The infected cells burst, the released parasites are again phagocytosed, and the process is repeated, producing a cutaneous lesion or visceral infection depending upon the species of parasite and the host response. The amastigotes are oval, $2-6 \times 1-3$ μm, with a laterally placed oval vesicular nucleus and a dark-staining, rodlike kinetoplast.

B. Culture and Growth Characteristics: In NNN or Tobie's medium, only the promastigotes are found. *L donovani* usually grows slowly, the promastigotes forming tangled clumps in the fluid. *L tropica* grows more quickly, promastigotes forming small rosettes attached by their flagella in the fluid, produc-

ing a fine granular appearance with a distinct surface film, while *L braziliensis* may produce a waxlike surface with fewer, smaller promastigotes. In contrast, *L mexicana* produces rapid growth of large organisms in simple blood agar medium. In tissue cultures, intracellular amastigotes may occur in addition to the extracellular promastigotes.

C. Variations: There are strain differences in virulence, tissue tropism, and biologic and epidemiologic characteristics.

Pathogenesis, Pathology, & Clinical Findings

L donovani, which causes kala-azar, spreads from the site of inoculation to multiply in reticuloendothelial cells, especially macrophages in spleen, liver, lymph nodes, and bone marrow. This is accompanied by marked hyperplasia of the spleen. Progressive emaciation is accompanied by growing weakness. There is irregular fever, sometimes hectic. Untreated cases with symptoms of kala-azar usually are fatal. Some forms, especially in India, develop a postcure florid cutaneous resurgence 1–2 years later (postkala-azar dermal leishmanoid).

L tropica, L major, L mexicana, and other dermotropic forms induce a dermal lesion at the site of inoculation by the sandfly: cutaneous leishmaniasis, Oriental sore, Delhi boil, etc. Mucous membranes are rarely involved. The dermal layers are first affected, with cellular infiltration and proliferation of amastigotes intracellularly and spreading extracellularly, until the infection penetrates the epidermis and causes ulceration. Satellite lesions may be found (hypersensitivity or anergy type of cutaneous leishmaniasis) that contain few or no parasites and do not respond to treatment.

L braziliensis braziliensis causes mucocutaneous or nasopharyngeal leishmaniasis in Amazonian South America. It is known by many local names. The lesions are slow-growing but extensive (sometimes 5–10 cm). From these sites, migration appears to occur rapidly to the nasopharyngeal or palatine mucosal surfaces, where no further growth may take place for years. After months to over 20 years, relentless erosion may develop, destroying the nasal septum and surrounding regions in an often intractable, fungating, polypoid course. In such instances, death occurs from asphyxiation due to blockage of the trachea, starvation, or respiratory infection. This is the classical clinical picture of espundia, most commonly found in the Amazon basin. At high altitudes in Peru, the clinical features (uta) resemble those of Oriental sore. *L braziliensis guyanensis* infection frequently spreads along lymphatic routes, where it appears as a linear chain of nonulcerating lesions. *L mexicana* infection is more typically confined to a single, indolent, ulcerative lesion that heals in about 1 year, leaving a characteristic depressed circular scar. In Mexico and Guatemala, the ears are frequently involved (chiclero ulcer), usually with a cartilage-attacking infection without ulceration and with few parasites.

Diagnostic Laboratory Tests

A. Specimens: Lymph node aspirates, scrapings, and biopsies are important in the cutaneous forms; lymph node aspirates, blood, and spleen, liver, or bone marrow puncture are important in kala-azar. Purulent discharges are of no value for diagnosis, although nasal scrapings may be useful.

B. Microscopic Examination: Giemsa-stained smears and sections may show amastigotes, especially in material from kala-azar and under the rolled edges of cutaneous sores.

C. Culture: NNN medium is the medium most generally used. A biphasic blood agar culture, Tobie's medium, is especially suitable. Blood culture is satisfactory only for *L donovani*. Lymph node aspirates are suitable for all forms; and tissue aspirates, biopsy material, scrapings, or small biopsies from the edges of ulcers are useful for the cutaneous forms and often for kala-azar also. However, only promastigotes can be cultivated in the absence of living cells.

D. Serology: The formol-gel (aldehyde) test of Napier is a nonspecific test that detects an elevated serum globulin level in kala-azar. The IHA (indirect hemagglutination antibody) test or the IFA (indirect fluorescent antibody) test may be useful, but they lack sufficient sensitivity and may cross-react with *T cruzi*. A skin test (Montenegro test) is epidemiologically important in indicating past exposure to any of the leishmanias.

Immunity

Recovery from cutaneous leishmaniasis confers a solid and permanent immunity, although it usually is species-specific and may be strain-specific as well. Natural resistance varies greatly among individuals and with age and sex. Vaccination significantly reduces the incidence of Oriental sore.

Immunity to kala-azar may develop but varies with the time of treatment and condition of the patient.

Treatment

Single lesions may be cleaned, curetted, treated with antibiotics if secondarily infected, and then covered and left to heal. Pentavalent antimony sodium gluconate (Pentostam, Solustibosan) is the drug of choice for all forms. Pentamidine isethionate (Lomidine) is useful for kala-azar resistant to antimony sodium gluconate. Cycloguanil pamoate in oil (Camolar) and amphotericin B (Fungizone) can be used for espundia, which is frequently quite unresponsive to treatment.

Epidemiology, Prevention, & Control

Kala-azar is found focally in most tropical and subtropical countries. Its local distribution is related to the prevalence of specific sandfly vectors. In the Mediterranean littoral and in middle Asia and South America, domestic and wild canids are reservoirs, and in the Sudan, various wild carnivores and rodents are reservoirs of endemic kala-azar. Control is aimed at destroying breeding places and dogs and protecting people from sandfly bites. Oriental sore occurs mostly in the Mediterranean region, North Africa, and the Middle and Near East. The "wet" type, caused by *L major,* is rural, and burrowing rodents are the main reservoir; the dry type, caused by *L tropica,* is urban, and humans are presumably the only reservoir. For *L braziliensis,* there are a number of wild but apparently no domestic animal reservoirs. Sandfly vectors are involved in all forms.

2. TRYPANOSOMA

Hemoflagellates of the genus *Trypanosoma* occur in the blood of mammals as mature elongated trypomastigotes. A multiplying epimastigote stage precedes the formation of infective trypomastigotes in the intermediate host (an insect vector) in all species of trypanosomes that infect humans. Trypanosomiasis is expressed as African sleeping sickness, Chagas' disease, and asymptomatic trypanosomiasis in humans. The parent form in Africa is *Trypanosoma brucei,* which causes nagana in livestock and game animals; the 2 human forms are *Trypanosoma brucei rhodesiense* and *Trypanosoma brucei gambiense*. The 3 forms are indistinguishable morphologically but differ ecologically and epidemiologically.

Morphology & Identification

A. Typical Organisms: African *T b gambiense* and *T b rhodesiense* vary in size and shape of the body and length of the flagellum (usually 15–30 μm) but are essentially indistinguishable. A "stumpy" short form is infective to the insect host and possesses a full battery of enzymes for energy metabolism. The elongated form requires host metabolic assistance and is specialized for rapid multiplication in the vertebrate bloodstream. The same forms are seen in blood as in lymph node aspirates. The blood forms of American *T cruzi* are present during the early acute stage and at intervals thereafter in smaller numbers. They are typical trypomastigotes, varying about a mean of 20 μm, frequently curved in a C shape when fixed and stained. A large, rounded terminal kinetosome in stained preparations is characteristic. The tissue forms, which are most common in heart muscle, liver, and brain, develop from amastigotes that multiply to form an intracellular colony after invasion of the host cell or phagocytosis of the parasite. *Trypanosoma rangeli* of South and Central America infects humans without causing disease and must therefore be carefully distinguished from the pathogenic species (Table 48–1).

B. Culture: *T cruzi* and *T rangeli* are readily cultivated (3–6 weeks) in the epimastigote form in fluid or diphasic media. Diagnosis of patients in the early, blood-borne phase of infection can be aided by using the multiplying powers of parasites in laboratory-reared, clean vector insects (kissing, or triatomine bugs) that have been allowed to feed on patients (see Xenodiagnosis, below).

C. Growth Requirements: *T cruzi* requires at

Table 48–1. Differentiation of *T cruzi* and *T rangeli.*

	T cruzi	*T rangeli*
Blood forms Size	20 μm	Over 30 μm
Shape	Often C-shaped in fixed preparations	Rarely C-shaped
Posterior kinetoplast	Terminal, large	Distinctly sub-terminal, small
Developmental stages in tissues	Amastigote to epi-mastigote	Not found (only trypomastigotes)
Triatomine bugs In salivary gland or proboscis (or both)	Always absent	Usually present
In hindgut or feces	Present	Present

least hemin, ascorbic acid, and certain dialyzable substances present in serum. The African forms require at least these for development, but neither these nor other known substances suffice to support development to the infective trypanosomal stage. The blood of some apparently uninfected persons inhibits growth of the African species.

D. Variation: There are variations in morphology (see above), virulence, and antigenic constitution. Antigenic variation occurs in characteristic waves and is due to genetically induced changes in the surface glycoprotein coat; it is viewed as a means of continuously escaping the host's antibody response by producing different antigenic membranes.

Pathogenesis, Pathology, & Clinical Findings

Infective trypanosomes of *T b gambiense* and *T b rhodesiense* are introduced through the bite of the tsetse fly and multiply at the site of inoculation to cause variable induration and swelling (the primary lesion), which may progress to form a trypanosomal chancre. They spread to lymph nodes, bloodstream, and, in terminal stages, to the central nervous system, where they produce the typical sleeping sickness syndrome: lassitude, inability to eat, tissue wasting, unconsciousness, and death. Infective forms of *T cruzi* pass to humans by rubbing infected triatomine bug feces into the conjunctiva or a break in the skin, *not* by the bite of the bug (which is the mode of entry of the nonpathogenic *T rangeli*). At the site of *T cruzi* entry, there may be a subcutaneous inflammatory nodule or chagoma. Chagas' disease is common in infants. Unilateral swelling of the eyelids (Romaña's sign) is characteristic at onset, especially in children. The primary lesion is accompanied by fever, acute regional lymphadenitis, and dissemination to blood and tissues. The parasites can usually be detected within 1–2 weeks as trypomastigotes in the blood. Subsequent developments depend upon the organs and tissues affected and on the nature of multiplication and release of toxins. The African forms multiply extracellularly as trypomastigotes in the blood as well as in the tis-

sues. *T cruzi* multiplies mostly within reticuloendothelial cells, going through a cycle starting with large agglomerations of amastigotes. In both African and American forms, multiplication in the tissues is punctuated by phases of parasitemia with later destruction by the host of the blood forms, accompanied by bouts of intermittent fever gradually decreasing in intensity. Parasitemia is more common in *T b rhodesiense* and is intermittent and scant with *T cruzi*.

The release of toxins explains much of the systemic and local reactions. The organs most seriously affected are the central nervous system and heart muscle. Interstitial myocarditis is the most common serious element in Chagas' disease. It is least evident in chronic Gambian infection. Central nervous system involvement is most characteristic of African trypanosomiasis. *T b rhodesiense* appears in the cerebrospinal fluid in about 1 month and *T b gambiense* in several months, but both are present in small numbers. *T b gambiense* infection is chronic and leads to progressive diffuse meningoencephalitis. The more rapidly fatal *T b rhodesiense* produces somnolence and coma only during the final weeks of a terminal infection. Other organs affected are the liver, spleen, and bone marrow, especially with chronic *T cruzi* infection.

Invasion or toxic destruction of nerve plexuses in the alimentary tract walls leads to megaesophagus and megacolon, especially in Brazilian Chagas' disease. Megaesophagus and megacolon are absent in Colombian, Venezuelan, and Central American Chagas' disease. All 3 trypanosomes are transmissible through the placenta, and congenital infections occur in hyperendemic areas.

Diagnostic Laboratory Tests

A. Specimens: Blood, preferably collected when the patient's temperature rises; cerebrospinal fluid; lymph node or primary lesion aspirates; or specimens obtained by iliac crest, sternal bone marrow, or spleen puncture are used.

B. Microscopic Examination: Fresh blood (or aspirated tissue in saline) is kept warm and examined immediately for the actively motile trypanosomes. Thick films may be stained with Giemsa's stain. Thin films stained with Giemsa's stain are necessary for confirmation. Centrifugation may be necessary. Tissue smears must be stained for identification of the pretrypanosomal stages. Centrifuged cerebrospinal fluid should be similarly examined; there is seldom more than one trypanosome per milliliter. The most reliable tests are smears of blood for *T b rhodesiense*, of gland puncture specimens for *T b gambiense*, and of cerebrospinal fluid for *T b rhodesiense* and advanced *T b gambiense*.

C. Culture: Any specimens may be inoculated into Tobie's, Wenyon's semisolid, NNN, or other media for culture of *T cruzi* or *T rangeli*. The organisms are grown at 22–24 °C and subcultured every 1–2 weeks. Centrifuged material is examined microscopically for trypanosomes. Culture of the African forms is unsatisfactory.

D. Animal Inoculation: *T cruzi* and *T rangeli* may be detected by inoculating blood intraperitoneally into mice (when available, pups and kittens are animals of first choice). *T b rhodesiense* is often detectable and *T b gambiense* sometimes detectable by this procedure. Trypanosomes appear in the blood in a few days after successful inoculation.

E. Serology: A positive indirect IHA, IFA, or CF (Machado's) test provides confirmatory support in *T cruzi* infection. African forms cause IFA reactions, but these are of limited diagnostic value.

F. Xenodiagnosis: This is the method of choice in suspected Chagas' disease if other examinations are negative, especially during the early phase of disease onset. *Because laboratory infection with* T cruzi *is a distinct hazard, the test should be performed only by workers trained in the procedure.* About 6 clean laboratory-reared triatomine bugs are fed on the patient, and their droppings are examined in 7–10 days for the various developmental forms. Defecation follows shortly after a fresh meal or may be forced by gently probing the bug's anus and then squeezing its abdomen. Xenodiagnosis is impracticable for the African forms.

G. Differential Diagnosis: *T b rhodesiense* and *T b gambiense* are morphologically identical but may be distinguished by their geographic distribution, vector species, and clinical disease in humans. The differentiation of *T cruzi* from *T rangeli* (Table 48–1) is important.

Immunity

Humans show some individual variation in natural resistance to trypanosomes. Strain-specific CF and protecting antibodies can be detected in the plasma, and these presumably lead to the disappearance of blood forms. Each relapse of African trypanosomiasis is due to a strain serologically distinct from the preceding one. Apart from such relapses, Africans free from symptoms may still have trypanosomes in the blood.

Treatment

There is no effective drug treatment for American trypanosomiasis, although Bayer-2502 (nifurtimox) may temporarily relieve some patients with trypomastigotes still present in the blood. African trypanosomiasis is treated principally with suramin sodium (Germanin) or pentamidine isethionate (Lomidine). Late disease with central nervous system involvement requires melarsoprol (Mel B), as well as suramin or tryparsamide.

Epidemiology, Prevention, & Control

African trypanosomiasis is restricted to recognized tsetse fly belts. *T b gambiense*, transmitted mostly by the streamside tsetse *Glossina palpalis*, extends from west to central Africa and produces a relatively chronic infection with progressive central nervous system involvement. *T b rhodesiense*, transmitted mostly by the woodland-savannah *Glossina morsitans*, is more restricted, being confined to the south and east of

Lake Tanganyika; it causes a smaller number of cases but is more virulent. Bushbuck and other antelopes may serve as reservoirs of *T b rhodesiense*, whereas humans are the principal reservoir of *T b gambiense*. Control depends upon searching for and then isolating and treating patients with the disease; controlling movement of people in and out of fly belts; using insecticides in vehicles; and instituting fly control, principally with aerial insecticides and by altering habitats. Contact with reservoir animals is difficult to control.

Chemoprophylaxis, eg, with suramin sodium, is difficult and short-lived.

American trypanosomiasis (Chagas' disease) is especially important in Central and South America, although infection of animals extends much more widely. A few autochthonous human cases have been reported in Texas. Certain triatomine bugs become as domiciliated as bedbugs, and infection may be brought in by rats, opossums, or armadillos—which may spread the infection to domestic animals. Since no effective treatment is known, it is particularly important to control the vectors with residual insecticides and habitat destruction and to avoid contact with animal reservoirs. Chagas' disease occurs largely among people in poor economic circumstances. An estimated 8 million persons harbor the parasite, and many of these sustain heart damage, with the result that their ability to work and their life expectancy are sharply reduced.

ENTAMOEBA HISTOLYTICA

Entamoeba histolytica is a common parasite in the large intestine of humans, certain other primates, and some other animals. Many cases are asymptomatic except in humans or among animals living under stress (eg, zoo-held primates).

Morphology & Identification

A. Typical Organisms: Three stages are encountered: the active ameba, the inactive cyst, and the intermediate precyst. The ameboid trophozoite is the only form present in tissues. It is also found in fluid feces during amebic dysentery. Its size is 15–30 μm. The cytoplasm is granular and may contain red cells (pathognomonic) but ordinarily contains no bacteria. Iron-hematoxylin or Gomori's trichrome staining shows the nuclear membrane to be lined by fine, regular granules of chromatin. Movement of trophozoites in fresh material is brisk and unidirectional. Pseudopodia are fingerlike and broad.

Cysts are present only in the lumen of the colon and in mushy or formed feces. Subspherical cysts of pathogenic amebas range from 10 to 20 μm. Smaller cysts ranging down to 3.5 μm are considered nonpathogenic *Entamoeba hartmanni*. The cyst wall, 0.5 μm thick, is hyaline. The initial uninucleate cyst may contain a glycogen vacuole and chromatoidal bodies with characteristic rounded ends (in contrast to splinter chromatoidals in developing cysts of *Entamoeba coli*). Nuclear division within the cyst produces the final quadrinucleate cyst, during which time the chromatoid bodies and glycogen vacuoles disappear. Diagnosis in most cases rests on the characteristics of the cyst, since trophozoites (see p 561) usually appear only in diarrheic feces in active cases and survive for only a few hours, though they may be excellently preserved in polyvinyl alcohol (PVA). Stools may contain cysts with 1–4 nuclei depending on their degree of maturation. (See Keys on pp 548–549.)

B. Culture: Trophozoites are readily studied in cultures; both encystation and excystation can be controlled.

C. Growth Requirements: Growth is most vigorous in various rich complex media or cell culture under partial anaerobiosis at 37 °C and pH 7.0—with a mixed flora or at least a single coexisting species.

D. Variation: Variations in cyst size are due to nutritional differences or to the presence of the small nonpathogenic form, *E hartmanni*.

Pathogenesis, Pathology, & Clinical Findings

The trophozoites multiply by binary fission. The trophozoite emerges from the ingested cyst (metacyst) after activation of the excystation process in the stomach and duodenum. The metacyst divides rapidly, producing 4 amebulae (one for each cyst nucleus), each of which divides again to produce 8 small trophozoites per infective cyst. These pass to the cecum and produce a population of lumen-dwelling trophozoites. Disease results (in about 10% of infections) when the trophozoites invade the intestinal epithelium. Mucosal invasion by amebas with the aid of proteolytic enzymes occurs through the crypts of Lieberkühn, forming discrete ulcers with a pinhead-sized center and raised edges, from which mucus, necrotic cells, and amebas pass. Pathologic changes are always induced by trophozoites; *E histolytica* cysts are not produced in tissues. The mucosal surface between ulcers typically is normal. Amebas multiply rapidly and accumulate above the muscularis mucosae, often spreading laterally. Healing may occur spontaneously with little tissue erosion if regeneration proceeds more rapidly than destruction, or the amebic trophozoites may break through the muscularis into the submucosa. Rapid lateral spread of the multiplying amebas follows, undermining the mucosa and producing the characteristic "flask-shaped" ulcer of primary amebiasis: a small point of entry, leading via a narrow neck through the mucosa into an expanded necrotic area in the submucosa. Bacterial invasion usually does not occur at this time, cellular reaction is limited, and damage is by lytic necrosis. Subsequent spread may coalesce colonies of amebas, undermining large areas of the mucosal surface. Trophozoites may penetrate the muscular coats and occasionally the serosa, leading to perforation into the peritoneal cavity. Subsequent enlargement of the necrotic area produces gross changes in the ulcer, which may develop shaggy overhanging edges, secondary bacterial invasion, and accumulation of neutrophilic leukocytes. Secondary intestinal lesions may develop as extensions from the primary lesion (usually in the cecum, appendix, or nearby portion of the ascending colon). The organisms may travel to the ileocecal valve and terminal ileum, producing a chronic infection. The sigmoid colon and rectum are favored sites for these later lesions. An amebic inflammatory or granulomatous tumor-like mass (ameboma) may form on the intestinal wall.

Factors that determine invasion of amebas include the number of amebas ingested, pathogenic capacity of the parasite strain, host factors such as gut motility and immune competence, and the presence of suitable enteric bacteria that enhance amebic growth. Most infected persons are not diseased but harbor only lumen-dwelling amebas that form cysts passed in the feces. Trophozoites, especially with red cells in the cytoplasm, found in liquid or semiformed stools are pathognomonic. Formed stools usually contain cysts only, while patients with active disease and liquid stools (flecked with blood and mucus strands containing numerous amebas) usually pass trophozoites only. Symptoms vary greatly depending upon the site and intensity of lesions. Extreme abdominal tenderness, fulminating dysentery, dehydration, and incapacitation occur in serious disease. In less acute disease, onset of symptoms is usually gradual, with episodes of diarrhea, abdominal cramps, nausea and vomiting, and an urgent desire to defecate. More frequently, there will be weeks of cramps and general discomfort, loss of appetite, and weight loss with general malaise. Symptoms may develop within 4 days of exposure, may occur up to a year later, or may never occur. However, a change in host resistance, malnutrition (especially protein deficiency), or immunosuppression predisposes asymptomatic carriers to develop the full syndrome.

Extraintestinal infection is metastatic and rarely occurs by direct extension from the bowel. By far the most common form is amebic hepatitis or liver abscess (4% or more of clinical infections), which is assumed to be due to microemboli, including trophozoites carried through the portal circulation. It is assumed that hepatic microembolism with trophozoites is a common accompaniment of bowel lesions but that these diffuse focal lesions rarely progress. A true amebic abscess is progressive, nonsuppurative (unless secondarily infected), and destructive without compression and formation of a wall. The contents are necrotic and bacteriologically sterile, active amebas being confined to the walls. A characteristic "anchovy paste" is produced in the abscess and seen on surgical drainage. More than half of patients with amebic liver abscess give no history of intestinal infection, and only one-eighth of them pass cysts in their stools. Rarely, amebic abscesses also occur elsewhere (eg, lung, brain, spleen, or draining through the body wall). Any organ or tissue in contact with active trophozoites may become a site of invasion and abscess.

Diagnostic Laboratory Tests

A. Specimens:

1. Fluid feces–

a. Fresh and warm for immediate examination for trophozoites.

b. Preserved in polyvinyl alcohol (PVA) or Merthiolate-iodine-formalin (MIF) fixative for mailing to a diagnostic laboratory (in a waterproofed or double mailing tube, the inner one of metal).

c. After a saline purge (or high enema after saline purge) for cysts and trophozoites.

2. Formed feces for cysts.

3. Scrapings and biopsies obtained through a sigmoidoscope.

4. Liver abscess aspirates collected from the edge of the abscess, not the necrotic center. Viscous aspirates should be treated with a liquifying enzyme such as streptodornase, then cultured or examined microscopically (see Beaver, Jung, & Cupp, 1984).

5. Blood for serologic tests and cell counts.

B. Microscopic Examination:

If possible, always examine fresh warm feces for trophozoites if the patient is symptomatic and has diarrheic stools. Otherwise, stain smears with trichrome or iron-hematoxylin stain. The stools in amebic dysentery can usually be distinguished from those in bacillary dysentery: the former contain much fecal debris, small amounts of blood with strings of nontenacious mucus and degenerated red cells, few polymorphonuclear cells or macrophages, scattered Charcot-Leyden crystals, and trophozoites. Although considerable experience is required to distinguish *E histolytica* from commensal amebas (see below and pp 561–562), it is necessary to do so because misdiagnosis often leads to unnecessary treatment, overtreatment, or a failure to treat.

Differentiation of *E histolytica* (H) and *E coli* (C), the most common other intestinal ameba, can be made in stained smears as follows:

1. Trophozoites–The cytoplasm in H is glassy and contains only red cells and spherical vacuoles. The cytoplasm in C is granular, with many bacterial and other inclusions and ellipsoid vacuoles. The nucleus of H has a very small central endosome and fine regular chromatin granules lining the periphery; the nucleus of C has a larger, eccentric endosome, and the peripheral chromatin is more coarsely beaded and less evenly distributed around the nuclear membrane. Moribund trophozoites and precysts of H and C are usually indistinguishable.

2. Cysts–Glycogen vacuoles disappear during successive divisions. Nuclei resemble those of the trophozoites. Rare cysts of H and C may have 8 and 16 nuclei, respectively. Cysts of H in many preparations contain many uninucleate early cysts; these are rarely seen with C. Binucleate developing cysts of C often show the nuclei pushed against the cell wall by the large central glycogen vacuole. Chromatoidal bodies in early cysts of H are blunt-ended bars; those of C are splinterlike and often occur in clusters.

C. Culture: Diagnostic cultures are made in a layer of fluid overlying a solid nutrient base in partial anaerobiosis. Dobell's diphasic and Cleveland-Collier media are most often used.

D. Serology: The CF test is not always satisfactory, because a good and highly specific antigen is not available. The IHA test is now used routinely and is of value when stool examinations are negative, as in extraintestinal amebiasis. Commercially available preparations employ the latex agglutination technique (Serameba); Ouchterlony double diffusion (ParaTek); and counterelectrophoresis (Amoebogen). Positive responses to several tests are of value in supporting a tentative diagnosis in doubtful cases of extraintestinal amebiasis.

Treatment

Metronidazole (Flagyl) is probably a drug of choice even though it is mutagenic in bacteria. Owing to varying cure rates when depending upon single-drug therapy and to the danger of undetected liver infections, the following combined drug therapy is currently recommended for symptomatic cases: (1) For mild to moderate intestinal disease: metronidazole plus diloxanide furoate or diiodohydroxyquin; *or* paromomycin followed by chloroquine; *or* diloxanide furoate or diiodohydroxyquin plus a tetracycline followed by chloroquine; (2) For severe intestinal disease (amebic dysentery): dehydroemetine (or emetine), oxytetracycline, and diloxanide furoate, followed by chloroquine; *or* metronidazole followed by diloxanide furoate. (3) For hepatic or other extraintestinal involvement, or for ameboma: metronidazole followed by diloxanide furoate, plus chloroquine; *or* dehydroemetine (or emetine) plus chloroquine and diloxanide furoate.

Epidemiology, Prevention, & Control

Cysts are usually ingested through contaminated water. In the tropics, contaminated vegetables and food are also important cyst sources; flies have been incriminated in areas of fecal pollution. Asymptomatic cyst passers are the main source of contamination and may be responsible for severe epidemic outbreaks where sewage leaks into the water supply or breakdown of sanitary discipline occurs (as in mental, geriatric, or children's institutions). A high-carbohydrate, low-protein diet favors the development of amebic dysentery both in experimental animals and in known human cases. Control measures consist of improving environmental and food sanitation. Treatment of carriers is controversial, although it is agreed that they should be barred from food handling. The danger of transformation from an asymptomatic lumen infection to an invasive tissue disease as well as possible environmental contamination should be considered in the treatment decision for an asymptomatic cyst passer. No fully satisfactory and safe drug is yet available for chemoprophylaxis, and the mix of drugs required for therapy attests to the problems of treating amebiasis.

OTHER INTESTINAL AMEBAS

Entamoeba histolytica must be distinguished from 4 other amebalike organisms that are also intestinal parasites of humans: (1) *Entamoeba coli,* which is very common; (2) *Dientamoeba fragilis,* the only intestinal parasite other than *E histolytica* that has been suspected of causing diarrhea and dyspepsia, but not by invasion; (3) *Iodamoeba bütschlii;* and (4) *Endolimax nana.* These organisms and their cysts are shown on pp 561–562. To facilitate detection, cysts should be concentrated by zinc sulfate flotation or a similar technique. Unstained, trichrome- or iron-hematoxylin-stained, and iodine-stained preparations should be searched systematically. Mixed infections may occur. Polyvinyl alcohol (PVA) fixation is especially valuable for preservation of trophozoites. The presence of nonpathogenic amebas is strongly indicative of poor sanitation or of accidental fecal contamination—both warnings of possible exposure to pathogenic *E histolytica*—or a possible pre-AIDS immunodeficient state (see Chapter 47).

Key for Identification of Amebic Trophozoites

If stools are liquid, examine a fresh, warm sample (within 30–60 minutes), or, if this is impracticable, one that has been promptly preserved while still fresh and warm. Include exudate and flecks of mucus in the specimen.

(1) If all trophozoites have one nucleus, see paragraph (2), below.

If more than half of trophozoites have 2 nuclei, the organism is

Dientamoeba fragilis–a small (mostly 5–15 μm), rounded, amebalike organism with nuclei containing a large chromatin mass in a clear space; no peripheral chromatin and no cysts. The prevalence of *D fragilis* is sometimes high in institutional populations.

(2) If nucleus has peripheral granules, see paragraph (3), below.

If the nucleus has no peripheral granules, has an endosome larger than the radius of the nucleus, and is surrounded by large light granules, the organism is

Iodamoeba bütschlii–an ameba with a characteristic cyst (see below). Its prevalence is usually very low.

(3) If the peripheral granules of the nucleus are regularly arranged and the endosome is small, see paragraph (4), below.

If the peripheral granules are scattered and scarce and the endosome is irregular and much larger than the radius of the nucleus, the organism is

Endolimax nana–a small organism that may be present in 15–20% of some populations.

(4) If the cytoplasm is not coarsely granular, nuclei are always invisible in saline preparations, trophozoites move steadily and in one direction by streaming into blunt pseudopods, and some contain erythrocytes undergoing digestion but not bacteria; or if in a trichrome-stained preparation the nuclear membrane is delicate and lined with a single layer of fine chromatin granules and the karyosome is minute and central, the organism is either

Entamoeba histolytica–The pathogenic trophozoites are present only in diarrheal fluid feces and are usually large (20–60 μm). (*Do not confuse with macrophages containing erythrocytes;* these may also contain bacteria, and they do not progress in one direction with single blunt pseudopods.) Verify identification by examining a series of stool specimens and searching for identifiable cysts. Pathogenic trophozoites are most often found in flecks of mucoid exudate.

or

Entamoeba hartmanni–nonpathogenic and present in fluid or formed feces, always small (8–12 μm). See Cysts, below.

If the cytoplasm is coarsely granular, nuclei are sometimes visible in saline preparation, trophozoites do not move progressively but protrude pseudopods in several directions simultaneously, and the cytoplasm contains bacteria but not erythrocytes; or if in trichrome preparations, the nuclear membrane is distinct and lined with large and irregular chromatin granules; or if larger than 15 μm, the organism is

Entamoeba coli–a normal commensal that may be almost impossible to differentiate from *E histolytica* in a fluid stool, except in the cystic state (see below).

Key for Identification of Amebic Cysts

No cysts are known for *Dientamoeba fragilis.*

(1) If mature cysts have 4 nuclei, see paragraph (2), below.

If mature cysts are often irregularly shaped, have 1–2 large nuclei with a large eccentric karyosome and an adjoining cluster of granules and a large iodine-staining vacuole, the organism is

Iodamoeba bütschlii.

If mature cysts have 8 nuclei, the organism is

Entamoeba coli.

(2) If quadrinucleate cysts are oval or ellipsoid and the nuclei have distinct large chromatin masses, the organism is

Endolimax nana.

If the cysts are spherical and the nuclei have regular peripheral chromatin granules and a small karyosome, the organism is

Entamoeba histolytica or *Entamoeba hartmanni* (mean diameters respectively above and below 10 μm).

FREE-LIVING AMEBAS

Primary amebic meningoencephalitis occurs in Europe and North America from amebic invasion of the brain. The free-living soil amebas *Naegleria fowleri, Acanthamoeba castellani,* and *Hartmanella* species have been implicated. Most cases have developed in children who were swimming in warm, soil-contaminated pools, either indoors or—usually—outdoors. The amebas apparently enter via the nose and the cribriform plate of the ethmoid, passing directly into brain tissue, where they rapidly form nests of amebas that cause extensive hemorrhage and damage, chiefly in the basilar portions of the cerebrum and the cerebellum. In most cases, death ensued in less than a week. Entry of *Acanthamoeba* into the central nervous system from skin ulcers has also been reported. Diagnosis is by microscopic examination of the cerebrospinal fluid, which contains the trophozoites and red cells but no bacteria. Amebas can be readily cultured on nonnutrient agar plates seeded with *Escherichia coli*. These soil amebas are distinguished by a large, distinct nucleus; by the presence of contractile vacuoles and mitochondria (absent in *Entamoeba*); and by cysts that have a single nucleus and lack glycogen or chromatoidal bodies. *Acanthamoeba* may encyst in invaded tissues, whereas *Naegleria* does not. Treatment with amphotericin B has been successful in a few cases, chiefly when diagnosis can be made quickly.

THE PLASMODIA

The sporozoan protozoa of the genus *Plasmodium* are pigment-producing ameboid intracellular parasites of vertebrates, with one habitat in red cells and another in cells of other tissues. Transmission to humans is by the bloodsucking bite of female *Anopheles* mosquitoes of various species.

Morphology & Identification

A. Typical Organisms: At least 5 species of plasmodia may infect humans: *Plasmodium vivax, Plasmodium ovale, Plasmodium malariae, Plasmodium falciparum,* and *Plasmodium knowlesi.* Natural transmission of *P knowlesi* to humans has only been demonstrated in Malaysia. The morphology and certain other characteristics of the 4 principal species that infect humans are summarized in Table 48–2 and illustrated on p 564. *P knowlesi* is morphologically distinct from the other species and is unique in having a 24-hour erythrocytic cycle.

B. Culture: Human malaria parasites have been successfully cultivated in fluid media containing serum, erythrocytes, inorganic salts, and various growth factors and amino acids. Continuous cultivation of the erythrocytic phase undergoing schizogony (asexual multiple division) has been achieved.

C. Growth Characteristics and Requirements: In host red cells, the parasites convert hemoglobin to globin and hematin, which becomes modified into the characteristic malarial pigment. Globin is split by proteolytic enzymes and digested. Oxygen, dextrose, lactose, and erythrocytic protein are also utilized. Growth requirements, in addition to carbohydrates, proteins, and fats, include methionine, riboflavin, ascorbic acid, pantothenic acid, and *p*-aminobenzoic acid.

D. Variation: Variations of strains exist within each of the 4 typical species that infect humans. Variations have been detected in morphology, pathogenicity, resistance to drug therapy, infectivity for mosquitoes, and other characteristics.

Pathogenesis, Pathology & Clinical Findings

Human infection results from the bite of an infected female *Anopheles* mosquito, in which occurs the sexual or sporogonic cycle of development (production of infective sporozoites). The first stage of development in humans takes place in parenchymal cells of the liver (the exoerythrocytic cycle), after which numerous asexual progeny, the merozoites, leave the ruptured liver cells, enter the bloodstream, and invade erythrocytes. Parasites in the red cells multiply in a species-characteristic fashion, breaking out of their host cells synchronously. This is the erythrocytic cycle, with successive broods of merozoites appearing at 48-hour intervals (*P vivax, P ovale,* and *P falciparum*) or every 72 hours (*P malariae*). The incubation period includes the exoerythrocytic cycles (usually 2) and at least one or 2 erythrocytic cycles. For *P vivax* and *P falciparum,* this period is usually 10–15 days, but it may be weeks or months. The incubation period of *P malariae* averages about 28 days. *P falciparum* multiplication is confined to the red cells after the first liver cycle. Without treatment, falciparum infection ordinarily will terminate spontaneously in less than 1 year unless

Table 48–2. Some characteristic features of the malaria parasites of humans (Romanowsky-stained preparations).

	P vivax (Benign Tertian Malaria)	P malariae (Quartan Malaria)	P falciparum (Malignant Tertian Malaria)	P ovale (Ovale Malaria)
Parasitized red cells	Enlarged, pale. Fine stippling (Schüffner's dots). Primarily invades reticulocytes, young red cells.	Not enlarged. No stippling (except with special stains). Primarily invades older red cells.	Not enlarged. Coarse stippling (Maurer's clefts). Invades all red cells regardless of age.*	Enlarged, pale. Schüffner's dots conspicuous. Cells often oval, fimbriated, or crenated.
Level of usual maximum parasitemia	Up to 30,000/μL of blood.	Less than 10,000/μL.	May exceed 200,000/μL; commonly 50,000/μL.	Less than 10,000/μL.
Ring stage trophozoites	Large rings (1/3–1/2 red cell diameter). Usually one chromatin granule; ring delicate.	Large rings (1/3 red cell diameter). Usually one chromatin granule; ring thick.	Small rings (1/5 red cell diameter). Often 2 granules; multiple infections common; ring delicate, may adhere to red cells.	Large rings (1/3 red cell diameter). Usually one chromatin granule; ring thick.
Pigment in developing trophozoites	Fine; light brown; scattered.	Coarse; dark brown; scattered clumps; abundant.	Coarse; black; few clumps.	Coarse; dark yellow-brown; scattered.
Older trophozoites	Very pleomorphic.	Occasional band forms.	Compact and rounded.*	Compact and rounded.
Mature schizonts (segmenters)	More than 12 merozoites (14–24).	Less than 12 large merozoites (6–12). Often in rosette.	Usually more than 12 merozoites (8–32). Very rare in peripheral blood.*	Less than 12 large merozoites (6–12). Often in rosette.
Gametocytes	Round or oval.	Round or oval.	Crescentic.	Round or oval.
Distribution in peripheral blood	All forms.	All forms.	Only rings and crescents (gametocytes).*	All forms.

*Ordinarily, only ring stages or gametocytes are seen in peripheral blood infected with P falciparum; post-ring stages make red cells sticky, and they tend to be retained in deep capillary beds except in overwhelming, usually fatal infections.

it ends fatally. The other 3 species continue to multiply in liver cells long after the initial bloodstream invasion, or there may be *delayed* multiplication in the liver. These exoerythrocytic cycles coexist with erythrocytic cycles and may persist as nongrowing resting forms after the parasites have disappeared from the peripheral blood. Resurgence of an erythrocytic infection (relapse) occurs when merozoites from the liver are not phagocytosed in the bloodstream and succeed in reestablishing a red cell infection (clinical malaria). Without treatment, *P vivax* and *P ovale* infections may persist for up to 5 years. *P malariae* infections lasting 40 years have been reported.

During the erythrocytic cycles, certain merozoites enter red cells and become differentiated as male or female gametocytes. The sexual cycle therefore begins in the vertebrate host, but then for its continuation into the sporogonic phase, the gametocytes must be taken up and ingested by bloodsucking female *Anopheles* as outlined in Fig 48–1.

P vivax, P malariae, and *P ovale* parasitemias are relatively low-grade, primarily because the parasites favor either young or old red cells but not both; *P falciparum* invades red cells of all ages, and parasitemia may be very high. *P falciparum* also causes parasitized red cells to agglutinate and adhere to the endothelial lining of blood vessels, with resulting obstruction, thrombosis, and local ischemia. *P falciparum* infections are therefore frequently more serious than the others, with a much higher rate of severe or fatal complications (cerebral malaria, malarial hyperpyrexia, gastrointestinal disorders, algid malaria, blackwater fever).

P malariae has also been implicated in a nephrotic syndrome in children—"quartan nephrosis"—with a peak incidence at about age 5 years. It is characterized by generalized edema, oliguria, massive proteinuria, and hypoproteinemia. Tubular degeneration is visible in renal biopsy specimens. Glomerular lesions include basement membrane thickening and sometimes fi-

Table 48–3. Time factors of the various plasmodia in relation to cycles.

	Length of Sexual Cycle (in mosquito at 27 °C)	Prepatent Period* (in humans) (preerythrocytic cycle)	Length of Asexual Cycle (in humans)
P vivax (tertian or vivax malaria)	8–9 days	8 days	48 hours
P malariae (quartan or malariae malaria)	15–20 days	15–16 days	72 hours
P falciparum (malignant tertian or falciparum malaria)	9–10 days	5–7 days	36–48 hours
P ovale (ovale malaria)	14 days	9 days	48 hours

*Preerythrocytic period only. Full incubation period before clinical malaria usually includes prepatent period (which ends 48 hours after infection of the erythrocytes) plus 2 or 3 erythrocytic schizogonic cycles and may extend over a much longer time.

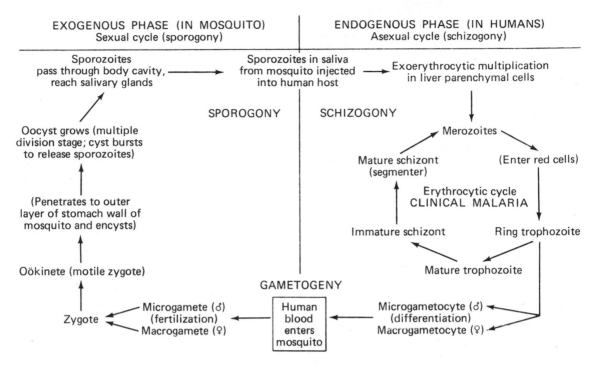

EXOGENOUS PHASE (IN MOSQUITO)
Sexual cycle (sporogony)

ENDOGENOUS PHASE (IN HUMANS)
Asexual cycle (schizogony)

Sporozoites pass through body cavity, reach salivary glands → Sporozoites in saliva from mosquito injected into human host → Exoerythrocytic multiplication in liver parenchymal cells

SPOROGONY

SCHIZOGONY

Oocyst grows (multiple division stage; cyst bursts to release sporozoites)

Merozoites

Mature schizont (segmenter)

(Enter red cells)

Erythrocytic cycle
CLINICAL MALARIA

(Penetrates to outer layer of stomach wall of mosquito and encysts)

Immature schizont

Ring trophozoite

Oökinete (motile zygote)

Mature trophozoite

GAMETOGENY

Zygote ← Microgamete (♂) (fertilization) / Macrogamete (♀) ← Human blood enters mosquito ← Microgametocyte (♂) (differentiation) / Macrogametocyte (♀)

Figure 48–1. Life cycle of the malaria parasites. Continuous cycling or delayed multiplication in the liver may cause periodic relapse over several years (2–3 years in *P ovale*, 6–8 years in *P vivax*), and a low-level blood infection may have a long-delayed resurgence of multiplication (recrudescence) in *P malariae*. However, relapse does not occur with *P falciparum*, though a long prepatent period may occur (perhaps drug-suppressed), resulting in initial symptoms appearing up to 6 months or more after exposure.

brosis. An antigen-antibody complex to quartan malaria or an autoimmune response to the sensitized kidney may be responsible. The response to antimalarial drugs given before irreversible renal changes occur is usually good.

Periodic paroxysms of malaria are closely related to events in the bloodstream. An initial chill, lasting from 15 minutes to 1 hour, begins as a generation of parasites rupture their host red cells and escape into the blood. Nausea, vomiting, and headache are common at this time. The succeeding febrile stage, lasting several hours, is characterized by a spiking fever that may reach 40 °C or more. During this stage, the parasites presumably invade new red cells. The third, or sweating, stage concludes the episode. The fever subsides, and the patient falls asleep and later awakes feeling relatively well. In the early stages of infection, the cycles are frequently asynchonous and the fever pattern irregular; later, paroxysms may recur at regular 48- or 72-hour intervals. As the disease progresses, splenomegaly and, to a lesser extent, hepatomegaly appear. A normocytic anemia also develops, particularly in *P falciparum* infections.

Diagnostic Laboratory Tests

A. Specimens and Microscopic Examination: The thick blood film stained with Giemsa's stain is the mainstay of malaria diagnosis. This preparation concentrates the parasites and permits detection even

of light infections. Examination of thin blood films stained with Giemsa's stain is necessary for species differentiation.

B. Other Laboratory Findings: Normocytic anemia of variable severity may be detected. During the paroxysms there may be transient leukocytosis; subsequently, leukopenia develops, with a relative increase in large mononuclear cells. Liver function tests may give abnormal results during attacks, but liver function reverts to normal with treatment or spontaneous recovery. The presence of protein and casts in the urine of children with *P malariae* is suggestive of quartan nephrosis. In severe *P falciparum* infections, renal damage may cause oliguria and the appearance of casts, protein, and red cells in the urine.

Immunity

The mechanisms of immunity in malaria are still not clearly understood. An acquired strain-specific immunity has been observed that appears to depend upon the presence of parasites in the bloodstream of the host. This so-called **premunition,** or **concomitant immunity,** is soon lost after the parasites disappear from the blood. Exoerythrocytic forms in the liver cannot alone support premunition, and they elicit no host inflammatory response. Hence, superinfection of the liver by homologous strains can continue to occur. Natural genetically determined partial immunity to malaria occurs in some populations, notably in Africa, where sickle cell disease, glucose-6-phosphate dehydrogenase deficiency, and thalassemia provide some protection against lethal levels of *P falciparum* infection. Most blacks in West Africa, where malaria is endemic, are totally resistant to *P vivax* malaria because they lack the Duffy antigen (FyFy), which acts as a receptor for *P vivax;* in its absence, *P vivax* cannot invade erythrocytes.

The gene responsible for the sporozoite antigen has been identified and cloned using monoclonal antibody and hybridoma techniques, and development of an antisporozoite vaccine is under way. However, a complete prophylactic vaccine would have to be active against both sporozoites and merozoites of the target species; this is many years in the future.

Treatment & Prevention

Chloroquine (Aralen) is the drug of choice for treatment of all forms of malaria during the acute attack; 1.5 g of chloroquine (base) is given over a 3-day period or 1.8 g over 4 days. There is no record of *P vivax* resistant to chloroquine. This drug will also terminate susceptible *P falciparum* infections, in which there are no exoerythrocytic forms. Primaquine, an 8-aminoquinoline, which disposes of the exoerythrocytic tissue forms, must be used in conjunction with chloroquine to achieve complete cure of other forms of malaria. Drug-resistant strains of *P falciparum* should be treated with quinine (intravenously in severe cases) or with pyrimethamine plus sulfadiazine, dapsone, or sulfadoxine.

Suppressive prophylaxis can be achieved with chloroquine diphosphate or amodiaquine except in chloroquine-resistant falciparum areas, eg, Southeast Asia, parts of South America, and Africa. In these areas, various combinations of quinine plus sulfonamides, or pyrimethamine plus dapsone (Maloprim) must be relied upon, though resistance to these combinations occurs in many areas of Southeast Asia. The problem is becoming more acute. Pyrimethamine plus sulfadoxine (Fansidar) is now recommended for therapeutic use only, owing to severe side effects that may occur with long-term prophylactic use. See Goldsmith (1986) for a current review of therapy and prophylaxis.

In pregnancy, continued prophylaxis with chloroquine (not pyrimethamine or a sulfonamide) is essential, because of the danger of transplacental transmission of malarial agents to the fetus.

Epidemiology & Control

Malaria today is generally limited to the tropics and subtropics, although recent outbreaks in Turkey attest to the capacity of this disease to reappear in areas cleared of the agent. Malaria in the temperate zones is relatively uncommon, although severe epidemic outbreaks may occur when the largely nonimmune populations of these areas are exposed; it is usually unstable and relatively easy to control or eradicate. Tropical malaria is usually more stable, difficult to control, and far harder to eradicate. In the tropics, malaria generally disappears at altitudes above 6000 feet. *P vivax* and *P falciparum,* the most common species, are found throughout the malaria belt. *P malariae* is also broadly distributed but considerably less common. *P ovale* is rare except in West Africa, where it seems to replace *P vivax.* All forms of malaria can be transmitted by blood transfusion or by needles shared among addicts when one is infected. Such cases of "needle malaria" do not develop a liver or exoerythrocytic infection; thus, relapse does not occur. Natural infection (other than transplacental transmission) takes place only through the bite of an infected female *Anopheles* mosquito.

Malaria control depends upon elimination of mosquito breeding places, personal protection against mosquitoes (screens, netting, repellents), suppressive drug therapy for exposed persons, and adequate treatment of cases and carriers. Eradication requires prevention of biting contact between *Anopheles* mosquitoes and humans for long enough to prevent transmission, with elimination of all active cases by treatment and by spontaneous cure. The results of massive efforts in highly endemic tropical areas have thus far been disappointing. Many costly eradication projects undertaken between 1955 and 1970 have been replaced with control programs specifically geared to the mosquito vector ecology and malaria epidemiology of each area, and these programs must be continued as *permanent* public health responsibilities.

ISOSPORA

Isospora belli, a sporozoan of the human intestine, causes coccidiosis in humans. Numerous species of intestinal sporozoa or coccidia occur in other animals and cause some of the most economically important diseases of domestic mammals and fowl. *I belli* is one of the few coccidia that multiply sexually in the human intestine—ie, in which humans are the definitive host.

Morphology & Identification

A. Typical Organisms: Only the elongated ovoid oocysts are known for *I belli.* Intestinal biopsies of patients with chronic isosporosis demonstrated both asexual schizogonic and oocyst-producing sexual phases. The oocyst of *I belli* is 25–33 × 12–16 μm and often has an asymmetric cyst wall.

B. Culture: These parasites have not been cultivated.

Pathogenesis & Clinical Findings

I belli inhabits the small intestine. Signs and symptoms of coccidiosis apparently are due to the invasion and multiplication of the parasites in the intestinal mucosa. Oocysts are shed into the intestinal lumen and pass out in the stools. Infections may be silent or symptomatic. About 1 week after ingestion of viable cysts, a low-grade fever, lassitude, and malaise may appear, followed soon by mild diarrhea and vague abdominal pain. The infection is usually self-limited after 1–2 weeks, but diarrhea, weight loss, and fever may last for 6 weeks to 6 months. Symptomatic coccidiosis is more common in children than in adults. Chronic infections occur in poorly nourished people living under unsanitary conditions where continued reinfection is more likely or in immunosuppressed persons.

Diagnostic Laboratory Tests

Diagnosis rests upon detection of oocysts in fresh stool specimens. Stool concentration techniques are usually necessary.

Immunity

Immunity to the coccidia following active infection is well documented in animals, although data from human infection are lacking. The many coccidia species are notably host-specific.

Treatment

Treatment of mild cases consists of bed rest and a bland diet for a few days. No specific treatment has been described for more severe and chronic cases.

Epidemiology

Human coccidiosis results from ingestion of cysts. It is usually sporadic and most common in the tropics and subtropics, although it occurs elsewhere, including the USA.

CRYPTOSPORIDIUM

Cryptosporidium species can infect the intestine in immunocompromised persons (eg, those with AIDS) and cause severe diarrhea. The organisms are coccidia related to *Isospora*. They have long been known as parasites of rodents, fowl, rhesus monkeys, and cattle and other herbivores and have probably been an unrecognized cause of self-limited, mild gastroenteritis and diarrhea in humans.

Morphology & Identification

The parasites are minute (2–5 μm) intracellular spheres found in great numbers just under the mucosal epithelium of the stomach or intestine. The mature trophozoite (schizont) divides into 8 arc-shaped merozoites, which are released from the parent cell to begin a new cycle. Oocysts measuring 4–5 μm and containing 4 sporozoites may be seen, but no sporocysts have been demonstrated. Oocysts passed into feces are presumed to be the infective agents.

Pathology & Clinical Findings

Cryptosporidium inhabits mucosal epithelial cells of the gastrointestinal tract, especially the villi of the lower small bowel. The prominent clinical feature of cryptosporidiosis is diarrhea, which is mild and self-limited (1–2 weeks) in normal persons but may be severe and prolonged in immunocompromised or very young or very old individuals.

Diagnostic Laboratory Tests

Diagnosis depends on detection of oocysts in fresh stool samples. Stool concentration techniques are usually necessary.

Treatment

Treatment is unnecessary for patients with normal immunity. For those receiving immunosuppressant drugs, cessation of immunosuppressants may be indicated; for those with AIDS or congenital immunodeficiency, only supportive therapy is available. Pyrimethamine plus sulfadiazine may temporarily be effective.

Epidemiology & Control

Cryptosporidiosis is acquired from infected animal or human feces or from feces-contaminated food or water. Mild cases are common in farm workers. For those at high risk (immunosuppressed and very young or old persons), avoidance of animal feces and careful attention to sanitation are required.

SARCOCYSTIS

Sarcocystis species are coccidia with a biphasic life cycle: an intestinal (sexual) stage in gut mucosal cells of carnivores, and an encysted tissue (asexual) stage in muscle or other cells of herbivores or other prey animals. Humans apparently serve as both intermediate and final hosts depending on the species of *Sarcocystis*. Human volunteers fed raw beef and pork with *Sarcocystis* cysts later passed *Isospora*-like oocysts in their stools; similar results have been obtained with dogs and cats.

Morphology & Identification

In the muscles, the parasites develop in elongated sarcocysts that range from less than 0.1 mm to several centimeters long. The sarcocysts, which may be divided by septa, are filled with trophozoites measuring 12–16 × 4–9 μm. When trophozoites are freed from a sarcocyst in the gut of a definitive host, they invade the cells of the intestinal mucosa and enter a sexual stage to produce the oocysts, which are later discharged in the host's feces. When ingested by an intermediate host, the oocysts open in the gut, each releasing 8 sporozoites. The sporozoites penetrate the gut wall, pass to tissue sites, and invade host cells, where each sporozoite develops into a new sarcocyst with numerous trophozoites.

Pathogenesis & Clinical Findings

Heavy *Sarcocystis* infections may be fatal in some animals (eg, mice, sheep, swine). Extracts of the parasite contain sarcocystin, a toxin that is probably responsible for the pathogenic effects. It is not clear that the parasite is pathogenic for humans. Fleeting subcutaneous swellings, eosinophilia, and heart failure have, however, been attributed to *Sarcocystis lindemanni*. Sarcocysts have been found in the human heart, larynx, and tongue as well as in skeletal muscles of the extremities.

Diagnostic Laboratory Tests

The infection ordinarily causes no symptoms or signs in humans. A reliable CF test has been developed for detection of suspected infections.

Treatment

There is no known effective treatment.

Epidemiology

Sarcocystis shows little host specificity; cross-infections between various hosts can easily be produced. Intestinal infections in humans result from ingestion of raw or poorly cooked infected lamb, beef, or other meats. *Sarcocystis* infections are common in sheep, cattle, and horses. Herbivores develop tissue cysts after eating grass contaminated with oocysts or sporocysts, and predators who consume infected herbivore tissue develop intestinal infections that result in production of infective cysts, which are passed in the feces.

TOXOPLASMA GONDII

Toxoplasma gondii is a coccidian protozoan of worldwide distribution that infects a wide range of animals and birds but does not appear to cause disease in them. The normal final hosts are the cat and related animals. The oocyst-producing sexual stage of *Toxoplasma* can only occur in these final hosts. Organisms (either sporozoites from oocysts or trophozoites from tissue cysts) invade the mucosal cells of the cat's small intestine, where they form schizonts and gametocytes. After sexual fusion of the gametes, oocysts develop, exit from the host cell into the gut lumen, and pass out via the feces. These infective, resistant oocysts resemble those of *Isospora;* each forms 2 sporocysts, and in about 48 hours, 4 sporozoites form within each sporocyst. The oocyst with its 8 sporozoites, when ingested, can either repeat its sexual cycle in a cat or—if ingested by a rodent or other mammal, including humans—establish an infection in which it reproduces asexually. In the latter case, the oocyst opens in the animal's duodenum and releases the 8 sporozoites, which pass through the gut wall, circulate in the body, and invade various cells, where they form viable trophozoites. These trophozoites multiply, break out, and spread the infection to lymph nodes and other organs (acute stage of disease); they later penetrate nerve cells, especially those of the brain and eye, multiply, and eventually form tissue cysts (chronic stage of disease). The tissue cysts are also infective when ingested by cats or other mammals.

The organism in humans produces either congenital or postnatal toxoplasmosis. Congenital infection, which develops only when nonimmune mothers are infected during pregnancy, is usually of great severity; postnatal toxoplasmosis is usually much less severe. Most human infections are asymptomatic.

Morphology & Identification

A. Typical Organisms: The trophozoites are boat-shaped, thin-walled cells that are $4–7 \times 2–4$ μm within tissue cells and somewhat larger outside them. They stain lightly with Giemsa's stain; fixed cells often appear crescentic. Packed intracellular aggregates are occasionally seen (see p 563). True cysts are found in the brain or certain other tissues. These cysts contain many thousands of sporelike trophozoites, which can initiate a new infection in a mammal ingesting the cyst-bearing tissues.

B. Culture: *T gondii* may be cultured only in the presence of living cells, in cell culture or eggs. Typical intracellular and extracellular organisms may be seen.

C. Growth Requirements: Optimal growth is at about 37–39 °C in living cells.

D. Variations: There is considerable strain variation in infectivity and virulence, possibly related to the degree of adaptation to a particular host.

Pathogenesis, Pathology, & Clinical Findings

The trophozoite directly destroys cells and has a predilection for parenchymal cells and those of the reticuloendothelial system. Humans are relatively resistant, but a low-grade lymph node infection resembling infectious mononucleosis may occur. Congenital infection leads to stillbirths, chorioretinitis, intracerebral calcifications, psychomotor disturbances, and hydrocephaly or microcephaly. In these cases, the mother was infected during pregnancy. Prenatal toxoplasmosis is a major cause of blindness and other congenital defects. Infection during the first trimester generally results in stillbirth or major central nervous system anomalies. Clinical manifestations of these infections may be delayed until long after birth, even beyond childhood. Neurologic problems or learning difficulties may be caused by the long-delayed effects of prenatal toxoplasmosis.

Diagnostic Laboratory Tests

A. Specimens: Blood, bone marrow, cerebrospinal fluid, and exudates; lymph node, tonsillar, and striated muscle biopsy material; and ventricular fluid (in neonatal infections) may be required.

B. Microscopic Examination: Smears and sections stained with Giemsa's stain may show the organism. The densely packed cysts, chiefly in the brain or other parts of the central nervous system, suggest chronic infection. Identification must be confirmed by isolation in animals.

C. Animal Inoculation: This is essential for definitive diagnosis. A variety of specimens are inoculated intraperitoneally into groups of mice that are free from infection. If no deaths occur, the mice are observed for about 6 weeks, and tail or heart blood is then tested for specific antibody. The diagnosis is confirmed by demonstration of cysts in the brains of the inoculated mice.

D. Serology: The Sabin-Feldman dye test depends upon the appearance in 2–3 weeks of antibodies that will render the membrane of laboratory-cultured living *T gondii* impermeable to alkaline methylene blue, so that organisms are unstained in the presence of positive serum. It is being replaced by the IHA, latex, IFA, and ELISA tests. None of these tests expose technologists to the danger of living organisms, as is required for the dye test. A CF test may be positive (1:8 titer) as early as 1 month after infection, but it is valueless in many chronic infections. The IFA and IHA tests are routinely used for diagnostic purposes. Frenkel's intracutaneous test is useful for epidemiologic surveys.

Immunity

Some acquired immunity may develop in the course of infection. Antibody titers in mothers, as detected in either blood or milk, tend to fall within a few months. Yet, the fact that prenatal infection is limited to infants born of mothers who were first exposed during their pregnancy strongly suggests that the presence of circulating antibodies is at least partially protective. Immune deficiency diseases (eg, AIDS), immunosuppressant drugs, or changes in host resistance may cause chronic infection with *Toxoplasma* to become a fulminating, acute toxoplasmosis.

Treatment

Acute infections can be treated with a combination of pyrimethamine, 25 mg/d for 3–4 weeks, and trisulfapyrimidines, 2–6 g/d for 3–4 weeks.

Epidemiology, Prevention, & Control

Transplacental infection of the fetus has long been recognized. Domestic cats have been incriminated in the transmission of the parasite to humans; the infection is transmitted by an *Isospora*-like oocyst found only in the feces of cats and related animals. Rodents play a role in transmission, since they harbor in their tissues infective cysts that may be ingested by cats. Avoidance of human contact with cat feces is clearly important in control, particularly for pregnant women with negative serologic tests. Since oocysts usually take 48 hours to become infective, daily changing of cat litter (*and* its safe disposal) can prevent transmission. However, pregnant women should avoid all contact with cats, particularly kittens. An equally important source of human exposure is raw or undercooked meat, in which infective tissue cysts are frequently found. Humans (and other mammals) can become infected *either* from oocysts in cat feces or from tissue cysts in raw or undercooked meat.

BABESIA MICROTI

Babesia species are widespread animal parasites, causing infectious jaundice of dogs and Texas cattle fever (redwater fever). Babesiosis, a red cell-infecting tick-borne piroplasmosis caused by *B microti*, is a human disease reported in increasing numbers from Massachusetts, the primary focus being Nantucket Is-

land. Recent outbreaks have been in healthy individuals with no record of splenectomy, corticosteroid therapy, or recurrent infection. The illness develops 7–10 days after the tick bite and is characterized by malaise, anorexia, nausea, fatigue, fever, sweats, myalgia, arthralgia, and depression. *Babesia* may be mistaken in humans for *Plasmodium falciparum* in its ring form in red cells. No pigment is produced, however. Human babesiosis is more severe in the elderly than in the young. Splenectomized individuals may develop progressive hemolytic anemia, jaundice, and renal insufficiency with prolonged parasitemia. Chloroquine provides clinical relief but is not curative. Good clinical results follow treatment with clindamycin and quinine.

BALANTIDIUM COLI

Balantidium coli, the cause of balantidiasis or balantidial dysentery, is the largest intestinal protozoan of humans. Morphologically similar ciliate parasites are found in swine and lower primates.

Morphology & Identification

A. Typical Organisms: The trophozoite is a ciliated, oval organism, 60×45 μm or larger. Its motion is a characteristic combination of steady progression and rotation around the long axis. The cell wall is lined with spiral rows of cilia. The cytoplasm surrounds 2 contractile vacuoles, food particles and vacuoles, and 2 nuclei—a large, kidney-shaped macronucleus and a much smaller, spherical micronucleus. When the organism encysts, it secretes a double-layered wall. The macronucleus, contractile vacuoles, and portions of the ciliated cell wall may be visible in the cyst, which ranges from 45–65 μm in diameter.

B. Culture: These organisms may be cultivated in many media used for cultivation of intestinal amebas.

Pathogenesis, Pathology, & Clinical Findings

When cysts are ingested by the new host, the cyst walls dissolve and the released trophozoites descend to the colon, where they feed on bacteria and fecal debris, multiply, and form cysts that pass out in the feces. Most infections are apparently harmless. However, rarely, the trophozoites invade the mucosa and submucosa of the large bowel and terminal ileum. As they multiply, abscesses and irregular ulcerations with overhanging margins are formed. The number of lesions formed depends upon intensity of infection and degree of individual host susceptibility. Chronic recurrent diarrhea, alternating with constipation, is the commonest clinical manifestation, but there may be bloody mucoid stools, tenesmus, and colic. Extreme cases may mimic severe intestinal amebiasis, and some have been fatal.

Diagnostic Laboratory Tests

The diagnosis of balantidial infection, whether symptomatic or not, depends upon laboratory detection of trophozoites in liquid stools or, more rarely, of cysts in formed stools. Sigmoidoscopy may be useful for obtaining material directly from ulcerations for examination. Culturing is rarely necessary.

Immunity

Humans appear to have a high natural resistance to balantidial infection. Factors underlying individual susceptibility are not known.

Treatment

A course of oxytetracycline may be followed by iodoquinol if necessary.

Epidemiology

B coli is found in humans throughout the world, particularly in the tropics, but it is a rare infection. Only a few hundred cases have been recorded. Infection results from ingestion of viable cysts previously passed in the stools by humans and possibly by swine. The strain found in swine was noninfective in volunteers. Outbreaks have been reported in crowded encampments, jails, or mental institutions.

PNEUMOCYSTIS CARINII

Pneumocystis carinii appears to be a sporozoan that is widely distributed among animals in nature—including rats, mice, and dogs—but usually without causing disease. It can be a cause of interstitial plasma cell pneumonitis in infants, the elderly, and immunosuppressed patients. It is a leading cause of death in patients with AIDS.

Morphology & Identification

A. Typical Organisms: The most characteristic stage is a rosette of 8 pear-shaped "sporozoites," each 1–2 μm, in a "cyst" 7–10 μm in diameter, as demonstrated in impression smears of specimens from tracheobronchial lavage or aspiration or lung biopsy stained with Giemsa's or methenamine silver stain. Rosettes are rarely seen in sputum.

B. Culture: The organism has been grown in various cell cultures.

Pathogenesis, Pathology, & Clinical Findings

Most infections in humans are probably inapparent. Excessive multiplication leading to blocking of the alveolar respiratory surface occurs after a 2- to 6-week incubation period, especially in premature or debilitated infants. The resulting disease is an interstitial plasma cell pneumonitis (seen in x-rays as a "ground glass" appearance), with alveoli filled with organisms and foamy material. The mortality rate is usually 30% or more. In patients with lowered resistance (eg, children and adults receiving corticosteroids or cytotoxic drugs, or those suffering from immunocompromised states), there is a febrile pneumonitis with cyanosis and a high mortality rate.

Diagnostic Laboratory Tests

Diagnosis rests on demonstration of organisms in specimens from lung biopsy or bronchial brushing or lavage using special stains. Serologic tests are rarely helpful except in infants, who may show a rise in antibody titer.

Treatment

Pentamidine isethionate or trimethoprim-sulfamethoxazole can be effective treatment.

Epidemiology, Prevention, & Control

The mode of infection is unknown, but cysts, presumably inhaled, may be derived from domestic rodents or pets or from carrier adults. Trimethoprim-sulfamethoxazole can be prophylactic in immunosuppressed persons.

HELMINTHS: OVA IN FECES & MICROFILARIAE IN BLOOD & TISSUES

Table 48–4 shows some diseases that are caused by helminths. Ova (pp 566 and 571) may be detected in feces (or urine, with *Schistosoma haematobium;* occasionally *Schistosoma mansoni*, especially with dual infections; and sometimes *Schistosoma japonicum*), preferably after concentration by zinc sulfate centrifugal sedimentation or other techniques (especially for operculated and schistosome eggs; see Garcia and Ash, Desowitz, and Melvin and Brooke references). Eggs of *Enterobius* may be collected directly from the anal margins with cellulose tape on the end of a spatula.

Microfilariae (see Table 48–5 and p 565) are the embryonic or prelarval stages of filariid worms in humans and are identified in blood smears or concentrate or (especially for *Onchocerca volvulus*) in a skin snip preparation.

Table 48–4. Diseases due to helminths.

C = cestode (tapeworm)		N = nematode (roundworm)		T = trematode (fluke)
Disease and Parasite	**Location in Host**	**Mode of Transmission**	**Geographic Distribution**	**Treatment of Choice**
Angiostrongyliasis; eosinophilic meningoencephalitis *Angiostrongylus cantonensis* (larval) (N), rat lungworm	Larvae in meninges.	Eating raw shrimps, prawns; raw garden slugs; aquatic and land snails; infested lettuce.	Local in Pacific, especially southwest.	Thiabendazole (experimental).
Angiostrongyliasis; intestinal angiostrongyliasis *Angiostrongylus costaricensis* (N), cotton rat arterial worm	Larval stages in bowel wall, especially appendix; also regional lymph nodes in mesenteric arteries.	Ingestion of infected snails, slugs, contaminated salad vegetables.	Central America, Brazil.	Surgical excision.
Anisakiasis *Anisakis, Phocanema,* other related genera (larval) (N)	Larvae in stomach or intestinal wall, rarely penetrate.	Eating raw or pickled marine fish.	Around Pacific basin (Japan, California, Hawaii) among people who eat raw fish.	Surgical excision. Usually short-lived.
Ascariasis *Ascaris lumbricoides* (N), common roundworm	Small intestine; larvae through lungs.	Eating viable eggs from feces-contaminated soil or food.	Worldwide, very common.	Pyrantel pamoate, mebendazole, levamisole, piperazine citrate.
Capillariasis *Capillaria philippinensis* (N)	Small intestine (mucosa).	Undercooked marine fish.	Philippines, Thailand.	Mebendazole.
Clonorchiasis *Clonorchis sinensis* (T), Chinese liver fluke	Liver (bile ducts).	Uncooked freshwater fish.	China, Korea, Indochina, Japan, Taiwan.	Praziquantel, chloroquine, bithionol.
Cysticercosis (bladder worm) *Taenia solium* (larval) (C)	Subcutaneous; eye, meninges, brain, etc.	Ingestion of eggs or regurgitation of gravid proglottid from lower GI tract.	Worldwide.	Surgical excision, mebendazole, praziquantel (experimental).
Dracontiasis *Dracunculus medinensis* (N), Guinea worm	Subcutaneous; usually leg, foot.	Drinking water with *Cyclops.*	Africa, Arabia to Pakistan; locally elsewhere in Asia.	Mechanical or surgical extraction, niridazole, metronidazole, thiabendazole.
Echinococcosis, hydatidosis *Echinococcus granulosus* (larval) (C), unilocular hydatid cyst	Liver, lung, brain, peritoneum, long bones, kidney.	Contact with dogs, foxes, other canids; eggs from feces.	Worldwide but local; sheep-raising areas.	Surgical aspiration and excision, praziquantel (experimental).
Echinococcus multilocularis (larval) (C), alveolar (multilocular) hydatid cyst	Liver.	Fox fur trappers.	Northern temperate areas with fox-vole cycle.	
Echinostomiasis *Echinostoma ilocanum* (T)	Small intestine.	Freshwater snails.	SE Asia.	Tetrachloroethylene, bithionol, hexylresorcinol (Crystoids).
Enterobiasis *Enterobius vermicularis* (N), pinworm	Cecum, colon (lumen).	Anal-oral; self-contamination and internal reinfection.	Worldwide.	Pyrantel pamoate, mebendazole, piperazine, pyrvinium pamoate.
Fascioliasis *Fasciola hepatica* (T), sheep liver fluke	Liver (bile ducts, after migration through parenchyma).	Watercress, aquatic vegetation.	Worldwide, especially sheep-raising areas.	Bithionol, emetine or dehydroemetine (subcutaneous).
Fasciolopsiasis *Fasciolopsis buski* (T), giant intestinal fluke	Small intestine.	Aquatic vegetation.	E and SE Asia.	Hexylresorcinol (Crystoids), bithionol, stilbazium iodide.
Filariasis *Wuchereria bancrofti, Brugia malayi* (N), human filarial worms	Lymph nodes; microfilariae in blood.	Bite of mosquitoes; several species.	Tropical and subtropical, very local but widespread.	Diethylcarbamazine.
Filariasis, occult *Dirofilaria* species (N), heartworm	Lungs (larvae).	Infected mosquitoes?	India, SE Asia.	Diethylcarbamazine or not treated.
Gnathostomiasis *Gnathostoma spinigerum* (N) rat stomach worm	Subcutaneous, migra-	Uncooked fish.	E and SE asia.	Surgical excision, diethylcarbamazine.

Table 48–4 (cont'd). Diseases due to helminths.

C = cestode (tapeworm)	N = nematode (roundworm)		T = trematode (fluke)	
Disease and Parasite	**Location in Host**	**Mode of Transmission**	**Geographic Distribution**	**Treatment of Choice**
Heterophyiasis *Heterophyes heterophes* (T), intestinal fish fluke of humans	Small intestine.	Uncooked fish (mullet).	China, Korea, Japan, Taiwan; Israel; Egypt.	Tetrachloroethylene, hexylresorcinol (Crystoids).
Hookworms *Ancylostoma duodenale, Necator americanus* (N)	Small intestine; larvae through lungs.	Through skin, infected soil, from drinking contaminated water (*Ancylostoma*).	Worldwide tropics and North America (*Necator*); temperate zones (*Ancylostoma*).	Mebendazole, pyrantel pamoate, bephenium hydroxynaphthoate, tetrachloroethylene.
Larva migrans: Cutaneous, creeping eruption *Ancylostoma braziliense* and other domestic animal hookworms (N)	Subcutaneous, migrating larvae.	Contact with soil contaminated by dog or cat feces.	Worldwide.	Thiabendazole, levamisole.
Visceral *Toxocara* species (N), cat and dog roundworms	Liver, lung, eye, brain, other viscera; migrating larvae.	Ingesting soil contaminated by dog or cat feces.	Worldwide.	Thiabendazole, levamisole, corticosteroids.
Loiasis *Loa loa* (N)	Subcutaneous, migratory; eye. Microfilariae in blood.	Bite of deer flies, *Chrysops*.	Equatorial Africa.	Surgical removal, diethylcarbamazine, or not treated.
Mansonelliasis *Mansonella ozzardi* (N), (nonpathogenic) Ozzard's filaria	Body cavities; microfilariae in blood.	Bite of gnat *Culicoides*.	Argentina, N coast of S America; Caribbean islands; Panama, Yucatan.	Not treated.
Mansonella perstans (N) (*Dipetalonema perstans*) (nonpathogenic?)	Peritoneal and other cavities; microfilariae in blood.	Bite of gnat *Culicoides*.	Equatorial Africa; N coast of S America, Argentina, Panama, Trinidad.	Not treated.
Metagonimiasis *Metagonimus yokogawai* (T), intestinal fish fluke of humans	Small intestine.	Uncooked fish.	As for *Heterophyes* plus USSR, Balkans, Spain.	Tetrachloroethylene, hexylresorcinol (Crystoids).
Onchocerciasis *Onchocerca volvulus* (N), nodular or blinding worm	Subcutaneous; microfilariae in skin, eyes.	Bite of black fly *Simulium*.	Equatorial Africa; C and S America.	Surgery, diethylcarbamazine, Ivermectin (experimental).
Opisthorchiasis *Opisthorchis felineus*, *Opisthorchis viverrini* (T), Asian liver flukes	Liver (bile duct).	Uncooked fish.	E Europe, USSR; Thailand.	Praziquantel.
Paragonimiasis *Paragonimus westermani* (T), lung fluke (several species)	Lung (paired worms in cyst), brain, other sites.	Raw crabs and other freshwater crustaceans.	E and S Asia; N central Africa; S America; animals in N America.	Bithionol, praziquantel.
Schistosomiasis *Schistosoma haematobium* (T), schistosomes or bilharzia worms, blood flukes; vesicular blood fluke	Venous vessels of urinary bladder, large intestine; liver.	Cercariae (larvae) penetrate skin in snail-infested water.	Africa, widely; Madagascar; Arabia to Lebanon.	Praziquantel, metrifonate.
Schistosoma japonicum (T), Japanese blood fluke	Venous vessels of small intestine; liver.	Cercariae (larvae) penetrate skin in snail-infested water.	China, Philippines, Japan; potentially Taiwan.	Praziquantel.
Schistosoma mansoni (T), Manson's blood fluke	Venous vessels of colon, rectum; liver.	Cercariae (larvae) penetrate skin in snail-infested water.	Africa to Near East; parts of S America; Caribbean tropics and subtropics.	Praziquantel, oxamniquine.

Table 48–4 (cont'd). Diseases due to helminths.

C = cestode (tapeworm)	N = nematode (roundworm)		T = trematode (fluke)	
Disease and Parasite	**Location in Host**	**Mode of Transmission**	**Geographic Distribution**	**Treatment of Choice**
Sparganosis *Spirometra mansonoides;* *Spirometra erinacei* (larval) (C), pseudophyllidean larva or spar- ganum from frogs, snakes, some birds and mammals (adult worms in felids or canids)	Intraorbital wound, other wounds or con- tusions if used as poultice; subcuta- neous tissues if from ingestion of procer- coid or sparganum.	Native poultices such as infected raw frog flesh; drinking water with infected copepods; ingestion of raw frogs, tadpoles, snakes.	Orient; occasionally other countries, in- cluding N and S America.	Surgical removal.
Strongyloidiasis *Strongyloides stercoralis* (N), threadworm	Duodenum, jejunum; larvae through skin, lungs.	Through skin and (rarely) by internal au- toreinfection.	Worldwide.	Thiabendazole, pyrvinium pamoate.
Tapeworm disease (see also Cysticercosis, Echinococcosis, Sparganosis); taeniasis *Diphyllobothrium latum* (C), broad fish tapeworm	Small intestine.	Uncooked freshwater fish.	Alaska, E Canada, Great Lakes area, NW Florida; parts of S America; N Europe; E Mediterranean, Asi- atic USSR, Japan; Australia.	Niclosamide, paromo- mycin; praziquantel.
Dipylidium caninum (C), dog tapeworm	Small intestine.	Ingestion of crushed fleas, lice from pets.	Worldwide.	Niclosamide, paromo- mycin, quinacrine.
Hymenolepis diminuta (C), rat tapeworm	Small intestine.	Indirectly from rats, mice via infected in- sects.	Worldwide.	Niclosamide, paromo- mycin, quinacrine, praziquantel.
Hymenolepis nana (C), dwarf tapeworm	Small intestine.	Anal-oral transfer of eggs or ingestion of in- fected insects; internal reinfection.	Worldwide.	Niclosamide, paromo- mycin, quinacrine, praziquantel.
Taenia saginata (C), beef tape- worm	Small intestine.	Uncooked beef.	Worldwide.	Niclosamide, paromo- mycin, quinacrine, praziquantel.
Taenia solium (C), pork tapeworm (see also Cysticercosis)	Small intestine.	Uncooked pork.	Worldwide.	Niclosamide, paromo- mycin, quinacrine, praziquantel.
Trichinosis *Trichinella spiralis* (N), trichina worm	Larvae in striated muscle (coiled within enlarged fiber cell).	Uncooked pork.	Worldwide.	Thiabendazole, corti- costeroids.
Trichostrongyliasis *Trichostrongylus* species (N)	Small intestine.	Ingestion of infective third stage from feces- contaminated food or soil; contact with herbi- vore feces.	E Europe, USSR, Iran.	Thiabendazole, pyran- tel pamoate.
Trichuriasis *Trichuris trichiura* (N), whipworm	Cecum; colon.	Ingestion of eggs from feces-contaminated soil.	Worldwide.	Mebendazole, hexylre- sorcinol enema.

Table 48–5. Microfilariae.

Filariid	Disease	Distribution	Vectors	Microfilariae		
				Sheath	Tail Nuclei	Periodicity*
Wuchereria bancrofti	Bancroftian and Malayan filariasis: lymphangitis, hydrocele, elephantiasis	Worldwide 41 N to 28 S	Culicidae (mosquitoes)	+	Not to tip	Nocturnal or non-periodic
Brugia malayi		Oriental region to Japan	Culicidae (mosquitoes)	+	Two distinct	Nocturnal or subperiodic
Loa loa	Loiasis; Calabar swellings; conjunctival worms	Western and central Africa	*Chrysops*, deer fly, mango fly	+	Extend to tip	Diurnal
Onchocerca volvulus	Onchocerciasis: skin nodules, blindness, dermatitis, hanging groin	Africa, Central and South America	*Simulium*, buffalo gnat, black fly	−	Not to tip	Nonperiodic in skin fluids
Mansonella (Dipetalonema) perstans	Mansonelliasis or dipetalonemiasis (minor disturbances)	Africa and South America	*Culicoides*, biting midge	−	Extend to tip	Nocturnal or diurnal or nonperiodic
Mansonella streptocerca	Usually nonpathogenic	Western and central Africa	*Culicoides*, biting midge	−	Extend to tip	In skin only
Mansonella ozzardi	Ozzard's mansonelliasis (benign), occasionally hydrocele	Central and South America	*Culicoides*, biting midge	−	Not to tip	Nonperiodic

*Microfilariae are found in peripheral blood (in blood smear) only at night (nocturnal periodicity), largely at night or during crepuscular hours (subperiodicity), largely during daylight hours (diurnal periodicity), or without clear distinction (nonperiodic). Periodicity appears to be correlated with the bloodsucking habits of the chief vector insect in the particular area of transmission of the filaria.

PROTOZOA IN FECES (× 2000)

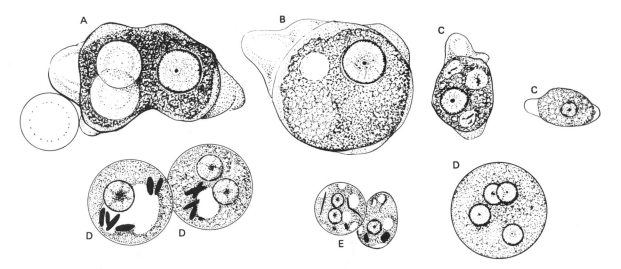

Entamoeba histolytica. A, B: Trophozoite (vegetative form) with ingested red cells in *A; C: Entamoeba hartmanni* trophozoite with food vacuoles, not red cells; *D:* cysts with 1, 2, and 4 nuclei and chromatoid bodies; *E: E hartmanni* binucleate cyst (left), uninucleate precyst (right).

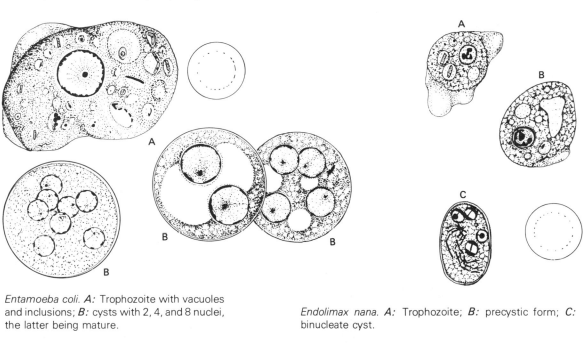

Entamoeba coli. A: Trophozoite with vacuoles and inclusions; *B:* cysts with 2, 4, and 8 nuclei, the latter being mature.

Endolimax nana. A: Trophozoite; *B:* precystic form; *C:* binucleate cyst.

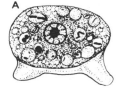
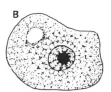
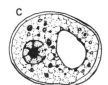
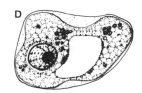

Iodamoeba bütschlii. A: Trophozoite; *B:* precystic form; *C* and *D:* cysts showing large glycogen vacuole (unstained in iron-hematoxylin preparation). Note variable shape of cysts.

[Simple double circles represent the size of red cells.]

PROTOZOA IN FECES (× 2000)*

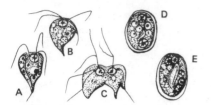

Enteromonas hominis. A, B, C: Trophozoites; *C:* dividing form; *D* and *E:* quadrinucleate cysts.

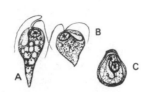

Retortamonas intestinalis. A and *B:* Trophozoites; *C:* cyst.

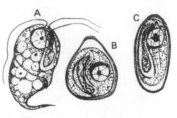

Chilomastix mesnili. A: Trophozoite; *B* and *C:* cysts.

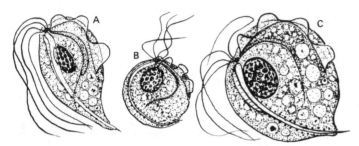

Trichomonas vaginalis. *A:* Normal trophozoite; *B:* round form after division; *C:* common form seen in stained preparation. **Cysts not found.**

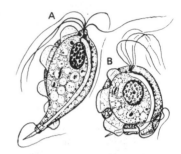

Trichomonas hominis. A: Normal and *B:* round forms of trophozoites, probably a staining artifact. **Cysts not found.**

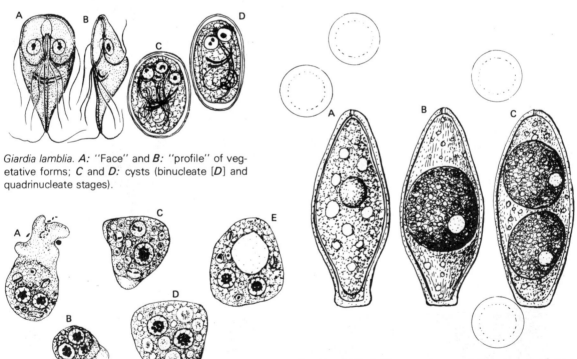

Giardia lamblia. A: "Face" and *B:* "profile" of vegetative forms; *C* and *D:* cysts (binucleate [*D*] and quadrinucleate stages).

Dientamoeba fragilis. Trophozoites (cysts not found). *A:* active; *B:* small; *C:* mononuclear; *D* and *E:* resting.

Isospora belli. A: Degenerate oocyst; *B:* unsegmented oocyst; *C:* oocyst segmented into 2 sporoblasts after passage with feces. Mature oocyst with sporoblasts developed into sporocysts, each containing 4 sporozoites, not shown.

[Simple double circles represent the size of red cells.]

Trichomonas vaginalis is found in vaginal and prostatic secretions.

PROTOZOA IN FECES (× 2000)

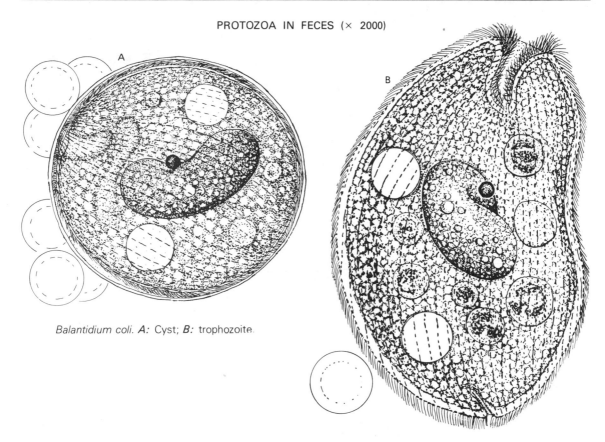

Balantidium coli. **A:** Cyst; **B:** trophozoite.

PROTOZOA IN BLOOD AND TISSUES (× 2000)

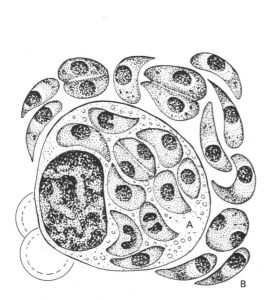

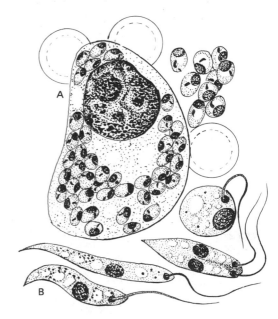

Toxoplasma gondii. **A:** Trophozoites in large mononuclear cell; **B:** free in blood. Not found within red cells, but parasitize many other cell types, particularly reticuloendothelial. Cyst not shown.

Leishmania donovani. **A:** Large reticuloendothelial cell of spleen with amastigotes. **B:** Promastigotes as seen in sandfly gut or in culture.

[Simple double circles represent the size of red cells.]

PROTOZOA IN BLOOD (× 1700)

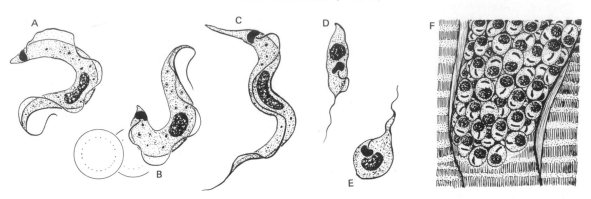

Trypanosoma cruzi. A, B, C: Trypomastigotes in blood; *D, E:* epimastigote (with short anterior undulating membrane); *F:* amastigote colony in heart muscle cell.

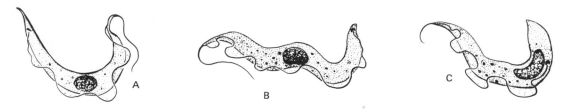

Trypanosoma brucei gambiense (or *Trypanosoma brucei rhodesiense,* indistinguishable in practice). *A, B:* Trypomastigotes in blood; *C:* epimastigote (intermediate type; kinetoplast not yet anterior to nucleus); found in tsetse fly, *Glossina* species.

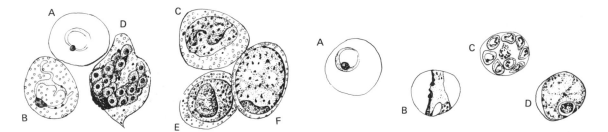

Plasmodium vivax. A: Young signet ring trophozoite; *B:* ameboid trophozoite; *C:* mature trophozoite; *D:* mature schizont, showing a distorted host cell; *E:* microgametocyte; *F:* macrogametocyte with compact nucleus. Note Schüffner's dots and enlarged host cells.

Plasmodium malariae. A: Developing ring form of trophozoite; *B:* band form of trophozoite (note absence of granules); *C:* mature schizont in "rosette" with 8 merozoites; *D:* mature gametocyte.

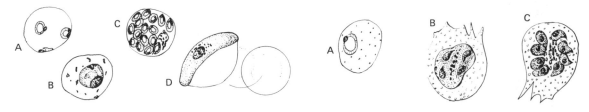

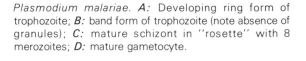

Plasmodium falciparum. A: Ring stage, or young trophozoites (triple infection); *B:* mature trophozoite showing clumped pigment in cytoplasm and Maurer's clefts in erythrocyte; *C:* mature schizont; *D:* mature gametocyte. *B* and *C* stages rarely seen in peripheral blood. Gametocytes in blood are diagnostic.

Plasmodium ovale. A: Young signet ring trophozoite and Schüffner's dots; *B:* ameboid trophozoite developing in fimbriated erythrocyte; *C:* mature schizont showing 8 merozoites.

[Simple double circles represent the size of red cells.]

MICROFILARIAE (× 600)
(in blood or tissue fluids)

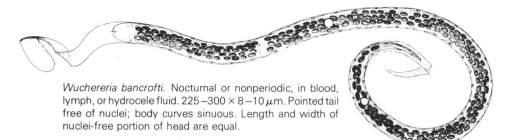

Wuchereria bancrofti. Nocturnal or nonperiodic, in blood, lymph, or hydrocele fluid. 225–300 × 8–10 µm. Pointed tail free of nuclei; body curves sinuous. Length and width of nuclei-free portion of head are equal.

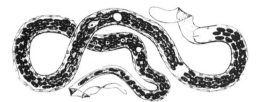

Loa loa. Diurnal periodicity, in blood. 250–300 × 6–9 µm. Nuclei extend to tip of tail; body curves angular or kinky.

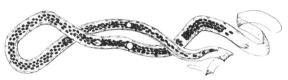

Brugia malayi. Nocturnal or subperiodic, in blood, lymph, or lymphocele fluid. 160–260 × 5–6 µm. Two nuclei in tip of tail; body curves angular or kinky; nuclei-free portion of head longer than it is wide.

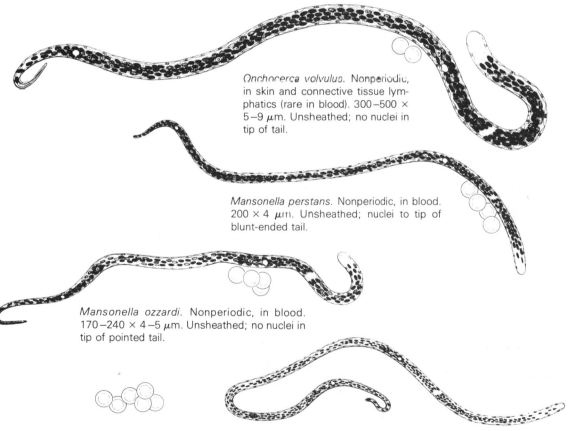

Onchocerca volvulus. Nonperiodic, in skin and connective tissue lymphatics (rare in blood). 300–500 × 5–9 µm. Unsheathed; no nuclei in tip of tail.

Mansonella perstans. Nonperiodic, in blood. 200 × 4 µm. Unsheathed; nuclei to tip of blunt-ended tail.

Mansonella ozzardi. Nonperiodic, in blood. 170–240 × 4–5 µm. Unsheathed; no nuclei in tip of pointed tail.

Mansonella streptocerca. Nonperiodic. 180 × 2–3 µm. Unsheathed; found in skin only, not in blood. Nuclei to tip of blunt-ended tail.

[Simple double circles represent the size of red cells.]

OVA OF TREMATODES (× 400)
(as seen in feces)

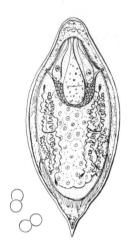

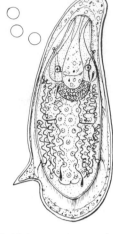

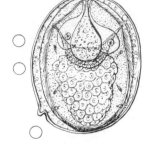

Schistosoma japonicum. Embryonated ovum with small lateral spine, often not visible.

Paragonimus westermani. Unembryonated operculated ovum.

Schistosoma haematobium. Terminally spined embryonated ovum (containing miracidium).

Schistosoma mansoni. Laterally spined embryonated ovum (containing miracidium).

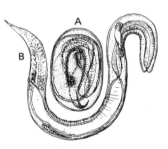

Clonorchis sinensis. Small operculated and embryonated ovum.

A: Heterophyes heterophyes or *B: Metagonimus yokogawai.* Minute embryonated operculated ova.

Fasciola hepatica or *Fasciolopsis buski.* Unembryonated operculated ovum.

OVA OF NEMATODES (× 400)

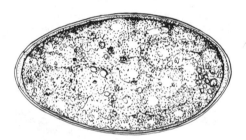

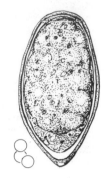

Ancylostoma duodenale or *Necator americanus.* Note shape, thin shell, 4- to 8-cell stage.

Ascaris lumbricoides. A: Fertilized unembryonated ovum; *B:* unfertilized ovum; *C:* fertilized decorticated ovum.

Strongyloides stercoralis. A: Embryonated ovum (rare in feces); *B:* rhabditiform larva (usually seen in feces).

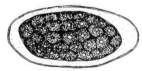

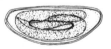

Trichostrongylus orientalis. Unembryonated ovum. (Rare in humans except in specific areas, eg, Iran.)

Trichuris trichiura. Unembryonated double-plug ovum.

Enterobius vermicularis. Embryonated ovum. Note flattening on one side, thin shell. Deposited on perianal skin.

[Simple circles represent the size of red cells.]

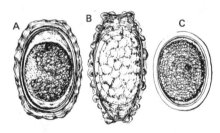

ADULT TREMATODES
(in intestine or tissues)

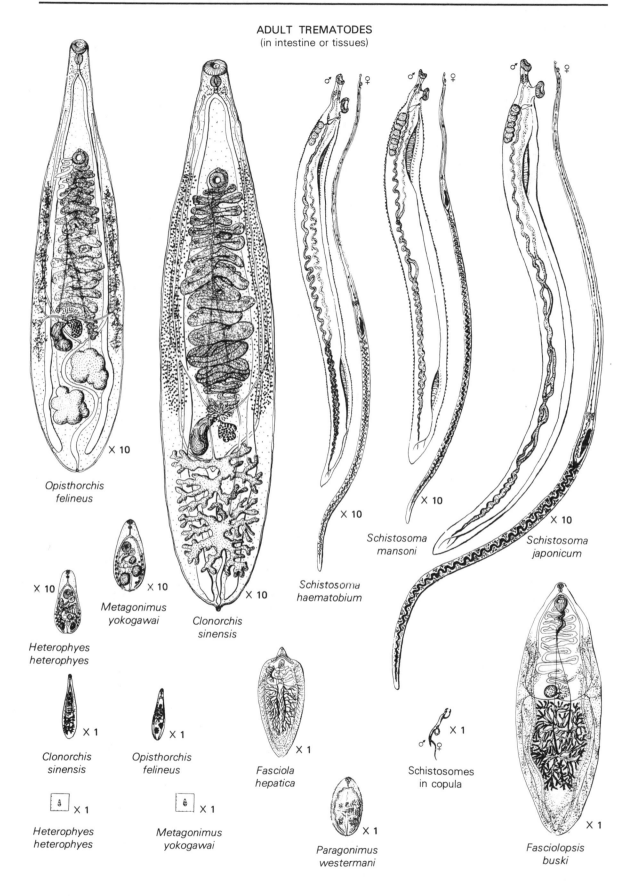

Opisthorchis
felineus
× 10

Heterophyes
heterophyes
× 10

Metagonimus
yokogawai
× 10

Clonorchis
sinensis
× 10

Schistosoma
haematobium
× 10

Schistosoma
mansoni
× 10

Schistosoma
japonicum
× 10

Clonorchis
sinensis
× 1

Opisthorchis
felineus
× 1

Fasciola
hepatica
× 1

Schistosomes
in copula
× 1

Heterophyes
heterophyes
× 1

Metagonimus
yokogawai
× 1

Paragonimus
westermani
× 1

Fasciolopsis
buski
× 1

INTESTINAL AND TISSUE NEMATODES

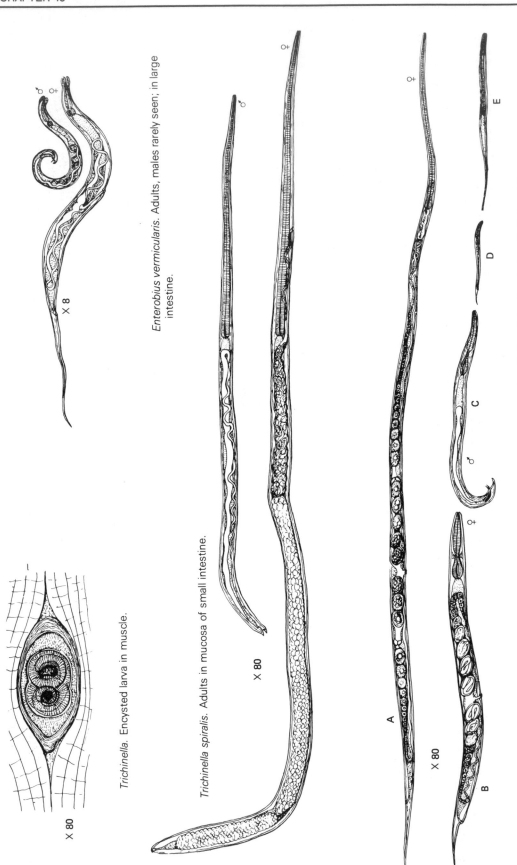

Trichinella. Encysted larva in muscle.

Trichinella spiralis. Adults in mucosa of small intestine.

Enterobius vermicularis. Adults, males rarely seen; in large intestine.

Strongyloides stercoralis. *A:* Parasitic female, lateral view, in human intestine; *B:* free-living female in soil; *C:* free-living male in soil; *D:* rhabditiform larva passed in feces or in free-living cycle in soil; *E:* filariform or infective larva in soil, ready to penetrate human skin.

INTESTINAL NEMATODES

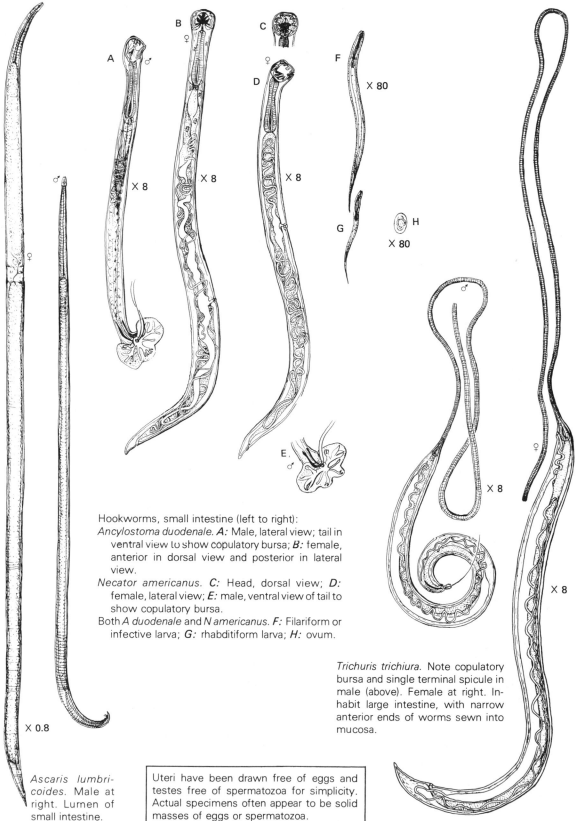

X 8

X 80

X 80

Hookworms, small intestine (left to right):
Ancylostoma duodenale. *A:* Male, lateral view; tail in
    ventral view to show copulatory bursa; *B:* female,
    anterior in dorsal view and posterior in lateral
    view.
Necator americanus. *C:* Head, dorsal view; *D:*
    female, lateral view; *E:* male, ventral view of tail to
    show copulatory bursa.
Both *A duodenale* and *N americanus*. *F:* Filariform or
    infective larva; *G:* rhabditiform larva; *H:* ovum.

X 8

Trichuris trichiura. Note copulatory
bursa and single terminal spicule in
male (above). Female at right. Inhabit large intestine, with narrow
anterior ends of worms sewn into
mucosa.

X 8

X 0.8

*Ascaris lumbri-
coides*. Male at
right. Lumen of
small intestine.

Uteri have been drawn free of eggs and
testes free of spermatozoa for simplicity.
Actual specimens often appear to be solid
masses of eggs or spermatozoa.

CESTODES (TAPEWORMS)

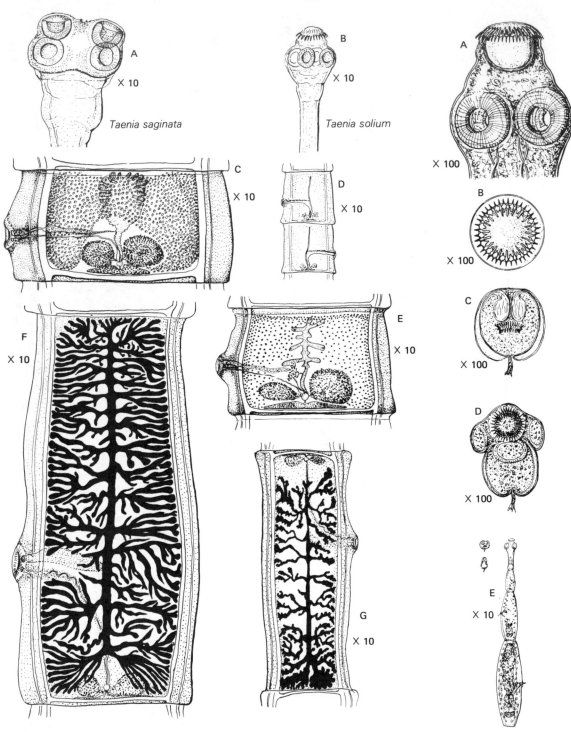

Taenia saginata and *Taenia solium*. **A:** Scolex of *T saginata*; **B:** scolex of *T solium* with beginning of strobila; **C:** mature proglottid of *T saginata*; **D:** immature proglottids of *T solium*; **E:** mature proglottid of *T solium*; **F:** gravid proglottid of *T saginata* with much more numerous uterine ramifications than in *T solium* (see at right); **G:** gravid proglottid of *T solium*.

Echinococcus granulosus. **A:** Scolex of adult; **B:** end view of rostellum, showing arrangement of 2 hook rows; **C:** larva from hydatid fluid, invaginated; **D:** same, evaginated; **E:** entire adult worm and larval scoleces (left).

CESTODES

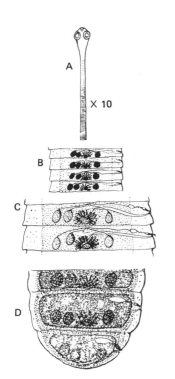

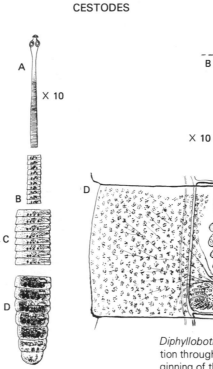

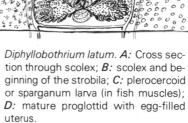

Hymenolepis diminuta. A: Unarmed scolex and beginning of strobila; *B:* some genitally mature proglottids; *C:* enlarged view; *D:* gravid proglottids.

Hymenolepis nana. A: Armed scolex and beginning of strobila; *B:* some genitally mature proglottids; *C:* enlarged view; *D:* gravid proglottids.

Diphyllobothrium latum. A: Cross section through scolex; *B:* scolex and beginning of the strobila; *C:* plerocercoid or sparganum larva (in fish muscles); *D:* mature proglottid with egg-filled uterus.

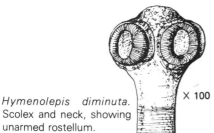

Hymenolepis diminuta. Scolex and neck, showing unarmed rostellum.

Hymenolepis nana. A: Scolex with hooked rostellum retracted; *B:* same with rostellum everted.

OVA OF CESTODES (× 400)

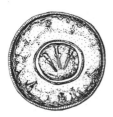

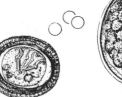

Hymenolepis diminuta

Hymenolepis nana

Taenia saginata, Taenia solium, or *Echinococcus*

Diphyllobothrium latum

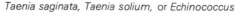

[Simple circles represent the size of red cells.]

Index

Lange Medical Books are available at medical bookstores within the United States.
To order directly from the publisher, complete and mail the postage-paid card below.

BASIC SCIENCE TEXTBOOKS

1. **Correlative Neuroanatomy & Functional Neurology, 19th Ed.**, *Chusid,* A0001-6, $21.50
2. **Biochemistry: A Synopsis,** *Colby,* A0033-9, $14.00
3. **Review of Medical Physiology, 13th Ed.,** *Ganong,* A8435-8, $24.00
4. **Physiology: A Study Guide,** *Ganong,* A0032-1, $13.00
5. **Review of Medical Microbiology, 17th Ed.,** *Jawetz et al.,* A8432-5, $22.00
6. **Basic Histology, 5th Ed.,** *Junquiera et al.,* A0570-0, $24.00
7. **Basic & Clinical Pharmacology, 3rd Ed.,** *Katzung,* A0553-6, $29.50
8. **Pharmacology: A Review,** *Katzung and Trevor,* A0031-3, $14.00
9. **Harper's Review of Biochemistry, 20th Ed.,** *Martin et al.,* A0003-2, $27.50
10. **Basic & Clinical Immunology, 6th Ed.,** *Stites et al.,* A0548-6, $29.00

CLINICAL SCIENCE TEXTBOOKS

11. **Principles of Clinical Electrocardiography, 12th Ed.,** *Goldman,* A0008-1, $22.00
12. **Review of General Psychiatry,** *Goldman,* A0030-5, $27.50
13. **Electrocardiography: Essentials of Interpretation,** *Goldschlager and Goldman,* A0029-7, $16.50
14. **Basic & Clinical Endocrinology, 2nd Ed.,** *Greenspan and Forsham,* A0547-8, $27.00
15. **General Urology, 11th Ed.,** *Smith,* A0009-9, $28.00

16. **Clinical Cardiology, 4th Ed.,** *Sokolow and McIlroy,* A0023-0, $26.50
17. **General Ophthalmology, 11th Ed.,** *Vaughan and Asbury,* A3108-6, $23.50

CURRENT CLINICAL REFERENCES

18. **Current Obstetric & Gynecologic Diagnosis & Treatment, 6th Ed.,** *Pernoll and Benson,* A1412-4, $31.50
19. **Current Pediatric Diagnosis & Treatment, 9th Ed.,** *Kempe et al.,* A1414-0, $31.50
20. **Current Medical Diagnosis & Treatment 1987, 26th Ed.,** *Krupp et al.,* A1413-2, $32.50
21. **Current Emergency Diagnosis & Treatment, 2nd Ed.,** *Mills et al.,* A0027-1, $29.50
22. **Current Surgical Diagnosis & Treatment, 7th Ed.,** *Way,* A0019-8, $34.00

HANDBOOKS

23. **Handbook of Obstetrics & Gynecology, 8th Ed.,** *Benson,* A0014-9, $13.00
24. **Handbook of Poisoning, 12th Ed.,** *Dreisbach and Robertson,* A3643-2 $16.50
25. **Physician's Handbook, 21st Ed.,** *Krupp et al.,* A0002-4, $16.50
26. **Handbook of Pediatrics, 15th Ed.,** *Silver et al.,* A3635-8, $16.50

ORDER CARD

Please send the books I've circled below on 30-day approval:

1. Chusid, A0001-6, $21.50
2. Colby, A0033-9, $14.00
3. Ganong, A8435-8, $24.00
4. Ganong, A0032-1, $13.00
5. Jawetz, A8432-5, $22.00
6. Junquiera, A0570-0, $24.00
7. Katzung, A0553-6, $29.50
8. Katzung, A0031-3, $14.00
9. Martin, A0003-2, $27.50

10. Stites, A0548-6, $29.00
11. Goldman, A0008-1, $22.00
12. Goldman, A0030-5, $27.50
13. Goldschlager, A0029-7, $16.50
14. Greenspan, A0547-8, $27.00
15. Smith, A0009-9, $28.00
16. Sokolow, A0023-0, $26.50
17. Vaughan, A3108-6, $23.50
18. Pernoll, A1412-4, $31.50

19. Kempe, A1414-0, $31.50
20. Krupp, A1413-2, $32.50
21. Mills, A0027-1, $29.50
22. Way, A0019-8, $34.00
23. Benson, A0014-9, $13.00
24. Dreisbach, A3643-2, $16.50
25. Krupp, A0002-4, $16.50
26. Silver, A3635-8, $16.50

☐ Payment enclosed. (Publisher pays postage & handling.)
  Please include your state sales tax.
☐ Bill me later.
Charge to: ☐ VISA ☐ Mastercard

Card #_____ Exp. Date_____

Signature_____

Prices and publication dates subject to change without notice. Prices advertised are applicable in the U.S., its territories and possessions only. For orders outside the U.S. and Canada contact: Prentice-Hall Intl., Englewood Cliffs, NJ 07632. In Canada, contact: Prentice-Hall Canada, Scarborough, Ontario, M1P 2J7.

NAME_____

ADDRESS_____

CITY/STATE/ZIP_____

APPLETON & LANGE
Combining the houses of Appleton-Century-Crofts
and Lange Medical Publications.
25 Van Zant St.
E. Norwalk, CT 06855

ACC604-9

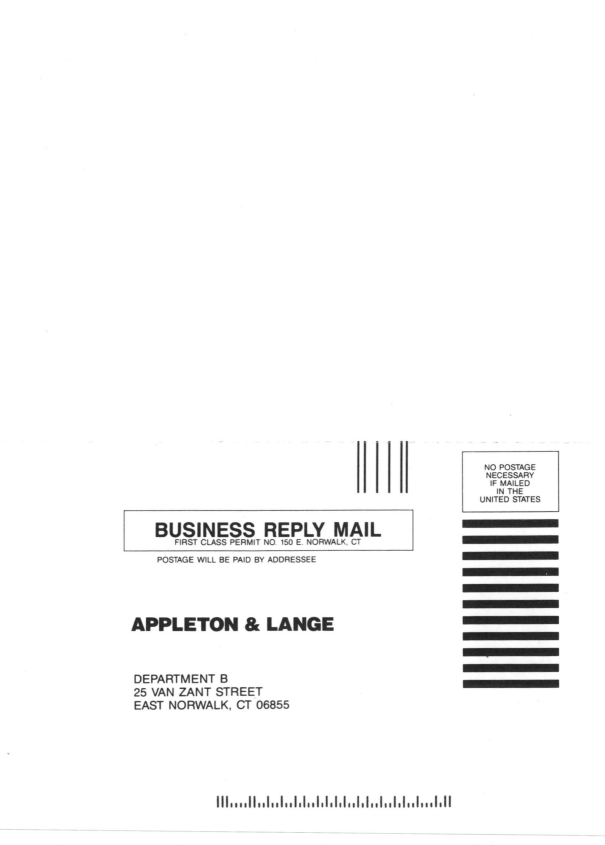

BUSINESS REPLY MAIL
FIRST CLASS PERMIT NO. 150 E. NORWALK, CT

POSTAGE WILL BE PAID BY ADDRESSEE

APPLETON & LANGE

DEPARTMENT B
25 VAN ZANT STREET
EAST NORWALK, CT 06855